Clinical Diabetes

Translating Research into Practice

Vivian A. Fonseca, MD
Professor of Medicine
Tullis-Tulane Alumni Chair in Diabetes
Chief, Section of Endocrinology, Department of Medicine
Tulane University Health Sciences Center
New Orleans, Louisiana

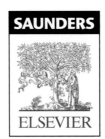

SAUNDERS

ELSEVIER

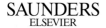

SAUNDERS
ELSEVIER

1600 John F. Kennedy Blvd.
Ste 1800
Philadelphia, PA 19103-2899

CLINICAL DIABETES

ISBN-13: 978-1-4160-0273-4
ISBN-10: 1-4160-0273-1

Notice

Knowledge and best practice in this field are constantly changing. As new research and experience broaden our knowledge, changes in practice, treatment, and drug therapy may become necessary or appropriate. Readers are advised to check the most current information provided (i) on procedures featured or (ii) by the manufacturer of each product to be administered, to verify the recommended dose or formula, the method and duration of administration, and contraindications. It is the responsibility of the practitioner, relying on their own experience and knowledge of the patient, to make diagnoses, to determine dosages and the best treatment for each individual patient, and to take all appropriate safety precautions. To the fullest extent of the law, neither the Publisher nor the Editor assumes any liability for any injury and/or damage to persons or property arising out of or related to any use of the material contained in this book.

The Publisher

Library of Congress Cataloging-in-Publication Data
Fonseca, Vivian A.
   Clinical diabetes: translating research into practice / Vivian A. Fonseca—1st ed.
      p. ; cm.
   ISBN 1-4160-0273-1
      1. Diabetes. I. Title.
      [DNLM: 1. Diabetes Mellitus—physiopathology. 2. Diabetes Mellitus—therapy.
   3. Evidence-Based Medicine. WK 810 F676c 2006]
   RC660.F66 2006
   616.4'62—dc22   2005047248

Acquisitions Editor: Rebecca Schmidt Gaertner
Developmental Editors: Marla Sussman, Agnes Byrne, Suzanne Flint
Publishing Services Manager: Frank Polizzano
Project Manager: Joan Nikelsky
Design Direction: Steve Stave

Printed in China

Last digit is the print number: 9 8 7 6 5 4 3 2

I dedicate this book to Sarita, Neil, and Adam, without whose support this book would not have been possible.

Vivian Fonseca

Contributors

Emily Lee Albertson, MD
Intern, Fellowship in Medical Research, Sansum Diabetes Research Institute, Santa Barbara, California
Diabetes and Pregnancy

Ahmad Aljada, PhD
Research Assistant Professor, Department of Medicine, State University of New York at Buffalo School of Medicine and Biomedical Sciences; Diabetes-Endocrine Center of Western NY, Buffalo, New York
Endothelial Disfunction in Diabetes

Jonathan Anolik, MD
Chief, Section of Endocrinology, Department of Medicine, Virtua-Memorial Hospital, Mount Holly; Endocrine Associates of South Jersey, Moorestown, New Jersey
Insulin-Sensitizing and Insulin-Sparing Drugs: Thiazolidinediones and Metformin

David G. Armstrong, MSc, DPM, PhD
Professor of Surgery, Chair of Research, and Assistant Dean, Dr. William M. Scholl College of Podiatric Medicine at Rosalind Franklin University of Medicine and Science; Director, Center for Lower Extremity Ambulatory Research (CLEAR), North Chicago, Illinois
The Diabetic Foot

Sunil Asnani, MD
Assistant Professor of Medicine, Department of Medicine/Endocrinology, Tulane University School of Medicine; Department of Medicine, Geriatrics and Endocrinology, Veterans Affairs Medical Center, New Orleans, Louisiana
Diabetes in Older Adults

George L. Bakris, MD
Professor and Vice-Chairman, Department of Preventive Medicine, Rush Medical College of Rush University; Director, Hypertension/Clinical Research Center, Rush University Medical Center, Chicago, Illinois
Diabetic Nephropathy

Salomon Banarer, MD
Assistant Professor, Department of Medicine, University of Louisville School of Medicine; Staff Physician, Department of Medicine, Louisville VA Medical Center, Louisville, Kentucky
Insulin Strategies in Type 1 and Type 2 Diabetes Mellitus

Lawrence Blonde, MD, FACP, FACE
Director, Ochsner Diabetes Clinical Research Unit, Section of Endocrinology, Diabetes, and Metabolic Diseases, and Associate Residency Program Director, Department of Internal Medicine, Ochsner Clinic Foundation, New Orleans, Louisiana
Using Computers and Technology for Diabetes Care

Zachary T. Bloomgarden, MD
Associate Clinical Professor, Division of Endocrinology and Metabolism, Department of Medicine, Mount Sinai School of Medicine, New York, New York
Pearls from Major Clinical Trials: Approaches to Improving Outcome of Persons with Diabetes

Andrew J. M. Boulton, MD, DSc(Hon), FRCP
Professor of Medicine, Department of Medicine, University of Manchester Faculty of Medicine; Consultant Physician, Department of Medicine, Manchester Royal Infirmary, Manchester, United Kingdom; Professor of Medicine, Department of Endocrinology, University of Miami College of Medicine, Miami, Florida
The Diabetic Foot

John B. Buse, MD, PhD, CDE
Associate Professor, Department of Medicine, University of North Carolina School of Medicine; Chief, Division of General Medicine and Clinical Epidemiology; Director, Diabetes Care Center, Chapel Hill, North Carolina
Scope of the Problem: The Diabetes and Metabolic Syndrome Epidemic

William T. Cefalu, MD
Douglas L. Manship Senior Professor in Diabetes, Louisiana State University School of Medicine; Chief, Division of Nutrition and Chronic Diseases, The Pennington Biomedical Research Center, Louisiana State University System, Baton Rouge, Louisiana
Pharmacologic Agents and Nutritional Supplements in the Treatment of Obesity

Manisha Chandalia, MD
Associate Professor, Department of Internal Medicine, Division of Endocrinology and Metabolism, The University of Texas Southwestern Medical Center at Dallas Southwestern Medical School; Staff Physician, Center for Human Nutrition, UT Southwestern Medical Center, Dallas, Texas
Diabetes and Inflammation

Ajay Chaudhuri, MBBS, MRCP(UK)
Assistant Professor, Department of Medicine, State University of New York at Buffalo School of Medicine and Biomedical Sciences; Associate Director/Attending Physician, Diabetes Endocrinology Center of Western NY, Kaleida Health, Buffalo, New York
Endothelial Disfunction in Diabetes

Brian E. Chavez, MD
Endocrinology Fellow, Department of Endocrinology, Diabetes and Metabolism, Veterans Affairs Medical Center, San Diego, California
Type 2 Diabetes: Insulin Resistance, Beta Cell Dysfunction, and Other Metabolic and Hormonal Abnormalities

Jean-Louis Chiasson, MD
Professor, Department of Medicine, University of Montreal Faculty of Medicine; Director, Endocrinology Laboratory, Hôtel-Dieu Hospital, Centre Hospitalier de l'Université de Montréal (CHUM), Montreal, Quebec, Canada
α-Glucosidase Inhibitors

David Conroy Yu Chua, MD, MS
Fellow, Internal Medicine, Division of Cardiovascular Disease, University of Virginia Medical Center, Charlottesville, Virginia
Diabetic Nephropathy

Ellie I. Chuang, MD
Endocrinologist, Joslin Diabetes Center, Southern New Hampshire Medical Center, Nashua, New Hampshire
Hypertension in Diabetes

Mandi D. Conway, MD
Professor of Ophthalmology, Tulane University School of Medicine; Director, Medical Retina and Uveitis Service, Department of Ophthalmology, Tulane University Hospital and Clinics and University Hospital of Medical Center of Louisiana; Attending Physician, Department of Ophthalmology, Lindy Boggs Medical Center, New Orleans, Louisiana
Diabetic Retinopathy

John Crean, PhD
Medical Science Liaison, Department of Medical Affairs, Amylin Pharmaceuticals, Inc., San Diego, California
Beyond Insulin Therapy

Samuel Dagogo-Jack, MD, MBBS, MSc, FRCP
Professor of Medicine and Endocrinology, Department of Medicine, University of Tennessee Health Science Center College of Medicine; Attending Physician, Department of Medicine, Methodist University Hospital, and Regional Medical Center; Associate Director, General Clinical Research Center, Memphis, Tennessee
Primary Prevention of Type 2 Diabetes Mellitus; New Drugs and Diabetes Risk: Antipsychotic and Antiretroviral Agents

Paresh Dandona, MD, PhD
UB Distinguished Professor of Medicine, Division of Endocrinology, Diabetes, and Metabolism, State University of New York at Buffalo School of Medicine and Biomedical Sciences; Staff, Millard Filmore Hospital, Buffalo, New York
Endothelial Disfunction in Diabetes

Jaime A. Davidson, MD, FACP, FACE
Clinical Associate Professor of Internal Medicine, The University of Texas Southwestern Medical Center at Dallas Southwestern Medical School; Physician on Staff, Medical City Dallas Hospital; Endocrine & Diabetes Associates of Texas, Dallas, Texas
Diabetes in Latin Americans

Stephen N. Davis, MD
Rudolph Kampmeier Professor of Medicine and Professor of Molecular Physiology and Biophysics, Vanderbilt University School of Medicine; Chief, Division of Diabetes, Endocrinology, and Metabolism, and Attending Physician, Department of Medicine, Division of Diabetes, Endocrinology and Metabolism, Vanderbilt University Medical Center; Attending Physician, Department of Diabetes, Tennessee Valley Health Care System, Veterans Affairs Medical Center, Nashville, Tennessee
Hypoglycemia in Diabetes

Prakash C. Deedwania, MD, FACC, FCCP, FACP, FAHA
Professor of Medicine, University of California, San Francisco, School of Medicine, San Francisco; Chief, Cardiology Division, Department of Medicine, VACCHCS/UCSF Program, Fresno, California
The Metabolic Syndrome and Its Effects on Cardiovascular Risks

Orlando Deffer, MD
Fellow, Non-Invasive Imaging, Department of Cardiology, Tulane University Health Sciences Center and Tulane University Hospital, New Orleans, Louisiana
Diagnostic Testing for Coronary Artery Disease in Diabetic Patients

Sridevi Devaraj, PhD
Associate Professor of Pathology, University of California, Davis, School of Medicine, Davis; Director of Toxicology, Laboratory for Atherosclerosis and Metabolic Research, UC Davis Medical Center, Sacramento, California
Diabetes and Inflammation

Jayant Dey, MD
Staff, Department of Endocrinology, Ochsner Clinical Foundation, New Orleans, Louisiana
Using Computers and Technology for Diabetes Care

Shehab A. Ebrahim, MD
Vitreoretinal Surgery Fellow, Department of Ophthalmology, Tulane University Health Sciences Center, New Orleans, Louisiana
Diabetic Retinopathy

Steven V. Edelman, MD
Founder and Director, Taking Control of Your Diabetes; Professor of Medicine, Division of Endocrinology and Metabolism, University of California, San Diego, School of Medicine; Staff, Veterans Affairs Medical Center, San Diego, California
Physiologic Insulin Replacement with Continuous Subcutaneous Insulin Infusion: Insulin Pump Therapy

Vivian A. Fonseca, MD, MRCP
Professor of Medicine and Director, Tullis-Tulane Alumni Chair in Diabetes, Chief, Section of Endocrinology, Department of Medicine, Tulane University Health Sciences Center, New Orleans, Louisiana
Erectile Dysfunction in Diabetes: An Endothelial Disorder

Om P. Ganda, MD
Associate Clinical Professor, Department of Medicine, Harvard Medical School; Attending Physician, Department of Medicine, Beth-Israel Deaconess Medical Center; Director, Lipid Clinic, Joslin Diabetes Center, Boston, Massachusetts
Lipid Management in Diabetes

Satish K. Garg, MD
Professor, Departments of Medicine and Pediatrics, University of Colorado School of Medicine; Staff Pediatrician, The Children's Hospital; Clinical Director, Adult Program, Endowed Clinical & Research Chairs, Barbara Davis Center for Childhood Diabetes at Fitzsimons, Aurora, Colorado
Glucose Monitoring of the Present and Future

John E. Gerich, MD
Professor of Medicine, University of Rochester School of Medicine and Dentistry; Staff Physician, Endocrinology & Metabolism Unit, Strong Memorial Hospital, Rochester, New York
Insulin Secretagogues

Barry J. Goldstein, MD, PhD
Professor of Medicine and Professor of Biochemistry and Molecular Pharmacology, Department of Medicine, Jefferson Medical College of Thomas Jefferson University; Director, Division of Endocrinology, Diabetes and Metabolic Diseases, Thomas Jefferson University Hospital, Philadelphia, Pennsylvania
Insulin-Sensitizing and Insulin-Sparing Drugs: Thiazolidinediones and Metformin

Dina E. Green, MD
Assistant Clinical Professor of Medicine, Department of Medicine, Columbia University College of Physicians and Surgeons; Staff Physician, The Naomi Berrie Diabetes Center at Columbia University Medical Center, New York, New York
Exercise in Diabetes

Frank Greenway, MD
Adjunct Professor, Department of Human Ecology, Louisiana State University School of Medicine; Medical Director, Clinical Trials, Pennington Biomedical Research Center, Baton Rouge, Louisiana
Pharmacologic Agents and Nutritional Supplements in the Treatment of Obesity

Gerald C. Groggel, MD
Professor of Medicine, Department of Internal Medicine, University of Nebraska College of Medicine; Chief of Nephrology, Department of Internal Medicine, Nebraska Medical Center, Omaha, Nebraska
Pancreas, Kidney, and Islet Transplantation: What Every Physician Needs to Know

Deanna L. Aftab Guy, MD
Assistant Professor of Pediatrics, Division of Pediatric Endocrinology, Vanderbilt University School of Medicine; Staff, Vanderbilt Children's Hospital, Nashville, Tennessee
Hypoglycemia in Diabetes

Robert R. Henry, MD
Professor of Medicine, University of California, San Diego, School of Medicine; Chief, Division of Diabetes and Endocrinology, Department of Endocrinology, Diabetes and Metabolism, Veterans Affairs Medical Center, San Diego, California
Type 2 Diabetes: Insulin Resistance, Beta Cell Dysfunction, and Other Metabolic and Hormonal Abnormalities

Irl B. Hirsch, MD
Professor, Division of Metabolism, Endocrinology and Nutrition, University of Washington School of Medicine; Medical Director, Diabetes Care Center, Seattle, Washington
Diabetes Management in the Hospital Setting

Silvio E. Inzucchi, MD
Professor, Section of Endocrinology and Metabolism, Department of Internal Medicine, Yale University School of Medicine; Director, Yale Diabetes Center, Yale–New Haven Hospital, New Haven, Connecticut
Type 2 Diabetes Therapy: Choosing Oral Agents

Deepika Israni, MHS, PT
University of Indianapolis Krannert School of Physical Therapy, Indianapolis, Indiana; Staff, Department of Rehab Services, Ochsner Clinic Foundation, New Orleans, Louisiana
Diabetes in Older Adults

Serge A. Jabbour, MD, FACP, FACE
Associate Professor of Clinical Medicine, Department of Medicine, Division of Endocrinology, Diabetes and Metabolic Diseases, Jefferson Medical College of Thomas Jefferson University; Staff, Thomas Jefferson Hospital, Philadelphia, Pennsylvania
Insulin-Sensitizing and Insulin-Sparing Drugs: Thiazolidinediones and Metformin

Ali Jawa, MD
Assistant Professor, Department of Medicine, Section of Endocrinology, Tulane University School of Medicine; Staff, Department of Medicine, Tulane University Hospital and Clinic, New Orleans, Louisiana
Erectile Dysfunction in Diabetes: An Endothelial Disorder

Ishwarlal Jialal, MD, PhD
Professor of Medicine and Pathology, University of California, Davis, School of Medicine, Davis; Staff, Laboratory for Atherosclerosis and Metabolic Research, UC Davis Medical Center, Sacramento, California
Diabetes and Inflammation

Lois Jovanovic, MD
Adjunct Professor, Bioengineering and Science, University of California, Santa Barbara, Santa Barbara; Clinical Professor of Medicine, University of Southern California, Los Angeles; Director and Chief Scientific Officer, Sansum Diabetes Research Institute, Santa Barbara, California
Diabetes and Pregnancy

Janet L. Kelly, PharmD, BC-ADM
Associate Clinical Professor, Department of Pharmacy, University of Washington School of Pharmacy; Outcomes & Cost Management Pharmacist, Department of Pharmacy, University of Washington Medical Center, Seattle, Washington
Diabetes Management in the Hospital Setting

Philip A. Kern, MD
Professor, Department of Internal Medicine, University of Arkansas for Medical Sciences; Associate Chief of Staff, Department of Research, Central Arkansas Veterans Healthcare System, Little Rock, Arkansas
The Pathogenesis and Treatment of High-Risk Obesity

Mehdi A. Khan, DO
Fellow, Vitreo-Retinal Surgery, Department of Ophthalmology, Tulane University Medical Center, and Lindy-Boggs Medical Center, New Orleans, Louisiana
Diabetic Retinopathy

Kristin E. Koenekamp, BS
Intern, Fellowship in Medical Research, Sansum Diabetes Research Institute, Santa Barbara, California
Diabetes and Pregnancy

Karmeen Kulkarni, MS, RD, BC-ADM, CDE
Adjunct Faculty, University of Utah College of Health Science, Salt Lake City; Nutrition Department, Utah State University, Logan; and Nutrition Department, Brigham Young University, Provo; Coordinator, St. Mark's Diabetes Center, Salt Lake City, Utah
Medical Nutrition Therapy for Type 1 and Type 2 Diabetes

Jennifer Larsen, MD
Professor, Department of Internal Medicine, University of Nebraska College of Medicine; Chief, Section of Diabetes, Endocrinology and Metabolism, Department of Internal Medicine, University of Nebraska Medical Center, Omaha, Nebraska
Pancreas, Kidney, and Islet Transplantation: What Every Physician Needs to Know

David G. Maggs, MD
Executive Director, Medical Affairs, Amylin Pharmaceuticals, Inc., San Diego, California
Beyond Insulin Therapy

Lawrence J. Mandarino, PhD
Professor and Chair, Department of Kinesiology, and Director, Center for Metabolic Biology, Arizona State University School of Life Sciences, Tempe, Arizona
Exercise in Diabetes

Glenn Matfin, BSc(Hons), MBChB, DGM, MFPM, MRCP(UK), FACE, FACP
Senior Medical Director, Global Diabetes Clinical Research, Novartis Pharmaceuticals, East Hanover, New Jersey
Erectile Dysfunction in Diabetes: An Endothelial Disorder

Roberta Harrison McDuffie, MSN, APRN, BC, CNS, CDE
Clinical Coordinator/Clinical Nurse Specialist, Endocrine Department, Tulane University School of Medicine; Clinical Coordinator/Clinical Nurse Specialist, General Clinical Research Center, Medical Center of Louisiana; Clinical Coordinator/Clinical Nurse Specialist, Endocrine Research, Veterans Administration Hospital, New Orleans, Louisiana; Clinical Nurse Specialist/CDE, Diabetes Wellness Company, Picayune, Mississippi
Diabetes Education

Viswanathan Mohan, MD, FRCP, PhD, DSc, FNASc
Visiting Professor, Department of Diabetology, Sri Ramachandra Medical College and Research Institute (Deemed University); Chairman and Diabetologist, Department of Diabetology, Dr. Mohans' M.V. Diabetes Specialities Centre and Madras Diabetes Research Foundation, Gopalapuram, Chennai, India
Diabetes in Asians

Priya Mohanty, MD
Clinical Assistant Professor, Department of Medicine, State University of New York at Buffalo School of Medicine and Biomedical Sciences; Attending Physician, Diabetes Endocrinology Center, Millard Fillmore Hospital, Buffalo, New York
Endothelial Disfunction in Diabetes

Mark E. Molitch, MD
Professor of Medicine, Division of Endocrinology, Metabolism and Molecular Medicine, Northwestern University Feinberg School of Medicine; Attending Physician, Department of Medicine, Northwestern Memorial Hospital, Chicago, Illinois
Hypertension in Diabetes

Kwame Osei, MD, FACE, FACP
Professor of Medicine, Department of Endocrinology, The Ohio State University College of Medicine and Public Health, Columbus, Ohio
Diabetes in African Americans

David Raymond Owens, CBE, MD, FRCP
Professor, Cardiff University College of Medicine; Consultant Diabetologist, Centre for Endocrine and Diabetes Sciences, Cardiff, South Wales; Professor and Consultant Diabetologist, Diabetes Research Unit, Landough Hospital, Penarth, Wales, United Kingdom
Insulin Strategies in Type 1 and Type 2 Diabetes Mellitus

Henri K. Parson, PhD
Director, Microvascular Biology, Strelitz Diabetes Institutes at Eastern Virginia Medical School, Norfolk, Virginia
Diabetic Neuropathies

Merri L. Pendergrass, MD, PhD
Associate Professor of Medicine, Harvard Medical School; Director of Clinical Diabetes and Interim Chief, Diabetes Section, Brigham and Women's Hospital, Boston, Massachusetts
Exercise in Diabetes

Anne L. Peters (Harmel), MD
Professor of Clinical Medicine, Department of Medicine, University of Southern California Keck School of Medicine; Director, USC Westside Center for Diabetes, Los Angeles, California
Running a Diabetes Clinic

Kevin Arthur Peterson, MD, MPH, FRCS(Ed), FAAFP
Assistant Professor, Department of Family Medicine and Community Health, University of Minnesota Medical School, Minneapolis, Minnesota
Using Computers and Technology for Diabetes Care

Nikolai Petrovsky, MD, PhD
Director, Department of Diabetes and Endocrinology Department, Flinders University Medical Centre, Adelaide, South Australia, Australia
Type 1 Diabetes: Immunology and Genetics

Raymond A. Plodkowski, MD
Chief of Endocrinology, Diabetes, and Metabolism Division, University of Nevada School of Medicine; Reno Veterans Affairs Medical Center, Reno, Nevada
Physiologic Insulin Replacement with Continuous Subcutaneous Insulin Infusion: Insulin Pump Therapy

Rajendra Pradeepa, MSc
Research Nutritionist, Department of Diabetology, Madras Diabetes Research Foundation, Gopalapuram, Chennai, India
Diabetes in Asians

Paolo Raggi, MD
Professor of Medicine, Division of Cardiology, Department of Medicine, Tulane University School of Medicine; Staff, Tulane University Hospital and Clinics, New Orleans, Louisiana
Diagnostic Testing for Coronary Artery Disease in Diabetic Patients

Neda Rasouli, MD
Assistant Professor, Division of Endocrinology and Metabolism, University of Arkansas for Medical Sciences, Little Rock, Arkansas
The Pathogenesis and Treatment of High-Risk Obesity

Ravi Retnakaran, MD, FRCPC
Endocrine Research Fellow, Division of Endocrinology and Metabolism, Department of Medicine, University of Toronto Faculty of Medicine, and Leadership Sinai Centre for Diabetes, Mount Sinai Hospital, Toronto, Ontario, Canada
The Biochemical Consequences of Hyperglycemia

Byron C. Richard, MS, RD, CDE
Director, Food Service, and Clinical Nutrition Manager, Houston Northwest Medical Center, Houston, Texas
Medical Nutrition Therapy for Type 1 and Type 2 Diabetes

Julio Rosenstock, MD
Clinical Professor of Medicine, The University of Texas Southwestern Medical Center at Dallas Southwestern Medical School; Staff Physician, Medical City Dallas Hospital/Dallas Diabetes and Endocrine Center, Dallas, Texas
Insulin Strategies in Type 1 and Type 2 Diabetes Mellitus

Richard R. Rubin, PhD
Associate Professor, Departments of Medicine and Pediatrics, Johns Hopkins University School of Medicine, Baltimore, Maryland
Stress and Depression in Disease

Darleen A. Sandoval, PhD
Research Associate Professor, Department of Psychiatry, University of Cincinnati College of Medicine, Cincinnati, Ohio
Hypoglycemia in Diabetes

Desmond A. Schatz, MD
Professor of Endocrinology and Associate Chairman, Department of Pediatrics, University of Florida College of Medicine; Medical Director, Diabetes Center of Excellence, Gainesville, Florida
Type 1 Diabetes: Immunology and Genetics

Dara P. Schuster, MD
Associate Professor, Department of Endocrinology, The Ohio State University College of Medicine and Public Health, Columbus, Ohio
Diabetes in African Americans

Leita Sharp, BA
Professional Research Assistant, Barbara Davis Center for Childhood Diabetes, University of Colorado Health Sciences Center, Aurora, Colorado
Glucose Monitoring of the Present and Future

Leslee J. Shaw, PhD
Director of Outcomes, American Cardiovascular Research Institute, Atlanta, Georgia
Diagnostic Testing for Coronary Artery Disease in Diabetic Patients

Dawn Smiley, MD
Endocrine Fellow, Internal Medicine, Division of Endocrinology, Emory University School of Medicine, Atlanta, Georgia
Diabetic Ketoacidosis and Hyperglycemic Hyperosmolar Syndrome

Tamar Smith, MD
Department of Internal Medicine, Franklin Square Hospital Center, Baltimore, Maryland
Insulin Secretagogues

R. Brian Stevens, MD, PhD
Associate Professor, Department of Surgery, University of Nebraska College of Medicine, Omaha, Nebraska
Pancreas, Kidney, and Islet Transplantation: What Every Physician Needs to Know

Mary Stults, PA-S
Barbara Davis Center for Childhood Diabetes, University of Colorado Health Sciences Center, Denver, Colorado
Glucose Monitoring of the Present and Future

William V. Tamborlane, MD
Professor, Department of Pediatrics, Yale University School of Medicine, Chief of Pediatric Endocrinology and Attending Physician, Department of Pediatrics, Yale–New Haven Children's Hospital, New Haven, Connecticut
Diabetes Mellitus in Children and Adolescents

Jagdeesh Ullal, MD, MS
Resident, Department of Internal Medicine, Eastern Virginia Medical School, Norfolk, Virginia
Diabetic Neuropathies

Guillermo Umpierrez, MD, FACP, FACE
Associate Professor of Medicine, Emory University School of Medicine; Director, Diabetes and Endocrinology, Grady Health Care System, Atlanta, Georgia
Diabetic Ketoacidosis and Hyperglycemic Hyperosmolar Syndrome

Aaron I. Vinik, MD, PhD
Director, Strelitz Diabetes Institutes at Eastern Virginia Medical School, Norfolk, Virginia
Diabetic Neuropathies

Natalia Volkova, MD
Assistant Professor, Department of Medicine, University of California San Francisco–Fresno, Fresno, California
The Metabolic Syndrome and Its Effects on Cardiovascular Risks

Stuart A. Weinzimer, MD

Associate Professor, Department of Pediatrics, Yale University School of Medicine; Attending Physician, Department of Pediatrics, Yale–New Haven Hospital, New Haven, Connecticut

Diabetes Mellitus in Children and Adolescents

Jeff D. Williamson MD, MHS

Director, Roena Kulynych Center for Memory and Cognition Research, J. Sticht Aging Center; Wake Forest University School of Medicine, Winston-Salem, North Carolina

Diabetes in Older Adults

William E. Winter, MD

Professor of Pathology and Pediatrics, Department of Immunology and Laboratory Medicine, University of Florida College of Medicine, Gainesville, Florida

Type 1 Diabetes: Immunology and Genetics

Kathleen Wyne, MD, PhD, FACE

Assistant Professor, Division of Endocrinology and Metabolism, Department of Internal Medicine, The University of Texas Southwestern Medical Center at Dallas Southwestern Medical School; Staff, Parkland Memorial Hospital; Medical Director, St. Paul Diabetes Management Institute, St. Paul University Hospital; Staff, Zale Lipshy University Hospital; Staff, Dallas Veterans Affairs Medical Center, Dallas, Texas

Managing Cardiovascular Disease and Events in the Patient with Diabetes

Bernard Zinman, MDCM, FRCPC, FACP

Professor of Medicine, Department of Medicine, University of Toronto Faculty of Medicine; Director, Leadership Sinai Centre for Diabetes, Mount Sinai Hospital; Samuel Lumenfeld Research Institute, Toronto, Ontario, Canada

The Biochemical Consequences of Hyperglycemia

Foreword

Diabetes mellitus has rapidly emerged as a major health problem in developed and developing countries throughout the world. The numerous factors contributing to this epidemic are related primarily to social, economic, technological, and scientific advances that have resulted in increased life expectancy, more adequate or abundant supplies of food, and a marked decrease in physical activity. These changes in environment and lifestyle interact with multiple, as-yet poorly understood genetic factors that predispose susceptible persons to what has been called the "dual epidemic" of obesity and diabetes. Type 1 diabetes, predominantly an autoimmune disease, also has been linked to environmental exposure to antigens that alter immune function and is increasing in prevalence, although not at the same rate as for type 2 diabetes.

Although the prevalence of diabetes is increasing rapidly in all age groups, in many parts of the world it is affecting younger segments of the population at alarmingly high rates. The need for early diagnosis and effective treatment is clear, and much emphasis is now being placed on identifying high-risk populations and implementing strategies for prevention.

There have been rapid advances in our understanding of the pathophysiology of both type 1 and type 2 diabetes, and of the long-term complications of diabetes. This achievement, combined with technological advances in self-monitoring of blood glucose, the development of new insulins and methods of insulin administration, and availability of new medications that target the underlying mechanisms of disease, has provided the possibility of and challenge for better, more effective care for people with diabetes.

This book provides comprehensive, up-to-date information on the pathophysiology of diabetes and its complications, and on the most current approaches to treatment. The chapters are written by leading authorities in the field, who present concise, easy-to-read discussions of practical, state-of-the-art approaches to diagnosis and management of this complex disease. In *Clinical Diabetes: Translating Research into Practice*, Dr. Vivian Fonseca has created an extremely valuable resource for health care professionals at all levels, from student to seasoned practitioner. I am sure that you will enjoy reading it, and that your patients will be grateful too.

Edward S. Horton, MD
VP and Director of Clinical Research
Joslin Diabetes Center
Professor of Medicine
Harvard Medical School
Boston, Massachusetts

Preface

Diabetes has reached epidemic proportions and is one of the most serious public health problems facing the world today. The problem is particularly acute, with the increase in obesity leading to type 2 diabetes in affluent countries, but is rapidly spreading to developing countries as well. Diabetes is one of the leading causes of morbidity and mortality and, because of its chronic nature, over time becomes one of the most expensive diseases, placing a tremendous financial burden on patients, as well as on health care systems. Over the last two decades, research in diabetes, obesity, and the metabolic syndrome has increased considerably and has led to a much-improved understanding of the pathophysiology of this condition. This has resulted in advances in prevention and management of both diabetes itself and its complications; however, many of these advances have not been translated into clinical practice.

With such a background, publication of a textbook of clinical diabetes, with a focus on translating recent research developments into practice, is timely and important. I am honored to be given the privilege of editing such a book written by a team of experts in the field, all of whom have made huge contributions to our understanding of both the pathophysiology and treatment of diabetes. All of the authors have played important roles in research, practice, and education and are published extensively in their areas of expertise.

The emphasis of the book is on translation of research into practice and highlighting lessons and clinical pearls from clinical trials that can be used by the practicing physician to improve patient outcomes. The book is divided into six sections, beginning with the basic pathophysiology of both type 1 and type 2 diabetes. Subsequent chapters in this section discuss the pathophysiology of diabetes complications, including microvascular complications and cardiovascular disease. The important new area of endothelial abnormalities and inflammation, as well as the pathogenesis and consequences of obesity, also has been incorporated into this section. The individual complications of diabetes, both acute and chronic, and complications of treatment such as hypoglycemia, are discussed in depth. Also included is a discussion of the strategies to screen for and manage these complications.

The next sections discuss management of patients, including the important and often neglected area of lifestyle management. Lifestyle management today must start before the onset of diabetes, so that the disease can be prevented. Continued emphasis on diet, exercise, and treatment of the psychological aspects is crucial. We are fortunate to have several new classes of medications that have become available in the past decade, necessitating separate chapters on the management of various agents to treat not only hypoglycemia but also hypertension and diabetes. Appropriate in this section is a discussion of new technologies for insulin delivery and glucose monitoring, as well as practical aspects of the management of patients following transplantation.

The next section discusses special populations and situations and includes the management of diabetes in pregnant women and children. The controversial topic of inpatient management of hyperglycemia during acute illness is discussed. In recognition of the fact that the pathophysiology of diabetes, insulin resistance, and obesity varies considerably across ethnic groups, and that different approaches are needed in these populations, these topics are addressed in separate chapters in this section.

The last two chapters of the book discuss the important area of organization and delivery of diabetes care, with suggestions on how to run a diabetes clinic, and how to use modern technology, including computers and the Internet, to deliver better care to our patients. Without such a systems approach, we may lack the ability to translate all of our research findings and new medications into improvement in outcomes.

Finally, there have been many major clinical trials that not only have helped us set goals for various parameters in patient management but also have taught us some lessons on the natural history of diabetes and how we can conquer it. For example, the United Kingdom Perspective Diabetes Study (UKPDS) and the Diabetes Control and Complications Trial (DCCT) both highlighted the importance of HbA$_{1C}$ as a surrogate marker for the development of long-term complications and also pointed out

the relative pros and cons of various treatment options. The UKPDS also clearly demonstrated the progressive nature of type 2 diabetes and, it is hoped, has led to increasing use of combination therapy at an earlier stage in the natural history. Major trials of hypertension and lipid-lowering therapy have helped us focus on a multiple-risk-factor approach, with lower and lower targets for the various risk factors. I am confident that if lessons learned from these trials are translated into practice, the burden of diabetes in our communities will be greatly alleviated, if not eliminated.

Although it may result in some overlap, each chapter stands on its own, being comprehensive from a practicing physician's viewpoint. The quality of the contributions to this book is outstanding, and it has been a pleasure to work with all of the authors. They all offer insights into how we can truly translate the enormous quantity of research that has been published and how to distill these findings into practical clinical applications that can be used by health care professionals every day.

Vivian Fonseca

Contents

Chapter 1

Scope of the Problem: The Diabetes and Metabolic Syndrome Epidemic

John B. Buse

KEY POINTS

- *The prevalence of diabetes is increasing rapidly, particularly in children and young adults.*
- *One third of cases of diabetes remain undiagnosed.*
- *The burden of death and disability from diabetes remains great despite broad advances in understanding and therapeutic techniques.*
- *Few patients with diabetes broadly achieve targets for blood pressure, lipid, or glucose management or take aspirin on a daily basis.*
- *Few patients with diabetes receive all the recommended annual screening evaluations for complications or preventive services.*
- *Organized systems of health care delivery can achieve better control of diabetes and its comorbidities.*

Diabetes is a dreadful affliction, not very frequent among men, being a melting down of the flesh and limbs into urine. The patients never stop making water and the flow is incessant. . . . Life is short, unpleasant and painful.

Aretaeus of Cappadocia

HISTORY

Modern clinicians can still identify with the eloquence of the sentiments expressed almost 2000 years ago by the second-century Greek physician Aretaeus of Cappadocia when he coined the term *diabetes* to describe an affliction with no known treatment.[1] By the end of the first millennium AD, writers in India, China, Japan, and the Middle East had described most of the salient features of the disease. They had noted that the polyuria of diabetes was sugary. Two forms of the disease were recognized, one afflicting older, overweight people and the other, more rapidly fatal, developing in younger, thin patients. Diabetes was recognized to be associated with chronic complications, specifically gangrene and impotence. Certain herbal preparations and dietary restrictions were thought to provide benefit.[1]

In the 17th century, the English physician Thomas Willis arguably first noted the onset of our current epidemic of diabetes, recognizing that diabetes had been a rare disease, "but in our age, given to good fellowship and gusling down chiefly of unallayed wine, we meet with examples and instances enough, I may say daily."[1] The roots of some of the trendiest lifestyle prescriptions for diabetes management were well described by the end of the 18th century as John Rollo attempted to treat patients with a diet rich in meats and restricted in carbohydrates, sometimes supplementing with anorectic compounds. Through the 19th and 20th centuries, dramatic advances have been made regarding our understanding of the etiology of the disorder, most importantly the identification of the role of the beta cell and insulin action.[1]

Particularly since the 1990s, a fundamental transformation has occurred in the principles of management of diabetes. Dozens of clinical trials involving hundreds of investigators and tens of thousands of patients with diabetes have documented improved outcomes associated with treatment of hyperglycemia, hypertension, dyslipidemia, and the hypercoagulable state of diabetes. These studies form the basis for the establishment of guidelines for treating diabetes.[2] Increasingly, adherence to these guidelines is monitored and in some cases enforced by insurers and health care systems.

Recognition of the increasing prevalence of diabetes combined with an understanding of the burden of costs associated with the treatment of complications of diabetes has led to a change in the level of concern about diabetes as a public health issue (Table 1–1). Through a broad-based public and professional education effort driven by public- and private-sector concerns, there have been changes in attitudes toward the treatment of diabetes among patients and providers. The spectrum of pharmacologic agents and monitoring technology to evaluate and titrate treatments as well as to recognize and slow complications at an asymptomatic stage has advanced dramatically. Increasingly since the turn of the 21st century, screening for diabetes, patient education, nutrition counseling, durable medical

Table 1–1. *The Burden of Diabetes in the United States, 2002.*

Factor	Amount
New cases of diabetes	1,300,000
Diabetes-related deaths	200,000
New cases of blindness due to diabetic retinopathy	24,000
New dialysis starts and kidney transplants	42,000
Nontrauma-related amputations	82,000
Direct costs	$92,000,000,000
Indirect costs	$40,000,000,000

From Centers for Disease Control and Prevention: National Diabetes Fact Sheet. Available at http://www.cdc.gov/diabetes/pubs/estimates.htm.

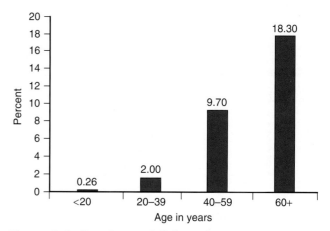

Figure 1–1. Prevalence of diabetes by age in the United States, 2002. (From Centers for Disease Control and Prevention: National Diabetes Fact Sheet. Available at http://www.cdc.gov/diabetes/pubs/estimates.htm.)

equipment, and pharmacotherapy for diabetes have become routinely covered benefits in the United States. These trends have made it possible to achieve excellent control of the metabolic derangements of diabetes and prevent or slow the complications of diabetes in the vast majority of cases. However, as a society, we are not achieving the full potential afforded by these advances due to inconsistent application of these resources.

In this chapter, the current state of diabetes is reviewed, focusing on the status of diabetes in the United States as documented by the Department of Health and Human Services' Centers for Disease Control and Prevention National Diabetes Fact Sheet.[3] The hope is that these alarming figures can motivate practitioners and patients to achieve the potential afforded by our understanding of the pathophysiology and natural history of diabetes and by the availability of robust technologies for treatment and prevention.

THE EPIDEMIC

In the United States, the prevalence of diabetes increases markedly as a function of age, increasing from 0.26% in those younger than age 20 years to more than 18% in those older than age 60 years (Fig. 1–1). Diabetes is more prevalent in all minority groups in the United States. As compared with non-Hispanic whites, African Americans have approximately 1.6 times the risk of diabetes. Among Latin Americans the prevalence is approximately 1.5 times the rate for non-Hispanic whites, though there are substantial differences based on country of origin: Mexican Americans are more than twice as likely to have diabetes as non-Hispanic whites of similar age. Native Americans exhibit a 2.2-fold increase in diabetes risk, and this risk is largest among those living in the southeastern United States and southern Arizona, where the risk is greater than three times that in non-Hispanic whites. There are more limited data on Asian Americans, but some groups certainly exhibit increased

risk of diabetes. These increased risks seem to be driven by both genetic and socioeconomic factors.[3] Other risk factors for diabetes include central obesity, hypertension, dyslipidemia, and cardiovascular disease, the core features of the metabolic syndrome.[4]

The prevalence of diagnosed diabetes in adults in the United States has risen substantially over time, increasing more than fourfold since the 1950s, with a particularly steep rise since the mid 1990s (Fig. 1–2). This epidemic is driven in part by changes in the diagnostic criteria for diabetes as well as increased efforts at disease detection. Superimposed secular trends in the prevalence and scale of obesity, coupled with increasing longevity and the aging of the population as well as growth in the percentage of ethnic minorities in the population, have produced a perfect storm of diabetes. The most disturbing of these trends is the rapid emergence since the 1990s of type 2 diabetes in children.[5]

The Centers for Disease Control and Prevention (CDC) estimates that in 2002, 18.2 million people in the United States (6.3% of the population) had diabetes. Approximately 13.0 million people had diagnosed diabetes, and another 5.2 million people were estimated to have undiagnosed diabetes. Despite greater emphasis on screening in the health care setting as a technique for making the diagnosis early, the fraction of persons with undiagnosed diabetes does not seem to have changed appreciably in recent years. In 2002, there were approximately 1.3 million new cases of diabetes in the United States.[3]

Current models suggest that the lifetime risk of developing diabetes by age 80 for a child born in 2000 in the United States is 33% for boys and almost 40% for girls, without accounting for those whose diabetes will remain undiagnosed.[6] Estimates suggest that between 2000 and 2050, the number of people in the United States with a diagnosis of diabetes will climb from 12 million to 39 million (a

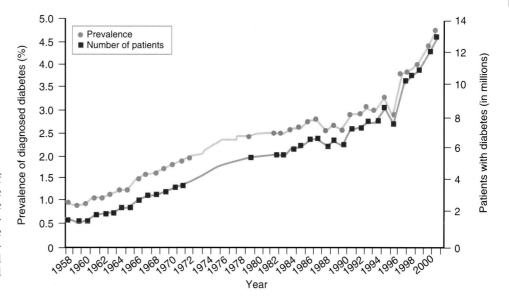

Figure 1-2. Prevalence of diagnosed diabetes and the number of patients in the United States. (From Engelgau MM, Geiss LS, Saaddine JB, et al: The evolving diabetes burden in the United States. Ann Intern Med 140:945-950, 2004.)

225% increase) and the prevalence from 4.4% to 9.7% (a 120% increase).[7]

DEATH AND DISABILITY

Coupled with the increase in the prevalence and incidence of diabetes is an increasing burden of death and disability associated with diabetes.[7] In 2000, diabetes was the sixth leading cause of death, contributing to the demise of more than 200,000 people, at least as reported on death certificates. This is likely a gross underestimate because only about 35% to 40% of those dying with diabetes have diabetes listed anywhere on the death certificate. Overall, the death rate for people with diabetes is about twice that of people without diabetes.[3] Estimates suggest that for those with diabetes at age 40, diabetes is associated with a 12- to 14-year reduction in life expectancy and 19- to 22-year reduction in quality-adjusted life-years.[6]

Heart disease accounts for the majority of diabetes-related deaths because people with diabetes exhibit heart disease at two to four times the rate of those without diabetes. Diabetic women are disproportionately affected and exhibit an age-adjusted risk of cardiovascular disease similar to that of men with diabetes. Vascular diseases in general, including stroke and peripheral vascular disease, account for more than 65% of deaths among people with diabetes.[3]

Microvascular complications of diabetes, namely eye, kidney, and nerve diseases, contribute substantially to the burden of disability. Diabetes is the leading cause of new cases of blindness among adults aged 20 to 74 years, with diabetic retinopathy contributing to 12,000 to 24,000 new cases of blindness each year.[3] Telephone survey data suggest that approximately 25% of people with diabetes have considerable visual impairment.[7]

Diabetes is the leading cause of end-stage renal disease, accounting for 44% of new cases in the United States. In 2001, more than 42,000 people with diabetes began treatment for end-stage renal disease and more than 140,000 people with diabetes were maintained on chronic dialysis or with a kidney transplant.

Current estimates suggest that at least 60% of people with diabetes have one or more forms of diabetic neuropathy associated with a wide range of symptoms. Severe peripheral neuropathy is the major contributor to diabetic foot ulcers and amputations; the majority of nontrauma-related amputations in the United States are performed on people with diabetes. About 82,000 nontrauma-related lower-limb amputations are performed annually among people with diabetes.[3] Estimates suggest that about 15% of people with diabetes will have a foot ulcer at some point in their lives and that 6% to 40% of them might require an amputation as part of treatment.[7]

Other complications of diabetes are legion. Poorly controlled diabetes before conception and during the first trimester of pregnancy causes major birth defects in 5% to 10% of pregnancies and spontaneous abortions in 15% to 20% of pregnancies. Later in pregnancy, poor glycemic control is associated with substantial complications during delivery for both mother and child. Almost one third of people with diabetes have severe periodontal disease.[3] Musculoskeletal disorders associated with decreased mobility and pain are more common in people with diabetes than in the general population.[8] Diabetes is even associated with an increased risk of many forms of cancer as well as overall cancer mortality.[9] Particularly in the setting of poorly controlled diabetes, issues such as hypercoagulability and poor immunologic defenses contribute to excess morbidity and mortality across the entire spectrum of human maladies from influenza

to recovery from surgery.[3] Finally, in the elderly, diabetes is associated with double the risk of dementia than in the general population.[7]

COSTS

The costs of diabetes are staggering. In 2002, direct medical costs of diabetes were estimated to be $92 billion, with an additional $40 billion in indirect costs due to disability, work loss, and premature mortality. This estimated $132 billion price tag is certainly a substantial underestimate because it omits costs incurred in persons with undiagnosed diabetes, intangibles such as pain and suffering, the cost of unreimbursed care such as that provided by family members and friends, and certain areas of health care spending for which data were not available and in which people with diabetes consume services at higher rates than the general population, such as care by optometrists and dentists. Overall health care costs for people with diabetes are more than double the costs for people who do not have diabetes.[10]

REPORT CARD

The real tragedy of diabetes in the early 21st century in the United States is that there is so much diabetes-related death and disability despite a rapid evolution in diagnostic and therapeutic technology as well as a robust understanding of the techniques required to minimize the risk of developing end-stage complications. The clinical trial basis for current guidelines regarding the management of people with diabetes suggests that the vast majority of complications of diabetes can be prevented. However, adherence with current guidelines is poor.

That is not to say that progress has not been made. Using data from the National Health and Nutrition Examination Survey (NHANES) for 1971 to 1974, 1976 to 1980, 1988 to 1994, and 1999 to 2000, 30-year trends in control of major cardiovascular risk factors have been evaluated in US adults older than the age of 20 years. Certainly the fraction of people with diabetes who exhibit high cholesterol, hypertension, and smoking has decreased substantially over the 30-year interval.[11] Nevertheless, estimates suggest that in 2000, 64% of people with diabetes had blood pressure higher than or 130/80 mm Hg; 63% had a hemoglobin A1c (HbA1c) greater than 7% and 37% had an HbA1c greater than 8%; 52% had a total cholesterol greater than or equal to 200 mg/dL; 16% smoked tobacco; and only 23% took aspirin on a nearly daily basis (Fig. 1–3).[12] Most disturbing, the odds of a patient with diabetes achieving an HbA1c less than 7% was 21% lower in NHANES 1999 to 2000 compared with NHANES 1988 to 1994.[13] Less than 5% of people with diabetes in the United States in 2000 achieved

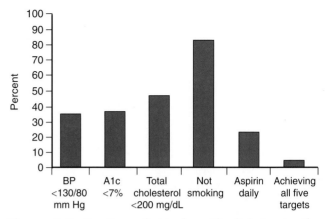

Figure 1–3. Fraction of people with diabetes in the United States achieving treatment targets, 2000. A1c, hemoglobin A1c fraction; BP, blood pressure. (From Saydah SH, Fradkin J, Cowie CC: Poor control of risk factors for vascular disease among adults with previously diagnosed diabetes. JAMA 291:335-342, 2004.)

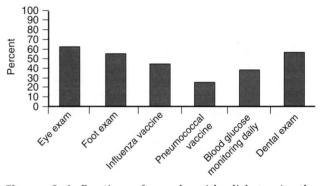

Figure 1–4. Fraction of people with diabetes in the United States who have had the appropriate screening and preventive services, 1995. (From Saaddine JB, Engelgau MM, Beckles GL, et al: A diabetes report card for the United States: Quality of care in the 1990s. Ann Intern Med 136:565-574, 2002.)

the five health care targets that are universally considered critical for controlling cardiovascular and microvascular risk.[12]

The results of surveys assessing process measures are equally disturbing. In 1995, a national telephone survey among diabetic patients between the ages of 18 and 75 found that 37% had not had an annual eye exam, 45% had not had an annual foot exam, 54% had not had an annual influenza vaccine, 74% had not had a pneumococcal vaccine, 62% were not self-monitoring blood glucose at least once daily, and 42% had not had an annual dental examination (Fig. 1–4).[14] Chart audits and patient interviews conducted across nine health care organizations demonstrated that highly organized processes of care, as have been implemented in the Veterans Affairs system, can result in 70% to 90% or more of patients receiv-

ing recommended individual screening evaluations and better control of cardiovascular risk factors than the looser organizational structure of most managed care organizations.[15]

CONCLUSION

Diabetes is an enormous burden on patients, families, and the health care system today. The epidemic increase in the numbers of people with diagnosed diabetes forecast year after year for the next half century, coupled with its enormous burden of cost, both fiscal and physical, threatens not only the health of tens of millions of individuals in our society but also the health of our society itself. Based on the knowledge and technology described in the following chapters, it should be routine to correct the metabolic abnormalities associated with diabetes in virtually every patient and to prevent or delay the onset of both diabetes and its complications. Whether that hope is realized will depend on clinicians and their patients carefully applying the principles described in subsequent chapters, and it will be judged in the years to come. But the need is urgent.

References

1. MacFarlane IA, Bliss M, Jackson JGL, Williams G: The history of diabetes mellitus. In Pickup JC, Williams G (eds): Textbook of Diabetes, vol 1. Oxford, Blackwell Science, 1991, pp 1-21.
2. American Diabetes Association: Standards of medical care in diabetes. Diabetes Care 28:S4-S36, 2005.
3. Centers for Disease Control and Prevention: National Diabetes Fact Sheet. Available at http://www.cdc.gov/diabetes/pubs/estimates.htm.
4. Grundy SM, Brewer HB Jr, Cleeman JI, et al: Definition of metabolic syndrome: Report of the National Heart, Lung, and Blood Institute/American Heart Association conference on scientific issues related to definition. Circulation109:433-438, 2004.
5. Pinhas-Hamiel O, Dolan LM, Daniels SR, et al: Increased incidence of non-insulin-dependent diabetes mellitus among adolescents. J Pediatr 128:608-615, 1996.
6. Narayan KM, Boyle JP, Thompson TJ, et al: Lifetime risk for diabetes mellitus in the United States. JAMA 290:1884-1890, 2003.
7. Engelgau MM, Geiss LS, Saaddine JB, et al: The evolving diabetes burden in the United States. Ann Intern Med 140:945-950, 2004.
8. Crispin JC, Alcocer-Varela J: Rheumatologic manifestations of diabetes mellitus. Am J Med 114:753-757, 2003.
9. Jee SH, Ohrr H, Sull JW, et al: Fasting serum glucose level and cancer risk in Korean men and women. JAMA 293:194-202, 2005.
10. Hogan P, Dall T, Nikolov P, for the American Diabetes Association: Economic costs of diabetes in the US in 2002. Diabetes Care 26:917-932, 2003.
11. Imperatore G, Cadwell BL, Geiss L, et al: Thirty-year trends in cardiovascular risk factor levels among US adults with diabetes. National Health and Nutrition Examination Surveys, 1971-2000. Am J Epidemiol 160:531-539, 2004.
12. Saydah SH, Fradkin J, Cowie CC: Poor control of risk factors for vascular disease among adults with previously diagnosed diabetes. JAMA 291:335-342, 2004.
13. Koro CE, Bowlin SJ, Bourgeois N, Fedder DO: Glycemic control from 1988 to 2000 among U.S. adults diagnosed with type 2 diabetes: A preliminary report. Diabetes Care 27:17-20, 2004.
14. Saaddine JB, Engelgau MM, Beckles GL, et al: A diabetes report card for the United States: Quality of care in the 1990s. Ann Intern Med 136:565-574, 2002.
15. Kerr EA, Gerzoff RB, Krein SL, et al: Diabetes care quality in the Veterans Affairs Health Care System and commercial managed care: The TRIAD study. Ann Intern Med 141:272-281, 2004.

Type 1 Diabetes: Immunology and Genetics

Nikolai Petrovsky, William E. Winter, and
Desmond A. Schatz

KEY POINTS

- *Type 1 diabetes mellitus results from immune-mediated destruction of pancreatic islet beta cells, although the precise mechanisms leading to the disease are unknown.*
- *Almost 90% of new cases occur without a family history of type 1 diabetes. However, relatives of patients with type 1 diabetes have a 15- to 20-fold increased risk of developing type 1 diabetes compared with the general population.*
- *Type 1 diabetes can be predicted in higher-risk relatives and in the general population by using a combination of genetic, immunologic, and metabolic testing.*
- *More than 90% of patients with type 1 diabetes have one or more autoantibodies directed against islet cells. These autoantibodies are the best predictors for subsequent development of type 1 diabetes.*
- *As many as 20 genes (and possibly more) influence susceptibility to type 1 diabetes, although the human leukocyte antigen gene complex, located on chromosome 6, has by far the strongest influence on diabetes susceptibility.*

Type 1 diabetes mellitus (T1DM) results from immune-mediated destruction of pancreatic islet beta cells. Most commonly, affected children and adolescents present with symptoms of hyperglycemia including polydipsia, polyuria, polyphagia, weight loss, and, in severe cases, ketoacidosis and coma. It is important to remember, however, that T1DM can occur at any age. It is estimated that approximately 5% to 10% of adult patients thought to have type 2 diabetes actually have a slowly progressive form of T1DM that is termed *latent autoimmune diabetes of adults* (LADA). Almost 90% of new cases of T1DM occur without a family history of T1DM. However, relatives of probands with T1DM have a 15- to 20-fold increased risk of subsequently developing T1DM compared with the general population.

Through the use of assays for immune markers such as islet cell autoantibodies (ICA) and autoantibodies to insulin (IAA), glutamic acid decarboxylase (GADA), and a tyrosine phosphatase (IA-2), we now know that T1DM has a variable preclinical phase that can last months to years or decades before clinical diabetes ensues. This discovery has raised the possibility of using immune interventions during this preclinical phase to prevent diabetes from developing. Although a cure has yet to be found, many immune-therapy approaches have been validated in animal models to prevent T1DM, and a number of these interventions have already progressed to human clinical trials.

Although much remains to be learned regarding the etiology and pathogenesis of this important autoimmune disorder, both genetic and environmental factors are known to contribute to susceptibility. As many as 20 or more genes influence susceptibility to T1DM, although the human leukocyte antigen (HLA) gene complex, located on the short arm of chromosome 6, has by far the strongest influence on diabetes susceptibility or resistance. Second in importance to HLA alleles is the insulin gene locus. Although many other susceptibility loci have been mapped, the responsible genes remain elusive. Recent research efforts have focused on better understanding of the immunoregulatory and immunoeffector mechanisms of pancreatic beta cell killing with a view to developing therapies to protect against T1DM.

NATURAL HISTORY OF TYPE 1 DIABETES

The first clue that T1DM was an immune-mediated disorder came in the mid 1970s with the identification of antibodies to islet cell cytoplasm (ICA) in the serum of patients with recently diagnosed T1DM and in patients with polyglandular autoimmune syndromes. Since that time the major target proteins to which these ICAs react have been characterized, the most important being GAD and IA-2

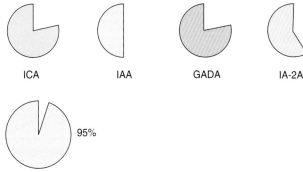

Islet Autoantibody Frequencies in New-Onset Children

ICA   IAA   GADA   IA-2A

95%

Figure 2–1. Ninety percent or more of new-onset subjects with type 1 diabetes are found to express one or more types of islet autoantibodies. Islet cell cytoplasmic autoantibodies (ICA) and glutamic acid decarboxylase autoantibodies (GADA) are the most common, being found in 70% to 80% of new-onset patients. Insulinoma-associated-2 autoantibodies (IA-2A) are less common (approximately 60% prevalence at disease onset). In children with new-onset disease, insulin autoantibodies (IAA) are present in about 50%. However, IAA are uncommon in adults.

(insulinoma-associated-2) autoantigen. More than 90% of patients with T1DM have one or more of these antibodies, or antibodies to insulin (IAA), or both (Fig. 2–1). These antibodies can be used diagnostically—for example, to distinguish type 1 from other forms of diabetes. They can also be used predictively—for example, to define persons at risk and thereby enhance the understanding of the natural history of prediabetes.[1-2]

T1DM develops in persons at increased genetic risk (Fig. 2–2). Although it still has to be confirmed, the prevailing hypothesis is that specific islet-directed autoimmunity is triggered by environmental agents. Islet-related antibodies, including ICA, IAA, GADA, and IA-2A, can often be detected long before diabetes manifests, indicating the presence of a prodromal preclinical phase during which beta cell destruction is taking place but there is still sufficient insulin capacity to maintain normoglycemia. It is not until the majority of beta cells are destroyed that hyperglycemia develops and clinical diabetes ensues. The rate of progression to T1DM is variable, being a lot faster in younger prepubertal subjects. Not all autoantibody-positive subjects go on to develop diabetes, indicating the relapsing-remitting nature characteristic of autoimmune diseases.

ICA and GADA are present in up to 70% to 80%, IA-2A in 50% to 60%, and IAA in about 40% of patients with newly diagnosed diabetes. IAAs are more commonly present in younger children with T1DM. Although the presence of any one autoanti-

body has a low predictive value for future diabetes development, the presence of two or more antibodies denotes a significant risk both in higher-risk relatives and the low-risk general population. With ongoing beta cell destruction, there is loss of insulin-secreting capacity that can be detected by intravenous glucose tolerance testing. Glucose intolerance determined during oral glucose tolerance testing occurs late in the T1DM process, predating the diagnosis of diabetes.

PANCREATIC ISLET HISTOLOGY

On rare occasions, postmortem and biopsy specimens from subjects with T1DM become available.[3] Such specimens reveal a characteristic histologic picture of early islet infiltration by macrophages, CD4 T cells, CD8 T cells, and B cells; hyperexpression of HLA class I and class II; the transporter associated with antigen processing (TAP); ICAM-1; and expression of inflammatory cytokines including interferon α (IFN-α) and IFN-γ (Fig. 2–3). Over time there is a complete loss of beta cells and relative preservation of the other islet cell types that secrete glucagon, somatostatin, and pancreatic polypeptide. Thus the destructive process that mediates T1DM is specifically targeted at beta cells. Islet-related autoantibodies are not thought to be pathogenic, rather acting as markers of ongoing beta cell destruction.

Considerable evidence in animal models of T1DM implicates T cells as key mediators of beta cell destruction. The disease can be transferred with splenocytes or purified T cells from acutely diabetic NOD mice when placed into young NOD mice. Additional support for the role of T cells comes from clinical studies where immunosuppressive therapies such as cyclosporine, azathioprine, and anti-CD3 monoclonal antibody administration have been able to at least temporarily preserve pancreatic beta cell function in subjects with recently diagnosed T1DM.

IMMUNE ABNORMALITIES IN HUMAN TYPE 1 DIABETES

A wide range of immune abnormalities[4,5] have been reported in humans and in animal models of T1DM (Table 2–1). Abnormalities in humans with T1DM include a deficiency of circulating natural killer and CD8 T cells, reduced theophylline sensitivity of peripheral blood lymphocytes, reduced autologous mixed lymphocyte response, defective generation of suppressor cell activity, reduced T-cell help for B-cell immunoglobulin production, and defective maturation and function of antigen-presenting cells. Peripheral blood analysis also reveals an increased percentage of HLA-DR, interleukin-2 (IL-2) receptor–positive T cells, and decreased percent-

Figure 2–2. A, The natural history of autoimmune beta cell destruction (type 1 diabetes mellitus; T1DM) begins with genetic susceptibility. This is predominantly supplied by specific human leukocyte antigen (HLA) alleles at the HLA-DRβ, HLA-DQα, and HLA-DQβ loci. The insulin gene locus also influences susceptibility to T1DM. In addition to the HLA complex and the insulin gene locus, more than 10 other loci influence susceptibility to T1DM. Genetics and environment interact to produce autoimmune beta cell destruction; however, the environmental triggers are still poorly described. Sometime after the environmental insult occurs, the first laboratory evidence of beta cell autoimmunity becomes evident in the finding of various islet autoantibodies such as islet cell cytoplasmic autoantibodies (ICA), insulin autoantibodies (IAA), glutamic acid decarboxylase autoantibodies (GADA), and insulinoma-associated-2 autoantibodies (IA-2A). With actual beta cell damage or cell death, beta cell mass declines (Y-axis) over time (X-axis). When the beta cell mass has declined approximately 50% from baseline, the first metabolic evidence of beta cell dysfunction is detected with a declining or deficient first-phase insulin response to the administration of intravenous glucose (i.e., the intravenous glucose tolerance test [IVGTT]). If beta cell destruction is progressive, the oral glucose tolerance test (OGTT) becomes abnormal, with the 2-hour glucose level equaling or exceeding 140 mg/dL and later equaling or exceeding 200 mg/dL. Fasting hyperglycemia follows postchallenge hyperglycemia. With the development of symptoms (e.g., polyuria, polydipsia, weight loss) or onset of ketoacidosis, the clinical diagnosis of T1DM is established. **B,** In this hypothetical model, the outcome of beta cell autoimmunity (beta mass: Y-axis) is depicted as one of several possible outcomes (time: X-axis). In the *red line,* progressive beta cell destruction is shown to cause classic type 1 diabetes mellitus near age 12 years. The *blue line* depicts a waxing-and-waning course, with eventual deterioration in beta cell function (e.g., relapse). The *yellow line* illustrates a decline in beta cell function followed by recovery. Some patients with islet autoantibodies do not experience a decline in beta cell function as shown in the *black dotted line.*

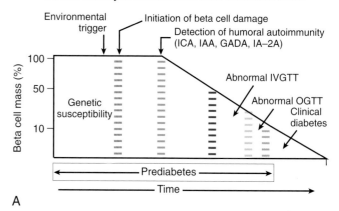

Natural History of Autoimmune Beta Cell Destruction

A

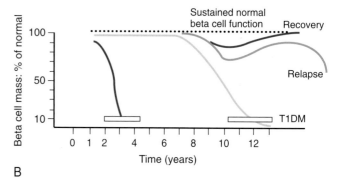

Beta Cell Autoimmunity: Possible Outcomes

B

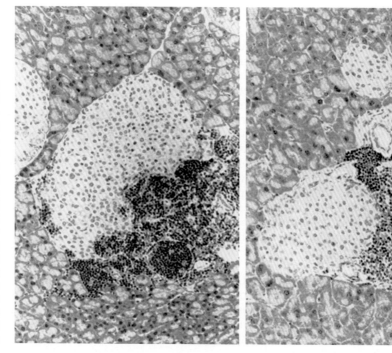

Figure 2–3. Experimental mice display insulitis and develop subsequent autoimmune diabetes that is similar to human type 1 diabetes. The best known mouse model of type 1 diabetes is the nonobese diabetic (NOD) mouse. These photographs display aspects of insulitis in experimental mice. **Left,** there is a heavy mononuclear cell infiltrate pressing into the mass of the islet. About 25% of the islet is infiltrated and there is also a heavy peri-islet infiltrate at the *lower right* portion of this photograph. **Right,** about 50% of the islet is infiltrated.

Table 2–1. *Type 1 Diabetes Mellitus in Humans and NOD Mice*

Characteristic	Humans	NOD Mice
Genetic predisposition, polygenetic trait	+	+
Environmental influence	yes	yes
Defective peripheral immunoregulation	yes	yes
Impaired DC maturation and function	yes	yes
Disease transmissible with BMT	yes	yes
Autoantigens	GAD65, IA-2, ins, 38k	GAD65, IA-2, ins, 38k
Delayed onset with immunosuppression	yes	yes
Endogenous retrovirus	?	yes
Diabetic ketoacidosis if not treated	yes	yes
T-cell driven insulitis	mild	severe
humoral reactivity to beta cells	GAD65, IA-2, insulin, ICA	insulin
Name	type 1 diabetes mellitus	autoimmune diabetes
IDDM-1 or *idd1*	multiple loci within MHC	one MHC locus (I-A^{g7})
Number of insulin genes	1	2
Incidence	0.25%-0.4%	>80%
Gender bias	no	females
Periinsulitis	no	yes
Lymphocyte infiltrates in other tissues	sometimes	always
Susceptibility of beta cells to STZ, NO	no	yes
Maternal autoantibodies	reduced risk	diabetogenic
B lymphocytes required	no	yes
Successful intervention therapies	?	multiple (A-Z)

BMT, bone marrow transplantation; DC, dendritic cells; GAD, glutamic acid decarboxylase; IA-2, insulinoma-associated-2 autoantigen; ICA, islet cell autoantibodies; NO, nitric oxide; MHC, major histocompatibility complex; NOD, nonobese diabetic; STZ, streptozotocin.

ages of CD4+ and CD45R+ T cells. It is unknown whether these differences in the peripheral blood actually reflect what is occurring in the islets or is secondary to underlying metabolic disturbances such as hyperglycemia and hyperlipidemia. However, some of these findings have been reported to predate hyperglycemia and therefore could represent immune abnormalities that confer susceptibility to T1DM.

Two distinct subgroups of T cells can be distinguished by their characteristic patterns of cytokine production. T helper 1 (Th1) cells produce IL-2, IFN-γ, and tumor necrosis factor β (TNF-β) and mediate cell-mediated immunity and delayed-type hypersensitivity (DTH) responses. T helper 2 (Th2) cells produce IL-4, -5, -6, and -10 and mediate humoral responses.

The histology of the insulitis lesion has the characteristics of a DTH lesion, and this has led to the hypothesis that T1DM is a Th1 disease. IFN-γ, TNF-α, and IL-1 have been reported to be elevated in the serum or plasma of patients with T1DM. However, although many mouse T-cell clones that successfully transfer diabetes produce IFN-γ, Th2 clones can also transfer diabetes, and both Th1 and Th2 cytokines are expressed in the mouse and human insulitis lesion. This suggests that both Th1 and Th2 cytokines play a role in diabetes pathogenesis.

Considerable effort has been expended over the years to develop an assay to detect autoreactive T cells in persons with T1DM. Readouts include T cell proliferation, cytokine production, or surface activation markers using ELISPOT (enzyme-linked immunospot technique), ELISA (enzyme-linked immunosorbent assay), or FACS (fluorescence-acti-

vated cell sorting) technologies. However, as yet no assay has been shown to reliably discriminate between persons who do and who do not have T1DM susceptibility. Thus, islet autoantibody assays remain the gold standard for identifying persons at risk for T1DM.

IMMUNOREGULATORY DEFECTS IN ANIMAL MODELS OF T1DM

The diabetes-prone BioBreeding (DP-BB) rat and the nonobese diabetic (NOD) mouse have been the most commonly used animal models of human T1DM.[6] Both rodent models exhibit major immune-system defects. The DP-BB rat exhibits severe lymphopenia, decreased cytotoxic T cells, increased susceptibility to infectious agents, and defective production of IL-1 and TNF. The NOD mouse has defects predominantly related to antigen-presenting cell function. NOD macrophages have a reduced ability to produce IL-1 and TNF-β, have abnormal prostaglandin (PGE$_2$) production, and respond poorly to the myeloid growth factors granulocyte-macrophage colony-stimulating factor (GM-CSF), IL-3, and IL-5. In addition, NOD macrophages aberrantly regulate mRNA transcripts that encode for CSF-1 and IFN-β receptors, and they fail to activate immunoregulatory cells in the syngeneic mixed lymphocyte reaction (MLR).

Collectively the animal data might argue that autoimmune susceptibility is a function of an underactive immune system rather than the more traditional view that autoimmunity is the conse-

Insulitis in NOD Mice

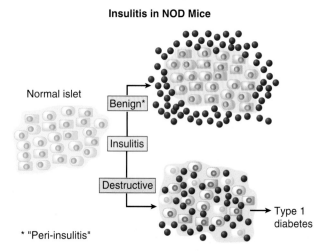

Normal islet

Benign*

Insulitis

Destructive

Type 1 diabetes

* "Peri-insulitis"

Figure 2–4. Insulitis, an inflammatory infiltration of the islets of Langerhans, is the pathognomonic histopathology of type 1 diabetes in both humans and nonobese diabetic (NOD) mice. In NOD mice, insulitis can appear in a variety of patterns. Nondestructive (benign) insulitis is characterized by peri-islet insulitis *(top right)*. In contrast, if the inflammatory cells invade the substance of the islet, beta cell destruction occurs *(bottom right)*.

quence of immune overactivity. This newer model is supported by the evidence that patients with immunodeficiency syndromes including AIDS also have a high incidence of autoimmune disease. Thus, autoimmune diseases such as T1DM might be amenable to treatment with immunostimulatory or immunoregulatory agents that have less potential for toxicity than traditional immunosuppressive drugs.

BENIGN VERSUS DESTRUCTIVE INSULITIS

Not all persons with islet-related autoantibodies progress to diabetes. This suggests that insulitis does not inevitably lead to beta cell destruction. Thus insulitis might exist in two states in humans: benign insulitis and destructive insulitis (Fig. 2–4).[7] In the NOD mouse model, beta cell destruction occurs late in the setting of chronic insulitis due to an unknown switch or trigger that leads to a failure of immune regulation or beta cell defense that culminates in rapid beta cell destruction. The switch from benign to destructive insulitis can be prevented or delayed in NOD mice by administering immunostimulants including OK-432 (a preparation derived from streptococci), Freund's complete adjuvant, bacillus Calmette-Guérin (BCG), or Q fever antigen (QFA). It is yet to be determined whether these promising immune intervention strategies will similarly be effective in preventing T1DM in prediabetic humans.

POTENTIAL MECHANISMS OF AUTOIMMUNITY

Autoimmunity is a process whereby the immune system attacks normal, healthy self-tissue instead of performing its normal function, which is to protect against pathogens and tumors. Thus, autoimmunity is a failure of normal self–nonself discrimination. The capacity of the immune system to avoid reacting against self is called *tolerance* (Fig. 2–5A).

Tolerance is predominantly a T-cell function. It is easier to tolerize experimental animals through prenatal or neonatal exposure to antigen than through exposure to antigen later in life. A prerequisite for autoimmunity is, therefore, a breakdown in tolerance (see Fig. 2–5B). Until recently it was believed that the primary mechanism of tolerance was the thymic deletion of all self-reactive T-cells. However, self-reactive T cells are found in the peripheral circulation of healthy persons, indicating that mechanisms other than thymic deletion prevent autoimmunity.

Central (thymic) tolerance occurs when developing double-positive T cells (i.e., positive for CD4 and CD8) strongly bind to major histocompatibility complex (MHC) molecules that express self-antigen peptides in the thymic cortex and subsequently undergo apoptosis. This is negative selection. In the periphery, when naive T cells encounter peptide without the necessary costimulatory molelcules (i.e., the T cell–B7 interaction with antigen-presenting cell CD28), the T cell is *anergized*. Anergized T cells do not undergo apoptosis; however they are unreactive to subsequent antigen peptide stimulation even if the normal costimulatory factors are present.

Tolerance is most likely a multitiered phenomenon encompassing numerous fail-safe mechanisms both at the level of the thymus and in the periphery. There is increasing evidence that unique populations of regulatory T cells (T regs)—which include discrete populations of natural killer (NK) T cells that secrete IL-4, T cells that secrete IL-10 or TGF-β, and CD4 T cells that bear the CD25 and CD62L markers—are involved in maintaining tolerance.

Autoimmunity can result from a failure to establish tolerance, allowing autoreactive cells to exit the thymus. Alternatively, tolerance might not be established because of a failure to develop peripheral tolerance upon autoantigen exposure.

A hypothetical model of autoimmune destruction of beta cells is shown in Figure 2–6. In this model, the environmental trigger damages the beta cell, releasing sequestered or altered self-antigens. Antigen-presenting cells, such as macrophages or dendritic cells, take up these self-antigens, process them, and present autoantigen peptides to naive CD4 T cells (Fig. 2–7). These cells differentiate into either Th1 or Th2 cells. Via IL-2, the Th1 cells help active naive CD8 T cells to become T killer (cytotoxic) cells that attack beta cells (Fig. 2–8). Simi-

Development of Tolerance to Self-Antigens

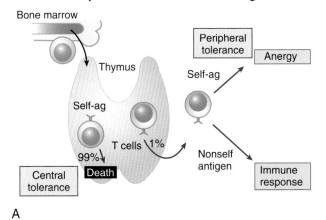

A

Autoimmunity: Failure of Tolerance to Self-Antigens

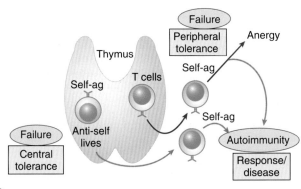

B

Figure 2–5. A, Normal tolerance pathways. All T cell precursors initially arise in the bone marrow *(top left)*. These progenitors enter the thymus and encounter self-antigen (self-ag). Strong self-antigen stimulation of developing T cells induces apoptosis, with approximately 99% of all developing T cells dying. This is central immunologic tolerance, where strongly anti-self T cells are eliminated. The mature, naive T cells that do leave the thymus can be subsequently tolerized to self-antigens not present in the thymus if these T cells encounter self-antigen without all of the normal costimulatory signals (e.g., B7–CD28 interactions, not shown). Induction of tolerance outside the thymus is termed *peripheral tolerance (top right)*, and it can be considered a backup or complementary mechanism to central tolerance. Peripheral tolerance is functionally expressed as anergy: Autoreactive cells are present but they are inactive *(top right)*. If the body confronts a nonself antigen, a normal immune response ensues *(bottom right)*. **B,** Autoimmunity develops because of a failure to establish tolerance or a loss of tolerance. With a failure of central tolerance *(bottom left)*, anti-self T cells survive that should not normally survive. When such anti-self T cells leave the thymus, they are able to produce autoimmunity *(green arrow)*. Alternatively, with a failure of peripheral tolerance *(top right, red arrow)*, if anergy does not occur after contact with self-antigen, an autoimmune response can occur *(green arrow)*.

larly, via IFN-γ release, the Th1 cells help active macrophages to release toxic cytokines that damage beta cells (see Fig. 2–8).

The details of CD8 T cell–target cell interaction are outlined in Figure 2–9. Activated CD8 T cells first recognize their target by the target's presentation of self-antigen peptide via class I MHC molecules. Next, one way that CD8 T cells kill targets is by introducing granzymes into the target cell cytoplasm; the granzymes induce apoptosis in the target cell. Granzymes enter the target cell via pores placed in the target cell plasma membrane by perforins. An alternative mechanism that CD8 T cells use to induce target-cell apoptosis is FAS/FAS ligand (Fig. 2–10). Fas ligand is expressed on the cytotoxic CD8 T cell, whereas FAS is expressed on the target cell. When B cells encounter antigen and receive help from activated Th2 cells (Fig. 2–11), these B cells can develop into plasma cells that produce islet autoantibodies (Fig. 2–12).

Several hypotheses have been proposed to explain the breakdown in tolerance leading to autoimmunity. Autoimmune diseases might occur because tolerance fails to develop early in life or tolerance to specific self-antigens is lost later in life. If self-antigen is not efficiently presented in the thymus, tolerance might not be established during T-cell education within the thymic cortex. For example, the diabetes susceptibility gene *IDDM2* maps to the insulin gene *VNTR* (variable number of tandem repeats). Variations in the number of tandem repeats in the insulin gene *VNTR*, approximately 500 base pairs upstream of the insulin gene promoter, influence the extent of insulin gene expression in the thymic cortex. Persons with the VNTR allele family linked to diabetes susceptibility have lower insulin mRNA expression in the thymus gland than those who have the allele family associated with diabetes protection. Low thymic insulin expression could thus result in a failure to delete autoreactive T cells directed against insulin, thereby predisposing to T1DM.

Central tolerance could also fail because an antigen might be sequestered intracellularly and therefore not come into contact with the immune system until there is a breakdown of anatomical barriers within the body. An example of this is the development of autoimmunity to the testes following testicular trauma. However, failure of thymic deletion alone does not explain T1DM susceptibility, because healthy persons harbor islet-antigen reactive T cells and yet do not develop diabetes.

Development of islet autoimmunity thus most likely reflects a failure of both central and peripheral tolerance. This could result, for example, from activation of autoreactive T cells by islet antigen in the context of potent T-cell costimulation. Peripheral tissues such as islets normally do not express T-cell costimulatory molecules. Aberrant expression of costimulatory molecules and up-regulation of HLA expression by islet cells in susceptible persons

Model of Autoimmune Beta Cell Destruction

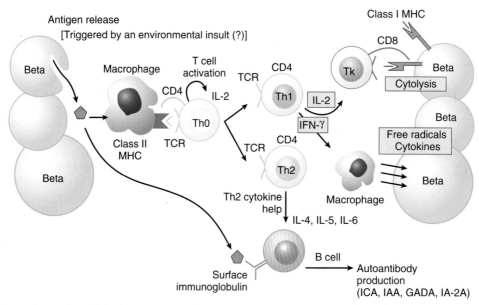

Figure 2–6. A hypothetical model of autoimmune beta cell destruction is illustrated. In this model, the environmental trigger damages the beta cell, releasing sequestered or altered self-antigens. Antigen-presenting cells such as macrophages or dendritic cells (not shown), take up these self-antigens, process the self-antigens, and present autoantigen peptides to naive CD4 T cells. These cells differentiate into either Th1 or Th2 cells. Via interleukin-2 (IL-2), the Th1 cells help activate naive CD8 T cells to become T killer (cytotoxic) cells that attack beta cells. Similarly, via interferon-γ (IFN-γ) release, the Th1 cells help activate macrophages to release toxic cytokines that damage beta cells. When B cells encounter antigen and receive help from activated Th2 cells, these B cells can develop into plasma cells that produce islet autoantibodies. GADA, glutamic acid decarboxylase autoantibodies; IAA, insulin autoantibodies; ICA, islet cell cytoplasmic autoantibodies; IA-2A, insulinoma-associated 2 autoantibodies; IL, interleukin; MHC, major histocompatibility complex; TCR, T cell receptor; Tk, T killer.

Figure 2–7. The pathogenesis of type 1 diabetes mellitus is controversial. In the sequestered-antigen hypothesis of initiation of beta cell autoimmunity, a yet-to-be described environmental trigger damages normal beta cells and releases self-antigens (autoantigens) to which the immune system lacks tolerance. These autoantigens are taken up by professional antigen-presenting cells (APCs). Via class II major histocompatibility complex (MHC) molecules located on the surface of the APCs, self-peptides are presented to naive CD4 T cells. Activation of the CD4 T cells of the Th1 variety is then able to initiate anti–beta cell cell-mediated autoimmunity.

Initial Activation of Anti-Beta Cell CD4 T Cells:
Sequestered Self-Antigen

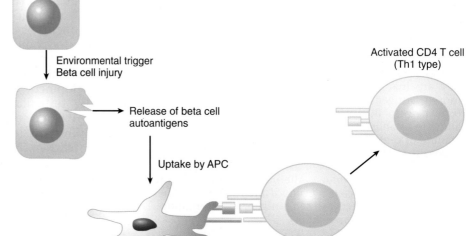

**CD4 T Cell (Th1 variety) Activates
Cell-Mediated Autoimmunity**

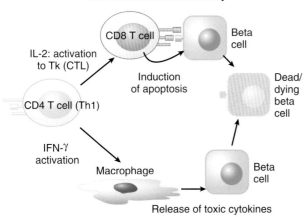

Figure 2–8. CD4 T cells of the Th1 variety can provide help to CD8 T cells via interleukin-2 (IL-2) elaboration. Activated CD8 T cells acquire cytotoxic T cell (CTL) activity as T killer (Tk) cells. Activated CD8 T cells traffic throughout the body. When these T killer cells encounter beta cells displaying self-peptides to which an autoimmune response has developed, the T killer cells induce apoptosis in the beta cells. As a complementary or alternative mechanism to CD8 T cell activation, via the release of interferon-γ (IFN-γ), Th1 cells can activate macrophages to locally release cytotoxic cytokines (e.g., IL-1) that damage or destroy beta cells. Both mechanisms—T killer cell attack on beta cells and macrophage attacks on beta cells—are manifestations of cell-mediated autoimmunity.

**CD8 T Cell (Tk) Induction of Apoptosis
in a Beta Cell via Perforin and Granzymes**

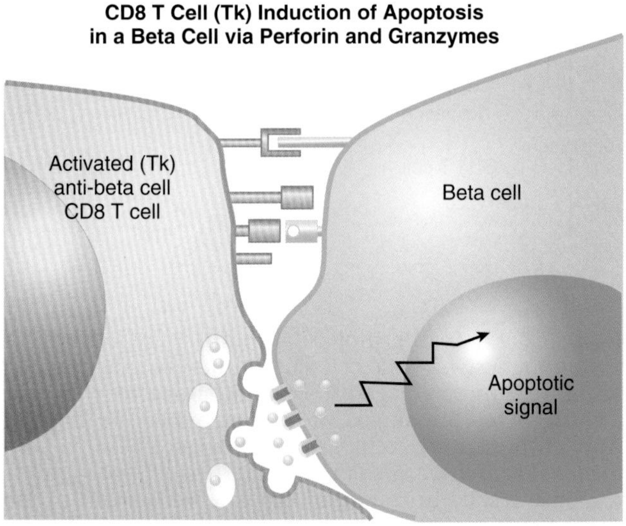

Figure 2–9. Beta cell killing via activated CD8 T cells (e.g., CTLs, Tks) is illustrated (the CD8 T cell is on the *left* and the beta cell is on the *right*). The T-cell receptor of the CD8 T cell recognizes peptide presented by class I MHC molecules on the beta cell surface. Supplemental molecular interactions strengthen this contact. The T killer cell membrane makes contact with the beta cell membrane, forming a cleft. The T killer cell secretes granules into the cleft. The granules contain granzymes (*yellow circles*) and perforins (*red rectangles*). The perforins place holes in the beta cell membrane, allowing the granzymes access to the beta cell cytoplasm. The granzymes activate intrinsic beta cell apoptotic mechanisms.

**CD8 T Cell (Tk) Induction of Apoptosis in a Beta Cell via
Fas Ligand–Fas Interaction**

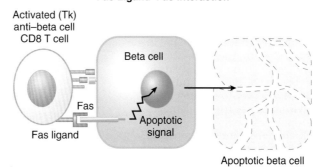

Figure 2–10. CD8 T cells can induce apoptosis via cell-surface contact interactions in addition to the perforin–granzyme pathway. The activated CD8 T cell (e.g., Tk or CTL) expresses Fas ligand on its surface. When Fas ligand contacts Fas on the beta cell target cell surface, intrinsic beta cell apoptotic mechanisms are engaged, causing apoptosis.

might, therefore, be an important contributor to breakdown of islet tolerance. This could happen in the context of viral infections that disturb cellular integrity and lead to simultaneous presentation of intracellular islet antigens on HLA class I and class II molecules and up-regulation of costimulatory molecules on the beta cell surface.

Alteration of self-antigens as a result of an environmental factor, such as an infection, could also underlie autoimmunity. Modification of self-proteins, for example by a virus, can result in a new antigen not normally part of the self-repertoire. An example of a neoantigen induced autoimmunity is autoimmune hemolytic anemia caused by drugs that bind to red blood cells.

Molecular mimicry is another popular theory for autoimmunity: An immune response originally directed against a dietary, viral, or bacterial antigen (e.g., infection) leads through cross reactivity to an immune response against a self-antigen (Fig. 2–13). For example, in rheumatic fever there is cross reactivity between streptococcal polysaccharide N-acetyl glucosamine and cardiac myosin.

Certain substances, termed *superantigens,* have the ability to cross link the T-cell receptor beta chain and HLA molecules. Autoimmunity could result when superantigens initiate an anti-self immune response as part of polyclonal immune activation. Endogenous retroviruses have been postulated as possible superantigens that could trigger autoimmunity in T1DM.

It is not known which mechanisms are relevant to T1DM, although clearly environmental and genetic factors are involved. Although environmental factors have been identified in other autoimmune diseases (e.g., wheat gliadin ingestion in celiac disease, penicillamine exposure in myasthenia gravis, and amiodarone in thyroiditis), the environmental factors involved in T1DM are currently not known.

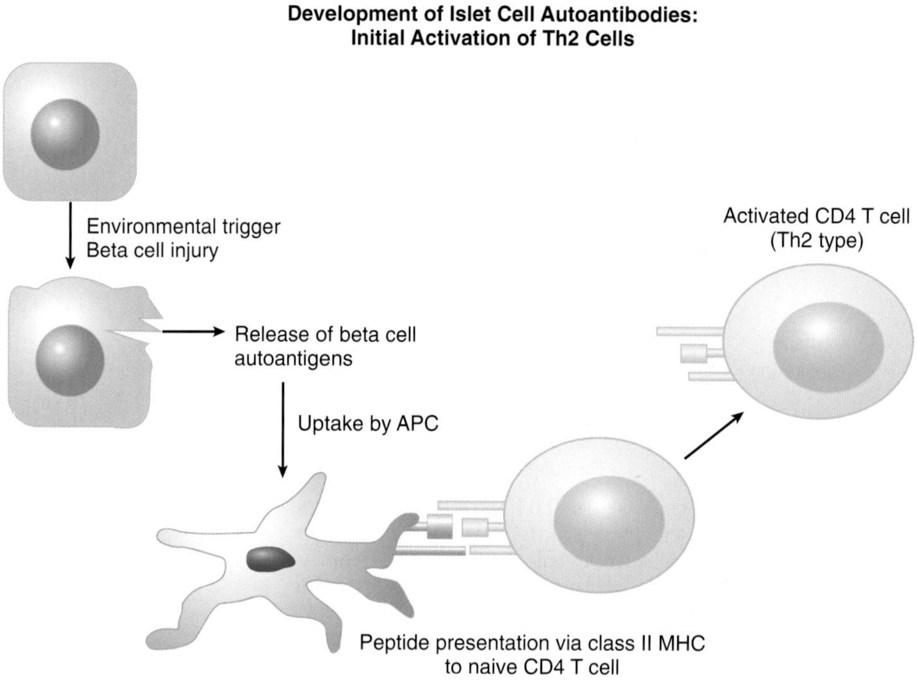

Figure 2–11. The hypothetical induction of islet cell humoral (antibody-mediated) autoimmunity is illustrated. As in figure 2-7, in the sequestered-antigen hypothesis of initiation of beta cell humoral autoimmunity, a yet-to-be described environmental trigger damages normal beta cells and releases self-antigens (autoantigens) to which the immune system lacks tolerance. These autoantigens are taken up by professional antigen-presenting cells (APCs). Via class II major histocompatibility complex (MHC) molecules located on the surface of the APCs, self-peptides are presented to naive CD4 T cells. Activation of the CD4 T cells of the Th2 variety is then able to initiate anti–beta cell humoral autoimmunity.

Development of Islet Cell Autoantibodies: Initial Activation of Th2 Cells

Environmental trigger
Beta cell injury

Release of beta cell autoantigens

Uptake by APC

Activated CD4 T cell (Th2 type)

Peptide presentation via class II MHC to naive CD4 T cell

Development of Islet Cell Autoantibodies: Activation of B Cells to Plasma Cells

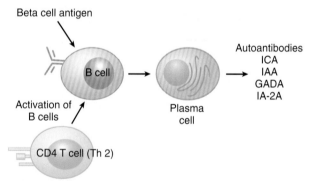

Beta cell antigen

B cell

Activation of B cells

Plasma cell

Autoantibodies
ICA
IAA
GADA
IA-2A

CD4 T cell (Th 2)

Figure 2–12. B cells that encounter self-antigen via B cell surface receptor (i.e., antibody) that also receive help from CD4 T cells and CD40–CD40 ligand interactions (not illustrated) become activated. CD4 T cells (Th2) include the cytokines interleukin (IL)-4, IL-5, and IL-6. Activated B cells undergo class switching and affinity maturation (not illustrated), eventually evolving into plasma cells that produce the islet autoantibodies islet cell cytoplasmic autoantibodies (ICA), insulin autoantibodies (IAA), glutamic acid decarboxylase autoantibodies (GADA) and insulinoma-associated 2 autoantibodies (IA-2A).

Molecular Mimicry in the Pathogenesis of Type 1 Diabetes

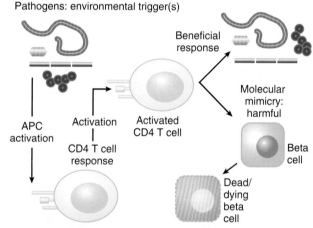

Pathogens: environmental trigger(s)

Beneficial response

Molecular mimicry: harmful

APC activation

Activation

CD4 T cell response

Activated CD4 T cell

Beta cell

Dead/ dying beta cell

Figure 2–13. In the molecular-mimicry hypothesis for the induction of beta cell autoimmunity, an immune response is initiated against an environmental pathogen: a virus, bacterium, fungus, protozoan, or parasite *(top left)*. Antigen-presenting cells (APCs) activate CD4 T cells *(bottom left to figure middle)*. A normal, beneficial immune response results in the clearance or containment of the pathogen *(top right)*. If cross reactivity exists between the beta cell antigens and the pathogenic antigens, a detrimental autoimmune attack on self occurs, destroying beta cells *(bottom right)*.

PATHWAYS OF BETA CELL DEATH

It appears that T cells are responsible for killing beta cells, and several mechanisms can account for beta cell destruction as discussed earlier (see Figs. 2–8 through 2–10). Beta cell death appears to be a complex process mediated by multiple pathways including the death receptors (Fas, TRAIL, TNF), cytokines (IL-1), IFN-γ, free radicals including nitric oxide (NO) and reactive oxygen species (ROS), cytotoxic factors (perforin, granzyme), metabolic insults (elevated free fatty acids and glucose), and endoplasmic reticulum stress. A key question is which

pathways are relevant to autoimmune destruction of beta cells.

During development of T1DM, the islet environment is modified by a progressive invasion of immune cells. This infiltrate is characterized by immune cells that produce cytokines, chemokines, nitric oxide (NO), and ROS. The nature of the beta cell response to this infiltrate involves a complex interaction of soluble mediators, receptor signaling, transcription factors, gene networks, and effector molecules. A recent important finding is that beta cells adapt in the presence of insulitis and actively protect themselves against cell death mediators such as ROS and NO.

At the same time, in response to cytokine stimulation, beta cells up-regulate expression of the death receptor, Fas, which is expressed on beta cells of persons with T1DM. On contacting Fas ligand expressed by activated autoreactive T cells, Fas triggers beta cell death.[8] Strategies that block Fas signaling can prevent diabetes development in the NOD mouse. A safe and effective method of blocking beta cell Fas expression has yet to be developed for humans. Another factor that might contribute to beta cell death is perforin, a product of CD8 T cells that damages the cell membrane of the target cell and thereby activates the caspase pathway, leading to cell death. It is possible that multiple pathways of beta cell death might need to be blocked, therefore, to completely prevent beta cell destruction and T1DM.

ASSOCIATION WITH OTHER AUTOIMMUNE DISORDERS

T1DM can occur in association other autoimmune diseases, including the autoimmune polyglandular syndromes (APS) (Fig. 2–14).[9] Associated conditions include adrenocortical insufficiency (Addison disease), autoimmune thyroid disease, and celiac disease. A gender bias is not present in patients with isolated T1DM, although there is a female predominance in APS type 2 patients.

Thyroid microsomal (thyroid peroxidase) or thyroglobulin autoantibodies, or both, identify thyroiditis in about 10% to 20% of patients with T1DM. Gastric parietal cell autoantibodies (PCA) are present in approximately 10% of female and 5% of male patients with T1DM, although progression to overt pernicious anemia rarely occurs before the age of 50 years. Adrenocortical autoimmunity is relatively uncommon among T1DM patients, with serologic evidence reported in 0.4% to 2.7% of cases. Celiac disease is present in 2% to 3% of patients with T1DM and should be suspected in patients with unexplained diarrhea, weight loss, failure to gain weight, or failure to thrive.

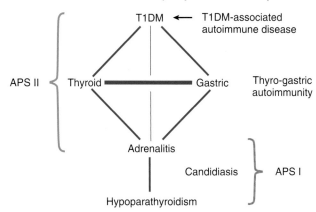

Autoimmune Endocrinopathy Interrelationships

Figure 2–14. Autoimmune endocrine and some nonendocrine disorders often occur in recognizable patterns. Autoimmune thyroid disease (thyroid autoimmunity, e.g., Hashimoto's thyroiditis or Graves' disease) is commonly present together with chronic lymphocytic gastritis (gastric autoimmunity) that can produce pernicious anemia. This forms the thyro-gastric association. In association with type 1 diabetes, thyroid, gastric, and adrenal autoimmunity can be observed. Adrenal autoimmunity can produce Addison's disease (i.e., primary adrenal insufficiency). Type I autoimmune polyglandular syndrome (APS) is the occurrence of chronic mucocutaneous candidiasis, hypoparathyroidism, and adrenal autoimmunity. Because of the frequent involvement of the skin and nails, this syndrome is also referred to as the autoimmune polyendocrinopathy, candidiasis, ectoderma dystrophy (APECED) syndrome. APS type I is inherited as an autosomal recessive trait and results from mutations in the autoimmune regulator *(AIRE)* gene. APS type I usually appears in childhood. APS type II is occurrence of adrenal autoimmunity and thyroid autoimmunity with or without type 1 diabetes mellitus ([T1DM] or islet autoantibodies). APS type II is polygenic and appears later than APS type I.

GENETICS OF TYPE 1 DIABETES

Familial aggregation and twin studies clearly demonstrate the importance of both genetic and environmental risk factors in T1DM.[10,11] Although there is a familial pattern of inheritance—first-degree relatives of patients with T1DM are 15 times more likely to become diabetic in their lifetimes—90% of patients with T1DM have no other affected family member. The concordance rate between monozygotic twins is approximately 30% to 50% and between dizygotic twins is 6% to 10%. The high discordance rate in monozygotic twins highlights the major role of environmental factors in diabetes pathogenesis plus the low penetrance of many T1DM susceptibility genes.

To date, more than 20 different T1DM susceptibility genes or gene regions have been described (Table 2–2). These genes are referred to as *diabetes susceptibility genes* because persons carrying the gene are more susceptible to T1DM than noncarriers.

None of these genes is either necessary or sufficient for the development of disease. Methods used for identifying or mapping of T1DM susceptibility genes include parametric (lod [linkage of the odds] score) linkage analyses, affected sib pair analyses, and association (linkage disequilibrium) analyses.

Human Leukocyte Antigens

The first human T1DM susceptibility locus to be identified was the HLA region (i.e., MHC) located on the short arm (p arm) of human chromosome 6. It is designated *IDDM1* and accounts for the greatest susceptibility to T1DM. The MHC region contains more than 200 genes and spans a 3.5-megabase region of chromosome 6, which is subdivided into three subregions (class I, II, and III) that contain the different HLA genes. The initial HLA associations were recognized among class I MHC, HLA-B locus alleles (e.g., HLA-B8), and T1DM (Fig. 2–15). The strongest linkage disequilibrium is between class II MHC alleles and T1DM region (Fig. 2–16).

The human MHC class II region genes encode for the α and β chains of the HLA class II molecules: HLA-DR, HLA-DQ, and HLA-DP, which are expressed on the surface of immune cells and present antigens to CD4+ T-lymphocytes. The HLA-DQA1, -DQB1, and -DRB1 loci in particular appear to be the most important genetic factors in T1DM susceptibility. The HLA-DQ molecule is a heterodimer consisting of two glycoprotein chains (α and β) that plays a role in immune recognition and antigen presentation. Both the α and β chains of the DQ locus are highly polymorphic.

In the white population, T1DM is positively associated with two combinations of DQα1 and DQβ1 alleles: DQα1*0501-DQβ1*0201 and DQα1*0301-DQβ1*0302, which encode the molecules DQ2 and DQ8, respectively. The HLA-DQ heterodimers DQα1*0501-DQβ1*0201 and DQα1*0301-DQβ1*0302 are in linkage disequilibrium with HLA-DR3 and HLA-DR4, respectively. Persons who are

Table 2–2. *Genetic Susceptibility to Type 1 Diabetes Mellitus*

Population	Absolute Risk (%)
General population	0.3-0.5
Twins	
Monozygotic	30-50
Dizygotic	5-10
Relatives	
Siblings	5
Offspring of affected father	8
Offspring of affected mother	5
Parents	3

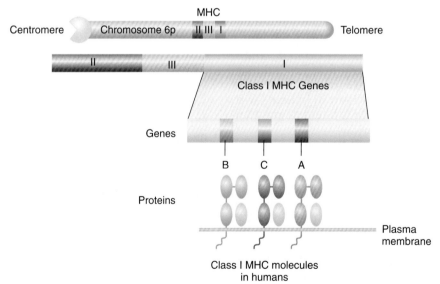

Major Histocompatibility Complex: Class I Region

Figure 2–15. The major histocompatibility complex (MHC) in humans is termed *human leukocyte antigen (HLA) complex*. Hundreds of genes are located in the MHC. The complex includes three regions. The class I MHC region encodes class I MHC heavy (or α) chains, the class II MHC region encodes class II MHC α and β chains, and the class III MHC region encodes several complement proteins and the enzyme 21-hydroxylase. Class I MHC molecules present cytoplasmic peptides to CD8 T cells. The class I MHC molecule is composed of a heavy or α chain and β2 microglobulin (orange ellipse), which is not encoded within the MHC. All nucleated cells of the body express class I MHC molecules. In humans, there are 3 types of class I MHC molecules: HLA-A (heavy chain in *green*), HLA-B (heavy chain in *violet*) and HLA-C (heavy chain in *gray*).

Major Histocompatibility Complex: Class II Region

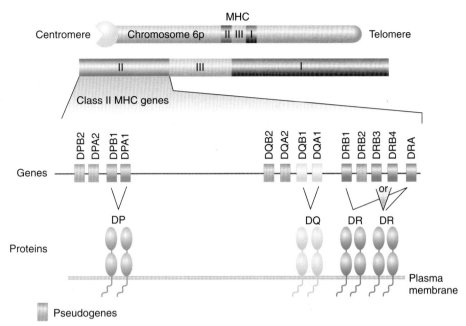

Figure 2–16. Class II major histocompatibility complex (MHC) molecules present extracellular and intravesicular peptides to CD4 T cells. The class II MHC molecule is composed of an α chain and a β chain. Specialized cells of the body, termed *antigen-presenting cells,* express class II MHC molecules. There are several nonexpressed genes within the MHC, which are depicted as *tan rectangles.* In humans, there are 3 types of class II MHC molecules: HLA-DR *(light blue),* HLA-DQ *(yellow),* and HLA-DP *(lavender).* HLA-DR β chains are encoded by 3 different loci (HLA-DRB1, HLA-DRB3, and HLA-DRB4). Per haplotype, all humans express one HLA-DR molecule formed by an α chain encoded by HLA-DRA and a β chain from HLA-DRB1. Most humans also express (per haplotype) a second HLA-DR molecule formed by an α chain encoded by HLA-DRA and a β chain from either HLA-DRB3 or HLA-DRB4. Thus there are usually 2 DR molecules expressed per haplotype. HLA-DRA is essentially nonpolymorphic, because more than 99% of the human population carries a single allele at this locus.

heterozygous for the DQ2 and the DQ8 molecules have the highest risk of disease, which suggests that the molecules act in synergy. Approximately 30% to 40% of T1DM patients are HLA-DQ2 and HLA-DQ8 heterozygotes. Interestingly, the degree of HLA susceptibility to or protection against type 1 diabetes correlates with key amino acid positions of the DQβ1 gene; DQβ1 alleles with an aspartic acid at DQβ residues 57*0301, 0303, 0401, 0402, 0503, 0601, and 0603 confer neutral to protective effects, and the two DQβ1 alleles with an alanine (DQβ1*0201 and DQβ1*0302) confer strong susceptibility to type 1 diabetes in all ethnic groups.

Using x-ray crystallography, investigators have described the three-dimensional structure of the DQ8 molecule (encoded by DQα1*0301-DQβ1*0302) linked with a peptide of the insulin molecule. The residue at position 57 of DQ8 contributes to the shaping of the HLA peptide binding pocket, suggesting that differences in antigen presentation by HLA DQ variants could explain their propensity to influence risk for type 1 diabetes.

On the other hand, some HLA molecules are associated with dominant T1DM protection. The HLA DR2 haplotype (DQα1*0102, DQβ1*0602,

DRβ1*1501) is negatively associated with T1DM and is found in less than 1% of T1DM patients in white (both European and North American), Asian, African-American, and Mexican-American populations. The DQβ1*0602 allele is the only class II allele exclusively found on protective DR2 haplotypes. This suggests that the diabetes-protective effect associated with DR2 haplotypes might be predominantly mapped to the DQβ1*0602 allele. Because DQβ1*0602 protects from T1DM even in the presence of high-risk HLA alleles, protection appears to be dominant.

Currently, the mechanism by which the HLA-DQ locus influences T1DM susceptibility is unknown.[12] Because HLA-DQ molecules participate in antigen presentation, it is possible that allelic variation at this locus affects the peptide binding and functional properties of HLA-DQ heterodimers and therefore the presentation of islet cell antigen-derived peptides to immunocompetent cells. Protective HLA molecules can have higher affinity for one or several peptides than predisposing HLA molecules. For example, the NOD mouse IA^{g7} molecule, homologous to the human DQ8 molecule, is generally a very poor peptide binder. It is possible, then, that predisposing HLA molecules are ineffective at

binding and presenting islet cell peptide-derived antigens.

One of the theories to explain HLA-associated susceptibility proposes that these HLA molecules bind and present specific self-peptides so as to induce pathogenic immune responses to pancreatic beta cell antigens. An opposing theory focuses on the inability of the immune system to maintain tolerance to pancreatic beta cell antigens. It proposes that protective HLA molecules have high binding affinity for certain beta cell peptides required to establish and maintain tolerance to beta cell antigens, and predisposing HLA molecules have a low affinity for tolerogenic peptides. Several observations indicate that class II MHC genes cannot explain all of the HLA association with T1DM. Recent reports suggest that HLA class I genes could influence susceptibility and clinical aspects of T1DM such as age of onset and the rate of beta cell destruction.

Non-HLA Susceptibility Genes

The IDDM2 locus has been mapped to a variable number of tandem repeats (VNTR) gene located about 0.5 kb upstream of the insulin gene (INS) in chromosome 11p15.5. It arises from tandem repetition of a 14– to 15–base pair oligonucleotide sequence. The number of tandem repeats varies from approximately 26 to more than 200, and VNTR alleles occur in three size classes: class I (26 to 63 repeats), class II (mean of 80 repeats), and class III (141 to 209 repeats). In white populations, class II alleles are almost absent, and the frequencies of class I and III alleles are 0.71 and 0.29, respectively.

In 1984, the VNTR polymorphism was reported to be associated with T1DM in a case-control study. Homozygosity for the short class I allele is associated with a two- to fivefold increase in risk of developing T1DM, whereas class III alleles seem to provide protection. The relative risk ratio of the I/I genotype versus I/III or III/III has been reported to be moderate (in the 3 to 5 range) and it accounts for about 10% of the familial clustering of T1DM. The supporting data for IDDM2 as a susceptibility locus comes from many disease-association studies in case-control and family-based cohorts. VNTR alleles are heterogeneous, differing in their ability to change disease susceptibility, and they probably reflect sequence differences within the VNTR that can affect its function and physical state.

Two studies have shown greater gene expression of the insulin gene in the thymus. This could explain the dominant protective effects of class III VNTR alleles, which might act by enhancing thymic tolerance to the preproinsulin protein. The insulin VNTR tandem repeat number also influences susceptibility to type 2 diabetes.

IDDM12 was originally described as a susceptibility gene in a study of a group of Italian families. The CTLA-4 (cytotoxic T lymphocyte–associated 4) and CD28 genes are located near the IDDM12 locus on chromosome 2q33. These genes encode two molecules that play an important role in regulating T cell function and hence in regulating immune responses. The interaction between B7 on antigen-presenting cells and CD28 on T cells provides the second signal necessary for naive T cells to become activated when presented with peptide to which such cells react. On the other hand, activated T cells down-regulate CD28 expression and up-regulate CTLA-4 expression. The interaction of CTLA-4 with B7 counters T-cell activation, acting to keep the immune response in check. Various studies have suggested that the IDDM12 locus could correspond to either CTLA4 itself or to or an unknown gene in very close proximity. A candidate gene has been identified in this region, ZNF236, which codes for a Kruppel-like zinc-finger protein. ZNF236 is expressed in all human tissues tested, including pancreas. IDDM7 on chromosome 2q31 was identified by linkage of D2S326 in one of the first genome scans.

Several genes have been proposed and investigated as candidate genes for the IDDM7 region, including the interleukin-1 gene cluster, HOXD8, GAD1, GALNT3, and NEUROD. Hox proteins are transcription factors that regulate developmental pathways along the vertebrate anteroposterior axis. GALNT3 encodes a glycosyltransferase that initiates mucin-type O-glycosylation. NEUROD is a transcription factor for the insulin gene.

A possible susceptibility locus on chromosome 14q24.3-q31, designated IDDM11, covers a region that includes two candidate genes; the ENSA gene (involved in regulation of the beta cell ATP channels) and the SEL1L gene (which regulates development of pancreatic endocrine cells). The IDDM13 locus maps to 2q34 and is linked to the D2S164 marker in white families from Australia and the United Kingdom. Possible candidate genes in this locus include IA-2, IGFBP2 (insulin-like growth factor binding protein-2), IGFBP5 (insulin-like growth factor binding protein-5), and NRAMP1 (natural resistance–associated macrophage protein).

In one study, North American and British families with more than two diabetic children were genotyped for IGH region microsatellites. The study suggested that a locus (assigned the symbol IDDM16) in the immunoglobulin heavy chain region (IGH), possibly an IGH gene, influenced susceptibility to T1DM. Other researchers have mapped IDDM18, a new susceptibility locus, to chromosome 5q31.1-q33.1. This locus is close to the gene IL12B (the interleukin 12 gene). Although the IL-12 gene is an important candidate in terms of immune function, several studies from other populations, including in Britain and the United States, have failed to confirm the finding.

Parental Effects on Inherited Gene Expression

The probable existence of parental effects acting on the transmission and expression of inherited genes further complicates the genetics of T1DM. Several studies, whose results have been debated, have shown that T1DM risk differs in the offspring of diabetic mothers and fathers, with an increased risk reported more commonly in children with affected fathers. Parental effects also influence the transmission of the VNTR alleles at the IDDM2 locus. Imprinting, a mechanism that regulates gene expression by silencing either the maternal or the paternal allele, could explain these observations. The insulin gene is located in a region of the human genome that is known to be subject to parental imprinting.

Acquired Genetic Factors

Environmental factors (viruses, diet) appear to play a role in determining progression to overt disease in persons carrying predisposing gene alleles for T1DM. Viruses could trigger autoimmune responses through mechanisms of molecular mimicry or by directly damaging the pancreatic beta cells. Retroviruses are unique viruses that can integrate into the human genome. These genes can be either inherited or acquired after birth, and different factors in a normal lifespan can activate dormant retroviruses. In turn, this awakening can trigger the development of diabetes in genetically predisposed persons.

Genetic Screening for At-Risk Persons

Two approaches currently exist for identifying T1DM-susceptible persons. One is primary antibody screening followed by quantification of risk by further antibody, genetic, and metabolic testing; the other is primary genetic screening (e.g., of neonates, using cord blood or dried blood spots placed on filter paper) with determination of high-risk HLA (DR3/4, DR4/4, DR3/3) gene alleles and subsequent quantification of risk by further antibody and metabolic testing. Depending on the population being considered, each approach has advantages and disadvantages.[13]

Primary antibody testing is based on the finding that the majority of patients with T1DM have islet-related autoantibodies in their serum.[14-16] ICA is the gold standard for autoantibody screening. However, better, more-sensitive, more-specific, and less-costly biochemical assays (GADA, IAA, and IA-2A) are now available. Screening with ICA, or with GADA

and IA-2A, has a high sensitivity, and when more than one antibody is present, specificity is markedly enhanced. Most studies have been done in high-risk relatives who have an overall risk of developing T1DM of approximately 5%. However, because 85% to 90% of patients with newly diagnosed type 1 diabetes have no family history of T1DM, the disease must ultimately be prevented in the at-risk general population.

Because the risk in the general population is only 1 in 300 (in the United States), or 15 to 20 times lower than in relatives, the low prevalence of the disease leads to a low positive predictive value and many false-positive results. Even a small false-positive rate identifies many subjects who will never get the disease (Bayes' theorem). Screening for the presence of two or more antibodies increases the positive predictive value but reduces sensitivity and markedly increases cost. Autoantibody screening has some further limitations, including the possible need to test more than once, because seroconversion is not uncommon in younger subjects.

Until recently, the most poorly defined part of the natural history of T1DM has been the time of life when the disease actually begins and the inductive events that trigger this process appear to act. Primary genetic infant screening programs help provide a more grounded understanding of which factors are responsible for the development of T1DM. HLA-DR3 in linkage disequilibrium with DQβ1*0201 and HLA-DR4/DQβ1*0302 are the highest risk alleles (Table 2–3), and HLA-DR2/DQβ1*0602 serve as protective gene alleles.

Primary genetic screening provides several advantages over autoantibody testing. Using primary genetic screening, infants can be followed from birth. Less than 5% of patients will require further antibody testing, and 60% to 80% of high-risk patients will be adequately identified. The ability to follow entire high-risk cohorts from birth to onset of T1DM should provide insight into the etiology and pathogenesis of T1DM and allow for the institution of primary prevention studies. Finally, the cost of primary genetic screening with follow-up autoantibody determination in high-risk subjects is approximately one third the cost of primary autoantibody testing.

Table 2–3. *Absolute Risk for Type 1 Diabetes According to DR/DQ Genotypes*

DR/DQ	First-Degree Relative	Population
DR 3/4, DQ 0201/0302	1/4 to 1/5	1/15
DR 4/4, DQ 0300/0302	1/6	1/20
DR 3/3, DQ 0201/0201	1/10	1/45
DR 4/X, DQ 0302/8 (X ≠ 0602)	1/15	1/60
X/X	1/125	1/600
DR 0403 or DQ 0602	1/15,000	1/15,000

PREVENTING OR REVERSING TYPE 1 DIABETES MELLITUS

Strategies to prevent or reverse T1DM development can be divided into those that focus on beta cell protection, immunomodulation, regeneration, or replacement.[17] Prevention of immune beta cell destruction involves either halting the immune attack directed against beta cells or making beta cells better able to withstand immune attack.

The recent identification of beta cell growth factors in combination with the development of stem-cell technologies provides an alternative route to the reversal of diabetes, namely beta cell regeneration. Stem cell–derived islets might be less sensitive to recurrent immune destruction than is normally seen in response to islet transplantation.

The last alternative is beta cell replacement or substitution. This covers a wide range of interventions including human whole pancreas transplantation, xenotransplantation, genetically modified beta cells, mechanical insulin sensing and delivery devices, and the artificial pancreas.

SUMMARY

T1DM is the end result of a long-standing process whereby T cells embark on a specific mission to locate, attack, and destroy pancreatic beta cells, which are the body's only source of insulin. Many genes influence susceptibility to T1DM, the major loci being HLA and other genes located in the MHC region of human chromosome 6. At least 20 other genes influence T1DM susceptibility. However, with the exception of the insulin gene, these other genes have yet to be definitively identified. T cells appear to be the major cause of beta cell death.

Persons at risk for T1DM can be identified through the presence in their serum of autoantibodies to beta cell proteins such as insulin, GADA, and IA-2A. A range of immunotherapies that were successful in preventing T1DM in animal models have now progressed to human clinical trials. To date, human studies of T1DM prevention have been disappointing. The large human trials of nicotinamide and trials of insulin tolerance failed to prevent T1DM. The challenge now is to use the substantial body of knowledge of the immunologic and genetic basis of T1DM to develop an effective preventive treatment for T1DM.

References

1. Atkinson MA, Eisenbarth GS: Type 1 diabetes: New perspectives on disease pathogenesis and treatment. Lancet 358:766-770, 2001.
2. Winter WE, Harris N, Schatz DA: Type 1 diabetes islet autoantibody markers. Diabetes Technol Ther 4:817-839, 2002.
3. Foulis AK, Liddle CN, Farquharson MA, et al: The histopathology of the pancreas in type 1 (insulin-dependent) diabetes mellitus: A 25-year review of deaths in patients under 20 years of age in the United Kingdom. Diabetologia 29:267-274, 1986.
4. Petrovsky N, Schatz DA: Immunology of insulin-dependent diabetes mellitus. In Williams G, Pickup J (eds): Textbook of Diabetes. Oxford, Blackwell Scientific, 2002, pp 1-14.
5. Roep BO: The role of T-cells in the pathogenesis of Type 1 diabetes: From cause to cure. Diabetologia 46:305-321, 2003.
6. Atkinson MA, Leiter EH: The NOD mouse model of type 1 diabetes: As good as it gets? Nat Med 5:601-604, 1999.
7. Dilts SM, Lafferty KJ: Autoimmune diabetes: The involvement of benign and malignant autoimmunity. J Autoimmun 12:229-232, 1999.
8. Suarez-Pinzon WL, Power RF, Rabinovitch A: Fas ligand-mediated mechanisms are involved in autoimmune destruction of islet beta cells in non-obese diabetic mice. Diabetologia 43:1149-1156, 2000.
9. Schatz DA, Winter WE: Autoimmune polyglandular syndromes. In Sperling M (ed): Pediatric Endocrinology. Philadelphia, W.B. Saunders, 2002, pp 671-688.
10. Melanitou E, Fain P, Eisenbarth GS: Genetics of type 1A (immune mediated) diabetes. J Autoimmun 21:93-98, 2003.
11. Morales A, She J-X, Schatz DA: Genetics of Type 1 diabetes. In Pescovitz OH, Eugster E (eds): Pediatric Endocrinology: Mechanisms, Manifestations, and Management. Philadelphia, Lippincott, Williams & Wilkins, 2004, pp 402-410.
12. Ridgway WM, Fathman CG: The association of MHC with autoimmune diseases: Understanding the pathogenesis of autoimmune diabetes. Clin Immunol Immunopathol 86:3-10, 1998.
13. Schatz DA, Krischer J, She J-X: To screen or not to screen for pre-type 1 diabetes? Horm Res 57(suppl 1):12-17, 2002.
14. Krischer JP, Cuthbertson DD, Yu L, et al: Screening strategies for the identification of multiple antibody positive individuals. J Clin Endocrinol Metab 88:103-108, 2003.
15. Winter WE, Harris N, Schatz DA: Type 1 diabetes islet autoantibody markers. Diabetes Technol Ther 4:817-839, 2002.
16. Bingley PJ, Christie MR, Bonifacio E, et al: Combined analysis of autoantibodies improves prediction of IDDM in islet cell antibody-positive relatives. Diabetes 43:1304-1310, 1994.
17. Winter WE, Schatz D: Prevention strategies for type 1 diabetes mellitus: Current status and future directions. BioDrugs 17:39-64, 2003.

Type 2 Diabetes: Insulin Resistance, Beta Cell Dysfunction, and Other Metabolic and Hormonal Abnormalities

Brian E. Chavez and Robert R. Henry

KEY POINTS

- *Pathophysiology of type 2 diabetes mellitus results from complex interplay of insulin resistance, beta cell dysfunction, and adipokines.*
- *Type 2 diabetes is a component of the metabolic syndrome (vascular inflammation, endothelial dysfunction, hypertension, dyslipidemia, central obesity, and a hypercoagulable state).*
- *Insulin resistance occurs primarily in muscle, adipose tissue, and the liver.*
- *Surrogate estimates of insulin resistance include the homeostasis model assessment of insulin resistance (HOMA IR) and quantitative insulin sensitivity check index (QUICKI).*
- *Decrease in beta cell mass could be due to increased beta cell apoptosis that exceeds islet neogenesis (formation of new islet cells).*
- *Potential insulin sensitizers are adiponectin and leptin.*
- *Potential insulin antagonists are resistin, tumor necrosis factor α, and interleukin-6.*

Patients with type 2 diabetes mellitus share a pathophysiology that involves the pancreatic beta cells, the liver, and peripheral target tissues, namely skeletal muscle and adipose tissue. A variable degree of beta cell dysfunction is present in these patients in addition to hepatic insulin resistance, resulting in glucose overproduction. Skeletal muscle is also resistant to the action of insulin via post–insulin-receptor binding defects. Glucose uptake into muscle cells requires insulin binding to cell-surface receptors and activation of the insulin signaling cascade, which in turn facilitates the movement of glucose across the cell membrane; ultimately the glucose is stored as glycogen or is used as an energy source via glycolysis to lactate or mitochondrial oxidation. Hormones and cytokines produced by adipose tissue (adipokines) have been discovered and appear to play a role in glucose and fat metabolism and likely contribute to the pathophysiology of type 2 diabetes. Free fatty acids also appear to play a role in the pathophysiology of type 2 diabetes by inducing insulin resistance and facilitating excessive rates of hepatic glucose production.

This chapter first reviews the normal physiology of glucose regulation and the natural history of type 2 diabetes. We focus on the mechanisms of insulin resistance, beta cell dysfunction, and the clinical means of estimating defects of insulin action (insulin resistance) and beta cell impairment. The role of adipokines is also discussed.

NORMAL PHYSIOLOGY OF GLUCOSE HOMEOSTASIS

Maintenance of normal glucose levels depends upon a closed feedback loop between the circulating glucose level and the pancreatic hormones, insulin and glucagon. In the fasting state, glucose is largely produced by the liver via glycogen breakdown and gluconeogenesis. Approximately 70% to 80% of the glucose produced by the liver is used by the brain (independent of insulin) and by other insulin-insensitive tissues, such as the gastrointestinal tract and erythrocytes. The insulin-sensitive tissues, principally muscle and fat, use only small quantities of glucose in the absence of increased insulin levels. Hepatic glucose output (HGO) in the short term (i.e., minutes to hours) is modulated by insulin, glucagon, catecholamines, and the glucose level itself. Growth hormone, thyroid hormone, and cortisol (glucocorticoids) serve as longer-term modulators (i.e., hours to days) of hepatic glucose production (Figure 3–1).

Insulin (from the pancreatic beta cell) exerts an inhibitory effect on hepatic glucose production. In contrast, glucagon (from the pancreatic alpha cell) stimulates hepatic glucose production. Thus, a reduction in insulin results in a slow rise in HGO. If the feedback loop is intact, as the serum glucose level rises, pancreatic insulin secretion would increase, and glucagon would decrease in order to maintain homeostasis. If peripheral insulin sensitivity changes, this would result in a change in serum glucose, which in turn would result in modulation of insulin and glucagon in order to maintain glucose levels. Complete adaptation actually

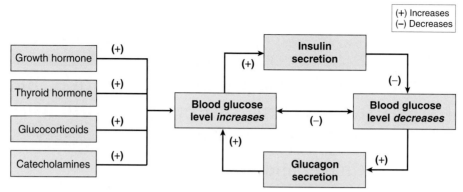

Figure 3–1. Normal glucose homeostasis. Maintenance of normoglycemia occurs via a closed-loop feedback system involving serum glucose level, insulin, and glucagon. Insulin lowers serum glucose by stimulating glucose uptake by insulin-sensitive tissues, namely skeletal muscle and adipose tissues. In contrast, glucagon increases serum glucose via stimulation of hepatic glycogenolysis and gluconeogenesis. In the short-term, hepatic glucose output is modulated by insulin, glucagon, catecholamines, and glucose itself. Long-term modulators of hepatic glucose output include growth hormone, thyroid hormone, and cortisol.

does not occur, and thus a new, higher, steady-state glucose level is reached. One must account for each variable that contributes to this regulatory system—hepatic glucose output, pancreatic endocrine function, and peripheral tissue glucose uptake—in order to appropriately evaluate abnormalities in glucose homeostasis.

At the cellular level, the mechanism of insulin action involves a cascade of biochemical interactions. The initial event begins with insulin binding to a cell surface receptor, which activates the receptor's intrinsic tyrosine kinase activity. Tyrosine kinases phosphorylate intracellular substrates, including themselves (autophosphorylation). The phosphorylation triggers a molecular phosphorylation/dephosphorylation signaling cascade as seen in Figures 3–1 and 3–2. Proteins such as IRS-1 (insulin receptor substrate-1) and IRS-2 are phosphorylated and ultimately result in the activation of three major pathways: the PI3 kinase (phosphatidylinositol-3 kinase) pathway, the CAP/Cbl/Tc10 pathway, and the ERK pathway.[1] Much research studies enzymes such as PTP-1B (protein tyrosine phosphatase 1B), PI-3 kinase, Akt, and GSK3 (glycogen synthase kinase 3), among others, in order to understand the nature of the postreceptor defects seen in type 2 diabetes.[2] The ultimate result of the signaling cascade is the recruitment and translocation of the GLUT4 protein from an intracellular pool to the cell membrane, which facilitates the influx of glucose into the cell for subsequent metabolism (see Fig 3–2 and Box 3-1).

NATURAL HISTORY AND EPIDEMIOLOGY OF INSULIN RESISTANCE

Insulin resistance is present in approximately 90% of patients with type 2 diabetes.[3] Insulin resistance is often associated with a cluster of metabolic

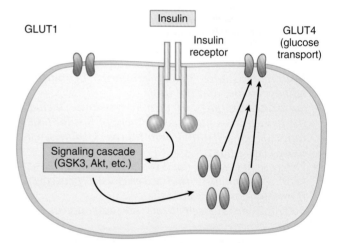

Figure 3–2. Concept of insulin signaling. The mechanism by which insulin exerts its actions occurs via a complex cascade of biochemical interactions. This illustration is a simplified representation of the insulin signaling cascade. Insulin first binds a transmembrane insulin receptor, which then activates the intrinsic receptor tyrosine kinase activity. This results in phosphorylation of the receptor itself and other molecules. The result is the activation of three known major pathways: the PI3 kinase pathway, CAP/Cbl/Tc10 pathway, and the ERK pathway. Activation of the PI3 kinase and CAP/Cbl/TC10 pathways results in recruitment of the GLUT4, a glucose transporter protein, to the cell membrane to allow glucose uptake into the cell. In contrast, the GLUT1 protein is involved in glucose uptake independent of increases of insulin. See Box 3-1, which lists some of the known molecules involved in the insulin signaling cascade. Many of these molecules may also be involved in the development of vascular inflammation and other aspects of the metabolic syndrome.

abnormalities (known as the metabolic syndrome, also known as the dysmetabolic syndrome, insulin resistance syndrome, syndrome X, and Reaven's syndrome). Glucose intolerance and hyperglycemia, hypertension, dyslipidemia, abdominal

Box 3-1. Components of the Insulin-Signaling Pathway[1]

Insulin receptor

IRS-1 and IRS-2 (liver)

PTP1B

p110-p85

PI3K pathway

- GSK3
- Akt
- PFK2 (liver)
- PEPCK gene (liver)
- p70S6K

CAP/Cbl/Tc10 pathway

ERK pathway

CAP, c-Cbl-associated protein; ERK, extracellular signal-regulated kinase; GSK, glycogen synthase kinase; IRS, insulin receptor substrate; PEPCK, phosphoenolpyruvate carboxykinase; PFK, phosphofructokinase; PTP, protein tyrosine phosphatase.
From Pirola L, Johnston AM, Van Obberghen E: Modulation of insulin action. Diabetologia 47:170-184, 2004.

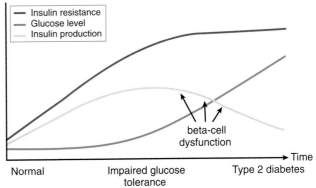

Figure 3-3. Natural history of type 2 diabetes. This diagram illustrates the progression from normal glucose tolerance to the development of overt hyperglycemia (type 2 diabetes) over a period of years. Insulin resistance worsens over a period of years, resulting in compensatory hyperinsulinemia. Initially, this compensation by the pancreatic beta cells is capable of maintaining a normal or near-normal glucose level. However, over time, beta cell dysfunction (burnout) occurs and insulin secretion begins to diminish, leading first to the development of hyperglycemia and then to overt diabetes. (From Henry RR: Type 2 diabetes care: The role of insulin-sensitizing agents and practical implications for cardiovascular disease prevention. Am J Med 105(1A):20S-26S, 1998.)

(central) obesity, endothelial dysfunction, impaired vascular reactivity, vascular inflammation, and a hypercoagulable state with impaired fibrinolysis compose the metabolic syndrome.[95] Some or all of these components may be present in any given patient.

The role of insulin resistance in the genesis of the metabolic syndrome remains controversial, but there is a strong association. Insulin resistance also occurs in persons who are not diabetic. Up to 25% of nondiabetic patients have a lower degree of insulin sensitivity, similar to those with type 2 diabetes who have good glycemic control.[4] The severity of insulin resistance is quite variable from person to person and is usually progressive over time.[5] Investigations of various populations in which insulin resistance, impaired glucose tolerance, and type 2 diabetes are prevalent have provided insight into the factors that influence the development and progression of these metabolic derangements.

A higher prevalence of glucose intolerance and type 2 diabetes has been observed among certain ethnic groups, such as Pima Indians and other Native Americans, Hispanic Americans, Pacific Islanders, and African Americans.[6] For example, the Pima Indians of Arizona have the highest rate of diabetes in the world. About 50% of the Pima Indian population between the ages of 30 and 64 years of age has type 2 diabetes. The severity of insulin resistance is one of the strongest predictors of type 2 diabetes in these high-risk groups.[7] Similar observations have been made in the Mexican American population and in children of diabetic parents who have signs of insulin resistance years before the onset of diabetes.[8,9] Additionally, the likelihood of

insulin resistance increases along with other cardiovascular risk factors, such as coagulation and fibrinolytic abnormalities, in first-degree relatives of patients with type 2 diabetes.[10,11]

Although more prevalent in older people, insulin resistance is not limited to adults. An increasing number of children and teenagers are found to have insulin resistance. Obese adolescents can manifest features of the metabolic syndrome, such as hypertension, dyslipidemia, acanthosis nigricans, and glucose intolerance, including frank type 2 diabetes. The natural history of type 2 diabetes is illustrated in Figure 3-3.

Generally, insulin resistance gradually progresses and worsens over a period of years.[5] With worsening insulin resistance, insulin is less able to dispose of glucose from the circulation. As a result, compensatory hyperinsulinemia ensues in order to maintain euglycemia. However, beta cell dysfunction gradually manifests, leading to inability to maintain a sufficient hyperinsulinemic state to overcome the insulin resistance, which eventually leads to prediabetes (impaired glucose tolerance) and then type 2 diabetes with overt hyperglycemia[12] (Fig. 3-4).

Although it is clinically challenging, our goal as clinicians should be to identify persons who are at risk as early as possible in the natural history, where interventions are likely to be most efficacious. Ethnicity, family history, features of the metabolic syndrome, and postprandial hyperglycemia even with

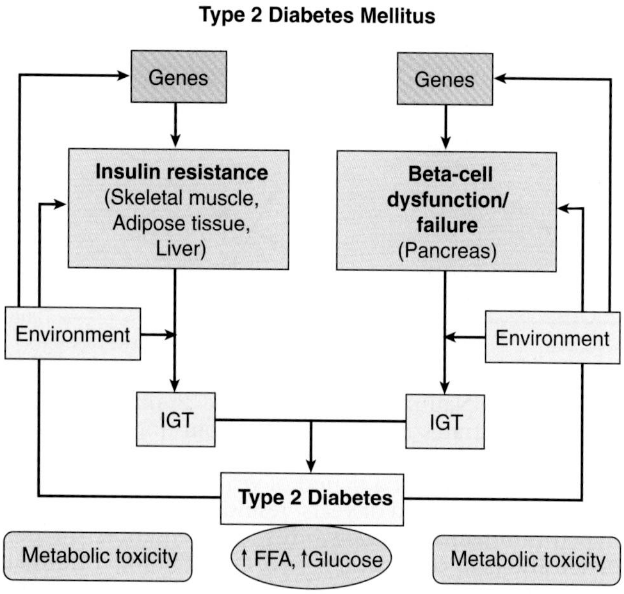

Type 2 Diabetes Mellitus

Figure 3–4. Pathogenesis of type 2 diabetes. This schematic illustrates the known factors involved in the pathogenesis of type 2 diabetes. Genetics certainly plays a role in predisposing the patient to developing type 2 diabetes. Multiple organs are involved. The combination of insulin resistance (at multiple tissues such as skeletal muscle, adipose tissue, liver) and beta cell dysfunction leads to impaired glucose tolerance (IGT). The environment (i.e., the modern sedentary lifestyle and overabundance of food) further contributes to this process. Eventually, type 2 diabetes ensues, and hyperglycemia and elevated free fatty acid (FFA) levels result in metabolic toxicity. The metabolic toxicity further exacerbates this process, and a vicious cycle occurs. Diabetes begets diabetes.

normal fasting glucose may be helpful in identifying these at-risk persons.

Patients with type 2 diabetes mellitus share a pathophysiology that involves the pancreatic beta cells, the liver, and the major insulin-sensitive peripheral target tissues, namely skeletal muscle and adipose tissue. We begin our review with an overview of insulin resistance in these major target tissues.

INSULIN RESISTANCE

Insulin resistance is defined as a condition of low insulin sensitivity in which the ability of insulin to lower circulating glucose is impaired. The genetic predisposition for the development of insulin resistance, while unquestionably present, is largely undefined, but observations of decreased insulin sensitivity among relatives of people with type 2 diabetes suggest a genetic association. Genetic determinants likely interact with other factors, such as obesity, aging, elevated free fatty acids, and hyperglycemia, to contribute to the development of

a pathologic, insulin-resistant state. The underlying biochemical and molecular basis of insulin resistance in most persons with type 2 diabetes remains to be determined.

Insulin resistance in muscle, adipose, and liver tissue arises from multiple complex metabolic abnormalities.[13] Biochemical defects that provoke insulin resistance involve impaired insulin signaling (a biochemical cascade of events) and reductions in glucose transport in insulin-sensitive tissue.

From a clinical standpoint, early insulin resistance results in compensatory hyperinsulinemia with the maintenance of euglycemia as discussed earlier in the natural history of type 2 diabetes. At this stage, measurement of fasting glucose and random glucose usually remains within normal limits, is asymptomatic, and thus is often undetected. On physical examination, one might detect acanthosis nigricans, which can occur in association with severe insulin resistance. Excessive skin tags may also be seen in association with insulin resistance (Fig. 3–5).

Hepatic Insulin Resistance

Basal rates of hepatic glucose output (HGO) have been described as increased or inappropriately normal in type 2 diabetes. The degree of abnormality in HGO positively and strongly correlates with the degree of fasting hyperglycemia. This suggests that the rate of HGO has a major role in contributing to fasting glucose levels.[14] The increased rate of HGO results from impaired effects of insulin and glucose to normally suppress glucose release from the liver. The insulin dose-response curve for suppression of HGO is right shifted in type 2 diabetic subjects studied at euglycemia. No reduction is seen in the maximum suppressive response at supraphysiologic insulin levels. In other words, the liver is insulin resistant, but given enough insulin, HGO can be completely suppressed. This is consistent with a decrease in hepatic insulin receptor number. However, other studies show that a defect in the ability of glucose to inhibit its own release from the liver is another factor contributing to hepatic glucose overproduction (Fig. 3–6).[15] Elevated glucagon can also contribute to reducing the suppressive effects of insulin and glucose on HGO.[16]

In the fed state, the liver continues to play a crucial role in maintaining glucose homeostasis. After a meal, glucose and insulin enter the liver via the portal circulation and change liver function from its role in the fasting state as a glucose-producing organ to that of storage. During feeding, glucose is stored in the form of glycogen in the liver. However, because there are defects in hepatic sensitivity to glucose and insulin, there is a delayed reduction in HGO suppression in the type 2 diabetic patient.[17] This is a major contributor to the postprandial hyperglycemia that is noted early in the

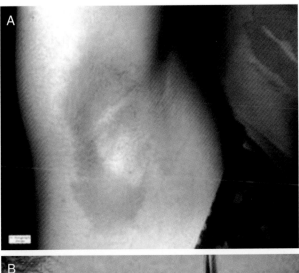

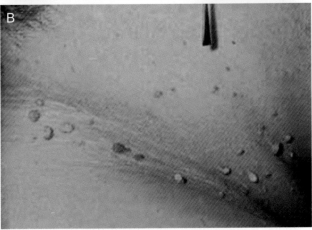

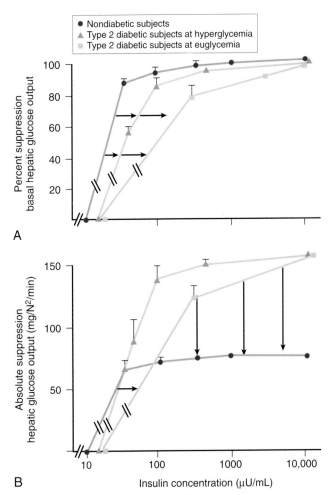

Figure 3–5. Physical examination findings associated with insulin resistance. **A,** Acanthosis nigricans in the axilla of a patient. Acanthosis nigricans is a velvety thickening and hyperpigmentation of the skin and is primarily found in the axilla and other body folds, neck, and back. **B,** Multiple acrodchordons (skin tags), which can also be associated with insulin resistance. Skin tags are skin-colored or tan or brown, round or oval, pedunculated lesions.

course of insulin resistance and the prediabetic state.

Peripheral Insulin Resistance

It is well established that subjects with type 2 diabetes exhibit peripheral insulin resistance in target tissues such as skeletal muscle. The hyperinsulinemic-euglycemic clamp technique, a research method for measuring peripheral insulin resistance, shows that the glucose disposal rate is usually reduced by at least 50% in subjects with type 2 diabetes.[15] Two abnormalities are observed in the insulin dose-response curve: a right shift (as seen in hepatic insulin resistance) and a decrease in maximal response (Fig. 3–7).

Figure 3–6. Hepatic insulin resistance (insulin-mediated suppression of hepatic glucose output). This figure demonstrates the effects of increased insulin and glucose on hepatic glucose output. Normal subjects are represented by *circles*, type 2 diabetes at hyperglycemia by *triangles*, and type 2 diabetes at euglycemia by *squares*. **A,** The insulin dose-response curve is right shifted in the diabetic subjects, which indicates insulin resistance. **B,** Again a right shift is noted consistent with insulin resistance in the diabetic subjects. Also of note, in the diabetic subjects at hyperglycemia, there is both a decrease in responsiveness (decreased maximal response) and a decrease in sensitivity to insulin. At extremely high concentrations of insulin (1000-10,000 μU/mL) hepatic glucose output is suppressed in all subjects. (Modified from Revers RR, Fink R, Griffin J, et al: Influence of hyperglycemia on insulin's in vivo effects in type II diabetes. J Clin Invest 73:664-672, 1984. Permission conveyed through Copyright Clearance Center, Inc.)

The rightward shift in the curve is consistent with a decreased number of insulin receptors. The decrease in maximal response implies a post-binding (intracellular) defect of insulin action. The exact underlying intracellular defects continue to be determined. Putative defects in IRS-1, (insulin receptor substrate 1), PI3 kinase (phosphoinositol-3-kinase), GSK3 (glycogen synthase kinase 3), and other factors have been demonstrated and are the subject of current research efforts.[18,19]

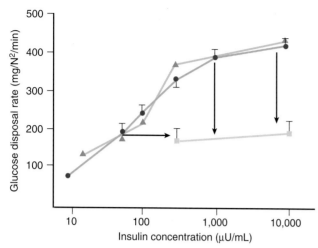

Figure 3-7. Peripheral insulin resistance. This figure depicts studies that characterize the insulin dose response curves for the peripheral tissue (i.e., muscle). Nondiabetic subjects are represented by *circles,* type 2 diabetes at hyperglycemia by *triangles,* and type 2 diabetes at euglycemia by *squares.* The key observation is the marked rightward shift and decreased maximal response in type 2 diabetes at euglycemia, which is consistent with a decrease in insulin receptor number and an intracellular defect in the insulin signaling cascade, respectively. Note that hyperglycemia normalizes insulin-stimulated glucose uptake in type 2 diabetes. (Modified from Revers RR, Fink R, Griffin J, et al: Influence of hyperglycemia on insulin's in vivo effects in type II diabetes. J Clin Invest 73:664-672, 1984. Permission conveyed through Copyright Clearance Center, Inc.)

The efficiency of peripheral glucose uptake after oral glucose ingestion is also defective in type 2 diabetic subjects. In normal subjects, after cellular uptake, glucose normally undergoes both oxidative and nonoxidative metabolism. At low insulin concentrations, the major route of peripheral glucose disposal is via glucose oxidation (i.e., using glucose as metabolic fuel). At higher insulin levels, an increasing fraction of disposal occurs via glycogen synthesis (i.e., glucose is removed from the circulation and stored). Glycogen synthesis is the major component of nonoxidative glucose metabolism. However, in type 2 diabetic subjects, the efficiency of glucose disposal by both these processes is reduced, primarily in the nonoxidative pathway.[20]

Glucose Resistance and Noninsulin-Mediated Glucose Uptake

Aside from insulin resistance and beta cell dysfunction, glucose uptake that is not mediated by insulin (insulin-independent glucose uptake or glucose-mediated glucose uptake) is important in determining glucose use. Noninsulin-mediated glucose uptake (NIMGU) plays an important role in the

rate of glucose disappearance. About 80% of tissue glucose uptake in the fasting state occurs via insulin-*independent* mechanisms, primarily in central nervous system tissue and to a much lesser degree in peripheral tissues, such as muscle and adipose tissue.

Baron and colleagues[23] found that in the fasting state, NIMGU is the major pathway for glucose disposal in both type 2 diabetic subjects and in normal controls. Furthermore, for a particular glucose level, the efficiency of NIMGU (defined as NIMGU–serum glucose) is equal in both type 2 diabetic subjects and normal controls. However, the absolute basal rate of NIMGU is higher in type 2 diabetic subjects compared with normal controls due to an elevated basal rate of glucose disposal. It is thought that this elevated basal rate of NIMGU in subjects with type 2 diabetes plays a role in the pathogenesis of type 2 diabetes.

A study by Revers and colleagues showed that in the presence of baseline hyperglycemia, physiologic insulin levels had a diminished ability to suppress HGO and to stimulate peripheral glucose disposal in type 2 diabetic subjects. As previously discussed, basal HGO is elevated in patients with type 2 diabetes, which might serve to maintain the level of hyperglycemia needed to compensate for this observed decrease in peripheral insulin action (e.g., mass action). Moreover, this study showed that fasting hyperglycemia exerted a suppressive effect on HGO, but it did not completely compensate for the decrease in hepatic insulin action seen in type 2 diabetic patients.[15] The exact underlying biochemical and cellular mechanisms behind these findings remain uncertain, but they likely involve multiple defects in the intracellular enzymes involved in glucose entry and use within the cell as well as abnormalities of the glucose transporter proteins.

Measurement of Insulin Resistance

The gold standard for assessing insulin resistance and insulin sensitivity is the hyperinsulinemic-euglycemic clamp technique. However, this procedure is too complex, labor intensive, time consuming, and costly for use in routine clinical practice.[3] Surrogate measures of insulin resistance include the Homeostasis Model Assessment of Insulin Resistance (HOMA IR) and the Quantitative Insulin Sensitivity Check Index (QUICKI), among many other methods.[25,30] Although these modeled measurements can have substantial limitations, they can be used easily in the office setting and provide gross approximations of insulin action. These measurements are calculated using the following formulas:

$$ HOMA = \frac{\text{fasting serum insulin} \times \text{fasting serum glucose}}{405} $$

$$QUICKI = \frac{1}{\log(\text{fasting serum insulin}) + \log(\text{fasting glucose})}$$

where fasting serum insulin is in microunits per milliliter (μU/mL) and fasting serum glucose is in milligrams per deciliter (mg/dL) in both equations. If the fasting glucose values in the HOMA equation are in SI units (mmol/L), the constant 405 must be replaced with 22.5.

Other tests of insulin sensitivity that are known to correlate with the hyperinsulinemic-euglycemia clamp technique include the modeled oral glucose tolerance test (OGTT; $r^2 = -0.67$, $P < 0.05$), continuous infusion of glucose with model assessment ($r^2 = 0.87$, $P < 0.001$), and the insulin-modified frequently sampled intravenous glucose tolerance test (FSIVGTT; $r = 0.84$, $P < 0.002$).[24-28] However, intravenous access or multiple venipunctures are the limitations of these alternative measurements, thus making them less desirable for clinic and office assessment. A triglyceride-to-HDL ratio greater than 3 has also been suggested as a reasonable estimate of insulin resistance (sensitivity 64%, specificity 68%).[29]

BETA CELL DYSFUNCTION

It is well accepted that the pathophysiology of type 2 diabetes involves progressive beta cell dysfunction. Conceivably, this could be due to a decrease in beta cell mass, to beta cell dysfunction, or to both abnormalities. Recent studies by Butler and colleagues support the hypothesis of a decrease in beta cell mass via beta cell apoptosis in the face of normal beta cell neogenesis. Frequency of beta cell neogenesis or beta cell apoptosis can be calculated with one equation:

$$\text{Frequency of beta cell replication or apoptosis} = \frac{\text{cells/islet}}{\% \text{ beta cell area}}$$

A study of human pancreatic tissue obtained from autopsies demonstrated that obese humans with impaired fasting glucose (110-125 mg/dL) had a 40% decrease in relative beta cell volume, and obese humans with type 2 diabetes had a 63% decrease in relative beta cell volume. Lean type 2 diabetic subjects had a 41% deficit in relative beta cell volume. Beta cell replication frequency was very low for all groups, on the order of 0.025 to 0.050. Beta cell neogenesis was found to be increased in all groups; however, patients with type 2 diabetes had a higher frequency of beta cell apoptosis. Compared with nondiabetic subjects (apoptosis frequency $\approx$ 0.05), there was a 10-fold increase in apoptosis in lean type 2 diabetic patients (apoptosis frequency $\approx$ 0.5),

and a 3-fold increase in obese type 2 diabetic patients (apoptosis frequency $\approx$ 0.15).[31]

A study in a mouse model examined beta cell mass in the setting of insulin resistance.[32] A transgenic mouse model that produces excess human islet amyloid polypeptide (IAPP) was used to model human IAPP effects. These mice develop islet pathology similar to that of humans who have type 2 diabetes. By 40 weeks of age, the obese nontransgenic mice did not develop diabetes. In response to insulin resistance, the transgenic mice adapted to excess IAPP by a ninefold increase in beta cell mass, which appeared to be accomplished by a 1.7-fold increase in islet *neogenesis* and a fivefold increase in beta cell replication per islet. On the other hand, despite increased beta cell mass, the obese transgenic mice developed diabetes and failed to adaptively increase beta cell mass even further. These transgenic mice had a 10-fold increase in *apoptosis*. The markedly increased frequency of beta cell apoptosis was related to the rate of increase of IAPP. Replicating islets seem to be more prone to apoptosis, which could account for the failure of beta cell mass to increase in response to type 2 diabetes.

Beta cell mass, islet size, and islet characteristics have all been studied postmortem in type 2 diabetic subjects. Some studies have found islet size to be reduced and the volume loss due purely to reduced beta cell mass, because no significant reduction of α, δ, or PP cells was found. As discussed earlier, increased IAPP is present in the postmortem pancreases of patients with type 2 diabetes, and it may be a factor in the pathogenesis of beta cell loss via induction of apoptosis. The mechanism of deposition of IAPP is unknown; however, a study by Butler and colleagues suggested that the mechanism of action of IAPP toxicity may be due to cell membrane destruction by "intermediate-sized toxic amyloid particles."[33] In humans, the beta cell deficiency in type 2 diabetes could be due, in part, to a failure to adaptively increase beta cell mass associated with an increased vulnerability (to IAPP) of replicating beta cells to undergo apoptosis.[34]

In vivo human studies to assess beta cell mass are difficult, but studies have been performed in animals. A 50% reduction in beta cell mass alone seems to be insufficient to induce fasting hyperglycemia and the insulin secretory abnormalities seen in type 2 diabetes. There appears to be a physiologic reserve built into the endocrine pancreas.

Other animal studies have looked at the extent of beta cell loss required to reproduce type 2 diabetes. Beta cell loss has been induced either surgically by partial pancreatectomy or chemically with streptozocin. Removal of two thirds of a dog's pancreas does not result in fasting hyperglycemia or the loss of first-phase insulin secretion that is typical in type 2 diabetes. In a rat model, 60% pancreatectomy had effects similar to those seen in the canine studies. It is only when beta cell mass is reduced by 90% or more that hyperglycemia and decrease in insulin secretion is seen similar to that in type 2 diabetes.

In streptozocin-treated animals, beta cell mass is also lost along with loss of first-phase insulin secretion, but beta cell response to arginine stimulation is different from that of type 2 diabetic patients. Thus, neither surgical nor chemical beta cell destruction produced models comparable to that present in human type 2 diabetic patients.[35]

Generally speaking, a relationship exists between the serum glucose and the loss of beta cell mass. From a clinical standpoint, when treating type 2 diabetes, a lack of significant glucose change with an insulin sensitizer (thiazolidinedione) might imply substantial beta cell dysfunction. Insulin sensitizers work primarily by improving the metabolic response to available circulating insulin (either secreted or exogenous insulin) and thus lower serum glucose. However, if the beta cell is unable to produce adequate insulin, a blunted or minimal change in serum glucose would be expected.

Several studies have shown that hyperglycemia itself can damage islets via structural damage and alterations of their secretory characteristics. For example, in a rat model after partial pancreatectomy, new islet tissue that is regenerated in the midst of this artificial hyperglycemic environment (surgically induced diabetes) includes disorganized and fibrotic tissue. These changes can be prevented by treatment with insulin.[35] Mild chronic hyperglycemia results in loss of glucose-stimulated insulin release, and as the severity of hyperglycemia increases, the potentiating effect of glucose is also lost. These studies suggest that hyperglycemia is somehow a beta cell toxin or that it leads to the suppression of islet function and likely contributes to the pathogenesis of type 2 diabetes.

What about the potential role of elevated free fatty acids (FFAs) and dietary fat on the pathogenesis of type 2 diabetes? A high-fat diet is associated with increased risk of developing diabetes. To some extent, this is due to increased weight (obesity) and associated insulin resistance, but it might also be due to alterations in beta cell function. The duration of increased dietary fat required to induce such changes is not known; however, reverting to a diet that is more balanced and contains more carbohydrates leads to improvement in glucose tolerance as quickly as within 3 days.[35] In vitro, FFAs also appear to impair islet function. Islets incubated in a high-FFA environment demonstrate reduced production of insulin.[35]

OTHER METABOLIC AND HORMONAL ABNORMALITIES

Adipokines and Adipose Tissue

Previously, adipose tissue was simply regarded as a simple site of fat deposition. However, adipose tissue is now also recognized as an active endocrine organ.

Box 3-2. Proteins Secreted by Adipocytes That Can Act as Signaling Molecules

Adiponectin

Leptin

Resistin

Tumor necrosis factor α

Interleukin-6

ASP (acylation stimulation protein, derived from adipsin, C2, and factor B)

Angiotensin

Glucocorticoids and sex hormones (modification)

PAI-1 (plasminogen activator inhibitor type 1)

Transforming growth factor β

The first hormone noted to originate from adipose tissue was leptin. Subsequently, studies revealed that numerous proteins, including tumor necrosis factor alpha (TNF-α), adiponectin, resistin, and adipsin, are produced by adipose tissue (Box 3-2). Collectively, these hormones are known as adipocytokines or adipokines.

We will focus on the adipokines that have potential insulin sensitizing properties (adiponectin and leptin) and on some of the potential insulin antagonists (resistin, TNF-α, IL-6).

Potential Insulin Sensitizers

Adiponectin

Adiponectin is a hormone secreted by adipose tissue; it was independently discovered by several research groups in 1995 and 1996. Formerly, it was called acrp30, GBP 28, adipoQ, and apMI, among other terms. It is a peptide composed of 247 amino acids with a collagenous domain at the N-terminus and a C-terminal globular domain.[36] Its globular domain has some structural similarity to that of TNF-α.[37]

In contrast to the other known adipokines, circulating adiponectin levels are reduced and inversely related to adipose tissue mass and type 2 diabetes.[38,39] In human cross-sectional studies, plasma adiponectin levels negatively correlate with obesity,[40] insulin resistance,[41] cardiovascular disease,[42] waist-to-hip ratio,[41] and diabetic dyslipidemia.[43] In case-control studies, low plasma adiponectin is an independent risk factor for the future development of type 2 diabetes[44,45] but not for obesity.[46] Adiponectin is also inversely associated with the traditional cardiac risk factors (e.g., blood pressure, heart rate, LDL cholesterol, and triglyceride levels). Adiponectin positively and strongly correlates with HDL cholesterol levels.[43,47,48]

A nested case-control study of participants of the Health Professional Follow-up Study demonstrated

tion in non-insulin-dependent diabetes. Diabetes 31: 333-338, 1982.

15. Revers RR., Fink R, Griffin J, et al: Influence of hyperglycemia on insulin's in vivo effects in type II diabetes. J Clin Invest 73:664-672, 1984.

16. Baron AD, Schaeffer L, Shragg P, Kolterman OG: Role of hyperglucagonemia in maintenance of increased rates of hepatic glucose output in type II diabetics. Diabetes 36:274-283, 1987.

17. Felig P, Wahren J, Hendler R: Influence of maturity-onset diabetes on splanchnic glucose balance after oral glucose ingestion. Diabetes 27:121-126, 1978.

18. Nikoulina SE, Ciaraldi TP, Mudaliar S, et al: Potential role of glycogen synthase kinase-3 in skeletal muscle insulin resistance of type 2 diabetes. Diabetes 49:263-271, 2000.

19. Beeson M, Dizon M, Grebenv D, et al: Activation of protein kinase C-zeta by insulin and phosphatidylinositol-3,4,5-$(PO_4)_3$ is defective in muscle in type 2 diabetes and impaired glucose tolerance: Amelioration by rosiglitazone and exercise. Diabetes 52:1926-1934, 2003.

20. Boden G, Ray TK, Smith RH, Owen OE: Carbohydrate oxidation and storage in obese non-insulin-dependent diabetic patients. Effects of improving glycemic control. Diabetes 32:982-987, 1983.

23. Baron AD, Kolterman OG, Bell J, et al: Rates of noninsulin-mediated glucose uptake are elevated in type II diabetic subjects. J Clin Invest 76:1782-1788, 1985.

24. Wallace TM, Matthews DR: The assessment of insulin resistance in man. Diabet Med 19:527-534, 2002.

25. Matthews DR, Hosker JP, Rudenski AS, et al: Homeostasis model assessment: Insulin resistance and beta cell function from fasting plasma glucose and insulin concentrations in man. Diabetologia 28:412-419, 1985.

26. Haffner SM, D'Agostino R Jr, Mykkanen L, et al: Insulin sensitivity in subjects with type 2 diabetes. Relationship to cardiovascular risk factors: The Insulin Resistance Atherosclerosis Study. Diabetes Care 22:562-568, 1999.

27. Ferrannini E, Mari A: How to measure insulin sensitivity. J Hypertens 16: 895-906, 1998.

28. Laakso M: How good a marker is insulin level for insulin resistance? Am J Epidemiol 137: 959-965, 1993.

29. McLaughlin T, Abbasi F, Cheal K, et al: Use of metabolic markers to identify overweight individuals who are insulin resistant. Ann Int Med 139: 802-809, 2003.

30. Katz A, Nambi SS, Mather K, et al: Quantitative insulin sensitivity check index: A simple, accurate method for assessing insulin sensitivity in humans. J Clin Endocrinol Metab 85:2402-2410, 2000.

31. Butler AE, Janson J, Bonner-Weir S, et al: Beta cell deficit and increased beta cell apoptosis in humans with type 2 diabetes. Diabetes 52:102-110, 2003.

32. Butler AE, Janson J, Soeller WC, Butler PC: Increased beta cell apoptosis prevents adaptive increase in beta cell mass in mouse model of type 2 diabetes: Evidence for role of islet amyloid formation rather than direct action of amyloid. Diabetes 52:2304-2314, 2003.

33. Janson J, Ashley RH, Harrison D, et al: The mechanism of islet amyloid polypeptide toxicity is membrane disruption by intermediate-sized toxic amyloid particles. Diabetes 48:491-498, 1999.

34. Ritzel RA, Butler PC: Replication increases β-cell vulnerability to human islet amyloid polypeptide-induced apoptosis. Diabetes 52:1701-1708, 2003.

35. Kahn SE, Porte D: The pathophysiology and genetics of type 2 diabetes mellitus, 6th ed. In Porte D Jr, Sherwin RS, Baron A (eds): Ellenberg and Rifkin's Diabetes Mellitus. New York, McGraw Hill, 2001, pp 331-365.

36. Stefan N, Stumvoll M: Adiponectin—its role in metabolism and beyond. Horm Metab Res 34:469-474, 2002.

37. Shapiro L, Scherer PE: The crystal structure of a complement-1q family protein suggests an evolutionary link to tumor necrosis factor. Curr Biol 8:335-338, 1998.

38. Statnick MA, Beavers LS, Corominola H, et al: Decreased expression of apM1 in omental and subcutaneous adipose tissue of humans with type 2 diabetes. Int J Exp Diabetes Res 1:81-88, 2000.

39. Hu E, Liang P, Spiegelman BM: AdipoQ is a novel adipose-specific gene dysregulated in obesity. J Biol Chem 271:10697-10703, 1996.

40. Arita Y, Kihara S, Takahashi M, et al: Paradoxical decrease of an adipose-specific protein, adiponectin, in obesity. Biochem Biophys Res Commun 257:79-83, 1999.

41. Weyer C, Funahashi T, Tanaka S, et al: Hypoadiponectinemia in obesity and type 2 diabetes: Close association with insulin resistance and hyperinsulinemia. J Clin Endocrinol Metab 86:1930-1935, 2001.

42. Hotta K, Funahashi T, Arita Y, et al: Plasma concentrations of a novel, adipose-specific protein, adiponectin, in type 2 diabetic patients. Arterioscler Thromb Vasc Biol 20:1595-1599, 2000.

43. Matsubara M, Maruoka S, Katayose S: Decreased plasma adiponectin concentrations in women with dyslipidemia. J Clin Endocrinol Metab 87:2764-2769, 2002.

44. Lindsay RS, Funahashi T, Hanson RL, et al: Adiponectin and development of type 2 diabetes in the Pima Indian population. Lancet 260:57-58, 2002.

45. Spranger J, Kroke A, Mohlig M, et al: Adiponectin and protection against type 2 diabetes mellitus. Lancet 361:226-228, 2003.

46. Vozarova B, Stefan N, Lindsay RS, et al: Low plasma adiponectin concentrations do not predict weight gain in humans. Diabetes 51:2964-2967, 2002.

47. Kazumi T, Kawaguchi A, Sakai K, et al: Young men with high normal blood pressure have lower serum adiponectin, smaller LDL size, and higher elevated heart rate than those with optimal blood pressure. Diabetes Care 25:971-976, 2002.

48. Cnop M, Havel PJ, Utzschneider KM, et al: Relationship of adiponectin to body fat distribution, insulin sensitivity and plasma lipoproteins: Evidence for independent roles of age and sex. Diabetologia 46:459-469, 2003.

49. Pischon T, Girman CJ, Hotamisligil GS, et al: Plasma adiponectin levels and risk of myocardial infarction in men. JAMA 291:1730-1737, 2004.

50. Combs TP, Wagner JA, Berger J, et al: Induction of adipocyte complement-related protein of 30 kilodaltons by PPAR-gamma agonists: A potential mechanism of insulin sensitization. Endocrinology 143:998-1007, 2002.

51. Fruebis J, Tsao TS, Javorschi S, et al: Proteolytic cleavage product of 30-kDa adipocyte complement-related protein increases fatty acid oxidation in muscle and causes weight loss in mice. Proc Natl Acad Sci 98:2005-2010, 2001.

52. Yamauchi T, Kamon J, Minokoshi Y, et al: Adiponectin stimulates glucose utilization and fatty acid oxidation by activating AMP-activated protein kinase. Nat Med 8:1288-1295, 2002.

53. Berg AH, Combs TP, Du X, et al: The adipocytes-secreted protein ACRP30 enhances hepatic insulin action. Nat Med 7:947-953, 2001.

54. Wu X, Motoshima H, Mahadev K, et al: Involvement of AMP-activated protein kinase in glucose uptake stimulated by the globular domain of adiponectin in primary rate adipocytes. Diabetes 52:1355-1363, 2003.

55. Yamauchi T, Kamon J, Ito Y, et al: Cloning of adiponectin receptors that mediate antidiabetic metabolic effects. Nature 423:762-769, 2003.

56. Yamauchi T, Kamon J, Waki H, et al: The fat-derived hormone adiponectin reverses insulin resistance associated with both lipoatrophy and obesity. Nat Med 7:941-946, 2001.

57. Shklyaev S, Aslanidi G, Tennant M, et al: Sustained peripheral expression of transgene adiponectin offsets the development of diet-induced obesity in rats. Proc Natl Acad Sci U S A 100:14217-14222, 2003.

58. Combs TP, Berg AH, Obici S, et al: Endogenous glucose production is inhibited by the adipose-derived protein Acrp30. J Clin Invest 108:1875-1881, 2001.

59. Pittas AG, Joseph NA, Greenberg AS: Adipocytokines and insulin resistance. J Clin Endocrinol Metab 89:447-452, 2004.

60. Saha AK, Schwarsin AJ, Roduit R, Masse F, et al: Activation of malonyl-CoA decarboxylase in rat skeletal muscle by contraction and the AMP-activated protein kinase activator 5-aminoimidazole-4-carboxamide-1-beta-D-ribofuranoside. J Biol Chem 275:24279-24283, 2000.

61. Chandran M, Phillips SA, Ciaraldi T, Henry RR: Adiponectin: More than just another fat cell hormone? Diabetes Care 26:2442-2450, 2003.

62. Considine RV, Sinha MK, Heiman ML, et al: Serum immunoreactive-leptin concentrations in normal-weight and obese humans. N Engl J Med 334:292-295, 1996.

63. Zhang Y, Proenca R, Maffei M, et al: Positional cloning of the mouse obese gene and its human homologue. Nature 372:425-432, 1994.

64. Minokoshi Y, Kim YB, Peroni OD, et al: Leptin stimulates fatty-acid oxidation by activating AMP-activated protein kinase. Nature 415:339-343, 2002.

65. Unger RH, Zhou YT, Orci L: Regulation of fatty acid homeostasis in cells: Novel role of leptin. Proc Natl Acad Sci U S A 96:2327-2332, 1999.

66. Montague CT, Farooqi IS, Whitehead JP, et al: Congenital leptin deficiency is associated with severe early-onset obesity in humans. Nature 387:903-908, 1997.

67. Farooqi IS, Matarese G, Lord GM, et al: Beneficial effects of leptin on obesity, T cell hyporesponsiveness, and neuroendocrine/metabolic dysfunction of human congenital leptin deficiency. J Clin Invest 110:1093-1103, 2002.

68. Clement K, Vaisse C, Lahlou N, et al: A mutation in the human leptin receptor gene causes obesity and pituitary dysfunction. Nature 392:398-401, 1998.

69. Heymsfield SB, Greenberg AS, Fujioka K, et al: Recombinant leptin for weight loss in obese and lean adults: A randomized, controlled, dose-escalation trial. JAMA 282:1568-1575, 1999.

70. Caro JF, Sinha MK, Kolaczynski JW, et al: Leptin: The tale of an obesity gene. Diabetes 45:1455-1462, 1996.

71. Wang MY, Lee Y, Unger RH: Novel form of lipolysis induced by leptin. J Biol Chem 274:17541-17544, 1999.

72. Banks WA, Farrell CL: Impaired transport of leptin across the blood-brain barrier in obesity is acquired and reversible. Am J Physiol Endocrinol Metab 285:E10-E15, 2003.

73. Bjorbaek C, El-Haschimi K, Frantz JD, Flier JS: The role of SOCS-3 in leptin signaling and leptin resistance. J Biol Chem 274:30059-30065, 1999.

74. Boden G, Shulman GI: Free fatty acids in obesity and type 2 diabetes: Defining their role in the development of insulin resistance and β-cell dysfunction. Eur J Clin Invest 32(S3):14-23, 2002.

75. Petersen KF, Oral EA, Dufour S, et al: Leptin reverses insulin resistance and hepatic steatosis in patients with severe lipodystrophy. J Clin Invest 109:1345-1350, 2002.

76. Steppan CM, Lazar MA: Resistin and obesity-associated insulin resistance. Trends Endocrinol Metab 13:18-23, 2002.

77. McTernan PG, McTernan CL, Chetty R, et al: Increased resistin gene and protein expression in human abdominal adipose tissue. J Clin Endocrinol Metab 87:2407-2410, 2002.

78. Heilbronn LK, Rood J, Janderova L, et al: Relationship between serum resistin concentrations and insulin resistance in nonobese, obese, and obese diabetic subjects. J Clin Endocrinol Metab 89:1844-1848, 2004.

79. Moller DE: Potential role of TNF-α in the pathogenesis of insulin resistance and type 2 diabetes. Trends Endocrinol Metab 11:212-217, 2000.

80. Fried SK, Bunkin DA, Greenberg AS: Omental and subcutaneous adipose tissues of obese subjects release interleukin-6: Depot difference and regulation by glucocorticoid. J Clin Endocrinol Metab 83:847-850, 1998.

81. Kern PA, Saghizadeh M, Ong JM, et al: The expression of tumor necrosis factor in human adipose tissue. Regulation by obesity, weight loss, and relationship to lipoprotein lipase. J Clin Invest 95:2111-2119, 1995.

82. Desfaits AC, Serri O, Renier G: Normalization of plasma lipid peroxides, monocyte adhesion, and tumor necrosis factor-α production in NIDDM patients after gliclazide treatment. Diabetes Care 21:487-493, 1998.

83. Hotamisligil GS, Shargill NS, Spiegelman BM: Adipose expression of tumor necrosis factor-α: Direct role in obesity-linked insulin resistance. Science 259:87-91, 1993.

84. Ofei F, Hurel S, Newkirk J, Sopwith M, Taylor R: Effects of an engineered human anti-TNF-α antibody (CDP571) on insulin sensitivity and glycemic control in patients with NIDDM. Diabetes 45:881-885, 1996.

85. Mohamed-Ali V, Goodrick S, Rawesh A, et al: Subcutaneous adipose tissue releases interleukin-6, but not tumor necrosis factor-α, in vivo. J Clin Endocrinol Metab 82:4196-4200, 1997.

86. Bruun JM, Lihn AS, Verdich C, et al: Regulation of adiponectin by adipose tissue-derived cytokines: In vivo and in vitro investigations in humans. Am J Physiol Endocrinol Metab 285:E527-E533, 2003.

87. Greenberg AS, McDaniel ML: Identifying the links between obesity, insulin resistance and β-cell function: Potential role of adipocyte-derived cytokines in the pathogenesis of type 2 diabetes. Eur J Clin Invest 32(Suppl 3):24-34, 2002.

88. Hotamisligil GS, Spiegelman BM: Tumor necrosis factor α: A key component of the obesity-diabetes link. Diabetes 43:1271-1278, 1994.

89. Miles PD, Romeo OM, Higo K, et al: TNF-α-induced insulin resistance in vivo and its prevention by troglitazone. Diabetes 46:1678-1683, 1997.

90. Peraldi P, Xu M, Spiegelman BM: Thiazolidinediones block tumor necrosis factor-α-induced inhibition of insulin signaling. J Clin Invest 100:1863-1869, 1997.

91. Souza SC, de Vargas LM, Yamamoto MT, et al: Overexpression of perilipin A and B blocks the ability of tumor necrosis factor alpha to increase lipolysis in 3T3-L1 adipocytes. J Biol Chem 273:24665-24669, 1998.

92. Vozarova B, Weyer C, Hanson K, et al: Circulating interleukin-6 in relation to adiposity, insulin action, and insulin secretion. Obes Res 9:414-417, 2001.

93. Kern PA, Ranganathan S, Li C, Wood L, Ranganathan G: Adipose tissue tumor necrosis factor and interleukin-6 expression in human obesity and insulin resistance. Am J Physiol Endocrinol Metab 280:E745-E751, 2001.

94. Pradhan AD, Manson JE, Rifai N, et al: C-reactive protein, interleukin-6, and risk of developing type 2 diabetes mellitus. JAMA 286:327-334, 2001.

95. Ridker PM, Rifai N, Stampfer MJ, Hennekens CH: Plasma concentration of interleukin-6 and the risk of future myocardial infarction among apparently healthy men. Circulation 101:1767-1772, 2000.

96. Bastard JP, Jardel C, Bruckert E, et al: Elevated levels of interleukin 6 are reduced in serum and subcutaneous adipose tissue of obese women after weight loss. J Clin Endocrinol Metab 85:3338-3342, 2000.

97. Gan SK, Kriketos AD, Poynten AM, et al:. Insulin action, regional fat, and myocyte lipid: Altered relationships with increased adiposity. Obes Res 11:1295-1305, 2003.

98. Carr DB, Utzschneider KM, Hull RL, et al: Intra-abdominal fat is a major determinant of the National Cholesterol Education Program Adult Treatment Panel III criteria for the metabolic syndrome. Diabetes 53:2087-2094, 2004.

99. Machann J, Haring H, Schick F, Stumvoll M: Intramyocellular lipids and insulin resistance. Diabetes Obes Metab 6:239-248, 2004.

100. Mori Y, Murakawa Y, Okada K, et al: Effect of troglitazone on body fat distribution in type 2 diabetic patients. Diabetes Care 22:908-912, 1999.

101. Miyazaki Y, Mahankali A, Matsuda M, et al: Effect of pioglitazone on abdominal fat distribution and insulin sensitivity in type 2 diabetic patients. J Clin Endocrinol Metab 87:2784-2791, 2002.

102. Gastaldelli A, Miyazaki Y, Pettiti M, et al: Metabolic effects of visceral fat accumulation in type 2 diabetes. J Clin Endocrinol Metab 87:5098-5103, 2002.

103. Dandona P, Aljada A, Chaudhuri A, Bandyopadhyay A: The potential influence of inflammation and insulin resistance on the pathogenesis and treatment of atherosclerosis-related complications in type 2 diabetes. J Clin Endocrinol Metab 88:2422-2429, 2003.

The Biochemical Consequences of Hyperglycemia

Ravi Retnakaran and Bernard Zinman

KEY POINTS

- *Four distinct pathways have been identified as biochemical mechanisms by which hyperglycemia can induce vascular damage: increased flux through the polyol pathway, formation of advanced glycation end products, activation of protein kinase C, and increased flux through the hexosamine biosynthesis pathway.*
- *Overproduction of superoxide by the mitochondrial electron transport chain has been proposed as a single hyperglycemia-induced process that activates all four of these pathways.*
- *New insight into molecular mechanisms by which hyperglycemia can induce vascular damage has led to the development of novel therapeutic strategies.*

Glucose metabolism can affect a wide variety of cellular functions and signaling pathways. Chronic hyperglycemia has been firmly established as a key factor in the development of diabetic microvascular disease affecting the retina, renal glomerulus, and vasa nervorum.[1,2] However, the specific mechanisms linking hyperglycemia to vascular damage have not been precisely defined. Substantial investigative efforts since the 1960s have led to the identification of four major biochemical pathways that could explain this association: increased flux through the polyol pathway, formation of advanced glycation end-products, activation of protein kinase C, and increased flux through the hexosamine pathway.

A unifying hypothesis has been formulated whereby these four seemingly unrelated pathways can be linked by a single hyperglycemia-driven process: the mitochondrial overproduction of reactive oxygen species.[3] This model has provided a new conceptual framework within which to consider the pathogenesis of diabetic vascular complications and has led to the development of novel therapeutic approaches. In this chapter, we review current insight into the molecular mechanisms by which hyperglycemia can induce vascular damage and the novel treatment strategies that have resulted from this understanding.

MECHANISMS OF HYPERGLYCEMIA-INDUCED VASCULAR DAMAGE

The Diabetes Control and Complications Trial (DCCT) and the United Kingdom Prospective Diabetes Study (UKPDS) provided incontrovertible evidence that chronic hyperglycemia is associated with an increased risk of microvascular complications in both type 1 diabetes mellitus (T1DM) and type 2 diabetes mellitus (T2DM) and that amelioration of hyperglycemia can modify this risk.[1,2] Although all tissues may be exposed to hyperglycemia, it is important to recognize that glucose-mediated damage is limited to cells that develop intracellular hyperglycemia. Under hyperglycemic conditions, vascular endothelial cells, in particular, are at risk for developing intracellular hyperglycemia because, unlike many other cell types, they are unable to down-regulate glucose uptake.[4] Glucose can pass freely through the endothelial cell membrane via the insulin-independent glucose transporter GLUT-1. In the setting of diabetes, the resultant intracellular hyperglycemia in endothelial cells can precipitate vascular damage that ultimately leads to microvascular complications.

Four distinct biochemical pathways have been identified as mechanisms by which intracellular hyperglycemia can induce vascular damage and contribute to the pathogenesis of diabetic complications. These mechanisms include increased flux through the polyol pathway, formation of advanced glycation end-products, activation of protein kinase C (PKC), and increased flux through the hexosamine pathway. In this section of the chapter, each of these biochemical mechanisms is considered in turn.

Increased Flux Through the Polyol Pathway

Mechanism

The polyol pathway is characterized by the action of aldose reductase (AR), a cytosolic enzyme that reduces toxic aldehydes generated from reactive oxygen species (ROS) to inactive alcohols and

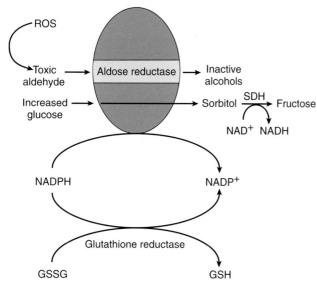

Figure 4–1. The polyol pathway. Hyperglycemia leads to increased shunting of glucose through the polyol pathway, resulting in increased aldose reductase activity and depletion of reduced glutathione. GSH, reduced glutathione; GSSG, glutathione disulfide; NAD$^+$, nicotinamide adenine dinucleotide; NADH, reduced NAD; NADP$^+$, nicotinamide adenine dinucleotide phosphate; NADPH, reduced NADP; ROS, reactive oxygen species; SDH, sorbitol dehydrogenase. (Adapted from Brownlee M, Aiello LP, Friedman E, et al: Complications of diabetes. In Larsen R, Kronenberg H, Melmed S, Polonsky K (eds): Williams Textbook of Endocrinology, 10th ed. Philadelphia, WB Saunders, 2003, p 1515.)

reduces glucose to the polyalcohol sorbitol in a reaction that requires nicotinamide adenine dinucleotide phosphate (NADPH) as a cofactor (Fig. 4–1). Because aldose reductase has a low affinity for glucose, this pathway accounts for a very small fraction of total glucose use at normal blood glucose concentrations. In the setting of hyperglycemia, however, the resultant increase in intracellular glucose concentration leads to increased flux through this pathway, such that up to 30% of glucose can be metabolized in this way.[5] Accordingly, there is increased conversion of intracellular glucose to sorbitol, which is subsequently oxidized to fructose by sorbitol dehydrogenase (SDH), the second enzyme in the polyol pathway.

Deleterious Effects

The main mechanism by which chronic hyperglycemia-induced flux through the polyol pathway can be harmful is not entirely clear, although several possible routes have been proposed. The most likely mechanism involves the consumption of NADPH in the reduction of glucose to sorbitol by aldose reductase and subsequent oxidative stress.[3] Because NADPH is also required for the regenera-

tion of reduced glutathione (see Fig. 4–1), depletion of NADPH can cause a decrease in the concentration of reduced glutathione. Given the role of glutathione as an important cellular antioxidant, a decline in its concentration can exacerbate intracellular oxidative stress.

In support of this theory, transgenic mice that overexpress aldose reductase in their lenses indeed exhibit decreased levels of reduced glutathione in that tissue.[6] Furthermore, in the setting of diabetes, aldose reductase knockout mice show neither the reduction in sciatic nerve glutathione concentration nor the decreased nerve conduction velocity observed in diabetic wild-type mice, consistent with a role for the polyol pathway as a source of hyperglycemia-induced oxidative stress in neuronal tissue.[7]

Another proposed deleterious effect of increased flux through the polyol pathway is the consumption of nicotinamide adenine dinucleotide (NAD$^+$) in the oxidation of sorbitol to fructose by sorbitol dehydrogenase (see Fig. 4–1). Researchers have hypothesized that a consequent increase in the cytosolic NADH/NAD$^+$ ratio could lead to inhibition of the enzyme glyceraldehyde 3-phosphate dehydrogenase (GAPDH) and subsequent elevated concentrations of triose phosphate.[8] Increased triose phosphate levels could lead to enhanced formation of both methylglyoxal, an advanced glycation end-product (AGE) precursor, and diacylglycerol (DAG), an activator of PKC (discussed later).[3] It should be recognized, however, that there is no direct evidence that increased flux through the polyol pathway leads to an increased cytosolic NADH/NAD$^+$ ratio. Furthermore, although hyperglycemia has been shown to increase the NADH/NAD$^+$ ratio in endothelial cells, this effect is due to consumption of NAD$^+$ by poly(ADP-ribose) polymerase (PARP) rather than conversion of NAD$^+$ to NADH.[9] ROS-induced activation of PARP (and subsequent inhibition of GAPDH) has in itself now emerged as a potential upstream mechanism underlying the deleterious activation of several pathways, including the polyol pathway (see PARP Activation and GAPDH Inhibition, later).

Two other, older proposed mechanisms, namely sorbitol-induced osmotic stress and decreased Na$^+$,K$^+$-ATPase activity, likely do not underlie the detrimental effects of flux through the polyol pathway. Because sorbitol does not readily diffuse across cell membranes, its intracellular accumulation via the polyol pathway had been suggested as a cause of osmotic damage to cells. However, with the recognition that sorbitol concentrations in diabetic vessels and nerves are much too low to cause such osmotic stress, this theory is now considered unlikely.[10] Decreased Na$^+$,K$^+$-ATPase activity, although initially linked to the polyol pathway, is now known to result from activation of PKC. Specifically, PKC activation leads to increased production of arachidonate and prostaglandin E$_2$ (PGE$_2$), two known inhibitors of Na$^+$,K$^+$-ATPase.[11]

Aldose Reductase Inhibition

Pharmacologic inhibition of aldose reductase has been studied as a means of reducing flux through the polyol pathway in diabetes. In animal models, aldose reductase inhibitors have prevented some of the pathologic changes associated with the microvascular complications of diabetes.[12,13] In general, in these studies, aldose reductase inhibitors have shown beneficial effects in the context of neuropathy but have been ineffective in preventing retinopathy or nephropathy. Clinical studies have shown a similar pattern, with positive results noted only in neuropathy.

In a meta-analysis of 19 clinical trials, aldose reductase inhibition provided modest reductions in the decline of motor nerve conduction velocity associated with diabetic neuropathy, although the clinical relevance of this effect remains unclear.[14] The relative lack of efficacy in human trials might reflect the inability to achieve adequate tissue concentrations of the drug or possibly a modest role for the polyol pathway in the pathogenesis of microvascular complications. The latter consideration, in particular, potentially points to the importance of considering the multifactorial nature of glucose-mediated cellular damage when designing therapeutic approaches to combat the effects of chronic hyperglycemia.

Formation of Advanced Glycation End-Products

Mechanism

In normal physiology, glucose reacts with free amino groups on proteins to form small amounts of early glycosylation products (stable Amadori products), through a nonenzymatic and reversible reaction. With normal aging, further processing causes irreversible glycation of proteins, leading to the formation of advanced glycation end-products. In diabetes, the process of irreversible, nonenzymatic glycation of proteins is markedly accelerated by chronic hyperglycemia, causing an accumulation of AGEs.[15,16] Furthermore, the presence of increased AGE concentrations in the extracellular matrix of retinal vessels and renal glomeruli in diabetes supports the suggestion that increased AGE formation could be a factor in the pathogenesis of vascular complications.[17,18]

Intracellular hyperglycemia is believed to be responsible for the enhanced AGE formation seen in diabetes. Intracellular hyperglycemia promotes production of reactive dicarbonyl precursors, including glyoxal, methylglyoxal, and 3-deoxyglucosone.[19] In the setting of hyperglycemia, these reactive precursors are formed from auto-oxidation of glucose to glyoxal, fragmentation of glyceraldehyde 3-phosphate to methylglyoxal, and decomposition of the Amadori product to 3-deoxyglucosone. The subsequent reaction of these precursors with amino groups of intracellular and extracellular proteins leads to the formation of AGEs.

Deleterious Effects

There are three general mechanisms by which AGE precursors can damage target tissues. AGE precursors can alter intracellular protein function and can modify matrix proteins and consequently disrupt normal matrix–matrix and matrix–cell interactions, and plasma AGEs can interact with specific AGE receptors on target cells, leading to the activation of pathologic signaling pathways (Fig. 4–2). Each of these mechanisms is considered in turn.

Intracellular modification of proteins by AGE precursors can disrupt protein and cellular function. For instance, endothelial cells cultured under hyperglycemic conditions exhibit a 13.8-fold increase in AGE-modified cytosolic proteins.[20] One such protein is basic fibroblast growth factor (bFGF). The observed 6.1-fold increase in AGE-modified bFGF was associated with a marked decrease in bFGF mitogenic activity, providing evidence of AGE alteration of intracellular protein function.[20] Similarly, macromolecular endocytosis is another cellular function affected by AGE formation. Specifically, the up-regulated endocytosis associated with increased intracellular AGE content when endothelial cells are cultured under hyperglycemic conditions can be reversed through over-expression of glyoxase I, an enzyme that decreases AGE formation by detoxifying methylglyoxal.[21]

AGE modification of important matrix proteins can change the structure and function of extracellular matrix. For example, AGE-mediated cross-linking of type I collagen can expand molecular packing of the protein and thereby decrease blood vessel elasticity.[22] AGE formation on type IV collagen undermines the ordered assembly of these molecules into their normal lattice-like structure on basement membranes.[23] Similar effects are observed with AGE formation on laminin.[23] Furthermore, AGE modification of these matrix proteins can interfere with matrix–cell interactions, as evidenced by the reduction in endothelial cell adhesion resulting from AGE-induced changes to the cell-binding domain of type IV collagen.[24]

A third mechanism by which AGEs can alter cellular function is through the binding of AGE-modified plasma proteins to specific AGE receptors on target cells. Specific receptors for AGE (RAGE) have been identified on endothelial cells.[25] Binding of AGE-modified proteins to RAGE induces cellular signal transduction, leading to generation of ROS and activation of signaling molecules such as nuclear factor κB (NF-κB), p21 ras, and PKC.[26,27] RAGE-mediated changes in gene expression contribute to vascular abnormalities in diabetes such as enhanced procoagulant activity (via thrombomodulin, tissue factor, and plasminogen activator inhibitor 1 [PAI-1]), proinflammatory changes (up-regulation of vascular cell adhesion molecule 1 [VCAM-1]), and increased vessel permeability (due

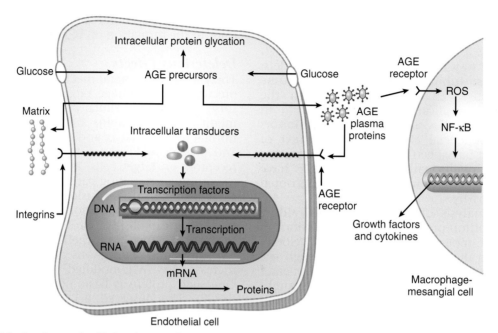

Figure 4–2. Mechanisms of cellular damage by intracellular production of advanced glycation end-products (AGEs). Accelerated AGE formation in the setting of hyperglycemia leads to disruption of intracellular proteins, modification of matrix proteins, and the interaction of plasma AGEs with AGE receptors on target cells, resulting in the activation of pathologic signaling pathways. mRNA, messenger RNA; NF-κB, nuclear factor κB; ROS, reactive oxygen species. (Adapted from Brownlee M: Biochemistry and molecular cell biology of diabetic complications. Nature 414:815, 2001. Copyright © 2001 Nature, www.nature.com.)

to up-regulation of vascular endothelial growth factor [VEGF]).[28-30]

Other AGE receptors identified on monocytes, macrophages, and glomerular mesangial cells include OST-48 80K-H, galectin-3, and macrophage scavenger receptor type II.[31-33] Binding of AGEs to these receptors stimulates expression of cytokines and growth factors, including tumor necrosis factor α (TNF-α), interleukin-1 (IL-1), insulinlike growth factor I (IGF-I), transforming growth factor β (TGF-β), granulocyte-macrophage colony-stimulating factor (GM-CSF), granulocyte colony-stimulating factor (G-CSF), and platelet-derived growth factor (PDGF).[3]

Inhibition of Advanced Glycation End-products

Further evidence supporting a role for AGEs in the pathophysiology of vascular complications in diabetes is provided by studies in which AGE formation has been inhibited. Aminoguanidine is one such AGE inhibitor, although its precise mechanism of action is unclear. In animal models of diabetes, treatment with aminoguanidine prevents AGE accumulation and has been associated with partial protection from retinopathy, nephropathy, and neuropathy.[34]

In a placebo-controlled, randomized trial in 690 patients with type 1 diabetes and nephropathy, aminoguanidine did not show a significant beneficial effect on the progression of overt nephropathy (primary outcome).[35] Nevertheless, this study provided clinical evidence that AGE inhibition may be associated with attenuation of some diabetic complications, including 24-hour proteinuria and progression of retinopathy (defined by an increase of three or more steps using the Early Treatment Diabetic Retinopathy Study score). Caution must be advised, however: These positive effects were noted only as secondary outcomes, and significant adverse events (including hepatic dysfunction and cardiovascular complications) interrupted a similar trial in patients with type 2 diabetes.[36]

A different approach to AGE inhibition is the use of a soluble form of the extracellular domain of RAGE to inhibit the interaction between AGEs and endogenous RAGE on endothelial cells. In an atherosclerosis-prone (apolipoprotein E (ApoE)–/–) diabetic mouse model, infusion of this construct suppressed the progression of atherosclerotic disease in a glycemia-independent manner.[37] Accordingly, RAGE blockade could emerge as a therapeutic approach in the future.

Activation of Protein Kinase C

Mechanism

The PKC family of cell-signaling enzymes contains at least 11 members.[38] Signaling pathways involving these enzymes regulate a variety of cellular functions including cell growth and differentiation, apoptosis, protein trafficking, cytoskeletal rearrangement, and cell polarity. Most PKC isoforms are activated by the lipid second messenger diacylglycerol (DAG), typically following DAG stimulation by

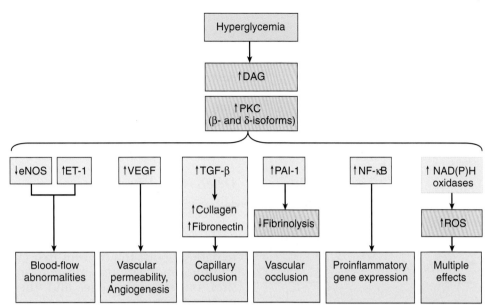

Figure 4–3. Deleterious effects of hyperglycemia-induced activation of protein kinase C (PKC). DAG, diacylglycerol; eNOS, endothelial nitric oxide synthase; ET-1, endothelin-1; NAD(P)H, reduced nicotinamide adenine dinucleotide (phosphate); NF-κB, nuclear factor κB; PAI-1, plasminogen activator inhibitor 1; ROS, reactive oxygen species; TGF-β, transforming growth factor β; VEGF, vascular endothelial growth factor. (Adapted from Brownlee M: Biochemistry and molecular cell biology of diabetic complications. Nature 414:815, 2001. Copyright © 2001 Nature, www.nature.com.)

ligand-receptor interactions at the cell membrane. In the setting of diabetes, however, intracellular hyperglycemia has been shown to stimulate de novo synthesis of DAG and thereby increase DAG content.[39]

Specifically, in the hyperglycemic state, there is increased metabolism of glucose to the glycolytic intermediate, glyceraldehyde 3-phosphate. Conversion of this intermediate through glycerol 3-phosphate subsequently drives de novo synthesis of DAG via increased substrate. Indeed, intracellular hyperglycemia increases DAG content both in cultured vascular cells and in target tissues (retina, glomerulus) of diabetic animals.[40,41] Furthermore, in both cases, increased DAG synthesis has been shown to activate PKC. Hyperglycemic stimulation of DAG principally activates the β and δ isoforms of PKC, though other isoforms can also be induced, including PKC-α and PKC-ε in the retina and glomerulus of diabetic rats.[39,42]

Deleterious Effects

PKC activation contributes to a wide variety of pathologic processes implicated in diabetic vasculopathy (Fig. 4–3). Activation of PKC-β has been associated with endothelial dysfunction. Contributing factors in this regard likely include PKC-mediated suppression of nitric oxide (NO) production via inhibition of endothelial nitric oxide synthase (eNOS) and PKC stimulation of endothelin-1 (ET-1) vasoconstrictor activity.[43-45] Activation of PKC signaling also contributes to other characteristic vascular abnormalities associated with diabetes, including increased vascular permeability (via induction of VEGF) and decreased fibrinolysis (via increased PAI-1).[46-48] In addition, PKC signaling stimulates accumulation of matrix proteins and mesangial expansion through induction of TGF-β, type IV collagen, and fibronectin.[49,50] Wide-ranging effects on gene expression may be mediated through PKC-mediated induction of the transcription factor NF-κB and via putative crosstalk with other signaling systems, including the mitogen-activated protein (MAP) kinase pathway and nuclear receptors.[51,52] Finally, pathologic PKC activation can stimulate NADPH oxidases and thereby generate ROS, leading to increased oxidative stress.[3]

Inhibition of Protein Kinase C

Because normal PKC signaling affects a wide variety of fundamental cellular processes, nonselective PKC inhibition is not likely a viable option. However, the recent development of a selective PKC inhibitor with high affinity for the β1 and β2 isoforms has provided the ability to block several of the pathologic effects associated with hyperglycemia-induced PKC activation.

Oral administration of this agent, ruboxistaurin mesylate (LY333531), has been shown to improve glomerular filtration rate, decrease albumin excretion, and reduce retinal circulation time in diabetic rats.[43] Other animal studies have confirmed a role for ruboxistaurin in attenuating early changes in retinopathy, nephropathy, and neuropathy.[13] In nondiabetic humans, a 7-day course of ruboxistaurin prevents the reduction in endothelium-dependent vasodilation induced by acute hyper-

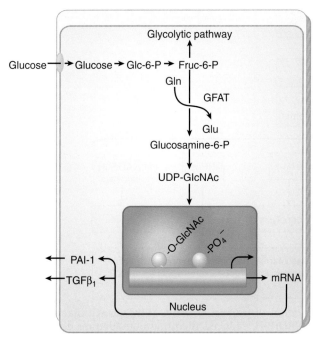

Figure 4–4. The hexosamine biosynthesis pathway. Increased shunting of glucose through the hexosamine pathway leads to increased O-GlcNAcylation (and decreased phosphorylation) of target proteins such as the transcription factor Sp1, leading to increased gene expression of PAI-1 and TGF-β. Fruc-6-P, fructose-6-phosphate; GFAT, glutamine:fructose-6-phosphate amidotransferase; Glc-6-P, glucosamine-6-phosphate; Gln, glutamine; Glu, glutamate; mRNA, messenger RNA; PAI-1, plasminogen activator inhibitor 1; PO_4^-, phosphate; TGF-β, transforming growth factor β; UDP-GlcNAc, UDP-N-acetylglucosamine. (Adapted fromBrownlee M, Aiello LP, Friedman E, et al: Complications of diabetes. In Larsen R, Kronenberg H, Melmed S, Polonsky K (eds): Williams Textbook of Endocrinology, 10th ed. Philadelphia, WB Saunders, 2003, p 1519.)

glycemia.[53] Clinical trials are currently in progress to evaluate the efficacy of this medication in patients with diabetic retinopathy and neuropathy.

Increased Flux Through the Hexosamine Pathway

Mechanism
In the setting of hyperglycemia, there is increased shunting of glucose into the hexosamine biosynthesis pathway. In the hexosamine pathway, the glycolytic intermediate fructose-6-phosphate (fruc-6-P) is converted to glucosamine-6-phosphate (glc-6-P) by the rate-limiting enzyme glutamine:fructose-6-phosphate amidotransferase (GFAT) (Fig. 4–4). Glc-6-P is subsequently converted to UDP-N-acetylglucosamine (UDP-GlcNAc). This product is then used by the enzyme O-GlcNAc transferase (OGT), which glycosylates serine and threonine residues of target proteins by the addition of N-

acetylglucosamine (GlcNAc). Like phosphorylation, this O-linked glycosylation can alter the functional properties of target proteins, many of which are transcriptional regulatory factors.[54,55] This system is partly regulated by the availability of UDP-GlcNAc. Thus, in the setting of hyperglycemia, it is apparent that increased flux through the hexosamine pathway can increase the concentration of UDP-GlcNAc and ultimately affect gene expression by modification of transcriptional regulators.

Deleterious Effects
The exact mechanism by which hyperglycemia-induced flux through the hexosamine pathway modulates gene expression in diabetes remains to be conclusively established. Nevertheless, evidence to date supports the concept that O-GlcNAcylation and phosphorylation compete to modify the same sites on target proteins and thereby modulate protein function.[56]

One such protein is the transcription factor Sp1. Hyperglycemia-induced activation of the hexosamine pathway has been shown to increase O-GlcNAcylation and decrease serine and threonine phosphorylation of Sp1.[56] The glycosylated form of Sp1 appears to exhibit greater transcriptional activity than the deglycosylated form.[57] Furthermore, the observation that hyperglycemia-induced activation of PAI-1 expression is dependent on Sp1 sites in the PAI-1 promoter has suggested a role for O-GlcNAcylation of Sp1 in the modulation of gene expression via the hexosamine pathway.[58]

Besides Sp1, most RNA polymerase II transcription factors are O-GlcNAcylated.[55] Thus, the proposed concept of competition between O-GlcNAcylation and phosphorylation on transcription factors can provide a generalized mechanism for modulation of glucose-responsive gene expression via the hexosamine pathway. In addition, many other nuclear and cytoskeletal proteins (besides transcription factors) are modified by O-GlcNAcylation, which provides a potential mechanism whereby the hexosamine pathway can also affect protein function in the development of diabetic vasculopathy.[55]

OXIDATIVE STRESS AS A COMMON INITIATING PROCESS

On the basis of substantial experimental evidence, hyperglycemia has been implicated as a causative factor in the generation of ROS, leading to increased oxidative stress in a variety of tissues. Oxidative stress is known to activate a host of stress-induced signaling pathways including NF-κB, p38 MAP kinase, and NH_2-terminal Jun kinase–stress-activated protein kinase (JNK/SAPK) signaling.[59] With increased ROS production, inappropriate activation of these pathways can have deleterious effects on cellular function. Accordingly, with the observation of increased levels of oxidized DNA,

proteins, and lipids in the setting of diabetes, oxidative stress has been proposed as a factor in the development of diabetic complications.[60] However, given the complex multitude of potential relationships between ROS and abnormal cellular functions in diabetes (as noted in the previous section), the precise role of oxidative stress in the development of diabetic complications has been subject to scientific debate.

Some resolution of this debate has been recently provided by Brownlee and colleagues in a series of elegant experiments that have led to their formulation of a new paradigm for the pathogenesis of diabetic vascular complications.[3] By identifying a mechanism whereby hyperglycemia-induced ROS generation can lead to activation of each of the four seemingly independent biochemical pathways discussed under Mechanisms of Hyperglycemia-Induced Vascular Damage, they have established a unifying hypothesis that integrates oxidative stress and the molecular mechanisms implicated to date. Specifically, the four pathways—increased flux through the polyol pathway, enhanced formation of AGEs, activation of PKC, and increased flux through the hexosamine pathway—share an underlying common denominator: the overproduction of the ROS superoxide by the mitochondrial electron transport chain.

Superoxide Overproduction by the Mitochondrial Electron Transport Chain

To understand how hyperglycemia-induced overproduction of mitochondrial superoxide can lead to vascular complications, it is helpful to first review glucose metabolism and the role of the mitochondrial electron transport chain.[61] Glucose metabolism begins with glycolysis, a cytoplasmic reaction yielding pyruvate and NADH. Pyruvate can be reduced to lactate (providing a substrate for hepatic gluconeogenesis) or it can be transported into the mitochondria. In the mitochondria, pyruvate is oxidized by the tricarboxylic acid (TCA) cycle to yield carbon dioxide, water, NADH, and $FADH_2$. Electron transfer from NADH and $FADH_2$ to molecular oxygen (O_2) via the electron transport chain generates an electrochemical proton gradient across the inner mitochondrial membrane. This transmembrane gradient provides the energy required for ATP synthesis in the inner mitochondrial membrane.

Electron flow through the mitochondrial electron transport chain involves the coordinated actions of four enzyme complexes associated with the inner membrane, cytochrome c, and ubiquinone or coenzyme Q (Fig. 4–5). Electrons accepted by complex I (NADH:ubiquinone oxidoreductase) from NADH and by complex II (succinate:ubiquinone oxidoreductase) from $FADH_2$ are ultimately transferred

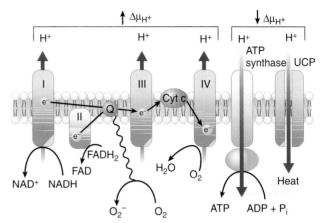

Figure 4–5. Superoxide production by the mitochondrial electron transport chain. Under hyperglycemic conditions, there is increased production of electron donors (NADH and $FADH_2$) from the tricarboxylic acid (TCA) cycle, leading to generation of a high mitochondrial membrane potential by the mitochondrial electron transport chain. The increased membrane potential inhibits electron transport at complex III, resulting in an increased half-life of superoxide-generating intermediates of coenzyme Q. ADP, adenosine diphosphate; ATP, adenosine triphosphate; $\Delta\mu_{H^+}$, mitochondrial membrane potential; e^-, electron; FAD, flavin adenine dinucleotide; $FADH_2$, reduced FAD; H^+, proton; NAD^+, nicotinamide adenine dinucleotide; NADH, reduced NAD; P_i, inorganic phosphate. (Adapted from Brownlee M: Biochemistry and molecular cell biology of diabetic complications. Nature 414:815, 2001. Copyright © 2001 Nature, www.nature.com.)

to ubiquinone. Electrons are then transferred from reduced ubiquinone to complex III (ubiquinol: cytochrome c oxidoreductase) via the Q cycle, which also generates free radical intermediates that can reduce O_2 to superoxide. From complex III, electron transport continues through cytochrome c, complex IV (cytochrome c oxidase), and ultimately O_2.

Protons pumped across the inner mitochondrial membrane by complexes I, III, and IV during electron transport generate a mitochondrial membrane potential that drives ATP production by ATP synthase. When the membrane potential generated by this proton gradient is high, electron transport is inhibited at complex III, increasing the half-life of superoxide-generating intermediates from the Q cycle. Indeed, superoxide production is significantly increased when the membrane potential exceeds a certain threshold.

Hyperglycemia leads to increased intracellular ROS by promoting overproduction of superoxide by the mitochondrial electron transport chain.[3,62] Specifically, by increasing flux through the TCA cycle and thereby increasing the supply of electron donors (NADH and $FADH_2$) to the electron transport chain, hyperglycemia causes the mitochondrial membrane potential to rise and, in fact, exceed its threshold value. As a result, overproduction of superoxide ensues.

Brownlee and colleagues showed that inhibition of superoxide overproduction by either collapsing the mitochondrial proton gradient (using uncoupling protein 1 [UCP-1]) or by overexpression of the antioxidant manganese superoxide disumutase (MnSOD) completely prevented hyperglycemia-induced increases in polyol pathway flux, AGE formation, PKC activation, and hexosamine pathway flux in endothelial cells.[56,62] Thus, hyperglycemia-induced superoxide overproduction was identified as an upstream initiator of all four of these pathologic processes.

PARP Activation and GAPDH Inhibition

The mechanism by which hyperglycemia-induced superoxide overproduction can activate four distinct biochemical pathways leading to vascular damage has recently been elucidated.[63] In the setting of hyperglycemia, increased superoxide production ultimately leads to DNA strand breakage. DNA strand breakage induces poly(ADP-ribose) polymerase (PARP), a nuclear enzyme involved in DNA repair.[64] Upon activation, PARP initiates an energy-consuming cycle by transferring ADP ribose units from NAD^+ to nuclear proteins in a process that depletes the cellular NAD^+ pool. One such protein affected by PARP activation is the glycolytic enzyme glyceraldehyde 3-phosphate dehydrogenase (GAPDH). PARP-mediated poly(ADP-ribosyl)ation of GAPDH causes inhibition of GAPDH activity.[63]

Du and colleagues have demonstrated that this hyperglycemia-induced inhibition of GAPDH can lead to increased intracellular AGE formation, PKC activation, and flux through the hexosamine pathway in aortic endothelial cells.[63] Furthermore, they have shown that inhibition of PARP (using the potent PARP inhibitor PJ34), like overexpression of UCP-1 or MnSOD, can prevent hyperglycemia-induced activation of these pathways (Fig. 4–6). Thus, a model has emerged wherein hyperglycemia-induced superoxide overproduction by the mitochondrial electron transport chain leads to DNA strand damage, which activates PARP. Activated PARP then inhibits GAPDH activity, which in turn leads to pathologic activation of AGE formation, PKC signaling, and hexosamine pathway flux (Fig. 4–7).

The mechanism by which GAPDH inhibition activates these pathways remains to be established. Researchers hypothesize that GAPDH inhibition causes upstream glycolytic metabolites to be diverted to these pathways of glucose overuse (Fig. 4–8).[3] Specifically, fragmentation of accumulated glyceraldehyde 3-phosphate (upstream of GAPDH) can produce the AGE precursor methylglyoxal. Similarly, increased flux of triose phosphate to DAG can lead to PKC activation. Increased diversion of fructose-6-phosphate to UDP-N-acetylglucosamine can amplify the effects of the hexosamine pathway, and increased glucose flux can augment the polyol pathway.

NOVEL THERAPEUTIC STRATEGIES

The new paradigm of hyperglycemia-induced oxidative stress at the level of the mitochondria as an upstream activator of the four classic biochemical pathways of diabetic vascular damage has yielded novel drug targets and therapeutic strategies for consideration. Interventions to date that have targeted individual pathways such as aldose reductase inhibitors and AGE inhibitors have met with limited success, but current insight into the shared upstream activators of these pathways has raised the possibility of therapeutic strategies that will simultaneously address multiple mechanisms. Specifically, therapy directed against processes such as superoxide overproduction, PARP activation, or shunting of glycolytic metabolites upstream of GAPDH into pathways of glucose overuse could theoretically block the activation of the biochemical mechanisms associated with hyperglycemia-induced vascular damage.

One such novel therapeutic approach is transketolase activation.[65] Transketolase, a thiamine-dependent enzyme, catalyzes the rate-limiting step in the nonoxidative branch of the pentose phosphate pathway. Two of the upstream glycolytic metabolites that are shunted toward the pathways of glucose overuse when GAPDH is inhibited—fructose-6-phosphate and glyceraldehyde 3-phosphate—are also end products of this pathway (see Fig. 4–8). Importantly, the direction and net flux of the transketolase reaction is dependent on substrate concentration.[66] Diabetes has been associated with reduced transketolase activity.[67] Therefore, in the setting of hyperglycemia-mediated inhibition of GAPDH, therapeutic up-regulation of transketolase activity could theoretically divert fructose-6-phospate and glyceraldehyde-3-phosphate away from the pathways of glucose overuse and into the pentose phosphate pathway.

This strategy has been tested using benfotiamine, a lipid-soluble thiamine derivative with greater bioavailability than its parent molecule.[68] Benfotiamine can activate transketolase and inhibit hyperglycemia-induced increases in AGE formation, PKC activation, and hexosamine pathway flux in endothelial cells and in the retinas of diabetic rats.[65] Furthermore, oral benfotiamine prevented the development of retinopathy over 36 weeks in a rodent model of diabetes.[65] Similarly, high-dose thiamine and benfotiamine treatment increased glomerular transketolase activity and inhibited the development of microalbuminuria over a 24-week period in diabetic rats.[69] These findings have supported the concept that transketolase activation

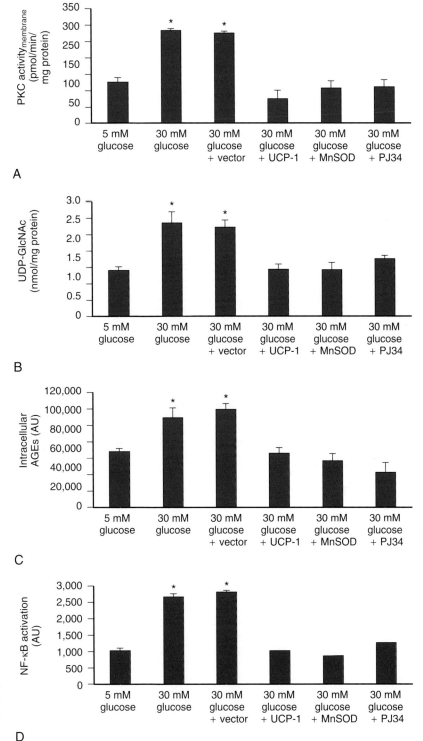

Figure 4–6. Inhibition of pathways of hyperglycemia-induced vascular damage. Inhibition of superoxide overproduction by collapsing the mitochondrial proton gradient (using uncoupling protein 1 [UCP-1]), overexpression of the antioxidant manganese superoxide dismutase (MnSOD) or PJ34-mediated poly(ADP-ribose) polymerase (PARP) inhibition can each block protein kinase C (PKC) activation, hexosamine pathway activation (UOP-GlcNAc), intracellular advanced glycation end-product (AGE) formation, and nuclear factor κB (NF-κB) activation in endothelial cells. AU, arbitrary units. (From Du X, Matsumura T, Edelstein D, et al: Inhibition of GAPDH activity by poly(ADP-ribose) polymerase activates three major pathways of hyperglycemic damage in endothelial cells. J Clin Invest 112:1055, 2003. Permission conveyed through Copyright Clearance Center, Inc.)

may be a useful strategy for preventing diabetic complications.

Inhibition of PARP activity is another novel strategy currently under study. By blocking PARP activation, it may be possible to prevent GAPDH inhibition and thereby avoid activation of pathways of glucose overuse. PJ34, the hydrochloride salt of N-(-oxo-5,6-dihydrophenanthridin-2-yl)-

N,N-dimethylacetamide, is a potent oral PARP inhibitor. As described earlier, PJ34 can prevent hyperglycemia-induced AGE formation, PKC activation, and hexosamine pathway flux in endothelial cells (see Fig. 4–6).[63] Furthermore, treatment with PJ34 for 2 weeks has been reported to correct deficits in motor and sensory nerve conduction velocity in diabetic rats.[70] The potential efficacy of

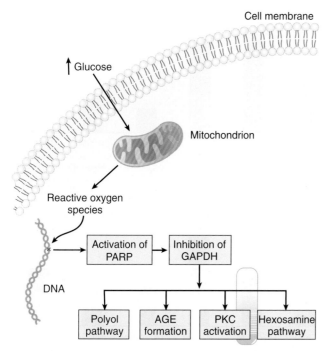

Figure 4–7. Proposed mechanism by which mito-chondrial overproduction of superoxide may lead to pathologic activation of pathways of glucose overuse. Hyperglycemia-induced oxidative stress leads to DNA damage, which activates PARP. Activated PARP inhibits GAPDH activity, which could lead to activation of pathways of glucose overuse. AGE, advanced glycation end-product; GAPDH, glyceraldehyde 3-phosphate dehy-drogenase; PARP, poly(ADP-ribose) polymerase; PKC, protein kinase C.

this compound in preventing the development and progression of microvascular complications is being studied.

A third approach under consideration is the use of antioxidant therapy to reduce the effects of superoxide overproduction by the mitochondrial electron transport chain.[71] To date, conventional antioxidant therapy has yielded disappointing results in regard to amelioration of diabetic com-plications. However, the development of low-molecular-weight catalytic antioxidants that act as superoxide dismutase (SOD) mimetics by selectively mimicking the catalytic activity of the endogenous enzyme could offer promise for continuous scav-enging of ROS. One such compound, tempol, is membrane permeable and exhibits both intra- and extracellular activity.[72] This agent has been reported to improve endothelial dysfunction in a rat model of diabetes.[72] Other antioxidant therapeutic agents under consideration include catalase mimetics and L-propionyl-carnitine.[71]

Peroxynitrite decomposition catalysts represent another novel therapeutic idea. Mitochondrial overproduction of superoxide can stimulate forma-tion of peroxynitrite, a strong initiator of single-strand DNA damage.[71,73] Because single-strand

breakage induces PARP activation, prevention of DNA damage might provide a means of avoiding the deleterious effects of PARP activity in diabetes. This strategy has led to the development of FP15, a compound that blocks peroxynitrite activity.[74] In limited study to date, FP15 has been reported to protect against endothelial dysfunction in diabetic mice.[74] As with all of the other novel agents that have thus far only been tested in animal models, further study is required to determine efficacy in human beings.

FUTURE PERSPECTIVES

Substantial scientific effort over several decades has documented a wide range of deleterious cellular effects associated with chronic hyperglycemia. With the recent formulation of a unifying hypothesis to reconcile the relationships between these varied effects, a new conceptual framework has emerged, providing fresh insight into the pathogenesis of dia-betic complications. Although this development represents a significant advance, many challenges remain, particularly because micro- and macrovas-cular disease continue to be a major source of mor-bidity and mortality associated with diabetes.

One area of interest is the role of genetic predis-position in the development of complications. Familial clustering has been noted in diabetic retinopathy and nephropathy.[75,76] These observa-tions suggest that genetic factors contribute to susceptibility to complications in patients with diabetes. Identification of these factors and their presumed interaction with hyperglycemia-induced biochemical changes will enhance understanding of the disease process and offer hope for potentially identifying (and treating) persons at the highest risk. In particular, modern molecular techniques may allow evaluation of the genome, transcriptome, and proteome profiles associated with enhanced cellular risk in the setting of hyperglycemia.

A second important challenge is the development of therapeutic strategies to ameliorate a patient's risk of diabetic complications. As just discussed, the paradigm of hyperglycemia-mediated biochemical changes has led to the identification of several novel therapeutic agents. Although these agents have shown promise in modifying key biochemical pathways in cell-based systems and in animal models, the ultimate measure of efficacy rests on their ability to modify the risk of complications in patients with diabetes. Such clinical trial evidence remains to be gathered.

Finally, despite our enhanced understanding of the hyperglycemia-induced pathophysiology of complications and the potential for novel thera-peutic interventions, it is important that we keep these advances in clinical context. Optimization of glycemic control has been clearly demonstrated to reduce the risk of microvascular complications in

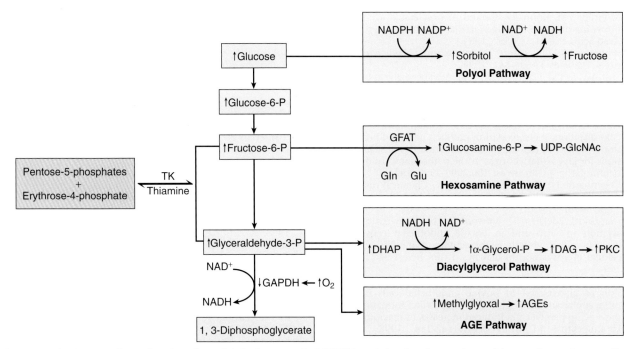

Figure 4–8. Potential mechanism by which decreased GAPDH activity in the setting of hyperglycemia can divert upstream glycolytic metabolites into pathways of glucose overuse. With hyperglycemia-induced inhibition of GAPDH, increased glyceraldehyde 3-phosphate can lead to activation of PKC and AGE formation. Similarly, increased glucose-6-phosphate and fructose-6-phosphate may be diverted to the polyol and hexosamine pathways, respectively. Activation of transketolase (TK) (e.g., by benfotiamine) can provide a means to divert these metabolites away from the pathways of glucose overuse and into the pentose phosphate pathway. AGEs, advanced glycation end-products; DAG, diacylglycerol; fructose-6-P, fructose-6-phosphate; GAPDH, glyceraldehyde 3-phosphate dehydrogenase; GFAT, glutamine:fructose-6-phosphate amidotransferase; Gln, glutamine; Glu, glutamate; glucose-6-P, glucose-6-phosphate; NAD$^+$, nicotinamide adenine dinucleotide; NADH, reduced NAD; NADP$^+$, nicotinamide adenine dinucleotide phosphate; PKC, protein kinase C; UDP-GlcNAc, UDP-N-acetylglucosamine. (From Hammes HP, Du X, Edelstein D, et al: Benfotiamine blocks three major pathways of hyperglycemic damage and prevents experimental diabetic retinopathy. Nat Med 9:295, 2003.)

both type 1 and type 2 diabetes.[1,2] Thus the primary clinical goal in the amelioration of hyperglycemic pathology must continue to be the achievement of long-term glycemic optimization.

References

1. The Diabetes Control and Complications Trial Research Group: The effect of intensive treatment of diabetes on the development and progression of long-term complications in insulin-dependent diabetes mellitus. N Engl J Med 329:977-986, 1993.
2. UK Prospective Diabetes Study (UKPDS) Group: Intensive blood-glucose control with sulphonylureas or insulin compared with conventional treatment and risk of complications in patients with type 2 diabetes (UKPDS 33). Lancet 352:837-853, 1998.
3. Brownlee M: Biochemistry and molecular cell biology of diabetic complications. Nature 414:813-820, 2001.
4. Kaiser N, Feener EP, Boukobza-Vardi N, et al: Differential regulation of glucose transport and transporters by glucose in vascular endothelial and smooth muscle cells. Diabetes 42:80-89, 1993.
5. Cheng HM, Gonzalez RG: The effect of high glucose and oxidative stress on lens metabolism, aldose reductase, and senile cataractogenesis. Metabolism 35(4 Suppl 1):10-14, 1986.
6. Lee AY, Chung SS: Contributions of polyol pathway to oxidative stress in diabetic cataract. FASEB J 13:23-30, 1999.
7. Chung SS, Ho ECM, Lam KSL, Chung SK: Contribution of the polyol pathway to diabetes-induced oxidative stress. J Am Soc Nephrol 14:S233-S236, 2003.
8. Williamson JR, Chang K, Frangos M, et al: Hyperglycemic pseudohypoxia and diabetic complications. Diabetes 42:801-813, 1993.
9. Garcia Soriano F, Virag L, Jagtap P, et al: Diabetic endothelial dysfunction: the role of poly(ADP-ribose) polymerase activation. Nat Med 7:108-113, 2001.
10. Brownlee M, Aiello LP, Friedman E, et al: Complications of Diabetes. In Larsen R, Kronenberg H, Melmed S, Polonsky K (eds): Williams Textbook of Endocrinology, 10th ed. Philadelphia, WB Saunders, 2003, p 1515.
11. Xia P, Kramer RM, King GL: Identification of the mechanism for the inhibition of Na$^+$,K$^+$-adenosine triphosphatase by hyperglycemia involving activation of protein kinase C and cytosolic phospholipase A2. J Clin Invest 96:733-740, 1995.
12. Engerman RL, Kern TS, Larson ME: Nerve conduction and aldose reductase inhibition during 5 years of diabetes or galactosemia in dogs. Diabetologia 37:141-144, 1994.
13. Sheetz MJ, King GL: Molecular understanding of hyperglycemia's adverse effects for diabetic complications. JAMA 288:2579-2588, 2002.
14. Airey M, Bennett C, Nicolucci A, Williams R: Aldose reductase inhibitors for the prevention of diabetic peripheral neuropathy. Cochrane Database Syst Rev (2):CD002182, 2000.

15. Monnier VM, Kohn RR, Cerami A: Accelerated age-related browning of human collagen in diabetes mellitus. Proc Natl Acad Sci U S A 81:583-587, 1984.

16. Brownlee M: Lilly Lecture: Glycation and diabetic complications. Diabetes 43:836-841, 1994.

17. Stitt AW, Li YM, Gardiner TA, et al: Advanced glycation end-products (AGEs) colocalize with AGE receptors in the retinal vasculature of diabetic and of AGE-infused rats. Am J Pathol 150:523-528, 1997.

18. Horie K, Miyata T, Maeda K, et al: Immunohistochemical colocalization of glycoxidation products and lipid peroxidation products in diabetic renal glomerular lesions: Implications for glycoxidative stress in the pathogenesis of diabetic nephropathy. J Clin Invest 100:2995-2999, 1997.

19. Degenhardt TP, Thorpe SR, Baynes JW: Chemical modification of proteins by methylglyoxal. Cell Mol Biol 44:1139-1145, 1998.

20. Giardino I, Edelstein D, Brownlee M: Nonenzymatic glycosylation in vitro and in bovine endothelial cells alters basic fibroblast growth factor activity. A model for intracellular glycosylation in diabetes. J Clin Invest 94:110-117, 1994.

21. Shinohara M, Thornalley PJ, Giardino I, et al: Overexpression of glyoxalase-I in bovine endothelial cells inhibits intracellular advanced glycation endproduct formation and prevents hyperglycemia-induced increases in macromolecular endocytosis. J Clin Invest 101:1142-1147, 1998.

22. Tanaka S, Avigad G, Brodsky B, Eikenberry EF: Glycation induces expansion of the molecular packing of collagen. J Mol Biol 203:495-505, 1988.

23. Charonis AS, Tsilbary EC: Structural and functional changes of laminin and type IV collagen after nonenzymatic glycation. Diabetes 41(Suppl 2):49-51, 1992.

24. Haitoglou CS, Tsilibary EC, Brownlee M, Charonis AS: Altered cellular interactions between endothelial cells and nonenzymatically glucosylated laminin/type IV collagen. J Biol Chem 267:12404-2407, 1992.

25. Neeper M, Schmidt AM, Brett J, et al: Cloning and expression of RAGE: A cell surface receptor for advanced glycosylation end products of proteins. J Biol Chem 267:14998-15004, 1992.

26. Schmidt AM, Hori O, Cao R, et al: RAGE: A novel cellular receptor for advanced glycation end products. Diabetes. 45(Suppl 3):S77-S80, 1996.

27. Schmidt AM, Stern DM: RAGE: A new target for the prevention and treatment of the vascular and inflammatory complications of diabetes. Trends Endocrinol Metab 11:368-375, 2000.

28. Schmidt AM, Hori O, Chen JX, et al: Advanced glycation end-products interacting with their endothelial receptor induce expression of vascular cell adhesion molecule-1 (VCAM-1) in cultured human endothelial cells and in mice: A potential mechanism for the accelerated vasculopathy of diabetes. J Clin Invest 96:1395-1403, 1995.

29. Lu M, Kuroki M, Amano S, et al: Advanced glycation end-products increase retinal vascular endothelial growth factor expression. J Clin Invest 101:1219-1224, 1998.

30. Yamagishi S, Fujimori H, Yonekura H, et al: Advanced glycation end-products inhibit prostacyclin production and induce plasminogen activator inhibitor-1 in human microvascular endothelial cells. Diabetologia 41:1435-1441, 1998.

31. Li YM, Mitsuhashi T, Wojciechowicz D, et al: Molecular identity and cellular distribution of advanced glycation end-product receptors: Relationship of p60 to OST-48 and p90 to 80K-H membrane proteins. Proc Natl Acad Sci U S A 93:11047-11052, 1996.

32. Sano H, Higashi T, Matsumoto K, et al: Insulin enhances macrophage scavenger receptor-mediated endocytic uptake of advanced glycation end products. J Biol Chem 273:8630-8637, 1998.

33. Vlassara H, Li YM, Imani F, et al: Identification of galectin-3 as a high-affinity binding protein for advanced glycation end-products (AGE): A new member of the AGE-receptor complex. Mol Med 1:634-646, 1995.

34. Friedman EA: Advanced glycosylated end products and hyperglycemia in the pathogenesis of diabetic complications. Diabetes Care 22(Suppl 2):B65-B71, 1999.

35. Bolton WK, Cattran DC, Williams ME, et al: Randomized trial of an inhibitor of formation of advanced glycation end products in diabetic nephropathy. Am J Nephrol 24:32-40, 2004.

36. Freedman BI, Wuerth JP, Cartwright K, et al: Design and baseline characteristics for the Aminoguanidine Clinical Trial in Overt Type 2 Diabetic Nephropathy (ACTION II). Control Clin Trials 20:493-510, 1999.

37. Park L, Raman KG, Lee KJ, et al: Suppression of accelerated diabetic atherosclerosis by the soluble receptor for advanced glycation endproducts. Nat Med 4:1025-1031, 1998.

38. Newton AC: Protein kinase C: Structure, function and regulation. J Biol Chem 270:28495-28498, 1995.

39. Koya D, King GL: Protein kinase C activation and the development of diabetic complications. Diabetes 47:859-866, 1998.

40. Shiba T, Inoguchi T, Sportsman JR, et al: Correlation of diacylglycerol level and protein kinase C activity in rat retina to retinal circulation. Am J Physiol 265(5 Pt 1):E783-E793, 1993.

41. De Rubertis FR, Craven PA: Activation of protein kinase C in glomerular cells in diabetes. Mechanisms and potential links to the pathogenesis of diabetic glomerulopathy. Diabetes 43:1-8, 1994.

42. Kikkawa R, Haneda M, Uzu T, et al: Translocation of protein kinase C alpha and zeta in rat glomerular mesangial cells cultured under high glucose conditions. Diabetologia 37:838-841, 1994.

43. Ishii H, Jirousek MR, Koya D, et al: Amelioration of vascular dysfunction in diabetic rats by an oral PKC beta inhibitor. Science 272:728-731, 1996.

44. Kuboki K, Jiang ZY, Takahara N, et al: Regulation of endothelial constitutive nitric oxide synthase gene expression in endothelial cells and in vivo: A specific vascular action of insulin. Circulation 101:676-681, 2000.

45. Schiffrin EL, Touyz RM: Vascular biology of endothelin. J Cardiovasc Pharmacol 32(suppl 3):S2-S13, 1998.

46. Williams B, Gallagher B, Patel H, Orme C: Glucose-induced protein kinase C activation regulates vascular permeability factor mRNA expression and peptide production by human vascular smooth muscle cells in vitro. Diabetes 46:1497-1503, 1997.

47. Aiello LP, Bursell SE, Clemont A, et al: Vascular endothelial growth factor-induced retinal permeability is mediated by protein kinase C in vivo and suppressed by an orally effective β-isoform-selective inhibitor. Diabetes 46:1473-1480, 1997.

48. Feener EP, Xia P, Inoguchi T, et al: Role of protein kinase C in glucose- and angiotensin II-induced plasminogen activator inhibitor expression. Contrib Nephrol 118:180-187, 1996.

49. Studer RK, Craven PA, De Rubertis FR: Role for protein kinase C in the mediation of increased fibronectin accumulation by mesangial cells grown in high-glucose medium. Diabetes 42:118-126, 1993.

50. Pugliese G, Pricci F, Pugliese F, et al: Mechanisms of glucose-enhanced extracellular matrix accumulation in rat glomerular mesangial cells. Diabetes 43:478-490, 1994.

51. Yerneni KK, Bai W, Khan BV, et al: Hyperglycemia-induced activation of nuclear transcription factor kappa B in vascular smooth muscle cells. Diabetes 48:855-864, 1999.

52. Tomlinson DR: Mitogen-activated protein kinases as glucose transducers for diabetic complications. Diabetologia 42:1271-1281, 1999.

53. Beckman JA, Goldfine AB, Gordon MB, et al: Inhibition of protein kinase C beta prevents impaired endothelium-dependent vasodilation caused by hyperglycemia in humans. Circ Res 90:107-111, 2002.

54. Kolm-Litty V, Sauer U, Nerlich A, et al: High glucose-induced transforming growth factor beta-1 production is mediated by the hexosamine pathway in porcine glomerular mesangial cells. J Clin Invest 101:160-169, 1998.

55. Hart GW: Dynamic O-linked glycosylation of nuclear and cytoskeletal proteins. Annu Rev Biochem 66:315-335, 1997.

56. Du X, Edelstein D, Rossetti L, et al: Hyperglycemia-induced mitochondrial superoxide overproduction activates the hexosamine pathway and induces plasminogen activator inhibitor-1 expression by increasing Sp1 glycosylation. Proc Nat Acad Sci U S A 97:12222-12226, 2000.

57. Kadonaga JT, Courey AJ, Ladika J, Tjian R: Distinct regions of Sp1modulate DNA binding and transcriptional activation. Science 242:1566-1570, 1988.

58. Chen YQ, Su M, Walia RR, et al: Sp1 sites mediate activation of the plasminogen activator inhibitor-1 promoter by glucose in vascular smooth muscle cells. J Biol Chem 273:8225-8231, 1998.

59. Evans JL, Goldfine ID, Maddux BA, Grodsky GM: Oxidative stress and stress-activated signaling pathways: A unifying hypothesis of type 2 diabetes. Endocr Rev 23:599-622, 2002.

60. Kuroki T, Isshiki K, King GL: Oxidative stress: The lead or supporting actor in the pathogenesis of diabetic complications. J Am Soc Nephrol 14:S216-S220, 2003.

61. Lodish H, Berk A, Zipursky LS, et al: Cellular energetics: Glycolysis, aerobic oxidation, and photosynthesis. In Lodish H, Baltimore D, Berk A, et al (eds): Molecular Cell Biology 4th ed. New York, WH Freedman, 2000, pp 618-641.

62. Nishikawa T, Edelstein D, Du XL, et al: Normalizing mitochondrial superoxide production blocks three pathways of hyperglycemic damage. Nature 404:787-790, 2000.

63. Du X, Matsumura T, Edelstein D, et al: Inhibition of GAPDH activity by poly(ADP-ribose) polymerase activates three major pathways of hyperglycemic damage in endothelial cells. J Clin Invest 112:1049-1057, 2003.

64. Garcia Soriano F, Virag L, Jagtap P, et al: Diabetic endothelial dysfunction: The role of poly(ADP-ribose) polymerase activation. Nat Med 7:108-113, 2001.

65. Hammes HP, Du X, Edelstein D, et al: Benfotiamine blocks three major pathways of hyperglycemic damage and prevents experimental diabetic retinopathy. Nat Med 9:294-299, 2003.

66. Schenk G, Duggleby RG, Nixon PF: Properties and functions of the thiamine diphospate dependent enzyme transketolase. Int J Biochem Cell Biol 30:1297-1318, 1998.

67. Saito N, Kimura M, Kuchiba A, Itokawa Y: Blood thiamine levels in outpatients with diabetes mellitus. J Nutr Sci Vitaminol (Tokyo) 33:421-430, 1987.

68. Loew D: Pharmacokinetics of thiamine derivatives especially of benfotiamine. Int J Clin Pharmacol Ther 34:47-50, 1996.

69. Babaei-Jadidi R, Karachalias N, Ahmed N, et al: Prevention of incipient diabetic nephropathy by high-dose thiamine and benfotiamine. Diabetes 52:2110-2120, 2003.

70. Li F, Szabo C, Pacher P, et al: Evaluation of orally active poly(ADP-ribose) polymerase inhibitor in streptozotocin-diabetic rat model of early peripheral neuropathy. Diabetologia 47:710-717, 2004.

71. Ceriello A: New insights on oxidative stress and diabetic complications may lead to a "causal" anti-oxidant therapy. Diabetes Care 26:1589-1596, 2003.

72. Nassar T, Kadery B, Lotan C, et al: Effects of the superoxide dismutase-mimetic compound tempol on endothelial dysfunction in streptozotocin-induced diabetic rats. Eur J Pharmacol 436:111-118, 2002.

73. Garcia Soriano F, Virag L, Szabo C: Diabetic endothelial dysfunction: Role of reactive oxygen and nitrogen species production and poly(ADP-ribose) polymerase activation. J Mol Med 79:437-448, 2001.

74. Szabo C, Mabley JG, Moeller SM, et al: Part I: Pathogenetic role of peroxynitrite in the development of diabetes and diabetic vascular complications: Studies with FP15, a novel potent peroxynitrite decomposition catalyst. Mol Med 8:571-580, 2002.

75. The Diabetes Control and Complications Trial Research Group: Clustering of long-term complications in families with diabetes in the diabetes control and complications trial. Diabetes 46:1829-1839, 1997.

76. Quinn M, Angelico MC, Warram JH, Krolewski AS: Familial factors determine the development of diabetic nephropathy in patients with IDDM. Diabetologia 39:940-945, 1996.

Chapter 5

Pathogenesis and Treatment of High-Risk Obesity

Philip A. Kern and Neda Rasouli

KEY POINTS

- *The prevalence of obesity is increasing at an alarming rate, and the obesity epidemic is driving the epidemic in type 2 diabetes.*
- *High-risk obesity is characterized by abdominal obesity with evidence of abnormal glucose and lipid metabolism and a state of heightened inflammation.*
- *With increasing body weight, lipid accumulation occurs not only in adipose tissue but also in other organs. This lipotoxicity in liver, muscle, islets, and elsewhere could account for many of the features of the metabolic syndrome.*
- *Adipose tissue produces many proteins. Some of these proteins are inflammatory cytokines, and others are anti-inflammatory or improve insulin sensitivity.*
- *Treatment of obesity requires identification of the high-risk patient and institution of lifestyle measures with a long-term outlook and with an avoidance of heavily marketed fads. Current research will likely lead to improved medications in the future.*

Obesity is among the most common diseases seen by physicians. It is a major cause of premature mortality and has an enormous economic impact on our society. A recent study estimated the annual cost of obesity in the United States at $93 billion per year, or 9.1% of all health care expenditures, of which about half is paid by federal funds.[1] As frightening as these numbers are, they are based on 1998 data on the prevalence of obesity, and more-recent studies have indicated that the obesity epidemic has continued unabated[2] and the percentage of adults with BMI greater than 30 kg/m² increased from 18.3% to 22.5% in the 4 years from 1998 to 2002.[3]

This chapter provides an overview of the pathogenesis of obesity, with particular emphasis on high-risk obesity, and gives recommendations for treatment interventions.

CLINICAL ASPECTS OF OBESITY

Definition and Incidence of Obesity

Obesity is defined as an excess of adipose tissue, although a useful classification of obesity is based not on adiposity alone but on excess adipose tissue leading to a spectrum of health consequences. These adverse effects on health usually occur when a patient exceeds normal body weight by 20% or more, although there is considerable variation among individual patients.

There are numerous approaches to measuring degree of obesity, and the body mass index (BMI) has gained widespread acceptance in a clinical setting. Although the terminology is imprecise, the *normal* weight range falls between a BMI of 20 and 25. A BMI range of 25 to 30 is often referred to as *overweight,* and a BMI greater than 30 is referred to as *obese. Severe obesity* is characterized by a BMI in excess of 35. Because some normal men have a muscular, stocky build, some studies define a normal BMI for men as less than 27.

In population studies, most of the complications of obesity, including overall mortality, begin to increase when the BMI exceeds 25 kg/m², with exponential increases at higher BMI levels.[4] For example, the relative risk of type 2 diabetes in relation to BMI is shown in Figure 5–1 using data from the Nurses' Health Study.[5] The risk of developing diabetes begins to increase at a BMI of 25, and this risk is threefold higher when the BMI reaches 30.

This relationship between obesity and diabetes (and other risk factors) has been known for many decades, and for many years the public has been advised to maintain a healthy lifestyle comprising moderation in food intake and regular exercise. Obesity has been a problem for many years, and the medical professional community has watched with great consternation as the prevalence of obesity has increased in an epidemic fashion. Figure 5–2 illustrates this epidemic, focusing on people with a BMI of greater than 30 kg/m², using data from the Behavior Risk Factor Surveillance System of the Centers for Disease Control and Prevention (CDC). In 1992, the prevalence of obesity (BMI greater than

30) was 15% to 19% in a few states and less than that in all others. By 2002, even the leanest 18 states had a prevalence of obesity of 15% to 19%, and the rest of the country had an obesity prevalence of greater than 20%; 3 states had a prevalence of greater than 25%. It is therefore not surprising that the prevalence of type 2 diabetes and impaired glucose tolerance has risen during this same period.[6,7]

Complications of Obesity

In addition to diabetes, there are many other health risks associated with obesity. These health problems include metabolic disturbances such as hyperlipidemia, insulin resistance, and hypertension, as well as sleep apnea, gallstones, arthritis, and an increased risk for several malignancies.[8,9] These medical problems are compounded by the social stigmata of obesity, depression, and the difficulties that obesity poses for the physical examination, diagnostic medical tests, and otherwise routine surgery. Box 5-1 lists many of the medical problems associated with obesity.

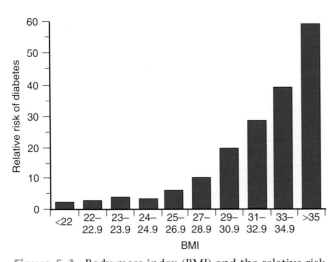

Figure 5–1. Body mass index (BMI) and the relative risk of type 2 diabetes from the Women's Health Study. The relative risk for the development of type 2 diabetes over 8 years for women 30 to 55 years of age in 1976 is shown. The data are adjusted for age, and the risk of diabetes at a BMI less than 22 kg/m^2 is adjusted to 1.0. (Data from Colditz GA, Willett WC, Stampfer MJ, et al: Weight as a risk factor for clinical diabetes in women. Am J Epidemiol 132:501-513, 1990. Redrawn with permission from Oxford University Press.)

Box 5-1. Medical Problems Associated with Obesity

Arthritis

Coronary artery disease

Depression

Diabetes, impaired glucose tolerance, insulin resistance, the metabolic syndrome

Gallstones

Gout

Hyperlipidemia, especially hypertriglyceridemia and low HDL (high-density lipoprotein)

Hypertension

Malignancies: uterine, colon, breast, prostate

Sleep apnea

Stroke

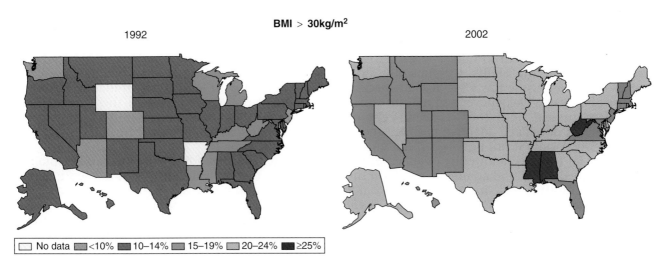

Figure 5–2. The prevalence of obesity in adults, 1992 and 2002. The data represent the percentage of subjects in each state with a BMI greater than 30 kg/m^2. (Data from Centers for Disease Control and Prevention: Behavioral Risk Factor Surveillance System Survey Data. Available at http://www.cdc.gov/brfss/.)

Etiology of Obesity

When discussing the etiology of obesity and the potential causal role of specific candidate genes, it is essential to bear in mind a number of important points. First, obesity represents an intake of more energy than is expended. This may seem trivial, but it is often lost in media hype, books written by "experts," and a market-driven weight-loss industry, which often imply that obese subjects are not subject to the laws of conservation of mass and energy. In addition, obesity is a complex condition that involves an interaction between both genetic and environmental factors. Obesity is not one disease, it is multifactorial, and it involves genetic, metabolic, and behavioral factors. Thus, any discussion of the etiology of obesity will likely prove correct in at least a small percentage of patients but will be incorrect in the rest.

Obesity can best be understood as the product of a rapidly changing environment on a genetic background that is adapted to a hunter-gatherer existence. There has been little change in the human gene pool since the appearance of *Homo sapiens sapiens* about 35,000 years ago, suggesting that modern humans are still genetically adapted to a preagricultural hunter–gatherer lifestyle.[10,11] The study of such a lifestyle has led to the suggestion that a number of modern chronic conditions, prominent among them obesity, may be due to a maladaptation of our lifestyle to our genome. The hunter–gatherer lifestyle involved a great deal of physical activity, coupled with a diet of unrefined foods that were high in protein and low in fat when food was available.[12] In addition, there were probably frequent periods of famine.[13] It is likely that many metabolic features of modern humans originally evolved as an adaptation to such a lifestyle. Prominent among these metabolic adaptations are the adaptations designed to maintain adipocyte lipid stores.

Through this long period of evolution as a hunter–gatherer, many adaptive systems developed to augment survival, and starvation was prominent among the threats to survival. Life was hard, the physical activity required to hunt and gather food was intense, and the ability to efficiently store energy in adipose tissue was a survival adaptation. Because obesity was likely never a significant threat to human survival until the late 20th century, humans never developed adaptive mechanisms to avoid obesity. Would it not be wonderful if an elevated body fat triggered a lowering of appetite, distaste for refined foods, and an urge to climb on the treadmill? Unfortunately, most humans do not respond to an elevated body fat with such useful measures.

A better understanding of these adaptive mechanisms, both the response to starvation and the opposite responses to obesity, will likely be forthcoming in the near future. An excellent example of this adaptation to starvation and the consequent

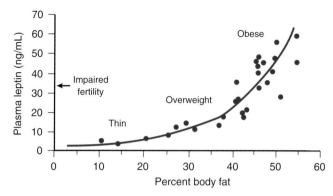

Figure 5–3. The relationship between obesity (using percentage of body fat) and plasma leptin levels in women.

implications for obesity are found in the adipose tissue hormone leptin, which was discovered in 1994.[14] Plasma leptin levels are directly correlated with adipose tissue mass, and leptin receptors are highly concentrated in the hypothalamus. Although leptin-deficient humans are rare, these persons are similar to leptin-deficient mice in terms of hyperphagia, extreme obesity, and inability to begin puberty, all of which is dramatically reversed by treatment with recombinant leptin.[15,16] Although complete leptin deficiency is rare, heterozygous leptin-deficient family members are more common, and they demonstrate plasma leptin levels that are lower than those of their ethnic counterparts, along with some obesity.[17]

On the other hand, common human obesity is associated with elevated plasma leptin levels.[18,19] In Figure 5–3, plasma leptin levels are shown in relation to percent body fat in 29 nondiabetic fasting women from our studies, covering a wide range of BMIs. The high level of leptin in obese subjects is clearly unable to signal anorexia of sufficient magnitude to result in leanness. These high levels of leptin in the face of obesity suggest that obesity is characterized by leptin resistance, which is analogous to the hyperinsulinemia and insulin resistance that is found in patients with type 2 diabetes. Clinical trials have been performed to determine whether or not leptin resistance could be overcome by treatment with leptin. Unfortunately, there was a minimal response to drug in these trials,[20] suggesting that this condition of leptin resistance could not be treated as readily as the insulin resistance of type 2 diabetes.

A better understanding of leptin can be obtained from the study of conditions with low leptin levels. In rodents and humans, very low leptin levels result in reproductive dysfunction. In humans, low body fat resulting from extreme leanness, extreme physical activity, or both, as is commonly seen in patients with anorexia nervosa and in some female athletes, results in low leptin levels and anovulation due to suppressed gonadotropin secretion. Several human children with homozygous leptin muta-

tions have been described, and these children were extremely obese and remained prepubertal until leptin was given. Following leptin administration, food intake was reduced, body weight returned toward normal, and puberty began according to a normal schedule.[15,21]

These data have led to much speculation concerning the precise role of leptin in normal human physiology. There was considerable evolutionary pressure to protect humans from starvation. Hence, low levels of leptin were an adaptive, protective mechanism to stimulate hunger and food-seeking behavior as well as to suppress reproduction during times of extreme leanness.[22] However, high levels of leptin do not effectively protect humans against obesity, because obesity has not been a threat to human survival until very recently.

Although the study of leptin and its receptors has not yet yielded any new treatments for the majority of obese patients, it has provided additional insight into the regulation of appetite and energy expenditure. As described in recent reviews,[22,23] the complex neurochemical pathways involve not only the leptin receptor–mediated *inhibition* of nerves that *stimulate* food intake but also *stimulation* of nerves that *inhibit* intake. Many other neuromodulators in the hypothalamus respond to leptin as well as to other hormonal and nutritional factors. Neuropeptide Y (NPY), agouti gene–related peptide (AGRP), melanin-concentrating hormone (MCH), ghrelin, and endogenous cannabanoids are examples of neuromodulators that stimulate feeding, whereas serotonin, norepinephrine, and α-MSH (alpha-melanocyte-stimulating hormone) are examples of anorexiant modulators. Because of the importance of feeding and energy expenditure in survival, it is perhaps not surprising that the regulatory mechanisms are so complex.

High-Risk Obesity

As described earlier, obesity leads to numerous medical problems, including features of the metabolic syndrome, which are powerful risk factors for atherosclerosis (Box 5-2), sleep apnea, structural problems with joints, and a higher risk for many malignancies. Body fat distribution is a particularly

Box 5-2. Features of the Metabolic Syndrome
Abnormal carbohydrate metabolism: type 2 diabetes, impaired glucose tolerance or impaired fasting glucose, insulin resistance
Hypertension
Hypertriglyceridemia
Increased visceral adipose tissue
Low HDL (high-density lipoprotein)

important factor in determining high risk obesity. Patients with abdominal obesity ("apples") are at greater risk for heart disease, diabetes, hypertension, and hyperlipidemia compared with patients who have more gluteal-fat distribution ("pears").[24] In one study, the removal of subcutaneous fat by liposuction, without any removal of visceral fat, resulted in no improvement in insulin resistance or inflammation, further highlighting the importance of the visceral adipose depot.[25] This difference in risk level with adipose tissue distribution is especially important for mildly obese persons. The reason for the association between abdominal obesity and the metabolic syndrome is not clear, but one leading concept maintains that visceral adipose tissue has a higher rate of lipolysis, resulting in elevated portal nonesterified fatty acids, which increase hepatic very-low-density lipid (VLDL) production, increase hepatic glucose production, and impair peripheral insulin sensitivity.[26]

Notwithstanding the strong statistical associations between visceral fat and the metabolic syndrome, these correlations leave many patients unexplained. Some patients are remarkably immune to the metabolic consequences of obesity, in spite of extreme obesity, whereas other patients develop the full spectrum of the metabolic syndrome with only a small weight gain. In any weight-control clinic, it is not uncommon to see patients who have a BMI greater than 40 kg/m^2 and normal glucose and lipid levels side by side with patients who have hyperlipidemia, diabetes, and coronary disease although their BMI is less than 30.

Ectopic Lipid Accumulation and the Metabolic Syndrome

Adipose tissue is the primary organ of lipid storage. However, with progressive obesity, lipid is deposited into other nonadipose organs, which is termed *ectopic lipid* (Fig. 5–4). This ectopic lipid is deposited in the liver, leading to the commonly observed hepatic steatosis, also known as nonalcoholic steatohepatitis (NASH), or fatty liver. Hepatic steatosis is very common in patients with the metabolic syndrome and is associated with elevated hepatic glucose production. The development of hepatic cirrhosis is more common in patients with NASH, although the precise pathogenesis of NASH-mediated cirrhosis is not known.

Obese subjects usually demonstrate hyperinsulinemia until the development of overt diabetes.[27] On the surface, this hyperinsulinemia might be interpreted as robust beta-cell function. However, when beta-cell function is examined in light of the reduced insulin sensitivity, it is apparent that deterioration of beta-cell function occurs early, long before the development of type 2 diabetes.[28-30] Much of this deterioration in beta-cell function is likely due to lipid accumulation in islets. Islet lipid

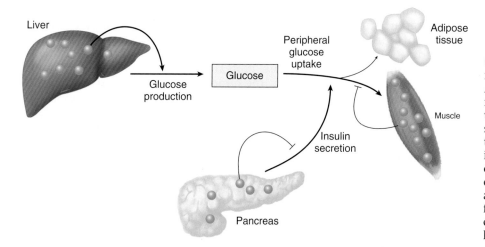

Figure 5–4. Ectopic lipid accumulation and insulin resistance. As obesity progresses, lipid accumulation occurs in organs other than adipose tissue (ectopic sites). The lipid accumulation in these ectopic sites leads to insulin resistance (impaired glucose uptake in muscle and increased glucose output in liver) and to impaired insulin secretion from the beta cells of the pancreas. *Blue circles* represent excess lipid.

accumulation results in apoptosis and in decreased beta-cell mass and function in Zucker diabetic fatty rats.[31] In addition, troglitazone and other peroxisome proliferator-activated receptor (PPAR) agonists lower islet lipid content and improve beta cell function in Zucker diabetic rats.[32-34] Thus, lipotoxicity is likely a phenomenon that is highly relevant to insulin secretion as well as to insulin action.

Because more than 70% of glucose disposal occurs in muscle,[35] this tissue is extremely important in understanding the mechanisms underlying peripheral insulin resistance. Insulin-resistant subjects consistently demonstrate a muscle phenotype characterized by increased intramyocellular lipid (IMCL), decreased proportion of the oxidative type I and type IIA muscle fibers, decreased oxidative capacity of each class of muscle fiber, and decreased capillary density.[36,37] Thus, the muscle of lean, nondiabetic, insulin-sensitive subjects tends to contain fibers with high numbers of mitochondria and high lipid-oxidative capacity and hence lower levels of stored triglyceride.

Muscle can obtain lipid from several sources. One source is albumin-bound nonesterified fatty acids (NEFA) derived from adipose tissue lipolysis; another is lipoprotein lipase (LPL)-mediated triglyceride-rich lipoprotein hydrolysis, which is especially important in reestablishing the intracellular triglyceride (IMTG) stores following exercise.[38] Regardless of how much lipid is available to the muscle cell, however, lipid catabolism requires transport of fatty acyl coenzyme A (FA-CoA) into mitochondria for fatty acid oxidation. Carnitine palmitoyltransferase 1 (CPT1) is the rate-limiting step in the metabolism of FA-CoA, and it catalyzes the transfer of long-chain FA-CoA into the mitochondria.[39] Through complex regulatory mechanisms, CPT1 activity is higher during fasting or glucose unavailability, thus allowing the efficient use of lipid as a fuel. The cause-and-effect relationship between muscle glucose uptake and muscle lipid metabolism is not well understood. However,

there is accumulating evidence that IMTG induces lipotoxicity, which affects peripheral insulin sensitivity and muscle glucose transport.[40-43]

Improvement in the IMTG and muscle oxidative capacity accompanies improvement in insulin resistance such as from weight loss.[44] In recent studies, subjects with impaired glucose tolerance have been treated with either metformin or pioglitazone, followed by muscle biopsies and the assessment of IMCL. There was no change in IMCL with metformin, but there was a significant decrease in IMCL with pioglitazone treatment, which accompanied an improvement in insulin sensitivity.[45] Therefore, a reduction in IMCL may be an attractive target for future drug therapies.

In summary, the development of obesity-related metabolic syndrome is strongly associated with, and likely directly related to, the deposition of lipid into skeletal muscle, liver, islets, and other organs. The accumulation of lipid in subcutaneous adipose tissue depots leads to excess weight and obesity, but it might not necessarily lead to obesity-related metabolic complications. Because the metabolic syndrome is controlled by complex genetics, these data suggest that the tendency to accumulate lipid in ectopic sites is also under genetic control. Based on the hunter–gatherer lifestyle during early human development and the survival advantage conferred upon a person with efficient fat storage, lipid deposition into ectopic sites might have been desirable as an adjunct to adipose tissue storage. Unfortunately, these evolutionary forces were designed for intermittent starvation in a setting of extreme physical activity, which is a far cry from the lifestyle of modern humans in developed countries.

Adipose Tissue Cytokine Expression and Inflammation

Understanding of the role of adipose tissue in the metabolic syndrome has continued to evolve with

CONTROVERSIES

- Postprandial glucose level is a better indicator of insulin resistance and should be used to identify patients with the metabolic syndrome.
- In special patient populations (e.g., South Asians) waist circumference as defined in ATP III criteria for the metabolic syndrome might not be appropriate. However, waist-to-hip ratio as described in WHO criteria will identify patients at risk.

mally. Insulin also plays a role in the vascular disorders, especially endothelial dysfunction. The abnormalities of fatty acid metabolism lead to accelerated atherosclerosis, increased risk of myocardial infarction, peripheral artery disease, and stroke.[57] Atherosclerosis is related to lipid metabolic abnormalities, which leads to cardiovascular disease.

The association among insulin resistance, hyperinsulinemia, and coronary disease is supported by a number of observational studies.[58-60] The strength of insulin resistance as a predictor of cardiovascular disease is substantially attenuated after adjustment for risk factors, which was reflected in review of studies examining both fasting and stimulated insulin concentrations; however, most recent trials revealed that insulin resistance could be an independent risk factor for coronary artery disease and stroke (Fig. 6–6).[60-65]

DYSLIPIDEMIA

Atherogenic dyslipidemia (see Box 6-1) is an integral component of the metabolic syndrome and is a major contributor to the cardiovascular risks in these patients. Combination of various risk factors seen in the metabolic syndrome can lead to a significant increase in the risks of cardiovascular disease. For example, hyperlipidemia in addition to diabetes or hypertension results in a 19-fold increased risk of myocardial infarction.[66] However, an abnormal lipid profile was found to be a more significant risk factor than either hypertension or diabetes alone.[66]

The typical lipid abnormalities defined in patients with the metabolic syndrome consist of a triad: increased small, dense low-density-lipoprotein (LDL) cholesterol; increased triglycerides; and decreased HDL cholesterol. However, several additional abnormalities might play an important role in atherosclerosis.

The role of LDL cholesterol in the development of cardiovascular disease is indisputable, but it is necessary to emphasize that patients with the metabolic syndrome have far more complex lipid abnormalities. The atherogenic lipid abnormalities

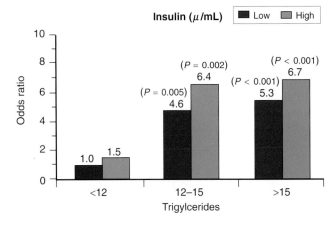

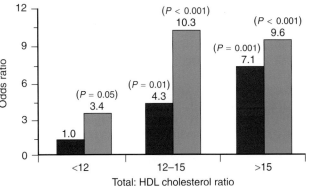

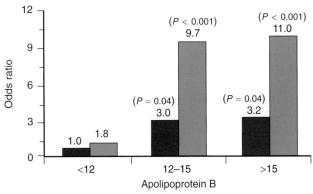

Figure 6–6. Odds ratios for ischemic heart disease according to plasma insulin and triglyceride concentrations, total cholesterol–to–HDL cholesterol ratios, and apolipoprotein B concentrations. Insulin was measured after subjects had fasted for 12 hours. The median triglyceride concentration (150 mg/dL [1.7 mmol/L]), total cholesterol–to–HDL cholesterol ratio (6.0), and apolipoprotein B concentration (119 mg/dL) were used to define men with either low levels (below the 50th percentile) or high levels (at or above the 50th percentile) for these variables. The results of tests for multiplicative interactions did not reach significance at the 0.05 level for any of the combinations. *P* values are for comparisons with the reference group, which was assigned an odds ratio of 1.0. To convert values for insulin to picomoles per liter, multiply by 6. HDL, high-density lipoprotein. (From Desperés J-P, Lamarche B, Mauriege P, et al: Hyperinsulinemia is an independent risk factor for ischemic heart disease. N Engl J Med 334:952-957, 1996. Copyright © 1996 Massachusetts Medical Society. All rights reserved.)

associated with the metabolic syndrome are comparable to dyslipidemia found in patients who have type 2 diabetes.

Low HDL cholesterol, high very-low-density lipoprotein (VLDL), and high triglycerides with a predominance of small, dense LDL cholesterol are typical dyslipidemic changes in the metabolic syndrome. In patients with the metabolic syndrome, suppression of the release of free fatty acids (FFAs) from adipose tissue is impaired secondary to insulin resistance.[67] This translates into increased influx of free fatty acids into the liver. The consequences of these additional FFAs in the liver are an increase in hepatic production and release of VLDL and triglycerides associated with decreased clearance of these substances, resulting in increase in VLDL and triglyceride levels. Transportation of cholesterol and triglyceride ester between HDL, LDL, and VLDL leads to formation of triglyceride-rich LDL and HDL particles, which become the preferred substrate for hepatic triglyceride lipase.

Due to the lack of hepatic lipase, there is poor clearance of small, dense particles of LDL cholesterol, which are more atherogenic and more susceptible to oxidation. Elevated levels of triglyceride-rich lipoproteins lower HDL cholesterol by inducing cholesterol exchange from HDL to VLDL via cholesteryl-ester transfer protein. A large fraction of small, dense LDL particles has been classified as LDL subclass B, or atherogenic lipoprotein phenotype.[68]

The atherogenic dyslipidemia of the metabolic syndrome is similar to combined hyperlipidemia, and these two phenotypes appear to overlap.[69] The cardiovascular outcomes associated with the atherogenic form of dyslipidemia typical in patients with the metabolic syndrome are much worse compared with clinical outcomes in patients who have isolated elevation of LDL cholesterol.[70] Patients who have this triad are also more likely to have other features of the metabolic syndrome, which puts them at greater risk for cardiovascular events.[71]

Another lipid abnormality that could contribute to increased risk of cardiovascular disease in patients with the metabolic syndrome is postprandial hyperlipidemia. After food digestion, plasma concentration of chylomicrons increases, and these triglyceride-rich remnant particles struggle to be cleared by the liver with endogenous triglyceride-rich proteins, for example, VLDL triglyceride. Due to high levels of VLDL triglyceride, clearance of chylomicrons is affected and leads to postprandial lipidemia. It is known that postprandial hyperlipidemia is associated with endothelial dysfunction, and this increase in triglyceride-rich remnant particles in the postprandial state in patients with the metabolic syndrome could play a major role in development of atherosclerosis and subsequent development of cardiovascular disease.[72] Despite the complex pathophysiology of the lipid abnormalities in the metabolic syndrome, it is crucial for clinicians to recognize and manage them effectively in an attempt to reduce increased risks of cardiovascular disease.

The 3-hydroxy-3-methylglutaryl coenzyme A reductase inhibitors (statins) have multiple indirect effects on the vasculature besides the direct cholesterol-lowering effect. These positive actions are commonly referred as pleotropic effects, and they include effects on inflammation, coagulability, and adhesion of cells to the vascular endothelium as well as effects on nitric oxide (NO) metabolism. Statins also can improve endothelial function; reduce vascular inflammation; reduce oxidative stress; decrease thrombosis, platelet aggregation, and adhesion of platelets and white cells to the vascular endothelium; stabilize vulnerable plaques; and promote new vessel formation.[73] These multiple beneficial effects of statins contribute to the reduction of cardiovascular events and stroke in patients with the metabolic syndrome and diabetes. Statins are therefore the vital part of treatment of the metabolic syndrome.

HYPERTENSION

An integral component of the metabolic syndrome is blood pressure greater than 130/85 mm Hg (see Box 6-1). Hypertension and the metabolic syndrome are so closely related that even lean hypertensive patients can manifest insulin resistance. Patients with hypertension are several times more likely to develop diabetes and cardiovascular disease over a three- to five-year period than are persons with normal blood pressure.[52,74-77] It is also evident that insulin resistance and hyperinsulinemia contribute to the increased propensity for development of hypertension. Researchers postulate that the direct effect of elevated insulin on sympathetic nervous system activity can lead to elevated blood pressure.[52]

Impaired insulin signaling through its phosphoinositol 3-kinase and downstream protein kinase B pathways is increasingly recognized as important for generation of NO and other vasodilatory factors when insulin-induced renal sodium retention is increased, which contributes to hypertension.[52] The generation of NO is important for insulin-mediated glucose use and vasodilation.[78-83]

Activation of the tissue renin-angiotensin system seems also to contribute to impaired insulin use in skeletal muscle and adipose tissue and decreases vasorelaxation.[52] Angiotensin II can also be produced by adipose tissue and has potent vasoconstrictive potential. In the vasculature, angiotensin II results in increased production of reactive oxygen species by stimulation of the NAD(P)H (reduced nicotinamide adenine dinucleotide [phosphate]) oxidase enzyme, which is expressed in endothelial cells, vascular smooth muscle cells, and vascular adventitial cells.[52,84-87] Increased production of reactive oxygen species in turn results in increased

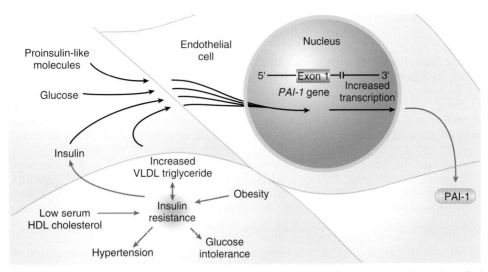

Figure 6–7. Relation between the synthesis of plasminogen-activator inhibitor type 1 (PAI-1) and the insulin resistance syndrome. The main feature of the insulin resistance syndrome is insulin resistance accompanied by hyperinsulinemia, abnormalities of glucose metabolism, hypertriglyceridemia with low serum concentrations of high-density lipoprotein (HDL) cholesterol, hypertension, and obesity. Insulin, proinsulin-like molecules, glucose, and very-low-density lipoprotein (VLDL) triglyceride directly stimulate PAI-1 transcription and secretion in endothelial cells. (From Kohler HP, Grant PJ: Mechanisms of disease: Plasminogen-activator inhibitor type 1 and coronary artery disease. N Engl J Med 342:1792-1801, 2000. Copyright © 2000 Massachusetts Medical Society. All rights reserved.)

NO turnover by its conversion to peroxynitrite, which also blocks vasodilation.[52,88] In hypertensive patients, increased local formation of angiotensin II in adipose tissue was noted and appears to be of considerable interest, given the close relationship that has been shown to exist between angiotensin II and insulin resistance.[89]

There is evidence confirming that insulin resistance and resulting hyperinsulinemia are related to hypertension and coronary artery disease. Untreated hypertensive patients often have higher fasting and postprandial insulin levels than normotensive persons regardless of body mass as well as direct correlation between plasma insulin concentrations and blood pressure levels.[52,75,76]

Genetic predisposition most likely contributes to coexistence of insulin resistance and hyperinsulinemia with hypertension. Changes in glucose metabolism in normotensive offspring of hypertensive parents could support the concept of genetic predisposition for this coexistence.[90,91] Increased plasma insulin levels predict elevated blood pressure in healthy children, which also supports this concept.[92]

The beneficial effects of renin-angiotensin system blockade by angiotensin enzyme inhibitor or angiotensin-receptor blocker on insulin sensitivity and the development of type 2 diabetes in several clinical trials further support a pathophysiologic role of the renin-angiotensin system in the metabolic syndrome and its cardiovascular complications (see Fig 6–5).[49,93-95]

FIBRINOLYTIC DYSFUNCTION

Patients with the metabolic syndrome have multiple abnormalities that lead to increased risk of thrombosis. Some of these abnormalities may be driven by adipokines.[96-98] Various associated coagulation abnormalities include increased platelet aggregation and activation and elevation of procoagulants, such as fibrinogen and von Willebrand factor. Defects of fibrinolysis include increased production and activity of plasminogen PAI-1 with low levels of tissue plasminogen activator (t-PA).[53,79] PAI-1 is elevated in patients with type 2 diabetes. This increase in PAI-1 is related to the complex interaction between the endothelial cell and glucose, insulin, and angiotensin II. Increased levels of PAI-1 have also been associated with visceral obesity and hyperinsulinemia.[99] Studies of the promoter region of the *PAI-1* gene have shown that hyperglycemia stimulates transcription of the gene, and reduction of blood glucose is expected to result in lowering PAI-1 and stimulating fibrinolytic activity (Fig. 6–7).[100]

Increased endogenous fibrinolytic inhibitor, such as PAI-1, and the associated elevation of endogenous tissue-type plasminogen activator (tPA) correlate with an increase in the risk of myocardial infarction.[101,102] Elevated PAI-1 and tPA can be viewed as a reflection of fibrinolytic dysfunction. Fibrinolytic dysfunction increases the propensity to develop arterial thrombosis, which leads to increased incidence of cardiovascular disease in

patients with the metabolic syndrome.[101] Plasma concentrations of PAI-1 are the highest at night and in the early morning hours, and the higher incidence of myocardial infarction in the early morning hours could be due to higher plasma PAI-1 concentrations, leading to lower fibrinolytic activity and an increased incidence of thrombosis at night.[102]

Diabetes and abdominal obesity are risk predictors for both venous thrombosis and an occlusive arterial disease most likely due to existence of an atherothrombotic syndrome secondary to insulin resistance and defective fibrinolysis. Patients with the metabolic syndrome have significantly more atherosclerosis compared with patients who do not have the metabolic syndrome, independent of their diabetes status.[101] These data suggest that the higher risk of cardiovascular events among patients with the metabolic syndrome could be related to impaired fibrinolysis and more advanced atherosclerosis.[101]

ENDOTHELIAL DYSFUNCTION

Current evidence emphasizes that endothelial function is compromised in patients with the metabolic syndrome. Endothelial dysfunction occurs in association with all the factors that predispose to the development of atherosclerosis and is the initial step in the development of vascular pathology. For clinical evaluation, endothelial cell function can be estimated by measuring changes in blood flow in response to physical or pharmacologic stimuli using invasive or noninvasive techniques. Increase of blood flow in the legs in response to metacholine, which is a stimulator of NO release, is impaired in nondiabetic insulin-resistant persons.[103]

In patients with insulin resistance, NO synthesis, which is partially mediated by insulin, is blunted and NO-mediated vasodilation is adversely affected.[103] NO also inhibits platelet aggregation, leukocyte migration, and cell adhesion to the endothelium, and it attenuates vascular smooth muscle cell proliferation and migration. Additional effects of NO include inhibition of release of cell adhesion molecules and reduced production of superoxide anions. Flow-mediated dilation of the brachial artery, which is NO dependent, was found to be impaired in metabolic syndrome patients with elevated and normal blood pressure.[104,105] Plasma adhesion molecules are also increased in proportion to the degree of insulin resistance in healthy volunteers, which could be related to the decreased NO production, which is associated with insulin resistance.[106]

The degree of endothelial dysfunction was found to be greater in patients with type 2 diabetes, compared to those with type 1 diabetes, suggesting that in addition to hyperglycemia and hyperinsulinemia, the associated dyslipidemia might play an important role.[107] Hyperglycemia was shown to be responsible for endothelial dysfunction in the metabolic syndrome. Acute or chronic hyperglycemia can produce impairment of endothelial-dependent vasodilation.[108]

Hyperglycemia-induced activation of protein kinase C (PKC) via increases in the synthesis of diacylglycerol (DAG), followed by activation of phospholipase A2, results in increased production of arachidonic acid metabolites, which have potent oxidizing effects. Reduced NO synthesis can result from activation of the polyol pathway, which increases the use of NADPH, an important cofactor in the biosynthesis of NO.[109] NADPH is essential for the regeneration of antioxidant molecules (such as glutathione, tocopherol, and ascorbate) and a cofactor of endothelial NO synthase (eNOS). Depletion of NADPH leads to depletion of NO.

Hyperglycemia is also associated with a variety of other molecular changes, including production of advanced glycation end products (AGEs), which can increase susceptibility of LDL cholesterol to oxidation as well as activate the receptors responsible for the release of IL-1, TNF-α, and growth factors that can stimulate the migration and proliferation of smooth muscle cells.[110]

Endothelium dysfunction plays a role in the development of coronary heart disease by inducing inflammation and thrombosis, especially in situations with elevated PAI-1 and tPA, which is typical for patients with the metabolic syndrome.

C-REACTIVE PROTEIN

The role of inflammation in the process of atherosclerosis is well established. C-reactive protein is an acute-phase reactant that is used clinically as a marker of inflammation in the body. Mild chronic elevations of CRP concentrations, even when within normal limits, are independently predictive of future cardiovascular events.[111,112]

CRP also correlates with every parameter of the metabolic syndrome, including adiposity, hyperinsulinemia, insulin resistance, hypertriglyceridemia, and low HDL cholesterol.[98,99] High levels of CRP are related to increased accumulation of visceral and subcutaneous fat depots measured by computed tomography scan.[113] In postmenopausal women and elderly patients, CRP can be used as a predictor of diabetes development and accordingly as a predictor of premature coronary artery disease.[97,114]

It has been proposed that the metabolic syndrome and diabetes mellitus are inflammatory conditions. For example, the risk of developing diabetes and the metabolic syndrome in relation to baseline CRP levels in 515 men and 729 women from the Mexico City Diabetes Study revealed that CRP was not a significant predictor of the development of the metabolic syndrome in men. However, inflammation was important in the pathogenesis of diabetes and metabolic disorders in women, which explains the correlation between CRP and cardiovascular disease.[115]

The West of Scotland Coronary Prevention Study, based on evaluation of 6447 participants, concluded that high concentrations of CRP among men with the metabolic syndrome can be an independent predictor of both coronary heart disease and diabetes.[116] CRP was found to add prognostic information on cardiovascular events when 14,719 initially healthy American women were followed for 8 years in the Women's Health Study.[98] These observations confirm again the role of inflammation in the processes critical to development of atherothrombosis leading to cardiovascular events.

MICROALBUMINURIA

Vasculature and the renal glomerulus have a lot in common structurally and functionally. They are derived from the same progenitor cell line. Vascular smooth muscle cells and mesangial cells produce growth factors (angiotensin II, insulin-like growth factor-1, and cytokines) as well as prostaglandins and NO to counterbalance many of the effects of growth factors. Microalbuminuria occurs due to the pathophysiologic changes of glomerulosclerosis. These changes ware very similar of those of atherosclerosis and include mesangial cell proliferation and hypertrophy, foam cell accumulation, build-up of extracellular matrix and amorphous materials, and evolving sclerosis. All of these would lead to matrix expansion, basement membrane abnormalities, and loss of basement membrane permoselectivity, resulting in proteinuria. As a parallel process, glomerulosclerosis and atherosclerosis are associated with enhanced oxidative stress, increased inflammation, impaired fibrinolysis, endothelial cell dysfunction, elevated systolic blood pressure, and lipid abnormalities.[52]

The association between microalbuminuria and cardiovascular risk has been extensively studied in diabetic patients and nondiabetic hypertensive patients. For example, the large study of 11,343 nondiabetic hypertensive patients with mean age 57 years old, from a general population sample in Germany, revealed that 51% were men and mean duration of hypertension was 69 months. Twenty-five per cent had coronary artery disease, 17% had left ventricular hypertrophy, 5% had had a stroke, and 6% had peripheral vascular disease. Microalbuminuria was present in 32% of men and 28% of women.

Comparison of patients who have microalbuminuria with patients who have normal albuminuria demonstrated an increase in coronary artery disease, left ventricular hypertrophy, stroke, and peripheral vascular disease.[117] Further, in patients with coronary artery disease, left ventricular hypertrophy, stroke, and peripheral vascular disease, microalbuminuria was significantly greater than in patients who did not have these complications. It was also shown in this study that microalbuminuria increased with age and with severity and dura-

tion of hypertension and hyperlipidemia, and it was associated with higher plasma creatinine values.[117]

It is well known that microalbuminuria is commonly occurs in patients with diabetes and is a marker of early stage nephropathy. It has been shown to be a strong predictor of cardiovascular events. The literature was systematically reviewed to evaluate the role of this phenomenon. The literature included 264 citations (in which 11 cohort studies were selected for inclusion in the overview) and a total of 2138 non–insulin-dependent diabetic patients with a mean of 6.4 years of follow-up. This study confirmed that microalbuminuria is the strong predictor of total and cardiovascular mortality and cardiovascular morbidity in patients with non–insulin-dependent diabetes mellitus, with an overall odds ratio for death of 2.4 and for cardiovascular morbidity or mortality of 2.0 (Fig. 6–8).[118]

The WHO definition of the metabolic syndrome has included microalbuminuria as one of the criteria (see Box 6-2). Microalbuminuria in association with obesity can also occur because high intake of food rich in protein can lead to renal hyperfiltration, renal impairment, and microalbuminuria, which also correlates with body mass index, waist-to-hip ratio, and insulin levels and becomes another cardiovascular risk factor in metabolic syndrome patients.[118]

Accelerated atherosclerosis and endothelial dysfunction can be recognized earlier if proteinuria is used as a marker. Patients with proteinuria have greater left ventricular mass, greater carotid medial thickening, and have endothelial dysfunction, which leads to greater risk of myocardial infarction and mortality (see Fig. 6–8).[119,120]

ABNORMAL URIC ACID METABOLISM

Elevated uric acid can be seen in patients who have the metabolic syndrome. The major component of the metabolic syndrome is insulin resistance, which influences protein metabolism; uric acid, as a product of protein metabolism, becomes elevated. In patients with the metabolic syndrome, excretion of uric acid via the kidneys is also impaired.

The precise role of hyperuricemia in coronary artery disease is controversial. The Framingham Heart Study demonstrated that uric acid does not have a causal role in the development of coronary artery disease or death from cardiovascular disease.[121] Contrary to the Framingham data, a cross-sectional population-based study in NHANES I from 1971-1975 (baseline) and the data from the NHANES I Epidemiologic Follow-up Study (NHEFS) suggest that increased serum uric acid levels are independently and significantly associated with risk of cardiovascular mortality.[122] In patients with essential hypertension, elevated uric acid levels were associated with increased cardiovascular disease and all-cause mortality.[123] Although no clear

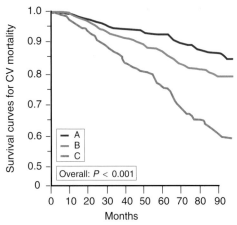

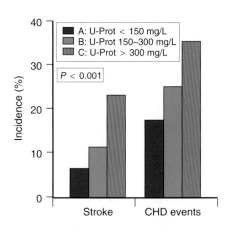

Figure 6–8. Proteinuria predicts stroke and coronary heart disease in type 2 diabetes patients. CHD, coronary heart disease; CV, cardiovascular; U-Prot, urinary protein concentration. (From Miettinen H, Haffner SM, Lehto S, et al: Proteinuria predicts stroke and other atherosclerotic vascular disease events in non-diabetic and non–insulin dependent diabetic subjects. Stroke 27:2033-2039, 1996.)

data exist reflecting the relationship between uric acid levels and cardiovascular risks in patients with the metabolic syndrome, elevated serum uric acid levels could have a role in increasing these risks.

SUMMARY

The metabolic syndrome represents a clustering of several risk factors linked with marked increase in cardiovascular disease and can be considered a coronary artery disease equivalent. Insulin resistance has been linked to each of the ATP III criteria needed for diagnosis of the metabolic syndrome (see Box 6-1). Even though insulin resistance is only one of the five criteria used by WHO to diagnose the metabolic syndrome (see Box 6-2), the available data indicate that insulin resistance and hyperinsulinemia, even in the absence of overt abnormalities of glucose tolerance, lead to increased cardiovascular disease. Insulin resistance is considered a continuous process in which progressive defects in insulin action and insulin release lead to more overt abnormalities of glucose homeostasis. Because insulin resistance is an independent risk factor for cardiovascular disease, its presence can lead to macrovascular complications long before other features of the metabolic syndrome are evident (the ticking clock hypothesis).[124]

Obesity is an important component of the metabolic syndrome. Visceral adipose tissue has been proposed as the major site of fat deposition associated with the metabolic consequences of obesity that have been related to the cytokine release by the adipocytes.[125] Currently, visceral (central) adiposity is the initial physical finding associated with insulin resistance. Increase in visceral adipose tissue leads to increase in FFA flux in portal and systemic circulations, which initiates the cascade of events that

are thought to be responsible for insulin resistance and atherogenic dyslipidemia. Visceral adipose tissue might also contribute to other causes of increased atherosclerotic risk, including inflammatory (C-reactive protein), prothrombotic, and fibrinolytic factors. Future assessment of adipose tissue hormonal activity might be helpful in predicting cardiovascular risks. Adiponectin is one of the hormones being intensively investigated in this area. Hypertension is also most likely related to adipocyte production of cytokines, including angiotensin II, leading to elevated blood pressure.

Atherogenic dyslipidemia is the central player in developing atherosclerosis, and specific features of lipid disorder in the metabolic syndrome put these patients at higher risk. The characteristic lipid disorders seen in this syndrome are hypertriglyceridemia, low levels of HDL cholesterol and, often, normal levels of small, dense LDL cholesterol.

The evidence described in this chapter from epidemiologic and observational studies highlights the importance of increasing awareness among clinicians regarding the strong relationship between the metabolic syndrome and cardiovascular disease. It also highlights the urgency to intervene and modify the fatal cascade of events that lead to significant increase in mortality and morbidity, which will have a major public health impact worldwide in the coming years.[126]

References

1. Reaven GM: Banting Lecture 1988: Role of insulin resistance in human disease. Diabetes 37:1595-1607, 1988.
2. Park Y, Shankuan Z, Palaniappan L et al: The metabolic syndrome. Arch Intern Med 163:427-436, 2003.
3. Fagan TC, Deedwania PC: The cardiovascular dysmetabolic syndrome. Am J Med 105(suppl1):77-82, 1998.

4. Caprio S: Insulin resistance in childhood obesity. J Pediatr Endocrinol Metab 15: (Suppl1):487-492, 2002.
5. Goran MI, Gower BA: Abdominal obesity and cardiovascular risk in children. Coron Artery Dis 9:483-487, 1998.
6. Weiss R, Dziura J, Burgert T, et al: Obesity and the metabolic syndrome in children and adolescents. N Engl J Med 350:2362-2374, 2004.
7. Sinha R, Fisch G, Teague B, et al: Prevalence of impaired glucose tolerance among children and adolescents with marked obesity. N Engl J Med 346: 802-810, 2002.
8. Strauss RS, Pollack HA: Epidemic increase in childhood overweight, 1986-1998. JAMA 286:2845-2848, 2001.
9. Ford ES, Giles WH, Dietz WH: Prevalence of metabolic syndrome among US adults: Findings from the third National Health and Nutrition Examination Survey. JAMA 287:356-359, 2002.
10. Isomaa B, Almgren P, Tuomi T, et al: Cardiovascular morbidity and mortality associated with the metabolic syndrome. Diabetes Care 24:683-689, 2001.
11. Fontaine KR, Redden DT, Wang C, et al: Years of life lost due to obesity. JAMA 289:187-193, 2003.
12. Cook S, Witzman M, Auinger P, et al: Prevalence of a metabolic syndrome phenotype in adolescents. Arch Pediatr Adolesc Med 157:821-827, 2003.
13. Malina R, Katzarzyk T: Validity of the body mass index as an indicator of the risk and presence of overweight in adolescents. Am J Clin Nutr 70(suppl):131S-136S, 1999.
14. Lakka HM, Laaksonen DE, Lakka TA, et al: The metabolic syndrome and total and cardiovascular disease mortality in middle-aged men. JAMA 25:2709-2716, 2002.
15. National Diabetes Data Group: Diabetes in America, 2nd ed. Washington, DC, National Institutes of Health, 1995.
16. Trevisan M, Liu J, Bahsas FB, et al: Syndrome X and mortality: A population-based study: Risk factor and life expectancy research group. Am J Epidemiol 148:958-966, 1998.
17. Wilson PW, Kannel WB, Silberschatz H, et al: Clustering of metabolic factors and coronary heart disease. Arch Intern Med 159:1104-1109, 1999.
18. Hu G, Qiao Q, Tuomilehto J, et al: Prevalence of the metabolic syndrome and its relation to all-cause and cardiovascular morality in nondiabetic European men and women. Arch Intern Med 164:1066-1076, 2004.
19. Resnick HE, Jones K, Ruotolo G, et al: Insulin resistance, the metabolic syndrome, and risk of incident cardiovascular disease in nondiabetic American Indians. The Strong Heart Study. Diabetes Care 26:861-867, 2003.
20. Alexander CM, Landsman PB, Teutsch S, et al: NCEP-defined metabolic syndrome, diabetes, and prevalence of coronary heart disease among NHANES III participants age 50 or older. Diabetes 52:1210-1214, 2003.
21. Ninomiya JK, L'Italien G, Criqui MH, et al: Association of the metabolic syndrome with history of myocardial infarction and stroke in the Third National Health and Nutrition Examination Survey. Circulation 109:42-46, 2004.
22. Kip KE, Marroquin OC, Kelley DE, et al: Clinical importance of obesity versus metabolic syndrome in cardiovascular risk in women. A report from the Women's Ischemia Syndrome Evaluation (WISE) study. Circulation 109:706-713, 2004.
23. Lawlor DA, Ebrahim S, Smith DG: The metabolic syndrome and coronary heart disease in older women: Findings from the British Women's Heart and Health Study. Diabetic Medicine 21: 906-913, 2004.
24. Janssen, I, Katzmarzyk P, Ross R: Body mass index, waist circumference and health risk. Arch Intern Med 162:2074-2079, 2002.
25. Grundy SM, Brewer HB, Cleeman JI et al: Definition of metabolic syndrome: Report of the National Heart, Lung, and Blood Institute/American Heart Association conference on scientific issues related to definition. Circulation 109:433-438, 2004.
26. Frayn KN: Adipose tissue and the insulin resistance syndrome. Proc Nutr Soc 60:375-380, 2001.
27. Yamauchi T, Kamon J, Waki H, et al: The fat-derived hormone adiponectin reverses insulin resistance associated with both lipoatrophy and obesity. Nat Med 7:941-946, 2001
28. Combs TP, Berg AH, Obici T, et al: Endogenous glucose production is inhibited by the adipose-derived protein Acrp30. J Clin Invest 108:1875-1881, 2001.
29. Hotta K, Funahashi T, Arita Y, et al: Plasma concentrations of novel, adipose-specific protein, adiponectin, in type 2 diabetic patients. Arterioscler Thromb Vasc Biol 20:1595-1599, 2000.
30. Weyer C, Funahashi T, Tanaka S et al: Hypoadiponectinemia in obesity and type 2 diabetes: Close association with insulin resistance and hyperinsulinemia. J Clin Endocrinol Metab 86:1930-1935, 2001.
31. Yamauchi T, Kamon J, Minakoshi Y, et al: Adiponectin stimulates glucose utilization and fatty acid oxidation by activating AMP activated protein kinase. Nat Med 8:1288-1295, 2002.
32. Stefan N, Vozarova B, Funahashi T, et al: Plasma adiponectin concentration is associated with skeletal muscle insulin receptor tyrosine phosphorylation, and low plasma concentration precedes a decrease in whole-body insulin sensitivity in humans. Diabetes 51(6):1884-1888, 2002.
33. Lindsay RS, Funahashi T, Hanson RL, et al: Adiponectin and development of type 2 diabetes in the Pima Indian population. Lancet 360:57-58, 2002.
34. Yang W-S, Lee W-J. Funahashi T, et al: Weight reduction increases plasma levels of adipose-derived antiinflammatory protein, adiponectin. J Clin Endocrinol Metab 86:2815-2819, 2001.
35. Pischon T, Girman CJ, Hotamisligil GS, et al: Plasma adiponectin levels and risk of myocardial infarction in men. JAMA 291:1730-1737, 2004.
36. Berg AH, Combs TP, Du X, et al: The adipocyte-secreted protein Acrp30 enhances hepatic insulin action. Nat Med 7:947-953, 2001.
37. Fruebis J, Tsao TS, Javorschi S, et al: Proteolytic cleavage product of 30-kDa adipocyte complement-related protein increases fatty acid oxidation in muscle and causes weight loss in mice. Proc Natl Acad Sci U S A 98:2005-2010, 2001.
38. Spranger J, Kroke A, Mohlig M, et al: Adiponectin and protection against type 2 diabetes mellitus. Lancet 361:226-228, 2003.
39. Maeda N, Shimomura I, Kishida K, et al: Diet-induced insulin resistance in mice lacking adiponectin/ACRP30. Nat Med 8:731-737, 2002.
40. Engeli S, Feldpausch M, Gorzelniak K, et al: Association between adiponectin and mediators of inflammation in obese women. Diabetes 52:942-947, 2003.
41. Ouchi N, Kihara S, Funahashi T, et al: Reciprocal association of C-reactive protein with adiponectin in blood stream and adipose tissue. Circulation 107:671-674, 2003.
42. Krakoff J, Funahashi T, Stehouwer CD, et al: Inflammatory markers, adiponectin, and risk of type 2 diabetes in Pima Indians. Diabetes Care 26:1745-1751, 2003.
43. Matsubara M, Namioka K, Katayose S: Decreased plasma adiponectin concentrations in women with low-grade C-reactive protein elevation. Eur J Endocrinol 148:657-662, 2003.
44. Kern PA, Di Gregorio GB, Lu T, et al: Adiponectin expression from human adipose tissue: Relation to obesity, insulin resistance, and tumor necrosis factor–α expression. Diabetes 52:1779-1785, 2003.
45. Ouchi N, Hihara S, Arita Y, et al: Adipocyte derived plasma protein, adiponectin, suppresses lipid accumulation and class A scavenger receptor expression in human monocyte-derived macrophages. Circulation 103:1057-1063, 2002.
46. Arita Y, Kihara S, Ouchi N, et al: Adipocyte-derived plasma protein adiponectin acts as platelet-derived growth factor-BB-binding protein and regulates growth factor-induced common postereceptor signal in vascular smooth muscle cell. Circulation 105:2893-2898, 2002.
47. Okamoto Y, Arita Y, Nishida M, et al: An adipocyte-derived plasma protein, adiponcectin, adheres to injured vascular walls. Horm Metab Res 32:47-50, 2000.

48. Kumada M, Kihara S, Sumitsuji S, et al: Association of hypoadiponectinemia with coronary artery disease in men. Arterioscler Thromb Vasc Biol 23:85-89, 2003.

49. Zoccali C, Mallamaci F, Tripepi G, et al: Adiponectin, metabolic risk factors, and cardiovascular events among patients with end-stage renal disease. J Am Soc Nephrol 13:134-141, 2002.

50. Okamoto Y, Kihara S, Ouchi N, et al: Adioncetin reduces atherosclerosis in apolipoprotein E–deficient mice. Circulation 106:2767-2770, 2002.

51. Yamauchi T, Kamon J, Waki H, et al: Globular adiopnectin protected ob/ob mice from diabetes and ApoE-deficient mice from atherosclerosis. J Biol Chem 278:2461-2468, 2003.

52. Sowers JR, Frohlich ED: Insulin and insulin resistance: Impact on blood pressure and cardiovascular disease. Med Clin N Am 88:63-82, 2004.

53. Klein S, Fontana L, Young L, et al: Absence of an effect of liposuction on insulin action and risk factors for coronary heart disease. N Engl J Med 350:2549-2557, 2004.

54. Reaven G: Metabolic syndrome: Pathophysiology and implications for management of Cardiovascular disease. Circulation 106:286-288, 2002.

55. DECODE Study Group, European Diabetes Epidemiology Group: Is the current definition for diabetes relevant to mortality risk from all causes and cardiovascular and noncardiovascular diseases? Diabetes Care 26:688-696, 2003.

56. Chiasson JL, Josse RG, Gomis R, et al: Acarbose treatment and the risk of cardiovascular disease and hypertension in patients with impaired glucose tolerance. The Stop-NIDDM trial. JAMA 290:486-494, 2003.

57. Coulston AM, Peragallo-Dittko V: Insulin resistance syndrome: A potent culprit in cardiovascular disease. J Am Diet Assoc 104:176-179, 2004.

58. Ducimentiere P, Eschwege E, Papoz L, et al: Relationship of plasma insulin level to the incidence of myocardial infarction and coronary heart disease. Diabetologia 19:205-210, 1989.

59. Fontbonne A, Charles MA, Thibault N, et al: Hyperinsulinemia as a predictor of coronary heart disease mortality in healthy population: The Paris Prospective Study, 15-year follow-up. Diabetologia 34:356-361, 1991.

60. Despres J-P, Lamarche B, Mauriege P, et al: Hyperinsulinemia as an independent risk factor for ischemic heart disease. N Engl J Med 1996;334:952-957.

61. Howard BV, Gray RS: Insulin resistance and cardiovascular disease. In Marshall SM, Home PD, Rizza RA (eds): The Diabetes Annual 12. Amsterdam, Elsevier Science, 1999, pp 305-316.

62. Bonora E, Formentine G, Calcaterra F: HOMA-estimated insulin resistance is an independent predictor of cardiovascular disease in type 2 diabetic subjects. Diabetes Care 25:1135-1141, 2002.

63. Salomaa V, Riley W, Kaark JD, et al: Non-insulin-dependent diabetes mellitus and fasting glucose and insulin concentrations are associated with arterial stiffness indexes. The ARIC Study. Atherosclerosis Risk in Communities Study. Circulation 91:1432-1443, 1995.

64. Suzuki M, Shinozaki K, Kanazawa A, et al: Insulin resistance as an independent risk for carotid wall thickening. Hypertension 28:593-598, 1996.

65. Shinozaki K, Naritomi H, Shimizu T, et al: Role of insulin resistance associated with compensatory hyperinsulinemia in ischemic stroke. Stroke 27:37-43, 1996.

66. Assmann G, Schulte H: The Prospective Cardiovascular Munster (PROCAM) study: Prevalence of hyperlipidemia in persons with hypertension and/or diabetes mellitus and relationship to coronary heart disease. Am Heart J 116:1713-1724, 1988.

67. Reynisdottir S, Angelin B, Landgin D, et al: Adipose tissue lipoprotein lipase and hormone-sensitive lipase. Contrasting finding in familial combined hyperlipidemia and insulin resistance syndrome. Arterioscler Thromb Vasc Biol 17: 2287-2292, 1997.

68. Davy BM, Melby LC: The effect of fiber-rich carbohydrates on features of Syndrome X. J Am Diet Assoc 103:86-96, 2003.

69. Eckel RH: Familial combined hyperlipidemia and insulin resistance: Distant relatives linked by intra-abdominal fat? Arterioscler Thromb Vasc Biol 21:469-470, 2001.

70. Castelli WP: Epidemiology of triglycerides: A view from Framingham. Am J Cardiol 70:3H-9H, 1992.

71. Ballantyne CM, Olsson AG, Cook TJ, et al: Influence of low high-density lipoprotein cholesterol and elevated triglyceride on coronary heart disease events and response to simvastatin therapy in 4S. Circulation 104:3046-3051, 2001.

72. Mamo JC, Yu KC, Elsegood CL, et al: Is atherosclerosis exclusively a postprandial phenomenon? Clin Exp Pharmacol Physiol 24:288-293, 1997.

73. Sowers JR: Effects of statins on the vasculature: Implications for aggressive lipid management in the cardiovascular metabolic syndrome. Am J Cardiol 91(suppl):14B-22B, 2003.

74. Ferrannini E, Buzzigoli C, Bonadonna R, et al: Insulin resistance in essential hypertension. N Engl J Med 317:350-357, 1987.

75. Shen DC, Shieh SM, Wu DA, et al: Resistance to insulin stimulated glucose uptake in patients with hypertension. J Clin Endocrinol Metab 66:580-583, 1998.

76. Gress TW, Niet FJ, Shahar E, et al: Hypertension and antihypertensive therapy as risk factors for type 2 diabetes mellitus. Atherosclerosis risk in community study. N Engl J Med 342:905-912, 1987.

77. Sowers JR, Bakris GL: Antihypertensive therapy and the risk of type 2 diabetes mellitus. N Engl J Med 342:969-970, 2000.

78. Sowers JR, Sowers PS, Peuler JD: Role of insulin resistance and hyperinsulinemia in development of hypertension and atherosclerosis. J Lab Clin Med 123:647-652, 1994.

79. Reaven GM, Lithell H, Landsberg L: Hypertension and associated metabolic abnormalities: The role of insulin resistance and sympathetic adrenal system. N Engl J Med 334:374-381, 1996.

80. Nolan JJ, Ludvik B, Baloga J, et al: Mechanisms of the kinetic defect in insulin action in obesity and NIDDM. Diabetes 46:494-500, 1997.

81. Sowers JR: Insulin and insulin-like growth factor in normal and pathological cardiovascular physiology. Hypertension 29:691-699, 1997.

82. Sowers JR: Effects of insulin and IGF-1 on vascular smooth muscle glucose and cation metabolism. Diabetes 45(Suppl 3):S47-S51, 1996.

83. Ren J, Samson WK, Sowers JR: Insulin-like growth factor 1 as a cardiac hormone: physiological and pathophysiological implications in heart disease. J Mol Cell Cardiol 31:2049-2061, 1993.

84. Wang HD, Xu S, Johns DG, et al: Role of NADH oxidase in the vascular hypertrophic and oxidative stress responses to angiotensin II in mice. Circ Res 88:947-953, 2001.

85. Huerta MG, Nadler JL: Role of inflammatory pathways in the development and cardiovascular complications of type 2 diabetes. Curr Diab Rep 2:396-402, 2002.

86. Griendling KK, Sorescu D, Ushio-Fukai M: NAD(P)H oxidase: Role in cardiovascular biology and disease. Circ Res 86:494-501, 2000.

87. Sowers JR: Hypertension, angiotensin II, and oxidative stress. N Engl J Med 346:1999-2001, 2002.

88. Kalinowksi L, Matjie T, Chabelsky E, et al: Angiotensin II AT1 receptor antagonists inhibit platelet adhesion and aggregation by nitric oxide release. Hypertension 40:521-527, 2002.

89. Katovich MJ, Pachori A: Effects of inhibition of the renin-angiotensin system on the cardiovascular actions of insulin. Diab Obes Metab 2:3-14, 2000.

90. Grunfeld B, Balzareti M, Romo H, et al: Hyperinsulinemia in normotensive offspring of hypertensive parents. Hypertension 23:112-115, 1994.

91. Beatty OL, Harper R, Sheridan B: Insulin resistance in offspring of hypertensive parents. BMJ 3017:92-96, 1993.

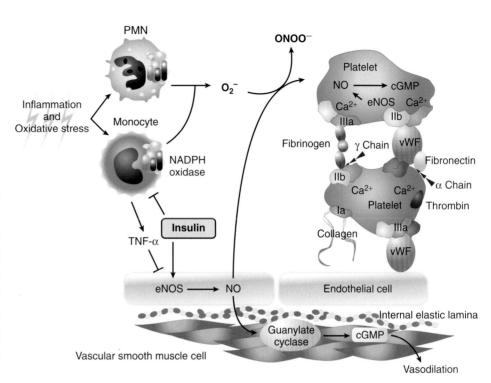

Figure 7–3. The pro-oxidative stress and proinflammatory state in obesity and diabetes results in a proconstrictive and proaggregatory state. This may be a result of insulin resistance, because insulin is unable to exert its vasodilatory and antiaggregatory properties. Ca^{2+}, calcium ion; cGMP, cyclic guanosine monophosphate; eNOS, epithelial nitric oxide synthase; NADPH, nicotinamide adenine dinucleotide phospate; NO, nitric oxide; O_2^-, superoxide; $ONOO^-$, peroxynitrite; PMN, polymorphonucleocyte; TNF-α, tumor necrosis factor α; vWF, von Willebrand factor.

TXA_2 in response to proaggregatory stimuli. TXA_2 is proaggregatory and is formed from arachidonic acid in phospholipids bound to the membrane. Phospholipase A2 in the platelet membrane hydrolyzes phospholipids to release arachidonic acid. The platelet-dense bodies contain norepinephrine and 5HT, which are vasoconstrictors and are proaggregatory to the platelets. Histamine, which is proinflammatory, is also contained in the dense bodies. The α-granules in the platelets contain proteins like β-thromboglobulin (β-TG), platelet factor 4, and CD40 ligand (CD40L). These proteins, especially CD40L, enhance vasoconstriction, platelet aggregation, and inflammation. The platelet attaches to the endothelium through the vWF expressed on the endothelium. vWF binds to IIb/IIIa receptor and fibrinogen. The platelet also binds to and is activated by collagen, which is contained in the vessel wall and is exposed when there is an erosion.

The monocyte is a key mediator of inflammation and responds to both acute and chronic inflammatory stimuli. It is a mediator of innate immunity while also activating adaptive immunity in its capacity as an antigen-presenting cell. It exposes and secretes a variety of proinflammatory and prothrombotic mediators. In obesity and diabetes, monocytes secrete an excess of proinflammatory cytokines, such as TNF-α, IL-6, migration inhibition factor (MIF), and matrix metalloproteinases (MMPs).[30] Upon challenge with high glucose concentrations, monocytes secrete these inflammatory mediators in greater amounts and induce activation of nuclear factor κB (NF-κB), activator protein (AP-1), and early growth response (Egr-1).[31,32] These proinflammatory transcription factors lead to the increased expression of the mediators mentioned earlier as well as TF and PAI-1.

The monocyte interacts with the platelet and the endothelium. Platelets activate the monocyte through CD40L release, and the monocyte activates the platelet through TF release. TF, in turn, activates factors VII and X, which results in the activation of prothrombin to thrombin. This reaction is of particular interest in the thrombus, which follows the rupture of the atherosclerotic plaque. Foam cells, which are derived from the monocyte-macrophage following the uptake of oxidized LDL, express thrombin formation near the foam cell surface. This triggers platelet aggregation and thrombosis.

Abnormalities in endothelial function might not only be due to the direct effect of oxidative stress and inflammation in obesity and diabetes; they may also result from the interaction of other cells in blood: the leukocyte (especially the monocyte) and the platelet. The monocyte and the platelet also have interactions that can affect endothelial function (Fig. 7–3).

INFLAMMATION IN OBESITY AND TYPE 2 DIABETES

The development of the concept that type 2 diabetes is an inflammatory condition is an exciting and novel approach to the understanding of this disease. It has implications for both the pathogenesis and the consequences (complications) of this condition.

The concept of inflammation in relation to metabolic conditions like obesity and insulin resistance started with a seminal study by Hotamisligil and colleagues, published in 1993, demonstrating that adipocytes constitutively express the proinflammatory cytokine TNF-α, that TNF-α expression in adipocytes of obese animals (ob/ob mouse, db/db mouse, and fa/fa Zucker rat) is markedly increased, and that neutralization of TNF-α by a soluble TNF-α receptor leads to a decrease in insulin resistance in these animals.[33] These observations provided the first link between an increase in the expression and the plasma concentration of a proinflammatory cytokine and insulin resistance.

Later data showed that adipose tissue in humans also expressed TNF-α constitutively and that its expression fell after weight loss.[34] Similar observations were made with respect to plasma TNF-α concentrations in the obese and their decrease after weight loss.[35] It was also shown that there was a significant correlation between body mass index (BMI) and plasma TNF-α concentrations. TNF receptor concentration has also been shown to be elevated in obese patients.[36]

Further work in the area of obesity has confirmed that obesity is a state of chronic inflammation as indicated by increased plasma concentrations of C-reactive protein (CRP),[37] IL-6,[38] and PAI-1.[39] However, attempts to reduce TNF-α activity by infusions of TNF-α antibody in humans have not been successful in restoring insulin sensitivity.[40] In some studies in the obese, TNF-α levels have not been shown to be elevated. These inconsistencies could be due to the assays used and the conditions in which the blood samples were obtained.

That obesity is a state of inflammation raises two important issues. Firstly, what is the pathogenesis of this inflammation? Secondly, is type 2 diabetes, another closely related insulin-resistant state, also an inflammatory condition? The answers to these questions are now beginning to emerge.

Pickup's group first proposed that type 2 diabetes was also an inflammatory condition characterized by elevated concentrations of acute-phase inflammatory reactants in the plasma: sialic acid and the proinflammatory cytokine IL-6.[41,42] These data have been confirmed by several studies, reinforcing the idea that type 2 diabetes is an inflammatory condition.

The observation that obesity (a major risk factor for type 2 diabetes) and diabetes are inflammatory conditions led to investigations exploring whether inflammatory mediators predict development of type 2 diabetes in populations at risk. Several such studies have now confirmed that the presence of inflammation predicts the development of type 2 diabetes. The first of these studies was by Schmidt and coworkers, in which the presence of inflammatory mediators predicted the future occurrence of type 2 diabetes in adults.[43] This was a part of the larger Atherosclerosis Risk in Communities Study (ARIC). A paper from the same study continues this theme by showing that elevated plasma concentrations of sialic acid, orosomucoid, IL-6, and CRP predict type 2 diabetes.[44] An overall inflammation score based on these four indices, the total leukocyte count, and plasma fibrinogen concentration provided an increased hazard ratio of 3.7 (when comparing the highest and the lowest quintiles) in white nonsmokers for the development of type 2 diabetes.[45]

At least three other prospective studies confirm that an increase in inflammatory indices at baseline predicts type 2 diabetes and insulin resistance.[46-49] Similarly, there is a correlation between fasting insulin concentrations and CRP concentrations in plasma,[37,50,51] indicating that insulin resistance and inflammatory processes are related and that in association with the other facts just mentioned there may be a causal link. Furthermore, there is a relationship between plasma FFA and CRP concentrations and the proinflammatory factors, including cytokines, that are expressed in circulating MNC in obesity. Similar studies are being conducted in diabetes.

So, what leads to inflammation in obesity and type 2 diabetes and what is the link between inflammation and insulin resistance? TNF-α causes an inhibition of autophosphorylation of tyrosine residues of the insulin receptor (IR) and an induction of serine phosphorylation of insulin receptor substrate-1 (IRS-1), which in turn causes serine phosphorylation of the IR in adipocytes and inhibits tyrosine phosphorylation.[52] In human aortic endothelial cells, TNF-α not only suppresses tyrosine phosphorylation, it also suppresses the expression of the insulin receptor itself.[53]

More recently, IL-6 has been shown to inhibit insulin signal transduction in hepatocytes.[54] This effect is related to SOCS-3, a protein that associates itself with the insulin receptor and inhibits its autophosphorylation and the tyrosine phosphorylation of IRS-1, the association of the p85 subunit of phosphoinositide 3 (PI3) kinase to IRS-1, and the subsequent activation of *Akt*. These effects of IL-6 were demonstrated in HepG-2 cells in vitro and in mice in vivo.[55] SOC-3 may also be the mediator of leptin resistance in obese humans.

As far as the association of inflammation with obesity is concerned, elevated concentrations of fibrinogen have a predictive value in the development of obesity itself,[45] and TNF-α concentration falls with dietary restriction and weight loss. There is also evidence that glucose intake induces acute oxidative stress and inflammation at the cellular and molecular level for 3 hours,[56,57] and a mixed fast food meal causes similar responses for 4 hours. Conversely, dietary restriction in the obese for a brief period of 4 weeks leads to a significant reduction in oxidative stress, which is markedly enhanced in the obese.[29] A 48-hour fast leads to a 50% reduction in reactive oxygen species (ROS) generation by leukocytes and a diminution in the expression of reduced nicotinamide adenine dinucleotide phosphate

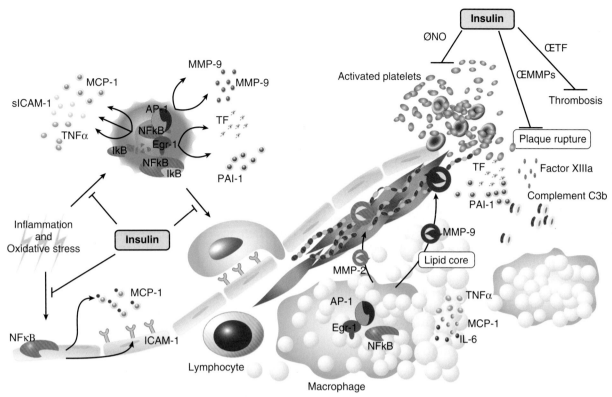

Figure 7–4. Abnormalities in endothelial function in obesity and diabetes are a result of oxidative stress and inflammation. Insulin, on the one hand, has antioxidative and anti-inflammatory effects, whereas glucose, on the other hand, exerts pro-oxidative and proinflammatory effects. All effects of insulin are matched by diametrically opposite effects of glucose. AP-1, activator protein-1; Egr-1, early growth response-1; ICAM-1, intercellular adhesion molecule-1; IκB, inhibitor of κB; IL-6, interleukin-6; MCP-1, monocyte chemoattractant protein; MMP, matrix metalloproteinase; NFκB, nuclear factor κB; PAI-1, plasminogen activator inhibitor-1; TF, tissue factor; TNFα, tumor necrosis factor α.

(NADPH) oxidase, the enzyme that converts molecular oxygen to the superoxide radical. The superoxide radical activates the redox-sensitive proinflammatory transcription factor NF-κB, which activates the transcription of most proinflammatory genes.

Thus, the pro-oxidant and proinflammatory effects of excessive macronutrient intake in normal subjects are similar to those found in obese subjects in their basal fasting state. It is likely that the proinflammatory state of obese persons is related to chronic excessive macronutrient intake. Indeed, increased concentrations of inflammation-sensitive proteins, fibrinogen, ceruloplasmin, orosomucoid, and α-antitrypsin are predictive of future weight gain.[58] Type 2 diabetes—the presence of hyperglycemia—further exacerbates the proinflammatory state.

Another possible reason that obesity and type 2 diabetes are associated with inflammation is that the state of insulin resistance promotes inflammation. This is because insulin has been shown to exert an anti-inflammatory effect at the cellular and molecular level both in vitro and in vivo. A low-dose infusion of insulin (2.0 IU/h) has been shown to reduce ROS generation by mononuclear cells, suppress NADPH oxidase expression and intranu-

clear NF-κB binding, induce expression of IκB (NF-κB inhibitor), and suppress plasma ICAM-1 and MCP-1 concentrations. It also suppresses intranuclear Egr-1, plasma tissue factor, PAI-1, and MCP-1 concentrations.[59,60] An interruption of insulin signal transduction would prevent the anti-inflammatory effect of insulin from being exerted (Fig. 7–4).

An important implication of the relationship among inflammation, obesity, insulin resistance, and type 2 diabetes is that atherosclerosis, which is responsible for the major cause of death (acute myocardial infarction) in this patient population, is itself an inflammatory process.[5] The activation of proinflammatory mechanisms and the accumulation of monocyte-macrophages in the intima, in addition to lipid infiltration, are characteristic of atherosclerosis. An increase in the plasma concentration of inflammatory mediators like CRP and IL-6 increases the risk of atherosclerotic complications like acute myocardial infarction. Thus, inflammation underlies both insulin resistance and atherosclerosis.

One mechanism that could connect these features is the anti-inflammatory and potential antiatherosclerotic effect of insulin, which, in the presence of insulin resistance, leads to a proinflammatory state. Insulin sensitizers of the thiazolidine-

dione (TZD) class have also been shown to be anti-inflammatory and potentially antiatherogenic.[61-63] Thus, insulin and TZDs exert a suppressive effect on ROS generation, NADPH oxidase expression, and intranuclear NF-κB binding, and they exert a stimulatory effect on IκB expression and reduce plasma concentrations of ICAM-1, MCP-1 chemokine, and PAI-1. TZDs also suppress the plasma concentrations of TNF and CRP. The suppressive effect of TZDs and insulin is relevant because PAI-1 concentration is elevated in proinflammatory states such as the metabolic syndrome, obesity, and type 2 diabetes, with an increase in the risk of atherosclerosis and its complications, which include acute myocardial infarction and stroke.[64]

Thus, obesity and type 2 diabetes are proinflammatory states in which inflammatory mechanisms might contribute to insulin resistance. Macronutrient intake might contribute to inflammation. Insulin resistance could itself promote inflammation by impairing the anti-inflammatory effect of insulin. Insulin and insulin sensitizers of the TZD class might therefore have a potential use as anti-inflammatory drugs in addition to their current use as antidiabetic drugs.

THE EFFECT OF DRUGS USED IN DIABETIC PATIENTS

With the establishment of the concept of the inflammatory nature of obesity and type 2 diabetes, and a probable causal relationship between inflammation and insulin resistance, it is of great interest that insulin has now been shown to exert an anti-inflammatory effect.[59] This would explain why insulin-resistant states are proinflammatory. It also suggests that drugs used in the treatment of type 2 diabetes should ideally have an anti-inflammatory activity, because this property can affect both insulin resistance and atherosclerosis. Atherosclerosis is the major cause of death in this condition through myocardial infarction and stroke.

We have considered insulin to be a metabolic hormone that lowers plasma glucose, fatty acid, and amino acid concentrations postprandially. Its secretion is regulated mainly by glycemic levels. However, insulin has now been shown to have a profound, acute anti-inflammatory effect. Thus, it suppresses intranuclear NF-κB binding, increases IκB expression, and suppresses ROS generation and the expression of p47^{phox}, a key protein component of NADPH oxidase.[59] It also suppresses intranuclear Egr-1 binding and the expression of the genes regulated by Egr-1: TF and *PAI-1*.[60] More recently, it has also been shown to suppress the plasma concentration of matrix metalloproteinase-9 (MMP-9) and vascular endothelial growth factor (VEGF).[65]

These data suggest that insulin is not only anti-inflammatory, it is also potentially antithrombotic and profibrinolytic. In addition, its ability to suppress MMP-9 may have a potential inhibitory effect on rupture of the vulnerable atherosclerotic plaque (see Fig. 7–4).[66] It was thus natural to ask whether these effects of insulin account for its profound beneficial effects in the clinical studies investigating acute myocardial infarction. Indeed, it has recently been shown that a low infusion of insulin causes a reduction of greater than 40% in the increase in CRP and serum amyloid A (SAA) following an acute myocardial infarction.[67] CRP and SAA are indices of inflammation and are known to increase following acute MI. The magnitude of their increase is related to the size of the infarct and is inversely related to the prognosis in acute MI.[68,69] Insulin also caused a suppression in the increase of PAI-1 and p47^{phox}; these effects indicate a profibrinolytic and an antioxidant effect. Finally, insulin caused a significant reduction in CK and CK-MB enzymes, indicating that insulin might have a cardioprotective effect.[67]

Thiazolidinediones

The thiazolidinediones were the first class of drugs shown to exert an anti-inflammatory effect in humans. Troglitazone, the first of these drugs to be used, suppresses ROS generation by peripheral blood mononuclear cells (MNC), intranuclear NF-κB binding activity, and p65 (Rel A) and p47^{phox} expression and enhances IκB expression in the same cells in obese patients and in obese diabetic patients.[61,70] Troglitazone also caused a fall in plasma concentrations of TNF-α, sICAM-1, MCP-1, CRP, and SAA when given at a dose of 400 mg daily.[61,70] Troglitazone also suppresses two other proinflammatory transcription factors (AP-1 and Egr-1) and their respective genes, the matrix metalloproteinases (MMP-2 and MMP-9), tissue factor (TF), and PAI-1.[71,72] Rosiglitazone given at a dose of 4 mg daily also suppressed ROS generation, p47^{phox}, and intranuclear NF-κB binding in addition to reducing plasma concentrations of sICAM-1, MCP-1, CRP, and SAA. Rosiglitazone also suppresses PAI-1.[73]

These anti-inflammatory effects at the cellular and molecular level become evident within a week of instituting treatment with TZDs, but the hypoglycemic effect of these drugs takes several weeks to develop. In addition, following TZD treatment, the fall in fasting insulin concentration starts much earlier than the fall in glucose levels. Thus, an investigation into the dynamics of the anti-inflammatory effects, insulin sensitization, and glucose-lowering induced by TZDs offers a potentially useful model for investigating the relationships among these processes. Based on the early onset of the anti-inflammatory effect of TZDs, one could hypothesize that inflammation and insulin resistance are probably related. As would be expected, TZDs normalize endothelial function.

Metformin

Although metformin is established as a potent antidiabetic drug that does not give rise to weight gain, it was only during the UKPDS that this drug was shown to cause a 40% reduction in cardiovascular mortality in type 2 diabetes.[74] More recently, metformin was also shown to be associated with a reduction in cardiovascular mortality by 40% in the retrospective Saskatchewan study based on pharmacy prescriptions.[75] Metformin might suppress the plasma concentrations of macrophage migration inhibition factor (MIF), a proinflammatory cytokine that might play a role in atherogenesis.[76] Metformin also improves endothelium-mediated postischemic vasodilation (Dandona P, Aljada A, Chaudhuri A, Mohanty P, unpublished data, 2004). This improvement is associated with a reduction in ROS generation. Such a reduction in oxidative stress could result in an increase in the bioavailability of NO, which in turn could cause an improvement in endothelium-dependent vasodilation; it might also, in the long term, result in an improvement in cardiovascular outcomes.

Sulfonylureas

Sulfonylureas are potent antidiabetic drugs, but there are no data showing either an anti-inflammatory effect or a beneficial effect in improving cardiovascular outcomes. Because the sulfonylureas lower plasma glucose concentrations rapidly, any potential anti-inflammatory effect would be extremely difficult to separate from their glucose-lowering effect. However, glucose has been shown to be proinflammatory, and therefore the lowering of blood glucose would have a potential anti-inflammatory effect.[31,56]

α-Glucosidase Inhibitors

Acarbose has been shown to be a mild antidiabetic drug that lowers HbA1c by 0.5% to 0.75%. It lowers postprandial glucose concentrations by reducing the rate of carbohydrate digestion in the small intestine through the inhibition of α-glucosidase.[77,78] In the Stop-NIDDM study, acarbose was effective in significantly reducing not only the incidence of type 2 diabetes but also the incidence of cardiovascular events.[79] Postprandial glucose concentrations are related to the frequency of cardiovascular events as shown in the Honolulu heart study.[80] A reduction in postprandial glycemia could reduce oxidative and inflammatory stress because the intake of glucose is associated with an increase in both. Repeated increase in postprandial oxidative and inflammatory stress could contribute to atherogenesis.

Cardiovascular Drugs Used in Diabetic Patients

β-Blockers have been shown to significantly reduce cardiovascular morbidity and mortality in the diabetic and nondiabetic populations.[81] They are antiarrhythmic and reduce oxygen requirements, which may be important in myocardial protection, but they also have a potent suppressive effect on ROS generation and thus may function as biologic antioxidants.[82,83] Such effects have been demonstrated for carvedilol and nadolol. This action can lead to an anti-inflammatory effect because ROS activate NF-κB and trigger inflammation, but such an effect is yet to be demonstrated.

Because angiotensin II has been shown to be a proinflammatory mediator, ACE inhibitors and ARBs may be expected to be anti-inflammatory. Indeed, the first reports demonstrating that ARBs are anti-inflammatory have now appeared. Valsartan suppresses ROS generation and intranuclear NF-κB binding, and it increases IκB expression and plasma CRP concentrations.[84] Candesartan induces a reduction in plasma concentrations of proinflammatory cytokines.[85] Definitive data on the anti-inflammatory effect of ACE inhibitors has yet to be shown in the human in vivo.

Statins are associated with a fall in plasma CRP concentrations in several large outcome studies.[86,87] They clearly have an anti-inflammatory effect as well as a long-term antiatherosclerotic effect, leading to a reduction in cardiovascular events. Fibric acid is associated with impressive reductions in cardiovascular morbidity and mortality, but there is no evidence that these drugs have either an ROS-suppressive effect or an anti-inflammatory action. Studies are currently under way to investigate the potential anti-inflammatory effect of statins and fibric acids. Similar studies should also be conducted for niacin and thiazides because they are commonly used in diabetic patients.

Use of statins, ACE-inhibitors, and ARBs in patients with established cardiovascular disease or cardiovascular risk leads to a reduction in the incidence of type 2 diabetes. This totally unexpected and seemingly unrelated outcome further fortifies the concept that inflammation underlies insulin resistance and that an anti-inflammatory drug can therefore potentially prevent type 2 diabetes.

References

1. Wu KK, Thiagarajan P: Role of endothelium in thrombosis and hemostasis. Annu Rev Med 47:315-331, 1996.
2. Gerritsen ME: Functional heterogeneity of vascular endothelial cells. Biochem Pharmacol 36:2701-2711, 1987.
3. Harrison DG: Cellular and molecular mechanisms of endothelial cell dysfunction. J Clin Invest 100:2153-2157, 1997.
4. Griendling KK, Alexander RW: Endothelial control of the cardiovascular system: Recent advances. FASEB J 10:283-292, 1996.

5. Ross R: Atherosclerosis—an inflammatory disease. N Engl J Med 340:115-126, 1999.

6. Repo H, Harlan JM: Mechanisms and consequences of phagocyte adhesion to endothelium. Ann Med 31:156-165, 1999.

7. Nicosia S, Oliva D, Bernini F, Fumagalli R: Prostacyclin-sensitive adenylate cyclase and prostacyclin binding sites in platelets and smooth muscle cells. Adv Cyclic Nucleotide Protein Phosphorylation Res 17:593-599, 1984.

8. Rovati GE, Giovanazzi S, Negretti A, Nicosia S: Prostacyclin effects on adenylate cyclase in platelets and vascular smooth muscle: Interaction with an inhibitory receptor or partial agonism? Adv Prostaglandin Thromboxane Leukot Res 23:263-265, 1995.

9. Furchgott RF, Zawadzki JV: The obligatory role of endothelial cells in the relaxation of arterial smooth muscle by acetylcholine. Nature 288:373-376, 1980.

10. Barrett ML, Willis AL, Vane JR: Inhibition of platelet-derived mitogen release by nitric oxide (EDRF). Agents Actions 27:488-491, 1989.

11. Grodzinska L, Marcinkiewicz E: The generation of TXA2 in human platelet rich plasma and its inhibition by nictindole and prostacyclin. Pharmacol Res Commun 11:133-146, 1979.

12. Boyko EJ, Ahroni JH, Stensel VL: Tissue oxygenation and skin blood flow in the diabetic foot: Responses to cutaneous warming. Foot Ankle Int 22:711-714, 2001.

13. Chin LC, Huang TY, Yu CL, et al: Increased cutaneous blood flow but impaired post-ischemic response of nutritional flow in obese children. Atherosclerosis 146:179-185, 1999.

14. Caballero AE, Arora S, Saouaf R, et al: Microvascular and macrovascular reactivity is reduced in subjects at risk for type 2 diabetes. Diabetes 48:1856-1862, 1999.

15. Griffith DN, Saimbi S, Lewis C, et al: Abnormal cerebrovascular carbon dioxide reactivity in people with diabetes. Diabet Med 4:217-220, 1987.

16. Dandona P, James IM, Newbury PA, et al: Cerebral blood flow in diabetes mellitus: Evidence of abnormal cerebrovascular reactivity. BMJ 2:325-326, 1978.

17. Menon RK, Grace AA, Burgoyne W, et al: Muscle blood flow in diabetes mellitus. Evidence of abnormality after exercise. Diabetes Care 15:693-695, 1992.

18. Johnstone MT, Creager SJ, Scales KM, et al: Impaired endothelium-dependent vasodilation in patients with insulin-dependent diabetes mellitus. Circulation 88:2510-2516, 1993.

19. Grover A, Padginton C, Wilson MF, et al: Insulin attenuates norepinephrine-induced venoconstriction. An ultrasonographic study. Hypertension 25:779-784, 1995.

20. Riddell DR, Owen JS: Nitric oxide and platelet aggregation. Vitam Horm 57:25-48, 1999.

21. Trovati M, Anfossi G: Influence of insulin and of insulin resistance on platelet and vascular smooth muscle cell function. J Diabetes Complications 16:35-40, 2002.

22. Forster W, Beitz J, Hoffmann P: Stimulation and inhibition of PGI₂ synthetase activity by phospholipids (PL), cholesterol esters (CE), unesterified fatty acids (UFA) and lipoproteins (LDL and HDL). Artery 8:494-500, 1980.

23. Sterin-Borda L, Borda ES, Gimeno MF, et al: Contractile activity and prostacyclin generation in isolated coronary arteries from diabetic dogs. Diabetologia 22:56-59, 1982.

24. van 't Veer C, Golden NJ, Kalafatis M, Mann KG: Inhibitory mechanism of the protein C pathway on tissue factor-induced thrombin generation. Synergistic effect in combination with tissue factor pathway inhibitor. J Biol Chem 272:7983-7994, 1997.

25. Podor TJ, Joshua P, Butcher M, et al: Accumulation of type 1 plasminogen activator inhibitor and vitronectin at sites of cellular necrosis and inflammation. Ann N Y Acad Sci 667:173-177, 1992.

26. Carmassi F, Morale M, Puccetti R, et al: Coagulation and fibrinolytic system impairment in insulin dependent diabetes mellitus. Thromb Res 67:643-654, 1992.

27. McGill JB, Schneider DJ, Arfken CL, et al: Factors responsible for impaired fibrinolysis in obese subjects and NIDDM patients. Diabetes 43:104-109, 1994.

28. Dandona P, James IM, Woollard ML, et al: Instability of cerebral blood-flow in insulin-dependent diabetics. Lancet 2:1203-1205, 1979.

29. Dandona P, Mohanty P, Ghanim H, et al: The suppressive effect of dietary restriction and weight loss in the obese on the generation of reactive oxygen species by leukocytes, lipid peroxidation, and protein carbonylation. J Clin Endocrinol Metab 86:355-362, 2001.

30. Ghanim H, Aljada A, Hofmeyer D, et al: Circulating mononuclear cells in the obese are in a proinflammatory state. Circulation 110:1564-1571, 2004.

31. Aljada A, Ghanim H, Mohanty P, et al: Glucose intake induces an increase in activator protein 1 and early growth response 1 binding activities, in the expression of tissue factor and matrix metalloproteinase in mononuclear cells, and in plasma tissue factor and matrix metalloproteinase concentrations. Am J Clin Nutr 80:51-57, 2004.

32. Aljada A, Ghanim H, Mohanty P, et al: Glucose activates nuclear factor–κB (NF-κB) pathway in mononuclear cells (MNC) and induces an increase in p47phox subunit in MNC membranes. Diabetes 51:A537, 2002.

33. Hotamisligil GS, Shargill NS, Spiegelman BM: Adipose expression of tumor necrosis factor-alpha: Direct role in obesity-linked insulin resistance. Science 259:87-91, 1993.

34. Kern PA, Saghizadeh M, Ong JM, et al: The expression of tumor necrosis factor in human adipose tissue. Regulation by obesity, weight loss, and relationship to lipoprotein lipase. J Clin Invest 95:2111-2119, 1995.

35. Dandona P, Weinstock R, Thusu K, et al: Tumor necrosis factor-alpha in sera of obese patients: Fall with weight loss. J Clin Endocrinol Metab 83:2907-2910, 1998.

36. Mantzoros CS, Moschos S, Avramopoulos I, et al: Leptin concentrations in relation to body mass index and the tumor necrosis factor-alpha system in humans. J Clin Endocrinol Metab 82:3408-3413, 1997.

37. Yudkin JS, Stehouwer CD, Emeis JJ, Coppack SW: C-reactive protein in healthy subjects: Associations with obesity, insulin resistance, and endothelial dysfunction: A potential role for cytokines originating from adipose tissue? Arterioscler Thromb Vasc Biol 19:972-978, 1999.

38. Mohamed-Ali V, Goodrick S, Rawesh A, et al: Subcutaneous adipose tissue releases interleukin-6, but not tumor necrosis factor-alpha, in vivo. J Clin Endocrinol Metab 82:4196-4200, 1997.

39. Lundgren CH, Brown SL, Nordt TK, et al: Elaboration of type-1 plasminogen activator inhibitor from adipocytes. A potential pathogenetic link between obesity and cardiovascular disease. Circulation 93:106-110, 1996.

40. Ofei F, Hurel S, Newkirk J, et al: Effects of an engineered human anti-TNF-alpha antibody (CDP571) on insulin sensitivity and glycemic control in patients with NIDDM. Diabetes 45:881-885, 1996.

41. Crook MA, Tutt P, Pickup JC: Elevated serum sialic acid concentration in NIDDM and its relationship to blood pressure and retinopathy. Diabetes Care 16:57-60, 1993.

42. Pickup JC, Mattock MB, Chusney GD, Burt D: NIDDM as a disease of the innate immune system: Association of acute-phase reactants and interleukin-6 with metabolic syndrome X. Diabetologia 40:1286-1292, 1997.

43. Schmidt MI, Duncan BB, Sharrett AR, et al: Markers of inflammation and prediction of diabetes mellitus in adults (Atherosclerosis Risk in Communities study): A cohort study. Lancet 353:1649-1652, 1999.

44. Duncan BB, Schmidt MI, Pankow JS, et al: Low-grade systemic inflammation and the development of type 2 diabetes: The Atherosclerosis Risk in Communities study. Diabetes 52:1799-1805, 2003.

45. Duncan BB, Schmidt MI, Chambless LE, et al: Fibrinogen, other putative markers of inflammation, and weight gain in middle-aged adults—the ARIC study. Atherosclerosis Risk in Communities. Obes Res 8:279-286, 2000.

46. Pradhan AD, Manson JE, Rifai N, et al: C-reactive protein, interleukin 6, and risk of developing type 2 diabetes mellitus. JAMA 286:327-334, 2001.

47. Barzilay JI, Abraham L, Heckbert SR, et al: The relation of markers of inflammation to the development of glucose disorders in the elderly: The Cardiovascular Health Study. Diabetes 50:2384-2389, 2001.

48. Han TS, Sattar N, Williams K, et al: Prospective study of C-reactive protein in relation to the development of diabetes and metabolic syndrome in the Mexico City Diabetes Study. Diabetes Care 25:2016-2021, 2002.

49. Pradhan AD, Cook NR, Buring JE, et al: C-reactive protein is independently associated with fasting insulin in nondiabetic women. Arterioscler Thromb Vasc Biol 23:650-655, 2003.

50. Hak AE, Stehouwer CD, Bots ML, et al: Associations of C-reactive protein with measures of obesity, insulin resistance, and subclinical atherosclerosis in healthy, middle-aged women. Arterioscler Thromb Vasc Biol 19:1986-1991, 1999.

51. Lemieux I, Pascot A, Prud'homme D, et al: Elevated C-reactive protein: Another component of the atherothrombotic profile of abdominal obesity. Arterioscler Thromb Vasc Biol 21:961-967, 2001.

52. Hotamisligil GS, Budavari A, Murray D, Spiegelman BM: Reduced tyrosine kinase activity of the insulin receptor in obesity-diabetes. Central role of tumor necrosis factor-alpha. J Clin Invest 94:1543-1549, 1994.

53. Aljada A, Ghanim H, Assian E, Dandona P: Tumor necrosis factor-alpha inhibits insulin-induced increase in endothelial nitric oxide synthase and reduces insulin receptor content and phosphorylation in human aortic endothelial cells. Metabolism 51:487-491, 2002.

54. Senn JJ, Klover PJ, Nowak IA, Mooney RA: Interleukin-6 induces cellular insulin resistance in hepatocytes. Diabetes 51:3391-3399, 2002.

55. Senn JJ, Klover PJ, Nowak IA, et al: Suppressor of cytokine signaling-3 (SOCS-3), a potential mediator of interleukin-6-dependent insulin resistance in hepatocytes. J Biol Chem 278:13740-13746, 2003.

56. Esposito K, Nappo F, Marfella R, et al: Inflammatory cytokine concentrations are acutely increased by hyperglycemia in humans: Role of oxidative stress. Circulation 106:2067-2072, 2002.

57. Mohanty P, Hamouda W, Garg R, et al: Glucose challenge stimulates reactive oxygen species (ROS) generation by leukocytes. J Clin Endocrinol Metab 85:2970-2973, 2000.

58. Engstrom G, Hedblad B, Stavenow L, et al: Inflammation-sensitive plasma proteins are associated with future weight gain. Diabetes 52:2097-2101, 2003.

59. Dandona P, Aljada A, Mohanty P, et al: Insulin inhibits intranuclear nuclear factor κB and stimulates IκB in mononuclear cells in obese subjects: Evidence for an anti-inflammatory effect? J Clin Endocrinol Metab 86:3257-3265, 2001.

60. Aljada A, Ghanim H, Mohanty P, et al: Insulin inhibits the pro-inflammatory transcription factor early growth response gene-1 (Egr-1) expression in mononuclear cells (MNC) and reduces plasma tissue factor (TF) and plasminogen activator inhibitor-1 (PAI-1) concentrations. J Clin Endocrinol Metab 87:1419-1422, 2002.

61. Ghanim H, Garg R, Aljada A, et al: Suppression of nuclear factor-κB and stimulation of inhibitor κB by troglitazone: Evidence for an anti-inflammatory effect and a potential antiatherosclerotic effect in the obese. J Clin Endocrinol Metab 86:1306-1312, 2001.

62. Haffner SM, Greenberg AS, Weston WM, et al: Effect of rosiglitazone treatment on nontraditional markers of cardiovascular disease in patients with type 2 diabetes mellitus. Circulation 106:679-684, 2002.

63. Dandona P, Aljada A, Mohanty P: The anti-inflammatory and potential anti-atherogenic effect of insulin: A new paradigm. Diabetologia 45:924-930, 2002.

64. Juhan-Vague I, Alessi MC, Mavri A, Morange PE: Plasminogen activator inhibitor-1, inflammation, obesity, insulin resistance and vascular risk. J Thromb Haemost 1:1575-1579, 2003.

65. Dandona P, Aljada A, Mohanty P, et al: Insulin suppresses plasma concentration of vascular endothelial growth factor and matrix metalloproteinase-9. Diabetes Care 26:3310-3314, 2003.

66. Galis ZS, Sukhova GK, Lark MW, Libby P: Increased expression of matrix metalloproteinases and matrix degrading activity in vulnerable regions of human atherosclerotic plaques. J Clin Invest 94:2493-2503, 1994.

67. Chaudhuri A, Janicke D, Wilson MF, et al: Anti-inflammatory and profibrinolytic effect of insulin in acute ST-segment-elevation myocardial infarction. Circulation 109:849-854, 2004.

68. Barrett TD, Hennan JK, Marks RM, Lucchesi BR: C-reactive-protein-associated increase in myocardial infarct size after ischemia/reperfusion. J Pharmacol Exp Ther 303:1007-1013, 2002.

69. Katayama T, Nakashima H, Yonekura T, et al: [Significance of acute-phase inflammatory reactants as an indicator of prognosis after acute myocardial infarction: Which is the most useful predictor?]. J Cardiol 42:49-56, 2003.

70. Aljada A, Garg R, Ghanim H, et al: Nuclear factor-κB Suppressive and inhibitor-κB stimulatory effects of troglitazone in obese patients with type 2 diabetes: Evidence of an anti-inflammatory action? J Clin Endocrinol Metab 86:3250-3256, 2001.

71. Aljada A, Garg R, Ghanim H, et al: Troglitazone reduces intranuclear activator protein (AP-1) in mononuclear cells (MNC) and plasma matrix metalloproteinase-9 (MMP-9) concentration. Diabetes 50 Suppl 2:A532, 2001.

72. Ghanim H, Aljada A, Mohanty P, et al: Troglitazone suppresses pro-inflammatory transcription factors, early growth response-1 (Egr-1) and activator protein (AP-1) in mononuclear cells: Further evidence of the anti-inflammatory effects of troglitazone. Diabetes 51(2):A97, 2002.

73. Mohanty P, Aljada A, Ghanim H, et al: Evidence for a potent antiinflammatory effect of rosiglitazone. J Clin Endocrinol Metab 89:2728-2735, 2004.

74. UK Prospective Diabetes Study (UKPDS) Group: Effect of intensive blood-glucose control with metformin on complications in overweight patients with type 2 diabetes (UKPDS 34). Lancet 352:854-865, 1998.

75. Johnson JA, Majumdar SR, Simpson SH, Toth EL: Decreased mortality associated with the use of metformin compared with sulfonylurea monotherapy in type 2 diabetes. Diabetes Care 25:2244-2248, 2002.

76. Dandona P, Aljada A, Ghanim H, et al: Increased plasma concentration of macrophage migration inhibitory factor (MIF) and MIF mRNA in mononuclear cells in the obese and the suppressive action of metformin. J Clin Endocrinol Metab 89:5043-5047, 2004.

77. Krause HP, Keup U, Puls W: Inhibition of disaccharide digestion in rat intestine by the α-glucosidase inhibitor acarbose (BAY g 5421). Digestion 23:232-238, 1982

78. William-Olsson T: α-Glucosidase inhibition in obesity. Acta Med Scand Suppl 706:1-39, 1985.

79. Chiasson JL, Josse RG, Gomis R, et al: Acarbose treatment and the risk of cardiovascular disease and hypertension in patients with impaired glucose tolerance: the STOP-NIDDM trial. JAMA 290:486-494, 2003.

80. Rodriguez BL, Curb JD, Burchfiel CM, et al: Impaired glucose tolerance, diabetes, and cardiovascular disease risk factor profiles in the elderly. The Honolulu Heart Program. Diabetes Care 19:587-590, 1996.

81. Chen J, Marciniak TA, Radford MJ, et al: Beta-blocker therapy for secondary prevention of myocardial infarction in elderly diabetic patients. Results from the National Cooperative Cardiovascular Project. J Am Coll Cardiol 34:1388-1394, 1999.

82. Magsino CH, Jr, Hamouda W, Bapna V, et al: Nadolol inhibits reactive oxygen species generation by leukocytes and linoleic acid oxidation. Am J Cardiol 86:443-448, 2000.

83. Dandona P, Karne R, Ghanim H, et al: Carvedilol inhibits reactive oxygen species generation by leukocytes and oxidative damage to amino acids. Circulation 101:122-124, 2000.

84. Dandona P, Kumar V, Aljada A, et al: Angiotensin II receptor blocker valsartan suppresses reactive oxygen species generation in leukocytes, nuclear factor-κB, in mononuclear cells

of normal subjects: Evidence of an antiinflammatory action. J Clin Endocrinol Metab 88:4496-4501, 2003.

85. Tsutamoto T, Wada A, Maeda K, et al: Angiotensin II type 1 receptor antagonist decreases plasma levels of tumor necrosis factor alpha, interleukin-6 and soluble adhesion molecules in patients with chronic heart failure. J Am Coll Cardiol 35:714-721, 2000.

86. Ridker PM: Connecting the role of C-reactive protein and statins in cardiovascular disease. Clin Cardiol 26:III39-44, 2003.

87. Ridker PM, Rifai N, Clearfield M, et al: Measurement of C-reactive protein for the targeting of statin therapy in the primary prevention of acute coronary events. N Engl J Med 344:1959-1965, 2001.

Chapter 8

Diabetes and Inflammation

Sridevi Devaraj, Manisha Chandalia, and Ishwarlal Jialal

KEY POINTS

- *Diabetes is associated with accelerated atherosclerosis.*
- *Hyperglycemia, oxidative stress, and inflammation play a key role in diabetic vasculopathies.*
- *Much evidence supports a role for inflammation in atherosclerosis.*
- *Diabetes is a proinflammatory state as evidenced by increased high-sensitivity C-reactive protein, fibrinogen, plasminogen activator inhibitor 1, soluble cell adhesion molecules, pro-inflammatory cytokines, and nuclear factor κB activity.*
- *C-reactive protein, the prototypical marker of inflammation, predicts the development of diabetes, confers increased cardiovascular risk, and is increased in diabetes.*

Diabetes currently affects an estimated 29 million people in the United States. For those born in 2000, the estimated lifetime risk of developing diabetes is 36%. People with diabetes have large reductions in life expectancy and in quality of life from diabetes-specific microvascular complications in the retina and kidney, from neuropathies, and from extensive atherothrombotic macrovascular disease affecting arteries that supply the heart, brain, and lower extremities.

The most common cause of morbidity and mortality among people with diabetes today is atherosclerotic cardiovascular disease. In fact, for patients with type 2 diabetes mellitus (T2DM) without prior myocardial infarction (MI), the risk of coronary artery disease (CAD) is as high as it is for patients without diabetes who have had an MI.[1,2] Most studies have indicated that only 25% of this excess risk for macrovascular complications can be explained on the basis of conventional risk factors such as dyslipidemia, hypertension, and smoking. Therefore, the diabetic state per se confers an increased propensity to accelerated atherogenesis; however, the precise mechanisms remain to be elucidated.

Hyperglycemia, oxidative stress, and inflammation contribute to the increased risk of diabetic vasculopathies (Box 8-1). Hyperglycemia leads to the formation of advanced glycation end-products (AGEs). AGEs are a heterogeneous class of molecules, including 3-deoxyglucosone derivatives and monolysyl adducts. AGEs are increased in diabetes, and microvascular lesions correlate with the accumulation of AGEs, as demonstrated in diabetic retinopathy. On endothelial cells, ligation of receptors for AGE (RAGE) by AGEs induces the expression of cell adhesion molecules (CAMs), tissue factor, cytokines such as interleukin-6 (IL-6), and monocyte chemoattractant protein 1 (MCP-1).

The role of AGEs will not be reviewed in this chapter, and the role of oxidative stress in diabetic vasculopathies has been reviewed by us previously.[3] In this review, we focus on the role of inflammation in diabetic vasculopathies.

ATHEROSCLEROSIS AND DIABETES

Much evidence supports a pivotal role for inflammation in all phases of atherosclerosis from the initiation of the fatty streak to the culmination in acute coronary syndromes (plaque rupture).[4-6] The earliest event in atherogenesis appears to be endothelial cell dysfunction. Various noxious insults, including diabetes, can result in endothelial cell dysfunction, which manifests primarily as deficiency of nitric oxide (NO) and prostacyclin and an increase in endothelin-1, angiotensin II, and plasminogen activator inhibitor-1 (PAI-1), among other aberrations.

Following endothelial cell dysfunction, mononuclear cells such as monocytes and T lymphocytes attach to the endothelium, initially loosely but thereafter adhering firmly, and then transmigrate into the subendothelial space. The rolling and tethering of leukocytes on the endothelium is orchestrated by adhesion molecules such as selectins (E-selectin, P-selectin), cell adhesion molecules (ICAM-1 [intercellular CAM-1], VCAM-1 [vascular CAM-1]), and integrins. Chemotaxis and entry of monocytes into the subendothelial space is

promoted by MCP-1 and interleukin-8 (IL-8). Thereafter, macrophage colony-stimulating factor (M-CSF) promotes the differentiation of monocytes into macrophages.

Macrophages incorporate lipids from oxidized low-density lipoprotein (LDL) via the scavenger receptor pathway (CD36, SR-A), becoming foam cells, the hallmark of the early fatty-streak lesion. Following development of the fatty-streak lesion, smooth muscle cells migrate into the intima, proliferate, and form the fibrous cap under the influence of platelet-derived growth factor (PDGF) and angiotensin II. Researchers hypothesize that lipid-laden macrophages and smooth muscle cells, during the process of necrosis and apoptosis, release matrix metalloproteinases, which cause a rent in the endothelium. Because the lipid-laden macrophage is rich in tissue factor, tissue factor is released from the macrophage and comes into contact with the circulating blood, resulting in thrombus formation and acute coronary syndromes (unstable angina and myocardial infarction). Thus, monocyte-macrophages are critical cells in all phases of atherosclerosis.

The importance of monocytes in atherosclerosis in T2DM is supported by a study by Moreno and colleagues,[7] which showed that coronary tissue from diabetic subjects exhibits a larger content of lipid-rich atheroma and macrophage infiltration than tissue from nondiabetic subjects. The risk of plaque rupture correlates poorly with the degree of stenosis: Half of all infarctions occur in arteries that have less than 50% luminal diameter narrowing, underscoring the role of other factors, such as inflammation, in atherosclerosis. Experiments on knockout and transgenic mice have underscored the importance of the various cytokines (e.g., IL-1), chemokines (e.g., MCP-1), and adhesion molecules (e.g., VCAM, P-selectin) in atherogenesis, emphasizing the importance of the inflammatory component (Table 8–1).

Numerous inflammatory markers have been shown to predict cardiovascular events. These include soluble cell-adhesion molecules, cytokines, chemokines, the CD40–CD40L dyad, acute phase reactants such as fibrinogen, serum amyloid A, and C-reactive protein.

Increasing evidence shows that interaction between CD40 and CD40 ligand (CD40L) plays a crucial role in the pathogenesis of atherosclerosis.[8-10] Disruption of CD40 signaling in hypercholesterolemic mice diminishes the formation and progression of atherosclerotic plaques. Furthermore, interference with CD40 ligation promotes changes in plaque composition that are associated in humans with lesions less prone to rupture, such as increased content of smooth muscle cells and collagen fibrils as well as decreased lipid and macrophage accumulation.

CD40L can occur in soluble form in plasma (sCD40L). Patients with unstable angina have higher levels of sCD40L than patients with stable angina or healthy volunteers. Also, there is a significant correlation between elevated levels of sCD40L and future cardiovascular events in apparently healthy middle-aged women.

Varo's group[11] demonstrated a significant ($P < 0.001$) association between plasma sCD40L and type 1 and type 2 diabetes. This association was independent of total cholesterol, high-density lipoprotein cholesterol, low-density lipoprotein cholesterol, triglycerides, blood pressure, body mass index, gender, C-reactive protein, and sICAM-1 (soluble ICAM-1). Furthermore, in a pilot study, administration of troglitazone (12 weeks, 600 mg/day) to patients with T2DM significantly diminished sCD40L plasma levels by 29%.[12] Lim and coworkers[13] showed similar results: Diabetic patients with microangiopathy had increased levels of plasma sCD40L compared with those who did not have microangiopathy and with matched controls. Jinchuan and coworkers[14] also showed that coronary heart disease patients with diabetes had increased levels of CD40 and CD40L coexpression on platelets as well as sCD40L compared with controls ($P < 0.01$). A positive correlation was found between serum AGE levels and CD40–CD40L interaction in patients with diabetes.

Table 8–1. Evidence Supporting the Pivotal Role of Inflammation in Atherosclerosis: Animal Models with Knockouts of the Inflammatory Cascade

Knockout	Atherosclerosis
eNOS	increased
VCAM, P-selectin	decreased
MCP-1, IL-8	decreased
CD40/40L	decreased
IL-1	decreased

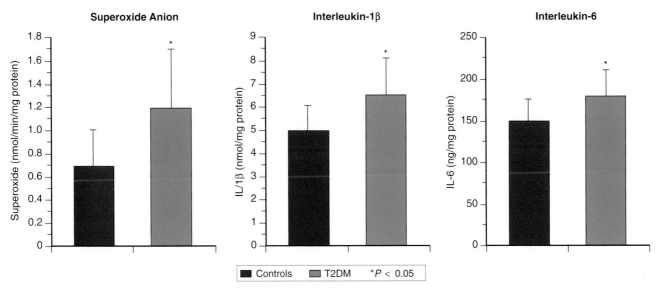

Figure 8–4. Superoxide anion and cytokine release from lipopolysaccharide-activated monocytes in type 2 diabetes. (From Devaraj S, Jialal I: Low-density lipoprotein postsecretory modification, monocyte function, and circulating adhesion molecules in type 2 diabetic patients with and without macrovascular complications: The effect of alpha-tocopherol supplementation. Circulation 102:191–196, 2000).

the IL-1β gene cluster is a potential candidate in the pathogenesis of diabetic nephropathy.[92] In vitro studies have shown that hyperglycemia can promote IL-1 release from monocytes and islet cells.[93] We have shown that human monocytes from T2DM subjects secrete more IL-1β compared with matched nondiabetic control subjects.[94]

TNF is another proinflammatory cytokine secreted by monocyte-macrophages, endothelial cells, and, to a large extent, by adipose tissue. Studies in mouse models of obesity have shown that adipose tissue in obese mice is characterized by macrophage infiltration, and these macrophages are an important source of inflammation in this tissue.[95,96] Thus it appears that obesity is associated with a local low-grade inflammation characterized by increased macrophage infiltration of adipose tissue and production of inflammatory cytokines, such as IL-6 and TNF-α.

TNF-α is a multifunctional cytokine that exerts pleiotropic biologic actions.[97] It activates endothelial cells and stimulates angiogenesis. Increased mRNA for TNF-α has been documented in carotid atherosclerotic plaques.[97-99] TNF-α processing via its receptor can promote apoptosis and contribute to the necrotic core of the atherosclerotic lesion. TNF-α also plays a role in the pathogenesis of obesity-linked insulin resistance.[97-99] Desfaits and coworkers have observed a significant increase in the level of lipopolysaccharide-stimulated TNF-α release from monocytes of T2DM.[100] In human subjects, TNF mRNA and protein positively correlate with body adiposity, and they decrease in obese subjects with weight loss.[101] Guha and coworkers[102] have shown that chronic hyperglycemia causes a dramatic increase in the release of TNF-α, through enhanced

TNF-α mRNA transcription, mediated by ROS via activation of transcription factors NF-κB and activating protein 1 (AP-1).

Hotamisligil and coworkers[97] first demonstrated that adipocytes constitutively express TNF. TNF expression in adipocytes of obese animals (ob/ob mouse, db/db mouse, and fa/fa Zucker rat) is markedly increased, and neutralization of TNF by soluble TNF receptor also leads to a decrease in insulin resistance in these animals. These observations provided the first link between an increase in the expression and the plasma concentration of a proinflammatory cytokine and insulin resistance.

APPROACHES TO ANTI-INFLAMMATION

IL-10 and Diabetes

The potential role of anti-inflammatory cytokines in diabetes is understudied. IL-10 is a potent anti-inflammatory cytokine. In the Leiden 85-Plus study, the odds ratio for T2DM was 2.7 (95% CI, 1.5-4.9) when subjects with the lowest IL-10 production capacity (in whole blood activated with lipopolysaccharide) were compared with subjects who had the highest IL-10 production capacity.[103] Esposito and colleagues[104] have shown that in both obese and nonobese women, IL-10 levels were lower in those with the metabolic syndrome than in women without the metabolic syndrome: In obese women the levels were 1.3 pg/mL versus 4.5 pg/mL (median; $P < 0.01$), respectively; in nonobese

women the levels were 0.9 pg/mL versus 1.3 pg/mL ($P < 0.05$), respectively.

Gunnett's group[105] has shown that maximum relaxation in vessels from diabetic IL-10–/– mice was significantly decreased (74 ± 5%) compared with nondiabetic IL-10–/– mice (93% ± 2%, $P < 0.05$). Thus, diabetes produces greater impairment of relaxation to acetylcholine in IL-10–/– mice than in IL-10+/+ mice. These findings provide direct evidence that IL-10 impedes mechanisms of endothelial dysfunction during diabetes.

Adiponectin and Diabetes

Adiponectin is another novel polypeptide that is very specific to adipose tissue, present in human plasma, and reported to be decreased in obesity, T2DM, and coronary heart disease.[106-109] Studies have demonstrated that body weight loss either by restrictive surgery[110] or with a very-low-calorie diet[111] increases plasma concentration of adiponectin. One study has observed that plasma concentration of adiponectin is inversely and more closely related to degree of insulin resistance than to the degree of adiposity.[108] We have shown lower plasma concentration of adiponectin in nonobese insulin-resistant South Asian men compared with white men (matched for age and body fat) who were not insulin resistant.[112] Higher plasma concentrations of adiponectin are associated with lower risk of myocardial infarction in men, and risk is independent of inflammation.[113]

Adiponectin attenuates TNF-α–mediated inflammatory response[114] and might modulate inflammatory response by inhibiting myelomonocytic cells, probably by inducing apoptosis.[115] Adiponectin modulates endothelial function and has an inhibitory effect on proliferation of vascular smooth muscle cells induced by growth factors.[116] These findings support the notion that adiponectin could have a protective effect against atherosclerosis, and it could be the link connecting obesity, T2DM, and atherosclerosis.

CONCLUSION

It is clear that diabetes is a proinflammatory state (Box 8-2). This is evidenced by increased levels of hsCRP, fibrinogen, and PAI-1 as well as sCAMs, sCD40, and proinflammatory cytokines. Studies are needed to answer the question of whether the diabetes begets inflammation or if a proinflammatory state precipitates the development of diabetic vasculopathies. Targeting inflammation with weight loss, statins, and peroxisome proliferator activated receptor-γ (PPAR-γ) agonists will lead to decreased cardiovascular disease and diabetes.

Box 8-2. Evidence Supporting Increased Inflammation in Diabetes

- Increased levels of hs-CRP
- Increased levels of plasma and monocytic cytokines, IL-1, TNF, IL-6
- Decreased levels of IL-10
- Increased levels of soluble cell adhesion molecules
- Increased levels of PAI-1 and fibrinogen
- Increased CD40 and sCD40L
- Decreased levels of adiponectin
- Increased activity of protein kinase C, NADPH oxidase, NF-κB

CRP, C-reactive protein; IL, interleukin; NADPH, nicotinamide adenine dinucleotide phosphate; NF-κB, nuclear factor κB; PAI, plasminogen activator inhibitor; TNF, tumor necrosis factor.

Acknowledgments

This work is supported by grants from the National Institutes of Health: NIH K24AT00596, NIH RO1 AT 00596, NIH DK69801; from the Juvenile Diabetes Foundation; from the American Diabetes Association; from the Centers for Disease Control and Prevention: H75/CCH523202; and from the American Heart Association: 0465017Y.

References

1. Stamler J, Vaccaro O, Neaton JD, Wentworth D: Diabetes, other risk factors, and 12-year cardiovascular mortality for men screened in the Multiple Risk Factor Intervention Trial. Diabetes Care 16:434-444, 1993.
2. Haffner SM, Lehto S, Ronemaa T, et al: Mortality from coronary heart disease in subjects with type 2 diabetes and in nondiabetic subjects with and without prior myocardial infarction. New Engl J Med 339:229-234, 1998.
3. Vega-Lopez S, Devaraj S, Jialal I: Oxidative stress and antioxidant supplementation in the management of diabetic cardiovascular disease. J Investig Med 52:24-32, 2004.
4. Libby P: Inflammation in atherogenesis. Nature 420:868-874, 2003.
5. Ross R: Atherosclerosis—an inflammatory disease. N Engl J Med 340:115-126, 1999.
6. Lusis AJ: Atherosclerosis. Nature 407:233-241, 2000.
7. Moreno PR, Murcia AM, Palacios IF, et al: Coronary composition and macrophage infiltration in atherectomy specimens from patients with diabetes mellitus. Circulation 102:2180-2184, 2000.
8. Schonbeck U, Libby P: CD40 signaling and plaque instability. Circ Res 89:1092-1103, 2001.
9. Schonbeck U, Libby P: The CD40/CD154 receptor/ligand dyad. Cell Mol Life Sci 58:4-43, 2001.
10. Mach F, Schonbeck U, Libby P: CD40 signaling in vascular cells: A key role in atherosclerosis? Atherosclerosis 137(Suppl):S89-S95, 1998.
11. Varo N, de Lemos JA, Libby P, et al: Soluble CD40L: Risk prediction after acute coronary syndromes. Circulation 108:1049-1052, 2003.
12. Varo N, Vicent D, Libby P, et al: Elevated plasma levels of the atherogenic mediator soluble CD40 ligand in diabetic patients: A novel target of thiazolidinediones. Circulation 107:2664-2669, 2003.

13. Lim HS, Blann AD, Lip GY: Soluble CD40 ligand, soluble P-selection, interleukin-6, and tissue factor in diabetes mellitus: Relationships to cardiovascular disease and risk factor intervention. Circulation 109:2524-2528, 2004.

14. Jinchuan Y, Zonggui W, Jinming C, Li L, et al: Upregulation of CD40–CD40 ligand system in patients with diabetes mellitus. Clin Chim Acta 339:85-90, 2004.

15. Jialal I, Devaraj S: Inflammation and atherosclerosis: The value of the high-sensitivity C-reactive protein assay as a risk marker. Am J Clin Pathol 116(Suppl):S108-S115, 2001.

16. Thompson D, Pepys MB, Wood SP: The physiological structure of human CRP and its complex with phospholipids. Structure 7:169-177, 1999.

17. Tracy RP: Inflammation markers and coronary heart disease. Curr Opin Lipidol 10:435-451, 1999.

18. Calabro P, Willerson JT, Yeh ET: Inflammatory cytokines stimulated C-reactive protein production by human coronary artery smooth muscle cells Circulation 108:1930-1932, 2003.

19. Kobayashi S, Inoue N, Ohashi Y, et al: Interaction of oxidative stress and inflammatory response in coronary plaque instability: Important role of C-reactive protein. Arterioscler Thromb Vasc Biol 23:1398-1404, 2003.

20. Yasojima K, Schwab C, McGeer EG, McGeer PL: Generation of C-reactive protein and complement components in atherosclerotic plaques. Am J Pathol 158:1039-1051, 2001.

21. Rifai N, Ridker OM: hsCRP—a novel and promising marker of CHD. Clin Chem 47:403-411, 2001.

22. Jialal I, Devaraj S: Role of C-reactive protein in the assessment of cardiovascular risk. Am J Cardiol 91:200-202, 2003.

23. Verma S, Yeh ET: C-reactive protein and atherothrombosis—beyond a biomarker: An actual partaker of lesion formation. Am J Physiol Regul Integr Comp Physiol 285:R1253-R1256, 2003.

24. Pasceri V, Cheng JS, Willerson JT, et al: Modulation of C-reactive protein–mediated monocyte chemoattractant protein-1 induction in human endothelial cells by anti-atherosclerosis drugs. Circulation 103:2531-2534, 2001.

25. Venugopal SK, Devaraj S, Yuhanna I, et al: Demonstration that C-reactive protein decreases eNOS expression and bioactivity in human aortic endothelial cells. Circulation 106:1439-1441, 2002.

26. Verma S, Wang CH, Li SH, et al: A self-fulfilling prophecy: C-reactive protein attenuates nitric oxide production and inhibits angiogenesis. Circulation 106:913-919, 2002.

27. Venugopal SK, Devaraj S, Jialal I: C-reactive protein decreases prostacyclin release from human aortic endothelial cells. Circulation 108:1676-1678, 2003.

28. Devaraj S, Xu DY, Jialal I: C-reactive protein increases plasminogen activator inhibitor-1 expression and activity in human aortic endothelial cells: Implications for the metabolic syndrome and atherothrombosis. Circulation 107:398-404, 2003.

29. Hattori Y, Matsumura M, Kasai K: Vascular smooth muscle cell activation by C-reactive protein. Cardiovasc Res 58:186-195, 2003.

30. Pickup JC, Mattock MB, Chusney GD, et al: NIDDM as a disease of the innate immune system: Association of acute-phase reactants and interleukin-6 with metabolic syndrome. Diabetologia 40:1286-1292, 1997.

31. Devaraj S, Jialal I: Alpha tocopherol supplementation decreases serum C-reactive protein and monocyte interleukin-6 levels in normal volunteers and type 2 diabetic patients. Free Radic Biol Med 29:790-792, 2000.

32. Ford ES: The metabolic syndrome and C-reactive protein, fibrinogen, and leukocyte count: Findings from the Third National Health and Nutrition Examination Survey. Atherosclerosis 168:351-358, 2003.

33. Tan KC, Chow WS, Tam SC, et al: Atorvastatin lowers C-reactive protein and improves endothelium-dependent vasodilation in type 2 diabetes mellitus. J Clin Endocrinol Metab 87:563-568, 2002.

34. Jager A, van Hinsbergh VW, Kostense PJ, et al: von Willebrand factor, C-reactive protein, and 5-year mortality in diabetic and nondiabetic subjects: The Hoorn Study. Arterioscler Thromb Vasc Biol 19:3071-3078, 1999.

35. Festa A, D'Agostino R, Howard G, et al: Chronic subclinical inflammation as part of the insulin resistance syndrome—The Insulin Resistance Atherosclerosis Study (IRAS). Circulation 102:42-47, 2000.

36. Chandalia M, Cabo-Chan AV Jr, Devaraj S, et al: Elevated plasma high-sensitivity C-reactive protein concentrations in Asian Indians living in the United States. J Clin Endocrinol Metab 88:3773-3776, 2003.

37. Folsom AR, Aleksic N, Catellier D, et al: C-reactive protein and incident coronary heart disease in the Atherosclerosis Risk In Communities (ARIC) study. Am Heart J 144:233-238, 2002.

38. Tracy RP, Lemaitre RN, Psaty BM, et al: Relationship of C-reactive protein to risk of cardiovascular disease in the elderly. Results from the Cardiovascular Health Study and the Rural Health Promotion Project. Arterioscler Thromb Vasc Biol 17:1121-1127, 1997.

39. Lindsay RS, Krakoff J, Hanson RL, et al: Gamma globulin levels predict type 2 diabetes in the Pima Indian population. Diabetes 50:1598-1603, 2001.

40. Bermudez EA, Rifai N, Buring J, et al: Interrelationships among circulating interleukin-6, C-reactive protein, and traditional cardiovascular risk factors in women. Arterioscler Thromb Vasc Biol 22:1668-1673, 2002.

41. Freeman DJ, Norrie J, Caslake MJ, et al, for the West of Scotland Coronary Prevention Study: C-reactive protein is an independent predictor of risk for the development of diabetes in the West of Scotland Coronary Prevention Study. Diabetes 51:1596-1600, 2002.

42. Thorand B, Lowel H, Schneider A, et al: C-reactive protein as a predictor for incident diabetes mellitus among middle-aged men: Results from the MONICA Augsburg cohort study, 1984-1998. Arch Intern Med 163:93-99, 2003.

43. Pradhan AD, Manson JE, Rifai N, et al: C-reactive protein, interleukin 6, and risk of developing type 2 diabetes mellitus. JAMA 286:327-334, 2001.

44. Muntner P, He J, Chen J, et al: Prevalence of non-traditional cardiovascular disease risk factors among persons with impaired fasting glucose, impaired glucose tolerance, diabetes, and the metabolic syndrome: Analysis of the Third National Health and Nutrition Examination Survey (NHANES III). Ann Epidemiol 14:686-695, 2004.

45. Hanley AJ, Festa A, D'Agostino RB Jr, et al: Metabolic and inflammation variable clusters and prediction of type 2 diabetes: Factor analysis using directly measured insulin sensitivity. Diabetes 53:1773-1781, 2004.

46. Magyar MT, Szikszai Z, Balla J, et al: Early-onset carotid atherosclerosis is associated with increased intima-media thickness and elevated serum levels of inflammatory markers. Stroke 34:58-63, 2003.

47. Liu S, Manson JE, Buring JE, et al: Relation between a diet with a high glycemic load and plasma concentrations of high-sensitivity C-reactive protein in middle-aged women. Am J Clin Nutr 75:492-498, 2002.

48. Kiechl S, Werner P, Egger G, et al: Active and passive smoking, chronic infections, and the risk of carotid atherosclerosis: Prospective results from the Bruneck Study. Stroke 33:2170-2176, 2002.

49. Cao JJ, Thach C, Manolio TA, et al: C-reactive protein, carotid intima-media thickness, and incidence of ischemic stroke in the elderly: The Cardiovascular Health Study. Circulation 108:166-170, 2003.

50. Verma S, Wang CH, Weisel RD, et al: Hyperglycemia potentiates the proatherogenic effects of C-reactive protein: Reversal with rosiglitazone. J Mol Cell Cardiol 35:417-419, 2003.

51. Devaraj S, Xu DY, Jialal I: C-reactive protein increases plasminogen activator inhibitor–1 expression and activity in human aortic endothelial cells: Implications for the metabolic syndrome and atherothrombosis. Circulation 107:398-404, 2003.

52. Sebestjen M, Zegura B, Guzic-Salobir B, et al: Fibrinolytic parameters and insulin resistance in young survivors of myocardial infarction with heterozygous familial hypercholesterolemia. Wien Klin Wochenschr 113:113-118, 2001.

53. Wiman B, Andersson T, Hallqvist J, et al: Plasma levels of tissue plasminogen activator/plasminogen activator inhibitor–1 complex and von Willebrand factor are significant risk markers for recurrent myocardial infarction in the Stockholm Heart Epidemiology Program (SHEEP) study. Arterioscler Thromb Vasc Biol 20:2019-2023, 2000.

54. Eren M, Painter CA, Atkinson JB, et al: Age-dependent spontaneous coronary arterial thrombosis in transgenic mice that express a stable form of human plasminogen activator inhibitor–1. Circulation 106:491-496, 2002.

55. Schafer K, Muller K, Hecke A, et al: Enhanced thrombosis in atherosclerosis-prone mice is associated with increased arterial expression of plasminogen activator inhibitor–1. Arterioscler Thromb Vasc Biol 23:2097-2103, 2003.

56. Eitzman DT, Westrick RJ, Xu Z, et al: PAI-1 deficiency protects against atherosclerosis progression in the mouse carotid artery. Blood 96:4212-4215, 2000.

57. Xiao Q, Danton MJ, Witte DP, et al: Plasminogen deficiency accelerates vessel wall disease in mice predisposed to atherosclerosis. Proc Natl Acad Sci U S A 94:10335-10340, 1997.

58. Fujii S, Goto D, Zaman T, et al: Diminished fibrinolysis and thrombosis: Clinical implications for accelerated atherosclerosis. J Atheroscler Thromb 5:76-81, 1998.

59. Alessi MC, Juhan-Vague I: Contribution of PAI-1 in cardiovascular pathology. Arch Mal Coeur Vaiss 97:673-678, 2004.

60. Festa A, D'Agostino R Jr, Mykkanen L, et al: Relative contribution of insulin and its precursors to fibrinogen and PAI-1 in a large population with different states of glucose tolerance. The Insulin Resistance Atherosclerosis Study (IRAS). Arterioscler Thromb Vasc Biol 19:562-568, 1999.

61. Fibrinogen Studies Collaboration. Collaborative meta-analysis of prospective studies of plasma fibrinogen and cardiovascular disease. Eur J Cardiovasc Prev Rehabil 11:9-17, 2004.

62. Bolibar I, Kienast J, Thompson SG, et al: Relation of fibrinogen to presence and severity of coronary artery disease is independent of other coexisting heart disease. The ECAT Angina Pectoris Study Group. Am Heart J 125:1601-1605, 1993.

63. Dotevall A, Johansson S, Wilhelmsen L: Association between fibrinogen and other risk factors for cardiovascular disease in men and women. Results from the Goteborg MONICA survey 1985. Ann Epidemiol 4:369-374, 1994.

64. Dunn EJ, Ariens RA. Fibrinogen and fibrin clot structure in diabetes. Herz 29:470-479, 2004.

65. Wilson PW. Insulin resistance syndrome and the prothrombotic state: A Framingham perspective. Endocr Pract 9(Suppl 2):50-52, 2003.

66. Van De Ree MA, De Maat MP, Kluft C, et al, for the DALI Study Group: Decrease of hemostatic cardiovascular risk factors by aggressive vs. conventional atorvastatin treatment in patients with type 2 diabetes mellitus. J Thromb Haemost 1:1753-1757, 2003.

67. Krieglstein CF, Granger DN: Adhesion molecules and their role in vascular disease. Am J Hypertens 14(6 Pt 2):44S-54S, 2001.

68. Kim JA, Berliner JA, Natarajan RD, et al: Evidence that glucose increases monocyte binding to human aortic endothelial cells. Diabetes 43:1103-1107, 1994.

69. Carantoni M, Abbasi F, Chu L, et al: Adherence of mononuclear cells to endothelium in vitro is increased in patients with NIDDM. Diabetes Care 20:1462-1465, 1997.

70. Hoogerbrugge N, Verkerk A, Jacobs M, et al: Hypertriglyceridemia enhances monocyte binding to endothelial cells in NIDDM. Diabetes Care 3:1122-1124, 1997.

71. Hwang S, Ballantyne CM, Sharrett AR, et al: Circulating adhesion molecules VCAM-1-1, ICAM-1, and E-selectin in Carotid atherosclerosis and incident coronary heart disease cases: The Atherosclerosis Risk In Communities (ARIC) Study. Circulation 96: 4219-4225, 1997.

72. Rohde LE, Lee RT, Jamocochian M, et al: Circulating CAMs are correlated with ultrasound measurement of carotid atherosclerosis. Arterioscler Thromb Vasc Biol 18:1765-1770, 1998.

73. Ridker PM, Hennekens CH, Roitman JB et al: Plasma concentration of soluble ICAM-1 and risks of future MI in apparently healthy men. Lancet 351:88-92, 1998.

74. Albertini JP. Valensi P. Lormeau B. et al: Elevated concentrations of soluble E-selectin and vascular cell adhesion molecule–1 in NIDDM. Effect of intensive insulin treatment. Diabetes Care 21:1008-1013, 1998.

75. Fasching P, Waldhausl W, Wagner OF: Elevated circulating adhesion molecules in NIDDM—potential mediators in diabetic macroangiopathy. Diabetologia 39:1242-1244, 1996.

76. Matsumoto K, Sera Y, Abe Y: Serum concentrations of soluble vascular cell adhesion molecule–1 and e-selectin are elevated in insulin-resistant patients with type 2 diabetes. Diabetes Care 24:1697-1698, 2001.

77. Hofmann MA, Schiekofer S, Isermann B, et al: Peripheral blood mononuclear cells isolated from patients with diabetic nephropathy show increased activation of the oxidative-stress sensitive transcription factor NF-κB. Diabetologia 42:222-232, 1999.

78. Black PH: The inflammatory response is an integral part of the stress response: Implications for atherosclerosis, insulin resistance, type II diabetes and metabolic syndrome X. Brain Behav Immun 17:350-364, 2003.

79. Tilg H, Dinarello CA, Mier JW: IL-6 and APPs: Anti-inflammatory and immunosuppressive mediators. Immunol Today 18:428-432, 1997.

80. Fantuzzi G, Dinarello CA: The inflammatory response in interleukin-1β–deficient mice: Comparison with other cytokine-related knock-out mice. J Leukoc Biol 59:489-493, 1996.

81. Olencki T, Finke J, Tubbs R, et al: Phase 1 trial of subcutaneous IL-6 in patients with refractory cancer: Clinical and biologic effects. J Immunother 23:549-556, 2000.

82. Dandona P, Aljada A, Bandyopadhyay A: Inflammation: The link between insulin resistance, obesity and diabetes. Trends Immunol 25:4-7, 2004.

83. Pickup JC, Chusney GD, Thomas SM, Burt D: Plasma interleukin-6, tumour necrosis factor alpha and blood cytokine production in type 2 diabetes. Life Sci 67: 291-300, 2000.

84. Devaraj S, Jialal I: Alpha tocopherol supplementation decreases serum C-reactive protein and monocyte interleukin-6 levels in normal volunteers and type 2 diabetic patients. Free Radic Biol Med 29:790-792, 2000.

85. Fasshauer M, Paschke R: Regulation of adipocytokines and insulin resistance. Diabetologia 46:1594-1603, 2003.

86. Arner P: Regional differences in protein production by human adipose tissue. Biochem Soc Trans 29(Pt 2):72-75, 2001.

87. Galea J, Armstrong J, Gadsdon P, et al: IL-1β in coronary arteries of patients with ischemic heart disease. Arterioscler Thromb Vasc Biol 16:1000-1006, 1996.

88. Bevilacqua M, Pober J, Wheeler M, et al: Interleukin 1 acts on cultured human vascular endothelium to increase the adhesion of polymorphonuclear leukocytes, monocytes, and related leukocyte cell lines. J Clin Invest 76:2003-2008, 1985.

89. Maziere C, Barbu V, Auclair M, Maziere JC: Interleukin 1 stimulates cholesterol esterification and cholesterol deposition in J774 monocytes-macrophages. Biochim Biophys Acta 1300:30-34, 1996.

90. Raines E, Dower S, Ross R: Interleukin-1 mitogenic activity for fibroblasts and smooth muscle cells is due to PDGF-AA. Science 243:393-395, 1989.

91. Kirii H, Niwa T, Yamada Y, et al: Lack of interleukin-1β decreases the severity of atherosclerosis in ApoE-deficient mice. Arterioscler Thromb Vasc Biol 23:656-660, 2003.

92. Loughrey BV, Maxwell AP, Fogarty DG, et al: An interleukin 1β allele, which correlates with a high secretor phenotype, is associated with diabetic nephropathy. Cytokine 10:984-988, 1998.

93. Orlinska U, Newton RC: Role of glucose in IL-1β production in LPS-activated human monocytes. J Cell Physiol 157:201-208, 1993.

94. Devaraj S, Jialal I: Low-density lipoprotein postsecretory modification, monocyte function, and circulating adhesion molecules in type 2 diabetic patients with and without macrovascular complications: The effect of alpha-tocopherol supplementation. Circulation 102:191-196, 2000.

95. Xu H, Barnes GT, Yang Q, et al: Chronic inflammation in fat plays a crucial role in the development of obesity-related insulin resistance. J Clin Invest 112:1821-1830, 2003.

96. Weisberg SP, McCann D, Desai M, et al: Obesity is associated with macrophage accumulation in adipose tissue. J Clin Invest 112:1796-1808, 2003.

97. Hotamisligil GS, Shargill NS, Spiegelman BM: Adipose expression of tumor necrosis factor-α: Direct role in obesity-linked insulin resistance. Science 259:87-91, 1993.

98. Arner P: The adipocyte in insulin resistance: Key molecules and the impact of the thiazolidinediones. Trends Endocrinol Metab 14:137-145, 2003.

99. Kern PA, Saghizadeh M, Ong JM, et al: The expression of tumor necrosis factor in human adipose tissue. Regulation by obesity, weight loss, and relationship to lipoprotein lipase. J Clin. Invest 95:2111-2119, 1995.

100. Desfaits AC, Serri O, Renier G: Normalization of plasma lipid peroxides, monocyte adhesion, and tumor necrosis factor-α production in NIDDM patients after gliclazide treatment. Diabetes Care 21:487-493, 1998.

101. Dandona P, Weinstock R, Thusu K, et al: Tumor necrosis factor-α in sera of obese patients: Fall with weight loss. J Clin Endocrinol Metab 83:2907-2910, 1998.

102. Guha M, Bai W, Nadler JL, et al: Molecular mechanisms of tumor necrosis factor alpha gene expression in monocytic cells via hyperglycemia-induced oxidant stress-dependent and -independent pathways. J Biol Chem 275:17728-17739, 2000.

103. van Exel E, Gussekloo J, de Craen AJ, et al, for the Leiden 85 Plus Study: Low production capacity of interleukin-10 associates with the metabolic syndrome and type 2 diabetes: The Leiden 85-Plus Study. Diabetes 51:1088-1092, 2000.

104. Esposito K, Pontillo A, Giugliano F, et al: Association of low interleukin-10 levels with the metabolic syndrome in obese women. J Clin Endocrinol Metab 88:1055-1058, 2003.

105. Gunnett CA, Heistad DD, Faraci FM: Interleukin-10 protects nitric oxide–dependent relaxation during diabetes: Role of superoxide. Diabetes 51:1931-1937, 2002.

106. Arita Y, Kihara S, Ouchi N, et al: Paradoxical decrease of an adipose-specific protein, adiponectin, in obesity. Biochem Biophys Res Commun 257:79-83, 1999.

107. Hotta K, Funahashi T, Arita Y, et al: Plasma concentrations of a novel, adipose-specific protein, adiponectin, in type 2 diabetic patients. Arterioscler Thromb Vasc Biol 20:1595-1599, 2000.

108. Weyer C, Funahashi T, Tanaka S, et al: Hypoadiponectinemia in obesity and type 2 diabetes: Close association with insulin resistance and hyperinsulinemia. J Clin Endocrinol Metab 86:1930-1935, 2000.

109. Kumada M, Kihara S, Sumitsuji S, et al, for the Osaka CAD Study Group: Coronary artery disease. Association of hypoadiponectinemia with coronary artery disease in men. Arterioscler Thromb Vasc Biol 23:85-89, 2003.

110. Yang WS, Lee WJ, Funahashi T, et al: Weight reduction increases plasma levels of an adipose-derived anti-inflammatory protein, adiponectin. J Clin Endocrinol Metab 86:3815-3819, 2001.

111. Xydakis AM, Case CC, Jones PH, et al: Adiponectin, inflammation, and the expression of the metabolic syndrome in obese individuals: the impact of rapid weight loss through caloric restriction. J Clin Endocrinol Metab 89:2697-2703, 2004.

112. Abate N, Chandalia M, Snell PG, et al: Adipose tissue metabolites and insulin resistance in nondiabetic Asian Indian men. J Clin Endocrinol Metab 89:2750-2755, 2004.

113. Pischon T, Girman CJ, Hotamisligil GS, et al: Plasma adiponectin levels and risk of myocardial infarction in men. JAMA 291:1730-1737, 2004.

114. Ouchi N, Kihara S, Arita Y, et al: Adiponectin, an adipocyte-derived plasma protein, inhibits endothelial NF-κB signaling through a cAMP-dependent pathway. Circulation 102:1296-1301, 2000.

115. Yokota T, Oritani K, Takahashi I, et al: Adiponectin, a new member of the family of soluble defense collagens, negatively regulates the growth of myelomonocytic progenitors and the functions of macrophages. Blood 96:1723-1732, 2000.

116. Matsuzawa Y, Funahashi T, Nakamura T: Molecular mechanism of metabolic syndrome X: Contribution of adipocytokines adipocyte-derived bioactive substances. Ann N Y Acad Sci 892:146-154, 1999.

Chapter 9

Diabetic Ketoacidosis and Hyperglycemic Hyperosmolar Syndrome

Guillermo E. Umpierrez and Dawn Smiley

KEY POINTS

- *Diabetic ketoacidosis is a triad of uncontrolled hyperglycemia, metabolic acidosis, and increased total body ketone concentration.*
- *Diabetic ketoacidosis is the initial manifestation of diabetes in approximately 25% to 40% of children and adolescents and 15% to 20% of adults; hyperglycemic hyperosmolar syndrome is the initial manifestation of diabetes in 20% of adults.*
- *Diabetic ketoacidosis is associated with a mortality rate of less than 5%, and hyperglycemic hyperosmolar syndrome is associated with a mortality rate of 5% to 25%.*
- *When insulin is deficient, hyperglycemia develops as a result of increased gluconeogenesis, accelerated glycogenolysis, and impaired glucose use by peripheral tissues. Ketoacidosis results from insulin deficiency and excess counterregulatory hormones.*
- *Management of diabetic ketoacidosis and hyperglycemic hyperosmolar syndrome consists of fluid replacement, correction of hyperglycemia and metabolic acidosis, electrolyte replacement, detection and treatment of precipitating causes, and proper conversion to maintenance insulin.*
- *Causes of DKA include infection, intercurrent illness, psychological stress, and noncompliance with therapy. Improved education regarding sick-day management is paramount.*

Diabetic ketoacidosis (DKA) is the most serious hyperglycemic emergency in patients with type 1 and type 2 diabetes mellitus. DKA is responsible for more than 100,000 hospital admissions and 500,000 hospital days per year in the United States at substantial expenditures related to direct medical expenses and indirect costs. In spite of advances in our understanding of its pathogenesis and more-uniform agreement about the diagnosis and treatment, DKA continues to be an important cause of morbidity and mortality among patients with diabetes. DKA is the leading cause of mortality in children with type 1 diabetes. In adult patients, recent controlled studies have reported a mortality rate less than 5%, with higher mortality observed in elderly subjects and in patients with concomitant life-threatening illnesses.

The triad of uncontrolled hyperglycemia, metabolic acidosis, and increased total body ketone concentration characterizes DKA. These metabolic derangements result from the combination of absolute or relative insulin deficiency and an increase in counterregulatory hormones (glucagon, catecholamines, cortisol, and growth hormone). Successful treatment of DKA requires frequent monitoring of patients, improvement of circulatory volume and tissue perfusion, correction of hypovolemia and hyperglycemia, replacement of electrolyte losses, and a careful search for the precipitating cause.

This chapter reviews recent advances in the epidemiology, diagnosis, and pathogenesis and the current recommendations for management of adult patients with DKA.

EPIDEMIOLOGY

Diabetic ketoacidosis is present in approximately 25% to 40% of diabetic children and adolescents[1] and in 15% to 20% of adult patients at the time of diagnosis of diabetes.[2,3] DKA is reported to be responsible for more than 100,000 hospital admissions per year in the United States,[4,5] and it accounts for 4% to 9% of all hospital discharge summaries among patients with diabetes.[2] In a Danish study, the incidence was 8.5 per 100,000 total population in the years 1975 to 1979.[6] A higher figure was reported by the EURODIAB (European diabetes) study, where 8.6% of 3,250 subjects with type 1 diabetes throughout Europe had been admitted with DKA in the previous 12 months.[7] Recent epidemiologic studies indicate that hospitalizations for DKA have increased since the mid 1980s, and the majority of cases occur as recurrent cases in the same subjects.[2,3]

In many reported series, women have been more likely than men to develop DKA, with a female-to-male ratio of 1.8:1.5[2,7]; however, recent reports suggest that this ratio is falling, particularly among the subgroup of patients with repeated admissions

in DKA.[3,8] In the United States, more than 60% of urban black patients with DKA are men.[3]

Most patients with DKA have autoimmune type 1 diabetes mellitus; however, patients with type 2 diabetes are also at risk during the catabolic stress of acute illness such as trauma, surgery, or infection. In contrast to popular belief, DKA is more common in adults than in children.[9] In community-based studies, more than 40% of patients with DKA are older than 40 years and more than 20% are older than 55 years.[10] Since the mid 1990s, an increasing number of ketoacidosis cases without precipitating cause have been reported in children, adolescents, and adult subjects with type 2 diabetes.[11-13]

More than half of obese African Americans with newly diagnosed diabetes manifesting with diabetic ketoacidosis have type 2 diabetes.[3] At presentation, they have markedly impaired insulin secretion and insulin action.[13,14] Intensified diabetic management results in significant improvement in beta cell function and insulin sensitivity sufficient to allow discontinuation of insulin therapy within a few months of follow-up.[15,16] One study showed that 10 years after diabetes onset, 40% of patients with ketosis-prone type 2 diabetes are still not insulin dependent.[14] This clinical presentation has been reported primarily in Africans and African Americans[12,13,16-18] but also in other minority ethnic groups,[19-21] and it has been referred to in the literature as idiopathic type 1 diabetes, atypical diabetes mellitus, type 1.5 diabetes, and more recently as ketosis-prone type 2 diabetes.[18,22-24]

Despite their presentation in DKA, because of the presence of obesity, a strong family history of diabetes, measurable insulin secretion, and a low prevalence of autoimmune markers of beta cell destruction, these patients appear to have type 2 diabetes. Although the mechanisms for beta cell dysfunction are not known, preliminary evidence suggests that patients with ketosis-prone type 2 diabetes display a unique propensity to glucose toxicity. Increased recognition of idiopathic or ketosis-prone type 2 diabetes has highlighted the difficulties in distinguishing the etiology of diabetes in some ethnic groups without sophisticated laboratory evaluation.

Treatment of patients with DKA uses significant health care resources. In 1983, the annual cost of hospitalization for DKA in Rhode Island was estimated to be $225 million.[2] More recently, it was estimated that treatment of DKA episodes accounts for one out of every four health care dollars spent on direct medical care for adult patients with type 1 diabetes and for one of every two dollars in patients experiencing multiple episodes of DKA.[25] Proportional costs are probably higher for children, adolescents, and inner-city minority populations. Based on an estimated number of 100,000 cases of DKA per year and estimated medical care charges of more than $10,000 per patient,[25,26] the annual hospital cost for patients with DKA in the United States may be greater than $1 billion.

Reported mortality from DKA in population-based studies and in studies using standardized written guidelines for therapy have demonstrated rates less than 5% in patients with DKA.[9,27-30] Complications related to DKA are the most common cause of death in children, teenagers, and young adults with diabetes, accounting for approximately 50% of all deaths in diabetic patients younger than 24 years of age.[31,32] In adult patients with diabetes, mortality increases substantially with aging, with mortality rates for those older than 65 to 75 years reaching 20% to 40%.[32,33] In the older age groups, the major cause of death relates to the underlying medical illness (i.e., trauma, infection) that precipitated the ketoacidosis,[28,33] but in younger patients, mortality is more likely to be due to the metabolic disarray.[31,34,35]

PRECIPITATING CAUSES

Diabetic ketoacidosis is the initial manifestation of diabetes in approximately 25% to 40% of children and adolescents[1] and in 15% to 20% of adult subjects at the time their diabetes is diagnosed.[2,3] In known diabetic patients, precipitating factors for DKA include infections, intercurrent illnesses, psychological stress, and noncompliance with therapy. Worldwide, infection remains the most common underlying cause, occurring in 30% to 50% of cases.[7,36] Urinary tract infection and pneumonia account for the majority of infections.[3,10,37] Other acute conditions that can precipitate DKA include cerebrovascular accident, alcohol abuse, pancreatitis, pulmonary embolism, myocardial infarction, and trauma. Drugs that affect carbohydrate metabolism such as corticosteroids, thiazides, sympathomimetic agents, and pentamidine can also precipitate DKA. A number of case reports indicate that the conventional antipsychotic as well as atypical antipsychotic drugs produce diabetes. Clozapine and olanzapine, in particular, have been implicated in producing diabetes as well as diabetic ketoacidosis.[38-40]

The evidence that psychological risk factors and insulin omission are the behavior precursors for recurrent DKA has been examined. Patients from families that show little support and adolescent patients whose parents are not involved in the adolescent's diabetes care are at higher risk of recurrent admissions with DKA.[41,42] Psychological problems complicated by eating disorders have been reported in up to 20% of recurrent episodes of ketoacidosis in young women.[43,44] Recently, it was estimated that up to one third of young women with type 1 diabetes have eating disturbances.[44] Omission of insulin can result from the desire or need to escape from the parental home, perhaps associated with sexual, physical, or emotional abuse or neglect[45] or the desire to be perceived as "normal" within their peer circle. In addition to patients' fears about

weight gain and hypoglycemia, diabetes management can be complicated by concomitant depression that is two to three times more prevalent in people with diabetes.

Poor compliance with therapy is a major precipitating cause for DKA in inner-city and medically indigent patients.[3,26,46] In a recent report,[46] the most common cause of DKA was stopping insulin therapy, which occurred in 67% of episodes. In this study, more than 50% of subjects stopped or reduced the dose of insulin because of lack of money or access to medical care; 21% did not know how to alter insulin dosage with change in appetite; 14% stopped insulin for behavioral or psychological reasons; and 14% stopped insulin because they did not know how to manage diabetes on sick days. Substance abuse may also represent an important factor for poor compliance with insulin therapy in inner-city patients with diabetes. We recently reported that a history of alcohol abuse was present in 35% and cocaine use in 13% of patients admitted with DKA.[3]

PATHOPHYSIOLOGY

DKA is a state of severe metabolic decompensation characterized by hyperglycemia, metabolic acidosis, and increased total ketone bodies or ketoacids. Ketoacidosis results from insulin deficiency and excess counterregulatory hormones including glucagon, catecholamines, cortisol, and growth hormone. The insulin deficiency of DKA can be absolute, as is usually the case in patients with autoimmune type 1 diabetes, or the insulin deficiency can be relative, as in patients with type 2 diabetes in the presence of stress or intercurrent illness that causes sudden worsening of insulin resistance and impairment of insulin secretion.[28,31]

The pathophysiology of hyperglycemia and ketoacidosis in DKA is shown in Figures 9-1 and 9-2. When insulin is deficient, hyperglycemia develops as a result of three processes: increased gluconeogenesis, accelerated glycogenolysis, and impaired glucose use by peripheral tissues.[47-51] Increased hepatic glucose production results from the high availability of gluconeogenic precursors, such as amino acids, lactate, and glycerol, and increased activity of gluconeogenic enzymes (phosphoenol pyruvate carboxykinase [PEPCK], fructose-1,6-bisphosphatase, and pyruvate carboxylase).[50,51] Amino acids (alanine and glutamine) increase as a result of accelerated proteolysis and decreased protein synthesis, lactate increases as a result of increased muscle glycogenolysis, and glycerol increases as a result of increased lipolysis.

In addition to insulin deficiency, increased counterregulatory hormones play an important role in glucose overproduction in DKA. Elevated glucagon and catecholamine levels lead to increased gluconeogenesis and glycogenolysis.[52-54] High cortisol

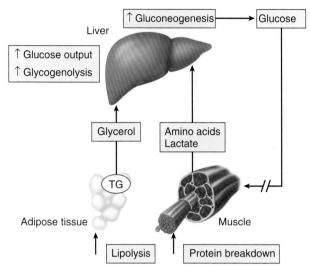

Figure 9–1. Mechanisms for increased glucose production in diabetic ketoacidosis. Hyperglycemia results from a relative or absolute insulin deficiency and excess counterregulatory hormones including glucagon, cortisol, catecholamines, and growth hormone. When insulin is deficient, hyperglycemia develops as a result of three processes: increased gluconeogenesis, accelerated glycogenolysis, and impaired glucose use by peripheral tissues. TG, triglycerides.

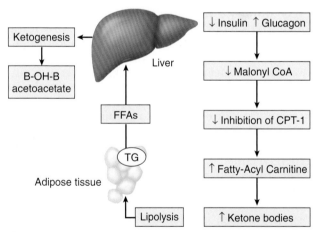

Figure 9–2. Mechanisms for increased ketone bodies in diabetic ketoacidosis. Accumulation of ketone bodies is caused by decrease in insulin levels combined with increase in counterregulatory hormones, particularly epinephrine, which causes the activation of hormone-sensitive lipase in adipose tissue. The increased activity of tissue lipase causes breakdown of triglyceride (TG) into glycerol and free fatty acids (FFAs). In the liver, FFAs are oxidized to ketone bodies, a process predominantly stimulated by glucagon. Increased concentration of glucagon lowers the hepatic levels of malonyl coenzyme A (CoA), which inhibits carnitine palmitoyl-transferase I (CPT I), the rate-limiting enzyme for transesterification of fatty acyl CoA to fatty acyl carnitine, allowing oxidation of fatty acid to ketone bodies.

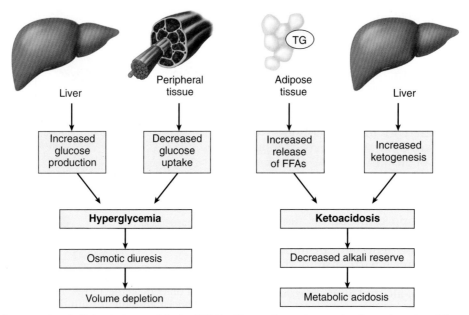

Figure 9–3. Pathogenesis of diabetic ketoacidosis (DKA). Hyperglycemia results from increased hepatic glucose production and impaired glucose use in peripheral tissues (primarily muscle). From a quantitative standpoint, increased hepatic glucose production represents the major pathogenic disturbance responsible for hyperglycemia in patients with DKA. Hyperglycemia causes osmotic diuresis that leads to hypovolemia, decreased glomerular filtration rate, and worsening hyperglycemia. Ketogenesis results in increased release of free fatty acids (FFAs) from adipose tissue. In the liver, free fatty acids are oxidized to ketone bodies. The two major ketone bodies are β-hydroxybutyrate and acetoacetic acid. Accumulation of ketone bodies leads to a decrease in serum bicarbonate concentration and metabolic acidosis. The ketosis and acidosis in DKA contribute to electrolyte disturbances, vomiting, and dehydration.

levels stimulate protein catabolism and increased concentration of circulating amino acids, providing precursors for gluconeogenesis.[48,55] In addition to increased glucose production, the combination of low insulin concentration and high levels of counterregulatory hormones impairs glucose uptake in peripheral tissues.[28,48,49,52,56] Hyperglycemia causes an osmotic diuresis that contributes to hypovolemia and decreases glomerular filtration rate, and this in turn increases the severity of the hyperglycemia.

The increased production of ketone bodies in DKA is caused by a decrease in effective circulating insulin associated with elevations in counterregulatory hormones, particularly epinephrine, which causes the activation of hormone-sensitive lipase in adipose tissue.[57,58] The increased activity of tissue lipase causes breakdown of triglyceride into glycerol and free fatty acids.[43] Once released, glycerol serves as a carbon skeleton for gluconeogenesis in the liver,[51,59] but it is the increased release of free fatty acids that constitutes the primary mechanism for ketoacid production[49,51] (Fig. 9-3). In the liver, free fatty acids are oxidized to ketone bodies, a process predominantly stimulated by glucagon.[52,60] Increased concentration of glucagon in DKA lowers the hepatic levels of malonyl coenzyme A (CoA), the first rate-limiting enzyme in de novo fatty acid synthesis. Malonyl CoA inhibits carnitine palmitoyl transferase 1 (CPT-1), the rate-limiting enzyme for transesterification of fatty acyl CoA to fatty acyl carnitine,[61,62] a step that subsequently allows oxidation of fatty acids to ketone bodies at the level of the mitochondria. The increased fatty acyl CoA and CPT-1 activity in DKA lead to increased ketogenesis in DKA.[51,62] In addition to increased production of ketone bodies, there is evidence that clearance of ketones is decreased in patients with DKA.[62,63]

We have reported that the hyperglycemia in patients with DKA is associated with a severe inflammatory state characterized by an elevation of proinflammatory cytokines, reactive oxygen species (ROS), and cardiovascular risk factors in the absence of obvious infection or cardiovascular pathology.[64] We reported that circulating levels of proinflammatory cytokines (tumor necrosis factor α [TNF-α], interleukin-6 [IL-6], IL-1β, and IL-8), products of ROS (thiobarbituric acid [TBA]-reacting material and dichlorofluorescein [DCF]), C-reactive protein (CRP), plasminogen activator inhibitor 1 [PAI-1]), free fatty acids (FFAs), cortisol, and growth hormone (GH) were significantly increased two- to fourfold on admission in patients with hyperglycemic crises compared with control subjects, and levels returned to normal after insulin treatment and resolution of the hyperglycemic crises.

In addition, in a different study we reported that in vivo activation of T cells in patients with DKA can exhibit de novo emergence of growth factor receptors (insulin, insulin-like growth factor I [IGF-I], and IL-2) in association with an increased level of lipid peroxidation (TBA-reacting material and

Box 9-1. Clinical Presentation of DKA

Symptoms

Abdominal pain

Nausea

Polydipsia

Polyuria

Vomiting

Weakness

Weight loss

Signs

Acetone breath

Altered sensorium

Hypothermia

Ileus

Kussmaul breathing

Tachycardia

Tachypnea

ROS such as DCF).[65] These studies in patients with DKA demonstrating in vivo activation of T cells led us to hypothesize that hyperglycemia or ketosis, or both, through production of ROS and generation of proinflammatory cytokines could result in de novo emergence of growth-factor receptor insulin, IGF-I, and IL-1β.[66] The initial activating event for T cells may be the presence of high levels of FFAs and glucose in patients with hyperglycemic crises,[64] which could result in the generation of ROS through diacylglycerol—and protein kinase C (PKC)-activated NAD(P)H (reduced nicotinamide adenine dinucleotide [phosphate]).[67]

DIAGNOSIS

Symptoms and Signs

Clinical features of DKA at presentation can be non-specific, but in general, patients complain of poly-dipsia and polyuria for several days prior to the development of ketoacidosis (Box 9-1). Type 1 diabetes patients with DKA tend to have a shorter pro-drome before presenting for medical attention due to the absolute lack of insulin. Generalized weakness, weight loss, and gastrointestinal symptoms including nausea, vomiting, and abdominal pain are usually present on admission.[68,69] Abdominal pain, sometimes mimicking an acute abdomen, is especially common in children.[70,71]

In a recent prospective study of 189 consecutive patients with DKA admitted to a large inner-city teaching hospital, we recently reported that abdominal pain was found in 86 of 189 patients with DKA (46%). The presence of abdominal pain was not related to the severity of hyperglycemia or dehydration; however, a strong association was observed between abdominal pain and metabolic acidosis. In DKA subjects with abdominal pain, the mean serum bicarbonate (9 mmol/L) and blood pH (7.12 ± 0.02) were lower than in patients without pain (serum bicarbonate 15 mmol/L, blood pH 7.24 ± 0.09). Abdominal pain was present in 86% of patients with serum bicarbonate lower than 5 mmol/L, in 66% of patients with levels 5 mmol/L to less than 10 mmol/L, in 36% of patients with levels 10 mmol/L to less than 15 mmol/L, and in 13% of patients with bicarbonate levels of 15 mmol/L to 18 mmol/L.

Although the cause of abdominal pain in DKA has not been elucidated, delayed gastric emptying and ileus induced by electrolyte disturbance and metabolic acidosis have been implicated as possible causes of abdominal pain.[69] Acute hyperglycemia has also been shown to impair gastrointestinal motility in diabetic patients and in normal subjects.[69,72] Similarly, acute hyperglycemia has adverse effects on esophageal motility and gallbladder contractility.[73] The abdominal pain in DKA has also been attributed to rapid expansion of the hepatic capsule, presumably secondary to fatty liver, or to bowel ischemia secondary to severe volume depletion and metabolic acidosis.[56,69] In the majority of patients, the abdominal pain spontaneously resolves once the metabolic disturbance is corrected; thus, in the absence of an overt cause for abdominal pain, allowing several hours to treat the underlying acidosis constitutes the best diagnostic tool to elucidate the etiology of abdominal pain in DKA.

Physical examination reveals signs of dehydration, including loss of skin turgor, dry mucous membranes, tachycardia, and hypotension. Most patients are normothermic or even hypothermic at presentation. Acetone on the breath and labored Kussmaul respirations may also be present on admission, particularly in patients with severe metabolic acidosis. Mental status can vary from full alertness to profound lethargy; however, less than 20% of patients are hospitalized with loss of consciousness.[74,75]

In a study of 144 consecutive patients with DKA, we found that 48% of patients were alert, 39% were lethargic, and only 13% presented in coma or with loss of consciousness.[3] Abnormalities in mental status correlated better with increased serum osmolality than with the severity of metabolic acidosis, patient's age, or duration of diabetes. The mean total serum osmolality was 311 ± 3 mmol/kg in noncomatose patients and 345 ± 4 mmol/kg in comatose patients.

Laboratory Findings

DKA consists of the biochemical triad of hyperglycemia, ketonemia, and metabolic acidosis. The

Table 9–1. *Diagnostic Criteria for Diabetic Ketoacidosis*

	Mild	Moderate	Severe
Glucose (mg/dL)	<250	>250	>250
pH	7.25-7.3	7.0-7.24	<7.0
HCO_3 (mEq/L)	15-18	10-14	<10
Ketones*	positive	positive	positive
Sensorium	alert	alert/drowsy	stupor/coma

* Nitroprusside reaction method.

Box 9-2. Useful Formulas for the Evaluation of DKA

Anion Gap

$$\text{Anion gap} = Na^+ - (Cl^- + HCO_3^-)$$

Total Serum Osmolality*

$$\text{Total serum osmolality} = \frac{2\,[Na^+] + \text{glucose}}{18} + \frac{BUN}{2.8}$$

Effective Serum Osmolality*

$$\text{Effective serum osmolality} = \frac{2\,[Na^+] + \text{glucose}}{18}$$

Corrected Serum Sodium*

$$\text{Corrected } [Na^+] = 1.6 \times \frac{\text{glucose} - 100}{100} + [\text{measured } Na^+]$$

Total Body Water Deficit*

$$\text{Total body water deficit} = [\text{weight} \times 0.6] - \left(\frac{[\text{corrected } Na^+] - 1}{140}\right)$$

*Blood urea nitrogen and glucose are measured in mg/dL; weight is measured in kilograms.
BUN, blood urea nitrogen.

most widely used diagnostic criteria for DKA have been blood glucose greater than 250 mg/dL, serum bicarbonate lower than 15 mEq/L, arterial pH lower than 7.3, an increased anion gap metabolic acidosis, and a moderate degree of ketonemia. Although these criteria served well for research purposes, they have significant limitations in clinical practice because the majority of patients with DKA present with mild metabolic acidosis[3,76] despite elevated serum glucose and β-hydroxybutyrate concentrations.

The biochemical criteria for diagnosis have been modified in the American Diabetes Association (ADA) guidelines for management of hyperglycemic crises.[77] The severity of DKA is now classified as mild, moderate, or severe based primarily on the severity of metabolic acidosis (blood pH, bicarbonate, ketones) and the presence of altered mental status (Table 9-1). Standards of care call for the use of arterial pH to assess the degree of acidosis; however, venous pH is a good alternative in clinical practice because it obviates a painful procedure and decreases the risk of vascular compromise. The venous pH is typically is 0.05 points less than the arterial pH. The severity of metabolic acidosis bears small relation to the degree of hyperglycemia, and cases of relative normoglycemic ketoacidosis (< 13.8 mmol/L or 250 mg/dL) have been reported.[78] This phenomenon has been reported during pregnancy, in patients with prolonged vomiting or starvation, and in those who present after receiving insulin. Similarly, relatively low glucose concentrations can occur in the presence of impaired gluconeogenesis, such as in patients with alcohol abuse or liver failure.[79,80]

The key diagnostic feature is the elevation in circulating total blood ketone concentration. Assessment of augmented ketonemia is usually performed by the nitroprusside reaction, which provides a semiquantitative estimation of acetoacetate and acetone levels. Although the nitroprusside test (both in urine and in serum) is highly sensitive, it can underestimate the severity of ketoacidosis because this assay does not recognize the presence of β-hydroxybutyrate, the main metabolic product in ketoacidosis.[51,81] Direct measurement of β-hydroxybutyrate is now available by finger-stick method[82] and may be a more accurate indicator of severity of ketoacidosis. In general, a positive nitroprusside reagent test (Ketostix) of at least 2+ represents a total serum ketone concentration of

approximately 3 mmol and indicates a moderate degree of ketonemia.[83] The mean admission serum β-hydroxybutyrate levels in patients with DKA are between 7.0 and 9.5 mmol/L.[3,56,80]

Accumulation of ketoacids results in an increased anion gap metabolic acidosis. The plasma anion gap is calculated by subtracting the major measured anions (chloride and bicarbonate) from the major measured cation (sodium), using the following formula:

$$\text{Anion gap} = Na^+ - (Cl^- + HCO_3^-)$$

(Box 9-2 gives formulas for the evaluation of DKA). The normal anion gap has been historically reported to be 12 ± 2 mEq/L.[20,29] Most laboratories, however, currently measure sodium and chloride concentrations using ion-specific electrodes, which measures plasma chloride concentration 2 to 6 mEq/L higher than with other methods.[84] Thus, the normal anion gap using the current methodology is between 7 and 9 mEq/L , and an anion gap greater than 10 to 12 mEq/L indicates increased anion gap acidosis.[77]

Although most subjects with DKA present with a high anion gap acidosis, it is important to keep in mind that patients may present with mixed acid–base disorders. It has been reported that 46% of patients admitted with DKA had predominant anion gap acidosis, 43% had mixed anion gap acidosis and hyperchloremic metabolic acidosis, and 11% had hyperchloremic metabolic acidosis.[85] More importantly, during treatment and resolution of DKA, most patients develop a transient nonanion-

gap hyperchloremic metabolic acidosis associated with fluid replacement.[80,86]

Assessment of total serum osmolality has traditionally been calculated with the formula:

$$\text{Total serum osmolality} = 2[Na^+] + (\text{glucose}/18) + (\text{blood urea nitrogen}/2.8)$$

where Na^+ concentration is in mEq/L and glucose and blood urea nitrogen (BUN) are in mg/dL. Normal values are 290 ± 5 mmol/kg H_2O. The effective serum osmolality rather than the total serum osmolality is now preferred for clinical use. Effective osmolality is calculated by:

$$\text{Effective serum osmolality} = 2[Na^+] + (\text{glucose}/18)$$

where Na^+ concentration is in mEq/L and glucose is in mg/dL. The urea concentration is not taken into account because it is freely permeable, and its accumulation does not induce major changes in intracellular volume or osmotic gradient across the cell membrane.[87] An effective serum osmolality greater than 320 mmol/kg characterizes a hyperosmolar state that is reported in approximately one third of patients with DKA.[3]

The admission serum sodium is usually low because of the osmotic flux of water from the intracellular to the extracellular space in the presence of hyperglycemia. An increase in serum sodium concentration in the presence of hyperglycemia indicates a profound degree of water loss. To assess the severity of sodium and water deficit, serum sodium may be corrected by adding 1.6 mg/dL to the measured serum sodium for each 100 mg/dL of glucose above 100 mg/dL.[28,49] Extreme hypertriglyceridemia, which may be present during DKA due to impaired lipoprotein lipase activity, can cause lipemic serum with spurious lowering of serum sodium (pseudohyponatremia).[88]

Serum potassium levels can also be low, normal, or high in patients with hyperglycemic crises, although normal to high levels tend to be the rule.[89] In one series,[3] the mean admission serum potassium in patients with DKA was 5.6 mEq/L. The shift of water from the intracellular to the extracellular space due to hyperosmolality causes a shift of potassium out to the extracellular space. Potassium shifts are further enhanced by the presence of acidosis and the breakdown of intracellular protein secondary to insulin deficiency. Furthermore, insulin deficiency results in a reduction in the activity of Na^+,K^+-ATPase, with reduced exchange of Na^+ and K^+ across the cell membrane. Hypokalemia at presentation (levels less than 3.5 mmol/L) is reported in less than 5% of DKA cases[90] and indicates severe total body potassium depletion. Hypokalemia can occur due to renal potassium losses as a result of osmotic diuresis and secondary hyperaldosteronism.[49]

The serum phosphate level in patients with DKA, like serum potassium, is usually elevated and does not reflect the actual body deficit that uniformly develops as intracellular phosphate shifts to the extracellular space.[75,91,92] Insulin deficiency, hypertonicity, and increased catabolism all contribute to the shift of phosphate out of cells.

On admission, leukocytosis with white blood cell (WBC) counts in the $10,000/mm^3$ to $15,000/mm^3$ range is the rule in DKA and might not indicate an infectious process. The admission mean WBC count in patients with uncomplicated DKA is $11,616 \pm 6$ per mm^3.[3] A leukocyte count on admission greater than $25,000/mm^3$ or the presence of greater than 10% neutrophil bands suggests bacterial infection.[93] In ketoacidosis, leukocytosis is attributed to stress, dehydration, and demargination of leukocytes.

Hyperamylasemia has been reported in 21% to 79% of patients with DKA.[94,95] There is little correlation between the presence, degree, or isoenzyme type of hyperamylasemia and the presence of gastrointestinal symptoms (nausea, vomiting, and abdominal pain), triglyceride concentration, or pancreatic imaging studies.[96] In some patients, the mean serum amylase concentration is significantly greater several hours after admission compared to at initial evaluation. The cause of hyperamylasemia in DKA is postulated to be multifactorial, the most important causes being existence of salivary amylase, reduced renal clearance of amylase, and increased leakage from acini secondary to neural and metabolic disturbance.[96] Nonspecific serum lipase elevation has also been noted in 29% to 41% of patients with DKA in the absence of clinical or radiologic evidence of acute pancreatitis.[97]

TREATMENT

Successful therapy of DKA depends on frequent monitoring of patients, replacement of fluid losses, correction of the hyperglycemia and metabolic acidosis, replacement of electrolyte losses, and careful scrutiny for precipitating factors for metabolic decompensation. Box 9-3 and Box 9-4 summarize our updated protocol for management of DKA.

There are no guidelines for determining the safety and cost effectiveness of treating patients with DKA in an intensive care unit (ICU) or in non-ICU settings. Several observational and prospective studies have indicated no clear benefits in treating DKA patients in the ICU compared to step-down units or general medicine wards.[29,98,99] The mortality rate, length of hospital stay, or time to resolve ketoacidosis are similar between patients treated in ICU and non-ICU settings. In addition, ICU admission has been shown to be associated with more testing and significantly higher hospitalization cost in patients with DKA.[25,98] In the United States, however, the majority of patients with DKA receive treatment in the ICU because of institutional policies and procedures that prevent use of intravenous

Box 9-3. Initial Clinical Evaluation of Patients with Suspected Diabetic Ketoacidosis

History and Physical Examination

Secure patient's airway, breathing, and circulation (ABCs)

Check mental status

Check cardiovascular and renal status

Look for source of infection

Evaluation of Volume and Hydration Status

Order laboratory studies

Measure arterial blood gases (ABGs)

Order complete blood count (CBC) with differential

Order comprehensive metabolic panel (CMP) (glucose, electrolytes, bicarbonate, phosphate, magnesium, blood urea nitrogen, creatinine)

Measure serum ketones

Order urinalysis

Order bacterial cultures (if clinically indicated)

Measure cardiac enzymes (if clinically indicated)

Box 9-4. Management of Patients with Diabetic Ketoacidosis

• Replacement of fluid losses
• Correction of hyperglycemia and metabolic acidosis
• Replacement of electrolytes losses
• Detection and treatment of precipitating causes
• Conversion to a maintenance insulin regimen (prevention of recurrence)

insulin infusion or insulin rate adjustment outside the ICU.[92]

In urban and medically indigent populations, poor compliance with insulin treatment is the most common precipitating cause, accounting for more than half of all DKA admissions.[3,26,46] Most patients with poor compliance are younger, are less critically ill, have lower disease severity scores, and have a lower rate of complications and mortality compared to non-DKA patients admitted to the ICU.[76,100] Although these patients should be candidates for early discharge, the length of hospitalization in mild DKA is similar to that for patients admitted with moderate or severe DKA.[28,98]

Based on these reports, it is our belief that ICU care is not required for successful treatment of uncomplicated DKA and that criteria for ICU admission should not be dictated by the severity of hyperglycemia or metabolic acidosis but by the severity of intercurrent medical illness that led to metabolic decompensation. Mentally obtunded patients and those with critical illness as the precipitating cause for DKA (e.g., myocardial infarction, gastrointesti-

nal bleeding, sepsis) require admission to an ICU or to a step-down unit where adequate nursing care and quick turnaround of laboratory tests are available. Most patients with mild to moderate DKA, especially those without an associated precipitating cause other than noncompliance, may be safely managed in step-down units or general medicine wards as long as quick turnaround of laboratory assessment is available and there is a knowledgeable team of health care providers on site.

Fluid Replacement

Patients with DKA and hyperglycemic hyperosmolar syndrome (HHS) are invariably volume depleted and have an estimated water deficit of approximately 100 mL/kg of body weight.[75] Expansion of extracellular fluid with intravenous fluids results in significant improvement of hyperglycemia, hypertonicity, and metabolic acidosis due to a decline in counterregulatory hormone levels.[101] The volume expansion also improves renal perfusion, which subsequently leads to increased urinary clearance of glucose.[102]

The severity of dehydration and volume depletion can be estimated by clinical examination. An orthostatic increase in pulse and a drop in blood pressure (more than 15/10 mmHg) indicates a 15% to 20% decrease in extracellular volume (i.e., 3 to 4 liters), and supine hypotension indicates a decrease of more than 20% in extracellular fluid volume (i.e., 5 to 8 liters).[92] The state of hydration can also be estimated by calculating plasma osmolality.[103,104] An effective plasma osmolality greater than 320 mOsm/kg H_2O is associated with large fluid deficits. The water deficit can be estimated, based on corrected serum sodium concentration, using the following equation:

$$\text{Water deficit} = (0.6 \times \text{body weight}) \times [(\text{corrected } [Na^+]/140) - 1]$$

where body weight is in kilograms.[105]

The initial fluid of choice is isotonic saline (0.9% NaCl) (Box 9-5, Intravenous Fluids). Generally 1 or 2 liters of saline at a rate of 500 to 1000 mL/h is sufficient to restore blood pressure and renal perfusion. Patients with severe hypovolemic shock should be given saline at a more rapid rate or should be given colloids (albumin or plasma) to maintain normal blood pressure. After intravascular volume depletion has been corrected, the rate of normal saline infusion should be reduced to 250 mL/h or changed to 0.45% saline, depending upon the serum sodium concentration and state of hydration. Hypotonic solutions are preferred when the corrected serum sodium exceeds 150 mEq/L[37,106] or when the calculated effective plasma osmolality is greater than 320 mOsm/kg.[102]

During treatment of DKA, hyperglycemia is corrected faster than ketoacidosis. The mean duration

Box 9-5. Treatment Protocol Management of Diabetic Ketoacidosis

Intravenous Fluids

0.9% saline at 500 to 1000 mL/h for 2 hours

0.45% saline at 250 to 500 mL/h until blood glucose is lower than 13.8 mmol/L (250 mg/dL)

Dextrose 5% in 0.45% saline at 150 to 250 mL/h until resolution of DKA

Potassium Replacement

K^+ > 5.5 mmol/L: Do not give K^+ but check serum K^+ every 2 hours

K^+ = 4 to 5.5 mmol/L: Add 20 mmol KCl to each liter of IV fluid

K^+ = 3 to < 4 mmol/L: Add 40 mmol KCl to each liter of IV fluid

K^+ < 3 mmol/L: Give 10 to 20 mmol KCl per hour until serum K^+ > 3 mmol/L, then add 40 mmol KCl to each liter of IV fluid

Insulin Therapy
Intravenous Regular Insulin

Initial IV bolus: 0.1 U/kg body weight, *followed by*

Continuous insulin infusion at 0.1 U/kg per hour

When blood glucose < 13.8 mmol/L (200 mg/dL), change IV fluids to D5% in 0.45% saline and reduce insulin infusion rate to 0.05 unit/kg per hour to keep glucose at approximately 11.1 mmol/L until resolution of DKA.

Subcutaneous Insulin (Lispro, Aspart) Every Hour

Initial dose SC: 0.3 U/kg body weight, *followed by*

SC lispro or aspart insulin at 0.1 U/kg every hour

When blood glucose < 13.8 mmol/L (200 mg/dL), change IV fluids to D5% saline and reduce lispro or aspart insulin to 0.05 U/kg per hour to keep glucose at approximately 11.1 mmol/L until resolution of DKA.

Subcutaneous Insulin (Lispro, Aspart) Every 2 Hours

Initial dose SC: 0.3 U/kg body weight, *followed by*

SC lispro or aspart insulin at 0.2 units 1 hour later and every 2 hours

When blood glucose < 13.8 mmol/L (200 mg/dL), change IV fluids to D5% in 0.45% saline and reduce SC lispro or aspart to 0.1 U/kg every 2 hours to keep glucose at approximately 11.1 mmol/l (200 mg/dL) until resolution of DKA.

Laboratory
Admission

Cell blood count with differential

Complete metabolic profile

Venous pH

Serum β-hydroxybutyrate

During Treatment

Basic metabolic profile (glucose, bicarbonate, sodium, potassium, chloride, urea, and creatinine)

Venous pH

Phosphorus

β-Hydroxybutyrate at 2 hours, at 4 hours, and then every 4 hours until resolution of DKA.

Glucose by Finger Stick

Check glucose every hour in patients receiving lispro or aspart insulin SC every hour.

Check glucose every 2 hours in patients receiving IV insulin or lispro or aspart insulin SC every 2 hours.

D5%, 5% dextrose; DKA, diabetic ketoacidosis; IV, intravenous; SC, subcutaneous.

of treatment until blood glucose is lower than 250 mg/dL and ketoacidosis (pH > 7.30, bicarbonate > 18 mmol/L) is corrected is 6 and 12 hours, respectively.[3,56] Once the plasma glucose is about 250 mg/dL, 5% to10% dextrose should be added to replacement fluids to allow continued insulin administration until ketonemia is controlled and to prevent hypoglycemia. An additional important aspect of fluid management is to replace the volume of urine losses, especially in subjects with excessive polyuria. Failure to adjust fluid replacement for urine losses can delay correction of the water deficit.

Insulin Therapy

The cornerstone of DKA management after initial hydration is insulin administration. Insulin increases peripheral glucose use and decreases hepatic glucose production, thereby lowering blood glucose concentration.[49] In addition, insulin therapy inhibits the release of free fatty acids from adipose tissue and decreases ketogenesis, both of which lead to the reversal of ketogenesis.[92]

Until 1972, large doses of intravenous, subcutaneous, or intramuscular insulin were used because of fears of insulin resistance.[107-109] In 1973, several reports demonstrated the effectiveness of small doses of insulin in patients with DKA.[110-114] Advantages over the previously used high-dose regimens include less frequent hypoglycemia and hypokalemia and a more predictable response to treatment.[109-113,115]

Although controlled studies in patients with DKA have shown that low-dose insulin therapy is effective regardless of the route of administration,[110,115-118] most medical centers and authorities recommend intravenous infusion because of the delayed onset of action and prolonged half-life of

subcutaneous regular insulin.[7,31,37,76,112,119,120] However, the ideal route of insulin therapy is still a matter of debate.

In a prospective randomized study in patients with DKA treated either with intramuscular or subcutaneous injections or with continuous intravenous infusion of regular insulin, Fisher and coworkers[116] reported that 30% to 40% of patients in the intramuscular and subcutaneous groups did not lower their plasma glucose by 10% in the first hour after insulin injection, and that the concentration of ketone bodies was lowered at a significantly faster rate in the first 2 hours in the intravenous group compared with the intramuscular or subcutaneous groups.

The delay in onset of action of regular insulin is substantiated by the report of Menzel and Jutzi,[120] who used frequent small subcutaneous injections and reported that only 4 of 24 patients showed a fall in blood glucose concentration in the first 3 hours of therapy. These differences in response can be explained by delays in reaching maximal circulating insulin concentration. Peak insulin concentration is achieved within the first hour in patients treated with intravenous insulin but not until the second or third hour of therapy in those treated with intramuscular or subcutaneous injections.[121]

Evidence indicates that new analogs of human insulin (aspart and lispro) with a rapid onset of action could represent alternatives to intravenous regular insulin in the treatment of DKA. With subcutaneous administration of these insulin analogs, the onset of action is in 10 to 20 minutes, peak of action is in 30 to 90 minutes, and duration of action is approximately 3 to 4 hours. These times are significantly shorter than those of regular insulin, which has an onset of action of 1 to 2 hours and a half-life of approximately 4 hours.[117,122]

We have reported that treating patients who have mild or moderate DKA with subcutaneous aspart insulin every 1 or 2 hours in non-ICU settings is as safe and effective as treatment with intravenous regular insulin in the ICU.[99,123] The rate of decline of blood glucose concentration and the mean duration of treatment until ketoacidosis is corrected were similar among patients treated with subcutaneous insulin analogs every 1 or 2 hours or with intravenous regular insulin. We observed no significant differences in the length of hospital stay, the total amount of insulin administered until resolution of hyperglycemia or ketoacidosis, or the number of hypoglycemic events among treatment groups. Until our preliminary studies are confirmed in clinical practice and outside the research arena, we believe that patients with severe DKA, hypotension, anasarca, or associated critical illness should be managed with intravenous insulin in the ICU or in a step-down unit. However, patients with mild DKA and uncomplicated DKA could be treated with subcutaneous rapid-acting insulin analogs in non-ICU settings.

A common and effective practice includes an initial intravenous (IV) bolus of regular insulin 0.1 U/kg of body weight, followed by a continuous infusion of regular insulin at a dose of 0.1 U/kg per hour (see Box 9-5, Insulin Therapy). The goal is to achieve a rate of decline of 50 mg to 100 mg per hour. Once the serum glucose has declined to about 250 mg/dL, an infusion of glucose (5% dextrose in 0.45% normal saline) should be started at 150 mL to 200 mL per hour, and the insulin infusion rate should be reduced to 0.05 U/kg per hour. Thereafter, the rate of insulin administration might need to be adjusted to maintain glucose levels at approximately 200 mg/dL and be continued until ketoacidosis is resolved.

Patients with DKA to be treated with subcutaneous rapid-acting insulin analogs (lispro or aspart) every hour should receive an initial priming dose of regular insulin of 0.2 U/kg of body weight, followed by 0.1 U/kg per hour until the blood glucose reaches 250 mg/dL. At that time, the insulin dose is reduced to 0.05 U/kg per hour, and the IV fluids can be changed to 5% dextrose and 0.45% saline to maintain blood glucose at about 200 mg/dL until DKA resolves. Patients treated with subcutaneous rapid-acting insulin analogs every 2 hours should receive an initial dose of 0.3 U/kg followed by 0.2 U/kg one hour later and then every 2 hours until the blood glucose reaches 250 mg/dL. At that time, insulin dose should be reduced to 0.1 U/kg every 2 hours, and the IV fluids can be changed to 5% dextrose and 0.45% saline to keep blood glucose at about 200 mg/dL until DKA resolves.

In most patients with DKA, insulin administration and intravenous saline can safely be started simultaneously; however, insulin therapy should be withheld in patients who have significant hypokalemia associated with dehydration and hyperglycemia. In patients admitted with serum potassium lower than 3.0 mEq/L, potassium replacement should be started immediately, and insulin therapy should be held for 1 or 2 hours until sufficient potassium is given.[28,124] Similarly, in hypotensive patients with severe hyperglycemia, insulin administration can be followed by vascular collapse due to a rapid reduction in plasma glucose concentration and shift of water from the extracellular to the intracellular space.[125] Such patients should be managed by aggressive hydration alone until blood pressure is stabilized.[11,24]

During therapy, capillary blood glucose should be determined every 1 to 2 hours at the bedside using a glucose oxidase reagent strip. Blood should be drawn at 2 hours and then every 4 hours during therapy for determination of serum electrolytes, glucose, BUN, creatinine, magnesium, phosphorus, and venous pH. Although serum β-hydroxybutyrate levels are usually lower than 1.5 mmol/L at resolution of DKA,[126] we do not recommend routine measurements of ketone levels during therapy. In some patients with mixed acid–base disorders, direct measurement of β-hydroxybutyrate levels may be

indicated to confirm the diagnosis and assess the response to therapy. The nitroprusside test, which measures acetoacetate and acetone levels but not β-hydroxybutyrate concentration, should be avoided during therapy because the fall in acetoacetate lags behind the resolution of DKA, and this test can remain positive several hours after resolution of metabolic acidosis.[56,126]

Potassium Therapy

Despite a total body potassium deficit of approximately 3 to 5 mEq/kg of body weight, most patients with DKA have a serum potassium level at or above the upper limits of normal.[86,89,90] With initiation of therapy, the extracellular potassium concentration invariably falls. Rehydration lowers the serum potassium level by exerting a dilutional effect and by increasing urinary potassium excretion.[49] Insulin therapy and correction of acidosis decrease serum potassium levels by stimulating cellular potassium uptake in peripheral tissues.[127] Therefore, to prevent hypokalemia, most patients require intravenous potassium during the course of DKA therapy.

We recommend replacement with potassium chloride (KCl, 20 to 30 mEq per liter of intravenous fluids) as soon as the serum potassium concentration falls below 5.5 mEq/L[77] (See Box 9-5, Potassium Replacement). The treatment goal is to maintain serum potassium levels within the normal range of 4 to 5 mEq/L. In some hyperglycemic patients admitted with severe potassium deficiency, insulin administration can precipitate profound hypokalemia, which can induce life-threatening arrhythmias and respiratory muscle weakness.[49,77,124] Thus, if the initial serum potassium is 3.0 mEq/L or lower, potassium replacement should begin immediately by an infusion of KCl at a rate of 20 mEq per hour. In such patients, one should consider withholding insulin therapy for 1 or 2 hours until sufficient intravenous potassium replacement is given.

Bicarbonate Therapy

Bicarbonate administration in patients with DKA remains controversial. Severe metabolic acidosis can lead to impaired myocardial contractility, cerebral vasodilation and coma, and gastrointestinal complications.[37,128,129] However, rapid alkalinization can result in hypokalemia, paradoxical central nervous system acidosis, and worsened intracellular acidosis as bicarbonate is ultimately converted to carbon dioxide.[130]

Several studies in the literature, however, support the notion that bicarbonate therapy for DKA offers no advantage in improving cardiac and neurologic functions or in the rate of recovery of hyperglycemia and ketoacidosis. Nine small studies have evaluated the effect of alkalinization in a total of 434 patients with diabetic ketoacidosis, 217 treated with bicarbonate and 178 patients without alkali therapy.[131-139] Several deleterious effects of bicarbonate therapy have been reported, such as increased risk of hypokalemia,[132] decreased tissue oxygen uptake,[140] and cerebral edema.[141]

Despite the lack of evidence in support of bicarbonate therapy in patients with DKA, some experts recommend that patients with severe metabolic acidosis (pH < 6.9 to 7.0) should be given 50 mEq of sodium bicarbonate as isotonic solution (in 200 mL of water) every 2 hours until pH rises to at least 7.0. In patients with arterial pH greater than 7.0, no bicarbonate therapy is necessary.

Phosphate Therapy

The serum phosphate level in patients with DKA is usually normal or elevated, but the admission serum phosphate does not reflect the actual body deficit that uniformly exists as shifts of intracellular phosphate to the extracellular space.[75,91,92] During insulin therapy and fluid replacement, phosphate reenters the intracellular compartment, leading to mild to moderate reductions in serum phosphate concentrations.

The clinical relevance and benefits of phosphate replacement therapy remain uncertain. Several studies have failed to show any beneficial effect of phosphate replacement on clinical outcome.[91,142] In fact, aggressive phosphate therapy may be potentially hazardous, as indicated in case reports of children with DKA who developed hypocalcemia and tetany secondary to intravenous phosphate administration.[31,143] Theoretical advantages of phosphate therapy include prevention of respiratory depression and increased generation of erythrocyte 2,3-diphosphoglycerate, which shifts the oxygen curve to the right to deliver more oxygen to tissues.[144,145]

Because of these potential benefits, careful phosphate replacement may be indicated in patients with cardiac dysfunction, anemia, or respiratory depression and in those with serum phosphate concentration lower than 1.0 to 1.5 mg/dL.[28,146] If phosphate replacement is needed, it should be administered as a potassium salt by giving two thirds as KCl and one third as potassium phosphate. In such patients, because of the risk of hypocalcemia, serum calcium and phosphate levels must be monitored during phosphate infusion.[31,146,147]

Transition to Subcutaneous Insulin

Patients with DKA should be treated with continuous intravenous insulin until ketoacidosis is resolved. Criteria for resolution of ketoacidosis include blood glucose lower than 200 mg/dL, a serum bicarbonate level at least 18 mEq/L, venous

pH greater than 7.3, and a calculated anion gap no more than 14 mEq/L.[13,56,77] When these criteria are met, subcutaneous insulin therapy may be started.

If the patient is able to eat, split-dose therapy with both regular (short-acting) insulin and intermediate-acting insulin may be given. Patients with known diabetes may be given insulin at the dosage they were receiving before the onset of DKA. In patients with newly diagnosed diabetes, an initial total insulin dose of 0.6 U/kg per day is usually sufficient to achieve and maintain metabolic control. Two thirds of this total daily dose should be given in the morning and one third in the evening as a split-mixed dose.

If the patient is not able to eat, we prefer to continue the intravenous insulin infusion protocol. However, the patient could receive a daily dose of baseline glargine (0.02 to 0.03 U/kg) plus subcutaneous regular or rapid-acting insulin analogs every 4 hours while an infusion of 5% dextrose in half-normal saline is given at a rate of 100 to 200 mL per hour.

It is easier to start subcutaneous insulin before breakfast or at dinner. To prevent recurrence of hyperglycemia or ketoacidosis during the transition period to subcutaneous insulin, it is important to allow an overlap of 1 to 2 hours between discontinuation of intravenous insulin and administration of subcutaneous regular insulin.

COMPLICATIONS

Hypoglycemia

The two most common complications associated with the treatment of DKA in adult subjects are hypoglycemia and hypokalemia. Despite the use of low-dose insulin protocols, hypoglycemia is reported in 10% to 25% of patients during insulin therapy.[3,4] Hypoglycemic events most commonly occur after several hours of insulin infusion (between 8 and 16 hours). The failure to reduce the insulin infusion rate and the failure to use dextrose-containing solutions when blood glucose levels reach 250 mg/dL are the two most common causes of hypoglycemia during insulin therapy.[3] Frequent blood glucose monitoring (every 1 to 2 hours) is mandatory for recognizing hypoglycemia because many patients with DKA who develop hypoglycemia during treatment do not experience adrenergic manifestations of sweating, nervousness, fatigue, hunger, and tachycardia.

Hypokalemia

Both insulin therapy and correction of acidosis decrease serum potassium levels by stimulating cellular potassium uptake in peripheral tissues and can lead to hypokalemia. The use of a low-dose insulin protocol and aggressive potassium replacement early in the management minimize the risk of hypokalemia.[115] To prevent hypokalemia, initiate replacement with intravenous potassium as soon as the serum potassium concentration falls below 5.5 mEq/L. In addition, in patients who present with normal or reduced serum potassium, aggressive intravenous potassium replacement should begin immediately and insulin therapy should be held until serum potassium rises above 3.3 mEq/L.[77]

Relapse

Relapse of DKA can occur after sudden interruption of IV insulin therapy, in patients not given concomitant subcutaneous insulin, or with lack of frequent monitoring. To prevent recurrence of ketoacidosis during the transition period to subcutaneous insulin, it is important to allow an overlap of 1 to 2 hours between administration of subcutaneous regular insulin and discontinuation of intravenous insulin. Other complications of diabetes include hyperchloremic acidosis with excessive use of NaCl or KCl, resulting in a nonanion-gap metabolic acidosis.[80,85,86] This acidosis has no adverse clinical effects and is gradually corrected over the subsequent 24 to 48 hours by enhanced renal acid excretion. The development of hyperchloremia can be prevented by reducing the chloride load with judicious use of hydration solutions.[85]

Cerebral Edema

Cerebral edema occurs in about 0.3% to 1% of all episodes of DKA, and its etiology, pathophysiology, and ideal method of treatment are poorly understood.[148-151] Cerebral edema is more common in children, is associated with a mortality rate of 20% to 40%,[151] and accounts for 57% to 87% of all DKA deaths in children.[150] Cerebral edema is rarely reported in adult patients with DKA. Symptoms and signs of cerebral edema are variable and include onset of headache, gradual deterioration in level of consciousness, seizures, sphincter incontinence, pupil changes, papilledema, bradycardia, elevated blood pressure, and respiratory arrest.[150,152] Cerebral edema typically occurs 4 to 12 hours after treatment is activated, but it can be present before treatment has begun or can develop any time during treatment for DKA.[152]

Although no single factor has been identified that can be used to predict the development of cerebral edema, a number of mechanisms have been proposed. These include cerebral ischemia or hypoxia, generation of various inflammatory mediators,[153] increased cerebral blood flow, disruption of cell

membrane ion transport, and rapid shift in extra-cellular and intracellular fluids that results in changes in osmolality.[151,154-156] Preliminary imaging studies in children with DKA, using ultrasound, computed tomography, or magnetic resonance imaging, indicate that some degree of cerebral edema may be present even in patients who do not have clinical evidence of elevated intracranial pressure.[157] Most studies show no association between the degree of hyperglycemia at presentation of DKA and the risk of cerebral edema after correcting for other covariates.

Data also suggest that cerebral edema in children may also be related to brain ischemia.[155] In children with diabetic ketoacidosis, both hypocapnia (which causes cerebral vasoconstriction) and extreme dehydration were associated with increased risk of cerebral edema. Prevention can include a gradual decrease in serum glucose and maintenance of serum glucose between 250 mg/dL and 300 mg/dL until the patient's serum osmolality is normalized and mental status is improved.

Treatment should be initiated as soon as the condition is suspected. The rate of fluid administration should be reduced and the patient should be transferred to the ICU for administration of mannitol and possibly mechanical ventilation. Intravenous mannitol should be given (0.25 to 1.0 g/kg over 20 minutes) in patients with signs of cerebral edema before they manifest respiratory failure.[158] Hypertonic saline (3%) 5 to 10 mL/kg over 30 minutes may be an alternative to mannitol.[27,151] There are no data regarding glucocorticoid use in DKA-related cerebral edema.

PREVENTION

The most common precipitating causes of DKA include infection, intercurrent illness, psychological stress, and noncompliance with therapy. Many episodes could be prevented through improved patient education and effective outpatient treatment programs. Paramount in this effort is improved education regarding sick-day management.[159] Sick-day management includes:

- Making early contact with the health care provider.
- Emphasizing the importance of insulin during an illness and the reasons to never discontinue it without contacting the health care team.
- Reviewing blood glucose goals and the use of supplemental short-acting or rapid-acting insulin.
- Having medications available to suppress a fever and treat an infection.
- Initiating an easily digestible liquid diet containing carbohydrates and salt when nauseated.
- Educating family members about sick-day management and record keeping, including assessing and documenting temperature, respiration, and pulse; testing blood glucose and urine and blood ketones; administering insulin; and monitoring and documenting oral intake and weight.

The use of home glucose–ketone meters can allow early recognition of impending ketoacidosis, which can help to guide insulin therapy at home, and it might prevent hospitalization for DKA. In addition, home blood ketone monitoring, which measures β-hydroxybutyrate levels on a finger-stick blood specimen, are now commercially available.[82] This system measures β-hydroxybutyrate levels in 30 seconds with a detection range of 0 to 6 mmol/L. Clinical studies have shown that elevated β-hydroxybutyrate levels are common in patients with poorly controlled diabetes, even in the absence of positive urinary ketones.[160]

Insulin discontinuation and poor compliance account for more than half of DKA admissions in inner city and minority populations.[3,26,46,56,161] Medically indigent patients face several cultural and socioeconomic barriers, such as low literacy rate, limited financial resources, and limited access to health care, and these barriers could explain the lack of compliance and why DKA continues to occur in such high rates in inner city patients. These findings suggest that the current mode of providing patient education and health care has significant limitations. Addressing health problems in the African American and other minority communities requires explicit recognition of the fact that these populations are probably quite diverse in their behavioral responses to diabetes.[162] To be successful, programs directed at improving diabetes care in minorities should involve implementation of health care and educational programs that incorporate cultural insight particular to minority groups.

HYPERGLYCEMIC HYPEROSMOLAR SYNDROME

Hyperglycemic hyperosmolar syndrome (HHS) is a serious complication of diabetes and has a high mortality rate. HHS is less common than DKA and accounts for 0.05% of all diabetes-related admissions.[3,56,75] Mortality attributed to HHS is considerably higher than in DKA. Recent mortality rates are 5% to 25%, and the higher rates are most likely secondary to the underlying illnesses in an older patient population.[28,87]

HHS occurs most commonly in older patients with type 2 diabetes, but it can be seen in younger and type 1 patients as well. The typical patient with HHS has undiagnosed diabetes, is between 55 and 70 years of age, and is often a nursing home resident with associated comorbid conditions (stroke, renal failure). Up to 20% of patients admitted with HHS do not have a previous diagnosis of diabetes.[3]

Causes

The most common precipitating causes are pneumonia and urinary tract infection, accounting for 30% to 50% of cases.[75,163,164] Other acute medical problems as precipitating causes include acute coronary syndromes, trauma, surgery, and cerebrovascular accidents that provoke the release of counterregulatory hormones or compromise access to water. Certain medications that cause DKA can also precipitate HHS, including glucocorticoids, thiazide diuretics, phenytoin (Dilantin), and β-blockers.[92,165]

Several case reports and retrospective studies suggest an increased risk of developing diabetes mellitus in patients treated with atypical antipsychotics compared with schizophrenic patients treated with conventional antipsychotics or those without treatment.[38-40] Clozapine and olanzapine, in particular, have been implicated in producing diabetes and hyperglycemic crises.[38-40] Possible mechanisms include the induction of peripheral insulin resistance and the direct influence on pancreatic beta cell function by 5-HT1A/2A/2C receptor antagonism, by inhibitory effects via α_2-adrenergic receptors, or by toxic effects.[166]

Clinical Features

HHS is characterized by severe hyperglycemia, hyperosmolality, and dehydration in the absence of significant ketoacidosis. The diagnostic criteria for HHS (Table 9-2) include plasma glucose concentration greater than 600 mg/dL, serum osmolality greater than 320 mOsm/kg, and absence of ketoacidosis (pH > 7.3, serum bicarbonate > 18 mEq/L, and negative or minimal ketonemia and ketonuria). Altered sensorium (lethargy, stupor, coma) is common[3] and correlates better with hyperosmolality than with the patient's age or with severity of the acid-base disturbance. Several reports have shown that the mean serum osmolality in patients who present with coma is greater than 340 mmol/kg.[3,87,167] Approximately 50% of patients with HHS have an increased anion gap metabolic acidosis as the result of concomitant ketoacidosis or an increase in serum lactate levels. BUN and creatinine levels are usually elevated, and initial azotemia may be due to both prerenal and renal causes.

As with DKA, HHS is characterized by insulinopenia and increased circulating counterregulatory hormones. Higher levels of circulating insulin and lower levels of counterregulatory hormones in patients with HHS might explain the absent or minimal ketosis, which is the key difference from DKA. Three major mechanisms have been proposed for the lack of ketoacidosis in HHS.[28,49,56,87,106,168,169] These include higher levels of endogenous insulin reserve in HHS (i.e., insulin concentration adequate to prevent lipolysis but inadequate to inhibit hepatic glucose production or stimulate glucose use), lower levels of counterregulatory hormones and free fatty acids, and inhibition of lipolysis by the hyperosmolar state, which thereby decreases ketogenesis.

Treatment

Therapeutic measures for HHS are similar to those recommended for patients with DKA. In general, treatment of HHS should be directed at replacing volume deficit, correcting hyperosmolality and electrolyte disturbances, and managing the underlying illness that may have precipitated metabolic decompensation.[170] Patients with HHS may be severely dehydrated, with an average fluid deficit of 8 to 10 liters. Aggressive fluid replacement with normal saline at a rate of 500 to 1000 mL per hour for the first 2 to 3 hours is the usual recommendation, followed by 0.45% saline at a rate of 200 to 500 mL per hour.

Insulin treatment does not have to be aggressive if fluid replacement is vigorously pursued. Insulin is administered by an initial bolus of 0.1 U/kg followed by a continuous intravenous infusion calculated to deliver 0.1 U/kg per hour, and continued at this rate until blood glucose has decreased to approximately 250 to 300 mg/dL. At this time, intravenous fluids should be changed to dextrose-containing solutions (D5%) and the insulin dose should be decreased by 50% (0.05 units/kg per hour), or to 2 to 3 units per hour. Thereafter, the rate of insulin administration is adjusted to maintain a blood glucose level of approximately 200 mg/dL. Using this protocol, we have reported that the mean duration of treatment in HHS for serum glucose levels to decrease into target range is about 11 hours.[3]

Intravenous insulin infusion is usually continued until the patient is hemodynamically stable, the level of consciousness is improved, and the patient is able to tolerate food. Although most patients require insulin therapy after recovery from HHS, some patients can be managed with diet alone or

Table 9–2. *Diagnostic Criteria for Hyperglycemic Hyperosmolar Syndrome*

Glucose (mg/dl)	>600
pH	>7.30
HCO$_3$ (mEq/L)	>15
Urine/serum ketones*	Small
Effective serum osmolality (mOsm/kg)†	>320
Sensorium/mental obtundation	Stupor/coma

* Nitroprusside reaction method
† Effective serum osmolality = 2[Na$^+$ (mEq/l)] + [glucose (mg/dl)/18]
Adapted from Kitabchi AE, Umpierrez GE, Murphy MB, et al: Hyperglycemic crises in patients with diabetes mellitus. Diabetes Care 26 (Suppl 1):S109-117, 2003.

diet plus an oral hypoglycemic agent during the initial admission or shortly after presentation.[87,171]

Increased serum potassium is commonly found in patients with HHS despite severe total body potassium depletion. Hyperglycemia and hyperosmolality cause a shift of potassium from the intracellular compartment into plasma,[87,171] and they can contribute to a false estimate of total body potassium. The serum potassium deficit in patients with HHS is estimated at about 4 to 6 mEq/kg of body weight.[87,171] The principles of potassium replacement in HHS are the same as in DKA. We recommend that potassium replacement be initiated after serum levels fall below 5.5 mEq/L, with the goal to maintain a serum potassium concentration within the normal range of 4 to 5 mEq/L.

REFERENCES

1. Smith CP, Firth D, Bennett S, et al: Ketoacidosis occurring in newly diagnosed and established diabetic children. Acta Paediatr 87:537-541, 1998.
2. Faich GA, Fishbein HA, Ellis SE: The epidemiology of diabetic acidosis: A population-based study. Am J Epidemiol 117:551-558, 1983.
3. Umpierrez GE, Kelly JP, Navarrete JE, et al: Hyperglycemic crises in urban blacks. Arch Intern Med 157:669-675, 1997.
4. Fishbein HA, Palumbo PJ: Acute metabolic complications in diabetes. In National Diabetes Data Group: Diabetes in America, 2nd ed. Bethesda, Md, National Institutes of Health, 1995, pp. 283-291. Downloadable pdf available at http://diabetes.niddk.nih.gov/dm/pubs/america/contents.htm.
5. Levetan CS, Passaro MD, Jablonski KA, Ratner RE: Effect of physician specialty on outcomes in diabetic ketoacidosis. Diabetes Care 22:1790-1795, 1999.
6. Geiss LS, Herman WH, Goldschmid MG, et al: Surveillance for diabetes mellitus—United States, 1980-1989. MMWR CDC Surveill Summ 42:1-20, 1993.
7. Ellemann K, Soerensen JN, Pedersen L, et al: Epidemiology and treatment of diabetic ketoacidosis in a community population. Diabetes Care 7:528-532, 1984.
8. Wright AD, Hale PJ, Singh BM, et al: Changing sex ratio in diabetic ketoacidosis. Diabet Med 7:628-632, 1990.
9. Graves EJ, Gillium BS: Detailed diagnosis and procedures: National Discharge Survey, 1995. National Center for Health Statistics. Vital Health Stat 13, Nov:1-146, 1997.
10. Johnson DD, Palumbo PJ, Chu CP: Diabetic ketoacidosis in a community-based population. Mayo Clin Proc 55:83-88, 1980.
11. American Diabetes Association: Type 2 diabetes in children and adolescents. Pediatrics 105:671-680, 2000.
12. Umpierrez GE, Woo W, Hagopian WA, et al: Immunogenetic analysis suggests different pathogenesis for obese and lean African-Americans with diabetic ketoacidosis. Diabetes Care 22:1517-1523, 1999.
13. Umpierrez GE, Casals MM, Gebhart SP, et al: Diabetic ketoacidosis in obese African-Americans. Diabetes 44:790-795, 1995.
14. Mauvais-Jarvis F, Sobngwi E, Porcher R, et al: Ketosis-prone type 2 diabetes in patients of sub-Saharan African origin: Clinical pathophysiology and natural history of beta-cell dysfunction and insulin resistance. Diabetes 53:645-653, 2004.
15. McFarlane SI, Chaiken RL, Hirsch S, et al: Near-normoglycaemic remission in African-Americans with Type 2 diabetes mellitus is associated with recovery of beta cell function. Diabet Med 18:10-16, 2001
16. Banerji MA, Chaiken RL, Huey H, et al: GAD antibody negative NIDDM in adult black subjects with diabetic ketoacidosis and increased frequency of human leukocyte antigen DR3 and DR4. Flatbush diabetes. Diabetes 43:741-745, 1994.
17. Sobngwi E, Vexiau P, Levy V, et al: Metabolic and immunogenetic prediction of long-term insulin remission in African patients with atypical diabetes. Diabet Med 19:832-835, 2002.
18. Kitabchi AE: Ketosis-prone diabetes—a new subgroup of patients with atypical type 1 and type 2 diabetes? J Clin Endocrinol Metab 88:5087-5089, 2003.
19. Maldonado M, Hampe CS, Gaur LK, et al: Ketosis-prone diabetes: Dissection of a heterogeneous syndrome using an immunogenetic and beta-cell functional classification, prospective analysis, and clinical outcomes. J Clin Endocrinol Metab 88:5090-5098, 2003.
20. Balasubramanyam A, Zern JW, Hyman DJ, Pavlik V: New profiles of diabetic ketoacidosis: Type 1 vs type 2 diabetes and the effect of ethnicity. Arch Intern Med 159:2317-2322, 1999.
21. Yamada K, Nonaka K: Diabetic ketoacidosis in young obese Japanese men. Diabetes Care 19:671, 1996.
22. Sobngwi E, Mauvais-Jarvis F, Vexiau P, et al: Diabetes in Africans. Part 2: Ketosis-prone atypical diabetes mellitus. Diabetes Metab 28:5-12, 2002.
23. Sobngwi E, Gautier JF: Adult-onset idiopathic type I or ketosis-prone type II diabetes: Evidence to revisit diabetes classification. Diabetologia 45:283-285, 2002.
24. Maldonado MR, Otiniano ME, Lee R, et al: Ethnic differences in beta-cell functional reserve and clinical features in patients with ketosis-prone diabetes. Diabetes Care 26:2469, 2003.
25. Javor KA, Kotsanos JG, McDonald RC, et al: Diabetic ketoacidosis charges relative to medical charges of adult patients with type I diabetes. Diabetes Care 20:349-354, 1997.
26. Maldonado MR, Chong ER, Oehl MA, Balasubramanyam A: Economic Impact of diabetic ketoacidosis in a multiethnic indigent population: Analysis of costs based on the precipitating cause. Diabetes Care 26:1265-1269, 2003.
27. Dunger DB, Sperling MA, Acerini CL, et al: European Society for Paediatric Endocrinology/Lawson Wilkins Pediatric Endocrine Society consensus statement on diabetic ketoacidosis in children and adolescents. Pediatrics 113:e133-e140, 2004.
28. Kitabchi AE, Umpierrez GE, Murphy MB, et al: Management of hyperglycemic crises in patients with diabetes. Diabetes Care 24:131-153, 2001.
29. Moss JM: Diabetic ketoacidosis: Effective low-cost treatment in a community hospital. South Med J 80:875-881, 1987.
30. Wagner A, Risse A, Brill HL, et al: Therapy of severe diabetic ketoacidosis. Zero-mortality under very-low-dose insulin application. Diabetes Care 22:674-677, 1999.
31. White NH: Diabetic ketoacidosis in children. Endocrinol Metab Clin North Am 29:657-682, 2000.
32. Basu A, Close CF, Jenkins D, et al: Persisting mortality in diabetic ketoacidosis. Diabet Med 10:282-284, 1993.
33. Malone ML, Gennis V, Goodwin JS: Characteristics of diabetic ketoacidosis in older versus younger adults. J Am Geriatr Soc 40:1100-1104, 1992.
34. Scibilia J, Finegold D, Dorman J, et al: Why do children with diabetes die? Acta Endocrinol Suppl 279:326-333, 1986.
35. White NH: Management of diabetic ketoacidosis. Rev Endocr Metab Disord 4:343-353, 2003.
36. Microvascular and acute complications in IDDM patients: The EURODIAB IDDM Complications Study. Diabetologia 37:278-285, 1994.
37. Lebovitz HE: Diabetic ketoacidosis. Lancet 345:767-772, 1995.
38. Ananth J, Parameswaran S, Gunatilake S: Side effects of atypical antipsychotic drugs. Curr Pharm Des 10:2219-2229, 2004.

39. Tavakoli SA, Arguisola MS: Diabetic ketoacidosis in a patient treated with olanzapine, valproic acid, and venlafaxine. South Med J 96:729-730, 2003.

40. Wilson DR, D'Souza L, Sarkar N, et al: New-onset diabetes and ketoacidosis with atypical antipsychotics. Schizophr Res 59:1-6, 2003.

41. Kovacs M, Charron-Prochownik D, Obrosky DS: A longitudinal study of biomedical and psychosocial predictors of multiple hospitalizations among young people with insulin-dependent diabetes mellitus. Diabet Med 12:142-148, 1995.

42. Dumont RH, Jacobson AM, Cole C, et al: Psychosocial predictors of acute complications of diabetes in youth. Diabet Med 12:612-618, 1995.

43. Polonsky WH, Anderson BJ, Lohrer PA, et al: Insulin omission in women with IDDM. Diabetes Care 17:1178-1185, 1994.

44. Rydall AC, Rodin GM, Olmsted MP, et al: Disordered eating behavior and microvascular complications in young women with insulin-dependent diabetes mellitus. N Engl J Med 336:1849-1854, 1997.

45. Skinner TC: Recurrent diabetic ketoacidosis: Causes, prevention and management. Horm Res 57 Suppl 1:78-80, 2002.

46. Musey VC, Lee JK, Crawford R, et al: Diabetes in urban African-Americans. I. Cessation of insulin therapy is the major precipitating cause of diabetic ketoacidosis. Diabetes Care 18:483-489, 1995.

47. Luzi L, Barrett EJ, Groop LC, et al: Metabolic effects of low-dose insulin therapy on glucose metabolism in diabetic ketoacidosis. Diabetes 37:1470-1477, 1988.

48. Felig P, Sherwin RS, Soman V, et al: Hormonal interactions in the regulation of blood glucose. Recent Prog Horm Res 35:501-532, 1979.

49. DeFronzo RA, Matsuda M, Barret E: Diabetic ketoacidosis: A combined metabolic-nephrologic approach to therapy. Diabetes Rev 2:209-238, 1994.

50. van de Werve G, Jeanrenaud B: Liver glycogen metabolism: An overview. Diabetes Metab Rev 3:47-78, 1987.

51. Foster DW, McGarry JD: The metabolic derangements and treatment of diabetic ketoacidosis. N Engl J Med 309:159-169, 1983.

52. Gerich JE, Lorenzi M, Bier DM, et al: Effects of physiologic levels of glucagon and growth hormone on human carbohydrate and lipid metabolism. Studies involving administration of exogenous hormone during suppression of endogenous hormone secretion with somatostatin. J Clin Invest 57:875-884, 1976.

53. Gerich JE, Lorenzi M, Bier DM, et al: Prevention of human diabetic ketoacidosis by somatostatin. Evidence for an essential role of glucagon. N Engl J Med 292:985-989, 1975.

54. Exton JH: Mechanisms of hormonal regulation of hepatic glucose metabolism. Diabetes Metab Rev 3:163-183, 1987.

55. Schade DS, Eaton RP: The temporal relationship between endogenously secreted stress hormones and metabolic decompensation in diabetic man. J Clin Endocrinol Metab 50:131-136, 1980.

56. Umpierrez GE, Khajavi M, Kitabchi AE: Review: Diabetic ketoacidosis and hyperglycemic hyperosmolar nonketotic syndrome. Am J Med Sci 311:225-233, 1996.

57. Arner P, Kriegholm E, Engfeldt P, Bolinder J: Adrenergic regulation of lipolysis in situ at rest and during exercise. J Clin Invest 85:893-898, 1990.

58. Jensen MD, Caruso M, Heiling V, Miles JM: Insulin regulation of lipolysis in nondiabetic and IDDM subjects. Diabetes 38:1595-1601, 1989.

59. Nurjhan N, Consoli A, Gerich J: Increased lipolysis and its consequences on gluconeogenesis in non-insulin-dependent diabetes mellitus. J Clin Invest 89:169-175, 1992.

60. Muller WA, Faloona GR, Unger RH: Hyperglucagonemia in diabetic ketoacidosis. Its prevalence and significance. Am J Med 54:52-57, 1973.

61. Cook GA, King MT, Veech RL: Ketogenesis and malonyl coenzyme A content of isolated rat hepatocytes. J Biol Chem 253:2529-2531, 1978.

62. Nosadini R, Avogaro A, Doria A, et al: Ketone body metabolism: A physiological and clinical overview. Diabetes Metab Rev 5:299-319, 1989.

63. Balasse EO, Fery F: Ketone body production and disposal: Effects of fasting, diabetes, and exercise. Diabetes Metab Rev 5:247-270, 1989.

64. Stentz FB, Umpierrez GE, Cuervo R, Kitabchi AE: Proinflammatory cytokines, markers of cardiovascular risks, oxidative stress, and lipid peroxidation in patients with hyperglycemic crises. Diabetes 53:2079-2086, 2004.

65. Kitabchi AE, Stentz FB, Umpierrez GE: Diabetic ketoacidosis induces in vivo activation of human T-lymphocytes. Biochem Biophys Res Commun 315:404-407, 2004.

66. Stentz FB, Kitabchi AE: Activated T lymphocytes in Type 2 diabetes: Implications from in vitro studies. Curr Drug Targets 4:493-503, 2003.

67. Itani SI, Ruderman NB, Schmieder F, Boden G: Lipid-induced insulin resistance in human muscle is associated with changes in diacylglycerol, protein kinase C, and IκB-α. Diabetes 51:2005-2011, 2002.

68. Umpierrez G, Freire AX: Abdominal pain in patients with hyperglycemic crises. J Crit Care 17:63-67, 2002.

69. Campbell IW, Duncan LJ, Innes JA, et al: Abdominal pain in diabetic metabolic decompensation. Clinical significance. JAMA 233:166-168, 1975.

70. Barrett EJ, DeFronzo RA: Diabetic ketoacidosis: Diagnosis and treatment. Hosp Pract (Off Ed) 19:89-95, 99-104, 1984.

71. Schindler AM, Kowlessar M: Prolonged abdominal pain in a diabetic child. Hosp Pract (Off Ed) 23:134-136, 1988.

72. Fraser RJ, Horowitz M, Maddox AF, et al: Hyperglycaemia slows gastric emptying in type 1 (insulin-dependent) diabetes mellitus. Diabetologia 33:675-680, 1990.

73. de Boer SY, Masclee AA, Lam WF, et al: Effect of hyperglycaemia on gallbladder motility in type 1 (insulin-dependent) diabetes mellitus. Diabetologia 37:75-81, 1994.

74. Wachtel TJ, Silliman RA, Lamberton P: Prognostic factors in the diabetic hyperosmolar state. J Am Geriatr Soc 35:737-741, 1987.

75. Kitabchi AE, Wall BM: Diabetic ketoacidosis. Med Clin North Am 79:9-37, 1995.

76. Freire AX, Umpierrez GE, Afessa B, et al: Predictors of intensive care unit and hospital length of stay in diabetic ketoacidosis. J Crit Care 17:207-211, 2002.

77. Kitabchi AE, Umpierrez GE, Murphy MB, et al: Hyperglycemic crises in patients with diabetes mellitus. Diabetes Care 26 Suppl 1:S109-117, 2003.

78. Jenkins D, Close CF, Krentz AJ, et al: Euglycaemic diabetic ketoacidosis: Does it exist? Acta Diabetol 30:251-253, 1993.

79. Munro JF, Campbell IW, McCuish AC, Duncan LJ: Euglycaemic diabetic ketoacidosis. BMJ 2:578-580, 1973.

80. Umpierrez GE, DiGirolamo M, Tuvlin JA, et al: Differences in metabolic and hormonal milieu in diabetic- and alcohol-induced ketoacidosis. J Crit Care 15:52-59, 2000.

81. Stephens JM, Sulway MJ, Watkins PJ: Relationship of blood acetoacetate and 3-hydroxybutyrate in diabetes. Diabetes 20:485-489, 1971.

82. Byrne HA, Tieszen KL, Hollis S, et al: Evaluation of an electrochemical sensor for measuring blood ketones. Diabetes Care 23:500-503, 2000.

83. Alberti KG, Hockaday TD: Rapid blood ketone body estimation in the diagnosis of diabetic ketoacidosis. BMJ 2:565-568, 1972.

84. Winter SD, Pearson JR, Gabow PA, et al: The fall of the serum anion gap. Arch Intern Med 150:311-313, 1990.

85. Adrogue HJ, Wilson H, Boyd AE 3rd, et al: Plasma acid–base patterns in diabetic ketoacidosis. N Engl J Med 307:1603-1610, 1982.

86. Adrogue HJ, Eknoyan G, Suki WK: Diabetic ketoacidosis: Role of the kidney in the acid–base homeostasis re-evaluated. Kidney Int 25:591-598, 1984.

87. Ennis ED, Stahl EJVB, Kreisberg RA: The hyperosmolar hyperglycemic syndrome. Diabetes Rev 2:115-126, 1994.

patients to calculate their actual food intake and dose their insulin much like the normal pancreatic insulin response in nondiabetic persons. In addition, the fast action of these analogs allows patients to inject immediately after a meal if they were unsure how much food was going to be consumed. This will also reduce postprandial hypoglycemia and may be useful in treating gastroparesis.

Traditional long-acting insulins (NPH, Ultralente, glargine) can contribute to an increased rate of hypoglycemia. This is due to their pharmacokinetics, with a rapid onset of action (1 to 2 hours and a broader peak at about 4 hours) that may rapidly decline within 8 to 16 hours.[16] Bedtime injections can lead to nocturnal hypoglycemia because action peaks at about 2:00 AM, when patients are more insulin sensitive.[16] Conversely, NPH action wanes in the early morning hours when patients are more insulin resistant (dawn phenomenon), making hyperglycemia a problem.[16] Ultralente action lasts 16 to 20 hours in most patients. The disadvantages to Ultralente are that it does have a peak in action, and the time course for peak action is unpredictable. Thus, if doses are given every 12 hours, one dose can overlap with the previous dose, increasing the risk of hypoglycemia.[17] Glargine, a new basal insulin analog, produces very little, if any, peak due to its lower solubility at the injection site.[18] Glargine action lasts up to 24 hours and provides the closest to physiologic basal insulin coverage of the long-acting insulins. Studies of patients with T1DM and T2DM have demonstrated that glargine insulin produces less hypoglycemia compared with NPH insulin.[19]

Iatrogenic Hypoglycemia with Oral Agents

Oral agents have lower reported rates of hypoglycemia compared with multiple doses of traditional insulins. However, the hypoglycemia experienced with oral agent therapy may impede the ability to achieve intensive control. Oral insulin secretagogues such as sulfonylurea agents or meglitinides are often used in the treatment of T2DM. The mechanism of action of these compounds is mediated by binding to the sulfonylurea receptor in the pancreatic beta cell, which causes insulin secretion. The onset and duration of action might not coincide with the ambient blood sugar either due to an inaccurate dose or a lack of carbohydrate intake, or both. This in turn leads to oversecretion of insulin in relation to the blood glucose, which causes relative hyperinsulinemia.

The incidence of hypoglycemia with first-generation and early second-generation sulfonylurea agents like chlorpropamide and glyburide are 16% and 38%, respectively.[2] Later second-generation oral sulfonylurea agents (glipizide and glimepiride) tend to demonstrate lower rates of

hypoglycemia, but certain formulations produce less insulin secretion than others.[20] Glimepiride is the newest of these agents. Reported rates of hypoglycemia in patients with T2DM are reported to be 7-fold to 10-fold lower with glimepiride as compared with glyburide.[21]

During hypoglycemia, an important protective mechanism is the ability to suppress endogenous insulin secretion. An ideal oral agent would stimulate insulin secretion in the face of hyperglycemia but allow the normal negative feedback upon endogenous insulin during hypoglycemia. During clamp studies, glimepiride has been shown to stimulate endogenous insulin secretion during euglycemia as evidenced by increased C-peptide levels but not during hypoglycemic conditions in healthy controls.[22] However, glyburide resulted in persistent insulin secretion despite the presence of hypoglycemia. Interestingly, glucagon and consequently endogenous glucose production responses to hypoglycemia were also reduced with glyburide, suggesting that the increased frequency of hypoglycemia reported previously[21] may be due to increased insulin secretion and reduced glucagon secretion during hypoglycemia.

Repaglinide is a nonsulfonylurea insulin secretagogue that has a similar incidence of hypoglycemia compared with earlier-generation sulfonylureas.[23] Nateglinide, which is also a glinitide, has a much lower incidence of hypoglycemia and has glucose-dependent insulin-secretory properties similar to those of glimepiride. Other oral agents that do not seem to be associated with an increased incidence of hypoglycemia include metformin, which reduces hepatic glucose production and enhances peripheral and hepatic insulin sensitivity,[24] acarbose, which delays absorption of carbohydrates within the small intestine and thus entry into the systemic circulation, and thiazolidinediones, which also enhance insulin sensitivity.[23]

HYPOGLYCEMIA-ASSOCIATED AUTONOMIC FAILURE

For T1DM patients, the loss of endogenous insulin regulation removes one of the major defense mechanisms against hypoglycemia. In patients with increased duration of T1DM (and, to some degree, advanced T2DM), the glucagon response to hypoglycemia is lost and might reflect an impaired alpha cell defect.[25] The lack of glucagon release results in an estimated 40% reduction in glucose recovery.[26] When glucagon responses to hypoglycemia are lost, the role of epinephrine in counterregulation becomes critical. Unfortunately, a prior episode of hypoglycemia blunts autonomic nervous system (norepinephrine and epinephrine), neuroendocrine (glucagon, cortisol, and growth hormone), and metabolic (endogenous glucose production) counterregulatory responses to subsequent episodes of

hypoglycemia in healthy persons and in patients with T1DM.[27-31] This cycle of episodes of hypoglycemia blunting counterregulatory, neuroendocrine, and metabolic responses to subsequent episodes of hypoglycemia has been termed *hypoglycemia associated autonomic failure* (HAAF; Fig. 10–2).[32] This blunting of counterregulatory responses can occur with antecedent hypoglycemia of as little as 70 mg/dL.[29] The blunting can occur within hours[33] and can last for up to 5 days. HAAF creates a situation whereby the patient is more susceptible to both deeper and more frequent episodes of hypoglycemia. The deficient counterregulatory responses of T1DM are illustrated in Figure 10–3.

T2DM patients are also susceptible to HAAF. We have found that in T2DM patients, after 6 months of intensive glucose control, autonomic (epinephrine and norepinephrine) and metabolic (endoge-nous glucose production and lipolysis) responses to hypoglycemia were significantly lower compared with responses before intensive glucose treatment.[34] Furthermore, antecedent hypoglycemia also causes blunting of autonomic (epinephrine) and metabolic (endogenous glucose production and lipolysis) responses to subsequent hypoglycemia.[35] These studies provide evidence that HAAF can also occur in T2DM. The deficient counterregulatory responses of T2DM are illustrated in Figure 10–3.

The mechanisms by which autonomic counterregulation is blunted by prior hypoglycemia is not clearly understood, but several hypotheses exist. Prior cortisol administration has been found to mimic the blunting effect of prior hypoglycemia in humans[36,37] and rats.[38] In addition, brain glucose uptake[39] and brain glycogen stores[40] might be enhanced after prior hypoglycemia and are theorized to lead to a lower threshold for autonomic activation during subsequent hypoglycemia. Establishing the mechanism for HAAF might lead to further understanding of how to prevent the vicious cycle of hypoglycemia and allow patients to achieve the long-term benefits of intensive glycemic control.

Thus, the cause of increased frequency of hypoglycemia with intensive glucose control is a complex interplay of relative and absolute insulin excess with a mismatch of carbohydrate intake and blunted counterregulation to falling glucose levels (HAAF).

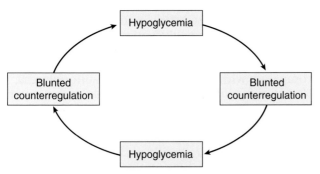

Figure 10–2. The cycle of hypoglycemia that causes hypoglycemia associated autonomic failure (HAAF). One episode of hypoglycemia blunts counterregulatory responses to subsequent episodes of hypoglycemia, leading to deeper and more frequent episodes of hypoglycemia.

HYPOGLYCEMIC SYMPTOMS

The onset of hypoglycemic symptoms (Box 10-1) in healthy subjects occurs at plasma glucose levels between 49 and 58 mg/dL.[41,42] Symptoms are categorized as neuroglycopenic or autonomic.[43] Neuro-

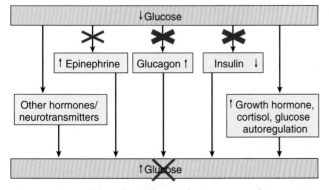

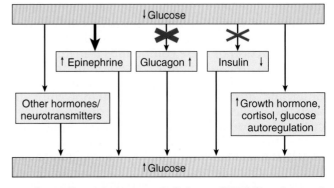

Figure 10–3. The physiology of counterregulatory responses to hypoglycemia in type 1 diabetes (T1DM) and type 2 diabetes (T2DM). In T1DM, as blood glucose falls, deficient changes in epinephrine, glucagon, and insulin prevent an increase in hepatic glucose production and also result in increased peripheral glucose disposal, contributing to further hypoglycemia. In intensively treated T2DM, deficient changes in glucagon and insulin may also prevent increases in hepatic glucose production. However, the exaggerated epinephrine responses may at least partially defend hepatic glucose production.

Box 10-1. Symptoms of Hypoglycemia

Neuroglycopenic Symptoms

- Coma
- Difficulty thinking
- Dizziness
- Fatigue
- Hunger
- Seizures
- Sleepiness
- Slurred speech
- Weakness

Autonomic Symptoms

- Anxiety
- Hunger
- Palpitations
- Paresthesias
- Sweating
- Tremulousness

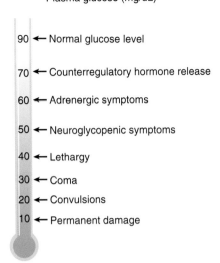

Responses to Falling Glucose Levels
Plasma glucose (mg/dL)

90 ← Normal glucose level

70 ← Counterregulatory hormone release

60 ← Adrenergic symptoms

50 ← Neuroglycopenic symptoms

40 ← Lethargy

30 ← Coma

20 ← Convulsions

10 ← Permanent damage

Figure 10–4. The physiologic and symptomatic changes as blood glucose falls. The body initiates a series of defense responses as blood glucose falls in order to prevent further hypoglycemia. If ignored and untreated, hypoglycemia can be detrimental.

glycopenic symptoms are caused by low cerebral glucose levels and include confusion or difficulty thinking, sleepiness, dizziness, weakness, fatigue, slurred speech, hunger, and eventually (if untreated) seizures and coma. Autonomic symptoms result from activation of the autonomic nervous system and include sweating, palpitations, tremulousness, anxiety, and paresthesias. There is a gradual order of symptoms as the blood glucose declines (Fig. 10–4).

The threshold of absolute plasma glucose that triggers these symptoms may be higher (conventional control) or lower (intensive control) depending upon the overall glycemic control of the patient. In other words, patients who tend to have a higher HbA1c percentage (overall higher ambient blood sugars) can perceive symptoms of hypoglycemia at a higher plasma glucose level than patients whose glycemia is more intensively controlled.[44] This is particularly true for patients with T2DM,[44,45] who can perceive hypoglycemic symptoms at blood glucose levels greater than 100 mg/dL, which is termed *relative hypoglycemia*. The converse is true in that patients whose glycemia is intensively controlled might not recognize low blood sugar until their plasma glucose is much lower.[46]

Recognizing symptoms of hypoglycemia allows patients to take corrective measures such as ingesting glucose-containing substances. This self-treatment during a mild episode prevents progression toward more severe hypoglycemia. Over time, patients exposed to recurrent hypoglycemia lose symptomatic response and become unaware of their hypoglycemia. Type 1 diabetic patients with

intensive glycemic control can develop hypoglycemic unawareness from 1 to 5 years after the diagnosis of the disease. Development depends on the frequency of hypoglycemia episodes; in other words, increased hypoglycemic episodes produce decreased awareness. Hypoglycemic unawareness greatly increases morbidity and mortality related to hypoglycemia. Fortunately, overt avoidance of hypoglycemia while maintaining intensive glucose control has been shown to reverse hypoglycemic unawareness to some extent within 3 days and fully within 3 to 4 weeks.[47]

Mild symptomatic hypoglycemia is usually easily recognized and treated by the patient. However, if it is unrecognized, as in hypoglycemic unawareness, mild hypoglycemia can lead to severe hypoglycemia, which can require external assistance for treatment and could even lead to seizures, coma, or death. Therefore, although it is critical to avoid severe hypoglycemia, the patient should be educated that asymptomatic or mild symptomatic hypoglycemia should be taken seriously as well in order to maintain awareness and prevent a more serious episode of hypoglycemia.

OTHER FACTORS INFLUENCING INCIDENCE OF HYPOGLYCEMIA

Exercise

Exercise is an important component of diabetes therapy. Regular exercise improves glycemic control by improving insulin sensitivity, helps maintain

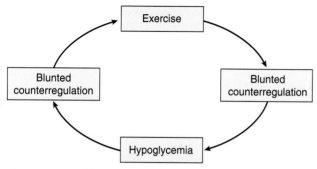

Figure 10–5. The cycle of hypoglycemia and exercise. A bout of exercise can blunt counterregulatory responses to subsequent exposure to hypoglycemia, which can also blunt counterregulatory responses to subsequent exercise, creating a vicious cycle of hypoglycemia.

body weight, and can reduce cardiovascular risk factors. However, acutely, exercise can increase glucose use for several hours after exercise. In the face of inadequate carbohydrate replacement or insulin excess, an acute exercise bout can lead to postexercise hypoglycemia. In addition, prior episodes of exercise and hypoglycemia can interact to blunt counterregulation, further contributing to hypoglycemia (Fig. 10–5). For example, prior hypoglycemia reduces both autonomic neuroendocrine and metabolic responses to subsequent prolonged exercise in both healthy subjects[48] and subjects with T1DM.[49] Conversely, prolonged exercise has been shown to also blunt autonomic and metabolic responses to subsequent hypoglycemia in nondiabetic[50,51] and T1DM subjects.[52] Furthermore, only one prolonged episode of exercise is needed to blunt counterregulatory responses to subsequent exercise[53] or hypoglycemia occurring later that day.[54]

Frequency, intensity, and duration of exercise may also be important factors to consider for preventing exercise-induced hypoglycemia. Increases in frequency, intensity, and duration can all independently increase carbohydrate requirements and deplete glycogen stores. In addition, in nondiabetic persons, insulin typically falls and glucose needs increase during exercise. Thus, a bolus of intermediate-acting or rapid-acting insulin can increase the risk of hypoglycemia during exercise.

For diabetic patients taking long-acting insulin analogs or oral hypoglycemic agents, decreasing insulin during exercise is not possible although glucose needs are still increasing. In this case, ingesting extra carbohydrate at 10 to 20 grams for each 30 minutes of exercise (depending on intensity) may also be recommended. An insulin pump is another method of insulin replacement for persons who exercise frequently so that insulin infusions can be lowered during exercise to prevent hypoglycemia. Short-acting insulin should be reduced both before and after a bout of exercise.

Carbohydrate should be consumed as soon after prolonged exercise as possible in order to replenish glycogen stores. Prolonged exercise (90 minutes), of either low or moderate intensity, blunts counterregulatory responses to subsequent hypoglycemia to the same degree in T1DM.[52] More research is needed to determine the impact of shorter-duration and higher-intensity exercise on counterregulatory function during subsequent hypoglycemia.

Thus, although beneficial as an adjunct therapy, regular exercise creates a difficult challenge for patients with diabetes in that the enhancement of insulin sensitivity (acutely and chronically) and the blunted counterregulation can increase depth and frequency of hypoglycemic episodes. More frequent and careful glucose monitoring, adjustment of insulin or oral medications, appropriate carbohydrate intake in anticipation of exercise, and, most importantly, patient education are critical to prevent hypoglycemia and allow patients to realize the benefits of exercise.

Gender

A patient's gender may also influence the ability to counterregulate in the face of hypoglycemia. It has been clearly demonstrated that healthy young women[55-57] and young women with T1DM[58] have reduced counterregulatory responses to hypoglycemia compared to men. Sympathetic nervous system, growth hormone, and endogenous glucose production responses were diminished with an enhanced autonomic symptom awareness and lipolytic response. This effect may be due to estrogen, because postmenopausal women taking estrogen-only hormone replacement were found to have blunted sympathetic nerve activity and epinephrine, glucagon, and endogenous glucose production responses compared with age-matched and BMI-matched men and compared with women not taking estrogen replacement.[59]

The Diabetes Control and Complications Trial did not find an increased incidence of hypoglycemia in women, but it did determine that women had a reduced risk of severe hypoglycemia when intensively treated as compared to men. Interestingly, when exposed to repeated episodes of hypoglycemia, women are more resistant to blunting of counterregulatory responses as compared to men.[60]

Thus, although gender differences in counterregulatory responses to hypoglycemia exist during the initial episode of hypoglycemia, the blunting that occurs with HAAF in men results in similar counterregulatory responses during subsequent episodes as compared to women. Thus, women are significantly more resistant to the deleterious effects of repeated hypoglycemia on counterregulatory responses as compared to men.

Age

Advanced age is a significantly increased risk for hypoglycemia.[61] In fact, hypoglycemia is an independent risk factor for morbidity in elderly subjects when hospitalized.[62] Although decreased clearance of hypoglycemic agents such as sulfonylureas and insulin could contribute to this risk,[61] impaired counterregulation[63] and decreased cognitive function[64] have also been implicated as causes.

One study demonstrated that older nondiabetic subjects had impaired insulin clearance and reduced glucagon, endogenous glucose production, and epinephrine responses to hypoglycemia as compared to younger nondiabetic subjects.[63] Another study found that cognitive function was more severely impaired in older (60 to 70 years) compared with younger (22 to 26 years) subjects, suggesting an impaired ability to recognize and potentially treat hypoglycemia.[64]

It is likely that many elderly patients have other concurrent illnesses and thus could be taking medications that interfere with or prolong the action of their diabetes medications.[61] For example, liver and renal function may be altered, leading to changes in clearance and metabolism of oral hypoglycemic agents. Thus, care must be taken when treating diabetes in older patients in order to prevent recurrent hypoglycemia.

Nighttime

The DCCT found that 40% of all severe episodes of hypoglycemia occur at night.[1] In fact, it is hypothesized that hypoglycemia can lead to cardiac (either thrombotic or arrhythmic) events during the night. QT interval is lengthened during both nighttime and daytime hypoglycemia, which supports this hypothesis.[65] However, the normal physiologic changes in insulin sensitivity that occur at night, the insulin regimen, and the potential lack of symptomatic and counterregulatory responses during sleep all contribute to the prevalence of nocturnal hypoglycemia. This last point has been the subject of recent studies that have determined that during sleep, patients with T1DM have significantly attenuated autonomic nervous system responses to hypoglycemia.[66] In addition, sleep prevents recognition and early intervention against hypoglycemia that can take place during the daytime.

Insulin sensitivity changes over the course of the night, increasing from 1 AM to 3 AM. Combined with different insulin regimens, this change can contribute to greater incidence of nocturnal hypoglycemia.[16] On the other hand, insulin requirements (by means of intravenous insulin) have been shown to increase by more than 20% in the early morning hours in order to maintain the same glycemic level in T1DM patients.[67] This effect, called the *dawn phenomenon,* is thought to occur because early morning increases in growth hormone and cortisol cause insulin resistance, thereby leading to early morning hyperglycemia.

The Somogyi phenomenon was also thought to cause an increase in morning hyperglycemia because of a rebound response to nocturnal hypoglycemia. However, studies in T1DM patients have demonstrated that nocturnally induced hypoglycemia did not cause higher plasma glucose levels in the morning, suggesting that the mechanism for early morning hyperglycemia is not due to a counterregulatory rebound from nocturnal hypoglycemia.[68]

Because of all of these factors, it is very important to modify treatment regimens to prevent nocturnal hypoglycemia. For example, glargine has been shown to reduce nocturnal hypoglycemia in both T1DM and T2DM.[69] Bedtime snacks that vary in composition and amount depending on the bedtime blood sugar may also prevent nocturnal hypoglycemia.[70] Overnight glucose monitoring is an important tool that is often underused in treating nocturnal hypoglycemia. The continuous glucose monitoring system (CGMS, Medtronic, Minneapolis, Minn) can give valuable information about undetermined hypoglycemia occurring during the night.

Ethanol

All diabetic patients are advised to moderate ethanol consumption because of the potential negative interaction with diabetic complications and because ethanol consumption is thought to cause hypoglycemia. In fact, two prospective studies have suggested that ethanol ingestion is responsible for a fifth of all severe hypoglycemic episodes in hospital emergency departments.[71,72] Other studies have shown that hypoglycemia is delayed after ethanol consumption[73-75] and that ethanol consumption impairs recovery from hypoglycemia in T1DM.[76]

Some research suggests that ethanol consumption blunts neuroendocrine counterregulatory responses leading to hypoglycemia. Growth hormone levels have been found to be reduced after ethanol consumption,[73] and growth hormone, cortisol, and glucagon levels were reduced during hypoglycemia following oral and intravenous ethanol.[77] Shirao and colleagues also demonstrated that ethanol administration attenuated stress-induced increases in norepinephrine release, suggesting decreased sympathetic nervous system drive.[78]

In addition to the potential for ethanol consumption to blunt counterregulation, various ethanol products can contain variable amounts of carbohydrate, leading to hyperglycemia and requiring an increased dose of insulin. Thus, limiting ethanol intake may also contribute to an avoidance of hypoglycemia.

TREATMENT AND PREVENTION OF HYPOGLYCEMIA

For some patients, poor glucose control is preferable to frequent hypoglycemic episodes. Thus, in order to improve glycemic control and compliance with intensive glucose control regimens, it is imperative to avoid hypoglycemia. This involves anticipatory guidance on the part of the patient and the diabetes care team.

Optimization of insulin or oral agent therapy to the patient's lifestyle can help decrease the incidence of hypoglycemia. The use of rapid-acting combined with long-acting insulin analogs can help prevent hypoglycemia in T1DM. some oral agents (glimepiride) have been shown to cause less hypoglycemia than others. Frequent glucose monitoring is also extremely important, especially in patients who are hypoglycemia unaware. Predetermined actions should be taken in response to glucose self-monitoring or when factors that increase the risk for hypoglycemia (exercise, aging, and ethanol consumption) are encountered.

To treat hypoglycemia, even mild relative hypoglycemia (blood sugar less than 80 mg/dL), all patients should have a rapidly available source of glucose with them at all times. The rule of 15 is a helpful treatment regimen: 15 grams of carbohydrate (rapidly absorbing forms of glucose as in glucose gel, sugar-containing soda, or glucose tablets) should raise the blood sugar by 15 mg/dL in about 15 minutes. In addition, when a patient has poor glucose control for an extended amount of time, symptoms of hypoglycemia can be felt at much higher glucose levels. To treat this relative hypoglycemia, patients can take 5 grams of carbohydrate for symptomatic hypoglycemia of greater than 70 mg/dL.

If a patient is unconscious, a 1-mg intramuscular glucagon injection may be given. Glucagon mobilizes glucose stores from the liver via glycogenolysis. Therefore, it may be less effective in a glycogen-depleted state than in prolonged starvation. The availability of a glucagon pen and education of use for family members or caregivers can also be helpful in treating serious hypoglycemia.

CONCLUSION

Limiting hypoglycemia in clinical practice is complex. It involves educating the patient about all the factors that can increase hypoglycemia, setting up predetermined actions to be taken when these factors are encountered, frequent glucose monitoring, and using medications and treatment regimens that cause less hypoglycemia and fit with the patient's schedule. With these objectives in place, patients will be able to maintain intensive glycemic control and thus prevent long-term complications associated with diabetes.

References

1. The Diabetes Control and Complications Trial Research Group: Epidemiology of severe hypoglycemia in the diabetes control and complications trial. Am J Med 90:450-459, 1991.
2. UK Prospective Study Group: Intensive blood-glucose control with sulphonylureas or insulin compared with conventional treatment and risk of complications in patients with type 2 diabetes [UKPDS 33]. Lancet 352:837-853, 1998.
3. The Diabetes Control and Complications Trial Research Group: Hypoglycaemia in the diabetes control and complication trial. Diabetes 46:271-286, 1997.
4. Bragd J, Adamson U, Lins PE, et al: A repeated cross-sectional survey of severe hypoglycaemia in 178 TYPE 1 diabetes mellitus patients performed in 1984 and 1998. Diabet Med 20:216-219, 2003.
5. Cryer PE: Hypoglycemia is the limiting factor in the management of diabetes. Diabetes Metab Res Rev 15:42-46, 1999.
6. Cryer PE: Hypoglycemia: Pathophysiology, Diagnosis and Treatment. New York, Oxford University Press, 1997.
7. Levin BE: Glucosensing neurons: The metabolic sensors of the brain? Diabetes Nutr Metab 15:274-280, 2002.
8. Towler DA, Havlin CE, Craft S, Cryer P: Mechanism of awareness of hypoglycemia. Perception of neurogenic (predominantly cholinergic) rather than neuroglycopenic symptoms. Diabetes 42:1791-1798, 1993.
9. Havel PJ, Parry SJ, Stern JS, et al: Redundant parasympathetic and sympathoadrenal mediation of increased glucagon secretion during insulin-induced hypoglycemia in conscious rats. Metabolism 43:860-866, 1994.
10. Hepburn DA, MacLeod KM, Pell AC, et al: Frequency and symptoms of hypoglycemia experienced by patients with type 2 diabetes treated with insulin. Diabet Med 10:231-237, 1993.
11. Dimitriadis GD, Gerich JE: Importance of timing of preprandial subcutaneous insulin administration in the management of diabetes mellitus. Diabetes Care 6 374-377, 1983.
12. Howey DC, Bowsher RR, Brunelle RL, Woodworth JR: [Lys(B28), Pro(B29)]-human insulin—a rapidly absorbed analog of human insulin. Diabetes 43:396-402, 1994.
13. Home P: Insulin aspart. Drugs 57:766-767, 1999.
14. Brunelle BL, Llewelyn J, Anderson JH Jr, et al: Meta-analysis of the effect of insulin lispro on severe hypoglycemia in patients with type 1 diabetes. Diabetes Care 21:1726-1731, 1998.
15. Home PD, Lindholm A, Hylleberg B, Round P: Improved glycemic control with insulin aspart: A multicenter randomized double-blind crossover trial in type 1 diabetic patients. Diabetes Care 21:1904-1909, 1998.
16. Bolli GB, Periello G, Fanelli CG, De Feo P: Nocturnal blood-glucose control in type-i diabetes-mellitus. Diabetes Care 16:71-89, 1993.
17. Gerich JE: Insulin glargine: Long-acting basal insulin analog for improved metabolic control. Curr Med Res Opin 20:31-37, 2004.
18. Dreyer M, Pein M, Schmidt C, et al: Comparison of the pharmacokinetics/dynamics of Gly[A21]-Arg[B31,B32]-human-insulin [HOE71GT] with NPH-insulin following subcutaneous injection by using euglycemic clamp technique. Diabetologia 37(suppl 1):A78, 1994.
19. Porcellati F, Bartocci L, Di Vincenzo A, et al: Glargine vs NPH as basal insulin in intensive treatment of T1DM given lispro at meals: One year comparison. Diabetes 51(suppl 2):A53, 2002.
20. Burge MR, Schmitz-Fiorentino K, Fischette C, et al: A prospective trial of risk factors for sulfonylurea-induced hypoglycemia in type 2 diabetes mellitus. JAMA 279: 137-143, 1998.
21. Campbell RK: Glimepiride: Role of a new sulfonylurea in the treatment of type 2 diabetes mellitus. Ann Pharmacother 32:1044-1052, 1998.
22. Aftab Guy D, Richardson A, Davis SN, et al: Counterregulatory responses to hypoglycemia differ between glimepiride and glyburide in healthy man. Diabetes 53:A165, 2004.

23. DeFronzo RA: Pharmacologic therapy for type 2 diabetes mellitus. Ann Intern Med 131:281-303, 1999.

24. Bailey CJ, Turner RC: Drug therapy: Metformin. New Engl J Med 334:574-579, 1996.

25. Gerich JE, Langlois M, Noacco C, et al: Lack of glucagon response to hypoglycemia in diabetes: Evidence for an intrinsic pancreatic alpha cell defect. Science 182:171-173, 1973.

26. Rizza RA, Cryer PE, Gerich JE: Role of glucagon, catecholamines, and growth hormone in human glucose counterregulation. J Clin Invest 64:62-71, 1979.

27. Davis MR, Mellman MJ, Shamoon H: Further defects in counterregulatory responses induced by recurrent hypoglycemia in IDDM. Diabetes 41:1335-1340, 1992.

28. Davis SN, Tate D: Effects of morning hypoglycemia on neuroendocrine and metabolic responses to subsequent afternoon hypoglycemia in normal man. J Clin Endocrinol Metab 86:2043-2050, 2001.

29. Davis SN, Shavers C, Mosqueda-Garcia R, Costa F: Effects of differing antecedent hypoglycemia on subsequent counterregulation in normal humans. Diabetes 46:1328-1335, 1997.

30. Heller SR, Cryer PE: Reduced neuroendocrine and symptomatic responses to subsequent hypoglycemia after one episode of hypoglycemia in nondiabetic humans. Diabetes 40:223-226, 1991.

31. Widom B, Simonson D: Intermittent hypoglycemia impairs glucose counterregulation. Diabetes 41:1597-1602, 1992.

32. Cryer PE: Hypoglycemia-associated autonomic failure in diabetes. Am J Physiol Endocrinol Metab 281:E1115-E1121, 2001.

33. Davis SN, Mann S, Galassetti P, et al: Effects of differing durations of antecedent hypoglycemia on counterregulatory responses to subsequent hypoglycemia in normal humans. Diabetes 49:1897-1903, 2000.

34. Davis SN, Galassetti P, Wasserman D, Tate D: The effects of 6 months intensive glucose control on counterregulatory responses to hypoglycemia in type 2 DM. Diabetes 49:A132, 2000.

35. Davis SN, Mann S, Tate DB, et al: Effects of antecedent hypoglycemia on counterregulatory response to subsequent hypoglycemia in patients with Type 2 diabetes. Diabetes 48:A363, 1999.

36. Davis SN, Shavers C, Costa F, Mosqueda-Garcia R: Role of cortisol in the pathogenesis of deficient counterregulation after antecedent hypoglycemia in normal humans. J Clin Invest. 98:680-691, 1996.

37. McGregor VP, Banarer S, Cryer PE: Elevated endogenous cortisol reduces autonomic neuroendocrine and symptom responses to subsequent hypoglycemia. Am J Physiol Endocrinol Metab 282:E770-E777, 2002.

38. Sandoval D, Ping L, Neill AR, et al: Cortisol acts through central mechanisms to blunt counterregulatory responses to hypoglycemia in conscious rats. Diabetes 52:2198-2204, 2003.

39. Boyle PJ, Kempers SF, O'Connor AM, Nagy RJ: Brain glucose uptake and unawareness of hypoglycemia in patients with insulin-dependent diabetes mellitus. N Engl J Med 333:1720-1731, 1995.

40. Choi IY, Seaquist ER, Gruetter R: Effect of hypoglycemia on brain glycogen metabolism in vivo. J Neurosci Res 72:25-32, 2003.

41. Mitrakou A, Ryan C, Veneman T, et al: Hierarchy of glycemic thresholds for counterregulatory hormone secretion, symptoms, and cerebral dysfunction. Am J Physiol 260:E67-E74, 1991.

42. Schwartz NS, Clutter WE, Shah SD, Cryer PE: Glycemic thresholds for activation of glucose counterregulatory systems are higher than the threshold for symptoms. J Clin Invest 79:777-781, 1987.

43. Cryer PE: Symptoms of hypoglycemia, thresholds for their occurrence, and hypoglycemia unawareness. Endocrinol Metab Clin North Am 28:495-504, 1999.

44. Boyle PJ, Schwartz NS, Shah SD, et al: Plasma glucose concentrations at the onset of hypoglycemic symptoms in patients with poorly controlled diabetes and in nondiabetics. N Engl J Med 318:1487-1492, 1988.

45. Spyer G, Hattersley AT, MacDonald IA, et al: Hypoglycaemic counter-regulation at normal blood glucose concentrations in patients with well-controlled type-2 diabetes. Lancet 356:1970-1974, 2000.

46. Amiel SA, Sherwin RS, Simonson DC, Tamorlane WV: Effect of intensive insulin therapy on glycemic thresholds for counterregulatory hormone release. Diabetes 37:901-907, 1988.

47. Dagogo-Jack S, Rattarasarn C, Cryer PE: Reversal of hypoglycemia unawareness, but not defective glucose counterregulation, in IDDM. Diabetes 43:1426-1434, 1994.

48. Davis SN, Galassetti P, Wasserman DH, Tate D: Effects of antecedent hypoglycemia on subsequent counterregulatory responses to exercise. Diabetes 49:73-81, 2000.

49. Galassetti P, Tate D, Neill RA, et al: Effect of antecedent hypoglycemia on neuroendocrine responses to subsequent exercise in type 1 diabetes. Diabetes 50:A54, 2001.

50. McGregor VP, Griewe JS, Banarer S, Cryer PE: Limited impact of vigorous exercise on defenses against hypoglycemia: Relevance to hypoglycemia-associated autonomic failure. Diabetes 50:A138, 2001.

51. Galassetti P, Mann S, Tate D, et al: Effect of antecedent prolonged exercise on subsequent counterregulatory responses to hypoglycemia. Am J Physiol 280:E908-E917, 2001.

52. Sandoval DA, Guy DL, Richardson MA, et al: Effects of low and moderate antecedent exercise on counterregulatory responses to subsequent hypoglycemia in type 1 diabetes. Diabetes 53:1798-1806, 2004.

53. Galassetti P, Mann S, Tate D, et al: Effect of morning exercise on counterregulatory responses to subsequent, afternoon exercise. J Appl Physiol 91:91-99, 2001.

54. Sandoval DA, Aftab-Guy D, Davis SN, et al: Effects of same day exercise on subsequent counterregulatory responses to hypoglycemia. Diabetes 53:A88, 2004.

55. Amiel SA, Maran A, Powrie JK, et al: Gender differences in counterregulation to hypoglycaemia. Diabetologia 36:460-464, 1993.

56. Diamond MP, Jones T, Caprio S, et al: Gender influences counterregulatory hormone responses to hypoglycemia. Metabolism 42:1568-1572, 1993.

57. Davis SN, Shavers C, Costa F: Differential gender responses to hypoglycemia are due to alterations in CNS drive and not glycemic thresholds. Am J Physiol Endocrinol Metab 279:E1054-E1063, 2000.

58. Davis SN, Fowler S, Costa F: Hypoglycemic counterregulatory responses differ between men and women with type 1 diabetes. Diabetes 49:65-72, 2000.

59. Sandoval DA, Ertl AC, Richardson MA, et al: Estrogen blunts neuroendocrine and metabolic responses to hypoglycemia. Diabetes 52:1749-1755, 2003.

60. Davis SN, Shavers C, Costa F: Gender-related differences in counterregulatory responses to antecedent hypoglycemia in normal humans. J Clin Endocrinol Metab 85:2148-2157, 2000.

61. Shorr RI, Ray WA, Daugherty JR, Griffin MR: Incidence and risk factors for serious hypoglycemia in older persons using insulin or sulfonylureas. Arch Intern Med 157:1681-1686, 1997.

62. Kagansky N, Levy S, Rimon E, et al: Hypoglycemia as a predictor of mortality in hospitalized elderly patients. Arch Intern Med 163:1825-1829, 2003.

63. Marker JC, Cryer PE, Clutter W: Attenuated glucose recovery from hypoglycemia in the elderly. Diabetes 41:671-678, 1992.

64. Matyka K, Evans M, Lomas J, et al: Altered hierarchy of protective responses against severe hypoglycemia in normal aging in healthy men. Diabetes Care 20:135-141, 1997.

65. Robinson RT, Harris ND, Ireland RH, et al: Changes in cardiac repolarization during clinical episodes of nocturnal hypoglycaemia in adults with type 1 diabetes. Diabetologia 47:312-315, 2004.

66. Banarer S, Cryer PE: Sleep-related hypoglycemia-associated autonomic failure in type 1 diabetes: Reduced awakening from sleep during hypoglycemia. Diabetes 52:1195-1203, 2003.

67. DeFeo P, Perriello G, Torlone E, et al: Contribution of adrenergic mechanisms to glucose counterregulation in humans. Am J Physiol 261:E725-E736, 1991.

68. Tordjman KM, Havlin CE, Levandoski LA, et al: Failure of nocturnal hypoglycemia to cause fasting hyperglycemia in patients with insulin-dependent diabetes-mellitus. N Engl J Med 317:1552-1559, 1987.

69. Chase HP, Dixon B, Pearson J, et al: Reduced hypoglycemic episodes and improved glycemic control in children with type 1 diabetes using insulin glargine and neutral protamine Hagedorn insulin. J Pediatr 143:737-740, 2003.

70. Kalergis M, Schiffrin A, Gougeon R, et al: Impact of bedtime snack composition on prevention of nocturnal hypoglycemia in adults with type 1 diabetes undergoing intensive insulin management using Lispro insulin before meals: A randomized, placebo-controlled, crossover trial. Diabetes Care 26:9-15, 2003.

71. Potter J, Clarke P, Gale EA, et al: Insulin-induced hypoglycaemia in an accident and emergency department: The tip of an iceberg: BMJ 285:1180-1182, 1982.

72. Nilsson A, Tideholm B, Kalen J, Katzman P: Incidence of severe hypoglycemia and its causes in insulin-treated diabetics. Acta Med Scand 224:257-262, 1988.

73. Turner BC, Jenkins E, Kerr D, et al: The effect of evening alcohol consumption on next-morning glucose control in type 1 diabetes. Diabetes Care 24:1888-1893, 2001.

74. Lange J, Arends J, Willms B: [Alcohol-induced hypoglycemia in type 1 diabetic patients]. Med Klin (Munich) 86:551-554, 1991.

75. Joffe BI, Shires R, Lamprey JM, et al: Effect of drinking bottled beer on plasma-insulin and glucose responses in normal subjects. S Afr Med J 62:95-97, 1982.

76. Avogaro A, Beltramello P, Gnudi L, et al: Alcohol intake impairs glucose counterregulation during acute insulin-induced hypoglycemia in IDDM patients. Evidence for a critical role of free fatty acids. Diabetes 42:1626-1634, 1993.

77. Kolaczynski JW, Ylikahri R, Harkonen M, Koivisto VA: The acute effect of ethanol on counterregulatory response and recovery from insulin-induced hypoglycemia. J Clin Endocrinol Metab 67:384-388, 1988.

78. Shirao I, Tsuda A, Ida Y, et al: Effect of acute ethanol administration on noradrenaline metabolism in brain-regions of stressed and nonstressed rats. Pharmacol Biochem Behav 30:769-773, 1988.

Advanced Glycation End Products

An intracellular increase in glucose results in the formation of AGEs, which, along with other factors, may initiate an inflammatory cascade.[66] AGEs are increased during aging as well as diabetes by autooxidation of glucose and its binding to proteins. The protein binding is initially reversible, and then irreversible, modifying the proteins and their structure[67] with glucose[68] via the Maillard reaction,[69,70] with initial formation of Schiff bases, then rearranging to form more stable Amadori products, resulting in end products such as glyoxal, methylglyoxal, 3-deoxyglucose, pentosidine, and pyralline.

These reactions are reversible and cause no damage, but they undergo a slow, complex series of chemical events to form AGEs. This last reaction is no longer reversible and is the basis of their damage potential. Formation of AGEs damages cells by altering cell surface interactions, which activates intracellular signaling pathways to alter endothelial function.[71,72] AGEs alter neurofilament subunits by cross-linking material in the cytoskeletal fractions of diabetic nerves.[73,74] In addition, AGEs are deposited in peripheral nerves[75] and the optic nerve head.[76]

AGEs can bind to cell surface receptor proteins called receptors for AGE (RAGE). These receptors cause cellular dysfunction through a cascade of events including overactivation of PKC-β, increased NF-κB, and increased MAP kinase.[77-79] The RAGE receptor gene has binding sites for NF-κB and thus results in amplification of RAGE, promoting a vicious cycle of damage and oxidative stress that leads to further damage.

RAGE are increased in glomeruli of patients with diabetes[80] and in vascular endothelial cells in mice.[81] The presence of AGEs and RAGE in patients with diabetes suggests that these metabolic end products are a part of the etiology of neuropathy.

Aldose Reductase (Polyol) Pathway

In patients with diabetes, excess glucose not metabolized by glycolysis enters the polyol pathway. There is increased flux through the polyol pathway, resulting in elevated nerve levels of glucose, fructose, and sorbitol, possibly due to enhanced aldose reductase and reduced sorbitol dehydrogenase.[82,83] Sorbitol accumulation leads to cellular and osmotic stress. Aldose reductase uses reduced nicotinamide adenine dinucleotide phosphate (NADPH) to reduce glucose to sorbitol, which is oxidized to fructose by sorbitol dehydrogenase using nicotinamide adenine dinucleotide (NAD+). NADPH is needed to regenerate the antioxidant glutathione, thus promoting oxidative stress.

Decreases in cellular NADPH caused by the flux in the polyol pathway is referred to as *pseudohypoxia* and decreases generation of nitric oxide in endothelial cells and alters redox balance[84] because NADPH is needed as a cofactor for nitric oxide synthase. This complex interaction causes alterations in the redox state, which lead to oxidative stress, increased PKC-β, altered ion transport, and neuron damage.[85] The increased NADH/NAD+ ratio can alter enzyme activities, which contribute to diabetic microvascular complications.[86]

Hexosamine Pathway

The hexosamine pathway is activated when excess intermediates are formed from increased glycolytic activity. These intermediates alter gene function and protein expression that contribute to diabetic microvascular complications. Many of the acylglycosylated proteins are transcription factors that increase the production of proteins such as TGF-β and plasminogen activator inhibitor 1 (PAI-1), which increase nephropathy and microvascular disease. This pathway is particularly important in type 2 diabetes, wherein the activity of glutamine acts via glucosamine fructose-6-phosphate amidotransferase (GFAT). GFAT converts fructose-6-phosphate to glucosamine-6-phosphate, and UDP-N-acetylglucosaminyltransferase (UDP-GlcNAc) induces transcription factors. Activation of the hexosamine pathway may cause insulin resistance and oxidative stress, probably by increasing intracellular H_2O_2 and PKC-β modulation of c-myc.

Oxidative Stress

Each of these pathways leads to oxidative stress and formation of reactive oxygen species (ROS) (see Fig. 11–2). The polyol pathway depletes antioxidant defense mechanisms, AGEs increase by generation of ROS and PKC activation, and increased hexosamine leads to tissue ischemia and oxidative stress. During hyperglycemia, oxidative stress is increased by superoxides, which occur at abnormally high levels due to increased glycolysis and lipolysis with impaired mitochondrial activity. Superoxide is metabolized to H_2O_2 by superoxide dismutase. H_2O_2 is freely diffusible and reacts with iron to form OH radicals that damage lipids. The resultant lipid peroxides cause cell death.

ROS react with NO to form $ONOO^-$, which disrupts proteins, and they react with lipids, which is also toxic to cells. Proteins and nucleic acids undergo peroxidation and nitrosylation and interfere with recycling mechanisms, damaging neurons. For example, there is a decrease in bcl-2, an increase in c-Jun-N-terminal kinase (JNK), poly(ADP-ribose) polymerase (PARP), and cyclooxygenase-2 (COX-2), and loss of the antiapoptotic mechanism, leading to an increase in the proapoptotic genes involved in determining cell survival. Mitochondria are particularly sensitive to the deleterious process, leading to loss of energy function.

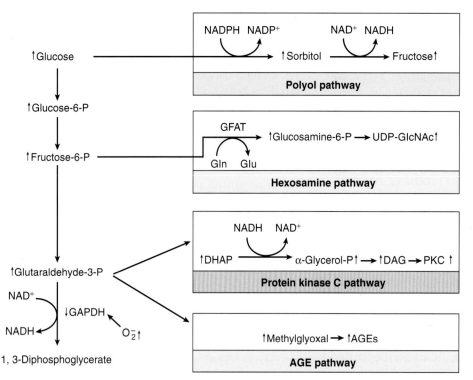

Figure 11–2. Hyperglycemia induces four pathways, including activation of protein kinase C. AGE, advanced glycated end product; DAG, diacylglycerol; DHAP, dihydroxyacetone phosphate; GAPDH, glyceraldehyde-3-phosphate dehydrogenase; GFAT, glucosamine-fructose-6-phosphate-aminotransferase 1; Gln, glutamine; Glu, glutamate; NAD+, nicotinamide adenine dinucleotide; NADH, reduced NAD; PKC, protein kinase C; UDP-GlcNAc, UDP-N-acetylglucosaminyltransferase.

Hyperglycemia induces oxidative stress by enhancing mitochondrial respiration, by redox alteration, and by uncoupling proteins, which leads to increased superoxide anions.[87,88] Oxidative stress and superoxides have detrimental effects on the cell. Human sural nerve biopsies indicate that oxidative stress is coupled with mitochondrial membrane depolarization and programmed cell death (apoptosis) of diabetic dorsal root ganglion neurons and Schwann cells, which is not observed in animals.[89] The oxidants produced can damage mitochondrial DNA[90,91] and cellular proteins[88,92] and can promote inflammation.[93,94] There is an increase in ROS during hyperglycemia that results in mitochondrial dysfunction, release of cytochrome *c*, and cleavage of caspases,[89] the enzymes involved in DNA destruction. Additionally, diabetic mice overexpressing superoxide dismutase—the enzyme that reduces the accumulation of ROS—are protected from renal injury, indicating a role of oxidative stress in pathogenesis of diabetic microvascular complications.[95,96]

Hyperglycemia and oxidative stress deplete NO within the peripheral nerves and endothelium of the microvasculature by reducing epithelial nitric oxide synthase (eNOS), which alters nerve perfusion.[97] Depletion of endothelial NO leads to low nerve blood flow, hypoxia, and mitochondrial dysfunction.[98,99] ROS down-regulates neuronal nitric oxide synthase (nNOS) during hyperglycemia. These observations suggest a role of NO repletion as a potential therapy in experimental diabetic polyneuropathy.

However, there is a biphasic response of NO to hyperglycemic and inflammatory damage to peripheral nerves. Under inflammatory conditions, inducible NOS (iNOS) increases, which leads to nanomolar quantities of NO, as opposed to the picomolar amounts produced with eNOS activation.[99,100] High levels of NO cause nerve damage via mitochondrial dysfunction and formation of peroxynitrite by interaction with ROS. Peroxynitrite nitrotyrosylates proteins, thereby impairing their function.

Although these changes in NO regulation depend on the cell type, there may be some benefit to up-regulation of endothelial-derived NO to improve vascular function.[101] Antioxidants typically defend the cell against damage. Some studies have shown that patients with diabetes have reduced levels of these antioxidants[102-104]; however, there is conflicting evidence in the literature.[105,106]

Another theory involves myoinositol. Decreased myoinositol levels play a role in nerve cells' ionic balance and nerve impulses. During hyperglycemia, glucose competitively inhibits myoinositol uptake and lowers levels within nerve cells. Inadequate myoinositol leads to sodium retention, edema, myelin swelling, and nerve degeneration.[107]

Vascular Mechanisms

Microvascular insufficiency, endoneural blood flow, and hemodynamic factors lead to nerve damage

in patients with diabetic polyneuropathy.[37,108-111] Although the sequence of events is not well understood, investigators propose that microvascular vasoconstriction, edema, and ischemia play a role in development of diabetic polyneuropathy. Endoneural edema increases endoneural pressure,[112] thereby causing capillary closure and subsequent nerve ischemia and damage.[113,114] Diminished regulation of the endoneural blood flow and ischemia can result from decreased nerve density and innervation of vessels[115] as measured with laser Doppler.[116] Nerve ischemia stimulates VEGF production, exacerbating diabetic polyneuropathy via overactivation of PKC-β.[117-122] As a result, ischemia and low blood flow reduce endothelial-dependent and nitric oxide–dependent vasorelaxation.[59,123,124] Vascular defects also result in changes in endoneural vessels.

Epineural changes include arteriolar attenuation, venous distension, and arteriovenous shunting that leads to new vessel formation.[125] Neural regulation of blood flow is complicated by arteriovenous anastomoses and shunting, which deviate the blood flow from the skin, creating an ischemic microenvironment.[97] There is thickening and deposition of substances in the vessel wall associated with endothelial cell growth, pericyte loss (in eyes), and occlusion.[126] Changes in blood flow correlate with changes in oxygen saturation[109,127] and reduced sural nerve endoneural oxygen tension.[128] These changes are followed by increased expression or action of vasoconstrictors such as endothelin and angiotensin and decreased activity of vasodilators such as prostacyclin, substance P, calcitonin gene-related peptide (CGRP), endothelium-derived hyperpolarizing factor (EDHF), and bradykinin.[129,130] Based on this theory, investigators have given oxygen and vasodilatory agents to patients; however, these therapies have not improved diabetic polyneuropathy.[131,132]

Methods of assessing skin blood flow have demonstrated that diabetes disturbs microvasculature, tissue PO_2, and vascular permeability. In particular, in patients with diabetic polyneuropathy there is disruption in *vasomotion,* the rhythmic contraction exhibited by arterioles and small arteries.[133,134] In type 2 diabetes, skin blood flow is abnormal and the loss of the neurogenic vasodilative mechanism in hairy skin might precede lower limb microangiopathic processes and C-fiber dysfunction.[134,135] Changes in endoneural blood flow often are reflected by changes in nerve conduction.[136-139] In addition, impaired blood flow can predict ulceration.[12,23,140-142] Therefore, both vascular and endoneural alterations can cause damage over time in the peripheral nerves of patients with diabetes.

Autoimmune Mechanisms

Autoimmunity plays a role in neuropathy. Antibodies develop that are directed against damaged nerves. Studies suggest that circulating autoantibodies against motor and sensory nerve structures are present in the serum of patients with diabetes.[143,144] In addition, antiphospholipid antibodies have been found in up to 88% of patients with diabetic neuropathy.[145] These antibodies are associated with a motor deficit that has electrophysiologic signs of demyelination and altered nerve function. Case studies have observed deposition of immunoglobulin M (IgM) and IgG in the nerves of patients with diabetic polyneuropathy, suggesting a role for autoimmunity.[146,147]

Additional studies indicate that neuropathy is a result of toxic factors in the blood in concert with hyperglycemia.[143] Serum from patients with diabetic polyneuropathy contains immunoglobulins that, in the presence of complement, bind to neuronal cells and increase calcium uptake, inducing Fas-mediated apoptosis of neurons in culture.[148] These studies suggest that autoimmunity and toxicity lead to nerve dysfunction.

Neurotrophic Factors

Neurotrophic factors are proteins that promote survival of neurons that regulate gene expression through second messenger systems. These proteins can induce morphologic changes, nerve differentiation, and nerve cell proliferation, and they can induce neurotransmitter expression and release. Subsequent reduction in levels of neurotrophic factors[149] can lead to neuron loss, possibly through activation of apoptosis.[150]

Many proteins have properties and characteristics of neurotrophic factors. These include cytokine-like growth factors, TGF-β, neurotrophin 3 (NT3), NGF, insulin-like growth factor-1 (IGF-I), and VEGF. Only a few neurotrophic factors have been extensively investigated, but a number of proteins have been identified as neurotrophic factors.[44,151] These proteins appear to have different expression in nerves of patients with diabetes.[126] For example, interleukin-6 (IL-6), a cytokine-like growth factor, may play a role in cell proliferation.[152] Often these growth factors are associated with changes in nerve structure via apoptosis or proliferation. The laminin B_2 gene is up-regulated in normal animals undergoing sciatic nerve regeneration following nerve section.[153] This process is impaired in diabetes. Other extracellular matrix proteins are altered in neuropathic nerves.[154] Therefore, understanding the role of neurotrophic factors has been the focus of much investigation.

Neurons affected in diabetic neuropathy are developmentally dependent on NGF. Therefore a decline in NGF synthesis in patients with diabetes plays a role in the pathogenesis of neuropathy, especially in small fibers.[155] More specifically, NGF has been shown to be trophic for sympathetic ganglion neurons and the neural crest–derived system.[151]

Other neurotrophic factors affect sympathetic neurons. Neurotrophins are trophic to large-diameter fiber sensory neurons.[156] These factors bind to the high-affinity receptor TRK (tropomyosin-related kinase)[157] or the low-affinity receptor p75[158]; both may activate different signaling cascades. Although their function is not well understood, IGF-I and IGF-II have been shown to regulate growth and differentiation of neurons.[159] IGF, NGF, and other neurotrophins are found in a number of proteins involved in growth of neurons.

Neurotrophic proteins are reduced in patients with diabetes. NGF protein levels in the serum of patients with diabetes are suppressed.[160] Additionally, diabetes can result in decreased serum IGF and increased IGF-I binding protein I,[161] thereby inhibiting the protein's downstream effects. Despite increasing evidence that growth factors are suppressed in patients with diabetes, no direct link has been found between neurotrophic factors and the pathogenesis of diabetic polyneuropathy,[151] and preliminary studies of NGF and NT3 treatment have met with limited success.

Our current view of the pathogenesis of diabetic neuropathy is summarized in Figure 11–2, which highlights multiple etiologies including metabolic, vascular, and autoimmune causes, oxidative stress, and neurohormonal growth-factor deficiency. Several articles highlight the most recent theories and provide an excellent review.[140,162,163] Research focus is on oxidative stress, AGEs, PKC, and the polyol pathways.

Diabetic neuropathy is a heterogeneous disease with various theories on its pathology, suggesting differences in pathogenic mechanisms for the different clinical syndromes. The production of treatments that prevent or reverse its development and progression will require the identification of these pathologic processes.

DIAGNOSIS

Difficulties

The San Antonio Consensus Conference has defined diabetic neuropathy as "a demonstrable disorder, either clinically evident or sub-clinical, that occurs in the setting of diabetes mellitus without other causes for peripheral neuropathy. The neuropathic disorder includes manifestations in the somatic and/or autonomic parts of the peripheral nervous system."[141] Neuropathy should therefore be diagnosed with a careful clinical examination, giving special consideration to the presence of symptoms and signs of peripheral nerve dysfunction after excluding causes other than diabetes.[142]

Diabetic neuropathy might not exhibit the typical symptoms, and in many cases it is asymptomatic. On the other hand, up to 10% of peripheral neuropathy was determined to be of nondiabetic origin in the Rochester Diabetic Neuropathy Study.[142] Consequently, it is generally recommended that diabetic neuropathy not be diagnosed on one symptom, sign, or test alone, but with a minimum of two abnormalities (from symptoms, signs, nerve conduction abnormalities, quantitative sensory tests, or quantitative autonomic tests).[164]

Due to the difficulty associated with the diagnosis, diabetic neuropathy is underdiagnosed, even by endocrinologists. One study, which assessed how often neuropathy is accurately diagnosed, identified the absence of neuropathy in 7000 patients but only accurately diagnosed the presence of mild neuropathy in a third of all cases.[165] Severe neuropathy was accurately diagnosed in 75% of the patients evaluated. Evidently there is a need for educating physicians in the art of correctly diagnosing diabetic neuropathy in a timely manner, so that they can employ preventive as well as therapeutic techniques.

Method

Patients with diabetes mellitus can have an extensive range of clinical neuropathic syndromes including dysfunction of almost every segment of the somatic peripheral and autonomic nervous system.[166] The pathophysiologic, therapeutic, and prognostic features of each syndrome are used as distinguishing factors.

A careful history is a prerequisite for the diagnosis of diabetic neuropathy. It is important to ascertain the positive and negative symptoms of neuropathy to provide an accurate diagnosis. Solely identifying neuropathic symptoms is not, however, useful in the assessment of diabetic neuropathy, as shown by Franse and coworkers.[167] One should be particularly wary of symptoms of painful neuropathy because they could arise from other nonspecific causes. It is crucial to thoroughly examine and evaluate both the central and peripheral nervous systems, with emphasis on the nerves most likely to be affected by diabetes, as shown in Figure 11–3.

Bedside neurologic examinations are quick and easy but only provide nominal or ordinal measures and contain substantial inter- and intraexaminer variation. Cranial neuropathies in diabetes are generally focal. Motor examinations usually focus on muscle weakness and muscle wasting resembling lower motor neuron palsy. Eliciting tendon reflexes accurately also assists in diagnosing neuropathy. Vibration perception should be measured with a tuning fork that has a frequency of 128 Hz because higher frequencies render the test insensitive.

Most diabetes clinics have 10-gram and 1-gram monofilaments for examination of touch sensation, using the 10-gram monofilament to predict foot ulceration, as in the Achilles reflex. However, both monofilament tests are insensitive in the early

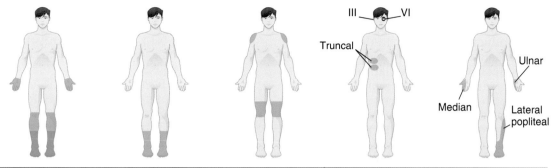

Large Fiber Neuropathy	Small Fiber Neuropathy	Proximal Motor Neuropathy	Acute Mono Neuropathies	Pressure Palsies
Sensory loss: 0 → +++ (touch, vibration) Pain: + → +++ Tendon reflex: N → ↓↓↓ Motor deficit: 0 → +++	Sensory loss: 0 → + (thermal, allodynia) Pain: + → +++ Tendon reflex: N → ↓ Motor deficit: 0	Sensory loss: 0 → + Pain: + → +++ Tendon reflex: ↓↓ Proximal motor deficit: + → +++	Sensory loss: 0 → + Pain: + → +++ Tendon reflex: N Motor deficit: + → +++	Sensory loss in nerve distribution: + → +++ Pain: + → +++ Tendon reflex: N Motor deficit: + → +++

Figure 11–3. Schematic illustration of the presentation of diabetic neuropathies. +, mild; +++, severe; ↓, decreased; ↓↓, very decreased; N, none.

detection of neuropathy. Using a 1-gram monofilament increases the sensitivity from 60% to 90%.[168]

Sensory evaluations should be performed on both sides of the feet and hands in order not to miss entrapment syndromes. Tinel's sign is evoked by tapping the nerve, which should produce a tingling sensation in the distribution of the nerve. Often patients with diabetes have carpal tunnel entrapments, and Tinel's sign is generally useful to diagnose carpal tunnel problems. It can be applied to the ulnar notch, the head of the fibula, and below the medial tibial epicondyle for ulnar, peroneal, and medial plantar entrapments, respectively.

The 1988 San Antonio conference on diabetic neuropathy and the 1992 conference of the American Academy of Neurology[162] recommended measuring at least one parameter from each of the following categories to classify diabetic neuropathy:

- Symptom profiles
- Neurologic examination
- Quantitative sensory tests
- Quantitative autonomic function tests
- Electromyography and nerve conduction studies.

Symptom Profiles

A number of simple symptom screening questionnaires are available to record symptom quality and severity. A simplified neuropathy symptom score used and validated in the European prevalence studies could also be useful in clinical practice.[5,169] The Michigan Neuropathy Screening Instrument (MNSI) is a 15-item questionnaire that can be administered to patients as a screening tool for neuropathy.[170] Other symptom-scoring systems have been described, and a number of questionnaires have now been developed by Boulton,[5] Dyck,[164] Vinik,[171] and others.[172,173] Simple visual analog or verbal descriptive scales can be used to follow

patients' responses to treatment of their neuropathic symptoms.[173,174,175] Identification of neuropathic symptoms should not be used as the sole diagnostic or screening tool in the assessment of diabetic neuropathy.[167]

Quantitative Sensory Tests

Objective indices of neurologic functional status are quantitative sensory tests and quantitative autonomic function tests (see next). The quantitative sensory tests consist of vibratory, proprioceptive, tactile, pain, and thermal sensation thresholds. These tests allow assessment of somatosensory function and are generally noninvasive and inexpensive. Findings can be easily correlated with specific nerve deficits.

Quantitative Autonomic Function Tests

Patients with diabetes who present with signs or symptoms of neuropathy should have a quantitative autonomic function test, which consists of a series of simple, noninvasive tests for detecting cardiovascular autonomic neuropathy.[176,177] The series includes tests of heart rate variability or R-R interval, expiration-inspiration ratios, and heart rate and blood pressure variability in response to a series of maneuvers consisting of inspiration and expiration, deep breathing, Valsalva's maneuvers, and supine or sitting versus standing. Other, more specific tests are used in evaluating disordered regulation of gastrointestinal, genitourinary, and pseudomotor function and peripheral skin blood flow induced by autonomic diabetic neuropathy.[168]

Nerve Conduction Studies

Whole-nerve electrophysiologic procedures (e.g., NCV, F-waves, sensory amplitudes, motor amplitudes) have emerged as an important method of tracing the onset and progression of diabetic

polyneuropathy.[178] An appropriate battery of electrophysiologic tests measures the speed of sensory and motor conduction, the amplitude of the propagating neural signal, the density and synchrony of muscle fibers activated by maximal nerve stimulation, and the integrity of neuromuscular transmission.[178,179] These are objective, parametric, non-invasive, and highly reliable measures. However, standard procedures, such as maximal NCV, reflect only a limited aspect of neural activity, and then only in a small subset of large-diameter and heavily myelinated axons. Even in large-diameter fibers, NCV is insensitive to many pathologic changes known to be associated with diabetic polyneuropathy.

A key role for electrophysiologic assessment is to rule out other causes of neuropathy or to identify neuropathies superimposed on polyneuropathy. Unilateral conditions, such as entrapments, are far more common in patients with diabetes.[180] The principal factors that influence the speed of NCV are the integrity and degree of myelination of the largest diameter fibers, the mean cross-sectional diameter of the responding axons, the representative internodal distance in the segment under study, and the microenvironment at the nodes, including the distribution of ion channels. Thus, demyelinating conditions affect conduction velocities, whereas diabetes primarily reduces amplitudes. Hence the finding of a profound reduction in conduction velocity strongly supports the occurrence of diabetic neuropathy in a diabetic patient with an alternative condition. Indeed, the odds of occurrence of chronic inflammatory demyelinating polyneuropathy (CIDP) were 11 times higher among diabetic than nondiabetic patients.[181]

NCV is only gradually diminished by polyneuropathy, with estimates of a loss of approximately 0.5 m/sec per year.[178] In a 10-year natural history study of 133 patients with newly diagnosed type 2 diabetes, NCV deteriorated in all six nerve segments evaluated, but the largest deficit was 3.9 m/sec for the sural nerve (from 48.3 m/sec to 44.4 m/sec), and peroneal motor NCV was decreased by 3.0 m/sec over the same period.[17] A similar slow rate of decline was demonstrated in DCCT. A simple rule is that a 1% fall in HbA1c improves conduction velocity about 1.3 m/sec.[182] There is, however, a strong correlation ($r = 0.74$; $P < 0.001$) between myelinated fiber density and whole-nerve sural amplitudes.[183]

Staging of Neuropathy

An international consensus has been reached with regard to management of diabetic peripheral neuropathy, and guidelines for physicians have been developed by an international group of experts in diabetic neuropathy.[142] This clinical staging is in general agreement with that proposed by Dyck[175] for use in both clinical practice and epidemiologic studies or controlled clinical trials. Using the scale Dyck developed, clinical "no neuropathy" is equivalent to N0 or N1a, "clinical neuropathy" is equivalent to N1b, N2a, or N2b, and "late complications" is equivalent to N3.

There have been a number of other relevant reports, including two on measures for use in clinical trials to assess symptoms[174] and QST.[184] The strengths of QST are well documented.[185] However, no matter what instrument or procedure is used, QST is only a semiobjective measure because it is affected by the subject's attention, motivation, and cooperation, as well as by anthropometric variables such as age, gender, body mass, and history of smoking and alcohol consumption. Expectancy and subject bias are additional factors that can exert a powerful influence on QST findings. Furthermore, QST is sensitive to changes in structure or function along the entire neuroaxis from nerve to cortex, and it is not a specific measure of peripheral nerve function.[185] The American Academy of Neurology has reported that the use of QST for clinical and research purposes[184] serves an ancillary role and should not be relied on for routine clinical use.

In the beginning of the 20th century, assessment of neuropathy in wounded soldiers was done using horsehairs as monofilaments. Since then, much progress has been made, and it has been particularly boosted by the development of the nylon fiber. Relatively inexpensive devices are now available that allow suitable assessment of somatosensory function, including perception of vibration, warmth, light touch, and pain.[185] Skin sensations can be assessed noninvasively, and results of the examination can be easily correlated to the type of nerve dysfunction. The Semmes-Weinstein monofilament is a simple and commonly used device in clinical practice.[186,187] The monofilament is designed to assess pressure perception. Gentle pressure is applied to the handle sufficient to buckle the nylon filament.

In clinical practice, the monofilament that exerts 10 grams of pressure is most commonly used to assess pressure sensation in the diabetic foot. However, there is an array of filaments of different pressures that can also be used. The filaments are calibrated to exert a force measured in grams that is 10 times the logarithm of the force exerted at the tip. For example, the logarithm of the force exerted by the 10-gram monofilament is 5.07, so the 10-gram monofilament is also referred to as the 5.07 monofilament.

A number of cross-sectional studies have been conducted to assess the sensitivity of the 10-gram monofilament to identify feet at risk of ulceration. Sensitivities vary from 86% to 100%.[174,184,187] There is no consensus on how many sites should be tested. The most common algorithm recommends four sites per foot, generally the hallux and metatarsal heads 1, 3, and 5.[186] There is little advantage gained, however, from multiple site assessments.[184] There is also no universal agreement on what constitutes an

abnormal result (i.e., 1, 2, 3, or 4 abnormal results from the sites tested). Despite these inconsistencies, the 10-gram monofilament is still widely used for the clinical assessment of risk for foot ulceration, and the 1-gram (or less) monofilament is used to detect neuropathy with a higher sensitivity.[186]

Booth and Young[190] determined that filaments manufactured by certain companies do not actually buckle at 10 grams of force. Indeed, several tested filaments buckled at less than 8 grams. Therefore, care should be taken to ensure that the right kinds of filaments are being used. Additionally, providing the patient with monofilaments helps in behavior modification and can reduce incidence of foot ulcers by more than half. Clinics can hand out monofilaments to their patients by cutting a 25 lb strain fishing line into 1-inch-long pieces. This yields 1000 pieces and costs about $5.00.

A graduated tuning fork is a valuable clinical tool to quantify loss of vibration sensations.[191] The Rydel-Seiffer tuning fork is used in screening and assessment of neuropathy.[192] This fork uses a visual optical illusion to allow the assessor to determine the intensity of residual vibration on a 0 to 8 scale at the point of threshold (disappearance of sensation). Liniger's group reported that results with this instrument correlated well with other QST measures.[193] Comparison of the neurothesiometer with the Rydel-Seiffer tuning fork has proved that it is equally helpful in detecting diabetic neuropathy.[194]

The tactile circumferential discriminator assesses the perception of calibrated change in the circumference of a probe (a variation of two-point discrimination). Vileikyte and coworkers reported 100% sensitivity in identifying patients at risk of foot ulceration.[187] This device also demonstrated good agreement with other measures of QST.

Neuropen is a clinical device that assesses pain using a Neurotip at one end of the pen and a 10-gram monofilament at the other end. This was shown to be a sensitive device for assessing nerve function when compared to the simplified nerve disability score.[169]

Differential Diagnosis of Neuropathy

Neuropathy associated with diabetes is diagnosed by the exclusion of other causes of neuropathy.[166,195] Biopsies of the nerve and skin are useful for excluding other causes of neuropathy and determining the optimal treatment.[196,197] Complex underlying pathologies are often unraveled with histopathologic examination.

PGP 9.5 is a neuron-specific marker that is used in staining and quantifying nerves in skin biopsies and has some clinical advantages in diagnosing small-fiber neuropathies when all other measures are negative.[22,198] It has now become apparent that

Box 11-2 Therapeutic Options for Controlling the Pathogenesis of Diabetic Polyneuropathy

- Glycemic control
- Aldose reductase inhibitors
- α-Lipoic acid
- γ-Linolenic acid (GLA)
- Protein kinase C inhibition
- Human intravenous gamma globulin (IVIg)
- Neurotrophic therapy

patients presenting with painful feet might have impaired glucose tolerance[199,200] or the metabolic syndrome.[201] PGP 9.5 has also been used to demonstrate the ability to induce nerve regeneration[202] and correlates with indices of neuropathy relevant to function of small unmyelinated C fibers.[201]

Malik and colleagues[203] reported the technique of confocal corneal microscopy in the assessment of diabetic polyneuropathy. This is a completely noninvasive technique that offers the future potential of assessing nerve structure in vivo without the need for biopsy.

MANAGEMENT

Treatment of neuropathy is directed toward preventing progression of neuropathy, reducing symptoms, and preventing complications of insensate extremities. A multipronged approach is used to successfully treat neuropathy, and the key lies in targeting individual pathogenic mechanisms (Box 11-2)

Glycemic Control

The outcome of the DCCT, the Kumamoto trials, and UKPDS has illuminated the significance of good glycemic control in the development of microvascular complications of diabetes. Pirart[7] followed 4400 diabetic patients over 25 years and showed an increase in prevalence of clinically detectable diabetic neuropathy from 12% of patients at the time of diagnosis of diabetes to almost 50% after 25 years. The highest prevalence occurred in the patients with poorest glycemic control.

Reports from the DCCT indicate that intensive insulin therapy has a profound effect on the prevention of neuropathy.[12] The DCCT involved 1400 subjects with type 1 diabetes who were stratified on the basis of microvascular disease at study entry, which established a primary and a secondary prevention cohort. Both cohorts were randomized to receive either conventional or intensive insulin therapy. The conventional cohort received twice-daily insulin with optional home glucose monitor-

ing; the intensive group received insulin three or four times a day, with mandatory home glucose monitoring and adjustment of insulin regimen with their health care provider. The prevalence rates for clinical or electrophysiologic evidence of neuropathy were reduced by 50% in those treated with intensive insulin therapy over 5 years. At that stage of the study, only 3% of the patients in the primary prevention cohort showed minimal signs of diabetic neuropathy, compared with 10% of those treated by the conventional regimen. In the secondary prevention cohort, intensive insulin therapy significantly reduced the prevalence of clinical neuropathy by 56% (7% prevalence in the intensive insulin therapy group versus 16% in conventional therapy group). The results of the DCCT study support the need for strict glycemic control, but the effect of insulin as a growth factor and immunomodulator, aside from its metabolic effects, must also be investigated.

The Kumomoto study followed the DCCT study design. The subjects were chosen from a population of thin Japanese patients with type 2 diabetes. The findings revealed that intensive insulin therapy reduced the HbA1c level to a mean of 7.1% (as compared with 9.3% in the standard treatment group) and sustained it for a period of 6 years. In the UKPDS, control of blood glucose was associated with improvement in vibration perception.[31,204,205]

In the Steno trial,[206] a reduction in ratio for the development of autonomic neuropathy of 0.32 was reported. The Steno trial used stepwise multifactorial intervention with pharmacologic therapy targeting hyperglycemia, hypertension, dyslipidemia, and microalbuminuria along with behavior modification. This confirms the multifactorial nature of the pathophysiology of neuropathy and the need to address all of the metabolic abnormalities that accompany diabetes.

Aldose Reductase Inhibitors

Diabetic patients often have abnormally high levels of intracellular glucose in noninsulin-dependent cells, causing stimulation of aldose reductase, which results in accumulation of sorbitol generated through the polyol pathway. Inhibition of the production of this enzyme reduces the flux of glucose through the polyol pathway, inhibiting tissue accumulation of sorbitol and fructose and preventing reduction of redox potentials.

In a placebo-controlled double-blind study of tolrestat, 219 diabetic patients with symmetrical polyneuropathy, as defined by at least one pathologic cardiovascular reflex, were treated for 1 year.[207] Patients who received tolrestat showed significant improvement in autonomic function tests and vibration-perception tests, whereas placebo-treated patients showed deterioration in most of the parameters measured.[208]

A 12-month study of zenarestat showed a dose-dependent improvement in nerve fiber density, particularly in small, unmyelinated nerve fibers.[209] This was accompanied by an increase in nerve conduction velocity, although the changes in NCV occurred at a dose of the drug that did not change the nerve fiber density.[209] Significant improvements in resting left ventricular ejection fraction, stroke volume, and cardiac output were observed with treatment with zopolrestat in diabetic neuropathy patients.[210]

In patients with a multitude of biochemical abnormalities, the use of aldose reductase inhibitors alone may be insufficient for achieving a desirable degree of metabolic enhancement. Therefore, in order to abate the relentless progress of diabetic neuropathy in these patients, it may become necessary to use aldose reductase inhibitors in combination with antioxidants.

α-Lipoic Acid

Lipoic acid (1,2-dithiolane-3-pentanoic acid), a derivative of octanoic acid, is present in food and is also synthesized by the liver. It is a natural cofactor in the pyruvate dehydrogenase complex, where it binds acyl groups and transfers them from one part of the complex to another. α-Lipoic acid, which is also known as thioctic acid, has generated considerable interest as a thiol-replenishing and redox-modulating agent. It is effective in ameliorating both somatic and autonomic neuropathies in diabetes.[211-213] It is currently undergoing extensive trials in the United States as an antidiabetic agent and as a treatment for diabetic neuropathy.

γ-Linolenic Acid

Linoleic acid, an essential fatty acid, is metabolized to dihomo-γ-linolenic acid, which serves as an important constituent of neuronal membrane phospholipids and as a substrate for prostaglandin E formation. It appears to be important for preservation of nerve blood flow. In diabetes, conversion of linoleic acid to γ-linolenic acid (GLA) and subsequent metabolites is impaired, possibly contributing to the pathogenesis of diabetic neuropathy.[214]

Evening primrose oil supplies GLA. Other commonly used sources of GLA are borage oil and flax seed oil, both of which are derived from plant seeds.

A multicenter double-blind placebo-controlled trial using GLA for 1 year demonstrated significant improvements in both clinical measures and electrophysiologic testing.[215] GLA improves vasodilator eicosanoid synthesis in diabetes, correcting nerve blood flow and NCV deficits. A combination of aldose reductase inhibitors and evening primrose oil produces a 10-fold amplification of nerve conduction velocities and blood flow responses.[216]

Human Intravenous Immunoglobulin

Immune intervention with intravenous immunoglobulin (IVIg) has become appropriate in some patients with forms of peripheral diabetic neuropathy that are associated with signs of antineuronal autoimmunity.[217,218] Chronic inflammatory demyelinating polyneuropathy associated with diabetes is particularly responsive to IVIg infusion. Treatment with immunoglobulin is well tolerated and is considered safe, especially with respect to viral transmission.[219]

The major toxicity of IVIg has been an anaphylactic reaction, but the incidence of these reactions is low and confined mainly to patients with immunoglobulin (usually IgA) deficiency. Patients can experience severe headache due to aseptic meningitis, which resolves spontaneously. In some instances, it may be necessary to combine treatment with prednisone or azathioprine, or both. Relapses can occur, requiring repeated courses of therapy.

Neurotrophic Therapy

There is considerable evidence in animal models of diabetes that decreased expression of NGF and its TRK A receptors reduces retrograde axonal transport of NGF and diminishes support of small unmyelinated neurons and their neuropeptides, such as substance P and CGRP, both of which are potent vasodilators.[220-222] Administration of rhNGF restores these neuropeptide levels toward normal and prevents manifestations of sensory neuropathy in animals.[223]

In a 15-center double-blind, placebo-controlled study of the safety and efficacy of rhNGF in 250 subjects with symptomatic small-fiber neuropathy,[18] rhNGF improved the neurologic impairment score of the lower limbs and improved small nerve fiber function cooling threshold (Aδ-fibers) and the ability to perceive heat pain (C-fibers) compared with placebo. These results were consistent with the postulated actions of NGF on TRK A receptors present on small-fiber neurons.

This led to two large multicenter studies conducted in the United States and the rest of the world. Results of these two studies were presented at the ADA meetings in June 1999.[19] Regrettably, rhNGF was not found to have beneficial effects over placebo. The reason for this dichotomy has not been resolved, but this has somewhat dampened the enthusiasm for growth factor therapy of diabetic neuropathy.

Box 11-3 Therapy for C-Fiber and Aδ-Fiber Pain

C-Fiber Pain
- Capsaicin
- Clonidine

Aδ-Fiber Pain
- Insulin
- Nerve blocking
- Tramadol and dextromethorphan
- Antidepressants
- Antiepileptics

THERAPEUTIC OPTIONS FOR CONTROLLING SYMPTOMS OF DIABETIC POLYNEUROPATHY

The most challenging aspect of diabetic neuropathy is the treatment and control of symptoms. Symptoms of pain necessitate treatment with antidepressants (including selective serotonin reuptake inhibitors), anticonvulsants, and other medications. In essence, simple measures are tried first. In pain syndromes, the numbers needed to treat (NNT) to reduce pain by 50% is 1.4 for optimal-dose tricyclic antidepressants, 1.9 for dextromethorphan, 3.3 for carbamazepine, 3.4 for tramadol, 3.7 for gabapentin, 5.9 for capsaicin, 6.7 for selective serotonin reuptake inhibitors, and 10.0 for mexiletine.[224] If, however, pain is divided according to its derivation from different nerve fiber types (Aδ-fiber or C-fiber), spinal cord, or cortical, then different types of pain respond to different therapies (Fig. 11–4), as listed in Box 11-3.[225]

C-Fiber Pain Therapy

C-fibers are slender nerve processes that are generally unmyelinated. Damage of these nerves results in pain that is described as burning or lancinating. This pain is of the dysesthetic type and is often accompanied by hyperalgesia and allodynia. Peripheral sympathetic nerve fibers are also small unmyelinated C-fibers.

Sympathetic blocking agents, such as clonidine, phenoxybenzamine, or regitine, might improve the pain. Loss of sympathetic regulation of sweat glands and A-V shunt vessels in the foot predisposes to bacterial infection by creating a favorable environment for bacteria to penetrate and multiply, giving rise to cellulitis and ulcers. These fibers use the neuropeptide substance P as their neurotransmitter, and depletion of axonal substance P (e.g., by capsaicin) often leads to amelioration of the pain.

However, when the destructive forces persist, the patient becomes pain free and develops impaired

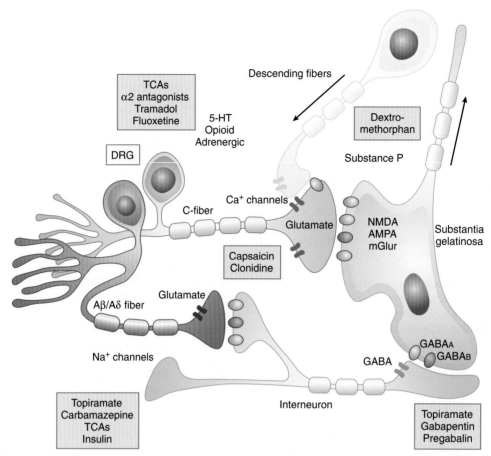

Figure 11–4. Schematic pathways of pain and sites of action of pain-relieving drugs. AMPA, alpha-amino-3-hydroxy-5-methyl-4-isoxazolepropionic acid; DRG, dorsal root ganglion; GABA, γ-amino butyric acid; 5-HT, serotonin; mGlur, metabotropic glutamate receptor; NMDA, N-methyl-D-aspartate; TCA, tricyclic antidepressant. (Modified from Vinik A, Mehrabyan A: Understanding diabetic neuropathies. Emerg Med 36:39-44. 2004.)

warm temperature and pain thresholds. Disappearance of pain in these circumstances should be hailed as a warning that the neuropathy is progressing.

Capsaicin

Capsaicin is a powerful alkaloid that is the pungent ingredient in chili peppers and is responsible for the heat associated with chilies. It has high selectivity for a subset of sensory neurons that have been identified as unmyelinated C-fiber afferent or thin-myelinated (Aδ) fibers. Prolonged application of capsaicin to the affected areas depletes stores of substance P, and possibly other neurotransmitters, from sensory nerve endings.

In practice, a simple cheap mixture is to add one to three teaspoons of cayenne pepper to a jar of cold cream and apply to the area of pain. This reduces or abolishes the transmission of painful stimuli from the peripheral nerve fibers to the higher centers.[226] Care must be taken to avoid eyes and genitals, and gloves must be worn. Because of capsaicin's volatility, it is safer to cover affected areas with plastic wrap. There is initial exacerbation of symptoms followed by relief in 2 to 3 weeks.

Clonidine

Clonidine is a central α_2-adrenergic agonist and can be used when there is an element of sympathetic-mediated C-fiber–type pain. Clonidine can be applied topically,[227] but the dose titration may be more difficult. If clonidine fails, the local anesthetic agent mexiletine warrants a trial. Phentolamine is another option in this line of treatment.

Aδ-Fiber Pain Therapy

Aδ-fiber pain is a more deep-seated, dull, and gnawing ache, which often does not respond to the previously described measures. A number of agents have been used for the pain associated with these fibers, with varying success.

Insulin

Continuous intravenous insulin infusion without resort to blood glucose lowering may be useful in patients who have Aδ-fiber pain. A response with reduction of pain usually occurs within 48 hours,[228]

GASTROPARESIS

Gastrointestinal motor disorders are frequent and debilitating complications in patients with diabetes mellitus, and they are often associated with retinopathy, nephropathy, peripheral neuropathy, and other forms of autonomic dysfunction. Although gastroparesis has been known clinically for more than 50 years, the pathophysiology is unknown.

Gastric dysfunction can cause nausea, vomiting, constipation, postprandial fullness, abdominal pain, belching, bloating, and weight loss. These symptoms can last days to months or occur in cycles and can cause poor blood glucose control. There is poor correlation between symptoms and objective evidence of functional or organic defects, making gastroparesis difficult to diagnose.

Gastroparesis affects both type 1 and type 2 diabetic patients and there is little evidence of a time correlation between diagnosis of diabetes and onset of gastroparesis. A proper diagnosis of gastroparesis requires identifying the correct symptom complex and ruling out other gastrointestinal problems such as peptic ulcer disease, rheumatologic diseases, and side effects of medications. A 4-hour gastric emptying study can be used to confirm the diagnosis.

The treatment options for gastroparesis are limited to diet modification, use of pharmaceutical agents, and in severe cases surgical or endoscopic placement of gastrostomies or jejunostomies. The first step in the management of diabetic gastroparesis requires placing the patient on a diet consisting of frequent small feedings. The patient should follow a low-fat diet because fatty foods can further delay gastric emptying. Although maintaining proper glycemic control can be difficult, attempts should be made to keep it under control.

Multiple pharmaceutical agents can be used to increase gastric motility and frequency of gastric contractions, including metoclopramide, domperidone, and erythromycin. Erythromycin is generally the most effective. It acts on the motilin receptor ("the sweeper of the gut") and shortens gastric emptying time. Unfortunately, erythromycin loses much of its stimulatory effects after just a few weeks and is therefore not usually an option for long-term treatment.

If treatment with medication fails, and the patient continues to suffer from severe gastroparesis, jejunostomy placement into normally functioning bowel may be necessary. Although some studies show that gastric pacing is effective at improving gastroparesis, its use is still extremely controversial.

SUMMARY

Diabetic neuropathy is a common and debilitating complication of diabetes. In spite of all the advances in modern medicine, much remains to be understood regarding the definition, pathophysiology, and measurement of this disorder. The key to management of diabetic neuropathy is primary prevention and achieving good metabolic control. This is often a challenging task to achieve because it involves many hands and many minds to work together, and it lies, for the most part, in the patient-physician relationship.

The vascular hypothesis and the role of oxidative stress and autoimmunity have opened up new possibilities in terms of treatment options. Differentiating different types of neuropathies helps in targeting appropriate therapies for specific fiber types. There has been a lot of progress in measurement of neuropathy and diagnostic tests. These tests must be validated and standardized to allow comparability between studies and a more meaningful interpretation of study results. Our ability to successfully manage the many different manifestations of diabetic neuropathy depends ultimately on our success in uncovering the pathogenic processes underlying this disorder.

References

1. Vinik AI, Mitchell BD, Leichter SB, et al: Epidemiology of the complications of diabetes. In Leslie RDG, Robbins DC (eds): Diabetes: Clinical Science in Practice. Cambridge, Cambridge University Press, 1994, pp. 221-287.
2. EURODIAB IDDM: Microvascular and acute complications in IDDM patients. Diabetologia 37:278-285, 1994.
3. Holzer SE, Camerota A, Martens L, et al: Costs and duration of care for lower extremity ulcers in patients with diabetes. Clin Ther 20:169-181, 1998.
4. Caputo GM, Cavanagh PR, Ulbrecht JS, et al: Assessment and management of foot disease in patients with diabetes. N Engl J Med 331:854-860, 1994.
5. Young MJ, Boulton AJM, MacLeod AF, et al: A multicentre study of the prevalence of diabetic peripheral neuropathy in the United Kingdom hospital clinic population. Diabetologia 36:1-5, 1993.
6. Dyck PJ, Kratz KM, Karnes JL, et al: The prevalence by staged severity of various types of diabetic neuropathy, retinopathy, and nephropathy in a population-based cohort: The Rochester Diabetic Neuropathy Study. Neurology 43:817-824, 1993.
7. Pirart J: [Diabetes mellitus and its degenerative complications: A prospective study of 4,400 patients observed between 1947 and 1973 (3rd and last part) (author's transl)]. Diabetes Metab 3:245-256, 1977.
8. Vinik A: Diabetic neuropathy: pathogenesis and therapy. Am J Med 107(2B):17S-26S, 1999.
9. Armstrong DG, Lavery LA, Harkless LB: Validation of a diabetic wound classification system. The contribution of depth, infection, and ischemia to risk of amputation. Diabetes Care 21:855-859, 1998.
10. Levitt NS, Stansberry KB, Wychanck S, Vinik AI: Natural progression of autonomic neuropathy and autonomic function tests in a cohort of IDDM. Diabetes Care 19:751-754, 1996.
11. Rathmann W, Ziegler D, Jahnke M, et al: Mortality in diabetic patients with cardiovascular autonomic neuropathy. Diabet Med 10:820-824, 1993.
12. DCCT Research Group: The effect of intensive treatment of diabetes on the development and progression of long-term complications in insulin-dependent diabetes mellitus. N Engl J Med 329:977-986, 1993.

13. DCCT Research Group: The effect of intensive diabetes therapy on the development and progression of neuropathy. Ann Intern Med 122:561-568, 1995.

14. Ziegler D, Cicmir I, Mayer P, et al: Somatic and autonomic nerve function during the first year after diagnosis of type 1 (insulin-dependent) diabetes. Diabetes Res 7:123-127, 1988.

15. Shaw JE, Zimmet PZ, Gries FA: Epidemiology of diabetic neuropathy. In Gries A, Cameron NE, Low PA, Ziegler D (eds): Textbook of Diabetic Neuropathy. New York, Thieme, 2003, pp 64-82.

16. Adler AI, Boyko EJ, Ahroni JH, et al: Risk factors for diabetic peripheral sensory neuropathy. Results of the Seattle Prospective Diabetic Foot Study. Diabetes Care 20:1162-1167, 1997.

17. Partanen J, Niskanen L, Lehtinen J, et al: Natural history of peripheral neuropathy in patients with non-insulin-dependent diabetes mellitus. N Engl J Med 333:89-94, 1995.

18. Apfel SC, Kessler JA, Adornato BT, et al, and the NGF Study Group: Recombinant human nerve growth factor in the treatment of diabetic polyneuropathy. Neurology 51:695-702, 1998.

19. Vinik AI: Treatment of diabetic polyneuropathy (DPN) with recombinant human nerve growth factor (rhNGF). (Abstract). Diabetes 48(Suppl 1):A54-A55, 1999.

20. Dyck PJ, Kratz KM, Lehman KA, et al: The Rochester Diabetic Neuropathy Study: Design, criteria for types of neuropathy, selection bias, and reproducibility of neuropathic tests. Neurology 41:799-807, 1991.

21. Oh SJ: Clinical electromyelography: Nerve conduction studies. In Oh SJ (ed): Nerve Conduction in Polyneuropathies, 2nd ed. Baltimore, Williams & Wilkins, 1993, pp 579-591.

22. Kennedy WR, Wendelschafer-Crabb G, Johnson T: Quantitation of epidermal nerves in diabetic neuropathy. Neurology 47:1042-1048, 1996.

23. Herrmann DN, Griffin JW, Hauer P, et al: Epidermal nerve fiber density and sural nerve morphometry in peripheral neuropathies. Neurology 53:1634-1640, 1999.

24. Pittenger GL, Ray M, Burcus NI, et al: Intraepidermal nerve fibers are indicators of small-fiber neuropathy in both diabetic and nondiabetic patients. Diabetes Care 27:1974-1979, 2004.

25. Vinik AI, Maser RE, Mitchell BD, Freeman R: Diabetic autonomic neuropathy. Diabetes Care 26, 1553-1579. 2003.

26. Karamitsos DT, Didangelos TP, Athyros VG, Kontopoulos AG: The natural history of recently diagnosed autonomic neuropathy over a period of 2 years. Diabetes Res Clin Pract 42:55-63, 1998.

27. Ziegler D: Diabetic cardiovascular autonomic neuropathy: Prognosis, diagnosis and treatment. Diabetes Metab Rev 10:339-383, 1994.

28. Maser RE, Mitchell BD, Vinik AI, Freeman R. The association between cardiovascular autonomic neuropathy and mortality in individuals with diabetes: A meta-analysis. Diabetes Care 26:1895-1901, 2003.

29. DCCT Research Group: Effect of intensive diabetes treatment on nerve conduction in the Diabetes Control and complications Trial. Ann Neurol 38:869-880. 1995.

30. Dyck PJ, Davies JL, Litchy WJ, O'Brien PC: Longitudinal assessment of diabetic polyneuropathy using a composite score in the Rochester Diabetic Neuropathy Study cohort. Neurology 49:229-239, 1997.

31. UK Prospective Diabetes Study (UKPDS) Group: Intensive blood-glucose control with sulphonylureas or insulin compared with conventional treatment and risk of complications in patients with type 2 diabetes (UKPDS 33). Lancet 352:837-853, 1998.

32. Gaede P, Vedel P, Larsen N, et al: Multifactorial intervention and cardiovascular disease in patients with type 2 diabetes. N Engl J Med 348:383-393, 2003.

33. Sima AA: C-peptide and diabetic neuropathy. Expert Opin Investig Drugs 12:1471-1488, 2003.

34. Hale PJ, Nattrass M, Silverman SH, et al: Peripheral nerve concentrations of glucose, fructose, sorbitol and myoinositol in diabetic and non-diabetic patients. Diabetologia 30:464-467, 1987.

35. Greene DA, Sima AA, Stevens MJ, et al: Complications: Neuropathy, pathogenetic considerations. Diabetes Care 15:1902-1925, 1992.

36. Vague P, Coste TC, Jannot MF, et al: C-peptide, Na$^+$,K$^+$-ATPase, and diabetes. Exp Diabesity Res 5:37-50, 2004.

37. Tesfaye S, Malik RA, Ward JD: Vascular factors in diabetic neuropathy. Diabetologia 37:847-854, 1994.

38. Mellor H, Parker PJ: The extended protein kinase C superfamily. Biochem J 332(Pt 2):281-292, 1998.

39. Way KJ, Chou E, King GL: Identification of PKC-isoform-specific biological actions using pharmacological approaches. Trends Pharmacol Sci 21:181-187, 2000.

40. Way KJ, Katai N, King GL: Protein kinase C and the development of diabetic vascular complications. Diabet Med 18:945-959, 2001.

41. Inoguchi T, Battan R, Handler E, et al: Preferential elevation of protein kinase C isoform beta II and diacylglycerol levels in the aorta and heart of diabetic rats: Differential reversibility to glycemic control by islet cell transplantation. Proc Nat Acad Sci U S A 89:11059-11063, 1992.

42. Nishizuka Y: Intracellular signaling by hydrolysis of phospholipids and activation of protein kinase C. Science 258:607-614, 1992.

43. Suzuma K, Takahara N, Suzuma I, et al: Characterization of protein kinase C beta isoforms action on retinoblastoma protein phosphorylation, vascular endothelial growth factor-induced endothelial cell proliferation, and retinal neovascularization. Proc Nat Acad Sci U S A 99:721-726, 2002.

44. Leinninger GM, Vincent AM, Feldman EL: The role of growth factors in diabetic peripheral neuropathy. J Peripher Nerv Syst 9:26-53, 2004.

45. Ishii H, Koya D, King GL: Protein kinase C activation and its role in the development of vascular complications in diabetes mellitus. J Mol Med 76:21-31, 1998.

46. Bohlen HG, Nase GP: Arteriolar nitric oxide concentration is decreased during hyperglycemia-induced beta II PKC activation. Am J Physiol Heart Circ Physiol 280:H621-H627, 2001.

47. Nonaka A, Kiryu J, Tsujikawa A, et al: PKC-β inhibitor (LY333531) attenuates leukocyte entrapment in retinal microcirculation of diabetic rats. Invest Ophthalmol Vis Sci 41:2702-2706, 2000.

48. Shiba T, Inoguchi T, Sportsman JR, et al: Correlation of diacylglycerol level and protein kinase C activity in rat retina to retinal circulation. Am J Physiol 265(5 Pt 1):E783-E793, 1993.

49. Aiello L, Bursell S, Clermont A, et al: Vascular endothelial growth factor-induced retinal permeability is mediated by protein kinase C in vivo and suppressed by an orally effective β-isoform-selective inhibitor. Diabetes 46:1473-1480, 1997.

50. Ishii H, Jirousek MR, Koya D, et al: Amelioration of vascular dysfunctions in diabetic rats by an oral PKC-β inhibitor. Science 272:728-731, 1996.

51. Bursell SE, Takagi C, Clermont AC, et al: Specific retinal diacylglycerol and protein kinase C beta isoform modulation mimics abnormal retinal hemodynamics in diabetic rats. Invest Ophthalmol Vis Sci 38:2711-2720, 1997.

52. Danis RP, Bingaman DP, Jirousek M, Yang Y: Inhibition of intraocular neovascularization caused by retinal ischemia in pigs by PKC-β inhibition with LY333531. Invest Ophthalmol Vis Sci 39:171-179, 1998.

53. Nakamura J, Kato K, Hamada Y, et al: A protein kinase C-β-selective inhibior ameliorates neural dysfunction in streptozotocin-induced diabetic rats. Diabetes 48:2090-2095, 1999.

54. Koya D, Haneda M, Nakagawa H, et al: Amelioration of accelerated diabetic mesangial expansion by treatment with a PKC-β inhibitor in diabetic db/db mice, a rodent model for type 2 diabetes. FASEB J 114:439-447, 2000.

55. Kelly DJ, Zhang Y, Hepper C, et al: Protein kinase C beta inhibition attenuates the progression of experimental diabetic nephropathy in the presence of continued hypertension. Diabetes 52:512-518, 2003.

56. Bohlen HG, Nase GP: Obesity lowers hyperglycemic threshold for impaired in vivo endothelial nitric oxide function. Am J Physiol Heart Circ Physiol 283:H391-H397, 2002.

57. Nakamura J, Koh N, Hamada Y, et al: Effect of a protein kinase C-β specific inhibitor on diabetic neuropathy in rats. Diabetes 47(Suppl 1):A70, 1998.

58. Cameron NE, Cotter MA: Effects of protein kinase C beta inhibition on neurovascular dysfunction in diabetic rats: Interaction with oxidative stress and essential fatty acid dysmetabolism. Diabetes Metab Res Rev 18:315-323, 2002.

59. Nangle MR, Cotter MA, Cameron NE: Protein kinase C beta inhibition and aorta and corpus cavernosum function in streptozotocin-diabetic mice. Eur J Pharmacol 475:99-106, 2003.

60. Efendiev R, Bertorello AM, Pedemonte CH: PKC-β and PKC-ζ mediate opposing effects on proximal tubule Na$^+$,K$^+$-ATPase activity. FEBS Lett 456:45-48, 1999.

61. Kowluru RA, Jirousek MR, Stramm L, et al: Abnormalities of retinal metabolism in diabetes or experimental galactosemia: V. Relationship between protein kinase C and ATPases. Diabetes 47:464-469, 1998.

62. Beckman J, Goldfine A, Gordon M, et al: Inhibiton of protein kinase Cβ prevents impaired endothelium-dependent vasodilation caused by hyperglycemia in humans. Circ Res 90:107-111, 2002.

63. Aiello L, Bursell S-E, Devries T, et al: Protein kinase Cβ inhibitor Ly333531 ameliorates abnormal retinal hemodynamics in patients with diabetes. Diabetes 48(suppl 2):A19, 1999.

64. Cotter M, Jack A, Cameron N: Effects of protein kinase Cβ inhibitor LY333531 on neural and vascular function in rats with streptozotocin-induced diabetes. Clin Sci 103:311-321, 2002.

65. Kim H, Sasaki T, Maeda K, et al: Protein kinase Cβ selective inhibitor LY333531 attenuates diabetic hyperalgesia through ameliorating cGMP level of dorsal root ganglion neurons. Diabetes 52:2102-2109, 2003.

66. King RH: The role of glycation in the pathogenesis of diabetic polyneuropathy. Mol Pathol 54:400-408, 2001.

67. Brownlee M: Advanced protein glycosylation in diabetes and aging. Annu Rev Med 46:223-234, 1995.

68. King GL, Brownlee M: The cellular and molecular mechanisms of diabetic complications. Endocrinol Metab Clin North Am 25:255-270, 1996.

69. Thorpe SR, Baynes JW: Maillard reaction products in tissue proteins: New products and new perspectives. Amino Acids 25:275-281, 2003.

70. Baynes JW: From life to death—the struggle between chemistry and biology during aging: The Maillard reaction as an amplifier of genomic damage. Biogerontology 1:235-246, 2000.

71. Chibber R, Molinatti PA, Kohner EM: Intracellular protein glycation in cultured retinal capillary pericytes and endothelial cells exposed to high-glucose concentration. Cell Mol Biol (Noisy-le-grand) 45:47-57, 1999.

72. Brownlee M: Negative consequences of glycation. Metabolism 49:9-13, 2000.

73. Ryle C, Leow CK, Donaghy M: Nonenzymatic glycation of peripheral and central nervous system proteins in experimental diabetes mellitus. Muscle Nerve 20:577-584, 1997.

74. Ryle C, Donaghy M: Non-enzymatic glycation of peripheral nerve proteins in human diabetics. J Neurol Sci 129:62-68, 1995.

75. Sugimoto K, Nishizawa Y, Horiuchi S, Yagihashi S: Localization in human diabetic peripheral nerve of Nε-carboxymethyllysine-protein adducts, an advanced glycation endproduct. Diabetologia 40:1380-1387, 1997.

76. Amano S, Kaji Y, Oshika T, et al: Advanced glycation end products in human optic nerve head. Br J Ophthalmol 85:52-55, 2001.

77. Basta G, Del Turco S, de Caterina R: [Advanced glycation endproducts and vascular inflammation: Implications for accelerated atherosclerosis in diabetes]. Recenti Prog Med 95:67-80, 2004.

78. Naka Y, Bucciarelli LG, Wendt T, et al: RAGE axis: Animal models and novel insights into the vascular complications of diabetes. Arterioscler Thromb Vasc Biol 24:1342-1349, 2004.

79. Hudson BI, Schmidt AM: RAGE: A novel target for drug intervention in diabetic vascular disease. Pharm Res 21:1079-1086, 2004.

80. Tanji N, Markowitz GS, Fu C, et al: Expression of advanced glycation end products and their cellular receptor RAGE in diabetic nephropathy and nondiabetic renal disease. J Am Soc Nephrol 11:1656-1666, 2000.

81. Yamamoto Y, Kato I, Doi T, et al: Development and prevention of advanced diabetic nephropathy in RAGE-overexpressing mice. J Clin Invest 108:261-268, 2001.

82. Oates PJ: Polyol pathway and diabetic peripheral neuropathy. Int Rev Neurobiol. 50:325-392, 2002.

83. Kasajima H, Yamagishi S, Sugai S, et al: Enhanced in situ expression of aldose reductase in peripheral nerve and renal glomeruli in diabetic patients. Virchows Arch 439:46-54, 2001.

84. Tesfamariam B: Free radicals in diabetic endothelial cell dysfunction. Free Radic Biol Med 16:383-391, 1994.

85. Nishikawa T, Edelstein D, Du XL, et al: Normalizing mitochondrial superoxide production blocks three pathways of hyperglycaemic damage. Nature 404:787-790, 2000.

86. Williamson JR, Chang K, Frangos M, et al: Hyperglycemic pseudohypoxia and diabetic complications. Diabetes 42:801-813. 1993.

87. Giugliano D, Ceriello A, Paolisso G: Oxidative stress and diabetic vascular complications. Diabetes Care 19:257-267, 1996.

88. Hunt JV, Dean RT, Wolff SP: Hydroxyl radical production and autoxidative glycosylation. Glucose autoxidation as the cause of protein damage in the experimental glycation model of diabetes mellitus and ageing. Biochem J 256:205-212, 1988.

89. Vincent AM, Russell JW, Low P, Feldman EL: Oxidative stress in the pathogenesis of diabetic neuropathy. Endocr Rev 25:612-628, 2004.

90. Suzuki S, Hinokio Y, Komatu K, et al: Oxidative damage to mitochondrial DNA and its relationship to diabetic complications. Diabetes Res Clin Pract 45:161-168, 1999.

91. Hinokio Y, Suzuki S, Hirai M, et al: Oxidative DNA damage in diabetes mellitus: Its association with diabetic complications. Diabetologia 42:995-998, 1999.

92. Baynes JW, Thorpe SR: Role of oxidative stress in diabetic complications: A new perspective on an old paradigm. Diabetes 48:1-9, 1999.

93. Esposito K, Nappo F, Marfella R, et al: Inflammatory cytokine concentrations are acutely increased by hyperglycemia in humans: Role of oxidative stress. Circulation 106:2067-2072, 2002.

94. Lum H, Roebuck KA: Oxidant stress and endothelial cell dysfunction. Am J Physiol Cell Physiol 280:C719-C741, 2001.

95. DeRubertis FR, Craven PA, Melhem MF, Salah EM: Attenuation of renal injury in db/db mice overexpressing superoxide dismutase: Evidence for reduced superoxide-nitric oxide interaction. Diabetes 53:762-768, 2004.

96. Craven PA, Melhem MF, Phillips SL, DeRubertis FR: Overexpression of Cu^{2+}/Zn^{2+} superoxide dismutase protects against early diabetic glomerular injury in transgenic mice. Diabetes 50:2114-2125, 2001.

97. Vinik A, Erbas T, Stansberry KB, Pittenger G: Small fiber neuropathy and neurovascular disturbances in diabetes mellitus. Exp Clin Endocrinol Diabetes 109(Suppl 2):S451-S473. 2001.

98. Stevens MJ: Nitric Oxide as a potential bridge between the metabolic and vascular hypothesis of diabetic neuropathy. Diabetic Med 12:292-295, 1995.

99. Hoeldtke RD: Nitrosative stress in early type 1 diabetes. David H. P. Streeten Memorial Lecture. Clin Auton Res 13:406-421, 2003.

100. Stevens MJ: Nitric oxide as a potential bridge between the metabolic and vascular hypotheses of diabetic neuropathy. Diab Med. 12:292-295, 1995.

101. Vinik A, Stansberry K, Barlow P: Rosiglitazone treatment increases nitric oxide production in human peripheral skin. A controlled clinical trial in patients with type 2 diabetes mellitus. J Diabetes Complications 17:279-285. 2003.

102. Jain SK, McVie R: Effect of glycemic control, race (white versus black), and duration of diabetes on reduced glutathione content in erythrocytes of diabetic patients. Metabolism 43:306-309, 1994.

103. Jennings PE, Chirico S, Jones AF, et al: Vitamin C metabolites and microangiopathy in diabetes mellitus. Diabetes Res. 6:151-154, 1987.

104. Karpen CW, Cataland S, O'Dorisio TM, Panganamala RV: Production of 12-hydroxyeicosatetraenoic acid and vitamin E status in platelets from type I human diabetic subjects. Diabetes 34:526-531, 1985.

105. Will JC, Ford ES, Bowman BA: Serum vitamin C concentrations and diabetes: Findings from the Third National Health and Nutrition Examination Survey, 1988-1994. Am J Clin Nutr 70:49-52, 1999.

106. Campoy C, Baena RM, Blanca E, et al: Effects of metabolic control on vitamin E nutritional status in children with type 1 diabetes mellitus. Clin Nutr 22:81-86, 2003.

107. Sundkvist G, Dahlin LB, Nilsson H, et al: Sorbitol and myo-inositol levels and morphology of sural nerve in relation to peripheral nerve function and clinical neuropathy in men with diabetic, impaired, and normal glucose tolerance. Diabet Med 17:259-268, 2000.

108. Malik RA, Tesfaye S, Thompson SD, et al: Transperineurial capillary abnormalities in the sural nerve of patients with diabetic neuropathy. Microvasc Res 48:236-245, 1994.

109. Tesfaye S, Harris N, Jakubowski J, et al: Impaired blood flow and arteriovenous shunting in human diabetic neuropathy: A novel technique of nerve photography and fluorescein angiography. Diabetologia 36:1266-1274, 1993.

110. Malik RA, Tesfaye S, Thompson SD, et al: Endoneurial localization of microvascular damage in human diabetic neuropathy. Diabetologia 36:454-459, 1993.

111. Eaton S, Harris ND, Ibrahim S, et al: Increased sural nerve epineurial blood flow in human subjects with painful diabetic neuropathy. Diabetologia 46:934-939, 2003.

112. Griffey RH, Eaton RP, Sibbitt RR, et al: Diabetic neuropathy. Structural analysis of nerve hydration by magnetic resonance spectroscopy. JAMA 260:2872-2878, 1988.

113. Dyck PJ, Hansen S, Karnes J, et al: Capillary number and percentage closed in human diabetic sural nerve. Proc Natl Acad Sci U S A 82:2513-2517, 1985.

114. Myers RR, Powell HC: Galactose neuropathy: Impact of chronic endoneurial edema on nerve blood flow. Ann Neurol 16:587-594, 1984.

115. Teunissen LL, Veldink J, Notermans NC, Bleys RL: Quantitative assessment of the innervation of epineurial arteries in the peripheral nerve by immunofluorescence: Differences between controls and patients with peripheral arterial disease. Acta Neuropathol (Berl). 103:475-480, 2002.

116. Theriault M, Dort J, Sutherland G, Zochodne DW: Local human sural nerve blood flow in diabetic and other polyneuropathies. Brain 120 (Pt 7):1131-1138, 1997.

117. Samii A, Unger J, Lange W: Vascular endothelial growth factor expression in peripheral nerves and dorsal root ganglia in diabetic neuropathy in rats. Neurosci Lett 262:159-162, 1999.

118. Schratzberger P, Walter DH, Rittig K, et al: Reversal of experimental diabetic neuropathy by VEGF gene transfer. J Clin Invest 107:1083-1092, 2001.

119. Schratzberger P, Schratzberger G, Silver M, et al: Favorable effect of VEGF gene transfer on ischemic peripheral neuropathy. Nat Med 6:405-413, 2000.

120. Oosthuyse B, Moons L, Storkebaum E, et al: Deletion of the hypoxia-response element in the vascular endothelial growth factor promoter causes motor neuron degeneration. Nat Genet 28:131-138, 2001.

121. Williams B, Gallacher B, Patel H, Orme C: Glucose-induced protein kinase C activation regulates vascular permeability factor mRNA expression and peptide production by human vascular smooth muscle cells in vitro. Diabetes 46:1497-1503, 1997.

122. Koya D, Jirousek MR, Lin YW, et al: Characterization of protein kinase C beta isoform activation on the gene expression of transforming growth factor–β, extracellular matrix components, and prostanoids in the glomeruli of diabetic rats. J Clin Invest 100:115-126, 1997.

123. Kihara M, Low PA: Impaired vasoreactivity to nitric oxide in experimental diabetic neuropathy. Exp Neurol 132:180-185, 1995.

124. Cameron NE, Cotter MA, Archibald V, et al: Anti-oxidant and pro-oxidant effects on nerve conduction velocity, endoneurial blood flow and oxygen tension in non-diabetic and streptozotocin-diabetic rats. Diabetologia 37:449-459, 1994.

125. Boulton AJ, Malik RA: Diabetic neuropathy. Med Clin North Am 82:909-929, 1998.

126. Boulton A, Malik T, Arezzo JC, Sosenko J: Diabetic somatic neuropathies: Technical review. Diabetes Care 27:1458-1486, 2004.

127. Ibrahim S, Harris ND, Radatz M, et al: A new minimally invasive technique to show nerve ischaemia in diabetic neuropathy. Diabetologia 42:737-742. 1999.

128. Newrick PG, Wilson AJ, Jakubowski J, et al: Sural nerve oxygen tension in diabetes. Br Med J (Clin Res Ed). 293:1053-1054, 1986.

129. Kakizawa H, Itoh M, Itoh Y, et al: The relationship between glycemic control and plasma vascular endothelial growth factor and endothelin-1 concentration in diabetic patients. Metabolism 53:550-555, 2004.

130. Schneider JG, Tilly N, Hierl T, et al: Elevated plasma endothelin-1 levels in diabetes mellitus. Am J Hypertens 15:967-972, 2002.

131. Aydin A, Ozden BC, Karamursel S, et al: Effect of hyperbaric oxygen therapy on nerve regeneration in early diabetes. Microsurgery 24:255-261, 2004.

132. Caselli A, Rich J, Hanane T, et al: Role of C-nociceptive fibers in the nerve axon reflex-related vasodilation in diabetes. Neurology 60:297-300, 2003.

133. Shapiro SA, Stansberry KB, Hill MA, et al: Normal blood flow and vasomotion in the diabetic Charcot foot. J Diabetes Complications 12:147-153, 1998.

134. Stansberry KB, Shapiro SA, Hill MA, et al: Impaired peripheral vasomotion in diabetes. Diabetes Care 19:715-721, 1996.

135. Stansberry KB: Primary nociceptive afferents mediate the blood flow dysfunction in non-glabrous (hairy) skin of type 2 diabetes. Diabetes Care 22:1549-1554, 1999.

136. Coppey LJ, Gellett JS, Davidson EP, et al: Changes in endoneurial blood flow, motor nerve conduction velocity and vascular relaxation of epineurial arterioles of the sciatic nerve in ZDF-obese diabetic rats. Diabetes Metab Res Rev 18:49-56, 2002.

137. Coppey LJ, Gellett JS, Davidson EP, et al: Effect of M40403 treatment of diabetic rats on endoneurial blood flow, motor nerve conduction velocity and vascular function of epineurial arterioles of the sciatic nerve. Br J Pharmacol 134:21-29, 2001.

138. Coppey LJ, Gellett JS, Davidson EP, et al: Effect of antioxidant treatment of streptozotocin-induced diabetic rats on endoneurial blood flow, motor nerve conduction velocity, and vascular reactivity of epineurial arterioles of the sciatic nerve. Diabetes 50:1927-1937, 2001.

139. Coppey LJ, Davidson EP, Dunlap JA, et al: Slowing of motor nerve conduction velocity in streptozotocin-induced diabetic rats is preceded by impaired vasodilation in arterioles that overlie the sciatic nerve. Int J Exp Diabetes Res 1:131-143, 2000.

140. Greene DA, Stevens MJ, Obrosova I, Feldman EL: Glucose-induced oxidative stress and programmed cell death in diabetic neuropathy. Eur J Pharmacol 375:217-223, 1999.

Diabetic Nephropathy

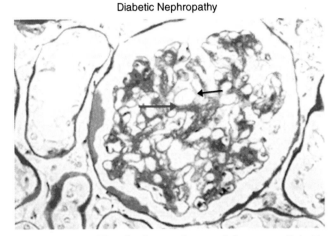

Figure 12–1. Histologic sections of human diabetic nephropathy. The *blue arrow* indicates mesangial expansion (the hallmark of diabetic nephropathy). The *black arrow* indicates glomerular capillary wall and location of foot processes, the area where the barrier to albumin breaks down and albuminuria occurs.

Table 12–1. *Stages and Clinical Features of Diabetic Kidney Disease*

Stage	Description	Clinical Features
	Increased risk	Diabetes mellitus, HBP, family history
1-2	Kidney damage	Microalbuminuria: Diabetes duration 5-10 years, retinopathy, rising BP Albuminuria: Diabetes duration 10-15 years, retinopathy, HBP
3-4	Decreased GFR	HBP, retinopathy, CVD, other diabetic complications
5	Kidney failure	Retinopathy, CVD, other diabetic complications, uremia

CVD, cardiovascular disease; GFR, glomerular filtration rate; HBP, high blood pressure

Table 12–2. *Prevalence of Hypertension in Diabetic Kidney Disease*

Clinical Feature	Prevalence (%)
Type 1 Diabetes	
Microalbuminuria	25-36
Macroalbuminuria	65-88
Type 2 Diabetes	
Microalbuminuria	40-83
Macroalbuminuria	78-96

Note: The prevalence in type 2 diabetes varies among ethnic populations and thus has a greater range.[7-11]

accelerated atherosclerosis and a more rapid progression of kidney disease.[4,12] A number of analyses show strong correlations between elevated BP and an increased risk of cardiovascular (CV) and renal events among diabetic subjects.[3,12,13] A higher systolic BP may be more predictive of kidney disease progression than diastolic blood pressure or pulse pressure.[12-15] Thus in diabetic patients, reducing BP to the goal of lower than 130/80 mm Hg, as recommended by guidelines from the Seventh Report of the Joint National Committee on Prevention, Detection, Evaluation, and Treatment of High Blood Pressure (JNC 7), the American Diabetes Association (ADA), and the National Kidney Foundation (NKF), is extremely important in reducing CV and renal morbidity and mortality.[4,16,17]

BENEFITS OF THERAPY

With time, the combination of diabetes and hypertension results in nephron loss. The remaining nephrons hypertrophy, with a concomitant decrease in renal arteriolar resistance and an elevation in glomerular plasma flow.[18,19] A further contribution is provided by angiotensin II, which mediates hypertension via arteriolar vasoconstriction, sodium retention, and sympathetic hyperactivity as well as effects on renal hemodynamics, constricting both afferent and efferent arterioles, with a resultant elevation in glomerular capillary hydraulic pressure and increased nephron filtration work; this leads to the loss of renal reserve and autoregulatory ability.[20-22] Ultimately, these compensatory changes result in renal demise.

Blockade of the renin-angiotensin system (RAS) improves glomerular permselectivity, a process that may be partially independent of changes in glomerular pressure. Angiotensin-converting enzyme (ACE) inhibitors and angiotensin-receptor blockers (ARBs) attenuate the glomerular actions of angiotensin II as well as the autoregulation of the GFR.[23,24] Post hoc analyses of more than a dozen trials in chronic kidney disease demonstrate a lower CV event rate and a slower decline in renal function in the groups with systolic BP lower than 140 mm Hg when compared to those with systolic BP 10 mm Hg higher.[25]

The ultimate goal of therapy is to reduce CV and renal morbidity and mortality. Timing is crucial in preventing the avalanche of progressive diabetic nephropathy. Interventions initiated during the earlier stages of kidney disease and that of associated CV risk factors (anemia, hypertension, and dyslipidemia) can effectively halt the progression to renal failure and prevent consequent systemic CV complications. This benefit has been demonstrated in different clinical trials involving ACE inhibitors and ARBs.[26-28] Several cost-effectiveness analyses concluded that the costs of more-intensive therapy with more frequent office visits are favorably offset

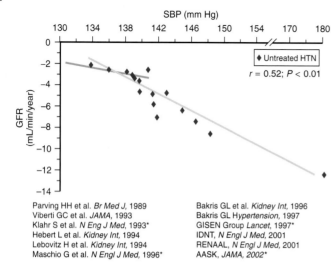

Figure 12–2. Impact of blood pressure level on progression of kidney disease. Trials were randomized to two levels of blood pressure on kidney outcomes. Note the 10 mm Hg lower BP slowest progression by 50% between 130 mm Hg and 140 mm Hg. (*) indicates nondiabetic renal disease. GFR, glomerular filtration rate; HTN, hypertension; SBP, systolic blood pressure.

by the significantly reduced risk of such high-cost complications as stroke, coronary artery disease, and heart and kidney failure.[29-31]

BLOOD PRESSURE GOALS

For patients with either diabetes or diabetic nephropathy, the recommended BP goal is systolic BP lower than 130 mm Hg and diastolic BP lower than 80 mm Hg.[16,17] In the United Kingdom Prospective Diabetes Study (UKPDS), 1148 subjects with type 2 diabetes were randomized to a BP target of either lower than 180/105 or lower than 150/85 mm Hg, with an average follow-up of 8.4 years. At the conclusion of the study, patients treated to the lower BP goal had BPs that were 10/5 mm Hg lower than patients in the other group, with a significant 24% reduction in diabetes-related endpoints in addition to other major CV benefits.[13]

Retrospective analyses demonstrate a markedly diminished risk of CV events and kidney disease progression among those with diabetes when a lower systolic BP (i.e., lower than 130 mm Hg) is achieved (Fig. 12–2).[4] Likewise, patients with diabetes randomized to diastolic goal BP of 80 mm Hg garnered the greatest benefit in terms of major CV events in the Hypertension Optimal Treatment (HOT) study.[32]

TREATMENT

Pharmacologic Interventions

Strict control of plasma glucose concentration (HbA1c goal <8.5%) can stabilize or reduce the degree of proteinuria in type 1 diabetic patients. This is best illustrated in the Diabetes Control and Complications Trial (DCCT), where the albumin excretion rate increased an average of 6.5% per year in patients receiving conventional insulin therapy versus no change in the intensive insulin therapy group.[29,33] Because diabetes itself is identified as a coronary risk equivalent, further CV benefit can be derived from aggressive lipid management, with a low-density liproprotein (LDL) cholesterol target lower than 100 mg/dL.[17,29,34]

The initial choice of the antihypertensive medication is probably the most important decision the clinician must make when treating diabetes and diabetic kidney disease. Special interests include the effects on glucose handling and insulin sensitivity. Because therapy is dependent upon renal excretory function, focus should be placed on agents that lower BP while reducing microalbuminuria or proteinuria, or both.[35-37] RAS blockade has been at the center of recent treatment strategies. ACE inhibitors and ARBs are two drug classes that effectively block circulating and tissue RAS, demonstrating unique capabilities and mechanisms of action that delay the progression of diabetic and nondiabetic renal diseases, reduce proteinuria, and provide renal protection independent of BP control.[26,38-40]

ACE inhibitors are an antihypertensive drug class effective in retarding the progression of nephropathy-associated diabetes, with clear evidence in type 1 diabetes. Data from the Collaborative Study Group trial of Captopril in Diabetic Nephropathy (Figure 12–3) and other randomized clinical trials indicate that ACE inhibitors are more effective than other agents in reducing albuminuria among subjects with renal disease and in retarding the decline in GFR and the onset of kidney failure even at similar levels of BP control, particularly in patients with type 1 diabetes.[26,39,41,42]

With regard to type 2 diabetes and renal disease, there are conflicting data on the efficacy of ACE inhibitors. Several studies demonstrate a vast reduction in albuminuria and decline in GFR, although the findings were beset by small sample sizes, use of surrogate outcomes, and inconsistent results in the surrogate outcomes. In contrast, large subgroup analysis of patients with type 2 diabetes and estimated GFR less than 60 mL/min per 1.73 m² who were enrolled in the ALLHAT study (Antihypertensive and Lipid-Lowering Treatment to Prevent Heart Attack Trial) showed no beneficial effects on GFR decline or onset of kidney failure over a 4-year period when the ACE inhibitor lisinopril was compared with the diuretic chlorthalidone.[42-45] Nonetheless, recent Kidney Disease Outcomes Quality Initiative (K/DOQI) clinical practice guide-

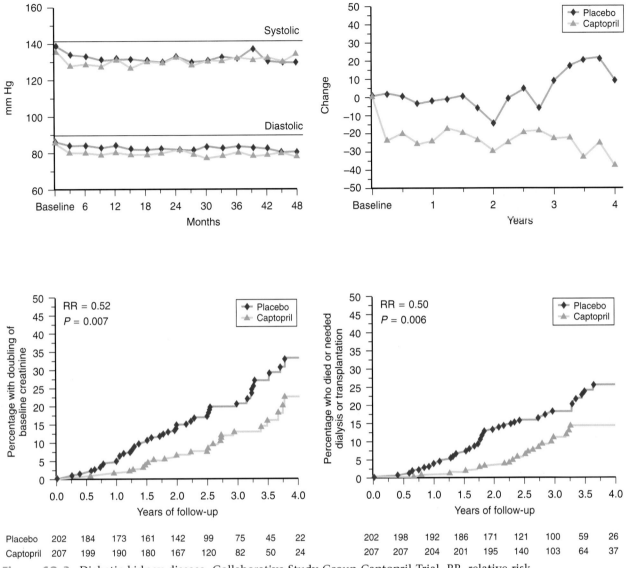

Figure 12–3. Diabetic kidney disease, Collaborative Study Group Captopril Trial. RR, relative risk.

lines recommend that ACE inhibitors be used to delay progressive nephropathy due to type 2 diabetes. Renal disease notwithstanding, this class of agents also has favorable effects upon plasma lipid concentrations.[46]

ARBs are more effective than other classes of antihypertensive agents tested (β-blockers, dihydropyridine calcium antagonists) in delaying the progression of nephropathy among type 2 diabetic patients with decreased GFR (<60 mL/min) and macroalbuminuria. In randomized, controlled trials, initial therapy with an ARB was more effective in preventing a composite renal endpoint than an initial placebo.[26,40,47] In both the Irbesartan Diabetic Nephropathy Trial (IDNT) and the Reduction of Endpoints in Non-Insulin Dependent Diabetes Mellitus with the Angiotensin II Antagonist Losartan (RENAAL) study, subjects randomized to irbesartan (or losartan in RENAAL) achieved a significant risk reduction in terms of dialysis, trans-

plantation, and death compared with placebo. In these trials an average of three antihypertensive agents were used, including the randomized drug. Although ARBs are of proven benefit in type 2 diabetes and there is no reason to think they would not also be effective in slowing nephropathy in type 1 diabetes, currently there is insufficient information regarding their use in the management of this disease.

Calcium antagonists (CAs) are established agents that effectively lower BP in patients who have renal disease that appears to be relatively resistant to antihypertensive therapy. However, the role of CAs in treatment of hypertension in diabetic patients has been controversial. CA subclasses show disparate effects on proteinuria, despite no statistically significant variance in systemic BP reductions due to differential effects on renal autoregulation, glomerular permeability, and tubular protein reabsorption.[48,49] Only the nondihydropyridine (nDHP)

CAs, verapamil and diltiazem, appear to be consistently effective in reducing proteinuria in advanced diabetic nephropathy, with evidence of reduced CV events in several outcome trials.[50,51] On the other hand, dihydropyridine (DHP) CAs, when used in the absence of blockers of the renin-angiotensin system, may be associated with increased risk of progressive diabetic kidney disease as noted in the IDNT.

Studies suggest that DHP CAs are less efficacious than ACE inhibitors, ARBs, and nDHP CAs in reducing albuminuria in diabetic kidney disease.[52] In IDNT, the group randomized to the DHP CA amlodipine had higher levels of proteinuria when compared to the ARB irbesartan, despite similar rates of GFR decline and need for dialysis.[26] However, when combined with ACE inhibitors or ARBs, or both, DHP CAs do *not* detract from the benefit of the RAS blockade. In fact, DHP CAs further lower BP with the resultant benefit of stroke reduction, as demonstrated in post hoc analyses of the RENAAL trial.[53] Thus, both the American Diabetes Association and the National Kidney Foundation recommend that DHP CAs not be used in diabetic nephropathy in the absence of ACE inhibitors or ARBs but rather as third-line therapy after diuretics and RAS blockers.[4,17]

Sodium retention is a major pathophysiologic consequence of hypertension in diabetic renal disease. Dietary sodium intake can strongly influence the BP and attenuate the protective effects of ACE inhibitors and ARBs. Salt restriction or treatment with a diuretic, or both, can potentiate the BP and the antiproteinuric response of RAS blockers.[54] Diuretics are the oldest class of antihypertensive agents and are excellent adjuncts, reducing CV mortality, even in patients with diabetes.[35,55] In general, if the GFR is less than 60 mL per minute or the serum creatinine is greater than 1.5 mg/dL in anyone older than 55 years, a loop diuretic should be used instead of a thiazide. Moreover, if furosemide is chosen it should be used twice daily for optimal BP-lowering effect.

Several clinical trials have demonstrated that the combination of agents that block RAS with thiazide diuretics is more effective than either agent alone for lowering blood pressure.[56-58] Appropriate use of diuretics mitigates the profound increases in serum potassium. Therapy with diuretics alone can adversely affect glucose handling and worsen insulin sensitivity primarily through reduced pancreatic insulin release secondary to the degree of potassium lowering.[36,37] Ideal serum potassium levels should be maintained at a minimum of between 3.9 and 4 mEq/L to ensure adequate insulin release.

β-Blockers are effective treatment adjuncts for diabetic patients, reducing CV events and retarding progression of nephropathy, although the progression is slowed less than with ACE inhibitors and ARBs. In the United Kingdom Prospective Diabetes Study (UKPDS) of patients with type 2 diabetes, the β-blocker atenolol was as effective as the ACE inhibitor captopril in lowering arterial pressure and protecting against macro- and microvascular disease.[13] Newer agents like carvedilol reduce CV and renal morbidity and mortality without an undesirable effect upon lipid profiles and insulin sensitivity.[59]

Lifestyle Modifications

All guideline statements highlight the need for lifestyle intervention as a primary mode of lowering blood pressure, although adherence to and compliance with such measures outside of formal trials has been unsatisfactory. Most guideline recommendations suggest weight loss for obese hypertensive patients, modification of dietary sodium intake to 100 mmol per day (2.4 g sodium or 6.0 g sodium chloride), modification of alcohol intake to no more than two drinks per day, and an increase in aerobic physical activity.[16,60,61] Dietary sodium intake can strongly influence the BP and attenuate the protective effects of RAS blockers.[54] Further improvement of CV health can be achieved with smoking cessation and tobacco avoidance.[16,62]

Lifestyle approaches are fraught with difficulties, including high rates of recidivism as shown in the Trials of Hypertension Prevention-2 (TOHP-2).[63] Nevertheless, the combination of antihypertensive medications and therapeutic lifestyle changes can potentially lower BP and thereby reduce morbidity and mortality even further than either successful lifestyle modifications or pharmacologic therapy alone.

RECOMMENDATIONS

There is no single method by which to achieve BP goals in diabetic kidney disease. Clinical trials indicate that the majority of patients require more than one agent to control BP, and most patients require an average of three antihypertensive agents to achieve the recommended goal BP of lower than 130/80 mm Hg (Fig. 12–4). Guidelines as outlined in JNC 7 and by the American Diabetes Association and the National Kidney Foundation state that all such patients should start taking an ACE inhibitor or an ARB while lifestyle modifications and dietary changes are addressed.[4,16,17] Figure 12–5 illustrates an algorithm integrating the JNC 7, ADA, and NKF guidelines for achieving the target BP of lower than 130/80 mm Hg in patients with kidney disease or diabetes.[4]

Evidence from clinical trials shows that the maximum approved doses for ACE inhibitors and ARBs should be used in all patients with renal disease whether or not they have proteinuria.[64,65] The concept of "maximal dosing strategy" is beset by inherent complexities due to large variable indi-

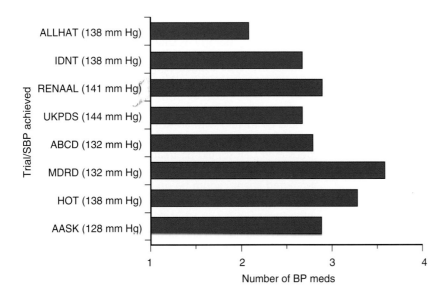

Figure 12–4. Number of antihypertensive medications required to achieve blood pressure (BP) goals in all clinical trials that randomized to two different levels of BP. SBP, systolic blood pressure. (From Bakris GL, William M, Dworkin L, et al. for The National Kidney Foundation Hypertension and Diabetes Executive Committees Working Group Preserving Renal Function in Adults with Hypertension and Diabetes. A Consensus Approach. Am J Kidney Dis 36:646-661, 2000. Reprinted with permission from National Kidney Foundation.)

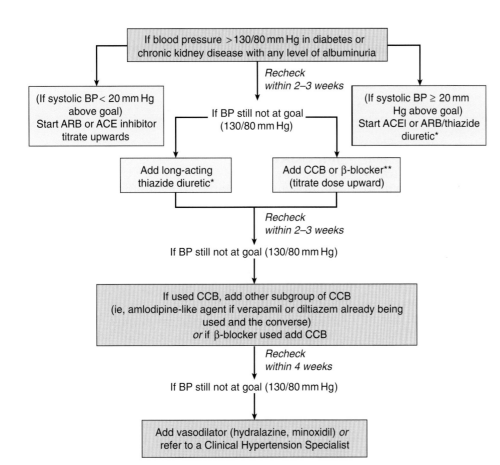

Figure 12–5. An approach to achieving blood pressure (BP) goals in the patient with microalbuminuria and chronic kidney disease (CKD).* Use of diuretics such as furosemide twice daily is needed if estimated glomerular filtration rate is <50 ml/min.** Of the beta blockers, carvedilol has been shown to reduce mortality from cardiovascular events in advanced kidney disease and minimize metabolic consequences. ACE, angiotensin-converting enzyme; ACEI, ACE inhibitor; ARB, angiotensin-receptor blocker; CCB, calcium channel blocker. (Courtesy of Bakris GL, Williams M, Dworkin L, et al, for The National Kidney Foundation Hypertension and Diabetes Executive Committees Working Group: Preserving renal function in adults with hypertension and diabetes: A consensus approach. Am J Kidney Dis 36:646-661, 2000.)

vidual responses to RAS blockade; it is difficult to ascertain the most effective means to retard proteinuria. Whether ACE inhibitors or ARBs should be discontinued because of elevations in serum creatinine above baseline is unclear. Both ACE inhibitors and ARBs generally raise both serum creatinine and potassium concentration. In general, serum potassium increases by 0.2 mEq/L in patients with rela-

tively normal renal function.[66] A 30% increase in serum creatinine (baseline less than 3 mg/dL) within the first 4 months of starting therapy or reducing BP toward the goal of lower than 130/80 with RAS blockade are positive prognostic signs that correlate with reduction of the progression of renal disease. Independent factors conducive to hyperkalemia are elevated creatinine level (greater

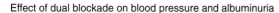

Effect of dual blockade on blood pressure and albuminuria

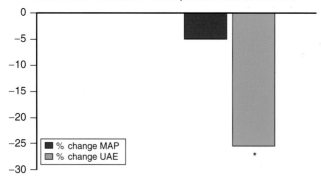

Dual blockade = ARB (300 mg irbesartan) was added to existing ACE
   inhibitor (100 mg captopril or 20 mg lisinopril) dosage.
n = 24 patients; Time = 8 weeks; baseline BP 131/74 mm Hg (Δ8/4)
mm Hg; baseline albuminuria = 519 mg/24 hours.

Figure 12–6. Percent change of blood pressure (BP) and albuminuria when a high-dose angiotensin-receptor blocker (ARB) was added to the maximally recommended dose of angiotensin-converting enzyme (ACE) inhibitor for diabetic nephropathy. *$P < 0.05$ compared to baseline. MAP, mean arterial pressure; UAE, urinary albumin excretion. (Adapted from Jacobsen P, Andersen S, Rossing K, et al: Dual blockade of the renin-angiotensin system versus maximal recommended dose of ACE inhibition in diabetic nephropathy. Kidney Int 63:1874-1880, 2003.)

Box 12-1 Summary of K/DOQI Recommendations on Pharmacologic Therapy in Diabetic Kidney Disease

- Patients with type 1 diabetes should be treated with an ACE inhibitor; an ARB can be substituted if the patient experiences cough or angioedema.
- Patients with type 2 diabetes and microalbuminuria should be treated with an ACE inhibitor or ARB.
- Patients with type 2 diabetes, macroalbuminuria, and decreased GFR should be treated with an ARB.
- Either agent can be used as an alternative agent, if the preferred agent cannot be used.
- Diuretics should be added as the second drug if target blood pressure is not achieved.
- Calcium channel blockers or β-blockers should be used as additional agents if target blood pressure is not achieved.
- Dihydropyridine calcium channel blockers should not be used without an ACE inhibitor or ARB.
- A systolic blood pressure goal even lower than under 130 mm Hg should be considered for patients with total protein-to-creatinine ratio greater than 1000 mg/g.

ACE, angiotensin-converting enzyme; ARB, angiotensin receptor blocker; GFR, glomerular filtration rate; K/DOQI, Kidney Disease Outcomes Quality Initiative.

than 1.6 mg/dL), congestive heart failure, and an increase in serum urea nitrogen level greater than 18 mg/dL.[67] Diuretics have been shown to ameliorate hyperkalemia.

Concomitant therapy of an ACE inhibitor with an ARB has been demonstrated to further reduce proteinuria and improve outcomes for diabetic renal disease as depicted in Figure 12–6.[68] If proteinuria persists despite high-dose single-therapy RAS blockade, an appropriate alternative strategy is an ACE inhibitor plus an ARB. It is generally difficult to determine the effectiveness of this approach due to a tendency for combining low to moderate doses of ACE inhibitors and ARBs without first maximally titrating the initial agent.[64,69]

Randomized clinical trials show that patients with diabetic nephropathy generally require an average of three antihypertensive agents to achieve the recommended goal BP of lower than 130/80 mm Hg (see Fig. 12–3). When an ACE inhibitor or an ARB does not produce the desired BP goal, antihypertensive medications with additive or synergistic effects on BP and proteinuria, such as diuretics or nDHP CAs, should be added. Diuretics potentiate RAS blockade, and nDHP CAs are superior to DHP CAs in reducing proteinuria despite the similar BP-lowering effects. A β-blocker should be added if goal BP has not been achieved and pulse rate is greater than 84 beats per minute.[4,70]

Box 12-1 provides a summary of current K/DOQI recommendations for pharmacologic therapy in diabetic kidney disease.[1]

IMPLICATIONS

Multiple interventions can retard the progression of nephropathy and reduce the risk of CV events in diabetic kidney disease: three or more antihypertensive medications, two drugs for glucose control, lipid-lowering therapy, and an emphasis on lifestyle modification including diet, aerobic exercise, and weight reduction.[28] One major obstacle to achieving adherence is the number of medications. Patients with renal disease, especially those on maintenance dialysis, take an average of 11 different medications daily. The selection of antihypertensive agents must also include considerations of cost, side effects, and convenience. Use of long-acting fixed-dose combination therapy, such as an ACE inhibitor or ARB combined with either a diuretic or a CA, can decrease the pill burden as well as copayments at managed-care pharmacies. Combination therapy is also likely to improve patient adherence to the medication regimen as well as improving BP control, resulting in a more consistent and cost-effective management of hypertension in diabetic nephropathy.

References

1. Kidney Disease Outcome Quality Initiative: K/DOQI clinical practice guidelines for chronic kidney disease: Evaluation, classification, and stratification. Am J Kidney Dis 43(Suppl 1):S1-S290, 2004.

2. Dalla VM, Saller A, Bortoloso E, et al: Structural involvement in type 1 and type 2 diabetic nephropathy. Diabetes Metab 26(Suppl 4):8-14, 2000.

3. Keane WF, Eknoyan G: Proteinuria, albuminuria, risk, assessment, detection, elimination (PARADE): A position paper of the National Kidney Foundation. Am J Kidney Dis 33:1004-1010, 1999.

4. Bakris GL, Williams M, Dworkin L, et al, for The National Kidney Foundation Hypertension and Diabetes Executive Committees Working Group: Preserving renal function in adults with hypertension and diabetes: A consensus approach. Am J Kidney Dis 36:646-661, 2000.

5. Scandling JD, Myers BD: Glomerular size-selectivity and microalbuminuria in early diabetic glomerular disease. Kidney Int 41:840-846, 1992.

6. Tamsma JT, van den Born J, Bruijn JA, et al: Expression of glomerular extracellular matrix components in human diabetic nephropathy: Decrease of heparan sulphate in the glomerular basement membrane. Diabetologia 37:313-320, 1994.

7. Go RC, Desmond R, Roseman JM, et al: Prevalence and risk factors of microalbuminuria in a cohort of African-American women with gestational diabetes. Diabetes Care 24:1764-1769, 2001.

8. Parving HH, Hommel E, Mathiesen E, et al: Prevalence of microalbuminuria, arterial hypertension, retinopathy and neuropathy in patients with insulin dependent diabetes. BMJ (Clin Res Ed) 296:156-160, 1988.

9. Wachtell K, Palmieri V, Olsen MH, et al: Urine albumin/creatinine ratio and echocardiographic left ventricular structure and function in hypertensive patients with electrocardiographic left ventricular hypertrophy: The LIFE study. Losartan Intervention for Endpoint Reduction. Am Heart J 143:319-326, 2002.

10. Tobe SW, McFarlane PA, Naimark DM: Microalbuminuria in diabetes mellitus. CMAJ 167:499-503, 2002.

11. de Court, Pettitt DJ, Knowler WC: Hypertension in Pima Indians: Prevalence and predictors. Public Health Rep 111(Suppl 2):40-43, 1996.

12. Gall MA, Rossing P, Skott P, et al: Prevalence of micro- and macroalbuminuria, arterial hypertension, retinopathy and large vessel disease in European type II (NIDDM) diabetic patients. Diabetologia 34:655-661, 1991.

13. UK Prospective Diabetes Study Group: Tight blood pressure control and risk of macrovascular and microvascular complications in type 2 diabetes: UKPDS 38. BMJ 317:703-713, 1998.

14. Perry HM Jr, Miller JP, Fornoff JR, et al: Early predictors of 15-year end-stage renal disease in hypertensive patients. Hypertension 25:587-594, 1995.

15. Bakris GL, Weir MR, Shanifar S, et al: Effects of blood pressure level on progression of diabetic nephropathy: Results from the RENAAL study. Arch Intern Med 163:1555-1565, 2003.

16. Chobanian A, Bakris GL, Black HR, et al: The Seventh report of the Joint National Committee on Prevention, Detection, Evaluation and Treatment of high blood pressure. JAMA. 289:2560-2572, 2003.

17. Summary of Revisions for the 2004 Clinical Practice Recommendations. Diabetes Care 27(Suppl 1):S1-S146, 2004.

18. Hayslett JP: Functional adaptation to reduction in renal mass. Physiol Rev 59:137-164, 1979.

19. Johnson HA, Vera Roman JM: Compensatory renal enlargement. Hypertrophy versus hyperplasia. Am J Pathol 49:1-13, 1966.

20. Johnston CI: Angiotensin receptor antagonists: Focus on losartan. Lancet 346:1403-1407, 1995.

21. Denton KM, Fennessy PA, Alcorn D, Anderson WP: Morphometric analysis of the actions of angiotensin II on renal arterioles and glomeruli. Am J Physiol 262:F367-372, 1992.

22. Yoshioka T, Shiraga H, Yoshida Y, et al: "Intact nephrons" as the primary origin of proteinuria in chronic renal disease. Study in the rat model of subtotal nephrectomy. J Clin Invest 82:1614-1623, 1988.

23. Ruggenenti P, Remuzzi G: The renoprotective action of angiotensin-converting enzyme inhibitors in diabetes. Exp Nephrol 4(Suppl 1):53-60, 1996.

24. Braam B, Koomans HA: Renal responses to antagonism of the renin-angiotensin system. Curr Opin Nephrol Hypertens 5:89-96, 1996.

25. Garg J, Bakris GL: Treatment of hypertension in patients with renal disease. Cardiovasc Drugs Ther 16:503-510, 2002.

26. Lewis EJ, Hunsicker LG, Clarke WR, et al, for The Collaborative Study Group: Renoprotective effect of the angiotensin-receptor antagonist irbesartan in patients with nephropathy due to type 2 diabetes. N Engl JMed 345:852-860, 2001.

27. Dahlof B, Devereux, RB, Kjeldsen SE, et al, for the LIFE study group: Cardiovascular morbidity and mortality in the Losartan Intervention for Endpoint reduction in hypertension study (LIFE): A randomized trial against atenolol. Lancet 359:995-1003, 2002.

28. Gaede P, Vedel P, Larsen N, et al: Multifactorial intervention and cardiovascular disease in patients with type 2 diabetes. N Engl J Med 348:383-393, 2003.

29. CDC Diabetes Cost-Effectiveness Group: Cost-effectiveness of intensive glycemic control, intensified hypertension control, and serum cholesterol level reduction for type 2 diabetes. JAMA 287:2542-2551, 2002.

30. Elliott WJ, Weir DR, Black HR: Cost-effectiveness of lowering treatment goal of JNC VI for diabetic hypertensives. Arch Intern Med 160:1277-1283, 2000.

31. Raikou M, Gray A, Briggs A, et al: Cost-effectiveness analysis of improved blood pressure control in hypertensive patients with type 2 diabetes: UKPDS 40. UK Prospective Diabetes Study Group. BMJ 317:720-726, 1998.

32. Hansson L, Zandretti A, Carruthers SG, et al: Effects of intensive blood pressure lowering and low-dose aspirin in patients with hypertension: Principal results of the Hypertension Optimal Treatment (HOT) randomised trial: The HOT Study Group. Lancet 351:1755-1762, 1998.

33. The Diabetes Control and Complications (DCCT) Research Group: Effect of intensive therapy on the development and progression of diabetic nephropathy in the Diabetes Control and Complications Trial. Kidney Int 47:1703-1720, 1995.

34. Executive Summary of the Third Report of the National Cholesterol Education Program (NCEP) Expert Panel on Detection, Evaluation, and Treatment of High Blood Cholesterol in Adults (Adult Treatment Panel III). JAMA 285:2486-2497, 2001.

35. Major outcomes in high-risk hypertensive patients randomized to angiotensin-converting enzyme inhibitor or calcium channel blocker vs diuretic: The Antihypertensive and Lipid-Lowering Treatment to Prevent Heart Attack Trial (ALLHAT). JAMA 288:2981-2997, 2002.

36. Gress TW, Nieto FJ, Shahar E, et al: Hypertension and anti-hypertensive therapy as risk factors for type 2 diabetes mellitus. Atherosclerosis Risk in Communities Study. N Engl J Med 342:905-912, 2000.

37. Sowers JR, Bakris GL: Antihypertensive therapy and the risk of type 2 diabetes mellitus. N Engl J Med 342:969-970, 2000.

38. Wright JT Jr, Bakris G, Greene T, et al, for the African American Study of Kidney Disease and Hypertension Study Group: Effect of blood pressure lowering and antihypertensive drug class on progression of hypertensive kidney disease: Results from the AASK Trial. JAMA 288:2421-2431, 2002.

39. Lewis EJ, Hunsicker LG, Bain RP, Rohde RD, for The Collaborative Study Group: The effect of angiotensin-converting-enzyme inhibition on diabetic nephropathy. N Engl J Med 329:1456-1462, 1993.

40. Brenner BM, Cooper ME, de Zeeuw D, et al: Effects of losartan on renal and cardiovascular outcomes in patients with type 2 diabetes and nephropathy. N Engl J Med 345:861-869, 2001.

41. Hebert LA, Bain RP, Verne D, for the Collaborative Study Group: Remission of nephrotic range proteinuria in type I diabetes. Kidney Int 46:1688-1693, 1994.

42. Parving HH, Hovind P: Microalbuminuria in type 1 and type 2 diabetes mellitus: Evidence with angiotensin converting enzyme inhibitors and angiotensin II receptor blockers for treating early and preventing clinical nephropathy. Curr Hypertens Rep 4:387-393, 2002.

43. Bakris GL, Weir M: ACE inhibitors and protection against kidney disease progression in patients with type 2 diabetes: What's the evidence? J Clin Hypertens (Greenwich) 4:420-423, 2002.

44. Bakris GL, Smith AC, Richardson DJ, et al: Impact of an ACE inhibitor and calcium antagonist on microalbuminuria and lipid subfractions in type 2 diabetes: A randomised, multi-centre pilot study. J Hum Hypertens 16:185-191, 2002.

45. Rahman M, Pressel S, Davis BR: Renal outcomes in high-risk hypertensive patients treated with an angiotensin-converting enzyme inhibitor or a calcium channel blocker vs. a diuretic: A report from the Antihypertensive Lipid-Lowering Treatment to Prevent Heart Attack Trial (ALLHAT). Arch Intern Med 165:936-946, 2005.

46. Ravid M, Neumann L, Lishner M: Plasma lipids and the progression of nephropathy in diabetes mellitus type II: Effect of ACE inhibitors. Kidney Int 47:907-910, 1995.

47. Molitch ME, DeFronzo RA, Franz MJ, et al: Diabetic nephropathy. Diabetes Care 26(Suppl 1):S94-S98, 2003.

48. Kloke HJ, Branten AJ, Huysmans FT, Wetzels JF: Antihypertensive treatment of patients with proteinuric renal diseases: Risks or benefits of calcium channel blockers? Kidney Int 53:1559-1573, 1998.

49. Hayashi K, Ozawa Y, Fujiwara K, et al: Role of actions of calcium antagonists on efferent arterioles—with special references to glomerular hypertension. Am J Nephrol 23:229-244, 2003.

50. Pepine CJ, Handberg EM, Cooper-DeHoff RM, et al: A calcium antagonist vs a non-calcium antagonist hypertension treatment strategy for patients with coronary artery disease. The International Verapamil-Trandolapril Study (INVEST): A randomized controlled trial. JAMA 290:2805-2816, 2003.

51. Black HR, Elliott WJ, Grandits G, et al: Principal results of the Controlled Onset Verapamil Investigation of Cardiovascular End Points (CONVINCE) trial. JAMA 289:2073-2082, 2003.

52. Bakris GL, Weir MR, Secic M, et al: Differential effects of calcium antagonist subclasses on markers of nephropathy progression. Kidney Int 65:1991-2002, 2004.

53. Bakris GL, Weir MR, Shanifar S, et al: Effects of blood pressure level on progression of diabetic nephropathy: Results from the RENAAL study. Arch Intern Med 163:1555-1565, 2003.

54. Buter H, Hemmelder MH, Navis G, et al: The blunting of the antiproteinuric efficacy of ACE inhibition by high sodium intake can be restored by hydrochlorothiazide. Nephrol Dial Transplant 13:1682-1685, 1998.

55. Curb JD, Pressel SL, Cutler JA, et al: Effect of diuretic-based antihypertensive treatment on cardiovascular disease risk in older diabetic patients with isolated systolic hypertension. Systolic Hypertension in the Elderly Program Cooperative Research Group. JAMA 276:1886-1892, 1996.

56. Weir MR, Smith DH, Neutel JM, Bedigian MP: Valsartan alone or with a diuretic or ACE inhibitor as treatment for African American hypertensives: Relation to salt intake. Am J Hypertens 14:665-671, 2001.

57. Bakris GL: The role of combination antihypertensive therapy and the progression of renal disease hypertension: Looking toward the next millennium. Am J Hypertens 11:158S-162S, 1998.

58. Melian EB, Jarvis B: Candesartan cilexetil plus hydrochlorothiazide combination: A review of its use in hypertension. Drugs 62:787-816, 2002.

59. Frishman WH: Carvedilol. N Engl J Med 339:1759-1765, 1998.

60. He J, Whelton PK, Appel LJ, et al: Long-term effects of weight loss and dietary sodium reduction on incidence of hypertension. Hypertension 35:544-549, 2000.

61. Whelton SP, Chin A, Xin X, He J. Effect of aerobic exercise on blood pressure: A meta-analysis of randomized, controlled trials. Ann Intern Med 136:493-503, 2002.

62. 2003 European Society of Hypertension-European Society of Cardiology guidelines for the management of arterial hypertension. J Hypertens 21:1011-1053, 2003.

63. The Trials of Hypertension Prevention Collaborative Research Group: Effects of weight loss and sodium reduction intervention on blood pressure and hypertension incidence in overweight people with high-normal blood pressure. The Trials of Hypertension Prevention, phase II. Arch Intern Med 157:657-667, 1997.

64. Rossing K, Christensen PK, Hansen BV, et al: Optimal dose of candesartan for renoprotection in type 2 diabetic patients with nephropathy: A double-blind randomized cross-over study. Diabetes Care 261:150-155, 2003.

65. Haas M, Leko-Hohr Z, Erler C, Mayer G: Antiproteinuric versus antihypertensive effects of high-dose ACE inhibitor therapy. Am J Kidney Dis 40:458-463, 2002.

66. Bakris GL, Weir MR: Angiotensin-converting enzyme inhibitor-associated elevations in serum creatinine: Is this a cause for concern? Arch Intern Med 160:685-693, 2000.

67. Reardon LC, Macpherson DS: Hyperkalemia in outpatients using angiotensin-converting enzyme inhibitors. How much should we worry? Arch Intern Med 158:26-32, 1998.

68. Jacobsen P, Andersen S, Rossing K, et al: Dual blockade of the renin-angiotensin system versus maximal recommended dose of ACE inhibition in diabetic nephropathy. Kidney Int 63:1874-1880, 2003.

69. Andersen NH, Mogensen CE: Angiotensin converting enzyme inhibitors and angiotensin ii receptor blockers: Evidence for and against the combination in the treatment of hypertension and proteinuria. Curr Hypertens Rep 4:394-340, 2002.

70. Tsuji H, Larson MG, Venditti FJ Jr, et al: Impact of reduced heart rate variability on risk for cardiac events. The Framingham Heart Study. Circulation. 94:2850-2855, 1996.

These had decreased expression of nNOS in the dorsal root ganglia and diminished withdrawal responses to noxious mechanical stimuli. Cyclic GMP levels paralleled nNOS expression. Insulin treatment led to improved nerve conduction and increased nNOS expression. This suggests that a decreased nNOS-cGMP system in the dorsal root ganglion could play a role in the pathogenesis of diabetic neuropathy.[42] It might provide a link between diabetic neuropathy and endothelial dysfunction in patients with diabetes and ED.

The ability to increase blood flow depends on an intact neurogenic vascular response. Diabetic autonomic neuropathy leads to impaired endothelium-dependent and endothelium-independent vasodilation even in the absence of clinical macrovascular disease.[43] The interaction between endothelial dysfunction and autonomic neuropathy results in an inability to increase blood flow under conditions of stress or increased demands.

Obesity

Cross-sectional studies have demonstrated that men with a BMI higher than 28.7 have a 30% higher risk for ED than those with a normal BMI (25).[44] The prevalence of obesity and its associated vascular risk factors in men reporting symptoms of ED is remarkably high.[45,46]

In the Massachusetts Male Aging Study, Derby and colleagues found that men who were overweight at baseline were at an increased risk of developing ED regardless of whether they lost weight during follow-up.[47] By contrast, men who initiated physical activity in midlife had a 70% reduced risk for ED relative to those who remained sedentary. In quantitative terms, this means that sedentary men may be able to reduce their risk of ED by adopting regular physical activity at a level of at least 200 kcal/day, which corresponds to walking briskly for 2 miles.

Results from the Health Professional Follow-up Study (31,742 men aged 50 to 93 with no history of prostate cancer) revealed that men who were most physically active (3 hours of running per week or the equivalent), had a 30% lower risk of ED when compared with men who reported little or no physical activity.[48] Conversely, watching more than 20 hours per week of television, smoking, and being overweight were associated with increased risk of ED.[48]

Lipids

Total cholesterol and HDL cholesterol are important predictors of ED. In a study of 3250 men (mean age 51 years) followed for a mean of 22 months, 71 developed ED during follow-up. Subjects with total cholesterol greater than 240 mg/dL had a 1.83 times increased risk of ED. An HDL greater than 60 mg/dL meant a 0.30 times risk for ED. This suggests that a high total cholesterol and a low HDL are risks for ED.[49]

INFLUENCE OF THERAPIES USED IN DIABETES AND IN THE METABOLIC SYNDROME ON ERECTILE DYSFUNCTION

Many drugs used in the treatment of diabetes and the various components of the metabolic syndrome can have an impact on ED.[2,3] Medication history is very important to consider in ED patients, especially in men with diabetes who are often taking multiple drugs to treat hypertension, dyslipidemia, depression, glaucoma, neuropathic pain, and diabetes itself (Box 13-2).

The major culprits that can induce ED are antihypertensives, especially nonselective β-blockers, sympatholytics, and diuretics. The main problem in diabetes and the metabolic syndrome is that often these agents cannot be replaced—β-blocker therapy is essential in patients with coronary artery disease or heart failure; depression and painful conditions should be adequately treated. All these problems are very real to the patient and can exacerbate ED if not adequately managed.

The clinician should try to optimize therapy using agents that are least likely to cause ED. Angiotensin-converting enzyme (ACE) inhibitors, angiotensin II receptor blockers (ARBs), statins, and thiazolidinediones (TZD) either enhance NO levels or block production of oxygen radicals, which quench NO and prevent vasodilation. However, other studies suggest that ACE inhibitors increase the incidence of ED (relative risk [RR], 2.78). This is still less than with diuretic therapy (RR, 3.86).

ERECTILE DYSFUNCTION AS A RISK MARKER OF CARDIOVASCULAR DISEASE

ED is associated with many of the traditional cardiovascular risk factors (aging, diabetes, hypertension, hyperlipidemia, and smoking). ED is also associated with nontraditional cardiovascular risk factors (such as endothelial dysfunction). The presence of ED, therefore, can be an early warning sign of underlying vascular disease (coronary, cerebrovascular, and peripheral), which in patients with diabetes may be asymptomatic.

Gazzaruso and colleagues evaluated the prevalence of ED in 133 men who had uncomplicated diabetes plus angiographically verified silent coronary artery disease (CAD) and in 127 diabetic men without myocardial ischemia at exercise ECG, 48-hour ambulatory ECG, and stress echocardiogra-

Box 13-2 Drug-Related Causes of Erectile Dysfunction*

Antihypertensive Medications

Thiazide Diuretics

- Spironolactone

Centrally Acting Antihypertensives

- Methyldopa
- Clonidine

β-Blockers:

- Propranolol
- Atenolol
- Metoprolol

Angiotensin-Converting Enzyme Inhibitors

- Lisinopril

Psychiatric Medications

Tricyclic Antidepressants (TCAs)

- Amitriptyline
- Doxepin
- Imipramine
- Protriptyline

Selective Serotonin Reuptake Inhibitors (SSRIs)

- Fluoxetine
- Paroxetine
- Sertraline

Monoamine Oxidase (MAO) Inhibitors

- Phenelzine
- Benzodiazepines

Antipsychotic Agents

- Chlorpromazine
- Thioridazine
- Risperidone

Anticonvulsants

- Phenytoin
- Carbamazepine

Anti-Parkinson Agents

- Levodopa

Lipid Regulators

- Gemfibrozil
- Clofibrate

Antiulcer Agents

- Cimetidine

Antiandrogens

- Flutamide
- Finasteride
- Cyproterone acetate
- Aminoglutethimide
- Leuprolide
- Estrogens

Miscellaneous

Agents of Abuse

- Alcohol
- Marijuana
- Cocaine

Other

- Ketoconazole
- Metochlopramide

*Approximately 25% of erectile dysfunction (ED) is causally related to drugs. Some drugs available over the counter (OTC), such as antihistamines and decongestants, can also cause ED.

phy.[50] Patients were screened for ED using the IIEF questionnaire. The prevalence of ED was significantly higher in patients with than in those without silent CAD (33.8% versus 4.7%). Multiple logistic regression analysis showed that ED, apolipoprotein(a) polymorphism, smoking, microalbuminuria, HDL, and low-density lipoprotein (LDL) were significantly associated with silent CAD; among these risk factors, ED appeared to be the most efficient predictor of silent CAD (odds ratio [OR], 14.8).

Thus there may be a strong and independent association between ED and silent CAD in patients with apparently uncomplicated type 2 diabetes, and ED may be a potential marker to identify diabetic patients who should be screened for silent CAD. Moreover, the high prevalence of ED among dia-

betic patients with silent CAD suggests the need to perform an exercise ECG before starting a treatment for ED, especially in patients with additional cardiovascular risk factors.

In the Detection of Ischemia in Asymptomatic Diabetics (DIAD) study, 1123 patients with type 2 diabetes, aged 50 to 75 years, with no known or suspected coronary artery disease, were randomly assigned to either stress testing (assessed by adenosine technetium-99m sestamibi single-photon emission computed tomography [SPECT] myocardial perfusion imaging) and 5-year clinical follow-up or to follow-up only.[51] A total of 113 out of 522 patients (22%) had silent ischemia, including 83 with regional myocardial perfusion abnormalities and 30 with normal perfusion but other abnormal-

ities (i.e., adenosine-induced ST-segment depression, ventricular dilation, or rest ventricular dysfunction). Moderate or large perfusion defects were present in 33 patients. The strongest predictors for abnormal tests were abnormal Valsalva (OR, 5.6), male sex (OR, 2.5), and diabetes duration (OR, 5.2).

Other traditional cardiac risk factors or inflammatory and prothrombotic markers were not predictive. Selecting only patients who met American Diabetes Association guidelines would have failed to identify 41% of patients with silent ischemia. Thus, silent myocardial ischemia occurs in more than one in five asymptomatic patients with type 2 diabetes, and cardiac autonomic dysfunction was a strong predictor of ischemia. These findings may have implications for guidelines for stress testing in diabetic patients. Further research is needed to clarify the importance of stress testing and its implications in patients with diabetes and ED who are free of cardiac symptoms.

Indeed, the severity of ED can correlate with the severity of coronary atherosclerosis.[52] In view of these findings, appropriate investigation and management of existing vascular disease should be undertaken by the health-care provider as part of the global care of the ED patient.[53,54]

Another consideration with respect to the presence of coexisting vascular disease in the ED patient is the safety of sexual activity itself. Expressed as a multiple of the metabolic equivalent (MET) of energy expenditure expanded in the resting state (MET = 1), sexual intercourse is typically associated with a workload of 2 to 3 METs before orgasm and 3 to 4 METs during orgasm. This workload is similar to walking one mile in 20 minutes on the flat, or climbing up two flights of stairs. If the ED patient can manage this level of workload, he should be safe from the cardiovascular standpoint (although more rigorous sexual activity can involve 5 to 6 METs or greater). If there is any doubt, a thorough cardiovascular workup should be considered.[53,54] Exercise testing can guide advice in the presence of reasonable concern (sexual workload is equivalent to 3 to 4 minutes on the standard Bruce treadmill protocol).

EVALUATION

A diagnosis of ED requires careful history (medical, sexual, and psychosocial), physical examination, and laboratory tests aimed at determining what other tests are needed to rule out organic causes of the disorder. Many medications, including prescribed, over-the-counter (OTC), and illicit drugs, can cause ED, and a careful drug history is therefore indicated (see Box 13-2). As well as potentially causing ED, many OTC agents are taken as therapies for ED and androgen replacement. For ED patients who do not respond to standard therapy, further evaluation is outlined in Box 13-3.

Box 13-3 Investigation of Nonresponders

Medication History*

- Antihypertensives: β-blockers, thiazide diuretics, clonidine, spironolactone, methyldopa. (*ACE inhibitors and α-blockers* are agents of choice.)
- Agents acting on the CNS: TCADs, SSRIs, phenothiazines, butyrophenones, atypical antidepressants. (*Trazodone* is agent of choice when indicated.)
- Agents affecting the endocrine system: Antiandrogens, GnRH agonists and antagonists, estrogens, cimetidine, metoclopramide, fibric acid derivatives, alcohol, marijuana. (Consider proton-pump inhibitors, *statins* when indicated)

Hormone Status

- Total (or free) testosterone
- Luteinizing hormone (LH), follicle-stimulating hormone (FSH), prolactin
- Ferritin

Autonomic Neuropathy

- Electrocardiogram (R-R variability); heart rate variability
- Orthostatic blood pressure readings
- Tilt-table studies

Vascular Disease

- Doppler studies of penile blood flow
- Pharmacodynamic testing using vasoactive compounds
- Pudendal angiography and cavernosometry

Psychosocial Assessment

- Combine with nocturnal penile tumescence (NPT) test
- Marital counseling

*Change agents that could contribute to the problem.

TREATMENT

ED is a distressing condition that can have a serious negative impact on not just the patient's sex life but also on his and his partner's overall quality of life. Despite this, up to 90% of sufferers are still reluctant to present to their doctor. One important aspect of ED that is sometimes underappreciated is that this is a disorder of the couple. Any attempt at therapy should be cognizant of the needs and desires of both parties.[2,3]

ED therapies may include psychosexual counseling, androgen replacement therapy (when deficiency is confirmed), oral and intracavernosal drug therapy, vacuum-tumescence devices, and surgical treatment (prosthesis and vascular surgery). Fortunately, the treatment options for ED have expanded in recent years, especially with the introduction of PDE5 inhibitors. However, a significant fraction of men with diabetes and ED are still frustrated by poor responses to the available treatment modalities.[55,56] This often leads to noncompliance and

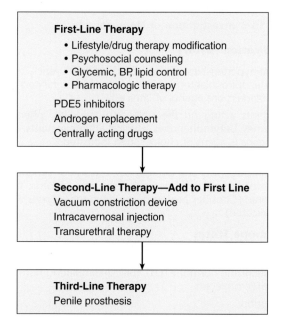

Figure 13–2. Proposed step-care approach to diabetic erectile dysfunction therapy. BP, blood pressure; PDE5, phosphoesterase 5.

Table 13–1. *Treatment Options and Response in Erectile Dysfunction*

Treatment Modality	Diabetic ED	Nondiabetic ED
PDE5 Inhibitors		
Sildenafil	59% T1DM 64% T2DM	74%
Tadalafil	64%	81%
Vardenafil	72%	85%
Other Treatments		
Intracavernosal PGE1 derivative (Alprostadil)	80%-85%	
Intraurethral PGE1 (MUSE)	70%	
Vacuum devices	75%	
Surgical implants	86%	
Androgen Therapy	17%	–
Combination injection therapy	84%	–

ED, erectile dysfunction.

increasing psychological distress as patients run out of therapeutic options.

It is the multifactorial etiology that makes ED in diabetes harder to treat. Most treatments deal with only one part of the ED equation, and this leads to partial or poor responses. Ongoing research is looking at agents, or combinations of agents, that will deal with all aspects of diabetic ED. The most promising therapeutic agents available so far are the PDE5 inhibitors.

Figure 13-2 suggests a stepped-care approach to treatment of ED in men with diabetes. Table 13-1

summarizes the data available for the different treatment options in erectile dysfunction. It also shows comparisons of success rates in men with and without diabetes, supporting the hypothesis that patients with diabetes have a lower rate of efficacy with treatment of ED.

Phosphodiesterase Type 5 Inhibitors

The treatment options for ED have expanded in recent years, especially with the introduction of PDE5 inhibitors. Sidenafil was the first drug in this class and has been extensively studied. Tadalafil and vardenafil are the newer generation of agents in this class and are potent and selective inhibitors of cGMP-specific PDE5.

An erection occurs when penile cavernosal smooth muscle relaxes under the influence of NO, which is released by cavernous nerves and vascular endothelial cells. Nitric oxide activates guanylyl cyclase, an enzyme that increases the concentration of cGMP, which in turn causes smooth muscle relaxation. PDE5 inhibitors act by preventing the breakdown of cGMP, thus facilitating the corporeal smooth muscle relaxation in response to sexual stimulation.

A meta-analysis of eleven randomized, double blind, placebo-controlled trials of sildenafil in patients with diabetes reported improved erections in 59% of those with type 1 diabetes and 63% in those with type 2 diabetes.[55] Improvement was noted regardless of age, race, ED severity and duration, or the presence of various comorbidities.[57] The response rate in men with diabetes is less than the 83% improvement in nondiabetic men with ED. Discontinuation rates range from 5% to 17% primarily because of insufficient clinical response.[55]

Vardenafil and tadalafil appear to be as effective as sildenafil. Tadalafil has the advantage of a longer duration of action. For tadalafil, 76% of men with diabetes taking the 20-mg dose had improved erections, and 58% of the total group had satisfactory erections to complete intercourse. In nondiabetic men the rates were 81% and 75%, respectively.[58]

In one of the few studies done exclusively in 216 patients with diabetes, treatment with tadalafil significantly improved all primary efficacy variables, regardless of baseline HbA1c level.[59] Therapy with tadalafil also significantly improved a number of secondary outcome measures, including changes in other IIEF domains, individual IIEF questions, and percentage of positive responses to a global assessment question measuring erection improvement. Tadalafil was well tolerated, with headache and dyspepsia being the most frequent adverse events with active treatment in this population.

A retrospective analysis of pooled data from 12 placebo-controlled trials was conducted to characterize the efficacy and safety of tadalafil for treating ED in men with diabetes compared with that in men without diabetes.[42] Despite more-severe baseline ED in men with diabetes, tadalafil was efficacious and well tolerated in this population. As reported for other PDE5 inhibitors, the response to tadalafil was slightly lower in men with diabetes compared to men without diabetes. Thus, tadalafil therapy significantly enhanced erectile function and was well tolerated by men with diabetes and ED.

Vardenafil led to similar results in nondiabetic men, with a 71% to 75% improvement in erections with 5-mg, 10-mg, and 20-mg doses. In men with diabetes the response to the 10-mg dose was 57% and to the 20-mg dose was 72%.[60]

One of the side effects of sildenafil is the visual complaint of seeing a bluish haze. This is due to an inhibition of PDE6, which is present in the retina. Tadalafil and vardenafil appear not to affect color vision due to a better PDE5/PDE6 selectivity ratio.[2]

Side effects common to this class of drugs include the typical vasomotor disturbances of headache, flushing, and rhinitis. All of the PDE5 inhibitors are generally well tolerated. Differences in efficacy and safety (which might be anticipated due to marked differences in potency and half-life) remain to be evaluated from further clinical trials, postmarketing studies, and surveillance.

The major concern regarding the use of PDE-5 inhibitors in ED is the concomitant use of nitrate therapy (such as sublingual nitroglycerin) and PDE5 inhibitors. This combination of agents is contraindicated due to the profound hypotension (and even death) that can occur. Hemodynamically, PDE5 inhibitors have mild nitrate-like activity (sildenafil was originally intended as an antianginal agent). In healthy volunteers, a single 100-mg dose of sildenafil transiently lowered blood pressure by an average of 10/7 mm Hg with a return to baseline at 6 hours post dose. Short-acting nitrates for angina should not be taken within 24 hours of PDE5 inhibitors and vice versa. Long-acting nitrates should not be taken within a week of PDE5 inhibitors. Concerns regarding the cardiovascular safety of sildenafil have largely been dispelled in consensus statements in the United States.[61]

Recent studies show that acute and chronic sildenafil therapy improves brachial artery flow-mediated dilation, an effect of intrinsic endothelial NO release (Fig. 13-3).[62] This enhanced dilation suggests that sildenafil directly improves endothelial function. Similar findings were noted in another study.[63] In addition, sildenafil dilates epicardial coronary arteries and inhibits platelet activation in patients with coronary artery disease.[64] Other studies are under way to test the hypothesis that chronic sildenafil use improves biochemical markers of endothelial dysfunction.

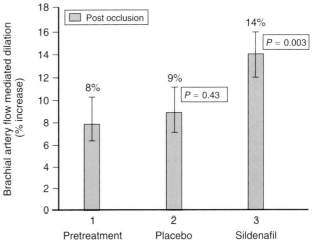

Figure 13–3. Effect of sildenafil taken for 2 weeks on endothelial function. (From DeSouza C, Parulkar A, Lumpkin D, et al: Acute and prolonged effects of sildenafil on brachial artery flow-mediated dilatation in type 2 diabetes. Diabetes Care 25:1336-1339, 2002.)

Intracavernosal Therapy

Several vasoactive substances can be used to stimulate the erectile process. These can be delivered directly into the corpus cavernosum by injection. When injected into one of the cavernosa, free diffusion into the opposite side occurs.

Papaverine (a nonspecific PDE) and alprostadil (a PGE₁ derivative) relax the smooth muscle of the corpus cavernosum. Phentolamine, a competitive inhibitor of α-adrenergic receptors, reduces sympathetic tone. Urologists have also combined these three agents.

Alprostadil is a synthetic prostaglandin related to PGE₁. It has α-blocking properties, is a vasodilator, and directly relaxes smooth muscle via a prostacyclin receptor. A number of studies have been reported using alprostadil in men with diabetes and ED. The largest study included 577 men. 69% of these men completed the 6-month injection therapy study. 87% reported satisfactory sexual function. The subjects who did not complete the study (31%) complained of pain at the injection sites and lack of efficacy. In all studies combined, 50% of men complained of pain at injection sites.

Although intracavernosal therapy has a success rate of 80% to 90% in neuropathic ED and 70% in vasculopathic ED, half of the men eventually discontinue because of pain, loss of effect, or lack of interest. As diabetic complications, including poor visual acuity from retinopathy and decreased manual dexterity, increase with age, it is not uncommon that men are excluded from this therapy or have a poor response.

Priapism is a prolonged (lasting more than 4 to 6 hours) and painful erection that is a true urologic

emergency because it can result in ischemia and fibrosis of the erectile tissue, with significant risk of subsequent impotence.[65] Currently, intracavernosal injection therapy for erectile dysfunction is one of the more common causes of priapism. Prolonged erections occur in 6% of men who use intracavernosal alprostadil and approximately 11% of those who use intracavernosal papaverine.

Intraurethral Prostaglandin Therapy

An intraurethral alprostadil suppository system (MUSE) was developed in an attempt to avoid the problems and issues of injection therapy.[66] This system is less effective and causes urethral pain in up to 30% of users but avoids the side effects of injection therapy. It is not effective in men who fail injection therapy. In the largest published study, 70% of men with diabetes were able to achieve an erection satisfactory for intercourse in 70% of the attempts. Only 2.4% discontinued the drug due to pain.[66]

Combination therapy could be used to augment the effect of MUSE. No clinical trial data support these combinations, but such treatment is available.

Vacuum Tumescence Devices

Vacuum tumescence devices work irrespective of the underlying etiology of ED. Reported success in men with diabetes is 75%.[67] Most find the technique acceptable, especially if they tried and failed oral or injection therapy. Some men consider it cumbersome, but other couples treat the application of the device as a form of sexual foreplay and therefore are more accepting of its use. It can also be added to one of the other treatment modalities to enhance a partial response.

Surgery

Penile prostheses are rarely recommended now that penile injection and vacuum therapy are widely available. However, the success rate is 86% at 5 years, and 91% of attainable erections are suitable for coitus.[68]

Men with diabetes are particularly prone to prosthesis-associated infection, which often necessitates prosthesis removal and possible worsening of the primary problem. Rarely, a severely compromised blood flow could be the reason for treatment failure. Revascularization might help some of these men, but it is difficult to select patients with a predictable, good outcome.[69] In other patients, venous incompetence prevails and ligation of the deep dorsal vein and any incompetent circumflex veins can improve venous leakage.

Unfortunately, the complexity of ED, such as underlying endothelial dysfunction and neuropathy, and the extent of vascular disease in patients with diabetes leads to less-successful outcomes for these surgical procedures. Surgery should be reserved for clear-cut cases of vascular or venous insufficiency in young patients with recent onset of diabetes.

α-Blockers

Yohimbine and phentolamine are α-adrenergic blockers. They are modestly effective in treating ED but are not widely used, especially in the United States, because of lack of availability or side effects, including palpitations and hypertension. A study of 18 nonsmoker men with ED had a 50% success rate (completion of intercourse) in more than 75% of attempts. The responders tended to have less-severe ED.[70] A meta-analysis of yohimbine use found it to be more effective than placebo.[71] However, one of the major difficulties when assessing new therapeutic agents for ED is the placebo response found in 30% to 35% of subjects.

Androgen Therapy

Hormonal causes of ED include a decrease in androgen levels due to both primary (hypergonadotropic) and secondary (hypogonadotropic) hypogonadism.[11] Investigation of ED should usually include a plasma testosterone level. If it is low, a prolactin level should be checked to rule out a central problem. Screening serum testosterone levels of 105 consecutive patients with ED showed that 37 patients had previously unsuspected disorders of the hypothalamic-pituitary-gonadal axis. Twenty patients had hypogonadotropic hypogonadism, seven had hypergonadotropic hypogonadism, eight had hyperprolactinemia, and two had occult hyperthyroidism. Once the specific defect was defined and treated, potency was restored in 33 patients.[72]

Obese men with type 2 diabetes are more prone to hypogonadotropic hypogonadism.[73] This is attributed to elevated levels of estrone and estradiol produced by aromatase in adipose tissue derived from adrenal (androstenedione) and testicular (testosterone) androgen. Serum testosterone concentration is inversely associated with carotid atherosclerosis in men with type 2 diabetes.[74]

Aging is also associated with a progressive decline in androgen levels. The term *andropause* has been used to describe an ill-defined collection of symptoms in aging men, typically those older than 50 years, who have a relative or absolute hypogonadism associated with aging.[11,73,75] It is uncertain if andropause contributes to ED, but it must be recognized and, if severe, treated with androgen replacement.

Testosterone monotherapy has had poor results in treatment of ED. Only 17% of 78 obese men with type 2 diabetes improved long-term sexual function when taking testosterone enanthate.

In a smaller study, 17 patients with ED due to hypogonadotropic hypogonadism received clomiphene citrate or placebo for 2 months each (cross-over design). Luteinizing hormone (LH), follicle-stimulating hormone (FSH), and total and free testosterone levels showed a significant elevation in response to clomiphene citrate over the response to placebo. However, sexual function, as monitored by questionnaires and nocturnal penile tumescence and rigidity testing, did not improve except for some limited parameters in younger and healthier men. The results confirmed that there can be a functional hypogonadotropic hypogonadism, but correction of the hormone level does not universally reverse the associated ED to normal. Closer scrutiny of claims of cause-and-effect relationships between hypogonadism and ED is required.[76]

The use of testosterone in men with normal testosterone levels is not recommended. Replacement therapy should be reserved for those who are androgen deficient, and especially if PDE5 inhibitor is under consideration. These agents require the presence of NO if they are to work, because neural NO production is androgen dependent. If androgen treatment is undertaken, the man should be screened before treatment and monitored during therapy for evidence of testosterone-dependent diseases.

Statin Therapy

Given the correlation of hyperlipidemia and ED, a recent small study showed improvement of ED by cholesterol lowering using daily atorvastatin for 4 months.[77] It is unclear whether this is a direct effect of lipid lowering or an indirect effect from improved endothelial function.[77]

Can Treating the Metabolic Syndrome Improve Erectile Dysfunction?

There is currently no approved pharmacologic therapy for the metabolic syndrome, and lifestyle change consisting of diet changes and exercise leading to weight loss are the cornerstone of therapy. Lifestyle change has been shown not only to prevent diabetes[78] but also to improve endothelial function and to decrease markers of inflammation.[79,80]

Ameliorating certain modifiable risk factors such as sedentary lifestyle or obesity might prevent the subsequent occurrence of ED or improve existing ED.[13] Esposito and coworkers tested this hypothesis in a randomized, controlled trial involving 110

obese men who had ED but no significant comorbid conditions (such as other features of the metabolic syndrome: hypertension, diabetes, and cardiovascular disease). Subjects were assigned to either an intensive weight loss group or usual general weight loss guidance.[36] After 2 years, almost one third of the obese men in the intensive group had reversed their ED after exercising more and losing weight (Fig. 13-4). Various measures of nontraditional cardiovascular risk factors were also evaluated. Change in CRP was independently associated with improvements in ED. Serum concentrations of CRP decreased more in the intervention group (from 3.3 mg/dL to 1.9 mg/L [mean decrease, 1.4 mg/dL]) than in the control group (from 3.4 mg/dL to 3.4 mg/dL [mean decrease, 0 mg/dL]) ($P = .02$).[36]

Other Management Strategies

Other therapies include use of rubber constricting devices at the base of the penis to maintain erections (with or without the prior use of a vacuum tumescence device). There are several OTC herbal remedies but no adequate scientific data to support their safety or efficacy.[81]

Apomorphine is available in several countries for treating ED. Apomorphine is a centrally acting agent that stimulates CNS dopamine receptors, particularly in the hypothalamus. The resulting increased parasympathetic outflow is thought to cause relaxation of corpus cavernosum smooth muscle, corporeal engorgement, and erection. Efficacy is less than with PDE5 inhibitors. The efficacy in diabetic patients remains to be clarified.

Animal experiments have shown that nitric oxide synthase can be restored by gene-transfer techniques, which physiologically improve erectile function.[82] This is an exciting field that could lead to the development of more therapeutic options in the treatment of ED.

As more understanding about the pathophysiology of ED is discovered, it is anticipated that drugs will be developed to specific targets.

CONCLUSION

The etiology of ED in patients with diabetes is multifactorial. Every effort should be made to correct or improve all causes of ED, whether organic, psychogenic, or iatrogenic. A multidisciplinary approach is recommended to deal with the comorbidities so as to ensure the best possible outcomes for patients with ED and diabetes.

Diabetes is a complex chronic disorder associated with various factors that could exacerbate ED (including other components of the metabolic syndrome): obesity, poor glycemic control, dyslipidemia, micro- and macrovascular disease, and

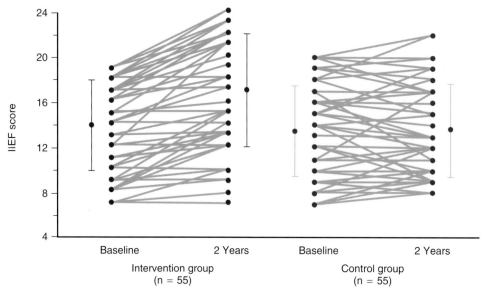

Figure 13–4. Effect of lifestyle changes on erectile dysfunction in obese men. IIEF, International Index of Erectile Function. (From Esposito K, Giugliano F, Di Palo C, et al: Effect of lifestyle changes on erectile dysfunction in obese men: A randomized controlled trial. JAMA 291:2978-2984, 2004. Copyright © 2004. American Medical Association. All rights reserved.)

autonomic neuropathy. All of these factors interact to some degree and exacerbate erectile failure.

Endothelial dysfunction is probably the major underscoring factor that makes ED in diabetes more difficult to treat. ED can be considered a risk marker for the presence of cardiovascular disease, the metabolic syndrome, and associated conditions.

References

1. NIH Consensus Development Panel on Impotence: NIH Consensus Conference. Impotence. JAMA 270:83-90, 1993.
2. Matfin G: New treatments for erectile dysfunction. Fertil Steril 80(Suppl 4):40-45, 2003.
3. Guay AT, Spark RF, Bansal S, et al: American Association of Clinical Endocrinologists medical guidelines for clinical practice for the evaluation and treatment of male sexual dysfunction: A couple's problem—2003 update. Endocr Pract 9:77-95, 2003.
4. Grundy SM, Brewer HB Jr, Cleeman JI, et al: Definition of metabolic syndrome: Report of the National Heart, Lung, and Blood Institute/American Heart Association conference on scientific issues related to definition. Circulation 109:433-438, 2004.
5. Guven S, Kuenzi J, Matfin G: Diabetes mellitus and the metabolic syndrome. In Porth CM (ed): Pathophysiology. Philadelphia, Lippincott Williams & Wilkins, 2005, pp 987-1015.
6. Romeo JH, Seftel AD, Madhun ZT, Aron DC: Sexual function in men with diabetes type 2: Association with glycemic control. J Urol 163:788-791, 2000.
7. McCulloch DK, Campbell IW, Wu FC, et al: The prevalence of diabetic impotence. Diabetologia 18:279-283, 1980.
8. Kaiser FE: Erectile dysfunction in the aging man. Med Clin North Am 83:1267-1278, 1999.
9. Feldman HA, Goldstein I, Hatzichristou DG, et al: Impotence and its medical and psychosocial correlates: Results of the Massachusetts Male Aging Study. J Urol 151:54-61, 1994.
10. Klein R, Klein BE, Lee KE, et al: Prevalence of self-reported erectile dysfunction in people with long-term IDDM. Diabetes Care 19:135-141, 1996.
11. Matfin G: The male genitourinary system. In Porth CM (ed): Pathophysiology. Philadelphia, Lippincott Williams & Wilkins, 2005, pp 1019-1030.
12. Lue TF: Erectile dysfunction. N Engl J Med 342:1802-1813, 2000.
13. Saigal CS: Obesity and erectile dysfunction: Common problems, common solution? JAMA 291:3011-3012, 2004.
14. Reaven GM: Banting lecture 1988. Role of insulin resistance in human disease. (Review) (71 refs). Diabetes 37:1595-1607, 1988.
15. McFarlane SI, Banerji M, Sowers JR: Insulin resistance and cardiovascular disease. J Clin Endocrinol Metab 86:713-718, 2000.
16. Fonseca VA: Risk factors for coronary heart disease in diabetes. Ann Intern Med 133:154-156, 2000.
17. Fonseca V, Desouza C, Asnani S, Jialal I: Nontraditional risk factors for cardiovascular disease in diabetes. Endocr Rev 25:153-175, 2004.
18. Stern MP: Diabetes and cardiovascular disease. The "common soil" hypothesis. Diabetes 44:369-374, 1995.
19. Calles-Escandon J, Cipolla M: Diabetes and endothelial dysfunction: A clinical perspective. Endocr Rev 22:36-52, 2001.
20. Richardson D, Vinik A: Etiology and treatment of erectile failure in diabetes mellitus. Curr Diab Rep 2:501-509, 2002.
21. Solomon H, Man JW, Jackson G: Erectile dysfunction and the cardiovascular patient: Endothelial dysfunction is common denominator. Heart 89:251-253, 2003.
22. Theuma P, Fonseca VA: Novel cardiovascular risk factors and macrovascular and microvascular complications of diabetes. Curr Drug Targets 4:477-486, 2003.
23. Baron AD: Insulin resistance and vascular function. J Diabet Complications 16:92-102, 2002.
24. Baron AD, Steinberg HO: Endothelial function, insulin sensitivity, and hypertension. Circulation 96:725-726, 1997.
25. Baron AD: Insulin and the vasculature—old actors, new roles. J Investig Med 1996; 44:406-412, 1996.
26. Steinberg HO, Chaker H, Leaming R, et al: Obesity/insulin resistance is associated with endothelial dysfunction. Impli-

cations for the syndrome of insulin resistance. J Clin Invest 97:2601-2610, 1996.

27. Steinberg HO, Paradisi G, Hook G, et al: Free fatty acid elevation impairs insulin-mediated vasodilation and nitric oxide production. Diabetes 49:1231-1238, 2000.

28. Grover A, Padginton C, Wilson MF, et al: Insulin attenuates norepinephrine-induced venoconstriction. An ultrasonographic study. Hypertension 25(4 Pt 2):779-784, 1995.

29. Aljada A, Dandona P: Effect of insulin on human aortic endothelial nitric oxide synthase. Metabolism 49:147-150, 2000.

30. Aljada A, Ghanim H, Assian E, Dandona P: Tumor necrosis factor–α inhibits insulin-induced increase in endothelial nitric oxide synthase and reduces insulin receptor content and phosphorylation in human aortic endothelial cells. Metabolism 51:487-491, 2002.

31. Zeng G, Quon MJ: Insulin-stimulated production of nitric oxide is inhibited by wortmannin. Direct measurement in vascular endothelial cells. J Clin Invest 98:894-898, 1996.

32. Caballero AE, Arora S, Saouaf R, et al: Microvascular and macrovascular reactivity is reduced in subjects at risk for type 2 diabetes. Diabetes 48:1856-1862, 1999.

33. Ross R: Atherosclerosis—an inflammatory disease. N Engl J Med 340:115-126, 1999.

34. De Angelis L, Marfella MA, Siniscalchi M, et al: Erectile and endothelial dysfunction in Type II diabetes: A possible link. Diabetologia 44:1155-1160, 2001.

35. Billups KL, Kaiser DR, Kelly AS, et al: Relation of C-reactive protein and other cardiovascular risk factors to penile vascular disease in men with erectile dysfunction. Int J Impot Res 15:231-236, 2003.

36. Esposito K, Giugliano F, Di Palo C, et al: Effect of lifestyle changes on erectile dysfunction in obese men: A randomized controlled trial. JAMA 291:2978-2984, 2004.

37. Chan NN, Chan JC: Asymmetric dimethylarginine (ADMA): A potential link between endothelial dysfunction and cardiovascular diseases in insulin resistance syndrome? Diabetologia 45:1609-1616, 2002.

38. Stuhlinger MC, Abbasi F, Chu JW, et al: Relationship between insulin resistance and an endogenous nitric oxide synthase inhibitor. JAMA 287:1420-1426, 2002.

39. Mass R, Schwedhelm E, Albsmeier J, Boger RH: The pathophysiology of erectile dysfunction related to endothelial dysfunction and mediators of vascular function. Vasc Med 7:213-225, 2002.

40. Masuda H, Tsujii T, Okuno T et al: Accumulated endogenous NOS inhibitors, decreased NOS activity, and impaired cavernosal relaxation with ischemia. Am J Physiol Regulatory Integrative Comp Physiol 282:R1730-R1738, 2002.

41. Cartledge JJ, Eardley I, Morrison JF: Impairment of corpus cavernosal smooth muscle relaxation by glycosylated human haemoglobin. BJU Int 85:735-741, 2000.

42. Fonseca V, Seftel A, Denne J, Fredlund P: Impact of diabetes mellitus on the severity of erectile dysfunction and response to treatment: Analysis of data from tadalafil clinical trials. Diabetologia. 47:1914-1923, 2004.

43. Veves A, Akbari CM, Primavera J, et al: Endothelial dysfunction and the expression of endothelial nitric oxide synthetase in diabetic neuropathy, vascular disease, and foot ulceration. Diabetes 47:457-463, 1998.

44. Bacon CG, Mittleman MA, Kawachi I, et al: Sexual function in men older than 50 years of age: Results from the Health Professionals Follow-up Study. Ann Intern Med 139:161-168, 2003.

45. Walczak MK, Lokhandwala N, Hodge MB, Guay AT: Prevalence of cardiovascular risk factors in erectile dysfunction. J Gend Specif Med 5:19-24, 2002.

46. Chung WS, Sohn JH, Park YY: Is obesity an underlying factor in erectile dysfunction? Eur Urol 36:68-70, 1999.

47. Derby CA, Mohr BA, Goldstein I, et al: Modifiable risk factors and erectile dysfunction: Can lifestyle changes modify risk? Urology 56:302-306, 2000.

48. Bacon CG, Mittleman MA, Kawachi I, et al: Sexual function in men older than 50 years of age: Results from the Health Professionals Follow-up Study. Ann Intern Med 139:161-168, 2003.

49. Wei M, Macera CA, Davis DR, et al: Total cholesterol and high density lipoprotein cholesterol as important predictors of erectile dysfunction. Am J Epidemiol 140:930-937, 1994.

50. Gazzaruso C, Giordanetti S, De Amici E, et al.: Relationship between erectile dysfunction and silent myocardial ischemia in apparently uncomplicated type 2 diabetic patients. Circulation 110:22-26, 2004.

51. Wackers FJ, Young LH, Inzucchi SE, et al: Detection of silent myocardial ischemia in asymptomatic diabetic subjects: The DIAD study. Diabetes Care 27:1954-1961, 2004.

52. Greenstein A, Chen J, Miller H, et al: Does severity of ischemic coronary disease correlate with erectile function? Int J Impot Res 9:123-126, 1997.

53. Russell ST, Khandheria BK, Nehra A: Erectile dysfunction and cardiovascular disease. Mayo Clin Proc 79:782-794, 2004.

54. Jackson G: Treatment of erectile dysfunction in patients with cardiovascular disease: Guide to drug selection. Drugs 64:1533-1545, 2004.

55. Fink HA, Mac DR, Rutks IR, et al: Sildenafil for male erectile dysfunction: A systematic review and meta-analysis. Arch Intern Med 162:1349-1360, 2002.

56. Guay AT, Perez JB, Velasquez E, et al: Clinical experience with intraurethral alprostadil (MUSE) in the treatment of men with erectile dysfunction. A retrospective study. Medicated urethral system for erection. Eur Urol 38:671-676, 2000.

57. Carson CC, Burnett AL, Levine LA, Nehra A: The efficacy of sildenafil citrate (Viagra) in clinical populations: An update. Urology 60:12-27, 2002.

58. Brock GB, McMahon CG, Chen KK, et al.: Efficacy and safety of tadalafil for the treatment of erectile dysfunction: Results of integrated analyses. J Urol 168:1332-1336, 2002.

59. Saenz de Tejada I, Anglin G, Knight JR, Emmick JT: Effects of tadalafil on erectile dysfunction in men with diabetes. Diabetes Care 25:2159-2164, 2002.

60. Porst H, Rosen R, Padma-Nathan H, E et al.: The efficacy and tolerability of vardenafil, a new, oral, selective phosphodiesterase type 5 inhibitor, in patients with erectile dysfunction: The first at-home clinical trial. Int J Impot Res 13:192-199, 2001.

61. Cheitlin MD, Hutter AM Jr, Brindis RG, et al.: Use of sildenafil (Viagra) in patients with cardiovascular disease. Technology and Practice Executive Committee. Circulation 99:168-177, 1999.

62. DeSouza C, Parulkar A, Lumpkin D, et al: Acute and prolonged effects of sildenafil on brachial artery flow-mediated dilatation in type 2 diabetes. Diabetes Care 25:1336-1339, 2002.

63. Katz SD, Balidemaj K, Homma S, et al: Acute type 5 phosphodiesterase inhibition with sildenafil enhances flow-mediated vasodilation in patients with chronic heart failure. J Am Coll Cardiol 36:845-851, 2000.

64. Halcox JP, Nour KR, Zalos G, et al: The effect of sildenafil on human vascular function, platelet activation, and myocardial ischemia. J Am Coll Cardiol 40:1232-1240, 2002.

65. Harmon WJ, Nehra A: Priapism: Diagnosis and treatment. Mayo Clinic Proceedings 72:350-355, 1997.

66. Padma-Nathan H, Hellstrom WJ, Kaiser FE, et al: Treatment of men with erectile dysfunction with transurethral alprostadil. Medicated Urethral System for Erection (MUSE) Study Group. N Engl J Med 336:1-7, 1997.

67. Price DE, Cooksey G, Jehu D, et al: The management of impotence in diabetic men by vacuum tumescence therapy. Diabet Med 8:964-967, 1991.

68. Carson CC, Mulcahy JJ, Govier FE: Efficacy, safety and patient satisfaction outcomes of the AMS 700CX inflatable penile prosthesis: Results of a long-term multicenter study. AMS 700CX Study Group. J Urol 164:376-380, 2000.

69. Benet AE, Sharaby JS, Melman A: Male erectile dysfunction assessment and treatment options. Compr Ther 20:669-673, 1994.

70. Guay AT, Spark RF, Jacobson J, et al: Yohimbine treatment of organic erectile dysfunction in a dose-escalation trial. Int J Impot Res 14:25-31, 2002.

71. Ernst E, Pittler MH: Yohimbine for erectile dysfunction: A systematic review and meta-analysis of randomized clinical trials. J Urol 159:433-436, 1998.

72. Spark RF, White RA, Connolly PB: Impotence is not always psychogenic. Newer insights into hypothalamic-pituitary-gonadal dysfunction. JAMA 243:750-755, 1980.

73. Tan RS, Pu SJ: Impact of obesity on hypogonadism in the andropause. Int J Androl 25:195-201, 2002.

74. Fukui M, Kitagawa Y, Nakamura N, et al: Association between serum testosterone concentration and carotid atherosclerosis in men with type 2 diabetes. Diabetes Care 26:1869-1873, 2003.

75. Leifke E, Gorenoi V, Wichers C, et al: Age-related changes of serum sex hormones, insulin-like growth factor-1 and sex-hormone binding globulin levels in men: Cross-sectional data from a healthy male cohort. Clin Endocrinol (Oxf) 53:689-695, 2000.

76. Guay AT, Bansal S, Heatley GJ: Effect of raising endogenous testosterone levels in impotent men with secondary hypogonadism: Double blind placebo-controlled trial with clomiphene citrate. J Clin Endocrinol Metab 80:3546-3562, 1995.

77. Saltzman EA, Guay AT, Jacobson J: Improvement in erectile function in men with organic erectile dysfunction by correction of elevated cholesterol levels: A clinical observation. J Urol 2004 172:255-258.

78. Knowler WC, Barrett-Connor E, Fowler SE, et al: Reduction in the incidence of type 2 diabetes with lifestyle intervention or metformin. N Engl J Med 346:393-403, 2002.

79. Esposito K, Di Palo C, Marfella R, Giugliano D: The effect of weight loss on endothelial functions in obesity: Response to Sciacqua et al. Diabetes Care 26:2968-2969, 2003.

80. Esposito K, Pontillo A, Di Palo C, et al: Effect of weight loss and lifestyle changes on vascular inflammatory markers in obese women: A randomized trial. JAMA 289:1799-1804, 2003.

81. Moyad MA, Hathaway S, Ni HS: Traditional Chinese medicine, acupuncture, and other alternative medicines for prostate cancer: An introduction and the need for more research. Semin Urol Oncol 17:103-110, 1999.

82. Bivalacqua TJ, Usta MF, Champion HC, et al: Gene transfer of endothelial nitric oxide synthase partially restores nitric oxide synthesis and erectile function in streptozotocin diabetic rats. J Urol 169:1911-1917, 2003.

Chapter 14

The Diabetic Foot

Andrew J. M. Boulton and David G. Armstrong

> ## KEY POINTS
>
> - *The neuropathic foot cannot be diagnosed by history alone. Always remove shoes and socks and examine the feet.*
> - *The key to healing a neuropathic foot ulcer is adequate offloading.*
> - *Assume that a warm, swollen, nonulcerated neuropathic diabetic foot is a Charcot foot until proven otherwise.*

Foot complications and amputation represent one of the most important of all the long-term problems of diabetes, medically, socially, and economically. Foot ulceration is the end-stage complication of neuropathy and vascular disease, and the risk of developing this end stage is much greater than the risk of reaching end-stage sequelae of retinopathy or nephropathy.

Progress has been made in our understanding of the pathogenesis and management of the diabetic foot since the 1980s. Published research on the diabetic foot has increased from 0.7% in 1980 to 1988 to at least 2.7% since 1999 as indexed in the National Library of Medicine's PubMed database. Councils and study groups have been formed in both the European Diabetes Association and the American Diabetes Association, and the International Working Group has published an international consensus booklet on the diabetic foot.[1]

The global term *diabetic foot* refers to a variety of pathologic conditions that affect the feet of people with diabetes. Neuropathy is a major contributory factor in the pathogenesis of foot ulceration and of Charcot's neuropathic arthropathy (CN). Often neuropathy can be implicated in the causal chain ultimately resulting in amputation.

This chapter includes discussion of the epidemiology of foot problems that result in ulceration and amputation and describes causal pathways that result in these major problems. The question of classification of foot ulcers is discussed as well as the investigation of patients with foot ulcers and wound healing in diabetes. Management of foot problems is described, including the role of footwear. Prevention of foot problems and recurrence of ulceration are covered, followed by a discussion of the increasingly common Charcot's neuropathic arthropathy.

EPIDEMIOLOGY OF ULCERS AND AMPUTATION

Foot problems remain a leading cause of hospital admission among people with diabetes mellitus in the United States. It is estimated that 15% of diabetic patients will develop a foot ulcer during their lifetime.[2-4] Diabetic foot problems are a major challenge to health care in developed countries, and they rank among the most frequent of diabetic complications in developing countries.[5,6]

The study of the epidemiology of diabetic foot disease has been beset by numerous problems relating to both diagnostic tests and populations selected.[7,8] Until proper population-based registers of people with diabetes are available, reliable data relating to accurate estimates of the prevalence and incidence of these late complications will remain limited. Foot ulcers and amputations remain common and serious complications of both main types of diabetes and are associated with significant mortality.[9-11]

Foot ulcers are lesions that involve a skin break with loss of epithelium; they can extend into the dermis and deeper layers, sometimes involving bone and muscle. *Amputation* is the removal of a terminal, nonviable portion of the limb.[9]

A selection of epidemiologic data on ulceration and amputation is listed in Table 14-1.[12-19] The incidence of foot ulcers in developed countries is approximately 2% per year in the general diabetes population.[13,14] Incidence data are lacking from developing countries, but it is clear that the prevalence of ulcers and amputations is much higher in these areas.[17-19] Ulceration is much more common in patients with predisposing risk factors; annual incidence rates in neuropathic patients vary from 5% to more than 7%.[20,21] It is likely that more than 5% of diabetic patients have a history of foot ulcers,[12] and the cumulative lifetime incidence may

Table 14–1. *Epidemiology of Diabetic Foot Ulceration and Amputation*

Author	Year	No	Ref	Country	Prevalence Ulcer	Prevalence Amputation	Incidence Ulcer	Incidence Amputation
Europe or North America								
Kumar et al	1994	811	11	UK	1.4	1.4	—	—
Abbott et al	2002	9710	12	UK	1.7	1.3	2.2	
Muller et al	2002	665	13	Netherlands	—	—	2.1	0.6
Lavery et al	2003	666	14	USA	—	—	6.8	0.6
Global								
Humphrey et al	1996	1564	15	Nauru Pacific region	—	—	—	0.76
Belhadj*	1998	865	16	Algeria	11.9	6.7	—	—
Pendsey*	1994	11300	17	India	3.6	—	—	—
Gulliford et al	2002	2106	19	Trinidad	12.0	4.0	—	—

*Clinic-based study (all others are population based or community based)

be as high as 15%.[9] Up to 85% of amputations are preceded by foot ulcers. Therefore, any successes in reducing foot ulcer incidence will be followed by a reduction in amputations.

Studies in Europe, with the exception of Sweden,[22] have been disappointing in this regard. Studies from Germany have shown no evidence of a decrease in amputation in the last decade,[23,24] whereas one report from the United Kingdom actually reported an increase.[25]

Ethnicity

Studies from the United Kingdom suggest that foot ulcers and amputations are less common in Asian patients of Indian subcontinent origin,[26,27] and Afro-Caribbean men, but not women, have lower amputation rates.[28] The possible explanation for the findings in South Asian patients relates to differences in limited joint mobility and better foot care in certain religious groups, such as Muslims. In contrast, Resnick and coworkers[29] reported that amputation rates were more common among African Americans with diabetes than among white Americans. Similarly, ulceration was much more common in Hispanic Americans and Native Americans than in non-Hispanic whites.[15]

Economic Consequences

The American Diabetes Association held a consensus conference on diabetic wound care in 1999 because of the vast cost of diabetic foot disease and the real need to develop cost-effective measures to treat and prevent ulcers.[3] Shearer and colleagues[30] confirmed that diabetic patients with neuropathic risk factors (reduced vibration perception) incur five times more direct medical costs for ulcers and amputations and live for two months less than non-

neuropathic diabetic subjects. Similarly, a Swedish study reported that an intensified prevention strategy involving education, foot care, and footwear would be cost effective and even cost saving if applied to patients with risk factors for foot problems.[31]

Average inpatient costs for lower limb complications in 1997 were $16,580 for foot ulcers, $25,241 for toe or toe and other distal amputations, and $31,436 for major amputations.[32] In the 1990s, the average outpatient cost for one diabetic foot ulcer episode was estimated to be $28,000 over 2 years.[33] The ongoing Global Lower Extremity Amputation Study will provide epidemiologic evidence on the world-wide incidence of lower extremity amputations, and it will enable a comparison of costs in this area.[34]

CAUSES OF FOOT ULCERATION

The breakdown of the diabetic foot does not occur spontaneously, and there are many warning signs that may be used to predict those at risk. Dr. Elliott Joslin recognized this more than 70 years ago when he stated that "diabetic gangrene is not heaven-sent but is earth-born."[35] Ulcers invariably occur as a consequence of an interaction between environmental hazards and specific pathologies of the lower limbs of diabetic patients. We cannot assume that a certain percentage of all diabetic patients will develop foot ulcers at some point in their life. A clear understanding of the pathogenesis of ulceration is essential if we are to succeed in reducing the incidence of foot ulceration and therefore amputation.

The breakdown of the diabetic foot was traditionally considered to result from peripheral vascular disease, peripheral neuropathy, and infection. More recently, other contributory causes such as psychosocial factors[36] and abnormalities of pres-

sures and loads under the foot[37] have been implicated. There is also no compelling evidence that infection is a direct cause of ulceration; it is likely that infection becomes established once the skin break occurs and thus is a consequence rather than a cause of ulceration. Neuropathy is the most important contributory cause in the pathway to ulceration,[38] especially in developing countries.[39]

Neuropathy

The association between somatic and autonomic neuropathy and foot ulceration has been recognized for many years.[40] It is only since the 1990s that prospective follow-up studies have confirmed the causative role of somatic neuropathy.[13,20,21] Patients with sensory loss appear to have up to a seven-fold increased risk of developing foot ulcers compared with non-neuropathic diabetic patients. Poor balance and instability are increasingly recognized as troublesome symptoms of peripheral neuropathy, presumably secondary to proprioceptive loss. The association of sway and postural instability with foot ulceration has been confirmed.[41,42]

Sympathetic autonomic neuropathy in the lower limb results in reduced sweating and therefore dry skin that is prone to crack and fissure as well as in increased blood flow in the absence of large vessel peripheral vascular disease. Increased blood flow results from the increase in arteriovenous shunting and causes a warm foot with distended dorsal foot veins, which are useful physical signs of an at-risk foot.

In clinical practice, peripheral neuropathy can usually be documented by a simple clinical assessment of large-fiber function and small-fiber function in the feet together with assessment of ankle reflexes.[13,43] Decrease in large-fiber function is indicated by loss of vibration perception as determined by a 128-Hz tuning fork, and small-fiber function can be tested with hot and cold rods or pin-prick sensation. A composite score of these clinical measures, the modified neuropathy disability score, is useful in predicting those at risk for future ulceration.[13]

The 10-gram monofilament is also commonly used in the United States to assess a patient's foot ulcer risk status.[44] This can be used to test several key areas on the foot[44] for the ability to perceive the sensation of pressure when the filament buckles (i.e., when a 10-gram force is applied). Although the test is simple to perform, care must be taken to ensure that the filaments are accurate in buckling with a 10-gram force.[45] One study confirmed that many filaments supposedly delivering a 10-gram force when buckling were in fact widely inaccurate.

As noted in Chapter 11, neuropathic symptoms correlate poorly with sensory loss, and their absence must never be equated with a lack of foot ulcer risk. In assessing foot ulcer risk, a careful examination of the feet after removal of shoes and socks *must always* be carried out, whatever the history of neuropathic symptoms.

Peripheral Vascular Disease

Peripheral ischemia resulting from proximal arterial disease was a component cause in the pathway to ulceration in 35% of cases in a two-center study of causal pathways.[38] A more-recent comparative study of peripheral arterial disease in diabetic and nondiabetic patients confirmed that diabetic patients had more distal disease and a poorer outcome with respect to both amputation and mortality.[46] The Framingham study[47] found that absence of foot pulses was more than 50% more common in diabetic men and women than in the general population.

The importance of obstructive vascular disease in the pathogenesis of diabetic foot problems has been confirmed in reports from both the United States and Europe.[48,49] Ultimately, however, ulceration results as a failure of the microcirculation, and occlusive disease of larger vessels can exacerbate preexisting microvascular abnormalities.[50]

Other Risk Factors

Of all the risk factors for ulceration (Box 14-1), one of the most important is a history of similar problems. In many series history of ulcers is associated with a 50% annual risk of reulceration. Other risk factors, as noted in Box 14-1, include the presence of peripheral edema, duration of diabetes, poor social background, and living alone.

Long-Term Complications
Patients with other late complications, particularly nephropathy, have an increased foot ulcer risk.

Box 14-1. Factors Increasing the Risk of Diabetic Foot Ulceration

- Peripheral neuropathy: somatic or autonomic
- Peripheral vascular disease
- Past foot ulcer history
- Plantar callus and elevated foot pressure
- Foot deformity
- Psychosocial factors
- Other microvascular complications, especially chronic renal failure
- Edema
- Ethnic background
- Living alone
- Poor social background

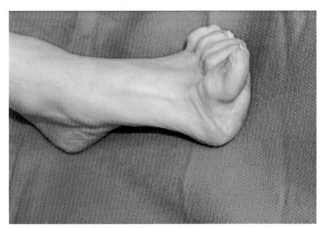

Figure 14–1. High-risk foot, showing prominent metatarsal heads and clawing of the toes.

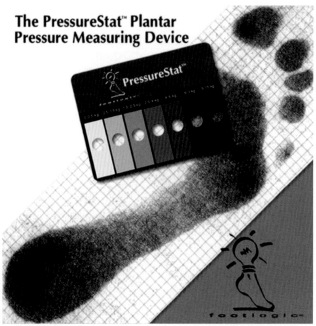

The PressureStat™ Plantar Pressure Measuring Device

Figure 14–2. The PressureStat device is a simple quantitative assessment: The darker the area, the higher the foot pressure. The calibration card is shown superimposed.

Retinopathy, with impaired vision, is a major risk for patients in whom laser therapy has restricted peripheral and dark vision. This defect, together with the reduced proprioception, might contribute to trips and falls that could result in insensitive injury or development of Charcot's neuropathic arthropathy.

Foot Deformity
A combination of motor neuropathy, cheiroarthropathy, and altered gait patterns are thought to result in the high-risk neuropathic foot, with clawing of toes, prominent metatarsal heads, high arch, and wasting of small muscles (Fig. 14–1).

Elevated Foot Pressures
Numerous studies have confirmed the contributory role that abnormal plantar pressures play in the pathogenesis of foot ulceration. After the original confirmation that plantar ulcers invariably occurred at sites of high pressure,[40] a prospective study confirmed that high foot pressures predict ulcer development in the insensate foot.[51] However, abnormalities of foot pressures should be considered in conjunction with other risk factors, especially neuropathy. When foot pressure is used alone, one study suggests that it is a poor tool for predicting ulceration.[52]

Although studies using sophisticated foot-pressure measurement systems have helped our understanding of foot ulcer pathogenesis,[53] they are not suited to day-to-day clinical practice in busy diabetic foot clinics. Thus a simple, inexpensive but reliable method for screening feet could be helpful to both physicians and patients. Such a semi-quantitative method was developed in the Netherlands: The Podotrack footprint system (Medical Gait Technology, Emmen, the Netherlands; PressureStat in the United States) is a semi-quantitative footprint mat that quantifies plantar pressure by visual comparison between the grayness of the footprint and the calibration card.[54]

In a comparative study with the gold standard, the optical pedobarograph, van Schie and colleagues confirmed that trained observers correctly identified high-pressure areas using the Podotrack or PressureStat system, which correlated well with the pedobarograph, suggesting that this system could be a useful screening tool.[54] Moreover, the visual impact on the patient (dark area indicates danger of ulceration) could be used as an educational aid (Fig. 14–2).

Plantar Callus
Plantar callus forms under weight-bearing areas as a consequence of dry skin (autonomic dysfunction), insensitivity, and repetitive moderate stress from high foot pressure. It acts as a foreign body and can cause ulceration.[55] The presence of callus in an insensate foot should alert the physician that this patient is at high risk for ulceration, and callus should be removed by a podiatrist or other trained health care professional.

Ethnicity
Foot ulceration appears to be more common in white and Hispanic patients compared with other groups such as Asians, although more work is required in this area.

Psychosocial Factors
Most of the causes of foot ulceration are physical factors. However, as discussed by Vileikyte and colleagues,[36] there have been few studies of psychosocial factors in the pathway to foot ulceration. It appears that patients' behavior is not driven by the

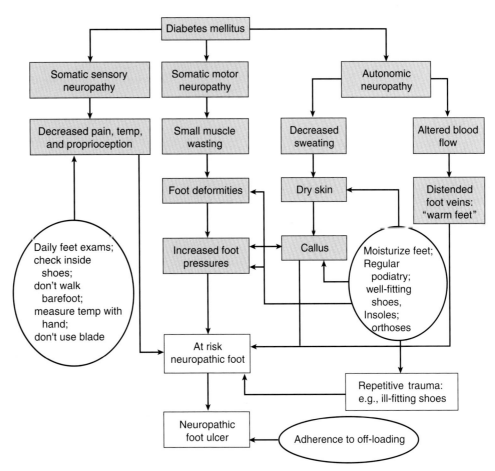

Figure 14–3. Causal pathways to ulceration, emphasizing the key role of the patient in ulcer prevention (*circles* and *arrows*). temp, temperature. (Reproduced with permission from Boulton AJ: The diabetic foot: From art to science. The 18th Camillo Golgi lecture. Diabetologia 47: 1343-1353, 2004.)

abstract designation of being at risk; it is driven by patients' perception of their risks. If patients do not believe that a foot ulcer lies on the path from neuropathy to amputation, are they likely to follow educational advice on how to reduce ulcer risk?[56] These observations might explain the finding of a systematic review of studies of preventive foot care education that was unable to confirm the usefulness of education.[57] There is, however, a suggestion that education and regular podiatric care could result in earlier presentation when ulceration does develop.[58]

PATHWAYS TO ULCERATION

As just discussed and as outlined in Figure 14–3, the pathway to ulceration is complex and involves an interaction of numerous factors. Reiber's group studied causal pathways that result in diabetic foot ulcers and applied the Rothman model of causation.[38] Component factors (such as neuropathy, peripheral vascular disease, plantar callus) are not sufficient by themselves to result in an ulcer, but the interaction of a number of component causes can be sufficient for ulceration.[38] In this study, the commonest component causes interacting to result in ulceration were neuropathy, deformity, and trauma;

this triad was present in 63% of the 150 patients studied.

A typical scenario is a patient with insensitive feet who buys shoes too small; the shoes traumatize the feet at maximum pressure points caused by the tight fit. Neuropathy was the most important component cause in this study,[38] and the vast majority of ulcers in this and other series were potentially preventable.

Other simple examples of two component pathways to ulceration are neuropathy and mechanical trauma (e.g. standing on a nail), neuropathy and thermal trauma, and neuropathy and chemical trauma (such as inappropriate use of over-the-counter chemical corn treatments).

CLASSIFICATION OF FOOT ULCERS

The management of diabetic foot ulceration is multidisciplinary, requiring communication between primary and secondary care practitioners as well as among a number of other health care professionals. Moreover, the increasing use of evidence-based practice, audit, and assessment of clinical effectiveness means that an accurate and concise ulcer description and classification is required to improve

Box 14-2. Traditional Meggitt-Wagner Ulcer Classification System

Grade 0

No ulcer, but high-risk foot (bony prominences, callus, deformities, etc.)

Grade 1

Superficial, full-thickness ulcer

Grade 2

Deep ulcer, may involve tendons, but without bone involvement

Grade 3

Deep ulcer with osteomyelitis

Grade 4

Local gangrene (toes or forefoot)

Grade 5

Gangrene of whole foot

Box 14-3. University of Texas Wound Classification System

Grade 0: Pre- or postulcerative lesion, completely epithelialized

Stage A: without infection or ischemia

Stage B: with infection

Stage C: with ischemia

Stage D: with infection and ischemia

Grade 1: Superficial wound not involving tendon, capsule, or bone

Stage A: without infection or ischemia

Stage B: with infection

Stage C: with ischemia

Stage D: with infection and ischemia

Grade 2: Wound penetrating to tendon or capsule

Stage A: without infection or ischemia

Stage B: with infection

Stage C: with ischemia

Stage D: with infection and ischemia

Grade 3: Wound penetrating to bone or joint

Stage A: without infection or ischemia

Stage B: with infection

Stage C: with ischemia

Stage D: with infection and ischemia

Adapted from Armstrong DG, Lavery LA, Harkless LB: Validation of a diabetic wound classification system. The contribution of depth, infection, and ischemia to risk of amputation [see comments]. Diabetes Care 21:855-859, 1998, and Armstrong DG, Peters EJ: Classification of wounds of the diabetic foot. Current Diabetes Rev 1:233-238, 2001.

multidisciplinary collaboration and communication.[3] Predicting clinical outcomes is also an important part of the initial assessment of patients presenting with new foot ulcers, but most wound classification systems have failed to assess and therefore provide evidence of the most important factors, such as infection and ischemia.[59,60]

Classification systems can include the presumed etiology; the location, size, or depth of the lesion; and the vascular and infection status. However, the most widely used foot ulcer classification is the Meggitt-Wagner grading, as shown in Box 14-2. One problem with this system is that it is not possible to assess the degree of ischemia in grade 1 through 3 wounds. However, the Meggitt-Wagner system has been shown to accurately predict amputation risk and has generally been regarded as the gold standard.

The University of Texas at San Antonio Wound Classification system (UT) (Box 14-3) is based upon the Meggitt-Wagner system, but it stages each grade of ulcer according to the presence or absence of infection or ischemia. This system has been validated in a longitudinal study, and outcomes deteriorate with the increasing stage and grade of wounds.[60] In a comparative prospective study across two centers, one in the United States and one in the United Kingdom, the University of Texas classification system was shown to be superior to the Meggitt-Wagner system at predicting outcome.[61] However, although this result suggests the benefit of adding grading for infection or ischemia to the traditional Meggitt-Wagner, this study also showed that the traditional Meggitt-Wagner system was itself generally accurate in predicting outcomes.

The American Diabetes Association and the International Working Group on the diabetic foot[1] are collaborating to establish a consensus on which wound classification systems to use for clinical practice and for research purposes. A preliminary discussion was published on a foot ulcer classification system for research purposes in 2004.[62]

For the purposes of further discussion of wound management in this chapter, the University of Texas wound classification system is used. Examples of a neuropathic ulcer (UT2A) and a neuroischemic ulcer (UT2C) are shown in Figures 14–4 and 14–5.

EVALUATION OF THE DIABETIC FOOT WOUND

Is Infection Present?

The definition of infection is not an easy one. Cultures, laboratory values, and subjective symptoms are all helpful. However, the diagnosis of an infec-

whereas deeper infections can require longer treatment together, on occasion, with surgical debridement.

For choice of antibiotic, refer to the international consensus on diagnosing and treating the infected diabetic foot.[99] Commonly used broad-spectrum antibiotics include clindamycin, cephalexin, ciprofloxacin, and amoxicillin–clavulanate potassium.[98,99] Intravenous antibiotic options for more serious infections (e.g., cellulitis) include imipenem-cilastatin, β-lactamase inhibitors (ampicillin-sulbactam and piperacillin-tazobactam), and broad-spectrum cephalosporins.

An increasing problem in diabetic foot clinics is the emergence of strains of bacteria that are resistant to many antibiotics.[100,101] Such multidrug-resistant organisms tend to be more common in those who have previously been hospitalized or have received long-duration antibiotic treatments. It does, however, seem likely that in the majority of cases the presence of such resistant organisms represents opportunistic colonization rather than true infection. For patients with infection by such organisms, a newer antibiotic, linezolid, which is active against gram-positive cocci including many resistant strains, has been shown in a randomized trial to be effective in such infections.[102]

Osteomyelitis

The diagnosis of osteomyelitis is a controversial topic. Contrary to traditional teaching, some cases of localized osteomyelitis, particularly in distal bones without involving joints, can be managed by long-term (10 to 12 weeks) antibiotic therapy that should cover organisms such as *Staphylococcus aureus,* which remains the commonest etiologic organism. Among the important therapeutic considerations for osteomyelitis are the anatomic site of the infection, the local vascular supply, the extent of soft tissue and bone destruction, and the presence of systemic illness. For detailed discussion of treatment algorithms, refer to the report from the International Consensus Group on the diagnosis and treatment of the infected diabetic foot.[99]

An alternative to prolonged use of antibiotics might be antibiotic-impregnated beads,[103] although controlled trials are still required in this area. Other cases of osteomyelitis, particularly involving joints, may require surgical debridement or even local amputation, (e.g., of a digit). Clearly, careful consideration must be given to the vascular status prior to any local surgery; proper assessment of the arterial tree is strongly recommended prior to surgical intervention.

Neuroischemic Ulcers

The percentage of patients with neuroischemic ulcers presenting to diabetic foot clinics in Western countries has been increasing. A neuroischemic ulcer is an ulcer occurring in a foot of a diabetic patient who has both a neuropathic deficit and impaired arterial inflow. In the UT classification these are 1C, 2C, or 3C in the absence of infection or 1D, 2D, or 3D in the presence of infection. Any patient with a new foot ulcer should be assessed for both neuropathic and ischemic deficits; the absence of foot pulses in a cold foot should suggest ischemia, which should prompt a noninvasive investigation of the peripheral circulation.

The principles of treatment are as described for the neuropathic or infected ulcers. Pressure offloading is equally important, and evidence suggests that antibiotics should be encouraged in any neuroischemic ulcer. Any patient with treatable peripheral vascular disease should undergo either angioplasty or arterial bypass surgery.

Adjunctive Treatments

A number of newer alternative approaches to treating diabetic foot ulcers have been described; however, none of these must detract from the three major principles of diabetic foot wound care, namely, keeping pressure off the wound, treating infection when present, and treating peripheral arterial disease when present.

Growth Factors

The recombinant platelet-derived growth factor becaplermin (Regranex; Johnson & Johnson, New Brunswick, NJ) was the first growth factor approved for treating neuropathic foot ulcers in diabetic patients. The most successful of four placebo-controlled trials of platelet-derived growth factor resulted in a moderate improvement in the rate of healing at 20 weeks.[104] A review of growth factors in the treatment of diabetic foot ulcers concluded that although other growth factors did not appear to improve healing, platelet-derived growth factor might be useful in chronic, nonhealing neuropathic ulcers that do not respond to conventional care.[105]

Tissue-Engineered Skin

Apligraf (Organogenesis, Canton, Mass) is tissue-engineered skin that comprises a cultured living dermis and sequentially cultured epidermis. Dermagraft (Smith and Nephew, La Jolla, Calif) is dermis derived from human fibroblasts. Both are derived from neonatal foreskin.[4] Engineered tissue improves the percentage of wounds healed at 12 weeks in randomized, controlled studies.[106,107] Both of these adjunctive therapies are limited by their substantial costs.

Larval Therapy

The use of sterile maggots, the larvae of the common green bottle fly, is not new. Indeed, early observations of the efficacy of maggots at wound

healing were made by one of Napoleon's surgeons, who noted that maggot-infested battle wounds did not become infected and healed faster! Today, sterile maggots are useful in desloughing wounds that are resistant to surgical debridement. It is believed that they secrete a broad spectrum of powerful enzymes that break down dead tissue. Limited evidence also suggests that they do not harm healthy tissue because the enzymes are inactivated by inhibitors present in normal skin.[108] A number of reports, predominantly case series, support their use in certain sloughy diabetic foot ulcers.[108]

Hyperbaric Oxygen

Despite the widespread use of hyperbaric oxygen in managing neuroischemic and ischemic ulcers in certain countries, particularly the United States, there is only limited controlled evidence to support its use.[109] However, it might have a place in the management of neuroischemic or ischemic ulcers in patients who have distal peripheral vascular disease that is not amenable to surgical reconstruction or angioplasty.

Intermittent Negative Pressure

Negative pressure wound therapy, also known as vacuum-assisted closure (VAC) therapy, is being used increasingly in the treatment of diabetic foot wounds.[110,111] The device (KCI, San Antonio, Texas) consists of a sterile open-foam cell dressing that is cut to fill a wound defect. The foam is then sealed to the wound at the side by an adhesive tape, and an evacuation tube is placed into the foam. The end of the tube not placed through the foam is attached to a pump outside of the wound so that subatmospheric (i.e., negative) pressure can be uniformly applied to all tissue within the wound.

This treatment stimulates the development of granulation tissue in a previously nonhealing wound, leading to epithelialization. Although this treatment may be used on an outpatient, it is particularly useful for inpatients with large wounds. Negative pressure therapy is also good at removing exudate and edema and stimulating angiogenesis.

PREVENTING FIRST AND RECURRENT ULCERS

More than 80% of ulcers should be potentially preventable, and the first step in prevention is identification of the high-risk foot. Similarly, because recurrent ulcer rates reach as high as 50%, and a past history of foot ulcers is the strongest predictor of new ulcers, much effort is also needed to prevent recurrent ulceration.

Many countries have adopted the principle of the annual review for patients with diabetes, whereby every patient is screened at least annually for evidence of diabetic complications. Such a review can be carried out either in primary care centers or at hospital clinics.[1] Patients identified with risk factors for foot ulceration and certainly those with a past history of foot ulceration should be considered for educational programs for reducing foot ulcer risk, regular podiatry, specialized footwear, and more frequent review. Research of foot ulcer recurrence suggests that these patients delay in reporting the symptoms and signs of reulceration, have poor glycemic control, and have more neuropathy.[112] Thus special attention should be paid to these facts in the education process.

Patient Education

Studies show that patients with foot ulcer risk lack knowledge and skills and consequently are unable to provide appropriate self-care.[113] Patients need to be informed of the risk of having sensory loss and the need for regular self-inspection, foot hygiene, and podiatry treatment as required. They must also be told what action to take in the event of injury or the discovery of a foot ulcer.[113,114] However, studies suggest that patients often have distorted beliefs about neuropathy, thinking that it is a circulatory problem, and link neuropathy directly to amputation.[36,56] Thus, an education program that focuses on reducing foot ulcers will be doomed to failure if patients do not believe that foot ulcers are on the path between neuropathy and amputation. Although a detailed systematic review of the role of patient education in preventing diabetic foot ulceration could not find much support for education as a means to reduce amputation,[57] it is clear that much more work is required in this area if appropriate education is to succeed in reducing foot ulceration and consequently amputations.

Footwear, Orthoses, and Hosiery

It has generally been accepted by the diabetes community that "good footwear" prevents foot ulcers. Indeed it is virtually an axiom of diabetes care that a patient with a history of foot ulceration is a footwear patient for life.[115] It is similarly accepted by most health care professionals that inappropriate (often tight) footwear is a major cause of ulceration. It has also been assumed that specialized footwear is perceived as unattractive, and the appearance has been a major cause of poor compliance when such footwear is prescribed.[116,117]

The question of whether good footwear actually prevents ulceration was addressed in a systematic review.[118] Because no studies have assessed footwear in the primary prevention of ulcers, this review focused on preventing ulcer recurrence. The researchers concluded that although protective benefit was found in some studies, a number of these reports may have been influenced by study-

design issues.[118] However, although firm, high-quality evidence might be lacking in confirming the role of good footwear in protecting the diabetic foot, appropriate footwear with sufficient depth and width should be considered for all patients who have risk factors for ulceration or a previous ulcer history.[117]

There is also some evidence that orthoses might also protect the insensate foot. One study that randomized patients to conventional podiatric care with or without custom-made plastic inserts showed that less callus formation was seen after a year in patients provided with the inserts.[119] Previous studies have also suggested that padded hosiery reduces high foot pressures and gives all-around protection to the high-risk diabetic foot provided that the shoes are fitted to accommodate the padded socks.[120]

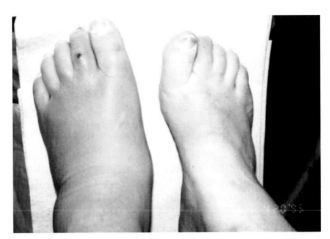

Figure 14–7. Dorsal view of a profoundly erythematous and edematous left foot characteristic of acute Charcot's neuropathic arthropathy.

Injected Liquid Silicone

Some podiatrists in the United States have injected small amounts of liquid silicone under high-pressure points and calluses of the plantar surface of the neuropathic foot, and there have been anecdotal reports of reduced ulcer incidence following this procedure. A randomized, double-blind trial of injected liquid silicone in the diabetic foot was later carried out and confirmed that silicone injections were associated with increased soft-tissue thickness under the metatarsal head, decreased foot pressure, and reduced callus formation.[121] Such an "injectable orthosis" might well be beneficial in high-risk patients.

Subsequent follow-up studies confirmed that patients at greatest risk of ulceration (those with higher baseline foot pressure) were most likely to benefit from silicone injections[122] but that after two years of follow-up, the benefits of injections, though still demonstrable, were reduced compared to baseline, suggesting that booster injections may periodically be needed.[123] This is an area of ongoing research.

CHARCOT'S NEUROPATHIC ARTHROPATHY

Charcot's neuropathic arthropathy (CN; Charcot's joint or Charcot's foot, Fig. 14–7) was first described in the mid 19th century by Jean-Martin Charcot, a Parisian neurologist. In the Western world, diabetes is now the commonest cause of this largely preventable condition. A generally acceptable definition of a Charcot joint is one in which there is simultaneous presence of bone and joint destruction, fragmentation, and remodeling. It is a relatively painless, progressive, and destructive arthropathy.[124]

The initiating event of the Charcot process is typically a seemingly trivial injury, which can result in a minor periarticular fracture or even a major fracture. Both somatic and autonomic peripheral neuropathy are believed to be prerequisites for the development of CN. Somatic neuropathy permits repeated insensate injury to go unnoticed, and autonomic dysfunction, in the absence of proximal arterial disease, results in increased peripheral blood flow with arterio-venous shunting, perhaps even in bone.[124] Although Young and colleagues[125] demonstrated reduced bone mineral density in the involved limbs of diabetic patients with CN, prospective studies are required to see whether localized osteopenia increases the risk of developing CN.

The treatment of CN depends upon the stage during which it is diagnosed. Although up to 50% of patients do experience pain or discomfort in the acute phase, the diagnosis is often made too late to arrest the destructive changes in bones and joints[124] (see Fig. 14–7). The presence of unilateral heat and swelling in a neuropathic diabetic patient should be presumed to be due to acute CN until proved otherwise. Management has been further hampered by the lack of any randomized trials at any stage of CN. The essence of treatment in the acute phase remains non–weight-bearing immobilization in a total contact or removable cast walker.

It was suggested that treatment with bisphosphonates might be useful in the management of acute CN, and a preliminary pilot study was conducted in 1994.[126] Bisphosphonates are potent inhibitors of osteoclast activation, and they might reduce disease activity in the acute phase when bone turnover markers are known to be increased.[127] In this early pilot study, symptoms improved and there was normalization of the skin temperature differential between acute and noninvolved feet, together with a decline of bone turnover as judged by alkaline phosphatase.[126] A

randomized trial of the bisphosphonate pamidronate versus placebo in acute CN confirmed that as well as reducing disease activity as measured by skin temperature differential, markers of bone turnover were also improved.[128] Trials of oral bisphosphonates in acute CN are in progress.

In the later stages, when the foot has maintained a stable shape for some time and the temperature differential has disappeared, surgery may be necessary to remove a bony lump or prominence, usually under the weight-bearing surface of the midfoot. Management should also include custom-molded footwear, frequent podiatry, and optimal self-care. The question of reconstructive surgery is controversial, but it might be considered in the chronic stage when conservative management has failed.

THE DIABETIC FOOT: NEED FOR A TEAM APPROACH

It should be clear that the spectrum of diabetic foot problems requires the involvement of professionals from many specialties. The diabetic foot cannot be regarded as the responsibility of the endocrinologist alone, and a number of reports have promoted the benefits of the multidisciplinary approach to diabetic foot care.[2,4,114] The team might include diabetologists, surgeons (both orthopaedic and vascular), specialist nurses, nurse educators, podiatrists, orthotists, pedorthotists, and often many other specialist health care professionals. Although many regard the nurse educator and podiatrists as key team participants, most agree that it is the high-risk or foot-ulcer patients themselves who must be regarded as the conductor of the diabetic foot orchestra. Without their willing participation, there is little that other team members can achieve to improve the overall outlook for the diabetic foot in the 21st century.

References

1. International Working Group on the Diabetic Foot. International Consensus on the Diabetic Foot. Amsterdam, International Diabetes Federation, 1999.
2. Mayfield JA, Reiber GE, Sanders LJ, et al: Preventive footcare in people with diabetes. Diabetes Care 21:2161-2177, 1998.
3. American Diabetes Association: Consensus development conference on diabetic wound care. Diabetes Care 22:1354-1360, 1999.
4. Boulton AJM, Kirsner RS, Vileikyte L: Neuropathic diabetic foot ulcers. N Engl J Med 351:48-55, 2004.
5. Morrison EY: Diabetes foot amputations as the most frequent diabetes complication in developing countries. IDF Bull 42:14-17, 1997.
6. Mbanya JC, Sobngwi E: Diabetes in Africa. Diabetes microvascular and macrovascular disease in Africa. J Cardiovasc Risk 10:97-102, 2003.
7. Shaw JE, Zimmett PZ: The epidemiology of diabetic neuropathy. Diabetes Rev 6:245-252, 1999.
8. Williams DRR, Airey M: The size of the problem: Epidemiological and economic aspects of the diabetic foot. In Boulton AJM, Connor H, Cavanagh PR (ed): The Foot in Diabetes, 3rd ed. Chichester, Wiley, 2000, pp 3-17.
9. Reiber GE, Ledoux WR: Epidemiology of diabetic foot ulcers and amputations: Evidence for prevention. In Williams R, Herman W, Kinmonth AL, Wareham NJ (eds): The Evidence Base for Diabetes Care. Chichester, Wiley, 2002, pp 641-665.
10. Carrington AL, Abbott CA, Griffiths J, et al: A foot care program for diabetic unilateral amputees. Diabetes Care 24:216-221, 2001.
11. Faglia E, Favales F, Moratibo A: New ulceration, new major amputation and survival rates in diabetic subjects hospitalised for foot ulceration from 1990-1993: A 6.5 year follow-up. Diabetes Care 24:78-83, 2001.
12. Kumar S, Ashe H, Fernando DJS, et al:. The prevalence of foot ulceration and its correlates in type 2 diabetic patients: A population-based study. Diabet Med 11:480-484, 1994.
13. Abbott CA, Carrington AL, Ashe H, et al: The North-West Diabetes Foot Care Study: incidence of, and risk factors for, new diabetic foot ulceration in a community-based patient cohort. Diabet Med 20:377-384, 2002.
14. Muller IS, de Grauw WJ, van Gerwen WH, et al: Foot ulceration and lower limb amputation in type 2 diabetic patients in Dutch primary health care. Diabetes Care 25:570-574, 2002.
15. Lavery LA, Armstrong DG, Wunderlich RP, et al: Diabetic foot syndrome: Evaluating the prevalence and incidence of foot pathology in Mexican Americans and non-Hispanic whites from a diabetes management cohort. Diabetes Care 26:1435-1438, 2003.
16. Humphrey ARG, Thomas K, Dowse GK, Zimmet PZ: Diabetes and non-traumatic lower extremity amputations. Incidence, risk factors and prevention: A 12 year follow-up study in Nauru. Diabetes Care 19:710-716, 1996.
17. Belhadj M: La place du pied diabetique. Diabete Metab 24(suppl 1):LXVII, 1998.
18. Pendsey S: Epidemiological aspects of the diabetic foot. J Diabetes Develop Countries 2:37-38, 1994.
19. Gulliford MC, Mahabir D: Diabetic foot disease in a Caribbean community. Diabet Res Clin Pract 56:35-40, 2003.
20. Young MJ, Veves A, Breddy JL, Boulton AJM: The prediction of diabetic neuropathic foot ulceration using vibration perception thresholds: A prospective study. Diabetes Care 17:557-560, 1994.
21. Abbott CA, Vileikyte L, Williamson S, et al: Multicentre study of the incidence of and predictive factors for diabetic neuropathic foot ulcers. Diabetes Care 21:1071-1075, 1998.
22. Larsson J, Apelqvist J, Agardh GD, Stenstrom A: Decreasing incidence of major amputation in diabetic patients: A consequence of a multidisciplinary foot care team approach? Diabet Med 12:770-776, 1995.
23. Trautner C, Haastert B, Spraul M, et al: Unchanged incidence of lower limb amputations in a German city 1990-1998. Diabetes Care 24:855-859, 2001.
24. Trautner C, Haastert B, Giani C, Berger M: Amputations and diabetes: A case-control study. Diabet Med 19:35-40, 2002.
25. Anonymous: An audit of amputations in a rural health district. Pract Diabet Int 14:175-178, 1997.
26. Toledano H, Young MJ, Veves A, Boulton AJM: Why do Asian diabetic patients have fewer foot ulcers than Caucasians? Diabet Med 10(suppl 1):539, 1993.
27. Chaturvedi N, Abbott CA, Whalley A, et al: Risk of diabetes-related amputation in south Asians vs Europeans in the UK. Diabet Med 19:99-106, 2002.
28. Leggetter SY, Chaturvedi N, Fuller JH, Edmonds ME: Ethnicity and risk of diabetes-related lower extremity amputation: A population-based, case-control study of Afro-Caribbeans and Europeans in the United Kingdom. Arch Int Med 162:73-78, 2001.
29. Resnick HE, Valsania P, Phillips CL: Diabetes mellitus and non-traumatic lower extremity amputation in black and white Americans: The National Health and Nutrition Examination Survey epidemiology follow-up study 1971-1992. Arch Int Med 159:2470-2475, 1999.

30. Shearer A, Scuffham P, Gordois A, Ogleshy A: Predicted costs and outcomes from reduced vibration detection in people with diabetes in the US. Diabetes Care 26:2305-2310, 2003.

31. Ragnarson-Tennvall G, Apelqvist J: Prevention of diabetes-related foot ulcers and amputations: A cost-utility analysis based on Markov model simulation. Diabetologia 44:2077-2087, 2001.

32. Assal JP, Mehnert H, Tritschler HS, et al: "On your feet" workshop on the diabetic foot. J Diabet Comp 16:183-194, 2002.

33. Ramsey SD, Newton K, Blough D, et al: Incidence outcomes and costs of foot ulcers in patients with diabetes. Diabetes Care 22:382-387, 1999.

34. LEA Study Group: Comparing the incidence of lower extremity amputation across the world: The global lower extremity amputation study. Diabet Med 12:14-18, 1995.

35. Joslin EP: The menace of diabetic gangrene. N Engl J Med 211:16-20, 1934.

36. Vileikyte L, Rubin RR, Leventhal H: Psychological aspects of diabetic neuropathic foot complications: An overview. Diabetes Metab Res Rev 20(suppl 1):S13-S18, 2004.

37. Boulton AJM: Pressure and the diabetic foot: Clinical science and offloading techniques. Am J Surg 187(5A):175-245, 2004.

38. Reiber GE, Vileikyte L, Boyko EJ, et al: Causal pathway for incident lower extremity ulcers in patients with diabetes from two settings. Diabetes Care 22:157-162, 1999.

39. Morbach S, Lutale JK, Viswanathan V, et al: Regional differences in risk factors and clinical presentation of diabetic foot lesions. Diabet Med 21:91-95, 2004.

40. Boulton AJM, Hardisty CA, Betts RP, et al: Dynamic foot pressure and other studies as diagnostic and management aids for diabetic neuropathy. Diabetes Care 6:26-33, 1983.

41. Katoulis EC, Ebdon-Parry M, Hollis S, et al: Postural instability in diabetic patients at risk of foot ulceration. Diabet Med 14:296-300, 1997.

42. Katoulis EC, Ebdon-Parry M, Lanshammar H, et al: Gait abnormalities in diabetic neuropathy. Diabetes Care 20:1904-1907, 1997.

43. Young MJ, Boulton AJM, MaCleod AF, et al: A multicentre study of the prevalence of diabetic peripheral neuropathy in the UK hospital clinic population. Diabetologia 36:150-154, 1993.

44. Mayfield JA, Sugarman JR: The use of the Semmes-Weinstein monofilament and other threshold tests for preventing foot ulceration and amputation in persons with diabetes. J Fam Pract 49(11 suppl):S17-S29, 2000.

45. Booth J, Young MJ: Differences in the performance of commercially available monofilaments. Diabetes Care 23:984-988, 2000.

46. Jude EB, Oyibo SO, Chalmers N, Boulton AJM: Peripheral arterial disease in diabetic and non-diabetic patients: A comparison of severity and outcome. Diabetes Care 24:1433-1437, 2001.

47. Abbott RD, Brand FN, Kannel WB: Epidemiology of some peripheral arterial findings in diabetic men and women: Experiences from the Framingham study. Am J Med 1990; 88:376-381.

48. Siitonen OI, Niskanen LK, Laasko M, et al: Lower extremity amputation in diabetic and non-diabetic patients: A population based study in Eastern Finland. Diabetes Care 16:16-20, 1993.

49. Pecoraro RE, Reiber GE, Burgess EM: Pathways to diabetic limb amputations: Basis for prevention. Diabetes Care 1990:13: 513-521.

50. Flynn MD, Tooke JE: Aetiology of diabetic foot ulceration: A role for the microcirculation? Diabet Med 9:320-329, 1992.

51. Veves A, Young MJ, Murray HJ, Boulton AJM: The risk of foot ulceration in diabetic patients with high foot pressures: A prospective study. Diabetologia 35:660-663, 1992.

52. Lavery LA, Armstrong DG, Wunderlich RP, et al: Predictive value of foot pressure assessment when part of a popula-tion-based diabetes disease management program. Diabetes Care 26:1069-1073, 2003.

53. Cavanagh PR, Ulbrecht JS, Caputo GM: What the practicing physician should know about diabetic foot biomechanics. In Boulton AJM, Connor H, Cavanagh PR (eds): The Foot in Diabetes, 3rd ed. Chichester, Wiley, 2000, pp 33-60.

54. Van Schie CHM, Abbott CA, Vileikyte L, et al: A comparative study of Podotrack, a simple semiquantitative plantar pressure measuring device and the optical pedobarograph in the assessment of pressures under the diabetic foot. Diabet Med 16:154-159, 1999.

55. Murry HJ, Young MJ, Boulton AJM: The association between callus formation, high pressures and neuropathy in diabetic foot ulceration. Diabet Med 13:979-982, 1996.

56. Vileikyte L: Psychological and behavioural issues in diabetic neuropathic foot ulceration. In Boulton AJM, Connor H, Cavanagh PR (eds): The Foot in Diabetes, 3rd ed. Chichester, Wiley, 2000, pp 121-130.

57. Valk GD, Kriegsman DM, Assendelf WJ: Patient education for reducing diabetic foot ulceration: A systematic review. Endocrinol Metab Clin N Am 31:633-658, 2002.

58. McCabe CJ, Stevenson RC, Dolan AM: Evaluation of a diabetic foot screening and prevention programme. Diabet Med 15:80-84, 1998.

59. Young MJ: Classification of ulcers and its relevance to ischemia. In Boulton AJM, Connor H, Cavanagh PR (eds): The Foot in Diabetes, 3rd ed. Chichester, Wiley, 2000, p 61.

60. Armstrong DG, Lavery LA, Harkless LB: Validation of a wound classification system. Diabetes Care 21:865-869, 1998.

61. Oyibo S, Jude EB, Tarawneh I, et al: A comparison of two diabetic foot ulcer classification systems: The Wagner and the University of Texas wound classification system. Diabetes Care 24:84-88, 2001.

62. Schaper NC: Diabetic foot ulcer classification system for research purposes: A progress report. Diabet Metab Res Rev 20(suppl 1):S90-S95, 2004.

63. Armstrong DG, Lipsky BA: Advances in the treatment of diabetic foot infections. Diabetes Technol Ther 6:167-177, 2004.

64. Edelman D, Hough DM, Glazebrook KN, et al: Prognostic value of the clinical examination of the diabetic foot ulcer. J Gen Intern Med 12:537-543, 1997.

65. Lavery LA, Armstrong DG, Quebedeaux TL, et al: Puncture wounds : The frequency of normal laboratory values in the face of severe foot infections of the foot in diabetic and non-diabetic adults. Am J Med 101:531-525, 1996.

66. Grayson ML, Balaugh K, Levin E, et al: Probing to bone in infected pedal ulcers. A clinical sign of underlying osteomyelitis in diabetic patients. JAMA 273:721-723, 1995.

67. Lipsky BA: Osteomyelitis of the foot in diabetic patients. Clin Infect Dis 25:1318-1326, 1997.

68. Hirsch AT, Gloviczki P, Drooz A, et al: Special communication: Mandate for creation of a national peripheral arterial disease public awareness program: An opportunity to improve cardiovascular health. Angiology 55:233-242, 2004.

69. Resnick HE, Lindsay RE, McDermott MM, et al: Relationship of high and low ankle brachial index to all cause and cardiovascular disease mortality: The Strong Heart Study. Circulation 109:733-739, 2004.

70. Thomas DW, Harding KG: Wound healing. Br J Surg 89:1203-1205, 2002.

71. Jeffcoate WJ, Price P, Harding KG: Wound healing and treatments for people with diabetic foot ulcers. Diabetes Metab Res Rev 20(suppl 1):S78-S89, 2004.

72. Kirsner RS, Bogensberger G: The wound healing process. In McColluch JM, Kloth LC, Feeder JA (eds): Wound Healing: Alternatives in Management, 3rd ed. Philadelphia, FA Davis, 1998, p 58.

73. Jeffcoate WJ, Harding KG: Diabetic foot ulcers. Lancet 361:1545-1551, 2003.

74. Jude EB, Blakytny R, Bulmer J, et al: Transforming growth factor-β 1, 2, 3 and receptor type 1 and 2 in diabetic foot ulcers. Diabet Med 19:440-447, 2002.

75. Lobmann R, Ambrosch A, Schultz G, et al: Expression of matrix-metalloproteinases and their inhibitors in the wounds of diabetic and non-diabetic patients. Diabetologia 45:1011-1016, 2002.

76. Nwomeh BC, Liang HX, Cohen IK, et al: MMP-8 is the predominant collagenase in healing wounds and non-healing ulcers. J Surg Res 81:189-195, 1999.

77. Blakytny R, Jude EB, Gibson JM, et al: Lack of insulin-like growth factor 1 (IGF-1) in the basal keratinocyte layer of diabetic skin and diabetic foot ulcers. J Pathol 190:589-594, 2000.

78. Jude EB, Boulton AJM, Ferguson MWJ, et al: The role of nitric oxide synthase isoforms and arginase in the pathogenesis of diabetic foot ulcers. Diabetologia 42:748-757, 1999.

79. Boulton AJM, Armstrong DG: Studies in plantar diabetic neuropathic ulcers: Time for a paradigm shift? Diabetes Care 26:2689-2690, 2003.

80. Boulton AJ: The diabetic foot: From art to science. The 18th Camillo Golgi lecture. Diabetologia 47:1343-1353, 2004.

81. Piaggesi A, Viacava P, Rizzo L et al: Semi-quantitative analysis of the histopathological features of the neuropathic foot ulcer—effects of pressure relief. Diabetes Care 26:3123-3128, 2003.

82. Badiavas EV, Falanga V: Gene therapy. J Dermatol 138:1079-1081, 2001.

83. Badiavas EV, Falanga V: Treatment of chronic wounds with bone marrow-derived cells. Arch Dermatol 139:510-516, 2003.

84. Delamaire M, Maugendre D, Moreno M, et al: Impaired leucocyte function in diabetic patients. Diabet Med 14:29-34, 1997.

85. Zacur H, Kirsner RS: Debridement: Rationale and therapeutic options. Wounds 14(suppl):2E-7E, 2002.

86. Steed DL, Donohoe D, Webster MW, et al: Effect of extensive debridement on the healing of diabetic foot ulcers. J Am Coll Surg 183:61-64, 1996.

87. Mueller MJ, Diamond JE, Sinacore DR, et al: Total contact casting in the treatment of diabetic plantar ulcers : Controlled clinical trial. Diabetes Care 12:384-388, 1989.

88. Armstrong DG, Nguyen HC, Lavery LA, et al: Offloading the diabetic foot wound: A randomized clinical trial. Diabetes Care 24:1019-1022, 2001.

89. Lavery LA, Vela SA, Lavery DC, Quebedeaux TL: Reducing dynamic foot pressures in high-risk diabetic subjects with foot ulcerations: A comparison of treatments. Diabetes Care 19:818-821, 1996.

90. Baumhauer JF, Wervery R, McWilliams J, et al: A comparison study of plantar foot pressure in a standardized shoe, total contact cast prefabricated pneumatic walking brace. Foot Ankle Int 18:26-33, 1997.

91. Armstrong DG, Lavery LA, Kimbriel HR, et al: Activity patterns of patients with diabetic foot ulceration: Patients with active ulceration may not adhere to a standard pressure offloading regimen. Diabetes Care 26:2595-2597, 2003.

92. Veves A, Sheehan P, Pham HT: A randomized controlled trial of Promogran vs standard treatment in the management of diabetic foot ulcers. Arch Surg 137:822-827, 2002.

93. Armstrong DG, Short B, Espensen EH, et al: Technique for fabrication of an 'instant total contact cast' for treatment of neuropathic diabetic foot ulcers. J Am Pod Med Assoc 92:405-408, 2002.

94. Katz I, Harlan A, Miranda-Palma B, et al: A randomised trial of two irremovable offloading devices in the management of plantar neuropathic diabetic foot ulcers. Diabetes Care 28:555-559, 2005.

95. Knowles EA, Armstrong DG, Hayat SA, et al: Offloading diabetic foot wounds using the Scotchcast boot: A retrospective study. Ostomy Wound Manage 48:50-53, 2003.

96. Williams DT, Harding KG: New treatments for neuropathic foot ulceration: Views from a wound healing unit. Curr Diab Rep 3:468-479, 2003.

97. Mason J, O'Keefe CO, Hutchinson A, et al: A systematic review of foot ulcers in patients with type 2 diabetes: II. Treatment. Diabet Med 16:889-909, 1999.

98. Lipsky BA, Berendt AR: Principles and practice of antibiotic therapy of diabetic foot infections. Diabet Metab Res Rev 16(suppl 1):542-546, 2000.

99. Lipsky BA: International consensus on diagnosing and treating the infected diabetic foot. Diabet Metab Res Rev 20(suppl 1):568-577, 2004.

100. Dang CN, Prasad YDM, Boulton AJM, et al: Methicillin-resistant staphylococcus aureus in the diabetic foot clinic: A worsening problem. Diabet Med 20:159-161, 2003.

101. Hartemann-Heurtier A, Robert J, Jacqueminet S, et al: Diabetic foot ulcer and multidrug-resistant organisms: Risk factors and impact. Diabet Med 21:710-715, 2004.

102. Lipsky BA, Itani K, Norden C: Treating foot infections in diabetic patients: A randomized, multicentre, open-labelled trial of linezolid versus ampicillin-sulbactam/amoxicillin-clavulanate. Clin Infect Dis 38:17-24, 2004.

103. Armstrong DG, Findlow AH, Oyibo S, et al: The use of absorbable antibiotic-impregnated calcium sulphate pellets in the management of diabetic foot infections. Diabet Med 18:942-943, 2001.

104. Weiman TJ, Smiell JM, Su Y: Efficacy and safety of a topical gel formulation of recombinant human platelet-derived growth factor—BB (Becaplermin) with chronic neuropathic diabetic ulcers: A phase III randomized placebo-controlled study. Diabetes Care 21:822-827, 1998.

105. Bennett SP, Griffiths GD, Schor AM, et al: Growth factors in the treatment of diabetic foot ulcers . Br J Surg 90:133-146, 2003.

106. Veves A, Falanga V, Armstrong DG, et al: Graft skin, a human skin equivalent, is effective in the management of non-infected neuropathic diabetic foot ulcers: A randomized multicenter clinical trial. Diabetes Care 24:290-295, 2001.

107. Marston WA, Hanft J, Norwood P, et al: The efficacy and safety of Dermagraft in improving the healing of chronic diabetic foot ulcers: Results of a prospective randomised trial. Diabetes Care 28:1701-1785, 2003.

108. Thomas S: Larval therapy. In Boulton AJM, Connor H, Cavanagh PR (eds): The Foot in Diabetes, 3rd ed. Chichester, Wiley, 2000, p 185.

109. Gill AL, Bell CAN: Hyperbaric oxygen: Its uses, mechanisms of actions and outcomes. QJM 97:385-396, 2004.

110. Armstrong DG: Guidelines regarding negative wound therapy (NPWT) in the diabetic foot. Ostomy Wound Manage 50(2 suppl):3S-27S, 2004.

111. McCallon SK, Knight CA, Valiulus JP, et al: Vaccum-assisted closure vs saline-moistened gauze in the healing of postoperative diabetic foot wounds. Ostomy Wound Manage 46:28-34, 2000.

112. Mantey I, Foster AN, Spencer S, et al: Why do foot ulcers recur in diabetic patients? Diabet Med 16:245-249, 1999.

113. Mason J, O'Keefe C, McIntosh A, et al: A systematic review of foot ulcers in patients with type 2 diabetics: I. Prevention. Diabetes Med 16:801-812, 1999.

114. Boulton AJM: Why bother educating the patient and the multi-disciplinary team? The example of prevention of lower-extremity amputation in diabetes. Patient Educ Couns 26:183-188, 1995.

115. Cavanagh PR: Can footwear help to protect the insensate diabetic foot? Int Diabetes Monitor 16:10-16, 2004.

116. Knowles EA, Boulton AJM: Do people with diabetes wear their prescribed footwear? Diabet Med 13:1064-1068, 1996.

117. Boulton AJM, Jude EB: Therapeutic footwear in diabetes: The good, the bad and the ugly. Diabetes Care 27:1832-1833, 2004.

118. Maciejewski ML, Reiber GE, Smith DG, et al: Effectiveness of diabetic therapeutic footwear in preventing reulceration. Diabetes Care 27:1774-1782, 2004.

119. Colagiuri S, Marsden LL, Naidu V, et al: The use of orthotic devices to arrest plantar callus in people with diabetes. Diabet Res Clin Pract 28:29-36, 1995.

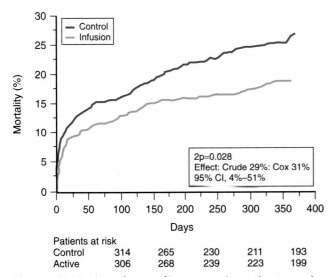

Figure 15–1. Actual mortality curves in patients receiving insulin-glucose infusion and in the control group during 1 year of follow-up in the DIGAMI (Diabetes Insulin-Glucose in Acute Myocardial Infarction) study. Numbers below the graph represent number of patients at different times of observation. Active, patients receiving infusion; CI, confidence interval. (From Malmberg K, Ryden L, Efendic S, Herlitz J, Nicol P, Waldenstrom A, et al. Randomized trial of insulin-glucose infusion followed by subcutaneous insulin treatment in diabetic patients with acute myocardial infarction (DIGAMI Study): Effects on mortality at 1 year. J Am Coll Cardiol 26:57-65, 1995. Reprinted with permission from American College of Cardiology Foundation.)

study have already affected clinical practice: Physicians were not willing to enroll their patients post-MI in a study that was not guaranteed to provide insulin as part of their regimen.

The infusion of insulin in the acute MI setting may have multiple benefits. In addition to preventing a rise in glucose it may be anti-inflammatory and thus may be clinically beneficial.[70]

Revascularization

Remarkable progress has been made in decreasing the morbidity and mortality associated with CVD through coronary artery bypass grafting (CABG), percutaneous transluminal coronary angioplasty (PTCA), and percutaneous interventions (PCI) including the use of atherectomy, stents, brachytherapy, and drug-eluting stents. The result has been a remarkable decrease in age-adjusted cardiovascular morbidity and mortality in the general population but not in persons with diabetes. Multiple studies have shown that revascularization improves survival over medical therapy alone in selected high-risk subsets of patients, including those with the most-severe forms of three-vessel disease and depressed left ventricular function or

left main coronary artery disease. However, these studies have not enrolled a large number of persons with diabetes.

In the Bypass Angioplasty Revascularization Investigation (BARI) study, the 19% of the randomized population (353 patients) who had diabetes had a better average 5.4-year survival with CABG as compared with PTCA, but this benefit was confined to those receiving at least one internal mammary artery graft.[71] The current BARI 2D trial, which uses a 2×2 factorial design to compare tight diabetic control with insulin-providing versus insulin-sensitizing therapy with and without a revascularization procedure of choice, will contribute significantly to our understanding of the appropriate revascularization strategy for diabetic patients.

Subsequent to these data being made available to practicing clinicians, a dramatic decrease in the use of PCI or increase in CABG in persons with diabetes has not been observed.[72] Practice patterns did not shift in response to the BARI data, probably because of the emerging widespread use of intracoronary stents during the mid to late 1990s. However, restenosis rates in persons with diabetes have remained high whether they undergo PTCA or PCI with a stent. The recent introduction of drug-eluting stents (DES) has reduced in-stent restenosis in the general population, but data in patients with diabetes is limited.

Meta-analysis of the results from six trials comparing DES (using sirolimus or paclitaxel) and bare metal stents (BMS) shows that the odds ratio (OR) of in-stent restenosis after a follow-up of 6 to 12 months was markedly lower when comparing DES with BMS and similar in both nondiabetic patients (OR, 0.16; 95% confidence intervals [CI], 0.12-0.20; $P < 0.00001$) and diabetic patients (OR, 0.16; CI, 0.11-0.24; $P < 0.00001$).[73] However, as compared to nondiabetic persons, the odds ratio of in-stent restenosis associated with diabetes still averaged 1.96 (CI, 1.28-3.01) in the groups receiving DES ($P = 0.002$), a figure quite similar (although less consistent between studies) to that observed with BMS (OR, 1.90; CI, 1.49-2.43; $P < 0.00001$).

The SIRIUS trial had a substudy devoted to diabetes, and in-lesion restenosis was significantly reduced with DES compared with BMS in the patients who did not require insulin (7.7% versus 49.3%, $P < 0.001$), but not in the insulin-requiring patients (35% versus 50%, $P = 0.38$).[74] These data are likely related to the fact that people treated with insulin have typically had many more years of uncontrolled diabetes than those not treated with insulin.

Based on these limited data it appears that DES are associated with a remarkable relative risk reduction of restenosis during the first year of follow-up in patients with diabetes as compared with BMS and that the restenosis rate now approaches that observed in patients without diabetes. However, despite the use of DES, diabetes mellitus still

remains an independent risk factor for restenosis, need for revascularization, and major adverse cardiac events. Prospective studies with highly effective DES need to be performed specifically in the population of persons with diabetes.

Stroke

Diabetes is known to increase the risk of ischemic stroke two- to fourfold.[1,75] Diabetes also confers a poor prognosis following stroke in terms of increased mortality, stroke recurrence, and impaired neurologic recovery.[76,77] A meta-analysis of 26 studies on stroke showed increased in-hospital mortality in patients with blood glucose levels of 110 to 126 mg/dL.[78] Stroke survivors with a blood glucose of 121 to 144 mg/dL without known diabetes showed worse functional recovery. Patients with known diabetes or newly discovered hyperglycemia (blood glucose > 140 mg/dL) had more severe strokes with greater mortality.[79]

The prevalence of recognized diabetes in acute stroke patients is between 8% and 20%, but between 6% and 42% of patients might have undiagnosed diabetes before presenting with stroke. When glucose tolerance testing was performed 12 weeks after the index stroke in the survivors of the Glucose Insulin in Stroke Trial (GIST), researchers found that almost two thirds of the patients who had poststroke hyperglycemia had recognized diabetes (21%), unrecognized diabetes (15%), or IGT (27%).[80] This is similar to the prevalence rates in post-MI patients.

The most effective strategies to prevent stroke among persons with diabetes include blood pressure control, antiplatelet therapy, and statin therapy. Tight glycemic control is recommended to prevent microvascular disease, but the effect on macrovascular disease, including stroke, has not been proved.

The initial management of patients with acute ischemic stroke includes reperfusion with intravenous recombinant tissue plasminogen activator (rtPA) if the patient can receive the medication within 3 hours of onset of stroke unless the patient has a contraindication. Hyperglycemia before reperfusion counterbalances, at least in part, the beneficial effect of tPA.[81] In stroke patients treated with rtPA, acute hyperglycemia is an independent predictor of early neurologic worsening and poor long-term outcome.[82,83]

The 2003 recommendations of the Stroke Council of the American Stroke Association stated that management of an elevated blood glucose level following stroke should be similar to that given to treatment of other acutely ill patients who have hyperglycemia, including monitoring of blood glucose and avoiding overly aggressive therapy to prevent fluid shifts, electrolyte abnormalities, and hypoglycemia, which can be detrimental to the brain. They suggested that a reasonable goal for the

Box 15-3. American Diabetes Association Recommendations for Cardiac Testing

Testing for CAD is warranted in patients with the following:

- Typical or atypical cardiac symptoms
- Resting electrocardiograph suggestive of ischemia or infarction
- Peripheral or carotid occlusive arterial disease
- Sedentary lifestyle, age 35 years, and plans to begin a vigorous exercise program
- Two or more of the following risk factors in addition to diabetes:
  - Total cholesterol 240 mg/dL, LDL cholesterol 160 mg/dL, or HDL cholesterol 35 mg/dL
  - Blood pressure 140/90 mm Hg
  - Smoking
  - Family history of premature coronary artery disease
  - Positive test for microalbuminuria or macroalbuminuria

Adapted from Consensus development conference on the diagnosis of coronary heart disease in people with diabetes: 10-11 February 1998, Miami, Florida. American Diabetes Association. Diabetes Care 21(9):1551-1559, 1998. Copyright © 1998 American Diabetes Association. Reprinted with permission from The American Diabetes Association.

management of hyperglycemia would be to lower markedly elevated glucose levels to less than 300 mg/dL.[84] They did recommend that fluids and insulin should be administered if the blood glucose concentrations are markedly elevated.

Studies in critically ill patients have shown that intensive glucose control (i.e., maintaining glucose around 100 mg/dL) decreases morbidity and mortality.[85,86] In fact, addressing glycemic control before reperfusion can improve the efficacy of thrombolytic therapy.[87] Poststroke management should include antiplatelet therapy and aggressive control of glucose, lipids, and blood pressure.

THE ROLE OF MULTIFACTORIAL MANAGEMENT

The management of the cardiovascular risk in a patient with diabetes begins with identifying who is at risk for CVD and determining who has clinically evident CVD. Application of the criteria for the metabolic syndrome allows identification of people who are at risk for CVD. Box 15-3 shows recommendations from the ADA consensus conference on the indications for cardiac testing in persons with diabetes.[88] The UKPDS established that microvascular complications associated with diabetes can be reduced with intensive glucose-lowering therapy.[59,89,90] However, lowering blood glucose had no statistically significant effect on macrovascular (i.e., cardiovascular) complications,

Table 15–3. *Treatment Goals for the Conventional-Therapy Group and the Intensive-Therapy Group*

Variable	Conventional Therapy		Intensive Therapy	
	1993-1999	2000-2001	1993-1999	2000-2001
Blood Pressure				
Systolic blood pressure (mm Hg)	<160	<135	<140	<130
Diastolic blood pressure (mm Hg)	<95	<85	<85	<80
Laboratory Values				
Glycosylated hemoglobin (%)	<7.5	<6.5	<6.5	<6.5
Fasting serum total cholesterol (mg/dL)	<250	<190	<190	<175
Fasting serum triglycerides (mg/dL)	<195	<180	<150	<150
Antihypertensive Therapy				
Treatment with ACE inhibitor irrespective of blood pressure	No	Yes	Yes	Yes
Aspirin Therapy				
For patients with known ischemia	Yes	Yes	Yes	Yes
For patients with peripheral vascular disease	No	No	Yes	Yes
For patients without coronary heart disease or peripheral vascular disease	No	No	No	Yes

although a positive trend toward reduction was observed. In fact, the modest decrease in blood pressure in the UKPDS has a very significant impact on macrovascular and microvascular complications. However, the question remains how one could maximally decrease all of the complications of uncontrolled diabetes.

Three studies have evaluated the impact of long-term intervention comprising combined behavior modification and polypharmacy specifically in patients with T2DM. Two of these studies have included patients with newly diagnosed T2DM, and the Steno-2 study required T2DM and microalbuminuria. The Diabetes Intervention Study was a randomized 5-year trial with the primary aim of testing the effect of intensified health education in improving metabolic regulation and reducing the level of CV risk factors and incidence of IHD.[91] They did not find a difference in the incidence of CVD among behavioral intervention, placebo, or clofibric acid.

A similar approach to multiple risk factor intervention was undertaken in the Danish study, Diabetes Care in General Practice, which was a randomized, controlled trial of structured personal care in T2DM.[92] At the end of follow-up after 6 years, the only differences between groups were seen for fasting plasma glucose, glycated hemoglobin, and systolic blood pressure. The primary outcome of the study of overall mortality, incidence of diabetic retinopathy, urinary albumin concentration higher than 15 mg/L, myocardial infarction, and stroke did not differ between groups. However, the Diabetes Care in General Practice study importantly demonstrated that an intensified and structured multifactorial intervention can be implemented at the general practitioner level, at least in a clinically controlled setting.

The Steno-2 study differed from the previous two studies by recruiting a high-risk group of type 2 diabetic patients with microalbuminuria, a marker of generalized vascular damage.[93,94] Patients were randomized to either conventional multifactorial treatment at their general practitioner following national guidelines or intensified multifactorial intervention integrating both behavior modification and polypharmacy by a diabetes team consisting of a doctor, a nurse, and a clinical dietitian at the Steno Diabetes Center in Copenhagen. As in the other two studies, patients in the intervention group were seen every third month. Targets for blood glucose, glycated hemoglobin A1c (HbA1c), systolic and diastolic blood pressure, and fasting values of serum total cholesterol, LDL cholesterol, and triglycerides were lower in the intervention group than with conventional therapy (Table 15-3). A stepwise, target-driven approach for drug treatment was used in order to achieve these goals.

Within one year the patients in the intervention group had lower values for glycosylated hemoglobin, fasting plasma glucose, fasting serum lipid, systolic and diastolic blood pressure, and urinary albumin excretion rate, and the differences in the values of these risk factors between the two groups were maintained throughout the 7.8 year follow-up period (Fig. 15–2). At the end of the study there was a significant relative risk reduction of 53% (absolute risk reduction 20%) for the composite end point with intensified multifactorial intervention (Fig. 15–3). The number of patients needed to treat to prevent one event was 5.0 for macrovascular complications, 5.3 for diabetic nephropathy, 6.2 for progression in retinopathy, and 4.2 for progression in autonomic neuropathy. These data conclusively show that multifactorial intervention can be done

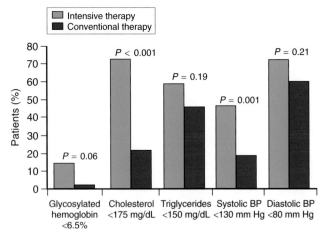

Figure 15–2. Percentage of patients in each group who reached the intensive-treatment goals at a mean of 7.8 years in the Steno-2 trial.

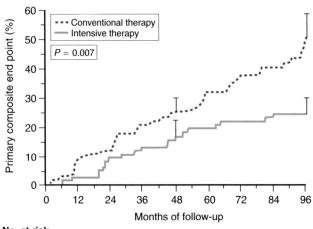

No. at risk

Conventional
therapy   80 72 70 63 59 50 44 41 13
Intensive
therapy   80 78 74 71 66 63 61 59 19

Figure 15–3. Kaplan-Meier estimates of the composite end point of death from cardiovascular causes, nonfatal myocardial infarction, coronary-artery bypass grafting, percutaneous coronary intervention, nonfatal stroke, amputation, or surgery for peripheral atherosclerotic artery disease in the conventional-therapy group and the intensive-therapy group in the Steno-2 trial. The P value was calculated with the use of the log-rank test. The bars show standard errors.

and that it can affect multiple complications in persons with diabetes at high risk for cardiovascular disease.

References

1. Kannel W, McGee D: Diabetes and cardiovascular disease: The Framingham Study. JAMA 24:2035-2038, 1979.
2. Kannel W, McGee D: Diabetes and glucose tolerance as risk factors for cardiovascular disease: The Framingham Study. Diabetes Care 2:120-126, 1979.
3. Pyörälä K, Laakso M, Uusitupa M: Diabetes and atherosclerosis: An epidemiologic view. Diabetes Metab Rev 3:463-524, 1987.
4. Bierman E: George Lyman Duff Memorial Lecture. Atherogenesis in diabetes. Arterioscler Thromb 12:647-656, 1992.
5. Donahue R, Orchard T: Diabetes mellitus and macrovascular complications: An epidemiological perspective. Diabetes Care 15:1141-1155, 1992.
6. Stratton IM, Adler AI, Neil HAW, et al: Association of glycaemia with macrovascular and microvascular complications of type 2 diabetes (UKPDS 35): Prospective observational study. BMJ 321:405-412, 2000.
7. Kleinman J, Donahue R, Harris M, et al: Mortality among diabetics in a national sample. Am J Epidemiol 128:389-401, 1988.
8. Butler W, Ostrander L Jr, Carman W, Lamphiear D: Mortality from coronary heart disease in the Tecumseh study. Long-term effect of diabetes mellitus, glucose tolerance and other risk factors. Am J Epidemiol 121:541-547, 1985.
9. Klein R: Hyperglycemia and microvascular and macrovascular disease in diabetes. Diabetes Care 18:258-268, 1995.
10. Kuller LH, Velentgas P, Barzilay J, et al: Diabetes mellitus: Subclinical cardiovascular disease and risk of incident cardiovascular disease and all-cause mortality. Arterioscler Thromb Vasc Biol 20:823-829, 2000.
11. The DECODE Study Group: Age, body mass index and glucose tolerance in 11 European population-based surveys. The DECODE Study Group, on behalf of the European Diabetes Epidemiology Group. Diabet Med 19:558-565, 2002.
12. Lloyd CE, Kuller LH, Ellis D, et al: Coronary artery disease in IDDM : Gender differences in risk factors but not risk. Arterioscler Thromb Vasc Biol 16:720-726, 1996.
13. Olson J, Edmundowicz D, Becker D, et al: Coronary calcium in adults with type 1 diabetes: A stronger correlate of clinical coronary artery disease in men than in women. Diabetes 49:1571-1578, 2000.
14. Barzilay JI, Spiekerman CF, Kuller LH, et al: Prevalence of clinical and isolated subclinical cardiovascular disease in older adults with glucose disorders: The Cardiovascular Health Study. Diabetes Care 24:1233-1239, 2001.
15. Pan W, Cedres L, Liu K, et al: Relationship of clinical diabetes and asymptomatic hyperglycemia to risk of coronary heart disease mortality in men and women. Am J Epidemiol 123:504-516, 1986.
16. Barrett-Connor E, Wingard D: Sex differential in ischemic heart disease mortality in diabetics: A prospective population-based study. Am J Epidemiol 118:489-496, 1983.
17. Sundquist J, Winkleby MA, Pudaric S: Cardiovascular disease risk factors among older black, Mexican-American, and white women and men: An analysis of NHANES III, 1988-1994. J Am Geriatr Soc 49:109-116, 2001.
18. Pinhas-Hamiel O, Dolan LM, Daniels SR, et al: Increased incidence of non-insulin-dependent diabetes mellitus among adolescents. J Pediatr 128(5, Part 1):608-615, 1996.
19. Martin M, Martin A: Obesity, hyperinsulinism, and diabetes mellitus in childhood. J Pediatr 82:192-201, 1993.
20. Jarvisalo MJ, Putto-Laurila A, Jartti L, et al: Carotid artery intima-media thickness in children with type 1 diabetes. Diabetes 51:493-498, 2002.
21. Sorof JM, Alexandrov AV, Cardwell G, Portman RJ: Carotid artery intimal-medial thickness and left ventricular hypertrophy in children with elevated blood pressure. Pediatrics 111:61-66, 2003.
22. Singh TP, Groehn H, Kazmers A: Vascular function and carotid intimal-medial thickness in children with insulin-dependent diabetes mellitus. J Am Coll Cardiol 41:661-665, 2003.
23. Raitakari OT, Juonala M, Kahonen M, et al: Cardiovascular risk factors in childhood and carotid artery intima-media thickness in adulthood: The cardiovascular risk in young Finns study. JAMA 290:2277-2283, 2003.
24. Knoflach M, Kiechl S, Kind M, et al: Cardiovascular risk factors and atherosclerosis in young males: ARMY Study (Atherosclerosis Risk-Factors in Male Youngsters). Circulation 108:1064-1069, 2003.

25. Pannacciulli N, De Pergola G, Ciccone M, et al: Effect of family history of type 2 diabetes on the intima-media thickness of the common carotid artery in normal-weight, overweight, and obese glucose-tolerant young adults. Diabetes Care 26:1230-1234, 2003.

26. Jarvisalo MJ, Raitakari M, Toikka JO, et al: Endothelial dysfunction and increased arterial intima-media thickness in children with type 1 diabetes. Circulation 109:1750-1755, 2004.

27. Krantz JS, Mack WJ, Hodis HN, et al: Early onset of subclinical atherosclerosis in young persons with type 1 diabetes. J Pediatr 145:452-457, 2004.

28. Mitsnefes MM, Kimball TR, Witt SA, et al: Abnormal carotid artery structure and function in children and adolescents with successful renal transplantation. Circulation 110:97-101, 2004.

29. Ford ES, Mokdad AH, Ajani UA: Trends in risk factors for cardiovascular disease among children and adolescents in the United States. Pediatrics 114:1534-1544, 2004.

30. Hardin DS, Hebert JD, Bayden T, et al: Treatment of childhood syndrome X. Pediatrics 100:E5, 1997.

31. Reaven P, Nader PR, Berry C, Hoy T: Cardiovascular disease insulin risk in Mexican-American and Anglo-American children and mothers. Pediatrics 101:E12, 1998.

32. Gower B: Syndrome X in children: Influence of ethnicity and visceral fat. Am J Hum Biol. 11:249-257, 1999.

33. Falkner B, Michel S: Obesity and other risk factors in children. Ethn Dis 9:284-289, 1999.

34. Chen W, Srinivasan SR, Elkasabany A, Berenson GS: Cardiovascular risk factors clustering features of insulin resistance syndrome (syndrome X) in a biracial (black-white) population of children, adolescents, and young adults: The Bogalusa Heart Study. Am J Epidemiol 150:667-674, 1999.

35. Chen W, Bao W, Begum S, et al: Age-related patterns of the clustering of cardiovascular risk variables of syndrome X from childhood to young adulthood in a population made up of black and white subjects: The Bogalusa Heart Study. Diabetes 49:1042-1048, 2000.

36. Sinaiko AR, Jacobs J, David R., et al: Insulin resistance syndrome in childhood: Associations of the euglycemic insulin clamp and fasting insulin with fatness and other risk factors. J Pediatrics 139:700-707, 2001.

37. Urrutia-Rojas X, Menchaca J, Wadley W, et al: Cardiovascular risk factors in Mexican-American children at risk for type 2 diabetes mellitus (T2DM). J Adolesc Health 34:290-299, 2004.

38. Turner RC, Millns H, Neil HAW, et al: Risk factors for coronary artery disease in non-insulin dependent diabetes mellitus: United Kingdom prospective diabetes study (UKPDS: 23). BMJ 1998;316:823-828.

39. Imperatore G, Cadwell BL, Geiss L, et al: Thirty-year trends in cardiovascular risk factor levels among US adults with diabetes: National Health and Nutrition Examination Surveys, 1971-2000. Am J Epidemiol 160:531-539, 2004.

39a. Bassuk SS, Rifai N, Ridker PM: High-sensitivity C-reactive protein: Clinical importance. Curr Probl Cardiol 29:439–493, 2004.

40. Caslake M, Packard C: Lipoprotein-associated phospholipase A2 (platelet-activating factor acetylhydrolase) and cardiovascular disease. Curr Opin Lipidol 14:347-352, 2003.

41. Haffner SM, Lehto S, Ronnemaa T, et al: Mortality from coronary heart disease in subjects with type 2 diabetes and in nondiabetic subjects with and without prior myocardial infarction. N Engl J Med 1998;339:229-234.

42. Malmberg K, Yusuf S, Gerstein HC, et al: Impact of diabetes on long-term prognosis in patients with unstable angina and non-Q-wave myocardial infarction: Results of the OASIS (Organization to Assess Strategies for Ischemic Syndromes) Registry. Circulation 102:1014-1019, 2000.

43. The Heart Outcomes Prevention Evaluation Study Investigators: Effects of an angiotensin-converting-enzyme inhibitor, ramipril, on cardiovascular events in high-risk patients. N Engl J Med 342:145-153, 2000.

44. Miettinen H, Lehto S, Salomaa V, et al: Impact of diabetes on mortality after the first myocardial infarction. The FIN-MONICA Myocardial Infarction Register Study Group. Diabetes Care 1998;21:69-75.

45. Svensson A, Abrahamsson P, McGuire D, Dellborg M: Influence of diabetes on long-term outcome among unselected patients with acute coronary events. Scand Cardiovasc J. 38:229-234, 2004.

46. Abbott R, Donahue R, Kannel W, Wilson P: The impact of diabetes on survival following myocardial infarction in men vs women. The Framingham Study. JAMA 260:3456-3460, 1988.

47. Herlitz J, Karlson B, Edvardsson N, et al: Prognosis in diabetics with chest pain or other symptoms suggestive of acute myocardial infarction. Cardiology 80:237-245, 1992.

48. Herlitz J, Wognsen G, Emanuelsson H, et al: Mortality and morbidity in diabetic and nondiabetic patients during a 2-year period after coronary artery bypass grafting. Diabetes Care 1996;19:698-703.

49. UKPDS Study Group: Effect of intensive blood-glucose control with metformin on complications in overweight patients with type 2 diabetes (UKPDS 34). Lancet 1998;352:854-865.

50. Pyörälä K, Pedersen T, Kjekshus J, et al: Cholesterol lowering with simvastatin improves prognosis of diabetic patients with coronary heart disease. A subgroup analysis of the Scandinavian Simvastatin Survival Study (4S). Diabetes Care 20:614-620, 1997.

51. Downs JR, Clearfield M, Weis S, et al: Primary prevention of acute coronary events with lovastatin in men and women with average cholesterol levels: Results of AFCAPS/TexCAPS. JAMA 279:1615-1622, 1998.

52. Goldberg RB, Mellies MJ, Sacks FM, et al: Cardiovascular events and their reduction with pravastatin in diabetic and glucose-intolerant myocardial infarction survivors with average cholesterol levels: Subgroup analyses in the Cholesterol And Recurrent Events (CARE) trial. Circulation 98:2513-2519, 1998.

53. The Long-Term Intervention with Pravastatin in Ischaemic Disease (LIPID) Study Group: Prevention of cardiovascular events and death with pravastatin in patients with coronary heart disease and a broad range of initial cholesterol levels. N Engl J Med 339:1349-1357, 1998.

54. Haffner SM, Alexander CM, Cook TJ, et al: Reduced coronary events in simvastatin-treated patients with coronary heart disease and diabetes or impaired fasting glucose levels: Subgroup analyses in the Scandinavian Simvastatin Survival Study. Arch Intern Med 159:2661-2667, 1999.

55. Colhoun HM, Betteridge DJ, Durrington PN, et al: Primary prevention of cardiovascular disease with atorvastatin in type 2 diabetes in the Collaborative Atorvastatin Diabetes Study (CARDS): Multicentre randomised placebo-controlled trial. Lancet 364:685-696, 2004.

56. Diabetes in Children and Adolescents Work Group of the National Diabetes Education Program: An update on type 2 diabetes in youth from the National Diabetes Education Program. Pediatrics 114:259-263, 2004.

57. American Diabetes Association: Type 2 diabetes in children and adolescents. Diabetes Care 23:381-389, 2000.

58. Rubins HB, Robins SJ, Collins D, et al: Gemfibrozil for the secondary prevention of coronary heart disease in men with low levels of high-density lipoprotein cholesterol. N Engl J Med 341:410-418, 1999.

59. UK Prospective Diabetes Study Group: Tight blood pressure control and risk of macrovascular and microvascular complications in type 2 diabetes: UKPDS 38. BMJ 317:703-713, 1998.

60. Hansson L, Zanchetti A, Carruthers SG, et al: Effects of intensive blood-pressure lowering and low-dose aspirin in patients with hypertension: Principal results of the Hypertension Optimal Treatment (HOT) randomised trial. The Lancet 351:1755-1762, 1998.

61. Yusuf S, Sleight P, Pogue J, et al: Effects of an angiotensin-converting-enzyme inhibitor, ramipril, on cardiovascular events in high-risk patients. N Engl J Med 342:145-153, 2000.

62. Blair S, Cheng Y, Holder J: Is physical activity or physical fitness more important in defining health benefits? Med Sci Sports Exerc 33(6 Suppl):S379-S399, 2001.

63. Church TS, Cheng YJ, Earnest CP, et al: Exercise capacity and body composition as predictors of mortality among men with diabetes. Diabetes Care 27:83-88, 2004.

64. Katzmarzyk PT, Church TS, Blair SN: Cardiorespiratory fitness attenuates the effects of the metabolic syndrome on all-cause and cardiovascular disease mortality in men. Arch Intern Med 164:1092-1097, 2004.

65. ETDRS Investigators: Aspirin effects on mortality and morbidity in patients with diabetes mellitus. Early Treatment Diabetic Retinopathy Study report 14. JAMA 268:1292-1300, 1992.

66. Yusuf S, Zhao F, Mehta SR, et al: Effects of clopidogrel in addition to aspirin in patients with acute coronary syndromes without ST-segment elevation. N Engl J Med 345:494-502, 2001.

67. Roffi M, Chew DP, Mukherjee D, et al: Platelet glycoprotein IIB/IIIA inhibitors reduce mortality in diabetic patients with non-ST-segment-elevation acute coronary syndromes. Circulation 104:2767-2771, 2001.

68. Meinert C, Knatterud G, Prout T, Klimt C: A study of the effects of hypoglycemic agents on vascular complications in patients with adult-onset diabetes. II. Mortality results. Diabetes 1970;19(Suppl):789-830.

69. Malmberg K, Ryden L, Efendic S, et al: Randomized trial of insulin-glucose infusion followed by subcutaneous insulin treatment in diabetic patients with acute myocardial infarction (DIGAMI Study): Effects on mortality at 1 year. J Am Coll Cardiol 26:57-65, 1995.

70. Chaudhuri A, Janicke D, Wilson MF, et al: Anti-inflammatory and profibrinolytic effect of insulin in acute ST-segment-elevation myocardial infarction. Circulation 109:849-854, 2004.

71. The BARI Investigators: Influence of diabetes on 5-year mortality and morbidity in a randomized trial comparing CABG and PTCA in patients with multivessel disease: The Bypass Angioplasty Revascularization Investigation (BARI). Circulation 96:1761-1769, 1997.

72. McGuire DK, Anstrom KJ, Peterson ED: Influence of the Bypass Angioplasty Revascularization Investigation National Heart, Lung, and Blood Institute Diabetic Clinical Alert on Practice Patterns: Results from the National Cardiovascular Network Database. Circulation 107:1864-1870, 2003.

73. Scheen AJ, Warzee F, Legrand VMG: Drug-eluting stents: Meta-analysis in diabetic patients. Eur Heart J 25:2167-2168, 2004.

74. Moussa I, Leon MB, Baim DS, et al: Impact of sirolimus-eluting stents on outcome in diabetic patients: A SIRIUS (SIRolImUS-coated Bx Velocity balloon-expandable stent in the treatment of patients with de novo coronary artery lesions) substudy. Circulation 109:2273-2278, 2004.

75. Fuller J, Shipley M, Rose G, et al: Mortality from coronary heart disease and stroke in relation to degree of glycaemia: The Whitehall study. Br Med J 287:867-870, 1983.

76. Olsson T, Viitanen M, Asplund K, et al: Prognosis after stroke in diabetic patients. A controlled prospective study. Diabetologia 33:244-249, 1990.

77. Toni D, Sacchetti M, Argentino C, et al: Does hyperglycaemia play a role on the outcome of acute ischaemic stroke patients? J Neurol 239:382-386, 1992.

78. Capes SE, Hunt D, Malmberg K, et al: Stress hyperglycemia and prognosis of stroke in nondiabetic and diabetic patients: A systematic overview. Stroke 32:2426-2432, 2001.

79. Kiers L, Davis S, Larkins R, et al: Stroke topography and outcome in relation to hyperglycaemia and diabetes. J Neurol Neurosurg Psychiatry 55:263-270, 1992.

80. Gray CS, Scott JF, French JM, et al: Prevalence and prediction of unrecognised diabetes mellitus and impaired glucose tolerance following acute stroke. Age Ageing 33:71-77, 2004.

81. Alvarez-Sabin J, Molina CA, Montaner J, et al: Effects of admission hyperglycemia on stroke outcome in reperfused tissue plasminogen activator-treated patients. Stroke 34:1235-1240, 2003.

82. Weir CJ, Murray GD, Dyker AG, Lees KR: Is hyperglycaemia an independent predictor of poor outcome after acute stroke? Results of a long term follow up study. BMJ 314:1303-1306, 1997.

83. Leigh R, Zaidat OO, Suri MF, et al: Predictors of hyperacute clinical worsening in ischemic stroke patients receiving thrombolytic therapy. Stroke 35:1903-1907, 2004.

84. Adams HP Jr, Adams RJ, Brott T, et al: Guidelines for the early management of patients with ischemic stroke: A scientific statement from the Stroke Council of the American Stroke Association. Stroke 34:1056-1083, 2003.

85. Van den Berghe G: Tight blood glucose control with insulin in "real-life" intensive care. Mayo Clin Proc 79:977-978, 2004.

86. Krinsley J: Effect of an intensive glucose management protocol on the mortality of critically ill adult patients. Mayo Clin Proc 79:992-1000, 2004.

87. Alvarez-Sabin J, Molina CA, Ribo M, et al: Impact of admission hyperglycemia on stroke outcome after thrombolysis: Risk stratification in relation to time to reperfusion. Stroke 35:2493-2498, 2004.

88. American Diabetes Association: Consensus development conference on the diagnosis of coronary heart disease in people with diabetes: 10-11 February 1998, Miami, Florida. Diabetes Care 21:1551-1559, 1998.

89. UK Prospective Diabetes Study Group: Efficacy of atenolol and captopril in reducing risk of macrovascular and microvascular complications in type 2 diabetes: UKPDS 39. BMJ 317:713-720, 1998.

90. UK Prospective Diabetes Study Group: Cost effectiveness analysis of improved blood pressure control in hypertensive patients with type 2 diabetes: UKPDS 40. BMJ 317:720-726, 1998.

91. Hanefeld M, Fischer S, Schmechel H, et al: Diabetes Intervention Study. Multi-intervention trial in newly diagnosed NIDDM. Diabetes Care 14:308-317, 1991.

92. Olivarius NdF, Beck-Nielsen H, Andreasen AH, et al: Randomised controlled trial of structured personal care of type 2 diabetes mellitus. BMJ 323:970-975, 2001.

93. Gaede P, Vedel P, Larsen N, et al: Multifactorial intervention and cardiovascular disease in patients with type 2 diabetes. N Engl J Med 348:383-393, 2003.

94. Gaede P, Vedel P, Parving H-H, Pedersen O: Intensified multifactorial intervention in patients with type 2 diabetes mellitus and microalbuminuria: The Steno type 2 randomised study. Lancet 353:617-622, 1999.

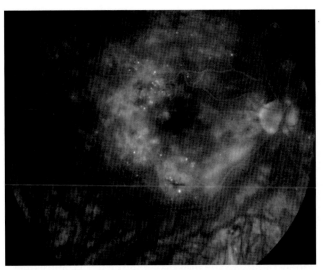

Figure 16–15. Retinal angiogram illustrating diffuse leakage within the macula. Subsequent edema threatening the anatomic fovea, or the retinal visual center, can greatly decrease visual acuity. (Photo courtesy of James LeBlanc, Tulane University Hospital and Clinic.)

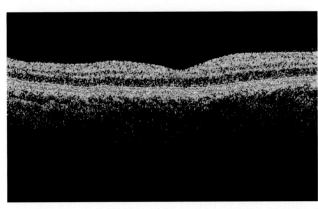

Figure 16–16. Optical coherence tomographic image of normal retinal cross-section showing the foveal depression centrally. Note the compact nature of retinal layers. (Photo courtesy of James LeBlanc, Tulane University Hospital and Clinic.)

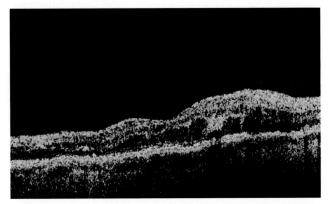

Figure 16–17. Optical coherence tomographic image of clinically significant macular edema showing diffuse edema and exudates around the central foveal depression. (Photo courtesy of James LeBlanc, Tulane University Hospital and Clinic.)

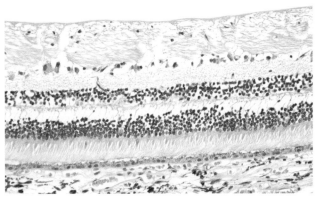

Figure 16–18. Histologic section (hematoxylin and eosin) of normal retina illustrating relationship of various layers.

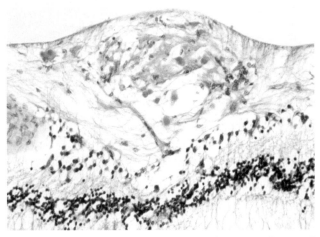

Figure 16–19. Histologic section (hematoxylin and eosin) of clinically significant macular edema illustrating thickening of retina and separation of layers by edema.

ischemic neurons due to cerebral ischemia after brain injury.[43] Cystoid macular edema is commonly seen in eyes that have other signs of severe NPDR, such as numerous hemorrhages or exudates. In severe persistent cystoid macular edema there is gross disruption of normal retinal anatomy (Figs. 16–20, 16–21, 16–22, and 16–23).

Patients with macular edema typically present with a gradual onset of blurred near and distant vision. They usually think they "need new glasses." However, on clinical fundus examination, they have evidence of retinal microvascular disease, such as hemorrhages and microaneurysms. Thus, diabetic patients with these complaints should be referred to an ophthalmologist for proper diagnosis and treatment.

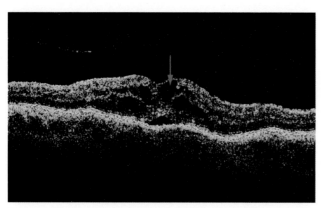

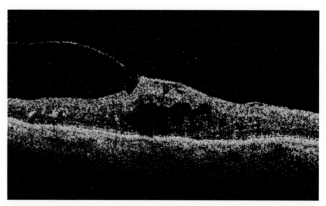

Figure 16–20. Optical coherence tomographic image of cystoid macular edema with intraretinal cystic spaces surrounding the central foveal depression. (Photo courtesy of James LeBlanc, Tulane University Hospital and Clinic.)

Figure 16–23. Optical coherence tomographic image of adhesive posterior hyaloid face, causing macular edema via traction on inner retinal layers. The face or cortex of the vitreous gel in the posterior segment of the eye can adhere tightly to the inner layer of the retina. Subsequent shrinking of the gel into the vitreous cavity can pull the retinal layers apart, contributing to intraretinal edema in a diabetic eye. (Photo courtesy of James LeBlanc, Tulane University Hospital and Clinic.)

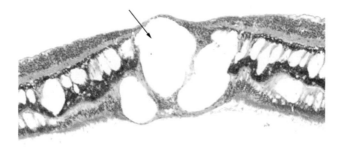

Figure 16–21. Histologic section (hematoxylin and eosin) of cystoid macular edema showing large intraretinal cystic spaces (*arrow*).

Advanced Nonproliferative Diabetic Retinopathy

In advanced NPDR, signs of increasing inner retinal hypoxia appear, including multiple retinal hemorrhages, cotton-wool spots, venous beading, loops of intraretinal microvascular abnormalities (IRMAs), and large areas of capillary nonperfusion depicted on fluorescein angiography.

Cotton-wool spots, also called soft exudates or nerve fiber infarcts, result from ischemia, not exudation. Local ischemia causes effective obstruction of axoplasmic flow in the normally transparent nerve fiber layer; the subsequent swelling of the nerve fibers gives cotton-wool spots their characteristic white fluffy appearance.[15] Fluorescein angiography shows no capillary perfusion in the area corresponding to a cotton-wool spot. Microaneurysms often surround the hypoxic area (Fig. 16–24).

Venous beading is an important sign of sluggish retinal circulation. Venous loops nearly always are adjacent to large areas of capillary nonperfusion. IRMAs are dilated intraretinal capillaries, which seem to function as collateral channels in ischemic areas.[15] IRMAs often are difficult to differentiate from surface retinal neovascularization on fundus examination but can be differentiated by fluorescein angiography, which demonstrates an absence of dye leakage from IRMA but profuse leakage from neovascularization. The new vessels grow at the vitreo-retinal interface devoid of capillary endothelial tight junctions. Hence, the fluorescein dye leaks from abnormal new vessels like water from a garden soaker hose. This increased interstitial fluid shows diffusion of nutrients and waste products sur-

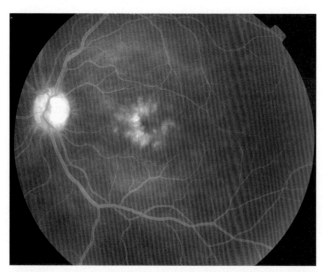

Figure 16–22. Retinal angiogram illustrating localized perifoveal leakage forming a petalloid pattern around the fovea. Extravasating dye from leaking vessels fills the cystic spaces noted in Figure 16-21. (Photo courtesy of James LeBlanc, Tulane University Hospital and Clinic.)

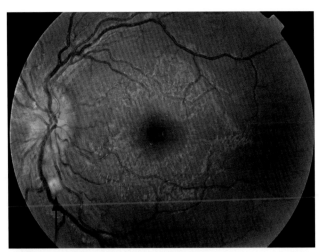

Figure 16–24. Retinal fundus photograph of an isolated cotton wool spot. (Photo courtesy of James LeBlanc, Tulane University Hospital and Clinic.)

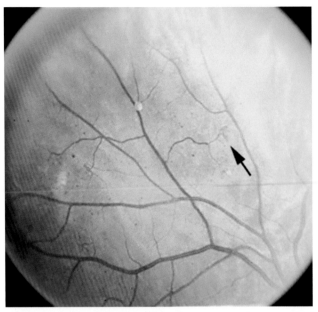

Figure 16–26. Retinal fundus photograph of intraretinal microvascular abnormalities (IRMAs) *(arrow)*. This collection of abnormal vessels is a precursor to frank neovascularization. IRMAs in just one quadrant of an eye indicate imminent progression to proliferative diabetic retinopathy, and panretinal photocoagulation laser therapy should be considered.

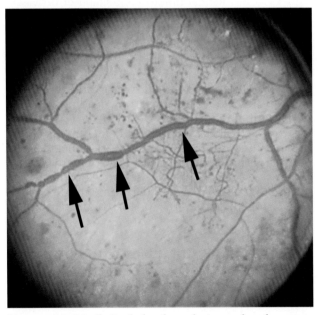

Figure 16–25. Retinal fundus photograph of venous beading *(arrows)*. Note alternating areas of venous constriction and dilation within a single retinal venule. Such a finding in two quadrants of the same eye indicates imminent progression to proliferative diabetic retinopathy and therefore is an indication for prophylactic panretinal photocoagulation laser therapy.

rounding the area of capillary leakage (Figs. 16–25 and 16–26).

The Early Treatment Diabetic Retinopathy Study (ETDRS) categorized nonproliferative diabetic retinopathy into mild, moderate, severe, and very severe. Severe and very severe NPDR was further defined by the "4:2:1" rule: diffuse intraretinal hemorrhages and microaneurysms in *4* quadrants, venous beading in *2* quadrants, and IRMA in *1* quadrant. The 4:2:1 rule assists the ophthalmologist

in identifying patients at greatest risk for progression from NPDR to PDR.[16] If one of the "4:2:1" criteria was fulfilled, the NPDR was designated severe and had a 15% chance of progression to PDR within one year. Very severe NPDR was defined by the presence of two or more of the "4:2:1" features and had a 45% chance of progression to PDR.[16] Due to increased risk of progression from severe and very severe NPDR to PDR, ETDRS recommended panretinal photocoagulation to reduce the risk of severe visual loss.[16]

The initial stage of cell death and increased capillary permeability may be followed by cycles of renewal and further cell death, leading to progressive microvascular obliteration, ischemic injury, and unregulated angiogenesis. More-severe ischemia results in vasoproliferation and in the formation of neovascularization or PDR. These new vessels can arise primarily from veins and can spread out within the retinal layers or push forward into the vitreous, becoming attached to the posterior cortical layer of the vitreous body. They are fragile and often form a lacelike pattern with a fine mesh of fibrous tissue connecting them. PDR can result in a vitreous hemorrhage or a retinal detachment, which severely impairs vision.

Approximately 45% of patients with very severe NPDR progress to proliferative retinopathy within 1 year.[16] Proliferative vessels usually arise from retinal veins and bud into fronds of multiple fine vessels (Figs. 16–27 and 16–28). When new vessels arise on or within one disc diameter of the optic nerve head

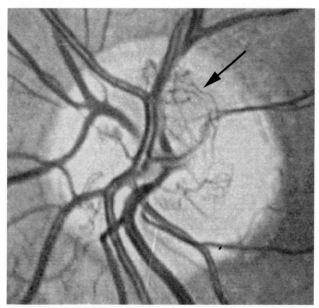

Figure 16–27. Retinal fundus photograph of neovascularization of the disc (NVD) *(arrow)*. The tortuous and fragile new vessels are growing on the head of the optic nerve secondary to retinal ischemia, which stimulates vasoproliferative factors.

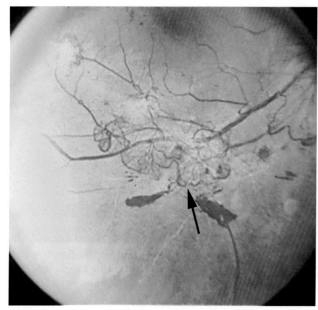

Figure 16–29. Retinal fundus photograph of neovascularization elsewhere (NVE) *(arrow)*. NVE arises via the same mechanism as neovascularization of the disc (NVD).

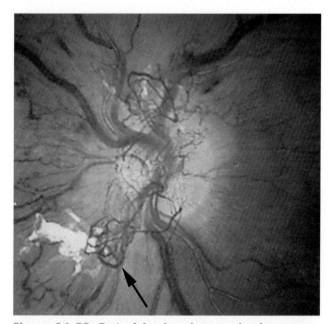

Figure 16–28. Retinal fundus photograph of neovascularization of the disc (NVD) *(arrow)*. This neovascularization extends beyond the nerve head and into the vitreous cavity.

more prominent. The collagen scaffold contracts and elevates the underlying retina, leading to a tractional retinal detachment.

Two types of diabetic retinal detachments occur: those caused by traction alone (nonrhegmatogenous) and those due to holes in the ischemic retina, which are caused by tissue breakdown and a rhegmatogenous retinal detachment (See Figs. 16–27, 16–28, 16–29, 16–30, 16–31, and 16–32).

OTHER OCULAR COMPLICATIONS OF DIABETES MELLITUS

Cornea

Corneal sensitivity is decreased in proportion to both the duration of the disease and the severity of the retinopathy.[17] Corneal abrasions are more common in people with diabetes, presumably because adhesion between the basement membrane of the corneal epithelium and the corneal stroma is not as firm as that found in normal corneas.[17]

Glaucoma

When severe retinal ischemia is present, new vessel proliferation, called *rubeosis,* can also occur on the surface of the iris (neovascularization of the iris) and in the anterior chamber.[18] These new vessels have incompetent tight junctions that leak proteins and blood products that can block the outflow path for aqueous humor from the eye, leading to acute

they are referred to as NVD (neovascularization of the disc). When they arise farther than one disc diameter away, they are called NVE (neovascularization elsewhere) (Fig. 16–29). Unlike normal retinal vessels, NVD and NVE both leak fluorescein into the vitreous as described previously. As the new vessels mature, the fibrous component becomes

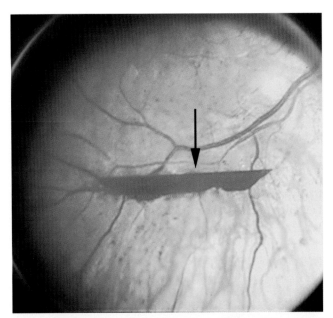

Figure 16–30. Retinal fundus photograph of preretinal hemorrhage *(arrow)*. The hemorrhage results from fragile neovascularization elsewhere (NVE). These boat-shaped hemorrhages settle into a pocket between the retina and a partially detached vitreous face, creating an appearance akin to an air fluid layer on a radiograph.

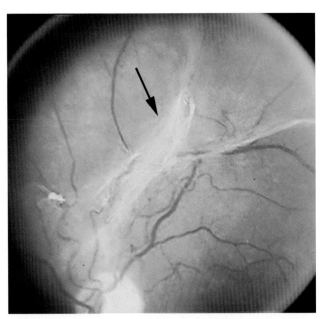

Figure 16–32. Retinal fundus photograph of a traction retinal detachment *(arrow)*. Neovascularization is a process of fibrovascular proliferation. In the natural progression, this fibrous proliferation can create traction on the retina, leading to retinal detachment.

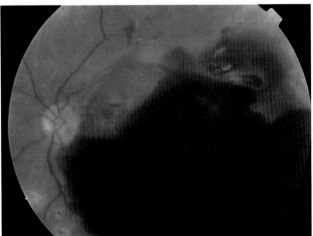

Figure 16–31. Retinal fundus photograph of more extensive vitreous hemorrhage, obscuring most of the retina. Such a hemorrhage limits both the patient's vision and the examiner's evaluation until it is either resorbed or surgically removed. (Photo courtesy of James LeBlanc, Tulane University Hospital and Clinic.)

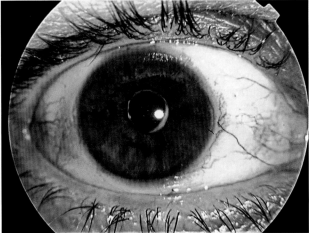

Figure 16–33. Anterior segment photograph of iris neovascularization (rubeosis). Vasoproliferative factors from untreated proliferative diabetic retinopathy (PDR) can lead to neovascularization in the anterior segment, causing neovascularization of the iris and drainage angle. These incompetent new vessels leak fluorescein dye on angiography. (Photo courtesy of James LeBlanc, Tulane University Hospital and Clinic.)

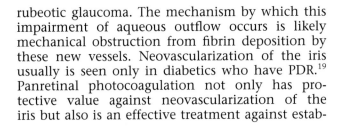

rubeotic glaucoma. The mechanism by which this impairment of aqueous outflow occurs is likely mechanical obstruction from fibrin deposition by these new vessels. Neovascularization of the iris usually is seen only in diabetics who have PDR.[19] Panretinal photocoagulation not only has protective value against neovascularization of the iris but also is an effective treatment against estab-

lished neovascularization of the iris (Figs. 16–33 and 16–34).[19]

Lens

Osmotic lens swelling changes the crystalline lens. The change in size leads to changes in refractive

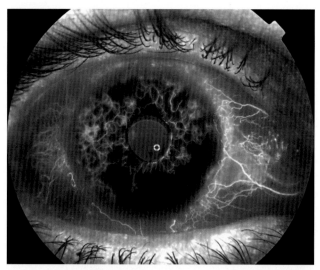

Figure 16–34. Angiogram of iris neovascularization (rubeosis) seen in Figure 16-33. Vasoproliferative factors from untreated proliferative diabetic retinopathy (PDR) can lead to neovascularization in the anterior segment, causing neovascularization of the iris and drainage angle. These incompetent new vessels leak fluorescein dye on angiography. (Photo courtesy of James LeBlanc, Tulane University Hospital and Clinic.)

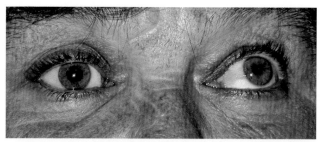

Figure 16–35. External photograph of a patient with cranial nerve III palsy of the left eye. Note that residual fourth and sixth cranial nerve innervation abducts and hyperdeviates the affected eye. (Photo courtesy of James LeBlanc, Tulane University Hospital and Clinic.)

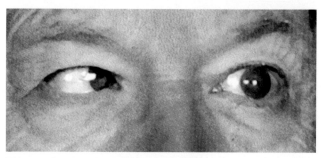

Figure 16–36. External photograph of a patient with cranial nerve VI palsy of the right eye. Note that residual third cranial nerve innervation adducts the affected eye. (Photo courtesy of James LeBlanc, Tulane University Hospital and Clinic.)

power. Therefore, diabetic patients with uncontrolled glycemia might need frequent spectacle changes. However, as the sorbitol slowly diffuses out of the lens, the lens returns to its previous shape, causing refractive power to return to baseline value. Repeated bouts of lens swelling lead to cataract formation. The risk of cataract is two to four times greater in diabetics than in nondiabetics and may be 15 to 25 times greater in diabetics younger than 40 years old.[20]

Patients with diabetes mellitus who have no retinopathy have excellent results from cataract surgery, with 90% to 95% having a final visual acuity of 20/40 or better, but chronic cystoid macular edema is about 14 times more common in diabetic patients than in nondiabetic persons.[21] The best-known predictor of postoperative success is the level of preoperative retinopathy.[22]

Postoperative complications of cataract surgery include macular edema, progression of proliferative retinopathy, new vitreous hemorrhage, and traction retinal detachment involving the macula.

Optic Neuropathy

Diabetic patients have an increased risk for anterior ischemic optic neuropathy (AION).[23] In addition, diabetic patients are susceptible to diabetic papillopathy, which is characterized by acute disc edema without the pallid swelling of anterior ischemic optic neuropathy. It is bilateral in one half of cases. Macular edema is a common concurrent finding

and is the most common cause of failure of visual recovery in these patients.[23] The visual prognosis is excellent: Most patients recover vision to 20/50 or better.[23]

Cranial Neuropathy

Extraocular muscle palsies may occur in diabetics secondary to neuropathy involving the third, fourth, or sixth cranial nerves. Recovery of extraocular muscle function in diabetic cranial nerve palsies generally takes place within 1 to 3 months.[24] When the third cranial nerve is involved, pupil function is usually normal. Sparing of the pupil in diabetic third cranial nerve palsy is an important diagnostic feature, helping to distinguish it from an intracranial tumor or aneurysm (Figs. 16–35 and 16–36).

DIAGNOSIS AND SCREENING

Intravenous fluorescein angiography (IVFA) provides a qualitative assessment of vascular leakage and nonperfusion and is the most widely used modality for the detection of ischemia and macular

leakage that needs treatment in diabetic retinopathy. Although fluorescein angiography is used to define specific areas of leakage, the clinical examination is initially performed to identify the disease. It is however, useful to quantitate both the extent of capillary nonperfusion and incompetence of macular capillaries causing macular edema.

Optical coherence tomography (OCT) offers a quantitative analysis as well as a cross-sectional view of retinal architecture. It is a novel, noninvasive, noncontact imaging technology that provides high-resolution images. OCT is analogous to ultrasound (B-scan) in that information is determined from time delays of reflected signals from various intraocular structures. Ultrasound uses low-frequency sound waves, but OCT uses light waves, yielding a very sensitive view of retinal architecture. The images produced by the OCT have an axial resolution of approximately 10 µm compared with 150 µm for ultrasound. OCT is a useful adjunct for diagnosing and managing macular edema.

Initial Screening

Type 2 diabetes is typically a disease with insidious onset, and some patients already have retinopathy at the time of diagnosis. Thus, these patients should have a comprehensive dilated examination by an ophthalmologist shortly after the diagnosis of type 2 diabetes is made.[25,26]

On the other hand, persons with type 1 diabetes who have not reached puberty rarely develop retinopathy. These patients will usually not develop retinopathy until 3 to 5 years after the onset of puberty.

Frequency of Examinations

The American Academy of Ophthalmology (AAO) recommends annual examinations for diabetic patients with no retinopathy and semiannual examinations for those with mild NPDR with good glucose control. The schedule for subsequent examinations must be correlated to the level of the risk to the eyes. A patient who has no retinopathy and poor glycemic control needs to be monitored closely (every 3 to 6 months) as does a patient with advanced retinopathy and good glucose control.

Method of Screening

The optimal method of screening for diabetic retinopathy is controversial. Seven-field stereoscopic photography through dilated pupils is the gold standard. This method was therefore compared to ophthalmoscopy by an experienced ophthalmologist, an optometrist, and an ophthalmic technician in the eyes of 1949 patients participating in the Wisconsin Epidemiology Study of Diabetic Retinopathy.[27]

There was almost complete agreement among the three observers in 86% of cases. Examiners were most likely to miss mild nonproliferative retinopathy and to overestimate the severity of retinopathy in patients with long-standing diabetes. Only one case of high-risk proliferative retinopathy was missed by direct ophthalmoscopy. The accuracy of ophthalmoscopy is substantially lower when performed by primary care physicians and optometrists.

Recommendations

Patients with type 1 diabetes usually do not develop retinopathy prior to puberty. Patients with type 1 diabetes should have a complete examination by an ophthalmologist within three to five years after the onset of the disease. Subsequent examinations should be determined by the presence and severity of retinopathy at the initial examination, but the minimum recommendation is an annual examination.

Patients with type 2 diabetes should have a complete examination by an ophthalmologist promptly at the time of diagnosis. Subsequent examinations or referral for treatment should be determined by the presence and severity of retinopathy at the initial examination, but the minimum recommendation is an annual examination.

Women with preexisting diabetes who become pregnant should have a complete examination by an ophthalmologist during the first trimester. Subsequent examinations or referral for treatment should be determined by the presence and severity of retinopathy at the initial examination, but the minimum recommendation is examination every three months until parturition. This recommendation does not apply to women with gestational diabetes, who rarely develop DR during pregnancy. Patients with macular edema, severe nonproliferative retinopathy, or proliferative retinopathy should be closely followed by an ophthalmologist experienced in managing DR.

DIFFERENTIAL DIAGNOSIS

The differential diagnosis of diabetic retinopathy is listed in Box 16-1.

TREATMENT

Medical Therapy

The ETDRS reported that aspirin, 650 mg daily, does not influence the progression of retinopathy, affect

Box 16-1 Differential Diagnosis of Diabetic Retinopathy

- Hypertensive retinopathy
- Retinal venous obstruction: central retinal vein occlusion, branch retinal vein occlusion
- Anemia of chronic disease
- Leukemia
- Radiation retinopathy
- Sickle cell retinopathy
- Coats' disease
- Ocular ischemic syndrome
- Age-related macular degeneration

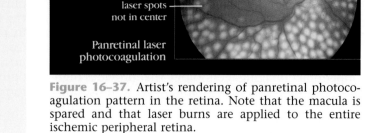

Figure 16–37. Artist's rendering of panretinal photocoagulation pattern in the retina. Note that the macula is spared and that laser burns are applied to the entire ischemic peripheral retina.

visual acuity, or influence the incidence of vitreous hemorrhages.[28] However, there was a significant decrease in cardiovascular morbidity in the aspirin-treated group compared with the placebo cohort.[28] Ticlopidine (Ticlid), like aspirin, inhibits adenosine diphosphate-induced platelet aggregation.[28] It has been shown to decrease the risk of stroke in patients with transient ischemic attacks, but there is no clear evidence showing an impact on diabetic retinopathy.

Surgical Therapy

Panretinal Photocoagulation

Photocoagulation is the primary treatment for proliferative diabetic retinopathy. Its efficacy was demonstrated in the Diabetic Retinopathy Study. The study proved that argon laser PRP significantly decreases the likelihood that an eye with high-risk characteristics will progress to severe visual loss.[29] High-risk characteristics are neovascularization in the eye, neovascularization on the optic nerve head (NVD), NVD covering one fourth to one third of the disc, and neovascularization elsewhere (NVE). Eyes with three or more high-risk factors should be considered for PRP. Any eyes with high-risk characteristics and with vitreous or preretinal hemorrhage need an immediate PRP (Figs. 16–37 and 16–38).

Vitrectomy in Diabetic Patients

Failure of laser therapy to stop new vessel proliferation can result in severe visual impairment due to extensive vitreous hemorrhage and subsequent fibrous contraction of mature collagen. The neovascularization contracts, causing a traction retinal detachment. Vitrectomy plays a vital role in the management of the severe complications of proliferative diabetic retinopathy. The major indications are nonclearing vitreous hemorrhage, macular-involving or macular-threatening tractional retinal detachment, and combined tractional-rhegmatogenous retinal detachment. Less-common indications are macular edema with a thickened and taut posterior hyaloid, epiretinal membrane, and severe pre-

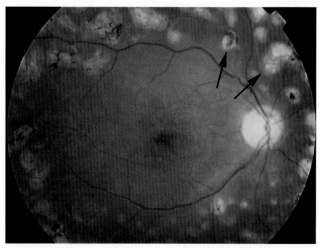

Figure 16–38. Retinal fundus photograph of panretinal photocoagulation scars applied as described in text. (Photo courtesy of James LeBlanc, Tulane University Hospital and Clinic.)

retinal macular hemorrhage. A relative indication is neovascular glaucoma with cloudy media.[32]

To evaluate whether early vitrectomy (in the absence of vitreous hemorrhage) might improve the visual prognosis by eliminating the possibility of later tractional macular detachment, the Diabetic Retinopathy Vitrectomy Study (DRVS) randomized 370 eyes with florid neovascularization and visual acuity of 20/400 or better to either early vitrectomy or to observation. This study was designed to ascertain which patients benefit most from vitrectomy. Patients with a recent and severe vitreous hemorrhage obstructing vision in one eye, particularly when there was already poor vision in the other eye had good benefit because vitrectomy sped up the rate of visual recovery and allowed these patients to function sooner. Patients with severe (high-risk) fibrovascular scar tissue due to PDR also had good benefit, even with good vision in the affected eye. In both these instances, vitrectomy resulted in better vision on the eye chart at 2 and 4 years of follow-up (Fig. 16–39).[33]

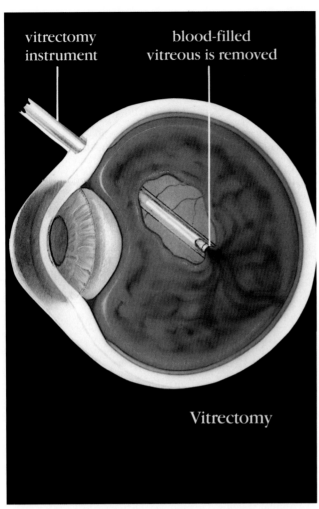

vitrectomy instrument

blood-filled vitreous is removed

Vitrectomy

Figure 16–39. Artist's rendering of vitrectomy performed to clear hemorrhage from the vitreous cavity.

Treatment of Macular Edema

The ETDRS defined clinically significant macular edema as:

- Retinal thickening involving the center of the macula
- Hard exudates within 500 μm of the center of the macula (if associated with retinal thickening)
- An area of macular edema greater than one disc area within one disc diameter of the center of the macula

The Diabetic Retinopathy Study and the ETDRS conclusively proved that timely focal laser photocoagulation of diabetic macular edema can reduce severe visual loss by 95%.[30] The goal of laser treatment is to help prevent moderate visual loss. From a cost-effectiveness point of view, ETDRS-style therapy saves an estimated $250 million to $500 million per year in the United States by enabling patients to avoid relying on disability or welfare support and to continue productive employment. Nevertheless, fully one half of Americans with diabetes do not receive annual eye examinations that include dilation.[31] This is despite a 6-year campaign by the AAO, called Diabetes 2000, to educate primary care physicians about the benefits of such screening.

CONCLUSION

Diabetic retinopathy afflicts the majority of patients with type 1 and type 2 diabetes over the course of a lifetime. Early detection and control of this disease process is essential for maintaining vision in these patients. Intensive systemic control of serum glucose levels is the central preventive treatment for these patients; without it, most ophthalmic treatments are insufficient. However, advances in the ocular detection, staging, and treatment of diabetic retinopathy in concert with systemic glucose control have greatly improved visual acuity outcomes in these patients.

Patients with type 1 diabetes should be referred to a general ophthalmologist or retinologist within 5 years of initial diagnosis or at onset of puberty. Patients with type 2 diabetes should be referred at the time of initial diagnosis, because they may manifest diabetic retinopathy at diagnosis. Through appropriate follow-up of mild to moderate nonproliferative diabetic retinopathy, many patients can receive sight-saving treatment without delay, as the systemic disease progresses in severity. Moreover, subtle macular edema can be detected and treated earlier in many diabetic patients before any substantial vision loss occurs if the patient is receiving regular ophthalmic follow-up.

Even patients manifesting proliferative diabetic retinopathy can be treated successfully with aggressive panretinal photocoagulation and operative procedures. Such treatments can often halt the progression of diabetic retinopathy and its sequelae, preventing any further loss of visual function.

The main emphasis for the prevention and treatment of diabetic retinopathy is frequent follow-up by the primary care physician or endocrinologist to facilitate intensive glycemic control. However, ophthalmic follow-up is critical to ensure that early stages of diabetic retinopathy are monitored and that treatment is administered at critical stages of disease progression.

References

1. Javitt, JC, Canner, JK, Frank, RG, et al: Detecting and treating retinopathy in patients with type 1 diabetes mellitus. Ophthalmology 97:483-494, 1990.
2. The Diabetes Control and Complications Trial Research Group: The effect of intensive treatment of diabetes on the development and progression of long-term complications in insulin-dependent diabetes mellitus. N Engl J Med 329:977-986, 1993.
3. Malone, JI, Morrison, AD, Pavan, PR, Cuthbertson, DD: Prevalence and significance of retinopathy in subjects with type 1 diabetes of less than 5 years' duration screened for the

Diabetes Control and Complications Trial. Diabetes Care 24:522-526, 2001.

4. Klein, R, Klein, BE: Vision disorders in diabetes. In Harris, MI, Hamman, RF (eds): Diabetes in America (DHHS publication number 85-1468). Washington, DC, United States Government Printing Office, 1985, p 1.

5. Klein, R, Klein, BE, Moss, SE, Cruickshanks, KJ: Association of ocular disease and mortality in a diabetic population. Arch Ophthalmol 117:1487-1495, 1999.

6. Klein R, Klein B, Moss S, et al: The Wisconsin epidemiologic study of diabetic retinopathy. XIV. Ten-year incidence and progression of diabetic retinopathy. Arch Ophthalmol 112:1217-1228, 1994.

7. Rosenn B, Miodovnik M, Kranias G, et al: Progression of diabetic retinopathy in pregnancy: Association with hypertension in pregnancy. Am J Obstet Gynecol 166:1214-1218, 1992.

8. Frank, RN: On the pathogenesis of diabetic retinopathy: A 1990 update. Ophthalmology 98:586-593, 1991.

9. Frank RN: The aldose reductase controversy. Diabetes. 43:169-172, 1994.

10. Maddux, BA, Sbraccia, P, Kumakura, S, et al: Membrane glycoprotein PC-1 and insulin resistance in non–insulin-dependent diabetes mellitus. Nature 373:448-451, 1995.

11. Karin, M: The AP-1 complex and its role in transcriptional control by protein kinase C. In Cohen, P, Foulkes, JG (eds): Molecular Aspects of Cellular Regulation. New York, Elsevier, 1991, p 235.

12. Pierce E, Foley E, Smith L: Regulation of vascular endothelial growth factor by oxygen in a model of retinopathy of prematurity. Ophthalmology 114:1219-1228, 1996.

13. Aiello L, Avery R, Arrigg P, et al: Vascular endothelial growth factor in ocular fluid of patients with diabetic retinopathy and other retinal disorders. N Engl J Med 331:1480-1487, 1994.

14. Adamis A, Shima D, Tolentino M, et al: Inhibition of VEGF prevents retinal ischemia associated iris neovascularization in non-human primate. Arch Ophthalmol 114:66-71, 1996.

15. Early Treatment Diabetic Retinopathy Study Research Group: Fundus photographic risk factors for progression of diabetic retinopathy. ETDRS Report No. 12. Ophthalmology. 98:823-833, 1991.

16. Early Treatment Diabetic Retinopathy Study Research Group: Early photocoagulation for diabetic retinopathy. ETDRS Report No. 9. Ophthalmology. 98: 766-785, 1991.

17. Schwartz D: Corneal sensitivity in diabetics. Arch Ophthalmol 91:174-178, 1974.

18. Klein B, Klein R, Jensen S: Open-angle glaucoma and older-onset diabetes: the Beaver Dam Eye Study. Ophthalmology. 101:1173-1177, 1994.

19. Jacobson D, Murphy R, Rosenthal A: The treatment of angle neovascularization with panretinal photocoagulation. Ophthalmology 86:1270-1275, 1979.

20. Bernth-Peterson P, Bach E: Epidemiologic aspects of cataract surgery. III: Frequencies of diabetes and glaucoma in a cataract population. Acta Ophthalmol 61:406-416, 1983.

21. Krupsky S, Zalish M, Oliver M, et al: Anterior segment complications in diabetic patients following extracapsular cataract extraction and posterior chamber intraocular lens implantation. Ophthalmic Surg 22:526-530, 1991.

22. Hykin P, Gregson R, Stevens J, et al: Extracapsular cataract extraction in proliferative diabetic retinopathy. Ophthalmology 100:394-399, 1993.

23. Regillo C, Brown G, Savino P, et al: Diabetic papillopathy: Patient characteristics and fundus findings. Arch Ophthalmol 113:889-895, 1995.

24. Burde R: Neuro-ophthalmic associations and complications of diabetes mellitus. Am J Ophthalmol 114:498-501, 1992.

25. American Diabetes Association: Position statement: Diabetic retinopathy. Diabetes Care 24(Suppl 1):S73, 2001.

26. American College of Physicians, American Diabetes Association, American Academy of Ophthalmology: Screening guidelines for diabetic retinopathy. Clinical Guideline. Ophthalmology 99:1626-1627, 1992.

27. Moss, SE, Klein R, Kessler SD, Richie KA: Comparison between ophthalmoscopy and fundus photography in determining severity of diabetic retinopathy. Ophthalmology 92:62-67, 1985.

28. Chew E, Klein M, Murphy R, et al: Effects of aspirin on vitreous/preretinal hemorrhage in patients with diabetes mellitus. ETDRS Report No. 20. Arch Ophthalmol 113:52-55, 1995.

29. Diabetic Retinopathy Study Research Group: Four risk factors for severe visual loss in diabetic retinopathy: The third report from the Diabetic Retinopathy Study. Arch Ophthalmol 97:654-665, 1979.

30. Ferris F: How effective are treatments for diabetic retinopathy? JAMA 269:1290-1291, 1993.

31. Javitt, JC, Aiello, LP, Chiang, Y, et al: Preventive eye care in people with diabetes is cost saving to the federal government. Implications for health-care reform. Diabetes Care 17:909-917, 1994.

32. Lewis H, Abrams G, Blumenkranz M, et al: Vitrectomy for diabetic macular traction and edema associated with posterior hyaloidal traction. Ophthalmology. 99:753-759, 1992.

33. Diabetic Retinopathy Vitrectomy Study Research Group: Early vitrectomy for severe proliferative diabetic retinopathy in eyes with useful vision. Results of a randomized trial—Diabetic Retinopathy Vitrectomy Study Report 3. Ophthalmology 95:1307-1320, 1988.

34. Peterson CA, Delamere NA: The lens. In Hart WM (ed): Adler's Physiology of the Eye. 2nd ed. St Louis, Mosby–Year Book, 1992, pp 361-381.

35. Gass JDM: Stereoscopic Atlas of Macular Diseases: Diagnosis and Treatment, 4th ed. St Louis, Mosby, 1997, p 4.

36. Heier JS, Sy JP, McCluskey E: RhuFabV2 (anti-VEGF-antibody) for treatment of exudative AMD. Program and abstracts of the American Academy of Ophthalmology 2002 Annual Meeting, Orlando, Fla, October 20-23, 2002.

37. Slakter J, Singerman L, Yanuzzi L, et al: Anecortave acetate administered as posterior juxtascleral injection in patients with subfoveal choroidal neovascularization. Program and abstracts of the American Academy of Ophthalmology 2002 Annual Meeting, Orlando, Fla, October 20-23, 2002.

38. Vlassara, H: Protein glycation in the kidney: Role in diabetes and aging. Kidney Int 49:1795-1804, 1996.

39. Brownlee, M: Glycation and diabetic complications. Lilly Lecture 1993. Diabetes 43:836-841, 1994.

40. Makita, Z, Radoff, S, Rayfield, EJ, et al: Advanced glycosylation end products in patients with diabetic nephropathy. N Engl J Med 325:836-842, 1991.

41. Rho DS: Treatment of acute pseudophakic cystoid macular edema: Diclofenac versus ketorolac. J Cataract Refract Surg 29:2378-2384, 2003.

42. Massin P, Audren F, Haouchine B, et al: Intravitreal triamcinolone acetonide for diabetic diffuse macular edema: Preliminary results of a prospective controlled trial. Ophthalmology 111:218-224, 2004; discussion 224-225.

43. Minami M, Satoh M: Chemokines and their receptors in the brain: Pathophysiological roles in ischemic brain injury. Life Sci 74:321-327, 2003.

44. Eyetech Pharmaceuticals: http://www.eyetk.com/clinical/clinical_index.asp.

Diagnostic Testing for Coronary Artery Disease in Diabetic Patients

Paolo Raggi, Orlando Deffer, and Leslee J. Shaw

KEY POINTS

- *Coronary artery disease remains asymptomatic in diabetic patients for several years and is often in advanced stages of development by the time it is discovered.*
- *Asymptomatic diabetic patients have the same cardiovascular risk as do nondiabetic subjects with known coronary artery disease, and diabetic patients have a poorer prognosis once a primary event has occurred.*
- *For cardiovascular disease, the mortality rate for diabetic patients has not declined, but the mortality rate for the general population has. Thus aggressive medical prevention and early detection of coronary artery disease are needed in the diabetic population.*
- *Imaging tests to diagnose obstructive coronary artery disease are very useful for risk stratifying diabetic patients. More frequent retesting should be considered in diabetic patients than in nondiabetic patients.*

SCOPE OF THE PROBLEM

Diabetes mellitus continues to run rampant throughout the world. A sedentary lifestyle and the increasing age and obesity of the population are the main culprits for an escalation in the prevalence of this disease.[1,2] In 1995, the prevalence of diabetes in the United States in adults older than 20 years was estimated to be 4%. Today 6.3% of the population is estimated to suffer from diabetes, and approximately 90% of diabetic patients have type 2 diabetes. As many as 5.2 million persons are not aware they have the disease.[3-5] Additionally, diabetes is diagnosed in about 1.3 million people aged 20 years or older every year.[3] As a result, the lifetime risk of diabetes for a 65-year-old is in the range of 15% to 30%, and the risk is higher in nonwhite populations. However, for men, the risk of diabetes accelerates beginning at age 40, while for women the risk accelerates beyond 30 years of age.[6]

Diabetes has long been recognized as an independent risk factor for cardiovascular disease (CVD). Epidemiologic studies, such as the Framingham, Honolulu, and San Antonio Heart Studies, have documented the excess CVD risk in patients affected by diabetes mellitus for many racial and ethnic groups.[4] The adverse influence of diabetes extends to all components of the cardiovascular system—the microvasculature and larger arteries, as well as the heart and kidneys—leading to frequent microvascular and macrovascular complications.[7] Microvascular and macrovascular complications start with the onset of hyperglycemia in the prediabetic phase of the disease (the "ticking clock" hypothesis).[7] As a result, it is estimated that the total (indirect and direct) annual cost in the United States for diabetes and its complications approaches $132 billion.[8]

Diabetic patients have a poorer prognosis than nondiabetic persons once a primary event has occurred. In fact, after suffering a first myocardial infarction (MI), diabetic patients have more frequent recurrent events and die from sudden death more often than nondiabetic patients.[9] Similarly, after a percutaneous coronary angioplasty, diabetic patients require recurrent procedures more often and suffer a myocardial infarction or die of myocardial infarction more often than nondiabetic subjects.[10-12] Mortality from coronary heart disease in diabetic patients has not decreased, even while such a trend has been recorded in the general population in the past several decades.[13] Hence, aggressive primary prevention of atherosclerotic heart disease and early detection of coronary artery disease (CAD) may be the only hope to improve survival in these patients.

The National Institutes of Health (NIH), through programs of the National Heart Lung and Blood Institute (NHLBI) and the National Institute of Diabetes and Digestive and Kidney Diseases, have noted the special risk of cardiovascular disease among diabetic patients in guidelines and educational programs.[2] The American Diabetes Association (ADA) and the Juvenile Diabetes Foundation International have long emphasized the importance of identifying and implementing interven-

tions to help diabetic patients reduce their risk of cardiovascular disease.[2] The growing importance of diabetes as a cause of CVD has led the American Heart Association (AHA) to formally designate diabetes a major risk factor for CVD[2] and the National Cholesterol Education Program III to name diabetes a cardiovascular disease risk equivalent.[14]

The diagnosis of CAD remains a difficult task, especially in its early and preclinical phases, when the disease may be more amenable to successful control. Hence, it is imperative to understand the utility of ancillary tests to assess the prevalence and extent of CAD. In this chapter, we discuss the current use of imaging techniques for diagnosing CAD in diabetes mellitus.

COMPUTED TOMOGRAPHY FOR CORONARY ARTERY CALCIUM SCREENING

Technical Considerations

Traditional noninvasive imaging methods used to diagnose the presence of CAD (electrocardiographic stress testing with and without imaging) are germane to the diagnosis of obstructive luminal disease, with very important consequences for revascularization therapy. However, the presence of an extensive atherosclerotic plaque burden in the vessel wall, even in the absence of obstructive disease, is responsible for the majority of acute coronary events.[15,16] Hence, there is an emerging interest in diagnosing atherosclerosis prior to the development of symptoms of CAD.

Cardiac computed tomography has been used to measure the extent of coronary artery calcium (Fig. 17–1) in asymptomatic and symptomatic patients with the intent of identifying subjects at increased risk of suffering a cardiac event. Calcium is deposited in the atherosclerotic plaque from its inception and grows in parallel with the growth of the plaque.[17] The deposition of calcium and phosphorus in the form of hydroxyapatite crystals is not due to a mere precipitation of crystals but occurs under the control of active processes of calcification similar to bone formation.[18-20] The processes are governed by vascular cells that turn into osteoblast-like cells and use enzymes normally found in healthy bone and necessary for the normal process of remodeling of bone.[20] The initiating event of such a cascade is not known, though multiple noxious stimuli (oxidized lipids, inflammatory mediators, hyperphosphatemia, vitamin D, end-products of glycation, etc.) are capable of inducing a phenotypic transformation of vascular smooth muscle cells to noncontractile and bonelike cells.[21-29]

Calcium accumulation in the coronary arteries can be detected by means of radiologic techniques such as plain X-rays and fluoroscopy. These tech-

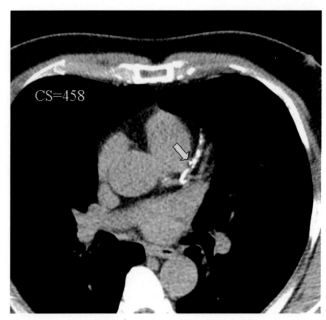

Figure 17–1. Cross-sectional image of the chest in a subject with dense calcification of the left anterior descending coronary artery indicated by the *yellow arrow.* CS, calcium score.

niques, however, do not allow a precise quantification of the calcium load. The calcium load can instead be calculated with computerized tomography technologies using high imaging speed. The speed of imaging is necessary to prevent image blurring due to continuous cardiac motion. The first CT developed for this purpose was the electron beam tomography (EBT) scanner (Fig. 17–2), followed more recently by spiral CT with simultaneous acquisition of multiple slices. In either case the extent of calcification is measured by means of a calcium score calculated by the computer software on the basis of plaque size and density.[30]

There is a relationship between calcium score and coronary artery lumen stenosis defined by angiography, with a greater likelihood of stenosis as the calcium score increases.[31-34] Nonetheless, this relationship is only modest ($r = \sim 50\%$), and the use of coronary calcium screening for predicting coronary artery stenosis cannot be recommended at this time. However, the main purpose of calcium screening is not to identify patients in need of revascularization but to detect vessel wall atherosclerosis. Indeed, the latter purpose may be as important as the former in that many acute coronary events occur on the basis of nonobstructive disease.[15,16]

Clinical Applications

There are now sufficient data showing the utility of coronary artery calcium (CAC) screening in nondiabetic populations. Indeed, in such populations the presence of CAC poses a significantly increased risk

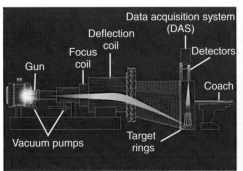
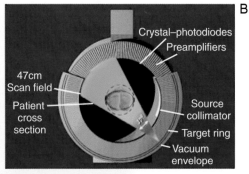
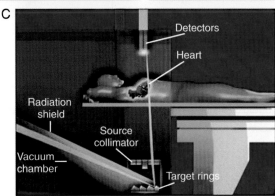

Figure 17–2. Schematic representation of an electron beam computed tomography scanner. **A,** A stationary source emits a beam of electrons. **B,** The beam impacts a tungsten ring lying below the patient, and a fan of X-rays is issued and accelerated along an arc of 210°. **C,** The patient holds his breath for 20 to 30 seconds and is moved in small increments (3 mm) through the fan.

of events proportional to the extent of calcification, and it adds incremental prognostic value to traditional risk factors for predicting hard cardiovascular events.[35-37] Whether screening for CAC could be useful in risk stratifying patients with diabetes mellitus is still being investigated, though evidence is accumulating.

Patients suffering from diabetes mellitus type 2 have been shown to harbor larger amounts of CAC than nondiabetic patients of similar age and with a similar risk factor profile.[38] Furthermore, the amount of CAC in patients with diabetes type 2 is similar to that of patients with established CAD but without diabetes, confirming the evidence provided by clinical data.[39] Finally, diabetic women harbor as much CAC as diabetic men, again confirming the clinical evidence that diabetes mellitus negates the well-known advantage of women over men in prevalence and extent of atherosclerosis.[40,41] Hoff and colleagues[42] used a large database to calculate the age and gender normative (percentile) distribution of calcium scores in asymptomatic (self-reported) diabetic patients. They showed that younger diabetic patients have a plaque burden comparable to that of older nondiabetic persons. It appears, therefore, that CAC mimics the epidemiology of CAD and tracks the pathologic findings of this disease.

Olson and coworkers[43] investigated the presence of CAC as well as the association with a history of CAD in patients with diabetes mellitus type 1. They recruited 302 subjects (146 men and 156 women) with a history of MI, angina, or evidence of ischemia on stress testing or surface electrocardio-

grams. Patients were participants in the Pittsburgh Epidemiology of Diabetes Complications (EDC) study, a 10-year prospective follow-up study of risk factors for complications of type 1 diabetes diagnosed before the age of 17. EBT imaging showed that the prevalence of CAC clearly increased with age (from 11% before age 30 to 88% in patients aged 50 to 55 years or older). CAC was detected in all patients 50 years and older with established CAD. Of the subjects who were free of clinical CAD, 5% had a CAC score higher than 400 (indicative of a large atherosclerosis burden),[31] as did 25% of subjects with angina and ischemia and 80% of patients with myocardial infarction or luminal stenosis. CAC showed a sensitivity of 84% and 71% for clinical CAD in men and women, respectively, and 100% sensitivity for MI or obstructive CAD. In multivariable regression analyses CAC was independently correlated with MI or obstructive CAD in both sexes and was the strongest independent correlate in men. This study, therefore, indicated that coronary calcium detected by EBT is strongly correlated with CAD in type 1 diabetes mellitus, particularly in men.

In the Coronary Artery Calcification in Type 1 Diabetes (CACTI) study,[44] type 1 diabetic subjects showed a high prevalence and severity of CAC, again with a disappearance of the known difference between men and women. The authors suggested that insulin resistance, associated with an android deposition of fat, may be somehow related to the increased prevalence of CAC in women with type 1 diabetes mellitus. According to Colhoun et al, the increased prevalence of CAC in women affected by

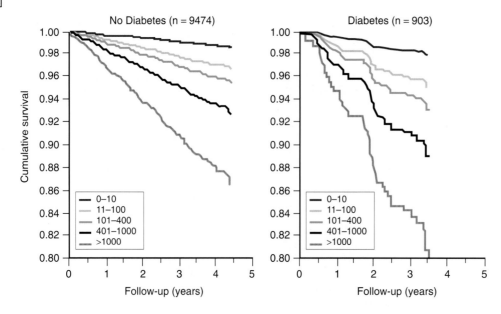

Figure 17–3. Survival curves in diabetic and non-diabetic subjects according to baseline coronary calcium score. Survival is lower in diabetic subjects at all levels of calcification but it is similar in all subjects with no or very low calcium amounts independent of the diagnosis of diabetes mellitus. This suggests that there is a great heterogeneity in risk among diabetic patients.

type 1 diabetes mellitus is not associated with traditional risk factors for atherosclerosis or the size and concentration of lipoproteins, but it may be related to the extent of inflammation.[45]

Few data exist on outcome related to CAC in diabetic patients. The potential impact of CAC as a predictor of events was analyzed in a small study by Hosoi and colleagues.[46] The authors studied a cohort of 101 diabetic and 181 nondiabetic patients who presented to the emergency department with angina pectoris and electrocardiographic findings suggestive of myocardial ischemia. Coronary angiography was performed in all patients, and EBT imaging was performed within 2 weeks of angiography. Among subjects without coronary luminal stenoses, diabetic patients showed more extensive CAC than nondiabetic subjects. In contrast, no significant difference in CAC burden was found between diabetic and nondiabetic patients in the presence of coronary luminal obstruction. A calcium score higher than 90 was associated with an equal sensitivity and specificity of 75% for coronary obstruction in diabetic patients, and a calcium score higher than 200 was associated with a sensitivity of 64% and a specificity of 83%. The authors concluded that CAC in symptomatic diabetic subjects is associated with the severity of coronary stenosis and the potential need for revascularization.

Two studies addressed the question of whether CAC constitutes a risk for events in asymptomatic patients but came to opposite conclusions. The South Bay Heart Watch was a prospective cohort study designed to determine the relation between radiographically detectable CAC and cardiovascular outcome in high-risk asymptomatic adults.[47] Researchers used mass mailing advertisements to recruit 1312 asymptomatic subjects older than 45 years with cardiac risk factors in the Los Angeles area; of these, 19% were diabetic patients. In a subanalysis of the main database after a mean follow-up of 6 years, Qu and coworkers[47] found an increased risk of cardiovascular events (death, myocardial infarction, stroke, and revascularizations) in diabetic patients compared to nondiabetic subjects in the presence of CAC. However, the risk did not increase as the calcium score increased.

These findings were in contrast with those published by another group. Raggi and colleagues[48] used data from a database of 10,377 asymptomatic subjects (903 diabetic patients), followed for an average of 5 years after having been referred by a primary care physician for an EBT screening for CAC. The primary end-point of the study was all-cause mortality. In this study, the risk of all-cause mortality was higher in diabetic patients than in nondiabetic subjects for any degree of calcification, and the risk increased as the calcium score increased (Fig. 17–3). Additionally, the absence of CAC predicted a low short-term risk of death (~1% at 5 years) for diabetic patients as well as subjects without diabetes. Hence, both the presence and absence of CAC were important modifiers of risk even in the presence of established risk factors for atherosclerosis such as diabetes mellitus. This suggests that there is a great heterogeneity among diabetes mellitus patients as well as any other risk cohort and that an evaluation of risk based on atherosclerosis visualization may be of benefit even in apparently high-risk persons.

The results presented by Raggi's group compare well with those reported by Giri and colleagues[49] in diabetic patients submitted to single-photon emission computed tomography (SPECT) testing. These investigators demonstrated that with increasing severity of myocardial perfusion abnormality, diabetic patients suffer an increasingly worse prognosis. Therefore, the presence of disease in the

vessel wall may be as serious a prognostic factor as obstructive luminal disease. However, in the study by Giri's group,[49] diabetic patients with a normal perfusion stress test had a fourfold higher morbidity and mortality during follow-up than nondiabetic subjects with normal stress nuclear scans, whereas in the study by Raggi's group,[48] patients with no or minimal CAC had the same outcome independent of the presence of diabetes.

Hence, an approach to the diagnosis of coronary artery disease that combines different techniques may be very helpful to the practicing physician faced with the dilemma of accurate patient risk assessment.

STRESS ECHOCARDIOGRAPHY

Technical Considerations

Both stress echocardiography and stress nuclear testing are highly sensitive tools for detecting obstructive CAD. Stress testing can be performed either on a treadmill or a bicycle ergometer or by means of pharmacologic agents. Because diabetic patients may be unable to exercise, pharmacologic stress echocardiography offers a commonly employed, safe, and sensitive alternative.[50] Vasodilator stress echocardiography testing with dipyridamole or adenosine is employed less often, although the results are reported to be similar to those obtained with the inotropic agent dobutamine.[51,52]

With vasodilative agents, the purpose is to induce a myocardial blood flow maldistribution favoring territories perfused by patent coronary arteries capable of vasodilation in response to pharmacologic stimulation. With inotropic agents, instead, perfusion abnormalities are induced by increasing oxygen demand due to increased heart rate and cardiac contractility, therefore inducing true ischemia in segments of the myocardium perfused by stenosed coronary arteries. Myocardial ischemia is considered present when stress induces segmental wall motion abnormalities, such as new or worsening hypokinesia, akinesia, or dyskinesia, develop during or soon after stress compared to baseline images (Figs. 17–4 and 17–5). Induction of abnormal wall motion is an appropriate method for assessing ischemia, because systolic and diastolic left ventricular dysfunction occur sooner than either chest pain or EKG changes in the cascade of ischemic events.

Due to poor acoustic windows, patient habitus, excessive respiratory motion artifacts, and limited technical experience of the operator, about 5% to 10% of the stress echocardiography tests are nondiagnostic. In comparison, the nondiagnostic rate with stress nuclear testing varies between 1% and 2%. However, stress echocardiography offers the advantage of easy portability, lower cost, and no radiation exposure compared with nuclear stress testing.

Clinical Applications

The diagnostic accuracy for obstructive CAD of stress echocardiography in diabetic patients is similar to that reported in nondiabetic subjects. Perfornis and coworkers[53] tested 56 asymptomatic subjects with electrocardiographic stress testing, dobutamine stress echocardiography (DSE), and exercise thallium-201 SPECT. All patients had a long history of diabetes (more than 15 years for 10 type 1 diabetic patients and more than 5 years for 46 type 2 diabetic patients) and carried at least three other risk factors for coronary artery disease, but they had no resting electrocardiographic abnormalities. Coronary angiography was performed on 26 patients with abnormal results on noninvasive testing, and 17 subjects demonstrated obstructive coronary luminal disease. The authors reported a positive predictive value for DSE, SPECT, and exercise electrocardiography of 69%, 75%, and 60%, respectively, for predicting obstructive CAD. Hence, DSE and SPECT demonstrated similar, albeit not excellent, diagnostic capabilities, and both were superior to electrocardiographic stress testing.

In a multicenter study,[54] 937 predominantly type 2 diabetic patients underwent exercise stress echocardiography or DSE for evaluation of known or suspected CAD. The primary end-point was all-cause mortality. Diabetic patients with resting or stress-induced wall motion abnormalities demonstrated very high mortality, and this was true for patients with and without prior CAD. Death during follow-up occurred in 115 of 232 patients (50%) who had exercise-induced wall motion abnormalities (i.e., ischemia), as well as 123 of 275 (45%) of those with resting left ventricular dysfunction (Fig. 17–6). In multivariable models, the strongest predictor of mortality was a referral for pharmacologic stress testing rather than exercise stress echocardiography, followed by the demonstration of ischemia during stress, presence of heart failure, and age. Hence, inability to exercise was an important predictor of a negative outcome. If the type of test performed was ignored in the statistical model, inducible ischemia and resting left ventricular dysfunction became the best predictors of a negative outcome followed by age.

The authors demonstrated that the presence of inducible ischemia on a stress echocardiogram adds incremental prognostic information for the prediction of all-cause death to a model based on clinical factors alone (age, heart failure, previous myocardial infarction, and referral for pharmacologic stress test). Similar information was reported in other studies that examined the value of stress echocardiography both for the prediction of all-cause mortality and more-specific cardiovascular events.[52,55-57]

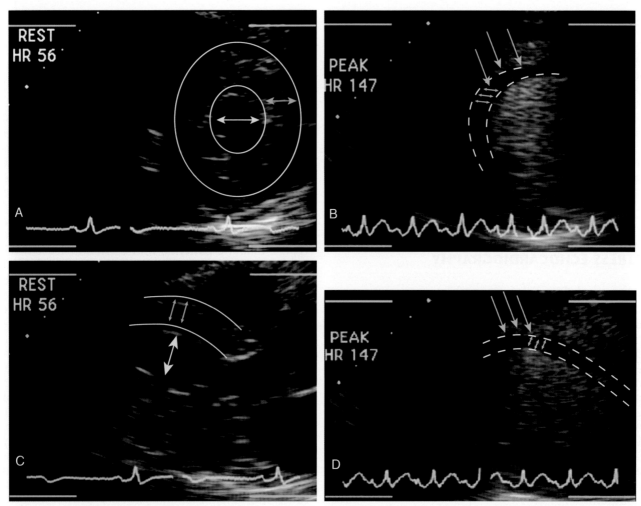

Figure 17–4. Echocardiographic systolic frames at rest (**A** and **C**) and after exercise (**B** and **D**) in a patient complaining of chest pain. The images in **A** and **B** were obtained in the short axis, and the images in **C** and **D** in the long axis parasternal view. There is an obvious area of dyskinesia (bulging) in the anterior wall of the left ventricle indicated by the *green arrows* and the *broken lines* in **B** and **D**. These segments were moving normally during the resting phase of the test (**A** and **C**). During the ischemic phase, the walls of the left ventricle do not contract and thicken as much as at rest. This is demonstrated by the *blue bidirectional arrows* in **A** through **D**. The *yellow bidirectional arrows* in **A** and **C** demonstrate that the left ventricular cavity is small at rest but it enlarges during the ischemic phase. Therefore ischemia is identified by the following three criteria: abnormal wall motion, abnormal wall thickening, and cavity enlargement.

Marwick[54] and other investigators[58] demonstrated that the mortality rate for patients with a negative stress echocardiogram averaged 4% per year in the first 5 years of follow-up. This is a much higher rate than that for nondiabetic subjects with a negative stress echocardiogram (~1% per year).

Two notations should be made with regard to this important observation. First, as was the case for the patients with a positive stress test result, the strongest predictor of death in diabetic subjects with a negative stress test was a physician referral for pharmacologic rather than exercise stress test, again underlining the importance of limited exercise tolerance in the prognosis of diabetic patients with suspected obstructive CAD. Further, the greater event rate in the presence of a negative stress

echocardiogram for diabetic than for nondiabetic subjects is probably related to the large number of comorbidities and the greater deconditioning demonstrated by diabetic patients, and it underlines the importance of not relying solely on tests for obstructive CAD to fully appreciate risk in diabetic patients. Techniques employed to directly visualize the atherosclerotic plaque burden could offer an opportunity to refine risk stratification in these patients and need to be further studied.

Stress echocardiography has also been employed for purposes other than diagnosing CAD in the diabetic population. It appears to constitute an optimal risk-stratification screening test prior to intra-abdominal organ transplant in diabetic subjects,[59] it can be used to exclude restenosis after the perfor-

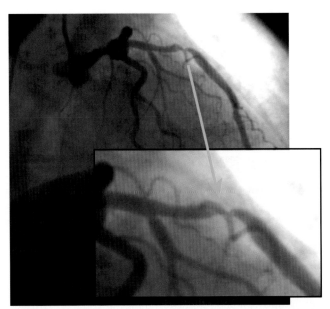

Figure 17–5. Coronary angiogram of the patient in Figure 17-4 showing a high-grade stenosis of the proximal left anterior descending coronary artery. The inset shows a magnification of the stenotic area *(arrow)*.

mance of coronary angioplasty,[60] and it provides accurate information on residual myocardial viability after myocardial infarction.[61,62]

Stress echocardiography is a safe, sensitive, and broadly available technique that can be employed without risk in a repetitive fashion in diabetic patients as an aid in the management of CAD. Furthermore, in spite of a slightly lower sensitivity compared to stress nuclear testing, stress echocardiography demonstrates a specificity superior to nuclear techniques with a smaller number of false positive tests and a lower operational and testing cost.

The limitations of stress echocardiography are the need for a highly skilled echocardiographer and adequately trained physician to interpret stress echocardiographic images, and its limited utility in detecting nonobstructive CAD that can constitute a prognostic factor as serious as obstructive disease. The latter is, of course, a limitation of all functional myocardial stress tests that do not provide information on the presence of atherosclerosis in the vessel wall.

NUCLEAR MYOCARDIAL PERFUSION STRESS TESTING

Technical Considerations

Among the different noninvasive tests used to diagnose obstructive CAD, nuclear myocardial perfusion imaging (MPI) has established itself as one of the most useful and informative tools. Obstructive

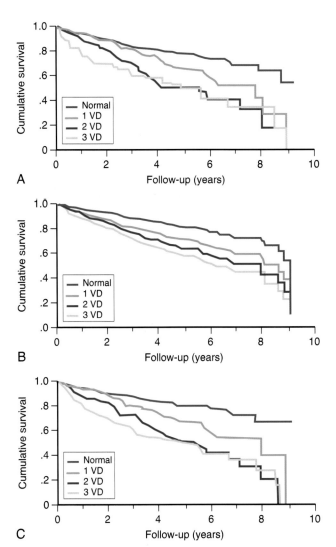

Figure 17–6. Cumulative cardiac survival for diabetic patients undergoing stress echocardiography. Survival is plotted by severity of abnormal wall motion, expressed as the number of involved vascular territories, at rest **(A)**, with stress **(B)**, and in combination **(C)**. VD, vessel disease. (Modified from Marwick TH, Case C, Sawada S, et al: Use of stress echocardiography to predict mortality in patients with diabetes and known or suspected coronary artery disease. Diabetes Care 25:1042-1048, 2002.)

CAD is demonstrated by detecting a reduced uptake of a radiotracer (i.e., a perfusion abnormality) in one or more areas of the myocardium perfused by a coronary artery with a significant (>50%) luminal stenosis (Fig. 17–7).[63] A perfusion defect is typically identified after the performance of a stress test (see Fig. 17–7), and the area of abnormal uptake may partially or completely normalize during subsequent rest imaging (reversible perfusion defect) or persist unchanged (fixed perfusion defect).

Reversible defects indicate ischemia of viable myocardium, whereas a fixed defect typically indicates a prior myocardial infarction and scar. Scoring systems are available to assess the extent and sever-

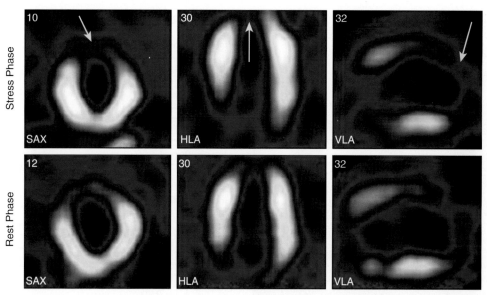

Figure 17–7. Example of single photon emission computed tomography (SPECT) perfusion image of the left ventricular myocardium. There is a moderate to large size defect in the anterior wall and apex of the left ventricle (indicated by the *yellow arrows*) during stress *(top row)*. The defect is partially reversible during rest *(bottom row)*. The tomographic projections are identified by the label in the left lower corner of each image. HLA, horizontal long axis image; SAX, short axis image; VLA, vertical long axis image.

ity of perfusion abnormalities, although in clinical practice sections corresponding to major vascular territories are interpreted for reduced perfusion (i.e., left anterior descending, right coronary, and left circumflex distributions). Recent advances in computer technology have rendered possible the analysis of rest and post-stress left ventricular ejection fraction and wall motion analysis, in combination with assessment of regional myocardial perfusion.[64] This provides a comprehensive examination of the extent and severity of myocardial perfusion and ventricular function.

The most commonly employed radiopharmaceutical agents are thallium-201 and technetium-99m-based tracers (Tc-99m sestamibi or Tc-99m tetrofosmin); each with different pharmacodynamic and pharmacokinetic characteristics. Thallium-201 has a long half-life (~73 hours), has a lower peak emission rate than technetium-99m, and recirculates in and out of viable cells using dynamics and channels similar to those of potassium.[63,65] Due to thallium-201's rapid redistribution, imaging must proceed quickly right after the injection of the tracer at peak exercise to detect stress-induced perfusion defects. Delayed imaging (usually 4 hours from stress imaging) is then performed to verify whether a difference in perfusion (tracer uptake) can be detected between the stress and rest phase in any region of the left ventricular myocardium. Technetium-99m has a higher peak emission and a shorter half-life (~6.5 hours) than thallium-201. It recirculates minimally in and out of viable cells and remains essentially trapped in the location of initial uptake, giving an instantaneous impression of the perfusion status at the time of injection. Due to technetium-99m's lack of redistribution, technetium-99m–based tracers must be injected at peak exercise and reinjected at rest to compare stress and rest images.[63,66]

Nuclear images are reconstructed with either a planar technique, very rarely performed now, or using the SPECT technique (see Fig. 17–7).[63] With SPECT it is possible to segment the left ventricle in several slices oriented along the three planes in space with spatial resolution and diagnostic quality superior to planar imaging.

MPI can be performed after treadmill or bicycle exercise or, as is the case with stress echocardiography, by means of pharmacologic stress agents. Indeed, diabetic patients often demonstrate poor exercise tolerance and are affected by peripheral vascular disease and cardiomyopathy that hinder their ability to achieve an optimal exercise workload. Hence, pharmacologic stress testing is often employed as an alternative to exercise stress testing to risk stratify diabetic patients for CAD.

The most commonly employed pharmacologic stress agents used with MPI are vasodilative agents (dipyridamole or adenosine),[67] whereas inotropic agents such as dobutamine are employed less frequently. With vasodilative agents, the purpose is to induce a myocardial blood flow maldistribution, favoring territories perfused by patent coronary arteries capable of vasodilation in response to pharmacological stimulation, over territories perfused by a coronary artery with a fixed stenosis.[67] Inotropic agents increase heart rate and contractility, and perfusion abnormalities are created by increasing oxygen demand and inducing ischemia in segments of the myocardium perfused by

stenosed coronary arteries that cannot supply as much oxygen as required to sustain the stress.[68]

Clinical Applications

Coronary artery disease is often silent in diabetes patients and typically in advanced stages of development by the time it manifests.[69] Hence, several investigators have used various forms of stress testing to detect CAD in its silent stages. Abnormal plain electrocardiographic stress tests have been reported in 12% to 31% of asymptomatic diabetic patients.[70-75] The wide variation in test results was likely due to the different criteria used by the investigators to define a positive test. Some authors were able to identify type 2 diabetic men as a variable independently associated with silent ischemia on exercise electrocardiography.[70,71,74] With the introduction of MPI following an electrocardiographic stress test, the fact that about 20% to 25% of asymptomatic diabetic patients suffer from unsuspected coronary artery disease was essentially confirmed.[76,77]

In the DIAD study,[76] 1124 type 2 diabetic patients were enrolled at 14 sites in the United States and Canada. Of the entire cohort, 502 underwent an adenosine-Tc-99m sestamibi stress test and the rest did not. In the imaging cohort, 22% of the subjects showed abnormal MPI results and 1 in every 18 subjects (5.5%) showed a moderate to severe perfusion defect indicative of poor prognosis. Because the entry criteria required an established diagnosis of diabetes type 2, a normal electrocardiogram, and no known CAD, the authors concluded that screening should be considered even in the absence of a minimum of two risk factors as recommended in the consensus statement of the ADA.[78] Indeed, the results of the DIAD trial indicate that silent coronary artery disease would have gone undetected in as many as 41% of type 2 diabetic patients if the ADA recommendations for screening were followed strictly.[78] In the DIAD trial there was no association between the inducibility of perfusion abnormalities and traditional or emerging (such as CRP) risk factors.

Similarly, De Lorenzo's group[77] submitted 180 asymptomatic adult-onset diabetic patients to stress MPI for detection of unsuspected obstructive coronary artery disease. A positive test result was reported in 26% of all subjects. During a follow-up of approximately 2 years, 34 patients suffered cardiac events: 7 cardiac deaths, 6 nonfatal myocardial infarctions, 10 coronary artery bypass surgeries, and 11 percutaneous angioplasties. Male gender and perfusion abnormalities were independent predictors of cardiac events, though inducible myocardial ischemia on MPI also added incremental prognostic value to clinical variables and exercise stress test variables.

Kang and colleagues published two consecutive series[78,79] analyzing the contribution of MPI to the management of CAD in diabetic patients. In the first and smaller series,[78] including 203 diabetic and 260 nondiabetic patients, they demonstrated similar sensitivity and specificity of MPI in diabetic and nondiabetic patients. The sensitivity was high in both patient groups (~90%), although the specificity was only moderate in either group (~50%). In the second series the authors investigated whether MPI adds incremental prognostic information over clinical data for predicting events in 1271 diabetic and 5862 nondiabetic patients. During an average follow-up period of 24 months, diabetic patients suffered almost twice as many hard (myocardial infarction and death) and hard and soft (coronary artery bypass or angioplasty) events as the nondiabetic subjects. Findings on MPI added significantly ($P < 0.001$) to the prognostic value provided by clinical and historical data in both subsets of patients.

A large multicenter study analyzed the value of MPI as a risk-stratification tool in symptomatic diabetic and nondiabetic subjects.[48] Giri and colleagues[48] followed 4755 patients (20% diabetic subjects) for an average of 2.5 years after a baseline MPI. Primary end points were the occurrence of cardiac death and nonfatal myocardial infarction (MI) or the performance of revascularization procedures. An abnormal MPI test was a significant predictor of cardiac death and MI in both diabetic and nondiabetic subjects. Using a simple scoring system reflecting the extent of myocardial ischemia by number of vascular territories, the total number of ischemic territories (ranging from none to three) was associated with a stepwise increment in the death rate of both diabetic and nondiabetic subjects. In diabetic patients, however, even a single vessel ischemia increased the risk of death in a very significant way compared to nondiabetic subjects.

Regardless of risk factors, in diabetic patients the presence of multivessel ischemia was the strongest predictor of total coronary events, whereas the presence of multiple fixed defects was the strongest predictor of cardiac death. The authors further showed that a normal MPI is associated with a very good event-free survival in subjects with and without diabetes in the short range. Nonetheless, the so-called protective effect of a normal MPI study in diabetic patients appeared to expire after about 2 years from the time of testing, when events started occurring very rapidly. Therefore the authors recommended retesting diabetic patients sooner than the rest of the population in the presence of a normal MPI due to faster disease progression. Notably, diabetic women showed the worst outcome for any given extent of reversible myocardial ischemia in this study, and this observation was also made in subsequent studies.

In a more recent single-center study, Berman and colleagues[80] reported on the incremental prognostic value of adenosine stress MPI in 6173 consecutively tested diabetic and nondiabetic patients. For the nondiabetic patients, a normal, mildly abnor-

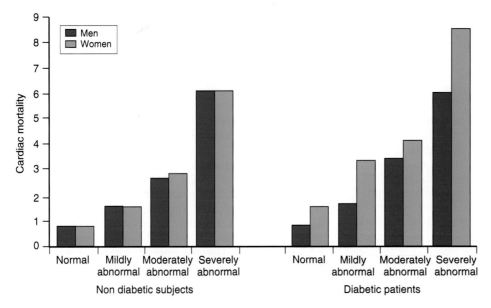

Figure 17–8. Cardiac mortality in diabetic and nondiabetic women and men according to severity of myocardial perfusion defects ranging from low to severely abnormal. (Modified from Berman DS, Kang X, Hayes SW, et al: Adenosine myocardial perfusion single-photon emission computed tomography in women compared with men: Impact of diabetes mellitus on incremental prognostic value and effect on patient management. J Am Coll Cardiol 41:1125-1133, 2003. Reprinted with permission from American College of Cardiology Foundation.)

mal, and moderately to severely abnormal SPECT study was associated with cardiac death rates ranging from 0.8% to 6.1% per year of follow-up. Though event rates were similar for nondiabetic men and women, diabetic women with perfusion defects demonstrated decidedly higher death rates than diabetic men (Fig. 17–8). For diabetic women, event rates were 1.5%, 3.3%, 4.1%, and 8.5% for normal, mildly abnormal, moderately abnormal, and severely abnormal MPI results, respectively (P < 0.0001). By comparison, the event rates ranged from 0.8% to 6% for diabetic men with normal to severely abnormal nuclear scans (P < 0.0001). The higher event rate in diabetic women with provocative ischemia confirmed the results of the previous study by Giri and colleagues.[48]

The reasons for the more unfavorable outcome for diabetic women than men are poorly understood and were recently reviewed in a meta-analysis of this subject (Fig. 17–9).[81] A further interesting finding in the study by Berman's group[80] was that in the presence of a normal MPI the cardiac death rate was higher for insulin-requiring diabetic patients than non–insulin-dependent diabetic patients and, obviously, nondiabetic subjects. Thus, in the setting of a normal MPI the death rate increased from approximately 0.6% for nondiabetic subjects to 1.8% for non–insulin-requiring and to 2.5% for insulin-requiring diabetic patients, respectively. In contrast, in the setting of an abnormal study, the annual cardiac death rates were approximately twofold higher for insulin-dependent diabetic patients as compared with non–insulin-requiring diabetic patients and nondiabetic subjects alike. These findings should alert the clinician to the serious risk posed by diabetes even in the absence of inducible perfusion defects and the need for further investigation of the vascular health status of these patients.

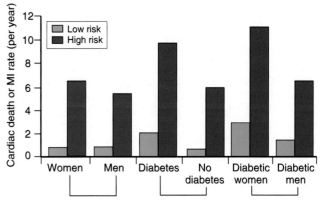

Figure 17–9. Annual risk of cardiac death or myocardial infarction in subjects identified by sex and diabetic status according to the results of a gated single-photon emission computed tomography (SPECT) imaging study. The terms *low risk* and *high risk* relate to the results of the SPECT study; low risk indicates normal perfusion; high risk indicates severely abnormal perfusion defects. As shown, diabetic women with high-risk scans suffered the highest rate of cardiac death and myocardial infarction. MI, myocardial infarction. (Modified from Shaw LJ, Iskandrian AE: Prognostic value of gated myocardial perfusion SPECT. J Nucl Cardiol 11:171-185, 2004.)

CURRENT RECOMMENDATIONS

There are currently almost 16 million patients with known diabetes mellitus in the United States alone. Of these, 3.5 million are known to have CAD. One can expect CAD to become clinically manifest in an additional 1.8 million of these patients each year. Who should be screened among the 12.5 million asymptomatic diabetic patients with subclinical CAD?

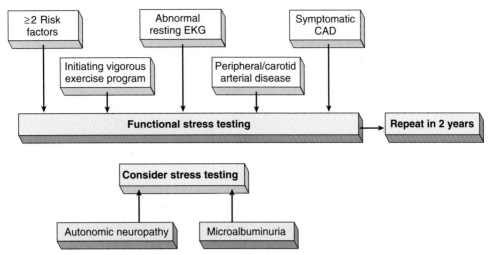

Figure 17–10. Guidelines proposed by the American Diabetes Association on performance of exercise stress testing, with or without an imaging modality associated with it, in diabetic patients. CAD, coronary artery disease; EKG, electrocardiogram. (Modified from American Diabetes Association Consensus development conference on the diagnosis of coronary heart disease in people with diabetes: Miami, Florida. Diabetes Care 21:1551-1559, 1998.)

The current recommendations of the ADA and American College of Cardiology (ACC) are summarized in Figure 17–10.[82] According to the ADA and ACC, exercise stress testing with or without imaging (i.e., functional stress testing) should be recommended in symptomatic patients and in asymptomatic subjects with abnormal resting electrocardiograms, patients with two or more risk factors for CAD, patients with peripheral or carotid arterial disease, and those beginning a vigorous exercise program.[78] Consideration should be given to testing diabetic patients older than age 35 with evidence of autonomic neuropathy and patients with microalbuminuria, because these two markers of disease have been associated with a high risk of cardiovascular events. Similarly, the French Diabetes Association[83] recommends stress testing in patients with peripheral vasculopathy, proteinuria, or multiple risk factors for cardiovascular disease or in patients older than age 65.

Contrary to these recommendations, the AHA recommends in its most recent guidelines against routine testing in asymptomatic diabetic patients.[84] This position was guided by the interpretation of diabetes mellitus as a cardiovascular disease equivalent that mandates aggressive therapy irrespective of findings on noninvasive imaging and the absence of solid data to demonstrate an improved outcome with interventional techniques in asymptomatic diabetic subjects.

CONCLUSIONS

If the current recommendations of the various clinical associations were strictly followed, significant but unsuspected coronary disease in many diabetic patients would remain undiagnosed. Although it is fairly obvious that diabetic patients should be treated very aggressively and considered at very high risk for CAD, each diabetic patient should be considered and treated as an individual patient and not as part of a group, given the heterogeneity among these patients. Indeed, to improve the cardiovascular prognosis it may become necessary to start testing diabetic patients with comorbidities more aggressively despite a normal resting electrocardiogram and absent anginal or anginal-equivalent symptoms. As a guide to choosing the right person to test, one could use clinical indicators of increased risk such as poor exercise tolerance, autonomic dysfunction, microalbuminuria, female sex, and insulin dependence.

Among the available noninvasive tests to diagnose obstructive CAD or derive a prognostic assessment of risk connected with established CAD, both stress echocardiography and SPECT imaging have been shown to be effective and to accurately risk stratify patients in low- to high-risk groups for major adverse events. The extent and severity of perfusion and wall motion abnormalities are at the core of effective risk stratification. A normal stress test confers a good prognosis, though the prognosis is worse than that of a normal stress test in nondiabetic subjects. This fact in addition to the more rapid development of symptoms in diabetic patients (about 2 years) with a normal test indicate the need for diabetic patients to undergo more frequent testing than nondiabetic persons.

The occurrence of a substantial number of events in the presence of a normal stress test raises the question of whether anatomic testing, such as measurement of atherosclerotic plaque burden with EBT or carotid intimal-media thickness (IMT), may improve risk prediction. The role of these tech-

niques is awaiting further clarification. Nonetheless, these methodologies allow a refinement of risk assessment in the general population and may eventually become useful in the diabetic population as well.

Acknowledgement

Dr. Orlando Deffer was partly supported for this work by CRC (Clinical Research Center) grant #5P20RR011104.

References

1. Grundy SM, Benjamin IJ, Burke GL, et al: Diabetes and cardiovascular disease: A statement for healthcare professionals from the American Heart Association. Circulation 100:1134-1146, 1999.
2. Grundy SM, Benjamin IJ, Burke GL, et al: Diabetes mellitus: A major risk factor for cardiovascular disease: A joint editorial statement by the American Diabetes Association; the National Heart, Lung, and Blood Institute; the Juvenile Diabetes Foundation International; the National Institute of Diabetes and Digestive and Kidney Diseases; and the American Heart Association. Circulation 100:1132-1133, 1999.
3. Diabetes Statistics. National Diabetes Information Clearinghouse. Bethesda, MD: National Institute of Diabetes and Digestive and Kidney Diseases, 1999, pp 99-326.
4. Nesto RW, Peter L: Diabetes mellitus and the cardiovascular system. In Braunwald E, Zipes DP, Libby P (eds): Heart Disease: a Textbook of Cardiovascular Medicine. Philadelphia, WB Saunders, 2001, pp 2133-2150.
5. King H, Aubert RE, Herman WH: Global burden of diabetes, 1995-2025: Prevalence, numerical estimates, and projections. Diabetes Care 21:1414-1431, 1998.
6. Venkat Narayan KM, Boyle JP, Thompson TJ, et al: Lifetime risk for diabetes mellitus in the United States. JAMA 290:1884-1890, 2003.
7. Haffner SM, Stern MP, Hazuda HP, et al: Cardiovascular risk factors in confirmed prediabetic individuals. Does the clock for coronary heart disease start ticking before the onset of clinical diabetes? JAMA 263:2893-2898, 1990.
8. American Diabetes Association: Diabetes Statistics. http://www.diabetes.org/diabetes-statistics.jsp. Accessed April 27, 2005.
9. Miettinen H, Lehto S, Veikko S, et al: Impact of diabetes on mortality after the first myocardial infarction. Diabetes Care 21:69-75, 1998.
10. Norhammar A, Malmberg K, Diderholm E, et al: Diabetes mellitus: the major risk factor in unstable coronary artery disease even after consideration of the extent of coronary artery disease and benefits of revascularization. J Am Coll Cardiol 43:585-591, 2004.
11. Mehran R, Dangas GD, Kobayashi Y, et al: Short- and long-term results after multivessel stenting in diabetic patients. J Am Coll Cardiol 43:1348-1354, 2004.
12. The BARI Investigators: Influence of diabetes on 5-year mortality and morbidity in a randomized trial comparing CABG and PTCA in patients with multivessel disease: The Bypass Angioplasty Revascularization Investigation (BARI). Circulation 96:1761-1769, 1997.
13. Gu K, Cowie CC, Harris MI: Diabetes and decline in heart disease mortality in US adults. JAMA 281:1291-1297, 1999.
14. Executive Summary of the Third Report of the National Cholesterol Education Program (NCEP) Expert Panel on Detection, Evaluation, and Treatment of High Blood Cholesterol in Adults (Adult Treatment Panel III). JAMA 285:2486-2489, 2001.
15. Naghavi M, Libby P, Falk E, et al: From vulnerable plaque to vulnerable patient: A call for new definitions and risk assessment strategies: Part I. Circulation 108:1664-1672, 2003.
16. Virmani R, Kolodgie FD, Burke AP, et al: Lessons from sudden coronary death: A comprehensive morphological classification scheme for atherosclerotic lesions. Arterioscler Thromb Vasc Biol 20:1262-1275, 2000.
17. Stary HC: The development of calcium deposits in atherosclerotic lesions and their persistence after lipid regression. Am J Cardiol 88:16E-19E, 2001.
18. Tintut Y, Demer LL: Recent advances in multifactorial regulation of vascular calcification. Curr Opin Lipidol 12:555-560, 2001.
19. Watson KE, Demer LL: The atherosclerosis-calcification link? Curr Opin Lipidol 7:101-104, 1996.
20. Bostrom KI: Cell differentiation in vascular calcification. Z Kardiol 89:69-74, 2000.
21. Parhami F, Basseri B, Hwang J, et al: High-density lipoprotein regulates calcification of vascular cells. Circ Res 91:570-576, 2002.
22. Parhami F, Morrow AD, Balucan J, et al: Lipid oxidation products have opposite effects on calcifying vascular cell and bone cell differentiation. A possible explanation for the paradox of arterial calcification in osteoporotic patients. Arterioscler Thromb Vasc Biol 17:680-687, 1997.
23. Tintut Y, Patel J, Parhami F: Tumor necrosis factor–α promotes in vitro calcification of vascular cells via the cAMP pathway. Circulation 102:2636-2642, 2000.
24. Shioi A, Katagi M, Okuno Y, et al: Induction of bone-type alkaline phosphatase in human vascular smooth muscle cells: roles of tumor necrosis factor–α and oncostatin M derived from macrophages. Circ Res 91:9-16, 2002.
25. Kizu A, Shioi A, Jono S, et al: Statins inhibit in vitro calcification of human vascular smooth muscle cells induced by inflammatory mediators. J Cell Biochem 93:1011-1019, 2004.
26. Jono S, McKee MD, Murry CE, et al: Phosphate regulation of vascular smooth muscle cell calcification. Circ Res 87:E10-17, 2000.
27. Jono S, Nishizawa Y, Shioi A, Morii H: 1,25-Dihydroxyvitamin D_3 increases in vitro vascular calcification by modulating secretion of endogenous parathyroid hormone–related peptide. Circulation 98:1302-1306, 1998.
28. Towler DA, Bidder M, Latifi T, et al: Diet-induced diabetes activates an osteogenic gene regulatory program in the aortas of low density lipoprotein receptor-deficient mice. J Biol Chem 273:27-34, 1998.
29. Mori S, Takemoto M, Yokote K, et al: Hyperglycemia-induced alteration of vascular smooth muscle phenotype. J Diabetes Complications 16:65-68, 2002.
30. Agatston AS, Janowitz AS, Hildner FJ, et al: Quantification of coronary artery calcium using ultrafast computed tomography. J Am Coll Cardiol 15:827-832, 1990.
31. Rumberger JA, Brundage BH, Rader DJ, et al: Electron beam computed tomographic coronary calcium scanning: A review and guidelines for use in asymptomatic persons. Mayo Clin Proc 74:243-252, 1999.
32. Bielak LF, Rumberger JA, Sheedy PF 2nd, et al: Probabilistic model for prediction of angiographically defined obstructive coronary artery disease using electron beam computed tomography calcium score strata. Circulation 102:380-385, 2000.
33. Rumberger JA, Sheedy PF, Breen JF, et al: Electron beam computed tomographic coronary calcium score cutpoints and severity of associated angiographic lumen stenosis. J Am Coll Cardiol 29:1542-1549, 1997.
34. Budoff MJ, Diamond GA, Raggi P, et al: Continuous probabilistic prediction of angiographically significant coronary artery disease using electron beam tomography. Circulation 105:1791-1796, 2002.
35. Raggi P, Callister TQ, Cooil B, et al: Identification of patients at increased risk of first unheralded acute myocardial infarction by electron-beam computed tomography. Circulation 101:850-855, 2000.

36. Shaw LJ, Raggi P, Schisterman E, et al: Prognostic value of cardiac risk factors and coronary artery calcium screening for all-cause mortality. Radiology 228: 826-833, 2003.

37. Greenland P, LaBree L, Azen SP, et al: Coronary artery calcium score combined with Framingham score for risk prediction in asymptomatic individuals. JAMA 29:210-215, 2004.

38. Schurgin S, Rich S, Mazzone T: Increased prevalence of significant coronary artery calcification in patients with diabetes. Diabetes Care 24:335-338, 2001.

39. Haffner SM, Lehto S, Ronnemaa T, et al: Mortality from coronary heart disease in subjects with type 2 diabetes and in nondiabetic subjects with and without prior myocardial infarction. N Engl J Med 339:229-234, 1998.

40. Mielke CH, Shields JP, Broemeling LD: Coronary artery calcium, coronary artery disease, and diabetes. Diabetes Res Clin Pract 53:55-61, 2001.

41. Khaleeli E, Peters SR, Bobrowsky K, et al: Diabetes and the associated incidence of subclinical atherosclerosis and coronary artery disease: Implications for management. Am Heart J 14:637-644, 2001.

42. Hoff JA, Quinn L, Sevrukov A, et al: The prevalence of coronary artery calcium among diabetic individuals without known coronary artery disease. J Am Coll Cardiol 41:1008-1012, 2003.

43. Olson JC, Edmundowicz D, Becker DJ, et al: Coronary calcium in adults with type 1 diabetes: A stronger correlate of clinical coronary artery disease in men than in women. Diabetes 49:1571-1578, 2000.

44. Dabelea D, Kinney G, Snell-Bergeon JK, et al: The Coronary Artery Calcification in Type 1 Diabetes Study. Effect of type 1 diabetes on the gender difference in coronary artery calcification: A role for insulin resistance? The Coronary Artery Calcification in Type 1 Diabetes (CACTI) Study. Diabetes 52:2833-2839, 2003.

45. Colhoun HM, Schalkwijk C, Rubens MB, et al: C-reactive protein in type 1 diabetes and its relationship to coronary artery calcification. Diabetes Care 25:1813-1817, 2002.

46. Hosoi M, Sato T, Yamagami K, et al: Impact of diabetes on coronary stenosis and coronary artery calcification detected by electron-beam computed tomography in symptomatic patients. Diabetes Care 25:696-701, 2002.

47. Qu W, Le TT, Azen SP, et al: Value of coronary artery calcium scanning by computed tomography for predicting coronary heart disease in diabetic subjects. Diabetes Care 26:905-910, 2003.

48. Raggi P, Shaw LJ, Berman DS, et al: Prognostic value of coronary artery calcium screening in subjects with and without diabetes. J Am Coll Cardiol 43:1663-1669, 2004.

49. Giri S, Shaw LJ, Murthy DR, et al: Impact of diabetes on the risk stratification using stress single-photon emission computed tomography myocardial perfusion imaging in patients with symptoms suggestive of coronary artery disease. Circulation 105:32-40, 2002.

50. Elhendy A, van Domburg RT, Poldermans D, et al: Safety and feasibility of dobutamine-atropine stress echocardiography for the diagnosis of coronary artery disease in diabetic patients unable to perform an exercise stress test. Diabetes Care 21:1797-1802, 1998.

51. Gaddi O, Tortorella G, Picano E, et al: Diagnostic and prognostic value of vasodilator stress echocardiography in asymptomatic type 2 diabetic patients with positive exercise thallium scintigraphy: A pilot study. Diabet Med 16:762-766, 1999.

52. Bigi R, Desideri A, Cortigiani L, et al: Stress echocardiography for risk stratification of diabetic patients with known or suspected coronary artery disease. Diabetes Care 24:1596-1601, 2001.

53. Penfornis A, Zimmermann C, Boumal D, et al: Use of dobutamine stress echocardiography in detecting silent myocardial ischaemia in asymptomatic diabetic patients: A comparison with thallium scintigraphy and exercise testing. Diabet Med 18:900-905, 2001.

54. Marwick TH, Case C, Sawada S, et al: Use of stress echocardiography to predict mortality in patients with diabetes and known or suspected coronary artery disease. Diabetes Care 25:1042-1048, 2002.

55. Elhendy A, Arruda AM, Mahoney DW, et al: Prognostic stratification of diabetic patients by exercise echocardiography. J Am Coll Cardiol 37:1551-1557, 2001.

56. Sozzi FB, Elhendy A, Roelandt JR, et al: Prognostic value of dobutamine stress echocardiography in patients with diabetes. Diabetes Care 26:1074-1078, 2003.

57. D'Andrea A, Severino S, Caso P, et al: Prognostic value of pharmacological stress echocardiography in diabetic patients. Eur J Echocardiogr 4:202-208, 2003.

58. Kamalesh M, Matorin R, Sawada S: Prognostic value of a negative stress echocardiographic study in diabetic patients. Am Heart J 143:163-168, 2002.

59. Bates JR, Sawada SG, Segar DS, et al: Evaluation using dobutamine stress echocardiography in patients with insulin-dependent diabetes mellitus before kidney and/or pancreas transplantation. Am J Cardiol 77:175-179, 1996.

60. Takeuchi M, Miura Y, Toyokawa T, et al: The comparative diagnostic value of dobutamine stress echocardiography and thallium stress tomography for detecting restenosis after coronary angioplasty. J Am Soc Echocardiogr 5:696-702, 1995.

61. Bigi R, Desideri A, Bax JJ, et al: Prognostic interaction between viability and residual myocardial ischemia by dobutamine stress echocardiography in patients with acute myocardial infarction and mildly impaired left ventricular function. Am J Cardiol 87:283-288, 2001.

62. Picano E, Sicari R, Landi P, et al: Prognostic value of myocardial viability in medically treated patients with global left ventricular dysfunction early after an acute uncomplicated myocardial infarction: A dobutamine stress echocardiographic study. Circulation 98:1078-1084, 1998.

63. Cullom SJ: Principles of cardiac SPECT imaging. In DePuey EG, Garcia EV, Berman DA (eds): Cardiac SPECT Imaging, 2nd ed. Philadelphia, Lippincott, Williams & Wilkins, 2001, pp 3-16.

64. Germano G, Kiat H, Kavanagh PB, et al: Automatic quantification of ejection fraction from gated myocardial perfusion SPECT. J Nucl Med 36:2138-2147, 1995.

65. Sharir T, Berman DS, Lewin HC, et al: Incremental prognostic value of rest-redistribution (201) Tl single-photon emission computed tomography. Circulation 100:1964-1970, 1999.

66. Taillefer R, Primeau M, Costi P, et al: Technetium-99m-sestamibi myocardial perfusion imaging in detection of coronary artery disease: Comparison between initial (1-hour) and delayed (3-hour) postexercise images. J Nucl Med 32:1961-1965, 1991

67. Taillefer R, Amyot R, Turpin S, et al: Comparison between dipyridamole and adenosine as pharmacologic coronary vasodilators in detection of coronary artery disease with thallium 201 imaging. J Nucl Cardiol 3:204-211, 1996.

68. Calnon DA, Glover DK, Beller GA, et al: Effects of dobutamine stress on myocardial blood flow, 99mTc sestamibi uptake, and systolic wall thickening in the presence of coronary artery stenoses: Implications for dobutamine stress testing. Circulation 96:2353-2360, 1997.

69. Alexander CM, Landsman PB, Teutsch SM: Diabetes mellitus, impaired fasting glucose, atherosclerotic risk factors, and prevalence of coronary heart disease. Am J Cardiol 86:897-902, 2000.

70. Milan Study on Atherosclerosis and Diabetes (MiSAD) Group: Prevalence of unrecognized silent myocardial ischemia and its association with atherosclerotic risk factors in noninsulin-dependent diabetes mellitus. Am J Cardiol 79:134-139, 1997.

71. Koistinen MJ, Huikuri HV, Pirttiaho H, et al: Evaluation of exercise electrocardiography and thallium tomographic imaging in detecting asymptomatic coronary artery disease in diabetic patients. Br Heart J 63:7-11, 1990.

72. Janand-Delenne B, Savin B, Habib G, et al: Silent myocardial ischemia in patients with diabetes: Who to screen. Diabetes Care 22:1396-1400, 1999.

73. May O, Arildsen H, Damsgaard EM, et al: Prevalence and prediction of silent ischaemia in diabetes mellitus: A population-based study. Cardiovasc Res 34:241-247, 1997.

74. Naka M, Hiramatsu K, Aizawa T, et al: Silent myocardial ischemia in patients with non–insulin-dependent diabetes mellitus as judged by treadmill exercise testing and coronary angiography. Am Heart J 123:46-53, 1992.

75. Koistinen MJ: Prevalence of asymptomatic myocardial ischaemia in diabetic subjects. BMJ 301:92-95, 1990.

76. Wackers FJ, Young LH, Inzucchi SE, et al: Detection of silent myocardial ischemia in asymptomatic diabetic subjects: The DIAD study. Diabetes Care 27:1954-1961, 2004.

77. De Lorenzo A, Lima RS, Siqueira-Filho AG, et al: Prevalence and prognostic value of perfusion defects detected by stress technetium-99m sestamibi myocardial perfusion single-photon emission computed tomography in asymptomatic patients with diabetes mellitus and no known coronary artery disease. Am J Cardiol 90:827-832, 2002.

78. Kang X, Berman DS, Lewin H, et al: Comparative ability of myocardial perfusion single-photon emission computed tomography to detect coronary artery disease in patients with and without diabetes mellitus. Am Heart J 137:949-957, 1999.

79. Kang X, Berman DS, Lewin HC, et al: Incremental prognostic value of myocardial perfusion single photon emission computed tomography in patients with diabetes mellitus. Am Heart J 138:1025-1032, 1999.

80. Berman DS, Kang X, Hayes SW, et al: Adenosine myocardial perfusion single-photon emission computed tomography in women compared with men: Impact of diabetes mellitus on incremental prognostic value and effect on patient management. J Am Coll Cardiol 41:1125-1133, 2003.

81. Shaw LJ, Iskandrian AE: Prognostic value of gated myocardial perfusion SPECT. J Nucl Cardiol 11:171-185, 2004.

82. American Diabetes Association Consensus development conference on the diagnosis of coronary heart disease in people with diabetes: Miami, Florida. Diabetes Care 21:1551-1559, 1998.

83. Passa P, Drouin P, Issa-Sayegh M, et al: Coronary disease and diabetes. Diabetes Metab 21:446-451, 1995.

84. Grundy SM, Garber A, Goldberg R, et al: Prevention Conference VI: Diabetes and Cardiovascular Disease: Writing Group IV: Lifestyle and medical management of risk factors. Circulation 105:e153-e158, 2002.

Box 19-1. Goals of Medical Nutrition Therapy for Diabetes

- Achieve and maintain optimal metabolic control:
  - Maintain normal blood glucose levels, or as close to normal as possible, to reduce or prevent the risk of acute and chronic complications of diabetes.
  - Reduce the risk of macrovascular disease with lipid and lipoprotein profiles as close to optimum as possible.
  - Maintain blood pressure values that reduce the risk for vascular disease.
- Prevent and treat diabetes chronic complications and modify the food intake as appropriate for the patient based on:
  - Health status
  - Ethnic and cultural preferences
  - The patient's willingness to change
  - Improve individual health through physical activity and healthy food choices.

Adapted from Franz MI, Bantle JP, Beebe CA, et al: Nutrition principles and recommendations in diabetes. Diabetes Care 27:S36-S46, 2004.

Box 19-2. Principles of Nutrition for Diabetes

- Eat meals and snacks (if necessary) at regular times of the day.
- Avoid missing meals or prolonged periods between meals.
- Eat approximately the same quantity of food daily and be consistent with the intake of carbohydrate at meals and snacks when using standard doses of insulin.
- Include high-fiber food choices such as whole grain breads and cereals, vegetables, dried beans and peas, and fruit.
- Enjoy a variety of foods from all the food groups: starches, fruits, vegetables, milk, and protein (meat and meat substitutes).
- Reduce the intake of fat, sugar, and salt (following specific recommendations).
- Control portion sizes for weight management.

emphasis on recommendations for optimal blood glucose levels. No special diet foods are essential, and the patient's family can also eat the same foods. The basic principles of nutrition for diabetes[3] are listed in Box 19-2.

MEDICAL NUTRITION THERAPY FOR TYPE 1 PATIENTS WITH DIABETES

Principles

Insulin Therapy

For people with type 1 diabetes whose diabetes is managed with conventional therapy (one interme-

diate- or long-acting insulin injection per day and two injections of short-acting insulin, one before breakfast and one before dinner), the goal is to integrate insulin with the lifestyle, which includes physical activity and food habits. Patients using this type of insulin regimen should eat at consistent times and synchronize meals with the time of action of their insulin dose, check their blood glucose levels, and have sufficient knowledge to adjust their rapid- or short-acting insulin dose based on the amount of carbohydrate to be consumed.

Those who use more intensive therapy, which is defined as three or more injections per day or insulin pump therapy, must learn to adjust their premeal insulin doses based on their premeal blood glucose levels. Adjustments include:

- Adjusting the insulin for variable carbohydrate intake
- Adjusting the premeal insulin when a meal is delayed or the fat content is high
- Taking additional insulin for snacks that are not part of the daily meal plan

Many people with type 1 diabetes select intensive insulin therapy because it provides more flexibility with their individual lifestyles and schedules. It is imperative to provide MNT not only for their macronutrient foundation but also for preventing and treating hypoglycemia, exercise-related blood glucose fluctuations, and diet during sick days.[2,3]

Carbohydrate

Many factors influence the glycemic response to foods; obviously, one factor is types of carbohydrates. The type of sugar—glucose, fructose, sucrose, lactose—and the nature of the starch (amylase, amylopectin, resistant starch) affect the glycemic response. Food processing and cooking, as well as other factors, such as the amount of fat in a meal, influence gastric emptying. Fasting and premeal blood glucose levels, the second meal, a delayed response to a meal high in fat, and a lente effect of carbohydrate are other variables that affect the glycemic response to foods. Franz and coworkers have shown that in subjects with type 1 diabetes, the ingestion of a variety of sugars or starches, for up to 6 weeks, did not result in a significant difference in blood glucose levels when the quantity of carbohydrate was the same.[2]

The total carbohydrate content of the meal and the premeal insulin dose affect the postprandial blood glucose response in people with type 1 diabetes. The premeal doses of insulin can be adjusted for the carbohydrate content of the meal. Patients taking fixed doses of insulin must be very careful to maintain day-to-day consistency of carbohydrate intake.[2]

There is no convincing evidence that planning meals according to the glycemic index can benefit patients with type 1 diabetes. Studies comparing low glycemic index diets with high glycemic index diets in patients with type 1 diabetes have been inconclusive.[1] This indicates that a diet based on

the glycemic index has limited value as a general recommendation. However, type 1 diabetic patients using intensive therapy and performing frequent blood glucose monitoring may establish their own personal glycemic index of foods based on their observations of various carbohydrates on their blood glucose values.

Fiber is encouraged in the daily food intake of people with type 1 diabetes, and a variety of fiber-containing foods, such as fruits and vegetables and whole-grain breads and cereals, should be worked into the daily meal plan. These foods also provide vitamins, minerals, and other essential nutrients that are beneficial to health. Short-term studies of small numbers of diabetic subjects whose diets included large amounts of fiber (50 g) found a beneficial effect on glycemic control. More-recent studies have indicated a mixed effect on glycemia.[2]

Protein

In the United States, the intake of protein is 15% to 20% of the total calories. People with type 1 diabetes typically consume about the same percentage of protein. There has been an assumption that in people with diabetes, abnormalities of protein metabolism are less affected by insulin deficiency and resistance than glucose metabolism is.

The effect of protein on satiety, energy intake, and long-term weight loss and management have not been studied in detail. The long-term safety and effectiveness of high-protein and low-carbohydrate diets are not known.[2]

Fat

The main goal for fat intake is to reduce saturated fat and dietary cholesterol. Saturated fat is the main dietary factor in the increase of plasma low-density lipoprotein (LDL) cholesterol. People with diabetes seem to be more sensitive to dietary cholesterol than persons who do not have diabetes. Recommendations for fat intake are given in Table 19-1. General recommendations[2,3] are:

- Reduce LDL and decrease saturated fat if weight loss or weight management is desired. The saturated fat in the meal plan can be replaced with carbohydrate or monounsaturated fat.
- Reduce or minimize the intake of *trans* fatty acids.
- Reduce overall fat intake; low-fat diets help improve dyslipidemia and produce a small amount of weight loss.
- Restrict polyunsaturated fat intake to approximately 10% of calories.

Effect of Macronutrients on Blood Glucose Levels

Carbohydrate has the greatest impact on postprandial blood glucose levels, and it is the basis for the meal-planning approach for carbohydrate count-

---

Box 19-3. Food Sources of Macronutrients

Carbohydrate

- Concentrated sweets such as cookies, candy, and regular soft drinks
- Dairy (milk, yogurt, ice cream)
- Fruits and juices
- Starches (breads, cereals, pasta, rice, lentils, dried beans and peas, crackers)

Protein*

- Cheese
- Eggs
- Fish
- Meat
- Milk
- Poultry

Fat*†

- Avocados
- Butter
- Lard
- Margarine
- Mayonnaise
- Nuts
- Oils
- Olives
- Peanut butter
- Salad dressings

*These foods have no direct effect on postprandial glucose.
†Large amounts of fat slow the absorption of other nutrients and delay gastric emptying.

ing. This meal-planning approach is just one of many approaches, and it was employed in the intensive therapy group for the Diabetes Control and Complications Trial (DCCT).[4]

All types of carbohydrates raise postprandial blood glucose levels. Sugar alcohols, which are heavily used in many foods that claim to be sugar free, also raise postprandial glycemia. Protein and fat have little or no impact on postprandial blood sugar, although it has been suggested, but not proved, that substantial additions of either protein or fat may delay, blunt, or both delay and blunt the postprandial blood glucose rise. Protein has no direct effect on postprandial glucose, and large amounts of fat slow the absorption of other nutrients and delay gastric emptying.[3]

Blood glucose levels should be checked two hours after any meal—straight carbohydrate or mixed meal—to evaluate the impact. Sources of macronutrients are listed in Box 19-3.

Table 19-1. *Recommendations for Nutrient Intake*

Factor	American Diabetes Association (2004)	American Association of Clinical Endocrinologists (2002)	*Recommendations* American Dietetic Association (2001)	Food and Nutrition Board, Institute of Medicine (2002)	American Heart Association (2000)	National Cholesterol Education Program (2001) TLC Diet
Target population	Persons with diabetes	Persons with diabetes	Persons with diabetes	Healthy persons	Healthy persons; addresses risk of heart disease and stroke	Persons with dyslipidemia
Carbohydrates (% of kcal)	60–70 CHO + monounsaturated fat	55–60	60–70 CHO + monounsaturated fat	45–65	Not specified: eat fruits, grains, vegetables	50–60
Sugar (added/refined)	Eaten in context of a healthy diet	NR	Not restricted, context of a healthy diet	<25% of total CHO	NR	NR
Glycemic index	Total CHO rather than sources more important	Total CHO rather than source seems to be critical factor	May reduce postprandial hyperglycemia; long-term benefits unclear	NR	NR	NR
Fiber (grams/day)	15–20 In T2DM, large amounts (50 g) needed to see benefit	"Starches with fiber may slow down glucose absorption"	15–20	≥50 y: men 38, women 25 <50 y: men 30, women 25	No specific target; recommended foods should provide >25	20–30
Protein (% of kcal)	15–20	10–20; with microalbuminuria, 10–15	15–20	10–35 (0.8 g/kg body weight)	15 (50–100 g/d should be adequate to meet most needs)	~15
Total fat (% of kcal)	≤30	≤30 As low as 15 in overweight or dyslipidemic persons	≤30	20–35	≤30 for weight loss	25–35
Saturated fat (% of kcal)	≤10 With ↑ LDL, <7	Avoid saturated fat with dyslipidemia	≤10 With ↑ LDL, <7	As little as possible	<7 for people with diabetes	<7
Monounsaturated fat (% of kcal)	Combined with CHO 60–70% of total kcal 60–70	NR	Combined with CHO 60–70% of total kcal	Reduce saturated fats	Substitute for saturated fat	Up to 20
Cholesterol (mg/day)	300 or less With ↑ LDL, 200 or less	NR	300 or less With ↑ LDL, 200 or less	As little as possible	200 or less for people with diabetes	Less than 200
Sodium (mg/day)	2400	NR	2400	1500 age 50–70 y, 1300 age 71+	Less than 2400	Less than 2400
Alcohol	One drink for women, two for men per day	Avoid or limit	One drink for women, two for men per day	Moderation	One drink for women, two for men per day	One drink for women, two for men per day

CHO, carbohydrate; LDL, low-density lipoprotein; qd, every day; NR, no recommendation; ↑, elevated

Carbohydrate Counting

Principles

Carbohydrate counting is a meal-planning system that focuses on consistent intake of foods that contain carbohydrate. It is used by clinicians as the basis for reviewing food, blood glucose, and physical activity records. All carbohydrates affect blood glucose levels in the same manner when they are consumed in the same quantity. The initial weighing and measuring of food is helpful for ensuring each meal contains the same amount of carbohydrate, and this helps the patient master quantification of carbohydrate amounts.

The basic level of carbohydrate counting can help diabetic patients achieve consistency in the amount of food they eat. (Carbohydrate counting may also assist type 2 patients in achieving portion control and thus maintain a reasonable caloric intake.) At the advanced level it is used to make adjustments

in food, insulin dose, and physical activity based on observed blood glucose patterns. It is the only method that can accurately recommend insulin-to-carbohydrate ratios when analyzed with preprandial and postprandial blood sugars. Persons with type 1 diabetes who use the advanced carbohydrate-counting method must understand how to make the food and insulin adjustments based on blood glucose results.[3]

Basic carbohydrate counting and advanced carbohydrate counting are explained in patient education booklets that provide step-by-step guidelines. These booklets are available from the American Diabetes Association and the American Dietetic Association.[5,6]

Intensive Therapy

Before the patient with type 1 diabetes begins intensive therapy with premeal rapid or short-acting insulin or with an insulin pump, the patient must demonstrate the skills necessary to adjust the insulin doses and meet the target blood glucose goals. This requires consistent use of food, insulin dose, blood glucose, and physical activity data for at least 2 weeks. This will help the clinician establish insulin-to-carbohydrate ratios for the patient to start with for calculating premeal insulin. An insulin-to-carbohydrate ratio is based on matching rapid or short-acting insulin to the carbohydrate content of the food to be consumed.[7]

There are many ways of determining insulin-to-carbohydrate ratios. Generally 50% of the total daily insulin dose is required for the basal or background insulin and 50% is required to cover the meal times. The meal-time or bolus dose is based on the grams of carbohydrate the person is planning to consume. One method for determining the insulin-to-carbohydrate ratio is given in Box 19-4.

This system is more flexible than the system using standard amounts of insulin. When the patient's carbohydrate intake varies, the insulin dose can be adjusted based solely on the carbohydrate content of the meal. Refining the insulin-to-carbohydrate ratio for physically active days versus sedentary days and for weekends versus work or school days is important to achieving optimal postprandial glycemia. Frequent record keeping of carbohydrate consumption along with premeal and postmeal blood glucose values allow for adjustments to the insulin-to-carbohydrate ratio and optimal blood sugar control. Accuracy of the portion sizes of carbohydrate foods and precise matching of insulin doses with the anticipated intake are also important for calculating this ratio.

Carbohydrate counting provides a great deal of flexibility to the person with diabetes. However, this flexibility also can result in weight management issues, because food choices can be high in calories and fat, and this system can cover any type of food. With carbohydrate counting, the patient also

---

Box 19-4. One Method for Determining the Insulin-to-Carbohydrate Ratio

- Using food records, determine the total amount of carbohydrate eaten, and then calculate the average daily intake of carbohydrate and the average amount for each meal and snack.
- Have the patient eat consistent amounts of carbohydrate at meals, and, if possible, include a variety of foods and resources to calculate the carbohydrate content of the meals or snacks. The nutrition facts panel of packaged food products is the most ubiquitous source of this information.
- Review blood glucose records with carbohydrate (grams), premeal and postmeal blood glucose results, and the amount of meal time insulin used.
- Calculate the insulin-to-carbohydrate ratio by dividing the number of grams of carbohydrate by the units of mealtime insulin used. For example: The patient consumes 60 grams of carbohydrate and takes 6 units of rapid-acting insulin administered.

$$60/6 = 10$$

---

has to pay attention to portions of protein and fat, even though the mealtime insulin coverage is not going to factor in the protein and fat content of the meal. If the patient is aware of fat intake and makes an effort to reduce it and also increases physical activity, the weight management can be effective.[8]

Because fat delays gastric emptying, a high-fat meal, such as pizza, can cause a delayed postprandial blood glucose rise. Frequent postprandial blood glucose checks will help in deciding if additional mealtime insulin is required either via injection or as a bolus from an insulin pump. Most insulin pumps either have a square wave or a dual or extended wave bolus feature and can be programmed to deliver the insulin bolus over a period of time to match the delayed rise in postprandial blood glucose from a high-fat meal.[8]

Paying attention to the fiber content of a meal is also important, because dietary fiber is not digested and absorbed like other carbohydrates. If the serving contains 5 or more grams of fiber, subtracting the total fiber from the total carbohydrate will provide the usable grams of carbohydrate per serving. This can help a person who is using an insulin-to-carbohydrate ratio to more accurately match up the insulin dose for the actual amount of carbohydrate that is being eaten. Meals that are high in carbohydrates, such as cooked dried beans or legumes, might require insulin during the meal: A patient using a pump should have the premeal insulin delivered right as the person is eating, and a patient using injections should take an injection halfway through the meal.[7]

People with type 1 diabetes may develop their own system of how various carbohydrates affect

Box 19-5. Meal-Planning Approaches

Basic Nutrition Guidelines

- Food Guide Pyramid (US Department of Agriculture)
- Guide to Good Eating (National Dairy Council)

Basic Diabetes Nutrition Guidelines

- Healthy Food Choices (American Diabetes Association, American Dietetic Association)
- The First Step in Diabetes Meal Planning (American Diabetes Association, American Dietetic Association)
- Eating Healthy Foods (American Diabetes Association, American Dietetic Association)

Menu Planning

- Individualized menus (American Diabetes Association)
- Month of Meals (American Diabetes Association)

Exchange Lists

- Exchange Lists for Meal Planning (American Diabetes Association)
- Healthy Food Choices (American Diabetes Association)

Counting Methods

- Carbohydrate Counting: Basic and Advanced (American Diabetes Association, American Dietetic Association)

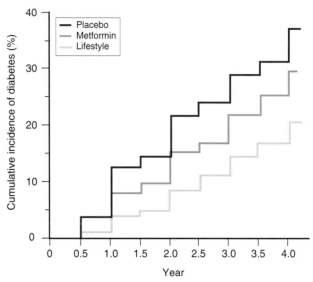

Figure 19-1. Cumulative incidence of diabetes according to study group ($P < 0.001$ for each group). (From Knowler WC, Barrett-Connor E, Fowler SE, et al, for the Diabetes Prevention Program Research Group: Reduction in the incidence of type 2 diabetes with lifestyle intervention or metformin. N Engl J Med 346:393-403, 2002. Copyright 2002 Massachusetts Medical Society. All rights reserved.)

their blood glucose levels, and this may be very individualized based on postprandial blood glucose levels.[7] Other meal-planning options are also available (Box 19-5).

MEDICAL NUTRITION THERAPY FOR PATIENTS WITH TYPE 2 DIABETES

Principles

Despite significant medical advances, the incidence of type 2 diabetes has reached epidemic proportions. Costacou and Mayer-Davis estimate that "up to 75% of the risk of type 2 diabetes is attributable to obesity."[9] Controlling obesity alone, no small task, would therefore sharply decrease the incidence of type 2 diabetes, the metabolic syndrome, and simple insulin resistance.

About 80% to 90% of those with type 2 diabetes are overweight, and the percentage is possibly higher in young people (who have less beta cell dysfunction). Therefore, diabetes education must be directed toward achieving weight loss and encouraging positive lifestyle changes. The American Academy of Pediatrics states, "prevention is one of the hallmarks of pediatric practice."[10] Diet, exercise, and behavior modification must be the first strategy for lifestyle changes that are needed for weight loss.[11] But prevention remains the "logical

first step in the management of the obese type 2 diabetic patient."[12]

Preventing Type 2 Diabetes

The Diabetes Prevention Program (DPP) Group study[13] provided evidence that treating patients who have impaired glucose tolerance (prediabetes) can prevent or delay the onset of type 2 diabetes. DPP data showed that a 7% reduction in body weight with moderate exercise (150 minutes a week) resulted in a 58% reduction in the incidence of diabetes. The lifestyle component of the DPP was shown to significantly reduce the incidence of diabetes (Fig. 19-1). This component employed several lifestyle interventions to achieve the 7% reduction in initial body weight (Box 19-6),[13] including a 16-lesson curriculum. The curriculum was taught by case managers on a one-to-one basis during the first 24 weeks after enrollment. It was "flexible, culturally sensitive and individualized." Behavioral change was reinforced through post-lesson individual and group sessions with the case managers. Data from Marion Franz (Fig. 19-2)[14] reveal similar findings with repeated intervention with a registered dietitian.

In a summary review[15] of the medical literature on screening and interventions for obesity in adults, McTigue and colleagues looked at more than 70 trials on counseling and behavioral intervention and more than 100 studies that included

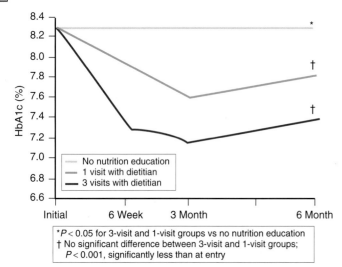

Figure 19–2. Effectiveness of medical nutrition therapy in management of type 2 diabetes. (From Franz MJ, Monk A, Barry B, et al: Effectiveness of medical nutrition therapy provided by dietitians in the management of non-insulin-dependent diabetes mellitus: A randomized, controlled clinical trial. J Am Diet Assoc 95:1009-1017, 1995.)

Box 19-6. Lifestyle Interventions

- Low-calorie, low-fat diet
- Moderate-intensity exercise, 150 minutes per week (brisk walking)
- Sixteen-lesson curriculum covering diet, exercise and behavior modification.

From Knowler WC, Barret-Connor E, Fowler SE, et al, for the Diabetes Prevention Program Research Group: Reduction in the incidence of type 2 diabetes with lifestyle intervention or metformin. N Engl J Med 346:393-403, 2002.

---

pharmacotherapy. Successful interventions typically included some combination of diet, exercise, or behavior therapy. High-intensity interventions (more than one contact per month) led to more weight loss than moderate-intensity interventions (one contact per month). Two of three low-intensity weight-loss interventions were ineffective. In 17 randomized, controlled trials, sibutramine promoted weight loss, but patients regained weight once the drug was removed (Fig. 19–3).[15] According to these studies, for the nearly two thirds of Americans who are overweight, multiple interventions should be promoted at the first physician visit.

Evidence-based recommendations, both in nutrition and medicine, require systematic literature reviews that identify and synthesize evidence of the effectiveness of intervention[16] and are more effective than consensus-based guidelines that have more limited research support. The clinical practice recommendations promoted by the American Diabetes Association use evidence-based protocols to develop the goals of MNT for diabetes.[17]

The American Dietetic Association position is similar to the American Diabetes Association's: Medical nutrition therapy is useful for preventing, delaying, and treating diabetes. Treatment should be individualized and metabolic parameters should be monitored.[18] The American Association of Clinical Endocrinologists (AACE) in their Diabetes Guidelines[19] concur that treatment should be individualized for providing MNT, normalizing blood glucose and lipid levels, and achieving a desirable weight. The AACE further states that reduction of insulin resistance, through weight loss and maintenance of weight loss, should be a goal for patients with type 2 diabetes. For the American Academy of Pediatrics[20] the goals of MNT are adequate metabolic control, prevention of microvascular and macrovascular complications, and maintaining a reasonable body weight. Obviously, there is consensus within these major organizations toward the goals of MNT; however, recommendations of macronutrient profiles vary.

Major medical scientific bodies recommend dietary practices, but only the American Dietetic Association, The American Diabetes Association, and the AACE address diabetes specifically. The dietary prescription offered by the American Dietetic Association is identical to that of the American Diabetes Association in macronutrient and fiber recommendations. A diet high in monounsaturated fat (40%) has been shown to have greater patient acceptance and improved lipid profile.[21] The American Academy of Pediatrics[20] encourages MNT delivered by a professional in diabetes or nutrition but offers no specific macronutrient detail. They promote broader diet changes such as increasing fruit and vegetable intake, limiting between-meal snacks and eating in front of the television, promoting "moderation rather than over-consumption, emphasizing healthful food choices rather than restrictive eating patterns."[10] The American Heart Association (AHA) and the National Cholesterol Education Program (NCEP) direct their diet recommendations toward cardiovascular risk factors and dyslipidemias, respectively. Their guidelines may be superimposed on, or used in conjunction with, prescribed diet patterns, because these guidelines predominantly address fat and fiber consumption. Table 19-1 summarizes the recommendations from these organizations.

Macronutrient Recommendations

Carbohydrate

Overall, recommendations for total carbohydrate range from 45% of calories alone up to 70% when combined with monounsaturated fats. The Institute of Medicine (IOM) is the only body to recommend limits on sugar, and no organization has yet approved use of the glycemic index in carbohydrate consumption, relying more on total carbohydrate intake rather than the source of carbohydrate.

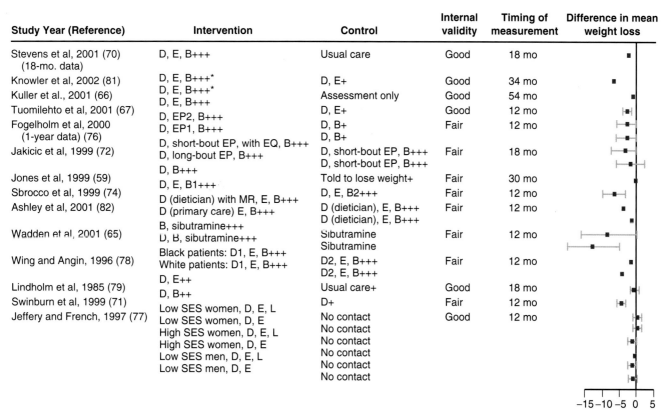

Study Year (Reference)	Intervention	Control	Internal validity	Timing of measurement
Stevens et al, 2001 (70) (18-mo. data)	D, E, B+++	Usual care	Good	18 mo
Knowler et al, 2002 (81)	D, E, B+++*	D, E+	Good	34 mo
Kuller et al., 2001 (66)	D, E, B+++*	Assessment only	Good	54 mo
Tuomilehto et al, 2001 (67)	D, E, B+++	D, E+	Good	12 mo
Fogelholm et al, 2000 (1-year data) (76)	D, EP2, B+++	D, B+	Fair	12 mo
	D, EP1, B+++	D, B+		
Jakicic et al, 1999 (72)	D, short-bout EP, with EQ, B+++	D, short-bout EP, B+++	Fair	18 mo
	D, long-bout EP, B+++	D, short-bout EP, B+++		
Jones et al, 1999 (59)	D, B+++	Told to lose weight+	Fair	30 mo
Sbrocco et al, 1999 (74)	D, E, B1+++	D, E, B2+++	Fair	12 mo
Ashley et al, 2001 (82)	D (dietician) with MR, E, B+++	D (dietician), E, B+++	Fair	12 mo
	D (primary care) E, B+++	D (dietician), E, B+++		
Wadden et al, 2001 (65)	B, sibutramine+++	Sibutramine	Fair	12 mo
	D, B, sibutramine+++	Sibutramine		
Wing and Angin, 1996 (78)	Black patients: D1, E, B+++	D2, E, B+++	Fair	12 mo
	White patients: D1, E, B+++	D2, E, B+++		
Lindholm et al, 1985 (79)	D, E++	Usual care+	Good	18 mo
Swinburn et al, 1999 (71)	D, B++	D+	Fair	12 mo
Jeffery and French, 1997 (77)	Low SES women, D, E, L	No contact	Good	12 mo
	Low SES women, D, E	No contact		
	High SES women, D, E, L	No contact		
	High SES women, D, E	No contact		
	Low SES men, D, E, L	No contact		
	Low SES men, D, E	No contact		

Figure 19–3. Differences in mean weight loss between intervention and control groups for counseling and behavioral interventions. Only studies for which the difference in mean weight loss could be calculated are included. Error bars represent 95% confidence intervals and are presented for studies in which those data were available. Data presented are as close as possible to 1-year follow-up. An asterisk indicates that the difference was statistically significant ($P < 0.05$) but there were insufficient data to calculate confidence intervals. B, behavioral therapy; D, diet; E, exercise; EP, exercise program; EQ, exercise equipment; L, lottery entry; MR, meal replacement; SES, socioeconomic status; +++, high intensity; ++, moderate intensity; +, low intensity.

Fiber

Total fiber recommendations range from 15 to 38 grams per day. The American Diabetes Association has acknowledged research that an amount of fiber intake that exceeded 50 grams might be beneficial for people with diabetes. Most of these organizations have recognized the benefits of fiber in slowing glucose absorption. The American Dietetic Association and the American Heart Association recommend consumption of fruit, vegetables, and grains, as in the Food Guide Pyramid, for increased fiber and nutrient intake.

Protein

Protein recommendations vary little from 10% to 20% of total calories for patients with or without microalbuminuria. The AACE recommends decreasing animal protein in the diet and keeping total protein intake between 10% and 15% in the presence of microalbuminuria. The IOM allows for a broader range of protein from 10% to 35% of total calories for healthy people. The RDA for protein is 0.8 gram per kilogram of body weight.

There is no strong evidence to suggest that an amount of protein less than the RDA will preserve renal function. With renal function deficit, the American Dietetic Association suggests 0.8 grams to 1.0 gram per kilogram of body weight. In one 5-week study of 12 patients with untreated type 2 diabetes, a high-protein diet (30% protein, 40% carbohydrate) significantly lowered the postprandial blood glucose, improved overall glucose control, and increased nitrogen retention when compared to a diet composed of 15% protein and 55% carbohydrate.[22,23]

Fat

Thirty percent of calories from fat is the most common recommendation for total fat intake. The range in recommendations for total fat is 20% to 35%, the same as the broader range established by the IOM. The AACE states that diabetic patients who are overweight or dyslipidemic could consume as little as 15% of calories from fat. The suggestion for saturated fat is 10% of calories or less. The American Diabetes Association and NCEP recommend

amounts of saturated fat less than 7% of calories for people with diabetes or elevated LDL. For people with diabetes, the AACE suggests avoiding saturated fat in the presence of dyslipidemia.

Both the American Diabetes Association and American Dietetic Association combine carbohydrate with monounsaturated fat intake for a total of 60% to 70% of calories. The NCEP recommends intake of monounsaturated fats up to 20% of calories, and the AHA suggests replacement of saturated fat with monounsaturated.

Dietary cholesterol recommendation is 300 mg/day or less. The AHA, NCEP, and American Diabetes Association suggest less than 200 mg/day for people with diabetes or elevated LDL. Omega-3 fats, not included in Table 19-1, may be of benefit. Reduction of *trans* fat should be considered.[24]

Other Nutrient Recommendations

Sodium intake, according to the American Diabetes Association, AHA, and NCEP, should be less than 2400 mg/day. The IOM recommends significantly lower levels at 1500 mg down to 1200 mg at age 71 and older.

The recommendation for alcohol consumption is generally one of moderation, but several bodies recommend no more than one drink per day for women and two drinks for men. Epidemiologic studies suggest that insulin sensitivity is increased[25] and risk of type 2 diabetes is reduced with light to moderate alcohol consumption.[26] Metformin, a common first-line medication for persons with type 2 diabetes, especially those who are overweight, can cause lactic acidosis with excessive alcohol intake; therefore, caution should be promoted in these patients.

Calories and Nutrients for Weight Loss

Calorie Requirements

Caloric needs are based on age, sex, weight, and height using a formula such as the Harris-Benedict equation. Macronutrient recommendations are then based on these calculated calorie levels. For overweight type 2 patients, a reduction in calories of 250 to 500 per day is suggested for gradual weight loss and consumption of a wide variety of foods with distribution of the carbohydrate load.[10] Similar reductions in caloric intake for the pediatric population would be well advised considering the need for linear growth and development. The National Institutes of Health recommends a reduction of 500 to 1000 daily calorie reduction from the usual intake or a total daily consumption of 1000 to 1200 kcal for overweight women and 1200 to 1600 kcal for overweight men. However, for the morbidly obese, who would benefit from such a low-calorie diet plan, a 1200 kcal diet would provide only 60 grams of protein per day (20% of calories). For a 300-pound (136 kg) person, this would provide only 0.44 g/kg of actual body weight or 55% of the RDA for protein.[27]

Calorie needs for obese adults can also be based on 15 to 25 kcal per kilogram of actual body weight. For a 300-pound (136 kg) woman, 15 kcal per kilogram is approximately 2000 calories a day. Given the macronutrient prescriptions discussed earlier, daily intake would be 1000 calories from carbohydrates (50%) or 250 grams, 600 calories from fat (30%) or 67 grams, and 400 calories from protein (20%) or 100 grams (barring any renal insufficiency); this amount of protein is only slightly less (0.73 g/kg) than the RDA for protein of 0.8 g/kg. Very-low-calorie diets as well as very-low-carbohydrate (Atkins) diets have met with short-term success, but in the longer term (12 months) the weight loss is not significant compared to standard low-fat formulas.[28-30]

Low-Carbohydrate Diets

For the obese and obese type 2 population, very-low-carbohydrate diets in the short term are proven methods for rapid weight loss without significant side effects and, in fact, can improve lipid profiles, insulin levels, and blood glucose control.[29] A study on the effect of the Atkins diet (21 g of carbohydrate daily versus 309 grams in the control group, and 125 g of protein daily in each group) in type 2 diabetes showed that the lost weight was from fat mass and water. Subjects had decreases in insulin levels and hemoglobin A1c and a 75% increase in insulin sensitivity. The study showed no changes in resting energy expenditure, total energy expenditure, or hormones.[31]

Patients following low-carbohydrate diets should have close medical supervision, particularly those taking sulfonylureas and insulin, because of the possibility of hypoglycemia. Equally important, patients need nutrition education to make the transition from these diets to sound, palatable, long-term methods of eating that will continue the process of weight loss or, in the least, stabilize the lower weight without regain. Rapid weight loss can be motivating for the obese, and low-carbohydrate and low-calorie diets, with medical supervision, should be given consideration.

Micronutrient Therapy

Recent and past evidence has mounted for the need for micronutrient therapy or adequacy in the weight-loss diet: vitamin C, chromium, and calcium. Vitamin C has been shown to be deficient in a set of obese type 2 patients. This deficiency might alter endothelial function and therefore increase insulin resistance.[32] Chromium deficiency can negatively affect glucose tolerance, fat mass, lean body mass, and blood pressure, and hyperglycemia can exacerbate the excretion of chromium.[33] Chromium picolinate, on the com-

mercial market, is the most absorbable chromium molecule.

Calcium in yogurt (~1200 mg/day) was shown to significantly improve weight, fat mass, and central obesity in groups of overweight adults.[34] Calcium is also associated with preventing osteoporosis and regulating blood pressure, which are more reasons for optimal calcium intake. In much of the population, especially adolescents, soft drinks have replaced milk as the beverage of choice. Approximately 80% to 90% of African Americans are known to have lactase insufficiency and might need alternative forms of calcium to meet the RDA.

US Department of Agriculture food intake research shows that Americans consume less than the recommended nine fruit and vegetable servings per day. Though only three micronutrients are mentioned here, getting patients to consume greater amounts of micro- and phytonutrients (antioxidants) lies in getting them to purchase and consume more plant matter.

Increasing fruit and vegetable intake is important, not only for weight maintenance, but also for reducing cardiopulmonary risk.[35] Increasing intake of plant matter also helps the patient to reduce calories, which is the most important part of a weight-reducing diet.[36] Vegetables are far less calorie dense and more nutrient dense than many processed starchy foods and animal products. Consuming plant matter can reduce caloric consumption and increase satiety.[37]

For the type 2 diabetic patient not using the carbohydrate counting method and multiple daily insulin injections, the plate method is easy to understand and is a generally healthy plan for patients (Fig. 19–4). The plate method can help patients achieve greater micronutrient intake. The addition of low fat yogurt or milk could optimize calcium intake as well.

SUMMARY

For many people with diabetes, the nutrition and meal planning part of the regimen is the most challenging. Health care providers should have a basic understanding of the nutrition recommendations and goals for type 1 diabetes. For individualizing the meal plan, the patient should be encouraged to see a dietitian for medical nutrition therapy and support in changing eating behavior.

Professional organizations provide guidelines for the nutritional needs of all diabetic patients. Generally, moderation in all macronutrients is key.[38,39] Box 19-7 illustrates some of the characteristics of the successful weight control registry members. Frequent contact with our patients, as well as education about diet, exercise, and behavior change, may be one of the most important factors in long-term success.

Plate Method

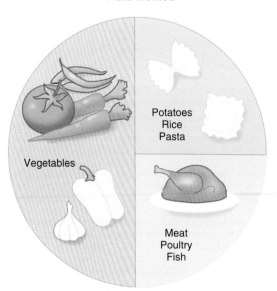

Figure 19–4. The plate method: Mark off half your dinner plate; this space is for vegetables. Divide the other half in two. One half of this half is for starch (potato, rice, or pasta). The other half is for lean protein (meat, poultry, or fish). This method is a quick and easy way of controlling your portions. Add one cup of milk or fruit if needed.

Box 19-7. Characteristics of Successful Weight Control Members

- Participants have made substantial changes in eating and exercise to lose and maintain weight.
- Nearly every participant used exercise and diet to lose weight and currently employs diet and exercise to maintain weight.
- About 50% of participants lost weight on their own without formal program help.
- Walking is the most frequently cited exercise.
- Diet consistency (consistent diet across the week) appears to be a strategy in long-term weight-loss maintenance.
- Eating breakfast: Breakfast eaters engage in more physical activity.
- As duration (time) of weight maintenance increases, effort toward weight maintenance decreases.
- Weight regain is in part due to failure to maintain dietary and exercise activity.
- Despite the method of weight loss (on their own, in an organized program, liquid), all use the same methods for weight maintenance.

Note: Successful members of the National Weight Control Registry have lost at least 30 pounds and have maintained a 30-pound weight loss for more than 1 year.

References

1. Bliss M: The Discovery of Insulin. Chicago, University of Chicago Press, 1982.
2. Franz MI, Bantle JP, Beebe CA, et al: Nutrition principles and recommendations in diabetes. Diabetes Care 27:S36-S46, 2004.
3. Austin MA, Kulkarni K, Powers MA: Blood Glucose Monitoring: Essential Skills for Health Care Professionals, 3rd ed. St. Paul, Minn, Peekytoe Productions, 2003.
4. The DCCT Research Group: Nutritional intervention for intensive therapy in the Diabetes Control and Complications Trial: Implications for clinical practice. J Am Diet Assoc 93:768-772,1993.
5. Daly A, Bolderman K, Franz M, Kulkarni K: Basic carbohydrate counting. Alexandria, Va, and Chicago, American Diabetes Association and American Dietetic Association, 2003.
6. Brooks AM, Kulkarni K: Insulin pump therapy and carbohydrate counting for pump therapy: carbohydrate to insulin ratios. In: Funnell MM, Hunt C, Kulkarni K, Rubin R (eds): A Core Curriculum for Diabetes Educators, 5th ed. Chicago, American Association of Diabetes Educators, 2003, pp 202-222.
7. Peters AL, Davidson MB: Protein and fat effects on glucose response and insulin requirements on subjects with insulin dependent diabetes mellitus. Am J Clin Nutr 58:555-600, 1993.
8. Strachan M, Frier B: Optimal time of administration of insulin lispro. Importance of meal composition. Diabetes Care 21:26-31, 1998.
9. Costacou T, Mayer-Davis EJ: Nutrition and prevention of type 2 diabetes. Annu Rev Nutr 23:147-170, 2003.
10. Krebs NF, Jacobson MS, and the American Academy of Pediatrics Committee on Nutrition: Prevention of pediatric overweight and obesity. Pediatrics 112:424-430, 2003.
11. Bedno SA: Weight loss in diabetes management. Nutr Clin Care 6:62-72, 2003.
12. Mannan MA, Rahman MS, Siddiqui NI. Obesity management in patients with type 2 diabetes mellitus. Mymensingh Med J 13:95-99, 2004.
13. Knowler WC, Barrett-Connor E, Fowler SE, et al, for the Diabetes Prevention Program Research Group: Reduction in the incidence of type 2 diabetes with lifestyle intervention or metformin. N Engl J Med 346:393-403, 2002.
14. Franz MJ, Monk A, Barry B, et al: Effectiveness of medical nutrition therapy provided by dietitians in the management of non-insulin-dependent diabetes mellitus: A randomized, controlled clinical trial. J Am Diet Assoc 95:1009-1017, 1995.
15. McTigue KM, Harris R, Hemphill B, et al: Screening and interventions for obesity in adults: Summary of the evidence for the U.S. Preventive Services Task Force. J Ann Intern Med 139:933-949, 2003.
16. Cooper MJ, Zlotkin SH: An evidence-based approach to the development of national dietary guidelines. J Am Diet Assoc 103(12 suppl 2):S28-S33, 2003.
17. Franz MJ, Bantle JP, Beebe CA, et al: Nutrition principles and recommendations in diabetes. Diabetes Care 27(Suppl 1):S36-S46, 2004.
18. American Dietetic Association: Nutrition Practice Guidelines for Type 1 and Type 2 Diabetes Mellitus. Chicago, American Dietetic Association, 2001. Available at http://guidelines.gov/summary/summary.aspx?doc_id=3296&nbr=2522.
19. The American Association of Clinical Endocrinologists: Medical guidelines for the management of diabetes. AACE Diabetes Guidelines. Endocr Pract 8(Suppl 1):41-63, 2002.
20. Gahagan S, Silverstein J, Committee on Native American Child Health and Section on Endocrinology: Prevention and treatment of type 2 diabetes mellitus in children, with special emphasis on American Indian and Alaska Native children. American Academy of Pediatrics: Clinical Report. Pediatrics 112:e328, 2003.
21. Rodriques-Villar C, Perez-Heras A, Mercade I, et al: Comparison of a high-carbohydrate and a high-monounsaturated fat, olive oil-rich diet on the susceptibility of LDL to oxidative modification in subjects with type 2 diabetes mellitus. Diabetes Med 21:142-149, 2004.
22. Nuttall FQ, Gannon MC, Saeed A, et al: The metabolic response of subjects with type 2 diabetes to a high-protein weight-maintenance diet. J Clin Endocrinol Metab 88:3577-3583, 2003.
23. Gannon MC, Nuttall FQ, Saeed A, et al: An increase in dietary protein improves the blood glucose response in persons with type 2 diabetes. Am J Clin Nutr 78:671-672, 2003.
24. Grundy SM, Abate N, Chandalia M: Diet composition and the metabolic syndrome: What is the optimal fat intake? Am J Med 113(Suppl 9B):25S-29S, 2002.
25. Van Dam RM. The epidemiology of lifestyle and risk for type 2 diabetes. Eur J Epidemiol 18:1115-1125, 2003.
26. Sierksma A, Patel H, Ouchi N, et al: Effect of moderate alcohol consumption on adiponectin, tumor necrosis, factor-α and insulin sensitivity. Diabetes Care 27:184-189, 2004.
27. National Institutes of Health/National Heart, Lung and Blood Institute, North American Association for the Study of Obesity: Practical Guide to the Identification, Evaluation and Treatment of Overweight and Obesity in Adults. Bethesda, Md, National Institutes of Health, 2000.
28. Volek JS, Westman EC: Very-low-carbohydrate weight-loss diets revisited. Cleve Clin J Med 69:849-862, 2002.
29. Samaha FF, Iqbal N, Seshadri P, et al: A low-carbohydrate as compared with a low-fat diet in severe obesity. N Engl J Med 348:2074-2081, 2003.
30. Foster GD, et al: A randomized trial of a low-carbohydrate diet for obesity. N Engl J Med. 348:2082-2090, 2003.
31. Guenther B, Sargrad K, Homko C, Davis E, Mozzoli M, Stein TP: Effects of the Atkins diet in type 2 diabetes: Metabolic balance studies. Paper presented at 64th Scientific Sessions, American Diabetes Association, Orlando, Fla, June 2004.
32. Quon MJ: Overview: The NCCAM perspective on diabetes. Paper presented at 64th Scientific Sessions, American Diabetes Association, Orlando, Fla, June 2004.
33. Anderson R: Chromium, glucose tolerance and diabetes. Paper presented at 64th Scientific Sessions, American Diabetes Association, Orlando, Fla, June 2004.
34. Zemel MB, Thompson W, Milstead A, et al: Calcium and dairy acceleration of weight and fat loss during energy restriction in obese adults. Obes Res 12:582-590, 2004.
35. Kumanyika SK, Van Horn L, Bowen D, et al: Maintenance of dietary behavior change. Health Psychol 19(1 suppl):42-56, 2000.
36. Rolls BJ, Bell EA: Dietary approaches to the treatment of obesity. Med Clin North Am 84:401-418, 2000.
37. Bell EA, Roe LS, Rolls BJ: Sensory-specific satiety is affected more by volume than energy content of a liquid food. Physiol Behav 78:593-600, 2003.
38. Klem ML, Wing RR, McGuire MT, et al: A descriptive study of individuals successful at long-term maintenance of substantial weight loss. Am J Clin Nutr 66:239-246, 1997.
39. Shick SM, Wing RR, Klem ML, et al: Persons successful at long-term weight loss and maintenance continue to consume a low-energy, low-fat diet. J Am Diet Assoc 98:408-413, 1998.

Chapter 21

Stress and Depression in Diabetes

Richard R. Rubin

KEY POINTS

- *Diabetes-related distress is common, and depression is also more common among patients with diabetes than it is in the general population.*
- *Diabetes-related distress and depression are associated with many negative outcomes, including lower levels of diabetes regimen adherence, elevated levels of glycemia, more diabetes-related complications, and much higher health care costs.*
- *Clinicians can identify patients in their practices who suffer from diabetes-related distress or depression.*
- *There are effective treatments for diabetes-related distress and depression; use of these treatments is also associated with improved diabetes outcomes.*

Diabetes outcomes depend substantially on patient behavior, because the vast majority of clinically relevant decisions are made by patients themselves. These decisions are made countless times each day, whenever patients make choices about eating, activity, monitoring blood glucose, taking medication, or contacting their health care providers.

There is abundant evidence that most people with diabetes do not make these choices in ways that maximize the likelihood of positive diabetes outcomes. A recent large-scale international survey of adults with diabetes and clinicians from 13 countries in Asia, Australia, Europe, and North America, called the Diabetes Attitudes, Wishes, and Needs (DAWN) study, found that patient-reported regimen adherence was poor and that clinician estimates of adherence were even lower.[1] For example, less than 40% of patients (with type 1 or type 2 diabetes) said they were completely successful following diabetes-related diet and exercise recommendations. Clinicians' estimates were less than 20% for patients with type 1 diabetes and less than 10% for their patients with type 2 diabetes. Patients reported higher levels of adherence to medical aspects of their self-care including taking medication (about 80% completely successful), self-monitoring of blood glucose (about 67% completely successful),

and keeping appointments with diabetes health care providers (about 72% completely successful). Again, clinician estimates of the percentage of patients who were completely successful were lower in these areas: about 60%, 30%, and 50% respectively.

Figures 21–1 and 21–2 summarize the rate of perception of compliance with recommendations by patients and health care providers for type 1 and 2 diabetes, respectively. Low adherence to treatment recommendations is a source of frustration to many clinicians, especially because poor adherence limits the potential benefits of efficacious new treatments, creating a widening gap between possible and actual outcomes for the majority of patients.

Why do so many of our patients manage their diabetes so poorly? Psychosocial factors, including stress and depression, seem to play a major role. Clinicians who responded to the multinational DAWN survey said that a substantial majority of their patients with diabetes suffered from psychological problems, and almost half the patients participating in the same survey reported poor psychological well-being according to the World Health Organization Well-Being Index (WHO-5) criteria.[2] Depression, the leading cause of disability in the world, and the third most common reason for seeing a primary care provider, is at least 1.5 times more common among people with diabetes than it is in the general population.[3-6]

Stress and depression can trigger a negative cascade (illustrated in Fig. 21–3) involving impaired concentration, energy, and self-efficacy; diminished motivation; less-active self-care; higher blood glucose levels; increased risk of complications; and poorer quality of life. Almost 70% of clinicians responding to the DAWN survey said that psychological problems (including stress and depression) affected regimen adherence among their patients with diabetes.[1] In a sample of primary care patients with diabetes, those who were in the upper third in terms of depression severity had twice as many days when they did not take oral hypoglycemic agents as prescribed, compared with those in the lowest third of depression severity (15% vs. 7%).[7] Depression in people with diabetes is also associated with

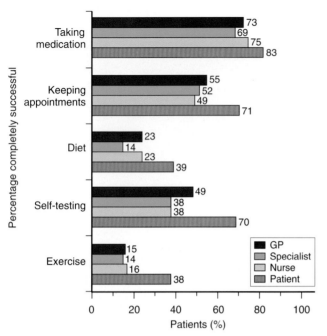

Figure 21–1. Compliance with recommendations for type 1 diabetes. GP, general practitioner.

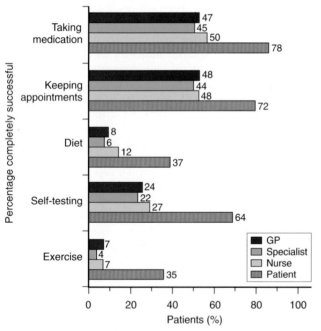

Figure 21–2. Compliance with recommendations for type 2 diabetes. GP, general practitioner.

higher hemoglobin A1c (HgA1c) levels,[8] increased complications rates,[7,9-11] and higher total health care costs.[7,12] Diabetes-specific emotional distress (frustration with the disease and its management) also appears to be directly related to self-care behavior and to long-term blood glucose control, even after adjusting for age, diabetes education, and general emotional distress.[13]

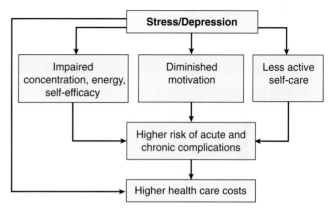

Figure 21–3. Effects of stress in patients with diabetes.

Unfortunately, despite their apparently substantial and widely recognized impact on medical and quality-of-life outcomes, psychological problems including stress and depression are rarely treated in patients with diabetes. In the DAWN survey almost half of patients reported poor psychological well-being and specific psychological problems, but only 10% said they received psychological treatment.[14] Only about 25% of diabetic patients suffering from depression receive adequate treatment for their psychological problems.[15]

This chapter is designed to help clinicians understand the association between psychosocial factors (especially stress and depression) and diabetes outcomes, identify patients whose diabetes care may be affected by psychological problems, and help these patients improve their psychological well-being and their self-care behavior and consequent health outcomes.

ASSOCIATION BETWEEN PSYCHOSOCIAL FACTORS AND DIABETES OUTCOMES

The association between psychological problems and diabetes outcomes has been a matter of interest for more than 300 years, since 1674. In that year Thomas Willis, the British physician who first identified glucosuria as a sign of diabetes, suggested that emotional problems *caused* diabetes. Willis said diabetes was the result of "sadness or long sorrow and other depressions and disorders."[16] This conjecture led to a fruitless search for the "diabetogenic personality," a search not abandoned until the 1970s, when attention turned from possible emotional *causes* of diabetes to emotional *consequences* of the disease.[17]

Life With Diabetes is Stressful

This shift made sense because life with diabetes is stressful and demanding for many patients. Living

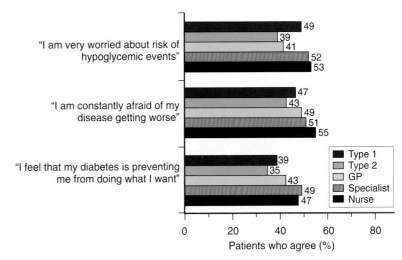

Figure 21–4. Diabetes-specific worries. GP, general practitioner.

with diabetes presents countless challenges ranging from the mundane to the monumental, from finding time to check your blood glucose in the middle of a busy day to learning to live with the reality of a major diabetes complication. Diabetes is there 24 hours a day, 365 days a year, and, as an 8-year-old patient with newly diagnosed diabetes pointed out to me a few years ago, 366 days in a leap year. Another patient noted that his diabetes was on his mind at least one time every 15 minutes, when he would stop briefly to check his "diabetes temperature," thinking about how he felt, how long it had been since he had eaten, how much insulin he had on board, what he thought his blood glucose level was, and whether he should check it.

Optimal diabetes care requires this kind of attention to the treatment regimen. That regimen involves essentially everything the person does, and for most people it also involves significant changes in lifestyle. All of our patients should monitor their blood glucose levels regularly, and many of them should take medication to help them keep their glucose, blood pressure, and cholesterol levels as close to normal as possible. A recent study found that half of a sample of people with type 2 diabetes took more than 7 different medications every day,[18] reminding us that the diabetes self-care regimen is complex, unremitting, and generally unpleasant, involving many restrictions and impositions. Few people would choose to eat as carefully and stay as active as people with diabetes are supposed to, and no one would choose to follow the regimen of medication taking, blood glucose monitoring, and medical follow-up recommended for most people with diabetes. Advances in diabetes treatment sometimes reduce the burden of diabetes self-care, but other times these advances are followed by recommendations for even more intensive self care.

Patients might find these demands more tolerable if their efforts were guaranteed to produce positive results, but this is not the case. Hard work increases the chances for good outcomes, but it does not guarantee these outcomes, and daily fluctuations in blood glucose levels when following the same regimen every day is a common experience.

High and low blood sugars themselves can add to the stress of living with diabetes. Hyperglycemia is associated with reduced levels of energy and poorer cognitive functioning, a combination of symptoms that contributes significantly to poorer quality of life.[19-20] The acute effects of hypoglycemia range from transient discomfort, to embarrassment when neuroglycopenia affects behavior, to emergencies when hypoglycemia is profound or it occurs when a person is driving. Chronic hypoglycemia can lead to cognitive impairment and physical limitations, and some people so fear hypoglycemia that they purposefully keep their blood glucose levels high enough to make low glucose levels—and avoiding acute and chronic diabetes complications—highly unlikely.[21]

Diabetes-Related Distress is Common

It is no wonder that people who have diabetes frequently say they feel frustrated, fed up, overwhelmed, or burned out by the demands of their disease. Many also report feeling chronically angry, guilty, or fearful. The DAWN study suggests that diabetes-related worries are very common among people with diabetes all over the world and that these problems are well-recognized by health care providers[1] (Fig. 21–4). Many patients who responded to the survey said they were constantly afraid their diabetes was getting worse (type 1, 46.5%; type 2, 42.5%), that diabetes was preventing them from doing what they wanted to do (type 1, 38.5%; type 2, 34.7%), that they were very worried that they would be unable to carry out their family responsibilities in the future because of their diabetes (type 1, 34.3%; type 2, 28.1%), that they were very anxious about their weight (type 1, 39.7%;

type 2, 55.1%), and that they were very worried about hypoglycemic events (type 1, 48.9%; type 2, 39.4%). Health care providers who participated in the DAWN study said they thought a larger fraction of patients experienced each of these diabetes-related worries, suggesting that clinicians know their patients are suffering from diabetes-related emotional distress. Potential sources of diabetes-related distress are listed in Box 21-1.

Studies by Polonsky and his associates reinforce the point that diabetes-related worries are common, leading to a condition sometimes labeled "diabetes burnout,"[22] or "diabetes overwhelmus."[23] Polonsky and his colleagues developed a questionnaire called the Problem Areas in Diabetes (PAID) Survey, designed to tap the breadth of emotional responses to diabetes.[13] For clinical purposes the PAID can be used to help providers identify patients experiencing high levels of diabetes-related emotional distress and formulate treatment interventions around specific problem areas.

The emotional reactions assessed by the PAID range from anger ("feeling angry when you think about having diabetes and living with diabetes") and interpersonal distress ("feeling that your family and friends are not supportive of your diabetes efforts") to frustration with aspects of the diabetes regimen ("feeling 'burned out' by the constant effort to manage diabetes"). The PAID has been shown to be a valid and reliable instrument for assessing diabetes-related emotional distress, and PAID scores were positively associated with other important outcomes, including general emotional distress, disordered eating, fear of hypoglycemia, and short- and long-term diabetes complications; PAID scores were negatively associated with reported self-care behavior and positively associated with hemoglobin A1c (HbA1c) levels. All of these associations strongly support the hypothesis that the PAID is tapping into the core concept of diabetes-related emotional distress.[13]

Polonsky and his associates found that approximately 60% of the respondents in their studies reported at least one serious diabetes-related distress; reports of no distress were rare, accounting for only 1.6% of all respondents.[13] The most strongly endorsed items were "worrying about the future and the possibility of serious complications" and "feeling guilty or anxious when you get off track with your diabetes management." It is clear that diabetes-related emotional distress is a common complaint among our patients with diabetes; it is also clear that this distress has negative consequences for diabetes self-care, metabolic control, and quality of life.

Psychological Disorders Are More Common among Those with Diabetes

According to a study in a national representative sample of adults with diabetes, the 12-month incidence of major depressive disorder (MDD) was 1.5 times the incidence in the general population (9.3% versus 6.0%).[3,5] These rates are lower for both populations than the results of a meta-analysis of 20 controlled studies that found the average rate of clinically significant depression symptoms was 20.5% among those with diabetes and 11.4% in those who did not have diabetes.[4] The lower rates reported in the national sample study could be explained by the fact that cases in this study were restricted to those with MDD—the most serious form of depression—and to the fact that cases in this study were established on the basis of a diagnostic interview, rather than the results of screening questionnaires that are known to identify a larger number of people as possibly depressed.

Regardless of how depression is assessed, it is clear that the condition is more common among patients with diabetes, and people with diabetes who get depressed often stay depressed. In one study,[24] 79% of patients who were depressed when they entered a study reported at least one recurrence of depression during the 5 years the study lasted; the average patient had 4.2 recurrences during that time. Risk factors for diabetes-related distress and depression are listed in Box 21-2, and common symptoms of depression are listed in Box 21-3.

When patients are depressed they often have trouble concentrating, they have little energy or self confidence, and they feel hopeless about the future. This probably explains why these patients are less adherent to diet, exercise, and medication recommendations.[7,25] The consequences of less-active self-care are seen in higher blood glucose levels and in higher complication rates. In a meta-analytic review of the literature, Lustman and colleagues found a small to moderate but significant association between depression and hyperglycemia in patients with type 1 and type 2 diabetes.[8] Another meta-analysis found an association of moderate effect size between depression and the presence of both macrovascular and microvascular complications,[9] and Ciechanowski and colleagues[7] found that in a population treated by primary care physicians,

Box 21-2. Risk Factors for Diabetes-Related Distress and Depression

- Difficulty following diabetes self-care recommendations
- Chronic hyperglycemia
- Reported diabetes symptoms inconsistent with blood glucose levels (over-reporting)
- Chronic pain
- Diabetes complications (especially neuropathy, cardiovascular disease, impotence)
- Smoking
- Obesity
- Female gender
- History of depression, anxiety disorder, or mental health treatment
- History of substance abuse
- Family history of depression or mental health treatment

Box 21-3. Symptoms of Depression

Cardinal Symptoms

- Depressed mood
- Loss of interest and pleasure

Secondary Symptoms: Physical

- Change in sleep
- Change in appetite
- Low energy or fatigue
- Psychomotor agitation or retardation

Secondary Symptoms: Cognitive or Mental

- Poor concentration
- Low self-esteem or guilt
- Recurrent thoughts of death or suicide

patients in the lowest tertile of depression severity had fewer complications than those in the two higher tertiles.

Some longitudinal studies suggest that depression is not simply associated with complications, but may contribute to the development and progression of at least some of them. For example, in one study, women with diabetes were followed for 10 years; those who were depressed at the beginning of the study had a fivefold increase in coronary artery disease (CAD) over the decade of the study compared with the women who were not depressed at baseline.[26] In another study of older adults with diabetes and CAD, the most powerful predictor of hospitalization or death during a 3-year follow-up period was a high depression screener score.[27] These findings suggest that effective depression treatment could dramatically reduce the toll taken by cardiovascular disease, the most common cause of death

in people with diabetes, accounting for about 70% of all deaths in this population.[28] Depression also seems to contribute to the development of other complications. Time spent in MDD predicted the development of retinopathy in a 10-year longitudinal study of children with type 1 diabetes.[29]

The association between depression and diabetes complications probably accounts for the dramatically higher health care costs associated with depression in people with diabetes. One study, based on health care costs in a nationally representative sample of people with diabetes in 1996, found these costs to be 4.5 times higher among patients who were depressed compared with those who were not depressed.[12] Another study also found elevated health care costs associated with depression, but the difference was smaller: total health care costs were 86% higher for those with high depression severity compared to those with low severity.[7] The economic toll of depression is probably not limited to excess health care costs; the lost productive work time attributable to depression in the United States is estimated to be more than $31 billion a year.[15,30]

MANAGEMENT

The management of patients with suspected diabetes related stress and depression is summarized in Figure 21–5.

How to Recognize Distressed or Depressed Patients

According to the best available estimates, almost 10% of patients with diabetes also suffer from major depressive disorder, at least 20% more suffer from milder forms of depression, and many more patients report significant diabetes-related emotional distress. All of these forms of emotional difficulty are known to be associated with less-active diabetes self-care and a cascade of negative physical and quality-of-life outcomes. These facts tell us why it is so important to recognize disease-specific distress and comorbid depression among our patients with diabetes and provide effective treatment to those who are distressed or depressed.

Patients at elevated risk for diabetes-related distress or depression can be identified through the medical history and clinical presentation, by asking specific questions, or through use of screening questionnaires. Patients at risk include those who have difficulty following diabetes self-care recommendations, especially those with high blood glucose levels.[13,19-20,31-34] Patients who report diabetes-related symptoms such as fatigue, blurred vision, thirst, and polyuria inconsistent with blood glucose levels, and those who report chronic pain out of proportion to the apparent physical basis are also at

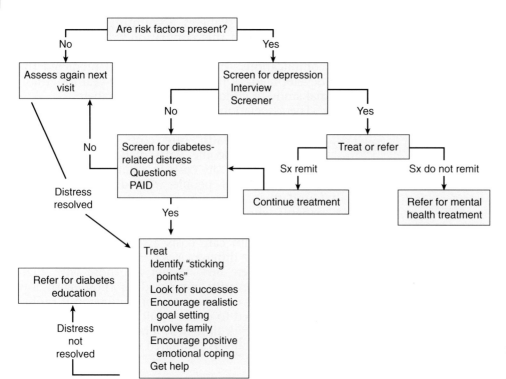

Figure 21–5. Comprehensive assessment and treatment of diabetes. PAID, Problem Areas in Diabetes Survey; Sx, symptoms.

increased risk for depression.[25] Patients who have diabetes complications, especially neuropathy, impotence, or cardiovascular disease, are also much more likely to suffer from diabetes-specific distress, depression, and anxiety disorder.[13,31,35-43] Smoking and obesity are associated with more depression in people with diabetes,[44] and women are more likely than men to report high levels of diabetes-related distress or to be depressed.[35-36,45-47] Patients with a history of depression, anxiety disorder, mental health treatment, or substance abuse are also at elevated risk for a current psychological problem, and so are those with a family history of depression or mental health treatment.

Once a patient who might be suffering from diabetes-related distress or depression is identified, the clinician must determine whether the patient has a problem, and if so what kind. The first objective is to see if the patient might be suffering from a frank psychological disorder such as depression, because this condition requires immediate medical attention, and effective treatment is associated with improved glycemic control.

Screening for Depression

According to the *Diagnostic and Statistical Manual*, 4th edition (DSM-IV),[48] nine symptoms are characteristic of depression. Two of these—depressed mood and loss of interest and pleasure—are called the cardinal symptoms, and at least one must be present for a diagnosis of major depression. It is important to recognize that people can be depressed and suffer the consequences of depression without reporting depressed mood; adhedonia, or lack of interest and pleasure, can be the primary symptom of depression in some patients. The clinician can identify patients likely to be depressed by asking two questions about mood and anhedonia (the DSM-IV cardinal diagnostic criteria): "During the past 2 weeks, have you felt down, depressed, or hopeless?" and "During the past 2 weeks, have you lost interest or pleasure in doing things?" Positive responses to one or both questions should trigger questions about the remaining seven DSM-IV symptoms.

Four of these symptoms are physical symptoms of depression—change in sleep, change in appetite or weight, low energy or fatigue, and psychomotor agitation or retardation—and can mimic medical symptoms that patients present with. The remaining three symptoms are cognitive or mental symptoms: poor concentration, low self-esteem or guilt, and recurrent thoughts of death or suicide. To make a diagnosis of major depressive disorder, *five or more* of these nine symptoms must be present (including *one or both* cardinal symptoms) nearly every day for at least 2 weeks and must cause significant distress or dysfunction. The clinician should verify the severity, frequency, and duration of any symptoms that are present.

Several forms of depression are commonly seen in medical practice. These include major depressive disorder, dysthymic disorder, adjustment disorder with depressed mood, and bipolar disorder II. *Major depressive disorder* (MDD) is the most serious and

of this 4-day program include improvements in several measures of emotional well-being (self-esteem, diabetes self-efficacy, depression, and anxiety), several aspects of self-care behavior (checking blood glucose, medication adherence and adjustment, diet, and exercise), as well as glycemic control.[70-72]

CONCLUSIONS

Helping patients resolve depression and diabetes-related distress can dramatically improve other diabetes outcomes. This chapter has offered guidelines and strategies for identifying patients who may be distressed or depressed, for helping patients resolve these problems, and for fostering positive emotional coping skills.

CONTROVERSIES

Some experts have begun to recommend chronic treatment for depression in the general population and in people with diabetes. Most clinicians still stop prescribing antidepressant medication once symptoms have remitted (and often before), but preliminary new evidence points to clear benefits for continuing treatment in patients with diabetes. Clinicians should be aware of this issue and consider the results of future research.

PITFALLS/COMPLICATIONS

Clinicians may doubt they have the time and other resources to screen for and treat diabetes-related distress and depression. Those who feel this way should keep two things in mind. First, these efforts are likely cost-effective if one considers the consequences of not treating these conditions; available data make it clear the toll is huge, including tremendous frustration for clinician and patient alike. Second, many of the strategies described in this chapter can be incorporated into practice without taking additional time. Clinicians should also consider having patients fill out screeners while they wait to be seen for visits, and involving office staff in scoring results and identifying patients who need more attention. Referrals for mental health treatment or diabetes self-management training should also be considered.

References

1. Rubin, R, Peyrot, M, Siminerio L: Predictors of diabetes self-management and control. Diabetes 51(Sup. 1):A437, 2002.
2. Bonsignore M, Barkow K, Jessen F, Heun R: Validity of the five-item WHO Well-Being Index (WHO-5) in an elderly population. Eur Arch Psychiatry Clin Neurosci 251(Suppl 2):II27-II31, 2001.
3. Egede LE, Zheng D: Independent factors associated with major depressive disorder in a national sample. Diabetes Care 26:104-111, 2003.
4. Anderson RJ, Freedland KE, Clouse RE, Lustman PJ: The prevalence of comorbid depression in adults with diabetes. Diabetes Care 24:1069-1078, 2001.
5. Kessler RC, Berglund P, Demler O, et al: The epidemiology of major depressive disorder: Results from the National Comorbidity Replication (NCS-R). JAMA 289:3095-3105, 2003.
6. Peyrot M, Rubin RR: Levels and risks of depression and anxiety symptomatology among diabetic adults. Diabetes Care 20:585-590, 1997.
7. Ciechanowski PS, Katon WJ, Russo JE: Depression and diabetes: Impact of depressive symptoms on adherence, function, and costs. Arch Intern Med 160:3278-3285, 2000.
8. Lustman, PJ, Anderson, RJ, Freedland, KE, et al: Depression and poor glycemic control: A meta-analytic review of the literature. Diabetes Care 23:934-942, 2000.
9. de Groot M, Anderson R, Freedland KE, et al: Association of depression and diabetes complications: A meta-analysis. Psychosom Med 63:619-630, 2001.
10. Rosenthal MJ, Fajardo M, Gilmore S, et al: Hospitalization and mortality of diabetes in older adults. A 3-year prospective study. Diabetes Care 21:231-235, 1998.
11. Clouse RE, Lustman PJ, Freedland KE, et al: Depression and coronary heart disease in women with diabetes. Psychosom Med 65:376-383, 2003.
12. Egede LE, Zheng D, Simpson K: Comorbid depression is associated with increased health care use and expenditures in individuals with diabetes. Diabetes Care 25:464-470, 2002.
13. Polonsky WH, Anderson BJ, Lohrer PA, et al: Assessment of diabetes-related distress. Diabetes Care 18:754-760, 1995.
14. Peyrot M, Rubin R, Siminerio L: Physician and nurse use of psychosocial strategies and referrals in diabetes. Diabetes 51(Suppl 2):A446, 2002.
15. Rubin RR, Ciechanowski P, Egede LE, et al: Recognizing and treating depression in patients with diabetes. Curr Diab Rep 4:119-125, 2004.
16. Willis T: Diabetes: A Medical Odyssey. New York, Tuckahoe, 1971.
17. Rubin RR, Peyrot MF: Psychosocial problems and interventions in diabetes: A review of the literature. Diabetes Care 15:1640-1657, 1992.
18. Piette JD, Heisler M, Wagner TH: Problems paying out-of-pocket medication costs among older adults with diabetes. Diabetes Care 27:384-391, 2004.
19. Van der Does FE, De Neeling JN, Snoek FJ, et al: Symptoms and well-being in relation to glycemic control in type II diabetes. Diabetes Care 19:204-210, 1996.
20. Mazze RS, Lucido D, Shamoon H: Psychological and social correlates of glycemic control. Diabetes Care 7:360-366, 1984.
21. Rubin RR: Hypoglycemia and quality of life. Can J Diab Care 26:60-63, 2002.
22. Hoover JW: Patient "burnout" can explain non-compliance. In Krall LP (ed): World Book of Diabetes in Practice, vol 3. New York, Elsevier Science, 1988, pp 321-324.
23. Rubin RR: Diabetes overwhelmus: Diagnosis, causes, and treatment. Practical Diabetology 19: 28-32, 2000.
24. Lustman PJ, Griffith LS, Clouse RE: Depression in adults with diabetes: Results of a 5-year follow-up study. Diabetes Care 11:605-612, 1988.
25. Ciechanowski PS, Katon WJ, Russo JE, Hirsch IB: The relationship of depressive symptoms to symptom reporting, self-care and glucose control in diabetes. Gen Hosp Psychiatry 25:246-252, 2003.
26. Clouse RE, Lustman PJ, Freedland KE, et al: Depression and coronary heart disease in women with diabetes. Psychosom Med 65:376-383, 2003.
27. Rosenthal MJ, Fajardo M, Gilmore S, et al: Hospitalization and mortality of diabetes in older adults. A 3-year prospective study. Diabetes Care 21:231-235, 1998.
28. Wingard DL, Barrett-Connor E: Heart disease and diabetes. In Harris MI (ed): Diabetes in America, 2nd edition. Bethesda, Md: National Institutes of Health, 1995, pp 429-448.

29. Kovacs M, Mukerji P, Drash A, Iyengar S: Biomedical and psychiatric risk factors for retinopathy among children with IDDM. Diabetes Care 8:1592-1599, 1995.

30. Stewart WF, Ricci JA, Chee E, et al: Cost of lost productive work time among US workers with depression. JAMA 289:3135-3144, 2003.

31. Trief PM, Grant W, Elbert K, and Weinstock RS: Family environment, glycemic control, and the psychosocial adaptation of adults with diabetes. Diabetes Care 21:241-245, 1998.

32. Saudek CD, Duckworth WC, Giobbie-Hurder A: Implantable insulin pump vs multiple dose insulin for non-insulin dependent diabetes mellitus. JAMA 276:1322-1327, 1996.

33. Hanestad BR, and Albrektsen G: Quality of life, perceived difficulties in adherence to diabetes regimen, and blood glucose control. Diabet Med 8:759-764, 1991.

34. Naess S, Midthjell K, Moum T, et al: Diabetes mellitus and psychological well-being. Results of the Nord-Trondelag health survey. Scand J Soc Med 23:179-188, 1995.

35. Peyrot M, Rubin RR: Levels and risks of depression and anxiety symptomatology among diabetic adults. Diabetes Care 20:585-590, 1997.

36. Peyrot M, Rubin RR: A new quality of life instrument for patients and families. Paper presented at the Psychosocial Aspects of Diabetes Study Group Third Scientific Meeting. Madrid, April 4-6, 1998.

37. Jacobson AM, de Groot M, and Samson JA: The evaluation of two measures of quality of life in patients with type I and type II diabetes. Diabetes Care 17:267-274, 1994.

38. Wuslin LR, Jacobson AM, Rand LI: Psychosocial aspects of diabetic retinopathy. Diabetes Care 10:367-373, 1987.

39. Wuslin LR, Jacobson AM: Visual and psychological function in PDR. Diabetes 38(Suppl 1):242A, 1989.

40. Whitehead ED, Klyde BJ, Zussman S, et al: Male sexual dysfunction and diabetes mellitus. N Y State J Med 83:1174-1179, 1983.

41. Lustman PJ, Clouse RE: Relationship of psychiatric illness to impotence in men with diabetes. Diabetes Care 13:893-895, 1990.

42. Cavan DA, Barnett AH, Leatherdale BA: Diabetic impotence: Risk factors in a clinic population. Diab Res 5:145-148, 1987.

43. Leedom LJ, Procci WP, Don D, Meehan WP: Sexual dysfunction and depression in diabetic women. Diabetes 35(Suppl 1):23A, 1986.

44. Katon W, Von Korff M, Ciechanowski P, et al: Behavioral and clinical factors associated with depression among individuals with diabetes. Diabetes Care 27:914-920, 2004.

45. Eiser C, Flynn M, Green E, et al: Quality of life in young adults with type 1 diabetes in relation to demographic and disease variables. Diabet Med 9:375-378, 1992.

46. Rubin RR, Peyrot M: Men and diabetes: psychosocial and behavioral issues. Diabetes Spectrum 11:81-87, 1998.

47. Ward J, Lin M, Heron G, Lajoie V: Comprehensive audit of quality-of-care and quality-of-life for patients with diabetes. J Qual Clin Pract 17:91-100, 1997.

48. American Psychiatric Association: Diagnostic and Statistical Manual of Mental Disorders, 4th ed. Washington, DC, American Psychiatric Association, 1994.

49. Lustman PJ, Harper GW: Nonpsychiatric physicians' identification of depression in patients with diabetes. Compr Psychiatry 28:22-27, 1987.

50. Spitzer RL, Kroenke K, Williams JBW, et al: Validation and utility of a self-report version of the PRIME-MD: The PHQ Primary Care Study. JAMA 282:1737-1744, 1999.

51. Beck AT, Beamesderfer A: Assessment of depression: The depression inventory. Med Probl Psychopharmacotherapy 7:151-169, 1974.

52. Radloff LS: The CES-D scale: A self-report depression scale for research in the general population. Appl Psych Meas 3:385-401, 1977.

53. Lustman PJ, Griffith LS, Clouse RE, et al: Effects of nortriptyline on depression and glycemic control in diabetes: Results of a double-blind, placebo-controlled trial. Psychosom Med 59:241-250, 1997.

54. Lustman PJ, Freedland KE, Griffith LS, Clouse RE: Fluoxetine for depression in diabetes: A randomized, double-blind, placebo-controlled trial. Diabetes Care 23: 618-623, 2000.

55. Lustman PJ, Griffith LS, Freedland KE, et al: Cognitive behavior therapy for depression in type 2 diabetes: A randomized controlled trial. Ann Intern Med 129: 613-621, 1998.

56. Katon WJ, Unutzer J, Simon G: The Pathways study: A randomized trial of collaborative care in patients with diabetes and depression. Arch Gen Psychiatry 61:1012-1049, 2004.

57. Williams JW Jr, Katon W, Lin EH, et al: The effectiveness of depression care management of diabetes-related outcomes in older patients. Ann Int Med 140:1015-1024, 2004.

58. Roose SP: Tolerability and patient compliance. J Clin Psychiatry 17(Suppl):14-17, 1999.

59. Montgomery SA, Reimitz PE, Zivkov M: Mirtazapine versus amitriptyline in the long-term treatment of depression: A double-blind placebo controlled study. Intl Clin Psychopharmacol 13:63-73, 1998.

60. Hinze-Selch D, Schuld A, Kraus T, et al: Effects of antidepressants on weight and on the plasma levels of leptin, TNF-α, and soluble TNF receptors: A longitudinal study in patients treated with amitriptyline or paroxetine. Neuropsychopharmacology 23:13-19, 2000.

61. Fava M, Judge R, Hoog SL, et al: Fluoxetine versus sertraline and paroxetine in major depressive disorder: Changes in weight with long-term treatment. J Clin Psychiatry 61:863-867, 2000.

62. Croft H, Houser TL, Jamerson BD, et al: Effect on body weight of bupropion sustained-release in patents with major depression treated over 52 weeks. Clin Ther 24:662-672, 2002.

63. Polonsky WH, Anderson BJ, Lohrer PA, et al: Assessment of diabetes-related distress. Diabetes Care 18:754-760, 1995.

64. Rubin RR, Peyrot M: Psychological issues and treatments for people with diabetes. J Clin Psychol 57:457-478, 2001.

65. Rubin RR: Facilitating self-care in people with diabetes. Diabetes Spectrum 14, 55-57, 2001.

66. Rubin RR, Biermann J, Toohey B: Psyching Out Diabetes: A Positive Approach to Your Negative Emotions, 3rd ed. Los Angeles, Lowell House, 1999.

67. Rubin RR, Peyrot M: Helping patients develop diabetes coping skills. In Anderson BJ, Rubin RR (eds): Practical Psychology for Diabetes Clinicians: How to Deal with the Key Behavioral Issues Faced by Patients and Health-Care Teams, 2nd ed. Alexandria, Va, American Diabetes Association, 2002.

68. Beck AT: Cognitive Therapy and Emotional Disorders. New York, International Universities Press, 1976.

69. Knowler WC, Barrett-Connor E, Fowler SE, et al: Reduction in the incidence of type 2 diabetes with lifestyle intervention or metformin. N Engl J Med 346:393-403, 2002.

70. Rubin RR, Peyrot M, Saudek CD: The effect of a diabetes education program incorporating coping skills training on emotional well-being and diabetes self-efficacy. Diabetes Educator 19:210-214, 1993.

70. Rubin RR, Peyrot M, Saudek CD: Differential effect of diabetes education on self-regulation and lifestyle behaviors. Diabetes Care 14:335-338, 1991.

72. Rubin RR, Peyrot M, Saudek CD: Effect of diabetes education on self-care, metabolic control, and emotional well-being. Diabetes Care 12:673-679, 1989.

Chapter 22

Exercise in Diabetes

Dina S. Green, Lawrence J. Mandarino, and Merri Pendergrass

KEY POINTS

- *Exercise in diabetes is potentially associated with risks as well as benefits.*
- *A well-planned program will optimize the likelihood of a safe and effective response by addressing what types of exercises can be performed and how much exercise is recommended.*
- *A pre-exercise evaluation should be performed to determine whether the patient has any long-term diabetes complications that could constitute a contraindication for certain exercises.*
- *For most patients, the exercise program should include both aerobic and resistance exercises.*
- *Aerobic exercise should consist of at least 150 minutes a week of moderate-intensity aerobic physical activity or at least 90 minutes a week of vigorous aerobic exercise distributed over at least 3 days a week and with no more than 2 consecutive days without physical activity.*
- *In the absence of contraindications, patients with diabetes should be encouraged to perform resistance exercise three times a week, including all major muscle groups.*

Regular physical activity is widely recognized as an essential component of the diabetes management plan. Because exercise in diabetes potentially is associated with risks (Box 22-1) as well as benefits (Box 22-2), health professionals who counsel patients on exercise should be familiar with potential adverse effects and how to prevent them. Each patient's unique characteristics (e.g., comorbid medical conditions, diabetes complications, medications) need to be carefully considered when a physician or other health care provider is formulating an exercise prescription. A well-planned program will optimize the likelihood of a safe and effective response by addressing what types of exercises can be performed and how much exercise is recommended.[1] It will also include appropriate monitoring to minimize the risk of complications and to increase the likelihood of adherence with the program.

Although advances in exercise physiology have facilitated the development of guidelines for developing exercise prescriptions in diabetes, the existing body of scientific information is not strong enough to warrant any rigid recommendations. Recommendations should be viewed as guidelines that should be applied to an individual patient in a flexible manner.

In this chapter we begin by reviewing the normal physiology of fuel metabolism during exercise. We highlight mechanisms by which exercise potentially ameliorates hyperglycemia and other metabolic abnormalities that occur in diabetes. We point out how diabetes-associated disruptions in normal physiology can pose potential exercise-associated risks. Next, we summarize potential benefits and risks of exercise in diabetes. We outline a pre-exercise evaluation to identify potential risks for certain types of exercise in some patients. We conclude by providing guidelines for formulating an exercise prescription. We use the terms "exercise" and "physical activity" interchangeably throughout the discussion.

PHYSIOLOGY OF FUEL METABOLISM DURING EXERCISE

Hormonal Events

Muscle glucose uptake is increased substantially by exercise. As long as the glucose uptake is balanced by increased glucose production, blood glucose remains relatively stable. In people with normal glucose tolerance, several compensatory hormonal changes occur during exercise to accomplish this. First, there is a decrease in endogenous insulin secretion. As insulin levels are suppressed, hepatic glucose production increases. Exercise also is associated with increases in counterregulatory

---

Box 22-1. Potential Risks of Exercise in Patients With Diabetes

- Cardiovascular events
- Musculoskeletal injury
- Vitreous hemorrhage or retinal detachment
- Foot ulcers
- Hypoglycemia
- Hyperglycemia
- Ketosis

Box 22-2. Potential Benefits of Exercise

- Delay or prevent the development of type 2 diabetes
- Reduce the need for medication in type 2 diabetes
- Lower blood glucose concentrations and hemoglobin A1c levels
- Improve lipid profiles
- Lower blood pressure
- Promote weight loss
- Improve cardiovascular conditioning
- Decrease overall mortality and cardiovascular mortality
- Reduce risk of cancer
- Reduce risk of depression
- Improve bone health
- Increase strength and flexibility
- Improve sense of well-being

---

hormones including glucagon, cortisol, and catecholamines. These hormones further augment hepatic glucose production.

If endogenous insulin levels cannot be suppressed during exercise, such as in patients treated with insulin or insulin secretagogues (sulfonylureas, meglitinides, or phenylalanine derivatives), the patient could be at risk for hypoglycemia. Sustained insulin levels not only inhibit hepatic glucose production but also stimulate peripheral glucose uptake. If the hepatic glucose production rate cannot match the rate of glucose uptake, the blood glucose concentration falls. This can actually be of benefit if the patient is hyperglycemic when exercise is initiated. However, if the patient has normal or near-normal glucose levels at the beginning of exercise, especially if the exercise is vigorous or prolonged, exercise can lead to hypoglycemia.

On the other hand, if a patient is underinsulinized, exercise-associated increases in hepatic glucose production could equal or exceed the fall in blood glucose. This can result in hyperglycemia, and it represents a particular risk with vigorous exercise, which is associated with larger increases in cortisol and catecholamines. In nondiabetic persons, insulin normally increases rapidly after the end of an intense exercise session, quickly restoring the glucose to baseline. In patients with deficient endogenous insulin production, hyperglycemia can last for several hours unless compensatory insulin is administered.

Glycemic decompensation is not the only metabolic risk the diabetic patient potentially faces during exercise. If there is concomitant insulin deficiency, hepatic ketone production also can be stimulated during exercise, and ketosis or ketoacidosis could ensue. This is most likely to occur in ketosis-prone patients with type 1 diabetes mellitus (T1DM).

Molecular Events

Exercise or muscle work has been known for many years to decrease the plasma glucose concentration in patients with T2DM. For example, during an exercise test to determine maximal aerobic capacity, which lasts about 15 minutes, the plasma glucose concentration in a patient with diabetes can decrease by 50 to 80 mg/dL.[2] Exercise can also have longer-term effects on glucose metabolism. For instance, a single bout of aerobic exercise improves insulin sensitivity for a period of 24 to 72 hours, depending on the duration and intensity of the activity.[3]

Many investigators have intensively studied the mechanisms that might be responsible for these effects. It has become apparent that the ability of muscle contraction to induce this immediate decrease in plasma glucose is directly related to a contraction-induced increase in the translocation of the GLUT4 glucose transporter to the sarcolemma, and this effect is largely independent of insulin.[4] Moreover, it is also clear that this effect of muscle contraction produces its effects by a signaling pathway that is independent of insulin signaling. Multiple laboratories have shown that muscle contraction does not activate the insulin receptor or its downstream signaling elements.[5,6] In addition, even moderate exercise decreases plasma insulin concentrations. Recent evidence points to activation of adenosine monophosphate (AMP)-dependent protein kinase as a requisite step in the increase in glucose uptake produced by muscle contraction.[7] Interestingly, both adiponectin and metformin also are AMP kinase activators.[8,9]

In addition to the acute glucose-lowering effects of exercise, more prolonged effects occur as well. Some of these effects can be mediated by prolonged (12 to 18 hours) activation of AMP kinase.[10] An additional factor is the decrease in muscle glycogen concentration produced by exercise, providing, in essence, a reservoir for plasma glucose. This decrease in glycogen content, along with other factors, also induces activation of skeletal muscle glycogen synthase, the rate-limiting enzyme in glycogen synthesis.[11] In the longer term, muscle

contraction also increases the protein abundance of hexokinase, specifically hexokinase II, which is the muscle-specific isoform.[12,13] Because this enzyme catalyzes the committed step in glucose uptake (phosphorylation of glucose), under certain conditions it can be a rate-limiting step for glucose uptake. Besides affecting muscle glucose uptake, acute exercise can also have effects on the liver. For example, a single 60-minute bout of moderate exercise undertaken by patients with type 2 diabetes (T2DM) lowers hepatic glucose production to near-normal levels.[11]

Chronic exercise, better termed *exercise training,* also produces long-term beneficial effects on plasma glucose concentrations and insulin sensitivity. For instance, 8 weeks of training increases insulin-stimulated glucose uptake in patients with T2DM.[14] In contrast to the acute effects of exercise, these long-term effects seem to be mediated mostly by changes in gene expression. The most consistent finding is that exercise training increases the protein expression of the GLUT4 glucose transporter.[4,14] However, there are also major increases in the protein abundance of glycogen synthase as well as the abundance of Akt, a key protein involved in insulin signaling.[14] Therefore, there seem to be multiple, coordinated changes in muscle, brought about by training, that lead to increased insulin signaling and glucose metabolism. Exercise training also improves endothelial function in patients with T2DM, which can be related to the improvement in insulin sensitivity or reduction in risk factors for cardiovascular disease.[15]

BENEFITS AND RISKS OF EXERCISE IN DIABETES

Exercise in T1DM does not improve the underlying pathogenetic defect. Nevertheless, patients with T1DM share the same benefits of exercise as do people with normal glucose tolerance (see Box 22-2) and should be counseled with this in mind.[16] On the other hand, as outlined in the preceding section, exercise in T2DM can improve molecular abnormalities associated with the disease. Exercise programs improve insulin sensitivity and can lower average blood glucose concentrations. The increased energy expenditure associated with exercise, in conjunction with caloric restriction, can improve weight reduction. Regular exercise also has been shown to be important for the prevention of T2DM.[17-19] Thus, regular exercise should be considered an integral component of the treatment regimen for T2DM.

Physical activity is a normal human function, and most people, including those with diabetes, should be safely able to participate in some kind of exercise program. However, exercise in diabetes also has risks (see Box 22-1). It is crucial that exercise programs be undertaken with the expectation that

---

Box 22-3. Pre-exercise Evaluation

A complete medical history, physical examination, and laboratory evaluation should be performed to determine

- Exercise history, including information about:
  - Readiness for change
  - Habitual level of activity
  - Type of exercise, frequency, duration, and intensity
- Presence of long-term diabetes complications that could constitute a contraindication for certain types of exercise, e.g.:
  - Autonomic neuropathy
  - Cardiovascular disease
  - Coronary heart disease
  - Hypertension
  - Microalbuminuria and nephropathy
  - Peripheral neuropathy
  - Peripheral vascular disease
  - Retinopathy
- Other medical information or conditions that require specific considerations
- Medications that might require adjustment (timing or dosing), in relation to the exercise program

---

potential benefits of exercise outweigh potential risks. It is therefore of prime importance that safety be the main concern in formulating the exercise prescription. Before advising a patient to increase the current level of physical activity, a pre-exercise evaluation should be performed.

PRE-EXERCISE EVALUATION

A pre-exercise evaluation is outlined in Box 22-3. A complete medical history, physical examination, and laboratory evaluation should be performed to determine whether the patient has any long-term diabetes complications or other medical condition that might constitute a contraindication for certain exercises. An exercise history that includes information on readiness for change, habitual level of activity, type of exercise, frequency, duration, and intensity should be obtained. Attention should be given to any medications that might need to be adjusted or timed in relation to the exercise regimen.

Because of the high prevalence of asymptomatic and symptomatic cardiovascular disease (CVD) in patients with diabetes, it seems prudent to include, as part of the pre-exercise evaluation, a formal evaluation for underlying cardiovascular disease. Unfortunately, there are no randomized trials or cohort studies evaluating the use of exercise stress testing specifically in people with diabetes. The American Diabetes Association previously recommended

testing all diabetic patients older than 35 years and all persons older than 25 years in the presence of even one additional CVD risk factor. Such a strategy would result in testing the majority of people with diabetes, including younger persons with a very low absolute risk of disease. This would be inconsistent with the US Preventive Service Task Force's (USPSTF) recent recommendation.[20,21] The USPSTF recommended that stress tests should not be performed to detect ischemia in asymptomatic persons who have a less than 10% risk of a cardiac event in the next 10 years because the risk of a false positive outweighed the expected benefits.

Although there are no proven benefits to screening for ischemia in low-risk, asymptomatic patients, there might be some value to performing a maximal aerobic exercise test in diabetic, as well as nondiabetic, persons. For example, it can provide useful information about maximal heart rate responses to different levels of exercise and initial performance status. This information can enable development of customized exercise prescriptions that might be safer and more beneficial for patients.

The American Diabetes Association's most recent technical review of exercise in diabetes concluded that available clinical evidence does not support any specific definitive recommendations regarding which patients should undergo stress testing.[22] In this context, the following revised criteria were proposed: In the absence of contraindications, maximal stress testing should be considered in diabetic patients to assess maximum heart rate, set exercise intensity limits, and assess functional capacity and prognosis. A graded exercise stress test with electrocardiographic monitoring should be considered before prescribing exercise with an intensity that exceeds the demands of everyday living in previously sedentary persons whose 10-year risk of a coronary event is greater than 10%. This corresponds to meeting any of the criteria listed in Box 22-4.

Box 22-4. Indications for Graded Exercise Testing With ECG Monitoring

- Age older than 40 years, with or without cardiovascular risk factors other than diabetes
- Age older than 30 years and
  - Diabetes of longer than 10 years duration
  - Hypertension
  - Cigarette smoking
  - Dyslipidemia
  - Proliferative or nonproliferative retinopathy
  - Nephropathy, including microalbuminuria
- Any of the following, regardless of age:
  - Known or suspected coronary artery disease, cerebrovascular disease, or peripheral vascular disease
  - Autonomic neuropathy
  - Advanced nephropathy with renal failure

EXERCISE IN THE PRESENCE OF DIABETES COMPLICATIONS

Unfortunately there is very little research on the risks and benefits of exercise in the presence of diabetes complications. The considerations discussed here primarily are based on expert opinion. Suggestions for selecting specific types of exercise for patients with diabetes complications are provided in Table 22–1.

Retinopathy

Neither resistance training nor aerobic training has been shown to have any adverse effects on vision or the progression of nonproliferative diabetic retinopathy or macular edema.[23] However, in the presence of proliferative or severe nonproliferative retinopathy, certain types of exercise (high-impact aerobic or heavy resistance exercises) may be contraindicated because of the risk of triggering hemorrhage or retinal detachment.[24] Following treatment by laser photocoagulation, a patient might need to wait several months before initiating or resuming this type of exercise. The appropriate time interval should be determined in conjunction with the treating ophthalmologist.

Peripheral Neuropathy

Common sense suggests that decreased pain sensation would result in increased risk of skin breakdown and infection, as well as Charcot joint destruction. In the presence of severe peripheral neuropathy it is probably best to encourage non–weight-bearing activities such as swimming or bicycling. It also is imperative to educate patients with diabetic neuropathy about foot care and regular foot inspection. In patients who have active foot ulceration, weight-bearing activity is absolutely contraindicated.[24] Patients with healed ulcers must use caution when performing weight-bearing exercise because of the vulnerability of scar tissue. Patients with evidence of Charcot's deformity should avoid weight-bearing activity.

Autonomic Neuropathy

Autonomic neuropathy can limit exercise capacity and can increase the risk of an adverse event during exercise.[25] Autonomic neuropathy is strongly suggestive of CVD in people with diabetes. People with this complication definitely should undergo cardiac investigation before beginning exercise at an intensity greater than their usual activities. Autonomic neuropathy also can increase the risk of exercise-induced injury associated with postural

Table 22–1. *Recommendations for Selecting Activities in Patients with Diabetes Complications*

Complication	Acceptable Activities	Discouraged Activities
Cardiovascular disease	Any	No specific restrictions on *mode* of exercise. Limitations on *intensity* should be dictated by cardiac status (see text).
Severe nonproliferative or proliferative retinopathy	Low-impact activities such as: Walking Step exercises Swimming Bicycling Rowing Chair exercises Arm exercises Tai Chi Yoga	Vigorous exercises that involve jarring, pounding, or Valsalva's maneuvers, such as: Boxing Heavy weight lifting Diving Jogging High impact aerobics Racquet sports Body contact sports Heavy trumpet playing
Peripheral neuropathy	Non–weight-bearing activities such as: Swimming Water aerobics Bicycling Rowing Chair exercises Arm exercises Tai Chi Yoga	Activities with repetitive stepping such as: Walking Step exercises Jogging
Autonomic neuropathy	See text	See text
Microalbuminuria and nephropathy	Any	No specific restrictions

hypotension, arrhythmias, impaired thermoregulation, anhidrosis with attendant dry skin prone to fissuring and ulceration, impaired night vision, impaired thirst, hypoglycemia from gastroparesis with unpredictable food delivery, hypoglycemic unawareness, hypoglycemic unresponsiveness, and incontinence.

If autonomic neuropathy is present, exercise programs should involve supervision by an exercise specialist with close attention to hemodynamic parameters. Patients with autonomic neuropathy also should pay special attention to foot care, including use of hydrating creams and wearing padded socks and appropriate footwear for exercise.

Microalbuminuria and Nephropathy

Physical activity can acutely increase urinary protein excretion, leading some experts to recommend that people with diabetic kidney disease perform only light or moderate exercise so that systolic blood pressure does not exceed 200 mm Hg.[26] However, there is no evidence from clinical trials or cohort studies demonstrating that vigorous exercise increases the rate of progression of diabetic kidney disease. The American Diabetes Association (ADA) technical review of exercise in diabetes does not recommend any specific exercise restrictions for people with diabetic kidney disease.[22]

However, because microalbuminuria and proteinuria are associated with an increased risk of CVD, it is important to perform a cardiac evaluation before beginning exercise that is more intense than the patient's current level of activity. Furthermore, screening for microalbuminuria should not occur in the aftermath of vigorous exercise, because exercise can transiently increase microalbumin excretion.

METABOLIC CONSIDERATIONS DURING EXERCISE

Patients with diabetes potentially are at risk for hypoglycemia, hyperglycemia, and ketosis, both during and after exercise. A general approach to glucose testing, nutrition supplementation, and medication adjustment related to exercise is shown in Figure 22–1.

In patients whose diabetes is well controlled and who are taking insulin or insulin secretagogues (sulfonylureas, meglitinides, phenylalanine derivatives), physical activity can precipitate hypoglycemia if the medication dose or carbohydrate consumption is not altered. This represents a particular risk when medication levels are at their peaks and during prolonged or particularly vigorous physical activity. Hypoglycemia is unlikely to occur in patients who are treated with diet alone, metformin, α-glucosidase inhibitors, or thiazolidinediones.

Patients who take insulin or insulin secretagogues should check their blood glucose before, during, and for several hours following an exercise session. This should be done on a regular and frequent basis until they know their own glycemic responses to

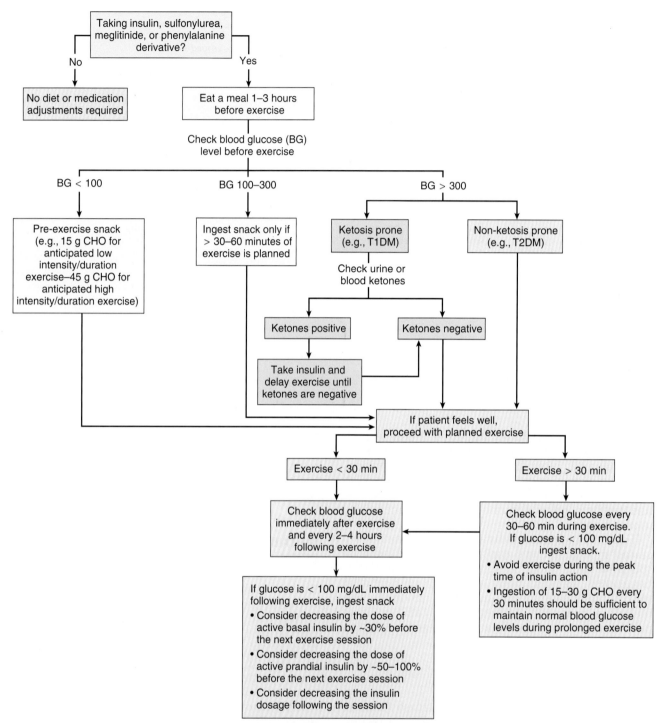

Figure 22–1. Approach to exercise-related glucose testing, nutrition supplementation, and medication adjustment. BG, blood glucose; CHO, carbohydrate; T1DM, type 1 diabetes mellitus; T2DM, type 2 diabetes mellitus.

specific exercise regimens. Patients predisposed to hypoglycemia might need to reduce doses of medications or consume extra carbohydrates before or during exercise.[27] After they become familiar with their own responses to exercise, they might be able to reduce the frequency of monitoring.

Unless ketosis is present, diabetic patients are unlikely to have problems when exercise is per-

formed in the presence of hyperglycemia. When glucose levels are elevated (greater than 300 mg/dL) before exercise, it would be prudent for patients with T1DM to check their urine or serum ketones. If ketones are negative and the patient feels well, it is probably unnecessary to postpone exercise strictly based on hyperglycemia. When glucose levels are elevated higher than 300 mg/dL in a patient with

Chapter 23

Insulin Secretagogues

Tamar Smith and John E. Gerich

KEY POINTS

- *Insulin secretagogues consist of two classes of drugs: sulfonylureas and meglitinides.*
- *In general, sulfonylureas are long acting (once-daily dosing), primarily target late insulin release, and reduce fasting plasma glucose levels without affecting postprandial plasma glucose increments. Meglitinides are short acting (preprandial dosing, 3 to 4 times daily), primarily target early insulin release, and reduce postprandial glucose excursions.*
- *With the exception of nateglinide, all secretagogues are equally efficacious in lowering hemoglobin A1c levels in people with type 2 diabetes and have similar major side effects.*
- *All secretagogues are biotransformed in the liver, and all except nateglinide need to be used with caution in patients with renal and hepatic failure.*

Type 2 diabetes (T2DM) is a heterogeneous disorder characterized by insulin resistance and impaired beta cell function.[1] Both genetic and environmental (i.e., acquired) factors are involved. Current evidence indicates that the primary genetic defect is impaired insulin release, whereas insulin resistance is largely an acquired defect secondary to obesity, physical inactivity, aging, high-fat diets, medications (e.g., steroids) and associated conditions (e.g., polycystic ovary syndrome).[2]

Defective beta cell function occurs early and can be detected in persons with normal glucose tolerance who have a first-degree relative with T2DM[3,4] and in persons with prediabetes (impaired glucose tolerance or impaired fasting glucose, or both).[2,5,6] Moreover, in genetically predisposed persons, beta cell function progressively deteriorates. Data from the United Kingdom Prospective Diabetes Study (UKPDS)[7] indicate that at the time of diagnosis, beta cell function is already reduced approximately 50% and decreases subsequently at a rate of about 6% per year, which is nearly 20-fold greater than the rate of about 0.3% per year that normally occurs

with aging.[8] Although people with prediabetes and T2DM have reductions in beta cell mass,[9] functional abnormalities, such as selective loss of first-phase or early insulin release,[10] also are present. Considering the fundamental importance of impaired insulin secretion in the pathogenesis of T2DM,[11] it is perhaps not surprising that the first oral agents demonstrated to be effective in treating this disorder were drugs that improved insulin secretion: the sulfonylureas.

Oral agents that improve insulin secretion—insulin secretagogues—are currently divided into two categories: sulfonylureas and nonsulfonylureas. The nonsulfonylureas, commonly called meglitinides, have been available for only a few years, whereas the sulfonylureas have been on the market since the 1950s. Although both meglitinides and sulfonylureas increase insulin secretion by fundamentally the same mechanism, they differ from each other in several aspects: structure (being either a benzoic acid [repaglinide] or a D-phenylalanine [nateglinide] derivative), efficacy, duration of action, beta cell binding characteristics, type of insulin response, and relative effects on fasting and postprandial hyperglycemia as well as the relative incidence of severe hypoglycemia, which is the major serious side effect of secretagogue therapy.

This chapter reviews key aspects of the major insulin secretagogues: their structures, mechanisms of action, pharmacology (onset, duration, routes of metabolism and pharmacokinetics, drug–drug interactions, and contraindications), efficacy, and adverse affects.

BACKGROUND

Sulfonylureas were the first oral hypoglycemic agents used to treat T2DM. They were initially developed as a result of studies in the 1920s and 1930s indicating that sulfonylamide antibiotics caused hypoglycemia.[12] By 1946, a series of classic experiments by Loubatieres[13-15] established that the sulfonamide group of these compounds was essential for hypoglycemic activity, that sulfonamides were effective in partially pancreatectomized—but

not totally pancreatectomized—dogs, and that pancreatecoduodenal vein effluents of a dog injected with a sulfonamide reduced plasma glucose levels in a cross-anastomosed totally pancreatectomized dog. These studies and subsequent ones showing no effect in type 1 diabetes (T1DM) patients lacking beta cells[16-18] established that these agents work predominantly, if not exclusively, by increasing insulin secretion.

The first sulfonylureas (carbutamide and tolbutamide) came to market in the early 1950s. Subsequent studies with these and other sulfonylureas suggested that these agents' antidiabetic action may also involve suppression of glucagon secretion (directly by acting on pancreatic alpha cells or indirectly by increasing intraislet insulin concentrations[19,20]) and improvement of insulin sensitivity. However, improvement of insulin sensitivity with these agents is most likely merely secondary to improved metabolic control rather than a direct effect on insulin target tissues, because sulfonylureas are ineffective in patients with type 1 diabetes who lack beta cells.[21]

Since the 1990s, use of the early sulfonylureas (tolbutamide, acetohexamide, tolazamide, chlorpropamide) has been superseded by use of the second-generation sulfonylureas (glyburide, glipizide, gliclazide, and glimepiride) because the newer drugs have convenient dosing, greater efficacy, and fewer side effects.[21] Of these agents, only glyburide, glipizide, and glimepiride are available for use in the United States. Consequently, only these sulfonylureas will be discussed in detail.

The structures of these sulfonylureas are shown in Figure 23–1. The basic sequence contained in all sulfonylureas is R_1-SO_2-NH-CO-NH-R_2. Differences in R_1 and R_2 lead to different pharmacokinetics, pharmacodynamics, and beta cell binding characteristics.

The meglitinides were developed as a result of screening amino acid derivatives[22] or modifications of meglitinide[23] (a compound related to the non-sulfonylurea portion of glyburide) for desirable effects on insulin secretion such as rapid and brief release of the hormone. Thus the meglitinides on the market in the United States (repaglinide and nateglinide) are characterized by a rapid onset and short duration of action. Their structures are shown in Figure 23–1.

These agents, like sulfonylureas, bind to sulfonylurea receptors on beta cells and stimulate insulin secretion by closing ATP-sensitive potassium channels. However, these agents apparently bind to different areas on the sulfonylurea receptor and have very rapid on and off kinetics so that they preferentially stimulate first-phase or early insulin release and do not apparently stimulate insulin release at subnormal glucose concentrations. These characteristics, in addition to their short duration of action in vivo (2 to 4 hours), result in their having their major action on postprandial glucose excursions.

BETACYTOTROPIC ACTIONS OF SULFONYLUREAS AND MEGLITINIDES

Adenosine triphosphate–sensitive potassium (K_{ATP}) channels play an essential role in the release of insulin (Fig. 23–2). Increases in intracellular ATP and ADP (adenosine diphosphate) levels as a result of metabolism of glucose close these channels. This causes depolarization of the beta cell membrane and an influx of calcium through voltage-sensitive calcium (Ca^{2+}) channels, which trigger the steps that lead to release of insulin.

K_{ATP} channels in beta cells consist of two components: the pore and a regulatory subunit that binds sulfonylureas and meglitinides (Fig. 23–3). The channel is actually an octomer containing four proteins that form the pore, called Kir6.2, and four proteins to which sulfonylureas and meglitinides bind, called the SUR (sulfonylurea receptor) (Fig. 23–4).[24]

Kir6.2 has a molecular weight of 43.5 kDa and contains 390 amino acids. It has two transmembrane domains, and both termini of the protein are intracellular. Another Kir protein—Kir6.1—with 70% homology has been identified in a variety of tissues and serves as part of the K_{ATP} channel in smooth muscle.[25]

The beta cell SUR, designated SUR1, has a molecular weight of 176 kDa and contains 1582 amino acids. It belongs to the ATP-binding cassette (ABC) family, has 17 transmembrane domains, and contains two nucleotide-binding domains. Binding of ATP to Kir6.2 closes the potassium channel, whereas binding of MgADP to SUR1 opens the channel. However, MgADP increases the efficacy of sulfonylureas and presumably meglitinides to close the channel.

Another SUR, existing as three splice variants termed SUR2A, SUR2B, and SUR2C, has been found in various tissues. SUR2A/Kir6.2 forms the potassium channel in heart and skeletal muscle. Both SUR2B/Kir6.2 and SUR2B/Kir6.1 exist in smooth muscle, whereas SUR1/Kir6.1 is found only in islets (alpha and beta cells) and neuronal tissue.

Sulfonylureas and meglitinides bind to intracellular domains of the K_{ATP} channel. There appear to be two binding sites—a high-affinity one on the SUR and a low-affinity one on the Kir. The latter is probably of no clinical significance because binding to it occurs only at supraphysiologic drug concentrations not observed in vivo. There is evidence that sulfonylureas such as glimepiride and glyburide interact with two segments on the SUR—one for the sulfonylurea moiety and one for the nonsulfonylurea moiety. Glyburide, glimepiride, and glipizide are thought to bind to both sites, whereas repaglinide and nateglinide bind only to the nonsulfonylurea site.

Sulfonylureas and meglitinides differ in their binding to the different SURs. For example, glyburide and glimepiride bind to SUR1 and SUR2 and are poorly reversible, whereas nateglinide, glic-

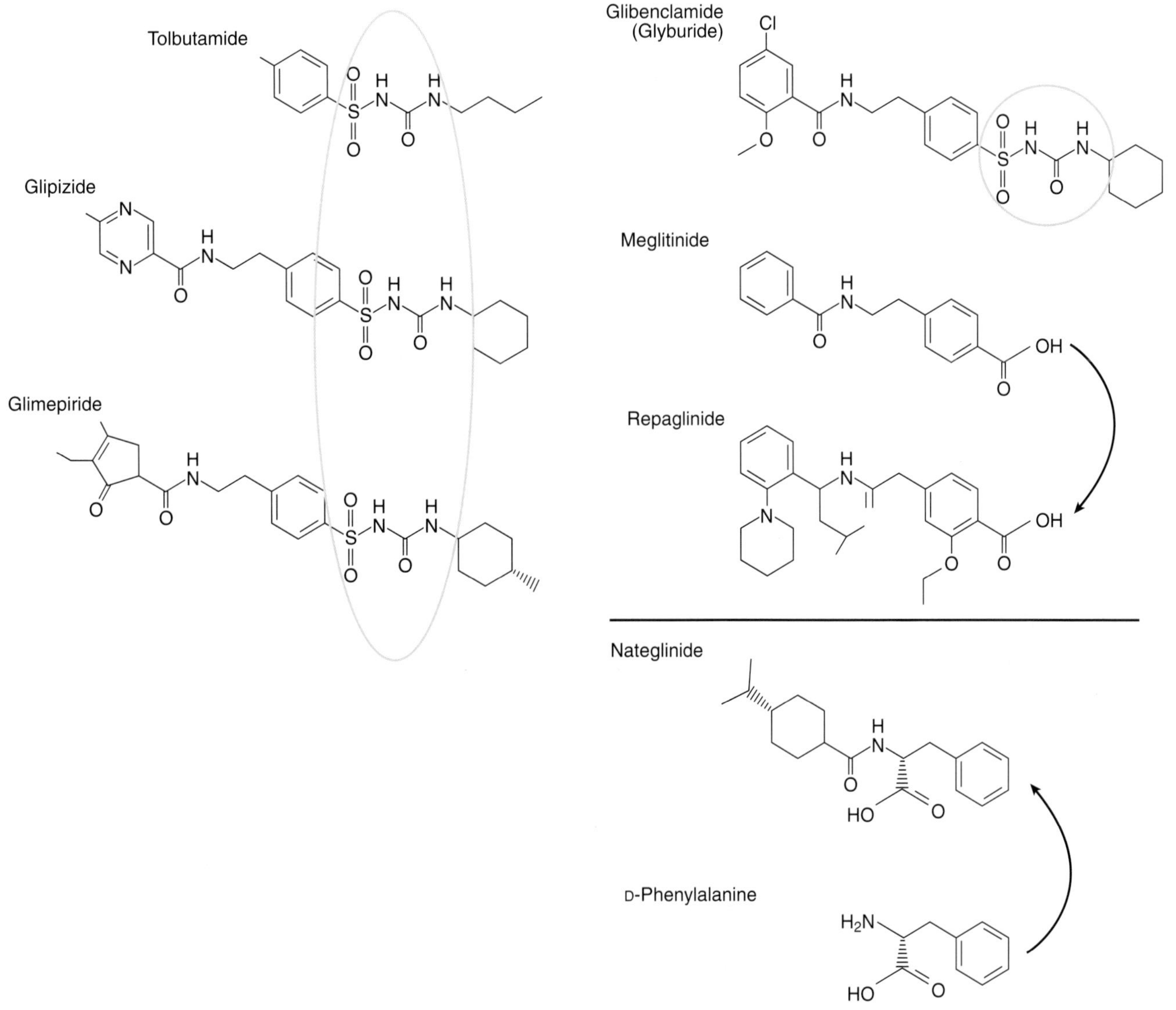

Figure 23–1. Structure of secretagogues. All sulfonylureas contain the basic structure R_1-SO_2-NH-CO-NH-R_2. Differences in R_1 and R_2 lead to different pharmacokinetics, pharmacodynamics, and beta cell binding characteristics. Nateglinide can be considered a phenylalanine derivative, whereas repaglinide is derived from the nonsulfonylurea portion of the glyburide molecule. Nevertheless, both are classified as meglitinides based on some structural similarities with meglitinide.

lazide, and glipizide essentially bind only to SUR1 and are reversible.[26] The relative order of displacement of labeled glyburide from cell membranes is glyburide > glimepiride > repaglinide > glipizide > nateglinide.[27]

The order of binding affinity of the sulfonylureas to their beta cell receptor parallels their relative potency.[28,29] Unlike glucose, sulfonylureas and meglitinides do not stimulate insulin synthesis. Although sulfonylureas can stimulate insulin secretion in vitro in the absence of glucose,[30] in vivo the main effect is to enhance the sensitivity of the beta cell to glucose. Thus greater increases in plasma insulin levels are observed at a given plasma glucose concentration.

Meglitinides and sulfonylureas also differ in their kinetics in closing the K_{ATP} channel.[31] The relative potency of inhibition of the K_{ATP} channel in patch clamp experiments has been reported to be repaglinide > glyburide > nateglinide, whereas in terms of onset of inhibition nateglinide was equal to glyburide but more rapid than repaglinide and glimepiride[27,31] and in terms of speed of reversibility nateglinide > glimepiride > glyburide > repaglinide. Finally, glyburide accumulates in islets whereas other sulfonylureas, repaglinide, and nateglinide are not appreciably internalized.[31]

These different interactions with K_{ATP} channels as well as differences in their pharmacokinetics may explain the differences in the patterns of insulin secretion observed when these agents are used therapeutically.

Secretion of insulin from beta cells is biphasic (Fig. 23–5). The first phase involves the fusion

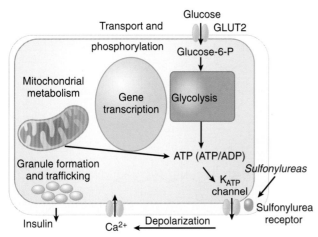

Figure 23–2. Mechanism of action of glucose and insulin secretagogues. When glucose is metabolized by beta cells, intracellular ATP/ADP ratios increase. This leads to closure of beta cell membrane ATP-sensitive potassium (K_{ATP}) channels. Binding of sulfonylureas and meglitinides to sulfonylurea receptors on beta cells also closes the potassium channel. This leads to depolarization of the cell membrane and the opening of voltage-sensitive calcium. The resultant increase in intracellular calcium triggers release of insulin. ADP, adenosine diphosphate; ATP, adenosine triphosphate; glucose-6-P, glucose-6-phosphate. (Modified and reproduced, with permission, from Boyd AE: Sulfonylurea receptors, ion channels, and fruit flies. Diabetes 37:847-850, 1988.)

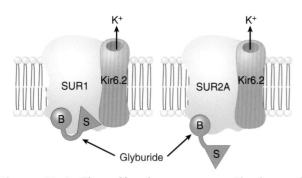

Figure 23–3. The sulfonylurea receptor. The beta cell sulfonylurea receptor (SUR1) has a molecular weight of 176 kDa, contains 1582 amino acids, and has 17 transmembrane domains and two nucleotide binding sites. (See Figure 23–4 for a description of Kir6.2 proteins.) (Modified from Babenko AP, Aguilar-Bryan L, Bryan I: A view of SUR/K_{IR}6.X, K_{ATP} channels. Annu Rev Physiol 60:667-687, 1998. Reprinted, with permission, from Annual Review of Physiology, Volume 60, © 1998 by Annual Reviews, www.annualreviews.org.)

of insulin-containing granules near the plasma membrane, the *immediately releasable pool*. The latter second phase of insulin release involves the transfer of insulin granules from a storage pool to the immediately releasable pool; the latter requires ATP. First-phase insulin release is believed to correspond to the early release of insulin after meal ingestion. This mechanism is defective in people with prediabetes and type 2 diabetes[10] and is a

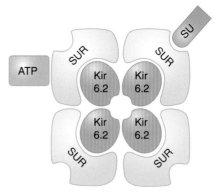

Figure 23–4. The tetrameric architecture of the K_{ATP} channel. The K_{ATP} channel is an octomer containing four sulfonylurea receptor (SUR) proteins and four pore proteins called Kir6.2. Kir6.2 has a molecular weight of 43.5 kDa, contains 390 amino acids, has two transmembrane domains, and forms the inner part (pore) of the K_{ATP} channel. (K_{ATP}, adenosine triphosphate–sensitive potassium. (Adapted and reproduced, with permission, from Clement JP 4th, Kunjilwar K, Gonzalez G, et al: Association and stoichiometry of K(ATP) channel subunits. Neuron 18:827-838, 1997).

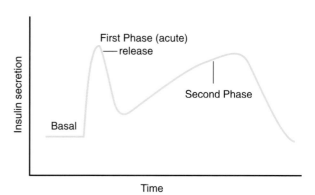

Figure 23–5. Schematic of biphasic insulin secretion. When insulin secretion is stimulated by square-wave hyperglycemia, both in vitro and in vivo, insulin is released in a biphasic pattern. The first phase consists of a spike lasting about 10 minutes. The first phase is followed by a slowly increasing release that reaches steady state after 1 to 2 hours depending on the degree of hyperglycemia. This is referred to as second-phase insulin release. First-phase insulin release is due to release of insulin from insulin-containing granules closely associated with the beta cell plasma membrane and constitutes a rapidly releasable pool. Second-phase insulin release involves the energy-dependent transfer of insulin-containing granules from a slowly releasable pool into the rapidly releasable pool. First-phase insulin release has been identified with the early (initial 30 minutes) increase in insulin secretion that occurs after food ingestion. First-phase, second-phase, and early insulin release are all impaired in people with impaired glucose tolerance and type 2 diabetes. A reduction in first-phase insulin release has been observed in people with normal glucose tolerance who have a first-degree relative with type 2 diabetes.[3] (Adapted and reproduced, with permission, from Pratley R, Weyer C: The role of impaired early insulin secretion in the pathogenesis of type II diabetes mellitus. Diabetologia 44:929-945, 2001.)

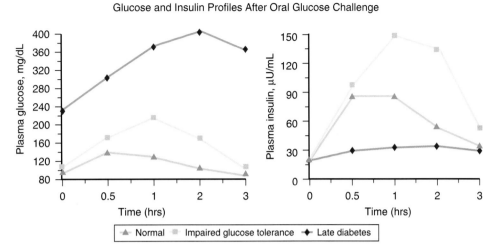

Figure 23–6. Comparison of plasma insulin levels during oral glucose tolerance tests in subjects with normal glucose tolerance *(blue triangles)*, impaired glucose tolerance *(yellow squares)*, and type 2 diabetes *(red lozenges)*. Note the reduced early (0.5 hour) levels in people with impaired glucose tolerance and type 2 diabetes despite greater hyperglycemia (i.e., a greater stimulus for insulin secretion). (Data from Mitrakou A, Kelley D, Mokan M, et al: Role of reduced suppression of glucose production and diminished early insulin release in impaired glucose tolerance. N Engl J Med 326:22-29, 1992, and Mitrakou A, Kelley D, Veneman T, et al: Contribution of abnormal muscle and liver glucose metabolism in postprandial hyperglycemia in noninsulin-dependent diabetes mellitus. Diabetes 39:1381-1390, 1990.)

Table 23–1. *Characteristics of Commonly Used Sulfonylureas and Meglitinides*

	Glyburide	Glipizide	Glimepiride	Repaglinide	Nateglinide
Half life (h)	10-16	3-5	4-6	~0.6	~1.5
Duration of action (h)	24-30	16-24	~24	4-5	5-6
Metabolism	Liver	Liver	Liver	Liver	Liver
Active metabolites	Yes	No	No	No	Yes
Elimination	Feces, kidney	Feces, kidney	Feces, kidney	Feces, kidney	Feces, kidney
Doses available (mg)	1.25, 2.5, 5	5, 10	1, 2, 4	0.5, 1.2	60, 120
Administration	Once or twice daily	Once or twice daily	Once daily	5-30 min before meals	5-30 min before meals
Maximum daily dose	10-15 mg	15-20 mg	4-8 mg	6-8 mg	120 mg

major cause of postprandial hyperglycemia (Fig. 23–6). Thus agents that improve first-phase insulin release, such as glimepiride,[32] repaglinide,[23] and nateglinide,[22] reduce postprandial increases in plasma glucose.[33]

CLINICAL PHARMACOLOGY

Sulfonylureas are rapidly and nearly completely absorbed after oral administration and circulate more than 99% bound to plasma proteins. Peak plasma levels of sulfonylureas occur at 2 to 4 hours after ingestion.[34-36] Food ingestion has little effect on their efficacy, but it is recommended that they be taken 15 to 30 minutes before consuming a meal. Repaglinide and nateglinide reach peak plasma levels earlier than sulfonylureas after oral administration (0.5 to 1 hour). Repaglinide is not significantly affected by food ingestion, but nateglinide is. Nevertheless, it is recommended that both these agents be taken immediately or shortly before meals. Like sulfonylureas, meglitinides circulate approximately 99% bound to plasma proteins.

Sulfonylureas and meglitinides are cleared from the circulation primarily by biotransformation in the liver and to a lesser extent by biliary and fecal excretion; their hepatic metabolites, of which some have hypoglycemic activity, are then primarily excreted by the kidney, mainly as carboxy- and hydroxy-derivatives.[21] Hepatic metabolism of these compounds involves the cytochrome P450 system and can thus be affected by genetic polymorphisms of these enzymes as well as drugs that alter the activity of these enzymes. Characteristics of sulfonylureas and meglitinides are summarized in Table 23–1.

Repaglinide[23] has a half-life of approximately 0.6 hours and thus a duration of action of 4 to 5 hours. It is biotransformed in the liver via the CYP3A4 enzyme system, with products excreted 90% fecally and 8% renally. Age and moderate renal insufficiency do not appreciably affect the pharmacoki-

netics of repaglinide, but chronic liver disease (Child Pugh grade B or C) increases its half-life and plasma concentrations twofold to threefold.[37] Repaglinide is available in doses of 0.5 mg, 1 mg, and 2 mg. For best results it should be taken immediately (5 to 30 minutes) before each meal. Although the maximum recommended premeal dose is 4 mg, maximum effects are generally achieved with the 2-mg dose.

Nateglinide[22] has a half-life of about 1.5 hours and thus a duration of action of 5 to 6 hours. It is metabolized by the hepatic mixed-function oxidase system, primarily via hydroxylation and glucuronide conjugation. About 90% of the drug is excreted renally as metabolites, some of which may be active. Age, mild to moderate renal insufficiency, and liver disease do not appreciably affect its pharmacokinetics.[38] The drug is available in doses of 60 and 120 mg to be taken before each meal (5 to 30 minutes). Titration of the drug is generally not necessary because the recommended starting and maintenance dose is 120 mg whether used singly or in combination with metformin or a thiazolidinedione.

Glipizide has a half-life of about 4 hours and an effective duration of action of 16 to 24 hours.[34,35,39,40] It can thus be given once daily but is usually given twice a day if the daily total exceeds 15 mg. An extended-release form with a similar efficacy and safety profile is available for once-a-day dosing.[41] Glipizide is converted in the liver to several inactive metabolites, most of which are excreted in the urine. About 15% of a dose is excreted in the feces.[42] According to the FDA-approved package insert, insufficient data are available to determine whether aging affects glipizide pharmacokinetics, and caution is urged in patients with hepatic and renal disease because they may prolong its effective half-life. Glipizide is more effective when administered 15 to 30 minutes before a meal than with a meal. It is available as 5-mg and 10-mg tablets. The maximum recommended daily dose is 40 mg, but maximum effects are generally achieved at 15 mg to 20 mg.[43]

Glyburide is the longest-acting insulin secretagogue; it has a half-life of about 10 hours and therefore an effective duration of action of well over 24 hours.[44,45] In practice, doses are usually divided when the daily total exceeds 10 mg, but there is no rational basis for this. Glyburide is converted in the liver to three major metabolites,[34,35,39,40] one of which (4-hydroxyglyburide) has about 15% of the potency of glyburide.[46] About 50% of a dose of glyburide is excreted in the feces and the remainder in the urine as metabolites, with only about 3% excreted as intact glyburide.[44,47] Although this excretion pattern should tend to lessen the influence of changes in renal function on glyburide's action, it is probably offset by the accumulation of the active metabolite 4-hydroxyglyburide in cases of renal failure.[45,48] In contrast, the accumulating metabolites of glimepiride and glipizide[49] are essentially inactive. Aging and hepatic and renal disease would be expected to prolong the duration of action and increase the effect of glyburide. Thus its use in these populations must be cautious. Glyburide is available as 1.25-mg, 2.5-mg, and 5-mg tablets. Daily doses higher than 20 mg are not recommended because the maximum effect is usually achieved at 10 mg to 15 mg daily.

Glimepiride[36] has a half-life of about 5 hours and is thus an effective duration of action of about 24 hours; it is therefore dosed once daily. It is completely metabolized in the liver by the cytochrome P450 system to essentially inactive metabolites that are eliminated renally and fecally. Neither aging nor renal insufficiency affects glimepiride pharmacokinetics; however, the impact of liver disease is unclear. The drug is available in 1-mg, 2-mg, and 4-mg denominations. It is usually given once daily in the morning shortly before breakfast (about 15 to 30 minutes). Although the maximum recommended dose is 8 mg per day, the maximum effect is usually achieved with 4 mg.

EFFICACY

The reader is referred to several reviews.[21-23,36,50,51]

Monotherapy

The clinical efficacy of sulfonylureas and meglitinides as antidiabetic agents has generally been assessed on the basis of their ability to reduce and maintain acceptable hemoglobin A1C (HbA1c) levels. Responses to both these groups of secretagogues are dependent on adequate beta cell function and the initial HbA1c. Patients with long-standing diabetes and little beta cell function generally fail to have a satisfactory response to secretagogue therapy, whereas patients with the highest HbA1c levels usually have the greatest decrements in HbA1c. In general, in drug-naive patients with initial HbA1c levels 8.5% to 9.5%, sulfonylureas can lower HbA1c levels by 1.5 to 2.0 percentage points.[51] Clinical trials indicate that there is no significant difference among glyburide, glipizide, or glimepiride, the most commonly used sulfonylureas.[52,53]

Compared to placebo, repaglinide appears to lower HbA1c levels to the same extent as the sulfonylureas (1.5 to 2.0 percentage points) as monotherapy,[54,55] whereas nateglinide produces somewhat lower decrements in HbA1c (0.6 to 1.2 percentage points).[56,57] In head-to-head comparisons with other agents, repaglinide has been reported to have efficacy equal to glyburide[58-60] and metformin.[61] In contrast, nateglinide has been reported to lower HbA1c levels approximately 0.3 percentage points less than metformin[57] and to reduce fasting plasma glucose levels less than gly-

buride (approximately 20 mg/dL versus approximately 50 mg/dL) while producing reductions in postmeal plasma glucose increments comparable to those of glyburide.[62] However, nateglinide was associated with less symptomatic hypoglycemia than glyburide,[62] whereas repaglinide has not been reported to produce significantly less symptomatic hypoglycemia than glyburide.[58-60]

If the target HbA1c level is less than 7.0% as recommended by the American Diabetes Association[63] or less than 6.5% as recommended by the American Association of Clinical Endocrinologists,[63] it stands to reason that a patient with an initial HbA1c higher than 9.0% is unlikely to achieve adequate glycemic control with sulfonylurea or meglitinide monotherapy.[21] This is commonly referred to as *primary sulfonylurea failure*. There is no evidence that switching such patients to another sulfonylurea (or a meglitinide) will improve glycemic control.

With prolonged sulfonylurea and meglitinide therapy, most patients who initially achieved adequate glycemic control eventually escape.[64] This is referred to as *secondary failure* and needs to be distinguished from transient deterioration in glycemic control due to acute stress such as infection, surgical procedure, or steroid treatment. The cause of secondary failure is progressive deterioration of beta cell function that is part of the natural history of the disease.

In the United Kingdom Prospective Diabetes Study (UKPDS),[64] beta cell function was already reduced by 50% in patients with newly diagnosed diabetes, and it decreased further at a rate of about 6% per year. A similar rate of decrease in beta cell function was observed in patients being treated by diet or metformin, indicating that sulfonylurea therapy does not uniquely lead to beta cell burnout and that the deterioration in beta cell function is part of the natural history of the disease. As a consequence, in the UKPDS at 3 years, only about 45% of patients who had initially achieved an HbA1c of 7% or less still had HbA1c levels below this point.[64] Thus it can be expected that patients initially treated with secretagogues as monotherapy will need a second oral agent of a different class and eventually some form of insulin therapy.

Combination Therapy

Sulfonylureas and meglitinides are approved for use with other oral antidiabetic agents that work via different mechanisms (insulin sensitizers such as metformin and thiazolidinediones; α-glucosidase inhibitors such as acarbose and miglitol) and insulin. Using secretagogues in combination with a sensitizer as initial therapy generally results in additive effects. For example, in a study comparing metformin alone, nateglinide alone, and nateglinide plus metformin in drug-naive patients who had an initial HbA1c of about 8.2%, metformin and nateglinide monotherapy reduced HbA1c levels by 0.8 percentage points, whereas combination therapy reduced it by 1.6 points.[65]

In general, adding sulfonylureas and meglitinides to other agents results in a reduction in HbA1c levels somewhat lower (1.0 points to 1.5 points) than that seen in drug-naive patients,[51] probably due to reduction in beta cell function at this stage of the disease. The reduction in HbA1c level expected upon adding another oral agent to sulfonylureas depends on which agent is added. In general, one can expect reductions of about 1.0 percentage point with metformin and thiazolidinediones and about 0.5 percentage points with α-glucosidase inhibitors. Adding a meglitinide to a sulfonylurea is ineffective because both secretagogues work by closing potassium channels; once potassium channels are closed, they cannot be closed more.

Using sulfonylureas and meglitinides with basal insulin (NPH or glargine) is superior to using insulin alone in producing more rapid improvements in glycemic control and perhaps diminishing the magnitude of hypoglycemia and weight gain, which are common side effects of insulin therapy.[66] The rationale for this approach is that the basal insulin reduces fasting plasma glucose levels and "rests the beta cell" so that the sensitization of beta cells to glucose levels by sulfonylureas can be taken advantage of to reduce postprandial glucose excursions.

SIDE EFFECTS

Sulfonylureas and meglitinides are generally well tolerated, with less than 2% of patients discontinuing treatment because of side effects.[21-23] Sulfonylureas and meglitinides are generally neutral with respect to plasma lipids and blood pressure. Their major side effects are weight gain, hypoglycemia, hypersensitivity reactions, and rarely hyponatremia.[21,67]

Weight Gain

The weight gain associated with sulfonylurea and meglitinide treatment is not inevitable[22,43,68] and can be attributed largely to three factors: retention of calories previously lost as glucosuria, reduction of resting energy expenditure as a result of reduced gluconeogenesis secondary to improved insulin secretion,[69] and overtreatment of mild hypoglycemia. Of these, the first and third are probably most important. The most weight gain is observed with agents most commonly associated with hypoglycemia (e.g., glyburide).[67] In some studies, little or no weight gain has been reported with nateglinide,[22] glipizide,[43] and glimepiride.[36,68]

Hypoglycemia

Hypoglycemia is the most serious side effect of secretagogue therapy. The incidence of severe sulfonylurea hypoglycemia (that producing coma or requiring the help of another person for recovery) is about 2 or 3 episodes per 1000 patient-years, with a mortality risk of 0.015 to 0.03 per 1000 patient-years.[70,71] About 10% of patients hospitalized because of sulfonylurea hypoglycemia die.[72] Mild episodes of hypoglycemia are more common. In the first 3 years of UKPDS,[73] for example, about 25% of the subjects treated with glyburide experienced hypoglycemic symptoms. Not unexpectedly, aging and impaired renal function increase the risk of severe hypoglycemia. In addition, some drugs can enhance the action of sulfonylureas (Box 23-1).

The frequency of hypoglycemia varies among sulfonylureas and meglitinides[67]: Glyburide is the agent associated with the highest frequency, and glimepiride and nateglinide are probably associated with the least. For example, in a population-based study, glyburide therapy was associated with an almost seven-fold greater frequency of severe hypoglycemia than was glimepiride therapy.[74]

The explanation for the differences in frequency of hypoglycemia among sulfonylureas (and meglitinides) is multifactorial and includes their relative potency, duration of action, presence or absence of active metabolites excreted renally, their relative effects on early and late insulin release, and their ability to stimulate insulin secretion inappropriately at low plasma glucose levels. Although detailed head-to-head comparisons are not available, the order of frequency of hypoglycemia among commonly used insulin secretagogues may be viewed as glyburide > glipizide ≥ repaglinide > glimepiride > nateglinide.

Other Side Effects

Uncommon side effects, which occur with about the same frequency with all agents, include dermatologic and hematologic reactions (less than 0.1%) such as rashes, pruritus, erythema nodosum, erythema multiforme, exfoliative dermatitis, hemolytic anemia, and bone marrow aplasia. These usually appear within the first 6 weeks of treatment.[21]

Chlorpropamide, which is not commonly used anymore, was often associated with Antabuse-like reactions similar to those produced by disulfiram and with the inappropriate secretion of antidiuretic hormone, which can cause severe hyponatremia. About 5% of the patients treated with chlorpropamide have serum sodium concentrations of less than 129 mmol/L, but they are usually asymptomatic.[70,75,76] Hyponatremia has also been reported with glyburide and glipizide, but not with glimepiride, repaglinide, or nateglinide. Other sulfonylureas, but not nateglinide or repaglinide,

---

Box 23-1. Pharmacokinetic and Pharmacodynamic Interactions That Augment the Hypoglycemic Action of Sulfonylureas and Meglitinides

Displace from Plasma Protein

Clofibrate

Nonsteroidal antiinflammatory drugs (NSAIDs)

Phenylbutazone

Salicylates

Sulfonamides

Reduce Hepatic Metabolism

Chloramphenicol

Dicumarol

Fluoroquinolone antibiotics

Gemfibrozil

H_2 blockers

Miconozole and related compounds

Monamine oxidase inhibitors

Phenylbutazone

Rifampin

Sulfaphenazole

Decrease Urinary Excretion of Metabolites

Allopurinol

Phenylbutazone

Probenecid

Salicylates

Sulfonamides

Intrinsic Hypoglycemic Activity

Alcohol

Angiotensin-converting enzyme (ACE) inhibitors

β-Adrenergic antagonists

Guanethidine

Monamine oxidase inhibitors

Insulin

Salicylates

---

are very rarely associated with Antabuse-like reactions.[39,40,70]

DRUG INTERACTIONS

Insulin secretagogues in general undergo biotransformation in the liver via the cytochrome P450 system to metabolites that may or may not be active. These metabolites may be further processed by glucuronidation or esterification and eliminated

135. Hookman P, Barkin J: Current biochemical studies of non-alcoholic fatty liver disease and nonalcoholic steatohepatitis suggest a new therapeutic approach. Am J Gastroenterol 98:2093-2097, 2003.

136. Marchesini G, Brizi M, Bianchi G, et al: Metformin in non-alcoholic steatohepatitis. Lancet 358:893-894, 2001.

137. Jones K, Arslanian S, Peterokova V, et al: Effect of metformin in pediatric patients with type 2 diabetes: A randomized controlled trial. Diabetes Care 25:89-94, 2002.

138. Lord J, Flight I, Norman R: Metformin in polycystic ovary syndrome: Systematic review and metaanalysis. BMJ 327:951, 2003.

139. Costello M, Eden J: A systematic review of the reproductive system effects of metformin in patients with polycystic ovary syndrome. Fertil Steril 79:1-13, 2003.

140. Harborne L, Fleming R, Lyall H, et al: Metformin or antiandrogen in the treatment of hirsutism in polycystic ovary syndrome. J Clin Endocrinol Metab 88:4116-4123, 2003.

141. Kazerooni T, Dehghan-Kooshkghazi M: Effects of metformin therapy on hyperandrogenism in women with polycystic ovarian syndrome. Gynecol Endocrinol 17:51-56, 2003.

142. Eagleson C, Bellows A, Hu K, et al: Obese patients with polycystic ovary syndrome: Evidence that metformin does not restore sensitivity of the gonadotropin-releasing hormone pulse generator to inhibition by ovarian steroids. J Clin Endocrinol Metab 88:5158-5162, 2003.

143. Maciel G, Soares Junior J, Alves da Motta E, et al: Nonobese women with polycystic ovary syndrome respond better than obese women to treatment with metformin. Fertil Steril 81:355-360, 2004.

144. Glueck CJ, Goldenberg N, Pranikoff J, et al: Pregnancy outcomes among women with polycystic ovary syndrome treated with metformin. Hum Reprod 17:2858-2864, 2002.

145. Glueck CJ, Goldenberg N, Wang P, et al: Metformin during pregnancy reduces insulin, insulin resistance, insulin secretion, weight, testosterone and development of gestational diabetes: Prospective longitudinal assessment of women with polycystic ovary syndrome from preconception throughout pregnancy. Hum Reprod 19:510-521, 2004.

146. Glueck CJ, Phillips H, Cameron D, et al: Continuing metformin throughout pregnancy in women with polycystic ovary syndrome appears to safely reduce first-trimester spontaneous abortion: A pilot study. Fertil Steril 75:46-52, 2001.

147. Gardiner S, Kirkpatrick C, Begg E, et al: Transfer of metformin into human milk. Clin Pharm Ther 73:71-77, 2003.

148. Misbin RI, Green L, Stadel BV, et al: Lactic acidosis in patients with diabetes treated with metformin. N Engl J Med 338:265-266, 1998.

149. Bailey CJ, Turner RC: Drug therapy: Metformin. N Engl J Med 334:574-579, 1996.

KEY POINTS

- *α-Glucosidase inhibitors competitively block the α-glucosidases in the brush border of the small intestine.*
- *The glucose-lowering effect of α-glucosidase inhibitors is observed within the first week of treatment and well maintained throughout the treatment, even after 3 years.*
- *Efficacy of α-glucosidase inhibitors is present no matter what other treatment the patients are taking.*
- *α-Glucosidase–inhibitor treatment is not associated with weight gain and can lead to a small but consistent weight loss.*
- *α-Glucosidase–inhibitor treatment is not associated with hypoglycemia when used as monotherapy.*

Type 2 diabetes mellitus (T2DM) is a major health problem associated with high morbidity, excess mortality, and substantial health care costs. Its prevalence is growing worldwide at an epidemic rate. It can be considered one of the major challenges of the 21st century.

It is now generally accepted that the diabetes-related complications are due, at least in part, to the prevailing hyperglycemia. The UKPDS (United Kingdom Prospective Diabetes Study) and the DCCT (Diabetes Control and Complications Trial) have shown that intensive glycemic treatment in subjects with T2DM and type 1 diabetes mellitus (T1DM), respectively, was associated with a significant reduction in the appearance or progression of microvascular complications.[1,2] Furthermore, it is suggested that such tight glycemic control could also have a beneficial impact on the incidence of cardiovascular disease associated with glucose intolerance.[3] For those reasons, it has been recommended that the treatment of type 2 diabetes should aim for plasma glucose levels as close to normal as possible.

Diet and exercise remain the cornerstone of treatment for T2DM. But when diet and exercise fail to achieve targeted blood glucose, oral hypoglycemic agents such as sulfonylureas, biguanides, or thiazolidinediones are added. All these agents are effective in decreasing fasting plasma glucose. In more than 60% of patients, however, persisting postprandial hyperglycemia can account for the sustained increase in glycated hemoglobin (HbA1c). It has now been shown that postprandial hyperglycemia accounts for a major portion of HbA1c, particularly at HbA1c lower than 8%.[4] Thus, postprandial hyperglycemia contributes significantly to the development of diabetes-specific complications, and it is probably involved in the development of cardiovascular disease as well.[5]

We now have oral hypoglycemic agents that specifically blunt the rise in postprandial plasma glucose: the meglitinides and the α-glucosidase inhibitors. This chapter discusses the α-glucosidase inhibitors. These compounds delay the digestion of complex carbohydrates, thus decreasing the rise in postprandial plasma glucose. By their novel mechanism of action, the α-glucosidase inhibitors significantly reduce both the postprandial glycemic and insulinemic excursion. Furthermore, these agents have an excellent safety profile.

MECHANISM OF ACTION

α-Glucosidase inhibitors competitively block the α-glucosidases in the brush border of the small intestine that are necessary to hydrolyze the oligo- and polysaccharides to monosaccharides for absorption.[6] Carbohydrates are usually absorbed rapidly within the first half of the small intestine. With the use of α-glucosidase inhibitors, carbohydrate digestion and absorption occur throughout the small intestine. This results in slower absorption of ingested carbohydrates and consequently in a blunting of the rise in postprandial plasma glucose and plasma insulin (Fig. 25–1).[7]

Three α-glucosidase inhibitors have been developed: acarbose, miglitol, and voglibose (Fig. 25–2). There are limited clinical trials of miglitol and voglibose,[8] and therefore this discussion is limited to acarbose.

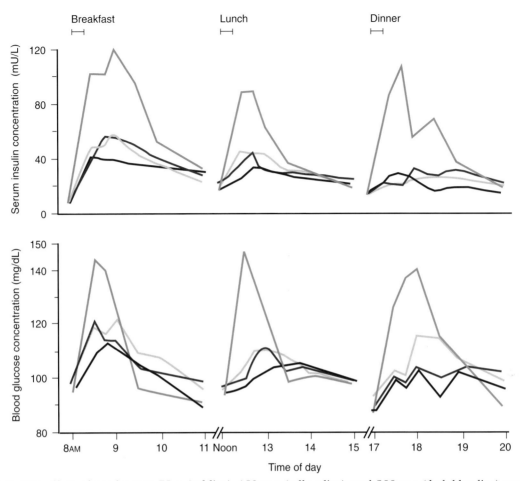

Figure 25–1. The effect of acarbose at 75 g *(red line)*, 150 mg *(yellow line)*, and 300 mg *(dark blue line)* versus placebo *(light blue line)* on diurnal blood glucose and insulin concentrations in healthy volunteers. (Reproduced with permission from Clissold SP, Edwards C: Acarbose. A preliminary review of its pharmacodynamic and pharmacokinetic properties, and therapeutic potential. Drugs 35:214-243, 1988.)

Acarbose is a pseudo-tetrasaccharide of microbial origin. Its chemical structure is analogous to that of oligosaccharides obtained from starch digestion. The active part of the molecule is an acarvosine unit that is linked to a maltose unit.[7] The nitrogen linkage of the acarvosine unit confers on the molecule its high affinity for the carbohydrate-binding site of various α-glucosidases, which exceeds the affinity of regular oligosaccharides from ingested carbohydrate by 10,000 to 100,000 times.[6] Because of its nitrogen linkage, acarbose cannot be hydrolyzed by the enzyme. However, this high affinity binding to α-glucosidases is reversible, and its inhibition kinetics is competitive.

Due to its specificity for α-glucosidases, acarbose does not inhibit β-glucosidases such as lactase. The digestion and absorption of lactose is therefore not affected by the drug. More importantly, it does not affect intestinal absorption of monosaccharides such as glucose.[6] The intact acarbose molecule is virtually unabsorbed by the gut (less than 1% to 2%) and can therefore exert its inhibitory action all along the small intestine up to the ileum.[6] However,

it is cleaved by bacterial enzymes in the large bowel into several metabolites, of which 35% can be found in the urine.[9]

If acarbose is to compete with oligosaccharide and disaccharide, it must be present at the site of enzymatic activity at the same time as carbohydrate. Therefore the drug should be taken with the first bite and not more than 15 minutes after the beginning of the meal.[10]

By delaying the digestion and absorption of carbohydrate in the small intestine, acarbose can increase the amount of fermentable carbohydrate reaching the colon. This can result in gastrointestinal symptoms such as flatulence and, sometimes, diarrhea. These side effects can be prevented or at least minimized by starting the drug at a low dose and titrating it up gradually.[9] It is recommended to start at 50 mg once daily (sometimes 25 mg once daily) and increase gradually by 50 mg per day every week until targeted blood glucose is achieved or to a maximum dose of 100 mg three times a day.

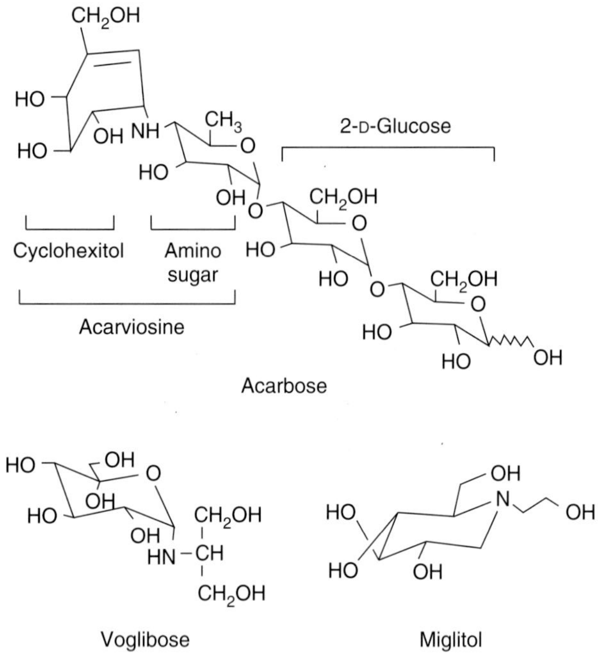

Figure 25–2. Structural formula of the α-glucosidase inhibitors acarbose, miglitol, and voglibose. (Reproduced with permission from Rabasa-Lhoret R, Chiasson J-L: α Glucosidase inhibitors. In DeFronzo RA, Ferranninni E, Keen H, Zimmet P: International Textbook of Diabetes Mellitus, 3rd ed. Chichester, John Wiley & Sons, 2004, pp 901-914.)

EFFICACY OF ACARBOSE IN TYPE 2 DIABETES MELLITUS

Much experience has been gained with the use of acarbose in the treatment of diabetes mellitus. Its efficacy in improving glycemic control has been demonstrated when acarbose was added or when compared to diet alone, to sulfonylureas, to metformin, to combined sulfonylureas and metformin, and to insulin in a number of double-blind, placebo-controlled, randomized clinical trials. These trials have revealed a number of constant features associated with acarbose treatment in diabetes (Box 25-1).

The randomized, controlled trials with acarbose in type 2 diabetes, with at least 12 weeks of follow-up and published in English medical journals, are reviewed. Altogether, 32 randomized, controlled trials were found in an exhaustive search of the literature (Table 25–1).

Drug-Naive and Diet-Treated Patients

Fourteen studies assessed the efficacy of acarbose in drug-naive or diet-treated patients (Table 25–2). Altogether, 1475 subjects with type 2 diabetes were randomized in a double-blind fashion to placebo or

Box 25-1. Efficacy of Acarbose in Treating Type 2 Diabetes

- A glucose-lowering effect is observed within the first week of treatment and is well maintained throughout the treatment, even after 3 years.
- Acarbose is effective no matter what other treatment the patients are taking.
- Acarbose seems to be more effective in patients with recent-onset diabetes and in drug-naive patients.
- Efficacy is independent of sex or racial origin.
- The higher the initial HbA1c, the greater the reduction with acarbose treatment.
- Acarbose is not associated with weight gain, and most studies have shown a small but consistent weight loss.
- Acarbose is not associated with hypoglycemia when used as monotherapy.
- The 100 mg tid dose evoked a near maximal response in glycemic control.

Table 25–1. Randomized, Controlled Trials Testing the Efficacy of Acarbose in Type 2 Diabetes

Selected Studies According to Treatment	No. of Studies
The effect of acarbose in diet-treated patients	14
The effect of acarbose in comparison to:	
Sulfonylurea	3
Metformin	1
The effect of acarbose in addition to:	
Sulfonylurea	3
Metformin	4
Insulin	3
Diet ± SU ± MF ± insulin	4
Total	**32**

MF, metformin; SU, sulfonylurea.

acarbose in doses ranging from 100 to 300 mg three times daily. A significant improvement in HbA1c was seen in all studies, with a reduction ranging from 0.3 percentage points to 2.5 points, with a mean of 0.74 points ± 0.15. The mean net effect of acarbose compared to placebo was 0.90 points ± 0.10 (Fig. 25–3).

Comparison to Sulfonylureas or Metformin

Three studies compared acarbose treatment to sulfonylurea treatment (Table 25–3). A total of 255 patients with type 2 diabetes were randomized head-to-head to acarbose, sulfonylurea, or placebo. Acarbose treatment resulted in an absolute reduction in HbA1c of 0.66 percentage points ± 0.28 compared to 0.88 points ± 0.28 for sulfonylureas

Table 25–2. *Efficacy of Acarbose in Patients with Type 2 Diabetes with Diet Alone*

Randomized, Controlled Trials	No. Pts	Change in HbA1c		
		Placebo (P)	Acarbose (A)	P–A
Hanefeld et al. (1991)[25]	94	–0.10	–0.70	–0.60
Hotta et al. (1993)[26]	37	–0.40	–1.40	–1.00
Santeusanio et al. (1993)[27]	64	+0.30	–0.77	–1.02
Chiasson et al. (1994)[28]	77	+1.40	–0.70	–2.10
Coniff et al. (1994)[29]	189	+0.53	–0.06	–0.59
Hoffmann et al. (1994)[30]	58	+0.10	–0.99	–1.09
Coniff et al. (1995)[31]	122	+0.33	–0.45	–0.78
Coniff et al. (1995)[32]	129	+0.04	–0.54	–0.58
Braun et al. (1996)[33]	86	–1.10	–2.50	–1.40
Hoffmann et al. (1997)[34]	64	+0.40	–1.10	–1.50
Chan et al. (1998)[35]	121	–0.27	–0.70	–0.43
Hasche et al. (1999)[36]	74	–0.60	–1.65	–1.05
Josse et al. (2002)[37]	192	+0.30	–0.30	–0.60
Fischer et al. (1998)[38]	168	+0.37	–0.72	–1.09
Totals	**1475**	**+0.16 ± 0.14**	**–0.74 ± 0.15**	**–0.90 ± 0.10**

HbA1c, hemoglobin A1c.

Table 25–3. *Efficacy of Acarbose Compared to Sulfonylurea and Metformin in Patients with Type 2 Diabetes*

Randomized Controlled trials Compared to Sulfonylurea (SU)	No. Pts	Change in HbA1c		
		Placebo	Acarbose	SU
Hoffmann et al. (1994)[30]	95	+0.10	–0.99	–0.80
Coniff et al. (1995)[32]	133	+0.04	–0.54	–0.93
Hanefeld et al. (2002)[39]	27	+0.90	–0.50	–1.70
Total	**255**	**+0.13 ± 0.28**	**–0.66 ± 0.16**	**–0.88 ± 0.28**
Compared to Metformin (MF)		Placebo	Acarbose	MF
Hoffmann et al. (1997)[34]	**96**	**+0.4 ± 0.20**	**–1.1 ± 0.13**	**–1.0 ± 0.10**

HbA1c, hemoglobin A1c.

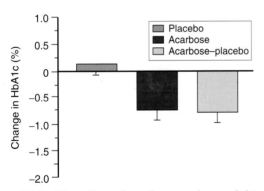

Figure 25–3. The effect of acarbose on hemoglobin A1c (HbA1c) in patients with type 2 diabetes treated with diet alone.

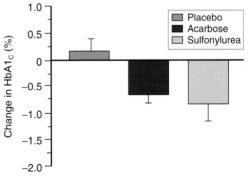

Figure 25–4. The effect of acarbose compared to sulfonylurea on hemoglobin A1c (HbA1c) in patients with type 2 diabetes.

(Fig. 25–4), for a net effect of 0.79 points versus 1.01 points, respectively. Only one study compared acarbose to metformin in 96 patients (see Table 25–3). Acarbose reduced HbA1c by 1.1 percentage points ± 0.13 compared to 1.0 percentage point ± 0.1 for metformin (Fig. 25–5). In these studies, it can be concluded that acarbose was slightly less effective than sulfonylureas in improving glycemic control but was similar to metformin.

Added to Sulfonylureas, Metformin, or Insulin

Three studies have compared acarbose to placebo in 227 patients whose diabetes was insufficiently controlled with sulfonylureas (Table 25–4). Acarbose treatment was associated with a reduction in HbA1c of 1.28 percentage points ± 0.46 compared with a decrease of 0.25 points ± 0.48 in the placebo group,

Table 25–4. *Efficacy of Acarbose Compared to Placebo in Patients with Type 2 Diabetes Insufficiently Controlled with Sulfonylurea, Metformin, or Insulin*

Randomized, Controlled Trials	No. Pts	Change in HbA1c		
		Placebo (P)	Acarbose (A)	A–P
In Addition to Sulfonylurea				
Lin et al. (2003)[40]	64	+0.13	−0.92	−1.06
Chiasson et al. (1994)[28]	103	+0.12	−0.90	−1.02
Willms et al. (1999)[41]	60	−1.3	−2.3	−1.0
Total	**227**	**−0.25 ± 0.48**	**−1.28 ± 0.46**	**−1.03 ± 0.02**
In Addition to Metformin				
Phillips et al. (2003)[42]	83	+0.6	−0.2	−0.8
Halimi et al. (2000)[43]	152	+78	−0.7	−0.9
Rosenstock et al. (1998)[44]	148	+0.08	−0.57	−0.65
Chiasson et al. (1994)[28]	83	+0.25	−0.55	−0.80
Total	**466**	**+0.24 ± 0.11**	**−0.54 ± 0.11**	**−0.79 ± 0.05**
In Addition to Insulin				
Coniff et al. (1995)[45]	207	−0.17	−0.57	−0.40
Hwu et al. (2003)[46]	107	+0.2	−0.50	−0.70
Chiasson et al. (1994)[28]	91	0	−0.50	−0.5
Total	**405**	**−0.04 ± 0.11**	**−0.54 ± 0.02**	**−0.50 ± 0.09**

HbA1c, hemoglobin A1c.

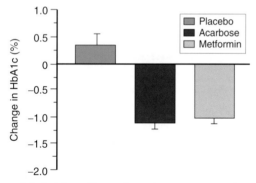

Figure 25–5. The effect of acarbose compared to metformin on hemoglobin A1c (HbA1c) in patients with type 2 diabetes.

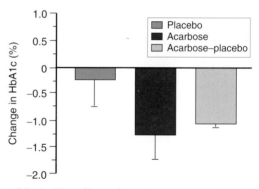

Figure 25–6. The effect of acarbose compared to placebo in patients with type 2 diabetes insufficiently controlled with sulfonylurea.

for a net effect for acarbose of 1.03 percentage points ± 0.02 (Fig. 25–6).

Acarbose was compared to placebo in four studies totaling 466 patients whose diabetes was insufficiently controlled with metformin (see Table 25–4). Acarbose resulted in a decrease in HbA1c of 0.54 percentage points ± 0.11 compared to an increase of 0.24 points ± 0.11 in the placebo group, for a net efficacy of 0.79 points ± 0.05 (Fig. 25–7).

Acarbose was added to insulin treatment in 405 patients whose type 2 diabetes was inadequately controlled and compared to placebo (see Table 25–4). Although placebo had no effect on glycemic control (HbA1c decreased by 0.04 percentage points ± 0.11), acarbose resulted in a reduction in HbA1c of 0.54 points ± 0.02 (Fig. 25–8).

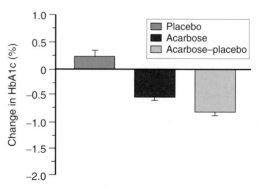

Figure 25–7. The effect of acarbose compared to placebo in patients with type 2 diabetes insufficiently controlled with metformin.

Table 25–5. *The Efficacy of Acarbose Compared to Placebo in Patients with Type 2 Diabetes Insufficiently Controlled with Diet Plus Sulfonylurea, Metformin, or Insulin*

Randomized, Controlled Trials	No. Pts	Change in HbA1c		
		Placebo (P)	Acarbose (A)	A–P
Lam et al. (1998)[47]	90	+0.10	–0.5	–0.6
Lindström et al. (2000)[48]	75	+0.30	–0.7	–1.0
Rosenbaum et al. (2002)[49]	40	+0.00	–0.8	–0.8
Total	**205**	**+0.15 ± 0.06**	**–0.63 ± 0.12**	**–0.79 ± 0.10**

HbA1c, hemoglobin A1c.

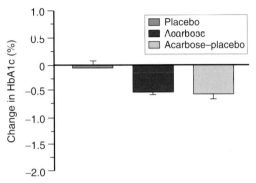

Figure 25–8. The effect of acarbose versus placebo in patients with type 2 diabetes insufficiently controlled with insulin.

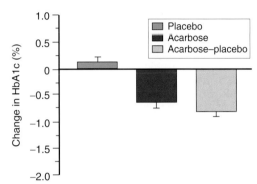

Figure 25–9. The effect of acarbose compared to placebo in patients with type 2 diabetes insufficiently controlled by diet with or without sulfonylurea, metformin, or insulin.

In summary, the addition of acarbose to the treatment of patients whose type 2 diabetes is suboptimally controlled will further reduce HbA1c, no matter what the current treatment is.

Added to Diet, Sulfonylureas, Metformin, or Insulin

Four studies have tested acarbose versus placebo in patients whose type 2 diabetes was insufficiently controlled with different treatment combinations. These include the UKPDS study, which deserves to be dealt with separately. The three others included 205 patients who were randomized to acarbose or placebo (Table 25–5). Acarbose treatment resulted in a reduction in HbA1c of 0.63 percentage points ± 0.12 compared to an increase of 0.15 points ± 0.06 in the placebo group, for a net effect of 0.79 points ± 0.1 (Fig. 25–9).

The UKPDS is discussed separately for two major reasons: The primary objective of the UKPDS was not the efficacy of acarbose but the effect of tight glycemic control on diabetes-related complications. Acarbose was added at the tail end of the study at a time when glycemic response was failing with other treatments, including various combinations of diet, sulfonylureas, metformin, and insulin.

Altogether, 1946 patients from the UKPDS were randomized to acarbose or placebo on top of the current treatment. Acarbose resulted in a slight but

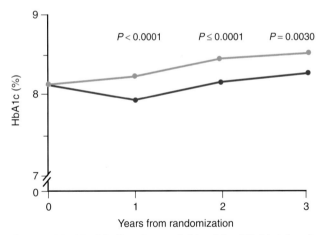

Figure 25–10. Median hemoglobin A1c (HbA1c) levels analyzed according to intention to treat at 1, 2, and 3 years after randomization. (Reproduced with permission from Holman RR, Cull CA, Turner RC: A randomized double-blind trial of acarbose in type 2 diabetes shows improved glycemic control over 3 years [UK Prospective Diabetes Study 44]. Diabetes Care 22:960-964, 1999.)

significant reduction in HbA1c at year 1 ($P < 0.001$) and then a gradual rise over the next 2 years. At all times, HbA1c remained significantly lower in the acarbose-treated group than in the placebo-treated group (0.2%; $P < 0.001$) (Fig. 25–10). Drug discontinuation was very high both for acarbose (61%)

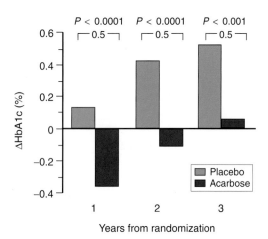

Figure 25–11. Mean change from baseline in hemoglobin A1c (HbA1c) analyzed according to actual therapy at 1, 2, and 3 years. (Reproduced with permission from Holman RR, Cull CA, Turner RC: A randomized double-blind trial of acarbose in type 2 diabetes shows improved glycemic control over 3 years [UK Prospective Diabetes Study 44]. Diabetes Care 22:960-964, 1999.)

and placebo (42%), mostly due to gastrointestinal symptoms (46% versus 20%) and partly due to the polypharmacy that far into the study. When analysis was done according to actual therapy, the difference in HbA1c at all times was 0.5 percentage points ($P < 0.001$) in favor of acarbose (Fig. 25–11). No matter how the analysis was done, acarbose had a significantly greater beneficial effect on HbA1c compared to placebo.

ACARBOSE IN THE PREVENTION OF DIABETES

It is generally accepted that insulin resistance and decrease in insulin secretion capacity are two major factors involved in the development of type 2 diabetes.[11] It is also believed that all subjects developing diabetes go through a prediabetic phase called *impaired glucose tolerance* (IGT). It has been shown in subjects with IGT that the higher the 2-hour plasma glucose following ingestion of 75 grams of glucose, the higher the risk of progressing to diabetes.[12,13]

Based on this information, it was postulated that reducing postprandial plasma glucose in subjects with IGT would decrease the risk of developing diabetes. This hypothesis was tested in the STOP-NIDDM (Study to Prevent Non–Insulin-Dependent Diabetes Mellitus) trial.[14] A total of 1429 subjects was randomized in a double-blind fashion to acarbose or placebo and followed for a mean period of 3.3 years. On the basis of a single oral glucose tolerance test (OGTT), acarbose treatment was associated with a relative risk reduction of 25%. If, however, we use two positive OGTTs to confirm the diagnosis as now recommended by the World Health Organization and the American Diabetes

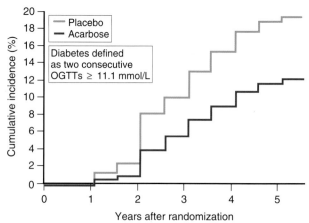

Figure 25–12. The effect of acarbose on the cumulative incidence of diabetes in subjects with impaired glucose tolerance based on two oral glucose tolerance tests (OGTTs). (Reproduced with permission from Rabasa-Lhoret, R, Chiasson, JL: α Glucosidase inhibitors. (In DeFronzo RA, Ferrannimni E, Keen H, Zimmet P: International Textbook of Diabetes Mellitus, 3rd ed. Chichester, John Wiley & Sons, 2004, pp 901-914. Copyright John Wiley and Sons Limited. Reproduced with permission.)

Association, the relative risk reduction was 35.6% (Fig. 25–12). This effect was independent of age, sex, and body mass index. This effect of acarbose in preventing or delaying the development of diabetes was similar to that for metformin but slightly less effective than that for intensive lifestyle modification.[15,16]

The efficacy of acarbose was also shown in a Chinese study published in 2001.[17] Altogether, 321 subjects with IGT were randomized to either no treatment ($n = 85$), diet and exercise ($n = 60$), acarbose ($n = 88$), or metformin ($n = 88$) and followed for 3 years. Acarbose treatment resulted in a relative risk reduction in the incidence of diabetes of 83% ($P < 0.001$), compared to 65% ($P < 0.001$) for metformin and 29% (P not significant) for diet and exercise (Fig. 25–13). It can therefore be concluded that in subjects with IGT, acarbose treatment is effective in preventing or delaying the progression to diabetes.

ACARBOSE IN THE PREVENTION OF CARDIOVASCULAR DISEASE

Cardiovascular disease (CVD) is the leading cause of death in subjects with diabetes. Although type 2 diabetes is often associated with hypertension and dyslipidemia as part of the metabolic syndrome, evidence is accumulating that supports hyperglycemia as an independent risk factor for CVD. A number of epidemiologic studies have shown that postprandial hyperglycemia was a much stronger risk factor than fasting hyperglycemia.[5] Hu and colleagues[18] have shown that cardiovascular events start years before the development of diabetes.

Several studies have now shown that IGT is associated with an increased risk of CVD.[19,20] The moderate increase in postprandial plasma glucose levels in patients with IGT was shown to be an independent risk factor for CVD. It was postulated that if postprandial plasma glucose is a risk factor for CVD, decreasing postprandial hyperglycemia in subjects with IGT should be associated with a reduction in the risk of CVD. This hypothesis was also tested in the STOP-NIDDM trial.[21] Treatment with acarbose in subjects with IGT resulted in a significant 49% risk reduction in cardiovascular events ($P < 0.03$) (Fig. 25–14). The most impressive reduction was in myocardial infarction, with only one event in the acarbose group compared to 12 in the placebo group ($P = 0.02$). Furthermore, the electrocardiograph reading identified eight silent myocardial infarctions, one in the acarbose group and seven in the placebo group, for a total of two in the acarbose group versus 19 in the placebo group ($P < 0.001$).

In a subgroup of IGT patients from the STOP-NIDDM trial ($n = 115$), carotid intima-media thickness (IMT), an accepted surrogate for atherosclerosis, was measured before randomization and at the end of the study.[22] Acarbose treatment significantly reduced the progression of the IMT of the carotids 50%, the first demonstration that decreasing postprandial hyperglycemia had a protective effect against atherosclerosis (Fig. 25–15; $P = 0.027$).

Hanefeld and colleagues[23] performed a meta-analysis of the long-term randomized, controlled trials on acarbose in type 2 diabetic subjects; the meta-analysis looked at cardiovascular events. Altogether, 2180 patients (1248 taking acarbose and 932 taking placebo) were included in the analysis. Using the Cox proportional analysis, acarbose treatment was associated with a risk reduction of 35% ($P = 0.006$) for any cardiovascular event and of 64% ($P = 0.012$) for myocardial infarction (Fig. 25–16). This is very similar to the observation made in subjects with IGT.

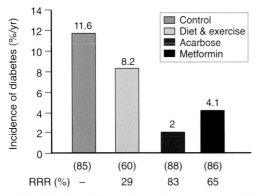

Figure 25–13. The effect of acarbose treatment in subjects with impaired glucose tolerance on the incidence of diabetes compared to diet and exercise, metformin, and no treatment (control). RRR, relative risk reduction. (Adapted from Yang W, Lin L, Qi J et al: The preventive effect of acarbose and metformin on the progression to diabetes mellitus in the IGT population: A 3-year multicenter prospective study. Chin J Endocrinol Metab 17:131-136, 2001.)

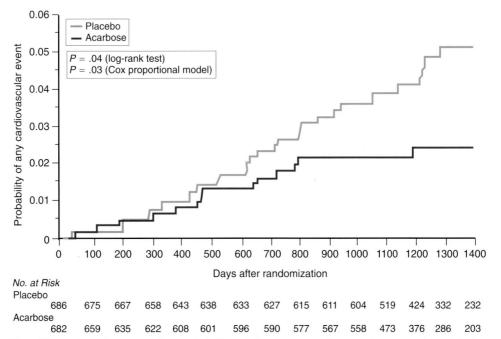

Figure 25–14. The effect of acarbose on the probability of having a cardiovascular event in subjects with impaired glucose tolerance. (Reproduced with permission from Chiasson J-L, Josse RG, Gomis R, et al: Acarbose treatment and the risk of cardiovascular disease and hypertension in patients with impaired glucose tolerance: The STOP-NIDDM trial. JAMA 290:486-494, 2003.)

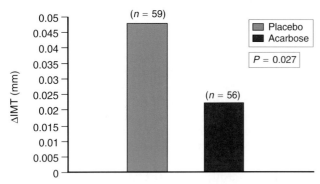

Figure 25–15. The effect of acarbose on the progression of the intima-media thickness (IMT) of the carotid artery in subjects with impaired glucose tolerance (IGT).

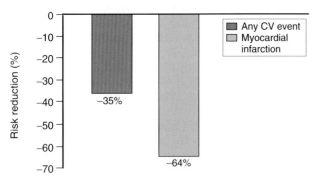

Figure 25–16. The effect of acarbose on the relative risk of developing any cardiovascular (CV) event or myocardial infarction.

All these observations suggest that acarbose treatment in both IGT and type 2 diabetes is associated with a reduction in the risk of CVD. This would support the hypothesis that postprandial plasma glucose is a risk factor for CVD.

CONCLUSION

Acarbose, with its novel mechanism of action, provides an interesting tool for treating and preventing type 2 diabetes, and it could be of potential benefit for preventing cardiovascular disease.

In subjects with type 2 diabetes, the published data consistently show a significant reduction in postprandial plasma glucose associated with a significant decrease in HbA1c (a mean of 0.7%). It is effective whether it is used as monotherapy or in combination with oral antidiabetic medications or insulin, and its effect is maintained over time. Although it can be associated with gastrointestinal side effects, it is not associated with any serious adverse effects, making it a particularly safe drug.

In subjects with IGT, both the STOP-NIDDM trial and the Chinese study have shown that acarbose treatment is associated with a significant reduction in the progression to diabetes. Based on these obser-

vations, the Canadian Diabetes Association recommends that subjects at risk should be screened for IGT and that acarbose treatment be considered.[24]

In subjects with IGT and type 2 diabetes, strong evidence has been presented suggesting that decreasing postprandial hyperglycemia with acarbose is associated with a risk reduction in CVD. This still needs to be confirmed in a well-designed prospective intervention trial powered to answer the question.

References

1. UK Prospective Diabetes Study Group: Intensive blood-glucose control with sulphonylureas or insulin compared with conventional treatment and risk of complications in patients with type 2 diabetes (UKPDS 33). Lancet 352:837-853, 1998.
2. DCCT Research Group: The effect of intensive treatment of diabetes on the development and progression of long-term complications in insulin-dependent diabetes mellitus. N Engl J Med 329:977-986, 1993.
3. Gaede P, Vedel P, Larsen N, et al: Multifactorial intervention and cardiovascular disease in patients with type 2 diabetes. N Engl J Med 348:383-393, 2003.
4. Monnier L, Lapinski H, Colette C: Contributions of fasting and postprandial plasma glucose increments to the overall diurnal hyperglycemia of type 2 diabetic patients: Variations with increasing levels of HbA1c. Diabetes Care 26:881-885, 2003.
5. The DECODE Study Group: Glucose tolerance and cardiovascular mortality: Comparison of fasting and 2-hour diagnostic criteria. Arch Intern Med 161:397-405, 2001.
6. Bischoff H: The mechanism of α-glucosidase inhibition in the management of diabetes. Clin Invest Med 18:303-311, 1995.
7. Rabasa-Lhoret R, Chiasson J-L: Potential of α-glucosidase inhibitors in elderly patients with diabetes mellitus and impaired glucose tolerance. Drugs Aging 13:131-143, 1998.
8. Vichayanrat A, Ploybutr S, Tunlakit M, Watanakejorn P: Efficacy and safety of voglibose in comparison with acarbose in type 2 diabetic patients. Diabetes Res Clin Pract 55:99-103, 2002.
9. Lebovitz HE: α-Glucosidase inhibitors as agents in the treatment of diabetes. Diabetes Rev 6:132-145, 1998.
10. Rosak C, Nitzsche G, König P, Hofmann U: The effect of the timing and the administration of acarbose on postprandial hyperglycaemia. Diabetic Med 12:979-984, 1995.
11. Kahn SE: The relative contributions of insulin resistance and beta-cell dysfunction to the pathophysiology of type 2 diabetes. Diabetologia 46:3-19, 2003.
12. Harris MI: Impaired glucose tolerance. Prevalence and conversion to NIDDM. Diabetic Med 13(Suppl 2):S9-S11, 1996.
13. Heine RJ, Nijpels G, Mooy JM: New data on the rate of progression of impaired glucose tolerance to NIDDM and predicting factors. Diabetic Med 13(Suppl 2):S12-S14, 1996.
14. Chiasson JL, Josse RG, Gomis R, et al: Acarbose for prevention of type 2 diabetes mellitus: The STOP-NIDDM randomised trial. Lancet 359:2072-2077, 2002.
15. Knowler WC, Barrett-Connor E, Fowler SE, et al: Reduction in the incidence of type 2 diabetes with lifestyle intervention or metformin. N Engl J Med 346:393-403, 2002.
16. Tuomilehto J, Lindstrom J, Eriksson JG, et al: Prevention of type 2 diabetes mellitus by changes in lifestyle among subjects with impaired glucose tolerance. N Engl J Med 344:1343-1350, 2001.
17. Yang W, Lin L, Qi J, et al: The preventive effect of acarbose and metformin on the progression to diabetes mellitus in the IGT population: A 3-year multicenter prospective study. Chin J Endocrinol Metab 17:131-136, 2001.

18. Hu FB, Stampfer MJ, Haffner SM, et al: Elevated risk of cardiovascular disease prior to clinical diagnosis of type 2 diabetes. Diabetes Care 25:1129-1134, 2002.

19. Saydah SH, Miret M, Sung J, et al: Postchallenge hyperglycemia and mortality in a national sample of U.S. adults. Diabetes Care 24:1397-1402, 2001.

20. Saydah SH, Loria CM, Eberhardt MS, Brancati FL: Subclinical states of glucose intolerance and risk of death in the U.S. Diabetes Care 24:447-453, 2001.

21. Chiasson JL, Josse RG, Gomis R, et al: Acarbose treatment and the risk of cardiovascular disease and hypertension in patients with impaired glucose tolerance. The STOP-NIDDM Trial. JAMA 290:486-494, 2003.

22. Hanefeld M, Chiasson JL, Koehler C, et al: Acarbose slows progression of intima-media thickness of the carotid arteries in subjects with impaired glucose tolerance. Stroke 35:1073-1078, 2004.

23. Hanefeld M, Cagatay M, Petrowitsch T, et al: Acarbose reduces the risk for myocardial infarction in type 2 diabetic patients: Meta-analysis of seven long-term studies. Eur Heart J 25:10-16, 2004.

24. Clinical Practice Guidelines Committee: Canadian Diabetes Association 2003 Clinical Practice Guidelines for the prevention and management of diabetes in Canada. Can J Diabetes 27:S1-S152, 2003.

25. Hanefeld M, Fischer S, Schulze J, et al: Therapeutic potentials of acarbose as first-line drug in NIDDM insufficiently treated with diet alone. Diabetes Care 14:732-737, 1991.

26. Hotta N, Kakuta H, Sano T, et al: Long-term effect of acarbose on glycaemic control in non-insulin-dependent diabetes mellitus: A placebo-controlled double-blind study. Diabet Med 10:134-138, 1993.

27. Santeusanio F, Ventura MM, Contadini S, et al: Efficacy and safety of two different dosages of acarbose in non-insulin-dependent diabetic patients treated by diet alone. Diabetes Nutr Metab 6:147-154, 1993.

28. Chiasson J-L, Josse RG, Hunt JA, et al, and collaborators: The efficacy of acarbose in the treatment of patients with non-insulin-dependent diabetes mellitus. A multicenter controlled clinical trial. Ann Intern Med 121:928-935, 1994.

29. Coniff RF, Shapiro JA, Seaton TB: Long-term efficacy and safety of acarbose in the treatment of obese subjects with non-insulin-dependent diabetes mellitus. Arch Intern Med 154:2442-2448, 1994.

30. Hoffmann J, Spengler M: Efficacy of 24-week monotherapy with acarbose, glibenclamide, or placebo in NIDDM patients. The Essen Study. Diabetes Care 17:561-566, 1994.

31. Coniff RF, Shapiro JA, Robbins D, et al: Reduction of glycosylated hemoglobin and postprandial hyperglycemia by acarbose in patients with NIDDM. Diabetes Care 18:817-824, 1995.

32. Coniff RF, Shapiro JA, Seaton TB, Bray GA: Multicenter, placebo-controlled trial comparing acarbose (BAY g5421) with placebo, tolbutamide, and tolbutamide-plus-acarbose in non-insulin-dependent daibetes mellitus. Am J Med 98:443, 1995.

33. Braun D, Schönherr U, Mitzkat H-J: Efficacy of acarbose monotherapy in patients with type 2 diabetes: A double-blind study conducted in general practice. Endocrinol Metab 3:275-280, 1996.

34. Hoffmann J, Spengler M: Efficacy of 24-week monotherapy with acarbose, metformin, or placebo in dietary-treated NIDDM patients: The Essen-II Study. Am J Med 103:483-490, 1997.

35. Chan JCN, Chan K-WA, Ho LLT, et al: For the Asian Acarbose Study Group. An Asian multicenter clinical trial to assess the efficacy and tolerability of acarbose compared with placebo in type 2 diabetes patients previously treated with diet. Diabetes Care 21:1058-1061, 1998.

36. Hasche H, Mertes G, Bruns C, et al: Effects of acarbose treatment in type 2 diabetic patients under dietary training: A multicentre, double-blind, placebo-controlled, 2-year study. Diabetes Nutr Metab 12:277-285, 1999.

37. Josse RG, Chiasson JL, Ryan EA, et al: Acarbose in the treatment of elderly patients with type 2 diabetes. Diabetes Res Clin Pract 59:37-42, 2003.

38. Fischer S, Hanefeld M, Spengler M, et al: European study on dose-response relationship of acarbose as a first-line drug in non-insulin-dependent diabetes mellitus: Efficacy and safety of low and high doses. Acta Diabetol 35:34-40, 1998.

39. Hanefeld M, Haffner SM, Menschikowski M, et al: Different effects of acarbose and glibenclamide on proinsulin and insulin profiles in people with type 2 diabetes. Diabetes Res Clin Pract 55:221-227, 2002.

40. Lin BJ, Wu HP, Huang HS, et al: Efficacy and tolerability of acarbose in Asian patients with type 2 diabetes inadequately controlled with diet and sulfonylureas. J Diabetes Complications 17:179-185, 2003.

41. Willms B, Ruge D: Comparison of acarbose and metformin in patients with type 2 diabetes mellitus insufficiently controlled with diet and sulphonylureas: A randomized, placebo-controlled study. Diabet Med 16:755-761, 1999.

42. Phillips P, Karrasch J, Scott R, et al: Acarbose improves glycemic control in overweight type 2 diabetic patients insufficiently treated with metformin. Diabetes Care 26:269-273, 2003.

43. Halimi S, Le Berre MA, Grange V: Efficacy and safety of acarbose add-on therapy in the treatment of overweight patients with type 2 diabetes inadequately controlled with metformin: A double-blind, placebo-controlled study. Diabetes Res Clin Pract 50:49-56, 2000.

44. Rosenstock J, Brown A, Fischer J, et al: Efficacy and safety of acarbose in metformin-treated patients with type 2 diabetes. Diabetes Care 21:2050-2055, 1998.

45. Coniff RF, Shapiro JA, Seaton TB, et al: A double-blind placebo-controlled trial evaluating the safety and efficacy of acarbose for the treatment of patients with insulin-requiring type II diabetes. Diabetes Care 18:928-932, 1995.

46. Hwu CM, Ho LT, Fuh MM, et al: Acarbose improves glycemic control in insulin-treated Asian type 2 diabetic patients: Results from a multinational, placebo-controlled study. Diabetes Res Clin Pract 60:111-118, 2003.

47. Lam KSL, Tiu SC, Tsang MW, et al: Acarbose in NIDDM patients with poor control on conventional oral agents. Diabetes Care 21:1154-1158, 1998.

48. Lindstrom J, Tuomilehto J, Spengler M: Acarbose treatment does not change the habitual diet of patients with type 2 diabetes mellitus. The Finnish Acargbos Study Group. Diabet Med 17:20-25, 2000.

49. Rosenbaum P, Peres RB, Zanella MT, Ferreira SR: Improved glycemic control by acarbose therapy in hypertensive diabetic patients: Effects on blood pressure and hormonal parameters. Braz J Med Biol Res 35:877-884, 2002.

Type 2 Diabetes Therapy: Choosing Oral Agents

Silvio E. Inzucchi

KEY POINTS

- *Different classes of oral agents have unique mechanisms of action, targeting different pathophysiologic derangements that characterize type 2 diabetes.*
- *Most oral agents are equally efficacious in lowering hemoglobin A1c, with the exception of the α-glucosidase inhibitors, which tend to be less potent.*
- *Each oral agent class has specific advantages and disadvantages, and a careful choice should incorporate patient, drug, and disease factors.*
- *Oral agent classes are effective in combination, with further lowering of hemoglobin A1c when compared to monotherapy.*
- *With time, patients with type 2 diabetes often require more intensive treatment regimens to maintain glycemic control. Due to progressive beta cell failure, many ultimately require insulin.*

BACKGROUND

The pharmacologic approach to type 2 diabetes mellitus (T2DM) has been transformed since the 1990s by the advent of several new drug classes, each of which addresses individual pathophysiologic defects of the disease. Since the 1950s, during a time in which there has been a steady increase in the number of classes of antihypertensive drugs, comparatively, the development of antihyperglycemic agents has lagged (Fig. 26–1). With the introduction of metformin in the United States in 1995, however, there has been a flurry of activity from the pharmaceutical industry. As of 2005, practitioners have five different oral agent categories available to them, each with distinct mechanisms of action. How to choose a specific drug class in an individual patient and how best to use these agents in combination is therefore a new challenge for clinicians managing diabetic patients. A full understanding of the metabolic defects at which these drugs are targeted is therefore of critical importance.

The natural history of T2DM begins with a period of insulin resistance with preserved, often augmented, insulin secretion, as the pancreas attempts to meet the increased peripheral insulin requirements and maintain euglycemia.[1] The relative insensitivity to insulin action in muscle and liver, the two major target organs of the hormone, is thereby initially overcome due to higher circulating insulin concentrations. As the disease progresses, however, pancreatic islet cell function fails, no longer able to meet demands. The nature of this failure is still not well understood, but it likely results from both genetic and environmental factors, the latter of which may be partially reversible.[2] As a result, insulin levels decline and hyperglycemia ensues, initially manifested in the postprandial phase, with fasting glucose typically preserved. Insulin levels at this point may be, if measured, actually still higher than those of nondiabetic persons. Subsequently, as beta cell function deteriorates further, fasting glucose levels climb, because insulin secretion persists to some extent in virtually all patients with T2DM. As a result, ketoacidosis is rare, and because of renal glucose clearance, plasma glucose levels usually plateau in the 250 to 350 mg/dL range, unless there is superimposed decline in renal function or severe dehydration.

Patients with insulin resistance as a rule exhibit a cluster of other clinical and biochemical features, which have been referred to as the insulin resistance syndrome or the metabolic syndrome.[3] These include central (i.e., visceral) adiposity, hypertension, dyslipidemia (high triglycerides, low high-density lipoprotein [HDL] cholesterol, and small, dense low-density lipoprotein [LDL] particles), and hyperuricemia. Other characteristics have also been identified, such as hypercoagulability, endothelial dysfunction, and vascular inflammation. As a result, patients with the metabolic syndrome are at increased risk for premature cardiovascular morbidity.[4] When superimposed upon the detrimental vascular effects of hyperglycemia, such as occurs in patients with T2DM, the propensity for atherosclerosis is further enhanced.

Angioedema with ACE inhibitors is a rare event (0.1% to 0.7%) that usually occurs within hours to several weeks of initiating therapy, but it can occur up to 1 year later. The risk appears to be greater in African Americans.[61] Angioedema is a contraindication to continued use, and patients should be switched to other antihypertensive agents.

Cough is a common (5% to 20%), irritating, but benign side effect of ACE inhibitors. It is more common in women than men and is thought to be related to inhibition of bradykinin breakdown. However, other evidence suggests the cough may be due to the increased synthesis of prostaglandins and thromboxane that follows from stimulating the arachidonic acid cascade. Cough can sometimes be treated by decreasing the dose, but usually complete discontinuation of the medication is necessary. Resolution of the cough usually occurs within a few days to a few weeks.[60,62] In some cases, cough may reoccur with ARB use.

Indications for Use
Given their specific benefit in patients with T1DM and known nephropathy, ACE inhibitors are indicated for treatment as first-line therapy in such patients, but only as second-line therapy in patients with T2DM and nephropathy. However, based on the data from the MICRO-HOPE study, ACE inhibitors have shown benefit in patients with T2DM who are older than 55 years and have additional cardiovascular risk factors (e.g., previous history of CVD, hyperlipidemia, smoking).

Because of these studies and their general efficacy and excellent adverse effect profiles, they can certainly be used as first-line treatment in other hypertensive patients, as well. There has been some question whether there is truly a class effect of ACE inhibitors in terms of the various beneficial outcomes that have been studied or if different effects might exist between specific ACE inhibitors, as suggested by small or observational studies.[63,64] Given the lack of good data regarding this issue, it seems prudent to attempt to use those ACE inhibitors that have been shown to be of benefit in large randomized trials of patients in specific clinical situations and at doses found effective in those trials (Table 28-1). It should be kept in mind, however, that likely there is indeed a class effect, and therefore choice of drug can also be based when appropriate on other factors such as cost and convenience. These basic principles can be applied in many cases to other drug classes.

Contraindications
ACE inhibitors are contraindicated in pregnancy due to the increased risk of fetal complications, namely oligohydramnios with use in the late second trimester and the third trimester.[65] ACE inhibitors should also be used with care in patients with any history of angioedema.

Angiotensin Receptor Blockers
Evidence of Benefit in Diabetic Subjects
For ARBs, more evidence of benefit in prevention of progression of nephropathy exists for T2DM than for T1DM. The Reduction of Endpoints in NIDDM with the Angiotensin II Antagonist Losartan (RENAAL) Study was a prospective, multicenter trial of 1513 hypertensive patients with T2DM who had albumin levels higher than 300 mg/g and serum creatinine levels of 1.3 to 3.0 mg/dL.[66] Patients were randomized to losartan or placebo, and the blood pressure was controlled (lower than 140/90) with other non–ACE inhibitor and non-ARB medications. In this study, losartan use resulted in a relative risk reduction of 16% compared to placebo in the composite end point of a doubling of the serum creatinine, end-stage renal disease, or death.

In a study of 1715 diabetic patients with similar baseline characteristics and a similar study design, the Irbesartan Diabetic Nephropathy Trial (IDNT) found that irbesartan treatment resulted in a 20% risk reduction of the same composite end point that was used in RENAAL, but no benefit was found with the dihydropyridine calcium channel blocker amlodipine.[67]

In a third study of 590 patients with nephropathy at the earlier stage of microalbuminuria with hypertension, irbesartan was found to decrease the rate of progression to albuminuria by 24% using a dose of 150 mg/day and by 38% using a dose of 300 mg/day.[68] The Microalbuminuria Reduction with Valsartan (MARVAL) trial of valsartan versus amlodipine demonstrated that valsartan decreased microalbuminuria and macroalbuminuria associated with type 2 diabetes more effectively than other antihypertensive classes.[69]

The question of whether an ACE inhibitor or an ARB is more effective for diabetic nephropathy remains open, as few data have been published from head-to-head trials. A small study by Muirhead's group comparing valsartan and captopril over 1 year in patients with type 2 diabetes and microalbuminuria showed similar efficacy of the two drugs in slowing progression of nephropathy, with the ARB better tolerated.[70] The 6-month Candesartan and Lisinopril Microalbuminuria (CALM) study has demonstrated similar effects of candesartan and lisinopril in lowering blood pressure and microalbuminuria in patients with type 2 diabetes,[71] as has the study by Lacourciere and colleagues comparing losartan and enalapril.[72] The large Diabetics Exposed to Telmisartan and Enalapril (DETAIL) study found that enalapril and telmisartan had similar effects on renal end points.[73] The Ongoing Telmisartan Alone and in Combination with Ramipril Global Endpoint Trial (ONTARGET) study will compare effects of ramipril and telmisartan on secondary renal end points.[74]

Despite the strong evidence for benefit of ARBs in slowing progression of type 2 diabetic nephropathy, evidence remains less clear-cut regarding their effects on CVD outcomes. The Losartan Interven-

Table 28–1. *Antihypertensive Medication Classes*

Drug Class and Examples	Specific Indications	Agents and Doses Used in Clinical Trials	Potential Side Effects	Contraindications	Monitoring; Other Comments
ACE inhibitors (ramipril, lisinopril, enalapril, fosinopril, benazepril, captopril, perindopril, quinapril, trandolapril, moexipril)	T1DM and nephropathy* and/or HTN T2DM and nephropathy,* intolerant of ARBs T2DM and HTN without nephropathy With other comorbidities such as CHF or decreased ejection fraction or in acute post-MI period	Ramipril 10 mg qd (HOPE study[127]) Enalapril 10–40 mg qd (ABCD, STOP-2[35,37]) Lisinopril 10 mg qd (STOP-2[37]) Fosinopril 20 mg qd (FACET[36]) Trandolapril 2-4 mg qd (TRACE[41])	Cough (5% to 20%), hyperkalemia (<3%), worsening of renal function, angioedema (0.1–0.7%), hypoglycemia (rare) in patients taking insulin or sulfonylurea	Pregnancy Use with care if any history of angioedema	Check serum K+ and creatinine 1 to 2 weeks after therapy start or any dose increase If hyperkalemia occurs, add loop diuretic or oral potassium-lowering agent; discontinue ACE inhibitor if K+ persistently >5.5 mEq/L despite these measures Discontinue ACE inhibitor if persistent decrease in GFR or increase in creatinine >30% at 4 mo
Angiotensin receptor blockers (losartan, valsartan, candesartan, irbesartan, telmisartan, olmesartan, eprosartan)	T2DM and nephropathy* T2DM and HTN without nephropathy T1DM and nephropathy,* intolerant of ACEIs With other comorbidities such as CHF or decreased ejection fraction or in acute post-MI period	Losartan 50-100 mg qd RENAAL,[66] LIFE[75] Irbesartan 300 mg qd (IDNT, IRMA-II[59,68]) Candesartan 16-32 mg qd (CHARM[73])	Hyperkalemia, worsening of renal function, angioedema	Pregnancy Use with care if any history of angioedema	Check serum K+ and creatinine 1-2 weeks after therapy start or any dose increase Other monitoring as for ACEIs
Diuretics (thiazides: hydrochloro-thiazide [HCTZ], chlorthalidone; loop: furosemide, torsemide, bumetanide; K-sparing: amiloride, triamterene)	Consider as first line in patients with edema and no nephropathy Add thiazide diuretics as supplemental therapy in DM with BP >130/80	Chlorthalidone 12.5-25 mg qd (ALLHAT, SHEP[5])[43]	Hyperglycemia (unlikely at thiazide doses ≤25 mg qd), hypokalemia, volume depletion, hyperkalemia (triamterene and amiloride), hyponatremia, worsened gout, hypomagnesemia	Avoid triamterene or amiloride when using ACEIs or ARBs in order to avoid hyperkalemia	Monitor K+ and serium creatinine 1-2 weeks after therapy start or dose change Thiazides are less effective with decreasing GFR and should be changed to loop diuretic when serum creatinine ≥2.0 mg/dL
β-Blockers (atenolol, metoprolol, timolol, carvedilol, labetolol)	Adjunctive (third- or fourth-line therapy) Consider if other comorbidities such as CHF or decreased ejection fraction or ischemic heart disease	Atenolol 50-100 mg qd (UKPDS[33])	Worsened glycemic control (nonselective and cardioselective agents, serious hypoglycemic events, bronchospasm, worsened peripheral vascular disease, bradycardia, postural hypotension, fatigue, impotence)	Active or severe asthma or COPD Severe peripheral vascular disease Bradycardia, second- or third-degree heart block Caution if CHF exacerbation Avoid in T1DM prone to hypoglycemia	Check pulse at every clinic visit Monitor glycemic control and hypoglycemic events closely

Table 28–1. *Antihypertensive Medication Classes—Cont'd*

Drug Class and Examples	Specific Indications	Agents and Doses Used in Clinical Trials	Potential Side Effects	Contraindications	Monitoring; Other Comments
Calcium channel blockers (dihydropyridine [DHCCB]: amlodipine, felodipine, nifedipine, nisoldipine; nondihydropyridine (NDHCCB). diltiazem, verapamil)	Supplemental (third-line) therapy in most cases Consider NDHCCB as second-line (with ACEI or ARB) if nephropathy and BP >130/80 Pregnant women with HTN or nephropathy	Amlodipine 2.5-10 mg qd (ALLHAT[43]) Verapamil SR 240 mg qd (INVEST[97]); verapamil ER 180-360 mg qd (CONVINCE[98])	DHCCBs: edema, headache, flushing, gingival hypertrophy NDHCCBs: constipation, headache, bradycardia, worsened systolic dysfunction	Caution in CHF Avoid NDHCCBs with second- or third-degree heart block	Check pulse at every clinic visit (NDHCCBs)
α-Adrenergic agents (α₁-blockers: erazosin, prazosin, doxazosin; centrally acting drugs: clonidine, methyldopa)	Supplemental fourth- or fifth-line therapy if BP >130/80 Consider in men with symptomatic BPH Methyldopa may be used in pregnant hypertensive women		Dry mouth, sedation, dizziness, rebound hypertension (with abrupt cessation)	Avoid methyldopa in liver disease	
Direct vasodilators (hydralazine, minoxidil)	Supplemental fourth- or fifth-line therapy Pregnant women with HTN (hydralazine)		Fluid retention, headache, drug-induced lupus (hydralazine)		
Aldosterone antagonists (spironolactone, eplerenone)	Add-on therapy with CHF or decreased ejection fraction	Spironolactone 25-50 mg qd (RALES[111]) Eplerenone 25-50 mg qd (EPHESUS[112])	Hyperkalemia, worsened renal function, gynecomastia (spironolactone), impotence (spironolactone), increased triglycerides (eplerenone)	Use with extreme caution with ACEIs and ARBs	Monitor K⁺ and creatinine closely, particularly with ACEIs and ARBs

*Including microalbuminuria, albuminuria, or overt renal failure.
ABCD, Appropriate Blood Pressure Control in Diabetes; ACEI, ACE inhibitor; ALLHAT, Antihypertensive and Lipid Lowering Treatment to Prevent Heart Attack; ARB, angiotensin II receptor blocker; BP, blood pressure; BPH, benign prostatic hyperplasia; CHARM, Candesartan in Heart failure Assessment of Reduction in Mortality and morbidity; CHF, congestive heart failure; CONVINCE, Controlled Onset Verapamil Investigation of Cardiovascular End Points; COPD, chronic obstructive pulmonary disease; DM, diabetes mellitus; EPHESUS, Eplerenone's Neurohormonal Efficacy and Survival Study; FACET, Fosinopril versus Amlopidine Cardiovascular Events Trial; GFR, glomerular filtration rate; HOPE, Heart Outcomes Prevention Evaluation; HTN, hypertension; IDNT, Irbesartan Diabetic Nephropathy Trial; INVEST, International Verapamil SR/trandolapril Study; IRMA-II, Irbesartan Microalbuminuria Type 2 Diabetes in Hypertensive Patients; LIFE, Losartan Intervention for Endpoint Reduction; RALES, Randomized Aldactone Evaluation Study; SHEP, Systolic Hypertension in the Elderly Program; STOP-2, Swedish Trial of Old Patients with Hypertension-2; T1DM, type 1 diabetes mellitus; T2DM, type 2 diabetes mellitus; TRACE, Trandolapril Cardiac Evaluation; UKPDS, United Kingdom Prospective Diabetes Study.

tion for Endpoint Reduction (LIFE) trial compared losartan to atenolol and showed a 24% reduction in cardiovascular morbidity and mortality, as well as all-cause mortality, with ARB treatment.[75]

The placebo-controlled Candesartan in Heart failure Assessment of Reduction in Mortality and morbidity (CHARM-Alternative) study of candesartan demonstrated decreased cardiovascular death and admissions for congestive heart failure (CHF) for the entire study group, but a subgroup analysis of the diabetic patients has not been published.[76] However, the RENAAL study of losartan versus placebo showed benefit only on rates of hospitalization for heart failure,[66] and the IDNT trial of irbesartan versus amlodipine versus placebo showed equivalence of the three treatment groups, again except for superiority of irbesartan in decreasing incidence of CHF.[77]

The Valsartan Antihypertensive Long-term Use Evaluation (VALUE) study of valsartan versus amlodipine did not find a significant difference in the effects on the composite cardiovascular end point in all subjects, although, notably, a lower blood pressure was achieved in the amlodipine group, and the approved effective dose range of valsartan was increased above that used in the trial.[78,79] The diabetic subgroup analysis has not yet been published. The results of the ABCD-V-2 trial looking at valsartan therapy in type 2 diabetic patients have not yet been published, and the ongoing ONTARGET and Telmisartan Randomized Assessment Study in ACEI Intolerant Patients with Cardiovascular Disease (TRANSCEND) studies will compare telmisartan, ramipril, telmisartan plus ramipril, and placebo effects on cardiovascular end points.[74]

On the issue of ARBs versus ACE inhibitors, the Valsartan in Acute Myocardial Infarction (VALIANT) study found that the ARB losartan was as effective as though not superior to captopril in improving survival of diabetic post-MI patients,[80] similar to the results of the Optimal Trial in Myocardial Infarction with Angiotensin II Antagonist Losartan (OPTIMAAL) trial[81] and the CHARM-Overall study, which showed no significant differences between the effect of candesartan or ACE-inhibitor therapy on cardiovascular death of admission for CHF in patients with ejection fractions no higher than 40%.[82]

Other Therapeutic Considerations

As with ACE inhibitors, there is evidence that ARBs increase insulin sensitivity. The LIFE trial, comparing losartan and atenolol, showed a reduced risk of new-onset diabetes with the ARB, as did the VALUE trial comparing valsartan and amlodipine and the CHARM trial of candesartan versus placebo.[82] Theoretically, there can be an increased risk of hypoglycemia, as can be seen with ACE inhibitors, but this has not been reported with ARBs. Worsening of renal function could still occur, but there is some suggestion that the risk of hyperkalemia might be lower with ARBs than with ACE inhibitors. ARBs do

not appear to induce cough, but cough can occur in patients who had a cough with ACE inhibitors. ARBs also appear to have a lower incidence of angioedema than is seen with ACE inhibitors.[60,83]

Indications for Use

Given their specific benefit in patients with T2DM and known nephropathy, ARBs are indicated for treatment as first-line therapy in such patients. Furthermore, based on the data from the LIFE study, ARBs are also indicated in type 2 diabetic patients older than 55 years who have additional cardiovascular risk factors. Because of these studies and because of the ARBs' general efficacy and excellent adverse effect profiles, they can certainly be used as first-line therapy in other hypertensive patients as well. Additionally, they can be used as alternative therapy in patients with T1DM who do not tolerate ACE inhibitors.

Contraindications

ARBs are contraindicated in pregnancy due to late second and third trimester risk of oligohydramnios. No other fetopathy has been reported. They should also be used with care in patients with any history of angioedema.

Combination Therapy with ACE Inhibitor plus ARB
Evidence of Benefit in Diabetic Subjects

Theoretically, the idea of dual blockade of the RAAS with agents of both classes is attractive because neither ACE inhibition nor angiotensin subtype 1 (AT_1) receptor blockade alone by pharmacologic agents leads to complete RAAS blockade, and clinical trials of each drug class alone have demonstrated slowing but not arrest of nephropathy progression. ACE inhibitors and ARBs block the RAAS at different levels, and combining the two would theoretically block the RAAS more completely. Therefore, combination ARB and ACE inhibitor therapy potentially has additive effects not only on decreasing blood pressure but also on vascular complications. This theory is supported by animal studies,[84] but few human clinical studies have been published.

A number of small studies have provided evidence that combination therapy may be of more benefit than monotherapy in slowing progression of diabetic nephropathy with respect to albuminuria levels.[85-89] In the largest, the CALM study of 199 diabetic subjects, candesartan plus lisinopril therapy for 6 months led to greater blood pressure reduction than with either agent alone, as well as greater reduction in microalbuminuria; however, it was not clear whether the latter effect was due to the greater blood pressure change or to more complete RAAS blockade.[71]

The Valsartan Heart Failure Trial (Val-HEFT) demonstrated the benefit of adding valsartan to patients with diabetes and heart failure already on an ACE inhibitor, but it raised concern that the combination of valsartan, ACE inhibitor, and β-

blocker might increase mortality and morbidity.[90] The CHARM-Added trial, however, while confirming increased benefit with the addition of candesartan to baseline ACE inhibitor therapy in heart failure patients, showed no adverse effects in those also taking a β-blocker.[91] The VALIANT study showed equivalence of valsartan to captopril in survival of diabetic post-MI patients; combination therapy with both agents did not significantly decrease mortality further, but it did increase the number of adverse drug effects.[80] The ONTARGET study is looking at the benefits of telmisartan, ramipril, or both together in high-risk patients.[74]

Other Therapeutic Considerations

The therapeutic benefits of an ACE inhibitor and an ARB together are presumed to be additive, so one would expect the adverse effects to be potentially increased, particularly effects on renal function and hyperkalemia. In a study of chronic renal failure patients with creatinine clearances of 20 to 45 mL/min treated with benazepril and valsartan, and in the CALM study of lisinopril and candesartan therapy in T2DM, similar side-effect profiles were found whether patients were taking an ACE inhibitor, an ARB, or both.[71,92] Conversely, the CHARM trial found a significantly greater incidence of treatment discontinuation due to increased creatinine or hyperkalemia in the patients taking candesartan rather than placebo in addition to an ACE inhibitor.[91] As with ACE inhibitor monotherapy, angioedema and cough remain possible adverse reactions. It should also be noted that both ACE inhibitors and ARBs (as well as diuretics, see later) can increase lithium levels.

Indications

Combination therapy with both an ACE inhibitor and an ARB may be indicated in the setting of diabetic nephropathy when there is uncontrolled blood pressure higher than 130/80 or continued proteinuria despite maximum therapy with one of the agents. It may also be indicated in diabetic patients with heart failure. In both clinical scenarios, referral to an appropriate subspecialist should be considered.

Diuretics
Evidence of Benefit in Diabetic Subjects

ALLHAT found no difference in progression to ESRD between groups treated with chlorthalidone, lisinopril, amlodipine, or doxazosin, although the lisinopril group had an overall higher achieved systolic blood pressure.[52] A subgroup analysis of diabetic subjects in ALLHAT similarly showed no difference in progression to ESRD or cardiovascular outcomes between these drugs[52a,52b]. The Systolic Hypertension in the Elderly Program (SHEP) trial showed that lowering systolic blood pressure to no higher than 160 mm Hg in older patients using low-dose chlorthalidone (a thiazide diuretic) as first-line therapy decreased multiple cardiovascular end

points, including major CVD events and all-cause mortality.[5] Benefits were greater in diabetic patients than in those without diabetes.

The ALLHAT study also found no difference between treatment groups in the primary end point (combined fatal coronary heart disease and nonfatal MI) or all-cause mortality, but the incidence of some secondary end points was lower in the total study population with chlorthalidone compared with lisinopril (stroke and combined CVD) or amlodipine (CHF). Although the authors stated "treatment effects for all outcomes were consistent across subgroups by . . . diabetic status," Table 6 in the report (illustrating relative risks with confidence intervals) showed the confidence intervals for the diabetic subgroup as crossing unity (1.0) for all outcomes except CHF.[52]

The much smaller ANBP2 study, consisting of 6083 subjects, suggested that thiazide diuretics were actually inferior to ACE inhibitors with respect to cardiovascular end points, although this was mainly in male subjects in a predominantly white, lower-risk population, and no subgroup analysis of the diabetic subjects has been published.[47]

Debate continues over perceived flaws in both of these studies; however, what ALLHAT at least seems to show is that diuretics are not harmful to diabetic patients (as seen also in STOP-2),[46] an important conclusion (see later). Furthermore, other studies have demonstrated the synergistic effect on lowering blood pressure of adding low-dose thiazide diuretic therapy to another antihypertensive agent, particularly an ACE inhibitor or ARB.[93]

Because loop diuretics and the potassium-sparing diuretics triamterene and amiloride have not been studied in large hypertension trials, their effects on reducing CVD risk or nephropathy are unknown.

Other Therapeutic Considerations

For years, arguments have been made that the cardiovascular benefits of diuretics had not been shown to outweigh their negative impact on insulin sensitivity and lipids, particularly in patients already known to have diabetes.[94,95] In fact, studies have now shown that the adverse effects (increased total and LDL cholesterol and triglycerides and increased insulin resistance with hyperinsulinemia) appear to be dose-dependent and unlikely to be significant except with higher doses (e.g., hydrochlorothiazide at doses greater than 25 mg).[96]

Because lower doses of thiazide diuretics (than the 50 to 100 mg daily used decades ago) are sufficient to cause significant blood pressure reduction, doses up to 25 mg daily are the most widely used. Even doses as low as 6.25 or 12.5 mg of hydrochlorothiazide daily have been shown to be effective add-on therapy for hypertension.[93] Such doses were safe and effective in preventing CVD in high-risk patients, including those with diabetes, in both the SHEP and ALLHAT trials,[5,52] despite evidence of greater incidence of new-onset diabetes and worsening of glycemic control in patients with

known diabetes. These were both relatively short-term studies (less than10 years), and it is not known how these metabolic effects might affect CVD adversely many years later.

Loop and potassium-sparing diuretics are of benefit in reducing extracellular fluid (ECF) volume and in helping to control either hyperkalemia or hypokalemia, respectively.

Potential adverse effects of diuretics include volume depletion, increase in uric acid (loop and thiazides), hypokalemia, hyperkalemia (triamterene and amiloride), hyponatremia (especially thiazides), and hypomagnesemia. Loop and thiazide diuretics can worsen gout. Rarely, pancreatitis or blood dyscrasias can occur. Potassium-sparing diuretics should be avoided in patients taking ACE inhibitors or ARBs to prevent hyperkalemia. Diuretics can also increase lithium levels in patients taking lithium.

Indications for Use

In hypertensive diabetic patients, low doses of thiazide diuretics are indicated primarily as second-line, add-on therapy in those who have not reached blood pressure goals. They could also be considered as primary therapy in patients with edema. Loop diuretics may be useful adjunctive therapy in patients with more severe edema, in those with decreased GFR (serum creatinine levels higher than 2.0 mg/dL), or to control hyperkalemia. Potassium-sparing diuretics may be useful adjuncts in patients with peripheral edema (though they are less effective than loop diuretics in this regard) and to treat or prevent hypokalemia associated with thiazide or loop diuretics. However, they should generally not be added when patients are already taking ACE inhibitors or ARBs.

β-Blockers
Evidence of Benefit in Diabetic Subjects

β-blockers are of benefit in reducing complications in diabetic subjects. The UKPDS showed that atenolol was as effective as captopril in lowering blood pressure and reducing microvascular and macrovascular complications.[42] Other studies of the vasodilating β-blocker carvedilol given as adjunctive therapy to an ACE inhibitor in CHF patients have shown benefit in decreasing mortality compared with placebo (the Carvedilol Post-Infarct Survival Control in Left Ventricular Dysfunction Study [CAPRICORN] study; no analysis of the diabetic subgroup was carried out).[97] Studies have also shown increased benefit compared with a cardio-selective β-blocker in terms of decreasing mortality and hospital admissions (the Carvedilol Or Metoprolol European Trial [COMET]).[98] However, in the COMET study, for the 731 diabetic subjects the hazard ratio was 0.85, with a confidence interval crossing unity (0.69-1.06). A meta-analysis of six other trials of β-blocker therapy in CHF concluded that the diabetic subjects derived benefit compared with placebo, although somewhat less magnitude

of benefit. Not all of the trials used a vasodilating β-blocker.[99]

Other Therapeutic Considerations

As with thiazide diuretics, there has been concern regarding the deleterious effects of β-blockers on insulin sensitivity and lipids and the possible attenuation, therefore, of cardiovascular benefit. Both nonselective and cardioselective β-blockers (including propranolol, pindolol, metoprolol, and atenolol) have been shown to reversibly decrease insulin sensitivity by 17% to 30%, as well as variably worsen lipid profiles. However, the newer, vasodilating β-blockers (such as carvedilol and celiprolol) have been demonstrated to actually improve insulin sensitivity (10% to 35%) and to have a neutral or possibly positive effect on lipids.[53]

Nonselective β-blockers can reduce awareness of hypoglycemia (by reducing sympathetically mediated symptoms) and reduce the ability of hypoglycemia-induced release of epinephrine to stimulate hepatic glucose release.[100] Through both of these mechanisms, the risk of serious hypoglycemic events may be increased.[101,102] Furthermore, with nonselective β-blockade during hypoglycemia, the unopposed α-adrenergic stimulation can cause an increase in blood pressure, and severe bradycardia has also been reported.[102,103] These adverse effects are primarily concerns in patients who are taking insulin and who are prone to hypoglycemia. Patients treated with oral agents, even sulfonylureas, or diet alone have not been found to have difficulties with the use of β-blockers.

Other potential adverse effects of β-blockers include bronchospasm, worsening of peripheral vascular disease, bradycardia, postural hypotension, fatigue, and impotence.

Indications for Use

β-Blockers remain a valuable adjunctive therapy in patients with diabetes because of their proven efficacy in lowering blood pressure and in improving outcomes in the presence of ischemic heart disease or chronic CHF. Thus, the diabetic patient who has ischemic cardiac disease is a special case because β-blockers have clearly been shown to be of substantial benefit in such patients both with and without diabetes.[104]

Contraindications

β-Blockers are contraindicated in active or severe asthma or chronic obstructive pulmonary disease and with severe peripheral vascular disease, bradycardia, or second- or third-degree heart block. They should be used with caution in the setting of CHF exacerbation. In patients with type 1 diabetes who are prone to hypoglycemia and especially in those with hypoglycemic unawareness, β-blockers are contraindicated. However, in the setting of an acute myocardial infarction in such a patient, the risks from not using β-blockers must be balanced against the necessity of increasing glycemic goals, and use

of a cardioselective β-blocking agent can decrease the risks discussed earlier. Frequent self-monitoring of blood glucose and scrupulous avoidance of hypoglycemia is critical when such patients are treated with β-blockers.

Calcium Channel Blockers
Evidence of Benefit in Diabetic Subjects
CCBs clearly are effective in lowering blood pressure, but for years debate has continued about the safety of this class due to studies that suggested they increase cardiovascular mortality.[105] Many think this issue has largely been put to rest after the publication of results from a number of large trials including ALLHAT (amlodipine), the International Verapamil SR/trandolapril Study (INVEST, with slow-release verapamil), and the Controlled Onset Verapamil Investigation of Cardiovascular End Points (CONVINCE, with extended-release verapamil).[52,106,107] Another issue is which subclass—dihydropyridine calcium channel blockers (DHCCBs, including amlodipine, nifedipine, felodipine, nicardipine) or nondihydropyridine calcium channel blockers (NDHCCBs: diltiazem, verapamil)—to use, especially because it is the DHCCB class that generally was implicated in possible adverse cardiovascular outcomes.

Studies have not shown DHCCBs to be of benefit in slowing progression of nephropathy (especially when compared to RAAS blockade), but NDHCCBs are potentially of benefit.[69,108,109] As reviewed by Bakris's group, trials of CCBs in renal disease have shown that both subclasses lower blood pressure equally but NDHCCBs have led to consistently greater reductions in proteinuria than DHCCBs whether they are used as monotherapy or combined with an ACE inhibitor or ARB.[108] This was true in diabetic renal disease with any level of proteinuria. The combination of an NDCCB and an ACE inhibitor has also been shown in a small study to decrease proteinuria in patients with diabetic nephropathy by a greater degree than either agent alone.[110]

In terms of CVD benefit, the large ALLHAT, INVEST, and CONVINCE studies each included either a DHCCB or NDHCCB and showed similar benefits of CCBs versus various other class agents on CVD or mortality, although there were higher rates of heart failure in the CCB-treated groups.[52,106,107] Analysis by Grossman and Messerli has shown that these results hold true for diabetic subjects.[111] However, as noted earlier, other smaller studies have shown DHCCBs to be inferior to ACE inhibitors with respect to CVD (FACET, ABCD).

Other Therapeutic Considerations
The CCBs appear to have neutral or positive effects on insulin sensitivity and lipid profiles.[53] One large randomized trial showed a lower incidence of new-onset diabetes with slow-release verapamil (versus a β-blocker).[106] Possible side effects of DHCCBs include edema, headache, flushing, and gingival hypertrophy. Side effects of NDHCCBs include constipation, bradycardia, headache, and worsened systolic dysfunction.

Indications for Use
CCBs clearly are effective at lowering blood pressure. However, given the specific benefits of several of the other classes of drugs, they appear to be best considered as third-line agents. One specific use might be in the pregnant patient who has diabetic nephropathy and hypertension. Diltiazem has been shown to be safe for use during pregnancy and reduces urinary albumin excretion and thus is a reasonable substitute for an ACE inhibitor or an ARB. An NDHCCB such as diltiazem or verapamil could also be a rational addition to an ACE inhibitor or ARB in a patient with nephropathy and blood pressure higher than 130/80.

Contraindications
CCBs should be used with caution in patients with congestive heart failure. NDHCCBs should be avoided in patients with second- or third-degree heart block.

α-Adrenergic Agents
Evidence of Benefit in Diabetic Subjects
There has not been much investigation of α-adrenergic agents in diabetic patients. A few small studies of α-blocker effects on diabetic nephropathy have not conclusively shown their equivalence to RAAS-blocking agents in this regard.[112-114] The ALLHAT study did include the α_1-blocker doxazosin in a treatment arm that was prematurely discontinued due to a significantly higher incidence of heart failure, although at the time of discontinuation there was no difference compared with chlorthalidone in terms of mortality or the primary composite cardiovascular end point.[52]

Other Therapeutic Considerations
α-Blockers (e.g., prazosin, terazosin, doxazosin) and central α-agonists (methyldopa, clonidine) have been shown to have either neutral or potentially beneficial effects on both insulin sensitivity and lipids.[115-117] Also, α-blockers might benefit men with symptomatic benign prostatic hyperplasia. However, as a group, the α-adrenergic agents tend to have a high side-effect profile that includes dry mouth, sedation, dizziness, and rebound hypertension with discontinuation.

Indications for Use
In hypertensive patients with diabetes, α-adrenergic agents are best used as adjunctive therapy, probably fourth- or fifth-line therapy, in patients who have not reached goal blood pressures. Methyldopa still finds occasional use in pregnant women with severe hypertension.

Contraindications
Avoid methyldopa with liver disease, because it is extensively hepatically cleared and can cause hepatic necrosis.

Peripheral Vasodilators
Evidence of Benefit in Diabetic Subjects
Peripheral vasodilators, which include minoxidil and hydralazine, have not been studied in large populations of diabetic patients.

Other Therapeutic Considerations
These agents are often used with β-blockers to minimize reflex tachycardia. Side effects can include fluid retention and headaches. Hydralazine has been implicated as a cause of drug-induced lupus.

Indications for Use
In diabetic patients, peripheral vasodilators are indicated as adjunctive (fourth- or fifth-line) therapy in those requiring additional blood pressure lowering. Minoxidil is usually reserved for patients with refractory hypertension and advanced renal insufficiency. Hydralazine still finds occasional use in pregnant patients with severe hypertension.

Aldosterone Antagonists
Evidence of Benefit in Diabetic Subjects
There are a couple of small studies suggesting that addition of an aldosterone antagonist to an ACE inhibitor may lead to a greater decrease in proteinuria.[118,119] The nonselective aldosterone antagonist spironolactone was studied in the placebo-controlled Randomized Aldactone Evaluation Study (RALES) trial, in which it led to a significant 30% decrease in mortality in heart failure patients; this study did not report separate data for the subjects with diabetes.[120]

The newer selective (for mineralocorticoid over glucocorticoid, progesterone, and androgen receptors) agent eplerenone has been studied in post-MI patients with low ejection fractions in the Eplerenone's Neurohormonal Efficacy and Survival Study (EPHESUS, which included more than 2000 patients with diabetes). Most of the subjects were already on conventional therapy including ACE inhibitor or ARB, β-blocker, aspirin, or diuretic, singly or in combination. The study demonstrated a reduction in mortality (similar between patients with or without diabetes) and in rates of hospitalization for heart failure.[121] However, there were significant increases in creatinine and incidences of hyperkalemia in the eplerenone-treated group.

Other Therapeutic Considerations
Both spironolactone and eplerenone demonstrate an increased risk of hyperkalemia and increased creatinine. Spironolactone can lead to gynecomastia and impotence, and eplerenone can increase triglycerides. Spironolactone is contraindicated in pregnancy because it can have feminizing effects on male fetuses.

Indications for Use
Aldosterone antagonists have been used in patients with persistent hypokalemia due to diuretic agents. This happens rarely when diuretics are added to ACE inhibitors or ARBs. They may also be beneficial in diabetic patients with CHF who have continued symptoms despite conventional therapy, and they are potentially beneficial in the post-MI period.

Contraindications
Aldosterone antagonists should be used with extreme caution in patients taking ACE inhibitors and ARBs because of the risk of hyperkalemia. Potassium levels should be checked frequently when such combinations are used.

Lifestyle Modifications

It is important not to neglect the potential benefits of changes in weight, diet, and exercise levels on blood pressure, in addition to pharmacologic therapy. Based on the described studies and others, the JNC VII guidelines have published the approximate potential reduction in systolic BP resulting from each lifestyle change. These approximations are included in Table 28–2.

Table 28–2. *Recommendations for Lifestyle Modifications in Patients with Diabetes and Hypertension**

Modification Type	Recommendations	Potential Decrease in BP
Weight	Decrease weight by diet and/or exercise, ideally to BMI <25 kg/m²	5–20 mm Hg reduction in systolic BP per 10 kg of weight lost
Diet	Dietary Approaches to Stop Hypertension (DASH) diet (high in fruits, vegetables, low-fat dairy products; low in red meat, sweets, saturated fats)	8–14 mm Hg reduction in systolic BP, mean 5.5 mm Hg reduction in diastolic BP[117]
Sodium	Dietary sodium <2.4 g/day	2–8 mm Hg reduction in systolic BP
Exercise	Aerobic exercise for at least 30 minutes most days of the week	4–9 mm Hg reduction in systolic BP, 4–8 mm Hg reduction in diastolic BP[122]
Alcohol	Men: ≤2 drinks** per day Women: ≤1 drink per day	2–3 mm Hg reduction in both systolic BP and diastolic BP[126]
Tobacco	Complete cessation	Up to 7 mm Hg reduction in systolic BP, 4 mm in diastolic BP[125]

*Data from JNC VII guidelines,[10] except where indicated.
**1 drink = 0.5 oz (15 mL) ethanol: 12 oz beer, 5 oz wine, or 1 oz 100-proof whiskey.
BP, blood pressure.

Weight Loss

Weight loss, in addition to decreasing insulin resistance, has been clearly shown to decrease BP.[122,123] Sustained, modest weight loss of 4.5 kg over 36 months led to decreases in systolic BP of 5 mm Hg and diastolic BP of 7 mm Hg in one large study of more than 1000 participants.[124]

In another study of 529 overweight or obese patients, diastolic blood pressure significantly dropped by 11.6 mm Hg at 6 months in those losing 4.5 kg or more by diet modification, a drop that was statistically equivalent to that achieved using either 25 mg of chlorthalidone (11.1 mm Hg) or 50 mg of atenolol (12.4 mm Hg).[125] Weight loss also potentiated drug effectiveness, so that a 4.5 kg or more weight loss in addition to use of atenolol led to an 18 mm Hg reduction, and a 2.25 kg or more weight loss in patients taking chlorthalidone led to a drop of 15.4 mm Hg.

Diet

Diet composition appears to affect blood pressure as well. The Dietary Approaches to Stop Hypertension (DASH) trial found that a diet high in fruits, vegetables, and low-fat dairy products and low in red meat, sweets, and saturated fats led to blood pressure reductions, particularly in hypertensive patients (systolic BP reduction 11.4, diastolic BP reduction 5.5 mm Hg).[126] The DASH diet also appeared to enhance blood pressure response to the ARB losartan in a study of 55 hypertensive patients.[127]

The DASH-Sodium study examined the effectiveness of reduction of dietary sodium in addition to application of the DASH diet; in hypertensive sub-

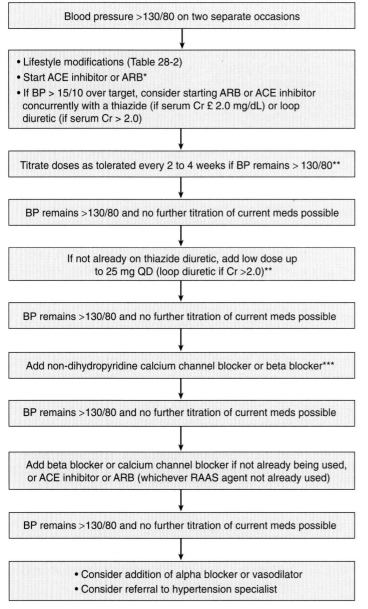

Figure 28–2. Algorithm for antihypertensive therapy in patients with diabetes. ACE, angiotensin-converting enzyme; ARB, angiotensin II receptor blocker; BP, blood pressure; Cr, creatinine; QD, once daily; RAAS, renin-angiotensin-aldosterone system. *Although ACE inhibitors and ARBs are often used interchangeably, we believe that given the current data as outlined in the text, choice of RAAS-blocking agent should be specific in two situations: If the patient has T1DM with nephropathy, an ACE inhibitor should be considered first-line therapy; if the patient has T2DM with nephropathy, an ARB should be considered first-line therapy. If a patient does not tolerate the first-line therapy, then an agent from the other class should be substituted. If there is no nephropathy, an agent from either class can be used. **Monitoring of K+ and serum creatinine should also be done, as outlined in Table 28-1. ***If the patient has nephropathy, use a nondihydropyridine calcium channel blocker (diltiazem or verapamil) preferably. *Note*: at each step, titration of medication doses should ideally occur approximately every 2 to 4 weeks.

jects, the DASH diet plus a low sodium intake (500 to 1000 mg/day) was found to lead to a further decrease in systolic BP of 11.5 mm Hg compared with that seen on the DASH diet and a high sodium intake (around 3600 mg/day).[128] These effects on blood pressure remained significant across subgroups but seemed greatest in hypertensive African Americans and persons older than 45 years.[129]

Reducing sodium intake appeared to potentiate the blood pressure effects of losartan in a small study of type 2 diabetic patients.[130] The JNC VII guidelines recommend daily intake of sodium less than 2.4 grams.[10]

Exercise

Increasing physical activity also lowers blood pressure (see Chapter 22); a meta-analysis of 9 randomized, controlled trials of hypertensive patients showed that aerobic exercise of 30 to 60 minutes 3 or 4 times per week led to average decreases in systolic BP of 7±5 mm Hg and in diastolic BP of 6±2 mm Hg.[131] Progressive resistance training also appears to lead to lower blood pressure.[132]

Other Factors

Tobacco and alcohol consumption can increase blood pressure.[133-135] It is important to counsel patients about the risks of either habit beyond causing hypertension and about strategies for cessation or reduction. For alcohol consumption, the JNC VII guidelines recommend no more than two drinks a day for men and one drink a day for women. One drink is equivalent to a total of 0.5 ounce (15 mL) of ethanol, such as 12 ounces (360 mL) of beer, 5 ounces (150 mL) of wine, or 1 ounce (30 mL) of 100-proof whiskey.[10] Reduction in alcohol consumption can lead to a 2 to 3 mm Hg drop in both systolic and diastolic BP.[135]

CONCLUSIONS

Hypertension is a serious comorbidity of diabetes and needs to be treated aggressively. The recommended blood pressure goals for such treatment have changed over the years based on the data that continue to flow from large clinical trials, and the current goal of less than 130/80 mm Hg could change yet again. Despite the significant risks of uncontrolled hypertension, many, if not most, diabetic patients in the United States are not reaching goal blood pressures. Although the reasons for this may be manifold and include factors such as noncompliance and lack of aggressive therapy titration, it is incumbent upon such patients' primary health care providers to work with them to change the situation.

As a guide and aid in achieving current blood pressure goals, we present our recommendations based on the best available evidence, outlined in the algorithm in Figure 28–2 (also see Table 28–1 for choices of agents and monitoring of therapy). Some

of the guiding principles are as follows: Blockade of the RAAS is clearly paramount in patients with diabetes; thiazide diuretics are valuable second-line agents, particularly because many patients have a component of volume overload; CCBs and β-blockers are safe and effective in diabetic patients and represent in most cases useful third-line add-on therapy. We make these recommendations despite the lack of superiority of RAAS blockade found in the ALLHAT study[52,52a,52b] and in the meta-analysis of the Blood Pressure Lowering Treatment Trialists' Collaboration[136] because of the wealth of other data for progression of ESRD and adverse prognostic significance of new diabetes in treated hypertensive subjects[137] coupled with the finding from ALLHAT that diuretics increase the incidence of diabetes.[52]

Health care providers also must not forget that many, if not most, patients with diabetes and hypertension require multiple drugs (potentially four or more) to achieve goal blood pressures, and escalation of dosage and of additional agents should be done in as timely a manner as possible (barring serious or intolerable side effects) so as to reach goal blood pressure as rapidly as possible. The algorithm provides a guide only; clinical judgment is always needed.

PITFALLS/COMPLICATIONS

ARB or ACE-Inhibitor Therapy

- ARBs or ACE inhibitors should not necessarily be discontinued if the patient is asymptomatic, has mild hyperkalemia, or has an increase in serum creatinine.
- Potassium levels up to 5.5 mEq/L can be tolerated in patients with diabetic kidney disease, and a loop diuretic or oral potassium-lowering agent may be added to achieve this range.
- A decrease in the creatinine clearance of less than 30% (or increase in serum creatinine of less than 30%) can also be tolerated without needing to discontinue therapy.

Thiazide Diuretics

- Thiazide diuretics should be considered earlier in antihypertensive therapy, especially in patients with an element of peripheral edema.
- Thiazides become less effective as the glomerular filtration rate (GFR) falls, and medication should therefore be changed to loop diuretics when the serum creatinine increases to more than 2.0 mg/dL.

β-Blocker Therapy

- β-Blockers should be avoided in patients with type 1 diabetes who are prone to hypoglycemia, because β-blockers can mask and worsen hypoglycemia.

References

1. National Institute of Diabetes and Digestive and Kidney Diseases: National Diabetes Statistics. Available at http://diabetes.niddk.nih.gov/dm/pubs/statistics/index.htm.
2. Collado-Mesa F, Colhoun HM, Stevens LK, et al: Prevalence and management of hypertension in type 1 diabetes mellitus in Europe: The EURODIAB IDDM Complications Study. Diab Med 16:41-48, 1999.
3. Jandeleit-Dahm K, Cooper ME: Hypertension and diabetes. Curr Opin Nephrol Hypertens 11:221-228, 2002.
4. Arauz-Pacheco C, Parrott MA, Raskin P: Hypertension management in adults with diabetes. Diabetes Care 27(Suppl 1):S65-S67, 2004.
5. Curb JD, Pressel SL, Cutler JA, et al: Effect of diuretic-based antihypertensive treatment on cardiovascular disease risk in older diabetic patients with isolated systolic hypertension. JAMA 276:1886-1892, 1996.
6. Tuomilehto J, Rastenyte D, Birkenhager WH, et al: Effects of calcium-channel blockade in older patients with diabetes and systolic hypertension. New Engl J Med 340:677-684, 1999.
7. Mogensen CE, Christensen CK: Predicting diabetic nephropathy in insulin-dependent patients. New Engl J Med 311:89-93, 1984.
8. Parving HH, Andersen AR, Smidt UM, et al: Diabetic nephropathy and arterial hypertension: The effect of antihypertensive treatment. Diabetes 32(Suppl 2):83-87, 1983.
9. Parving HH, Andersen AR, Smidt UM, et al: Early aggressive antihypertensive treatment reduces rate of decline in kidney function in diabetic nephropathy. Lancet 1:1175-1179, 1983.
10. Chobanian AV, Bakris GL, Black HR, et al: The Seventh Report of the Joint National Committee on Prevention, Detection, Evaluation, and Treatment of High Blood Pressure: The JNC 7 report. JAMA 289:2560-2572, 2003.
11. Adler AI, Stratton IM, Neil HA, et al: Association of systolic blood pressure with macrovascular and microvascular complications of type 2 diabetes (UKPDS 36): Prospective observational study. BMJ 321:412-419, 2000.
12. Bakris GL: The importance of blood pressure control in the patient with diabetes. Am J Med 116:30S-38S, 2004.
13. UK Prospective Diabetes Study Group: Tight blood pressure control and risk of macrovascular and microvascular complications in type 2 diabetes: UKPDS 38. BMJ 317:703-713, 1998.
14. Snow V, Weiss KB, Mottur-Pilson C: The evidence base for tight blood pressure control in the management of type 2 diabetes mellitus. Ann Intern Med 138:587-592, 2003.
15. Hansson L, Zanchetti A, Carruthers SG, et al: Effects of intensive blood-pressure lowering and low-dose aspirin in patients with hypertension: Principal results of the Hypertension Optimal Treatment (HOT) randomised trial. Lancet 351:1755-1762, 1998.
16. Estacio RO, Jeffers BW, Gifford N, et al: Effect of blood pressure control on diabetic microvascular complications in patients with hypertension and type 2 diabetes. Diabetes Care 23:B54-B64, 2000.
17. Schrier RW, Estacio RO, Esler A, et al: Effects of aggressive blood pressure control in normotensive type 2 diabetic patients on albuminuria, retinopathy and strokes. Kidney Int 61:1086-1097, 2002.
18. Parving HH, Andersen AR, Smidt UM, et al: Effect of antihypertensive treatment on kidney function in diabetic nephropathy. Brit Med J Clin Res Ed 294:1443-1447, 1987.
19. Bakris GL, Copley JB, Vicknair N, et al: Calcium channel blockers versus other antihypertensive therapies on progression of NIDDM associated nephropathy. Kidney Int 50:1641-1650, 1996.
20. Bakris GL, Mangrum A, Copley JB, et al: Effect of calcium channel or beta-blockade on the progression of diabetic nephropathy in African Americans. Hypertension 29:744-750, 1997.
21. The GISEN group (Gruppo Italiano di Studi Epidemiologici in Nefrologia): Randomised placebo-controlled trial of effect of ramipril on decline in glomerular filtration rate and risk of terminal failure in proteinuric, non-diabetic nephropathy. Lancet 349:1857-1863, 1997.
22. Hebert LA, Bain RP, Verme D, et al: Remission of nephrotic range proteinuria in type I diabetes. Collaborative Study Group. Kidney Int 46:1688-1693, 1994.
23. Klahr S, Levey AS, Beck GJ, et al, for the Modification of Diet in Renal Disease Study Group: The effects of dietary protein restriction and blood-pressure control on the progression of chronic renal disease. N Engl J Med 330:877-884, 1994.
24. Lebovitz HE, Wiegmann TB, Cnaan A, et al: Renal protective effects of enalapril in hypertensive NIDDM: Role of baseline albuminuria. Kidney Int 45(Suppl):150-155, 1994.
25. Maschio G, Alberti D, Janin G, et al: Effect of the angiotensin-converting-enzyme inhibitor benazepril on the progression of chronic renal insufficiency. The Angiotensin-Converting-Enzyme Inhibition in Progressive Renal Insufficiency Study Group. N Engl J Med 334:939-945, 1996.
26. Parving HH, Hommel E, Damkjaer Nielsen M, Giese J: Effect of captopril on blood pressure and kidney function in normotensive insulin dependent diabetics with nephropathy. BMJ 299:533-536, 1989.
27. Viberti G, Mogensen CE, Groop LC, Pauls F: Effect of captopril on progression to clinical proteinuria in patients with insulin-dependent diabetes mellitus and microalbuminuria. European Microalbuminuria Captopril Study Group. JAMA 271:275-279, 1994.
28. National Kidney Foundation Kidney Disease Outcomes Quality Initiative (K/DOQI): Guideline 8: Pharmacological therapy: Diabetic kidney disease. Am J Kidney Dis 43:S58-S142, 2004.
29. Turnbull F: Effects of different blood-pressure-lowering regimens on major cardiovascular events: Results of prospectively-designed overviews of randomised trials. Lancet 362:1527-1535, 2003.
30. Berlowitz DR, Ash AS, Hickey EC, et al: Hypertension management in patients with diabetes: The need for more aggressive therapy. Diabetes Care 26:355-359, 2003.
31. Zatz R, Anderson S, Meyer TW, et al: Lowering of arterial blood pressure limits glomerular sclerosis in rats with renal ablation and in experimental diabetes. Kidney Int 20(Suppl):S123-S129, 1987.
32. Zatz R, Dunn BR, Meyer TW, et al: Prevention of diabetic glomerulopathy by pharmacological amelioration of glomerular capillary hypertension. J Clin Invest 77:1925-1930, 1986.
33. Goa KL, Haria M, Wilde MI: Lisinopril. A review of its pharmacology and use in the management of the complications of diabetes mellitus. Drugs 53:1081-1105, 1997.
34. ACE Inhibitors in Diabetic Nephropathy Trialist Group: Should all patients with type 1 diabetes mellitus and microalbuminuria receive angiotensin-converting enzyme inhibitors? A meta-analysis of individual patient data. Ann Intern Med 134:370-379, 2001.
35. Lewis EJ, Hunsicker LG, Bain RP, et al: The effect of angiotensin-converting-enzyme inhibition on diabetic nephropathy. New Engl J Med 329:1456-1462, 1993.
36. Ravid M, Lang R, Rachmani R, et al: Long-term renoprotective effect of angiotensin-converting enzyme inhibition in non-insulin-dependent diabetes mellitus: A 7-year follow-up study. Arch Intern Med 156:286-289, 1996.
37. Ravid M, Brosh D, Levi Z, et al: Use of enalapril to attenuate decline in renal function in normotensive, normoalbuminuric patients with type 2 diabetes mellitus: A randomized, controlled trial. Ann Intern Med 128:982-988, 1998.
38. Heart Outcomes Prevention Evaluation Study Investigators: Effects of ramipril on cardiovascular and microvascular outcomes in people with diabetes mellitus: Results of the HOPE study and MICRO-HOPE substudy. Lancet 355:253-259, 2000.

39. Mogensen CE, Cooper ME: Diabetic renal disease: From recent studies to improved clinical practice. Diabet Med 21:4-17, 2004.

40. Agardh CD, Garcia-Puig J, Charbonnel B, et al: Greater reduction of urinary albumin excretion in hypertensive type II diabetic patients with incipient nephropathy by lisinopril than by nifedipine. J Hum Hypertens 10:185-192, 1996.

41. Nielsen FS, Rossing P, Gall MA, et al: Impact of lisinopril and atenolol on kidney function in hypertensive NIDDM subjects with diabetic nephropathy. Diabetes 43:1108-1113, 1994.

42. UK Prospective Diabetes Study Group: Efficacy of atenolol and captopril in reducing risk of macrovascular and microvascular complications in type 2 diabetes: UKPDS 39. BMJ 317:713-720, 1998.

43. Niskanen L, Hedner T, Hansson L, et al: Reduced cardiovascular morbidity and mortality in hypertensive diabetic patients on first-line therapy with an ACE inhibitor compared with a diuretic/beta-blocker-based treatment regimen: A subanalysis of the Captopril Prevention Project. Diabetes Care 24:2091-2096, 2001.

44. Estacio RO, Jeffers BW, Hiatt WR, et al: The effect of nisoldipine as compared with enalapril on cardiovascular outcomes in patients with non–insulin-dependent diabetes and hypertension. New Engl J Med 338:645-652, 1998.

45. Tatti P, Pahor M, Byington RP, et al: Outcome results of the Fosinopril Versus Amlodipine Cardiovascular Events Randomized Trial (FACET) in patients with hypertension and NIDDM. Diabetes Care 21:597-603, 1998.

46. Hansson L, Lindholm LH, Ekbom T, et al: Randomised trial of old and new antihypertensive drugs in elderly patients: Cardiovascular mortality and morbidity the Swedish Trial in Old Patients with Hypertension–2 study. Lancet 354:1751-1756, 1999.

47. Wing LM, Reid CM, Ryan P, et al: A comparison of outcomes with angiotensin-converting-enzyme inhibitors and diuretics for hypertension in the elderly. New Engl J Med 348:583-592, 2003.

48. Pfeffer MA, Braunwald E, Moye LA, et al: Effect of captopril on mortality and morbidity in patients with left ventricular dysfunction after myocardial infarction. New Engl J Med 327:669-677, 1992.

49. The Acute Infarction Ramipril Efficacy (AIRE) Study Investigators: Effect of ramipril on mortality and morbidity of survivors of acute myocardial infarction with clinical evidence of heart failure. Lancet 342:821-828, 1993.

50. Gustafsson I, Torp-Pedersen C, Kober L, et al: Effect of the angiotensin-converting enzyme inhibitor trandolapril on mortality and morbidity in diabetic patients with left ventricular dysfunction after acute myocardial infarction. J Am Coll Cardiol 34:83-89, 1999.

51. Jong P, Yusuf S, Rousseau MF, et al: Effect of enalapril on 12-year survival and life expectancy in patients with left ventricular systolic dysfunction: A follow-up study. Lancet 361:1843-1848, 2003.

52. ALLHAT Officers: Major outcomes in high-risk hypertensive patients randomized to angiotensin-converting enzyme inhibitor or calcium channel blocker vs diuretic: The Antihypertensive and Lipid-Lowering Treatment to Prevent Heart Attack Trial (ALLHAT). JAMA 288:2981-2997, 2002.

52a. Rahman M, Pressel S, Davis R, et al for the ALLHAT Collaborative Research Group: Renal outcomes in high-risk hypertensive patients treated with an angiotensin-converting enzyme inhibitor or a calcium channel blocker vs. a diuretic. Arch Intern Med 165:936-946, 2005.

52b. Whelton PK, Barzilay J, Cushman WC, et al for the ALLHAT Collaborative Research Group: Clinical outcomes in antihypertension treatment of type 2 diabetes, impaired fasting glucose concentration, and normoglycemia. Arch Intern Med 165:1401-1409, 2005.

53. Jacob S, Rett K, Henriksen EJ: Antihypertensive therapy and insulin sensitivity: Do we have to redefine the role of car-dioselective beta-blocking agents? Am J Hypertension 11:1258-1265, 1998.

54. Hansson L, Lindholm LH, Niskanen L, et al: Effect of angiotensin-converting-enzyme inhibition compared with conventional therapy on cardiovascular morbidity and mortality in hypertension: The Captopril Prevention Project (CAPPP) randomised trial. Lancet 353:611-616, 1999.

55. Yusuf S, Sleight P, Pogue J, et al: Effects of an angiotensin-converting-enzyme inhibitor, ramipril, on cardiovascular events in high-risk patients. New Engl J Med 342:145-153, 2000.

56. Morris AD, Boyle DI, McMahon AD, et al: ACE inhibitor use is associated with hospitalization for severe hypoglycemia in patients with diabetes. Diabetes Care 20:1363-1367, 1997.

57. Herings RM, de Boer A, Stricker BH, et al: Hypoglycaemia associated with use of inhibitors of angiotensin converting enzyme. Lancet 345:1195-1198, 1995.

58. Pedersen-Bjergaard U, Agerholm-Larsen B, Pramming S, et al: Activity of angiotensin-converting enzyme and risk of severe hypoglycaemia in type 1 diabetes mellitus. Lancet 357:1248-1253, 2001.

59. The Euclid Study Group: Randomised placebo-controlled trial of lisinopril in normotensive patients with insulin-dependent diabetes and normoalbuminuria or microalbuminuria. Lancet 349:1787-1792, 1997.

60. Mangrum AJ, Bakris GL: Angiotensin-converting enzyme inhibitors and angiotensin receptor blockers in chronic renal disease: Safety issues. Semin Nephrol 24:168-175, 2004.

61. Cicardi M, Zingale LC, Bergamaschini L, et al: Angioedema associated with angiotensin-converting enzyme inhibitor use: outcome after switching to a different treatment. Arch Intern Med 164:910-913, 2004.

62. Israili ZH, Hall WD: Cough and angioneurotic edema associated with angiotensin-converting enzyme inhibitor therapy: A review of the literature and pathophysiology. Ann Intern Med 117:234-242, 1992.

63. Pilote L, Abrahamowicz M, Rodrigues E, et al: Mortality rates in elderly patients who take different angiotensin-converting enzyme inhibitors after acute myocardial infarction: A class effect? Ann Intern Med 141:102-112, 2004.

64. Foy S, Crozier I, Turner J, et al: Comparison of enalapril versus captopril on left ventricular function and survival three months after acute myocardial infarction (the "PRACTICAL" study). Am J Cardiol 73:1180-1186, 1994.

65. Shotan A, Widerhorn J, Hurst A, et al: Risks of angiotensin-converting enzyme inhibition during pregnancy: Experimental and clinical evidence, potential mechanisms, and recommendations for use. Am J Med 96:451-456, 1994.

66. Brenner BM, Cooper ME, de Zeeuw D, et al: Effects of losartan on renal and cardiovascular outcomes in patients with type 2 diabetes and nephropathy. New Engl J Med 345:861-869, 2001.

67. Lewis EJ, Hunsicker LG, Clarke WR, et al: Renoprotective effect of the angiotensin-receptor antagonist irbesartan in patients with nephropathy due to type 2 diabetes. New Engl J Med 345:851-860, 2001.

68. Parving HH, Lehnert H, Brochner-Mortensen J, et al: The effect of irbesartan on the development of diabetic nephropathy in patients with type 2 diabetes. New Engl J Med 345:870-878, 2001.

69. Viberti G, Wheeldon NM for the MicroAlbuminuria Reduction with VALsartan (MARVAL) Study Investigators: Microalbuminuria reduction with valsartan in patients with type 2 diabetes mellitus: A blood pressure-independent effect. Circulation 106:672-678, 2002.

70. Muirhead N, Feagan BF, Mahon J, et al: The effects of valsartan and captopril on reducing microalbuminuria in patients with type 2 diabetes mellitus: A placebo-controlled trial. Curr Ther Res Clin E 60:650-660, 1999.

71. Mogensen CE, Neldam S, Tikkanen I, et al: Randomised controlled trial of dual blockade of renin-angiotensin

system in patients with hypertension, microalbuminuria, and non-insulin dependent diabetes: The candesartan and lisinopril microalbuminuria (CALM) study. BMJ 321:1440-1444, 2000.

72. Lacourciere Y, Belanger A, Godin C, et al: Long-term comparison of losartan and enalapril on kidney function in hypertensive type 2 diabetics with early nephropathy. Kidney Int 58:762-769, 2000.

73. Barnett AH, Bain SC, Bouter P, et al for the Diabetics Exposed to Telmisartan and Enalapril Study Group: Angiotensin-receptor blockade versus converting-enzyme inhibition in type 2 diabetes and nephropathy. N Engl J Med 351:1952-1961, 2004.

74. Yusuf S: From the HOPE to the ONTARGET and the TRANSCEND studies: Challenges in improving prognosis. Am J Cardiol 89:18A-25A; discussion 25A-26A, 2002.

75. Lindholm LH, Ibsen H, Dahlof B, et al: Cardiovascular morbidity and mortality in patients with diabetes in the Losartan Intervention For Endpoint reduction in hypertension study (LIFE): A randomised trial against atenolol. Lancet 359:1004-1010, 2002.

76. Granger CB, McMurray JJ, Yusuf S, et al: Effects of candesartan in patients with chronic heart failure and reduced left-ventricular systolic function intolerant to angiotensin-converting-enzyme inhibitors: The CHARM-Alternative trial. Lancet 362:772-776, 2003.

77. Berl T, Hunsicker LG, Lewis JB, et al: Cardiovascular outcomes in the Irbesartan Diabetic Nephropathy Trial of patients with type 2 diabetes and overt nephropathy. Ann Intern Med 138:542-549, 2003.

78. Weber MA, Julius S, Kjeldsen SE, et al: Blood pressure dependent and independent effects of antihypertensive treatment on clinical events in the VALUE Trial. Lancet 363:2049-2051, 2004.

79. Julius S, Kjeldsen SE, Weber M, et al: Outcomes in hypertensive patients at high cardiovascular risk treated with regimens based on valsartan or amlodipine: The VALUE randomised trial. Lancet 363:2022-2031, 2004.

80. Pfeffer MA, McMurray JJ, Velazquez EJ, et al: Valsartan, captopril, or both in myocardial infarction complicated by heart failure, left ventricular dysfunction, or both. New Engl J Med 349:1893-1906, 2003.

81. Dickstein K, Kjekshus J: Effects of losartan and captopril on mortality and morbidity in high-risk patients after acute myocardial infarction: The OPTIMAAL randomised trial. Lancet 360:752-760, 2002.

82. Pfeffer MA, Swedberg K, Granger CB, et al: Effects of candesartan on mortality and morbidity in patients with chronic heart failure: The CHARM-Overall programme. Lancet 362:759-766, 2003.

83. Gavras I, Gavras H: Are patients who develop angioedema with ACE inhibition at risk of the same problem with AT1 receptor blockers? Arch Intern Med 163:240-241, 2003.

84. Taal MW, Brenner BM: Renoprotective benefits of RAS inhibition: From ACEI to angiotensin II antagonists. Kidney Int 57:1803-1817, 2000.

85. Jacobsen P, Andersen S, Rossing K, et al: Dual blockade of the renin-angiotensin system in type 1 patients with diabetic nephropathy. Nephrol Dial Transp 17:1019-1024, 2002.

86. Rossing K, Jacobsen P, Pietraszek L, et al: Renoprotective effects of adding angiotensin II receptor blocker to maximal recommended doses of ACE inhibitor in diabetic nephropathy: A randomized double-blind crossover trial. Diabetes Care 26:2268-2274, 2003.

87. Laverman GD, Navis G, Henning RH, et al: Dual renin-angiotensin system blockade at optimal doses for proteinuria. Kidney Int 62:1020-1025, 2002.

88. Hebert LA, Falkenhain ME, Nahman NS Jr, et al: Combination ACE inhibitor and angiotensin II receptor antagonist therapy in diabetic nephropathy. Am J Nephrol 19:1-6, 1999.

89. Kuriyama S, Tomonari H, Tokudome G, et al: Antiproteinuric effects of combined antihypertensive therapies in patients with overt type 2 diabetic nephropathy. Hypertens Res 25:849-855, 2002.

90. Cohn JN, Tognoni G: A randomized trial of the angiotensin-receptor blocker valsartan in chronic heart failure. New Engl J Med 345:1667-1675, 2001.

91. McMurray JJ, Ostergren J, Swedberg K, et al: Effects of candesartan in patients with chronic heart failure and reduced left-ventricular systolic function taking angiotensin-converting-enzyme inhibitors: The CHARM-Added trial. Lancet 362:767-771, 2003.

92. Ruilope LM, Aldigier JC, Ponticelli C, et al: Safety of the combination of valsartan and benazepril in patients with chronic renal disease. J Hypertens 18:89-95, 2000.

93. Neutel JM, Black HR, Weber MA. Combination therapy with diuretics: An evolution of understanding. Am J Med 101:61S-70S, 1996.

94. Warram JH, Laffel LM, Valsania P, et al: Excess mortality associated with diuretic therapy in diabetes mellitus. Arch Intern Med 151:1350-1356, 1991.

95. Weir MR, Flack JM, Applegate WB: Tolerability, safety, and quality of life and hypertensive therapy: The case for low-dose diuretics. Am J Med 101:83S-92S, 1996.

96. Neutel JM: Metabolic manifestations of low-dose diuretics. Am J Med 101:71S-82S, 1996.

97. Dargie HJ: Effect of carvedilol on outcome after myocardial infarction in patients with left-ventricular dysfunction: The CAPRICORN randomised trial. Lancet 357:1385-90, 2001.

98. Poole-Wilson PA, Swedberg K, Cleland JG, et al: Comparison of carvedilol and metoprolol on clinical outcomes in patients with chronic heart failure in the Carvedilol Or Metoprolol European Trial (COMET): Randomised controlled trial. Lancet 362:7-13, 2003.

99. Haas SJ, Vos T, Gilbert RE, et al: Are beta-blockers as efficacious in patients with diabetes mellitus as in patients without diabetes mellitus who have chronic heart failure? A meta-analysis of large-scale clinical trials. Am Heart J 146:848-853, 2003.

100. Kleinbaum J, Shamoon H: Effect of propranolol on delayed glucose recovery after insulin-induced hypoglycemia in normal and diabetic subjects. Diabetes Care 7:155-162, 1984.

101. Trost BN, Weidmann P, Beretta-Piccoli C: Antihypertensive therapy in diabetic patients. Hypertension 76:II102-II108, 1985.

102. Kendall MJ: Impact of beta 1 selectivity and intrinsic sympathomimetic activity on potential unwanted noncardiovascular effects of beta blockers. Am J Cardiol 59:44F-47F, 1987.

103. Ryan JR, LaCorte W, Jain A, et al: Hypertension in hypoglycemic diabetics treated with beta-adrenergic antagonists. Hypertension 7:443-446, 1985.

104. Jonas M, Reicher-Reiss H, Boyko V, et al: Usefulness of beta-blocker therapy in patients with non–insulin-dependent diabetes mellitus and coronary artery disease. Bezafibrate Infarction Prevention (BIP) Study Group. Am J Cardiol 77:1273-77, 1996.

105. Eisenberg MJ, Brox A, Bestawros AN: Calcium channel blockers: An update. Am J Med 116:35-43, 2004.

106. Pepine CJ, Handberg EM, Cooper-DeHoff RM, et al: A calcium antagonist vs a non-calcium antagonist hypertension treatment strategy for patients with coronary artery disease. JAMA 290:2805-2816, 2003.

107. Black HR, Elliott WJ, Grandits G, et al: Principal results of the Controlled Onset Verapamil Investigation of Cardiovascular End Points (CONVINCE) trial. JAMA 289:2073-2082, 2003.

108. Bakris GL, Weir M, Secic M, et al: Differential effects of calcium antagonist subclasses on markers of nephropathy progression. Kidney Int 65:1991-2002, 2004.

109. Bakris GL, Weir MR, Sowers JR: Therapeutic challenges in the obese diabetic patient with hypertension. Am J Med 101:33S-46S, 1996.

110. Bakris GL, Weir MR, DeQuattro V, et al: Effects of an ACE inhibitor/calcium antagonist combination on proteinuria in diabetic nephropathy. Kidney Int 54:1283-1289, 1998.

111. Grossman E, Messerli FH: Are calcium antagonists beneficial in diabetic patients with hypertension? Am J Med 116:44-49, 2004.

112. Rachmani R, Levi Z, Slavachevsky I, et al: Effect of an alpha-adrenergic blocker, and ACE inhibitor and hydrochlorothiazide on blood pressure and on renal function in type 2 diabetic patients with hypertension and albuminuria: A randomized cross-over study. Nephron 80:175-182, 1998.

113. Holdaas H, Hartmann A, Berg KJ, et al: Contrasting effects of angiotensin converting inhibitor and alpha-1-antagonist on albuminuria in insulin-dependent diabetes mellitus patients with nephropathy. J Intern Med 237:63-71, 1995.

114. Giordano M, Sanders LR, Castellino P, et al: Effect of alpha-adrenergic blockers, ACE inhibitors, and calcium channel antagonists on renal function in hypertensive non–insulin-dependent diabetic patients. Nephron 72:447-453, 1996.

115. Giordano M, Matsuda M, Sanders L, et al: Effects of angiotensin-converting enzyme inhibitors, Ca^{2+} channel antagonists, and alpha-adrenergic blockers on glucose and lipid metabolism in NIDDM patients with hypertension. Diabetes 44:665-671, 1995.

116. Huupponen R, Lehtonen A, Vahatalo M: Effect of doxazosin on insulin sensitivity in hypertensive non-insulin dependent diabetic patients. Eur J Clin Pharmacol 43:365-368, 1992.

117. Lithell HO, Andersson PE: Antihypertensive treatment in insulin resistant patients. Hypertens Res 19:S75-S79, 1996.

118. Epstein M, Buckalew VJ, Martinez F, et al: Antiproteinuric efficacy of eplerenone, enalapril and eplerenone/enalapril combination therapy in diabetic hypertensives with microalbuminuria. Am J Hypertens 15:24A, 2002.

119. Chrysostomou A, Becker G: Spironolactone in addition to ACE inhibition to reduce proteinuria in patients with chronic renal disease. N Engl J Med 345:925-926, 2001.

120. Pitt B, Zannad F, Remme WJ, et al: The effect of spironolactone on morbidity and mortality in patients with severe heart failure. N Engl J Med 341:709-717, 1999.

121. Pitt B, Remme W, Zannad F, et al: Eplerenone, a selective aldosterone blocker, in patients with left ventricular dysfunction after myocardial infarction. New Engl J Med 348:1309-1321, 2003.

122. Reisin E, Frohlich E, Messerli F, et al: Cardiovascular changes after weight reduction in obesity hypertension. Ann Intern Med 98:315-319, 1983.

123. Stamler R, Stamler J, Grimm R, et al: Nutritional therapy for high blood pressure: Final report of a four-year randomized controlled trial—the Hypertension Control Program. JAMA 257:1484-1491, 1987.

124. Stevens V, Obarzanek E, Cook N, et al: Long-term weight loss and changes in blood pressure: Results of the Trials of Hypertension Prevention, phase II. Ann Intern Med 134:1-11, 2001.

125. Wassertheil-Smoller S, Blaufox M, Oberman A, et al: The Trial of Antihypertensive Interventions and Management (TAIM) study: Adequate weight loss, alone and combined with drug therapy in the treatment of mild hypertension. Arch Intern Med 152:131-136, 1992.

126. Appel LJ, Moore TJ, Obarzanek E, et al: A clinical trial of the effects of dietary patterns on blood pressure. New Engl J Med 336:1117-1124, 1997.

127. Conlin P, Erlinger T, Bohannon A, et al: The DASH diet enhances the blood pressure response to losartan in hypertensive patients. Am J Hypertens 16:337-342, 2003.

128. Sacks FM, Svetkey LP, Vollmer WM, et al: Effects on blood pressure of reduced dietary sodium and the Dietary Approaches to Stop Hypertension (DASH) diet. N Engl J Med 344:3-10, 2001.

129. Vollmer W, Sacks FM, Ard J, et al: Effects of diet and sodium intake on blood pressure: Subgroup analysis of the DASH-Sodium Trial. Ann Intern Med 135:1019-1028, 2001.

130. Houlihan C, Allen T, Baxter A, et al: A low-sodium diet potentiates the effects of losartan in type 2 diabetes. Diabetes Care 25:663-671, 2002.

131. Kelley G, McClellan P: Antihypertensive effects of aerobic exercise: A brief meta-analysis of randomized control trials. Am J Hypertens 7:115-119, 1994.

132. Kelley G, Kelley K: Progressive resistance exercise and resting blood pressure: A meta-analysis of randomized control trials. Hypertension 35:838-843, 2000.

133. Groppelli A, Giorgi DM, Omboni S, et al: Persistent blood pressure increase induced by heavy smoking. J Hypertens 10:495-499, 1992.

134. Verdecchia P, Schillaci G, Borgioni C, et al: Cigarette smoking, ambulatory blood pressure and cardiac hypertrophy in essential hypertension. J Hypertens 13:1209-1215, 1995.

135. Xin X, He J, Frontini MG, et al: Effects of alcohol reduction on blood pressure: A meta-analysis of randomized controlled trials. Hypertension 38:1112-1117, 2001.

136. Blood Pressure Lowering Treatment Trialists Collaboration: Effects of different blood pressure-lowering regimens on major cardiovascular events in individuals with and without diabetes mellitus. Results of prospectively designed overviews of randomized trials. Arch Intern Med 165:1410-1419, 2005.

137. Verdecchia P, Reboldi G, Angeli F, et al: Adverse prognostic significance of new diabetes in treated hypertensive subjects. Hypertension 43:963-969, 2004.

Chapter 29

Insulin Strategies in Type 1 and Type 2 Diabetes Mellitus

Julio Rosenstock, Salomon Banarer, and David Owens

KEY POINTS

- *Near-normal glycemic diabetes control can be achieved with the use of flexible insulin-replacement strategies designed to mimic physiologic basal or bolus insulin secretory patterns for fasting and postprandial glucose control.*
- *Insulin analogs with improved pharmacokinetic profiles allow simpler and more predictable insulin replacement aimed at achieving glycemic targets with fewer episodes of hypoglycemia.*
- *Multiple daily insulin injection strategies with long-acting analogs such as insulin glargine and detemir provide a more physiologic means of replacing basal insulin in conjunction with prandial rapid-acting insulin analogs (insulin lispro, aspart, and glulisine) for persons with type 1 diabetes.*
- *Early insulin replacement is an emerging strategy for optimal metabolic control of type 2 diabetes, rather than being reserved as a last resort.*
- *Implementation of early insulin replacement can potentially attain target hemoglobin A1c of less than 7% in 50% to 60% of patients with type 2 diabetes.*
- *Combination oral agents with early basal insulin supplementation can be subsequently advanced if the hemoglobin A1c remains higher than 7% by adding a second injection of a rapid-acting insulin analog at the main meal.*
- *Hypoglycemia remains the main barrier to achieving glycemic targets with insulin.*

MATCHING PHYSIOLOGY WITH INSULIN KINETICS

Exogenous insulin has been available for more than 80 years and remains the most powerful diabetes agent, limited only by hypoglycemia. Insulin therapy is required by all patients with type 1 diabetes mellitus (T1DM) and eventually by most patients with type 2 diabetes (T2DM) as glycemic targets become more stringent in an attempt to forestall the development and progression of long-term complications. Throughout its history, the aim of insulin therapy has been to emulate the physiologic patterns of insulin secretion in response to ambient blood glucose profiles throughout both daytime and nighttime in pursuit of near-normal glycemic control.

Normoglycemic control can potentially be achieved with the use of flexible insulin-replacement strategies, which are designed to mimic the physiologic insulin secretory patterns that occur in normal persons in the basal (postabsorptive) and the prandial (postprandial) periods. This strategy is referred to as the *basal–bolus regimen* because it combines both the basal and meal-induced components of normal insulin secretion. In general, 50% of the daily insulin secretion is required as basal insulin, which serves to balance the rate of hepatic glucose production and the peripheral uptake by glucose-dependent tissues overnight and during prolonged periods between meals. The remainder of the insulin requirement is provided as bolus insulin and is used to control postprandial hyperglycemia in response to food intake.

The pharmacokinetic limitations of the old animal and human insulin preparations invariably led to periods of relative insulin excess or insulin lack, resulting in episodes of hypoglycemia or hyperglycemia, respectively. These limitations have largely been overcome by the advent of the new fast-acting and long-acting insulin analogs. As the paradigm of insulin replacement continues to evolve, hypoglycemia remains the most feared and the critical limiting factor in the management of diabetes.[1,2] This remains true despite advances in insulin preparations with improved pharmacokinetics for simpler and more predictable insulin strategies aimed at achieving near-normal glycemic control with fewer episodes of hypoglycemia.

This chapter focuses on achieving safe, effective, and more practical intensive insulin replacement strategies based on the activity profiles of the rapid-acting and long-acting insulin analogs and their potential for improving glycemic control with a more physiologic insulin replacement regimen (Fig. 29–1).

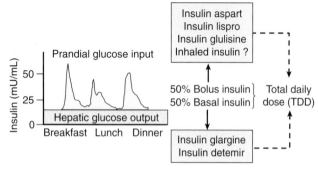

Mimicking Nature in Diabetes:
24-Hour Insulin Secretion and Replacement

Figure 29–1. Insulin replacement is designed to mimic normal endogenous insulin production, in which insulin is secreted to dispose of prandial glucose input and hepatic glucose production. Bolus insulin and basal insulin cover each of these insulin secretory patterns, respectively.

Table 29–1. *Pharmacokinetics of Human Insulin and Analogs*

Treatment	Onset of Action (h)	Peak (h)	Duration (h)
Conventional Human Insulin			
NPH	2-4	4-6	12-16
Lente	2-4	4-12	12-18
Ultralente	6-10	10-16	18-20
Regular	30-60 min	2-4	6-8
Analogs			
Glargine (Lantus)	2	flat	~24
Detemir (Levemir)	2	flat	~14-16
Lispro (Humalog)	5-15 min	60 min	4-5
Aspart (Novolog)	5-15 min	60 min	4-5
Glulisine (Apidra)	5-15 min	60 min	4-5

The time course of action can vary between patients and can vary at different times in the same patient. Consequently, the table data should be considered only as general guidelines.

PHARMACOKINETICS OF CURRENT INSULIN PREPARATIONS

Mimicking normal patterns of insulin secretion has been most challenging due to the highly variable pharmacokinetics and pharmacodynamics of subcutaneously administered conventional insulin preparations. These animal and human insulin preparations fail to meet the two fundamental features of normal insulin secretion: the immediate response to nutrient challenges during the day and a consistent and even insulin secretory response during the postabsorptive state, especially overnight. In attempting to attain and maintain near-normal glycemia with the aid of close glucose monitoring, the contributions of diet, exercise, and intra- and interindividual variations in insulin absorption and action must all be taken into consideration and balanced against the need to prevent the most feared complication of insulin therapy: hypoglycemia.

Insulin preparations are simply classified as short-, intermediate-, or long-acting types when they are injected subcutaneously.[3] The activity profiles of these insulins diverge significantly from the normal insulin secretory response seen in nondiabetic healthy persons, resulting in suboptimal glycemic control despite complex multiple injection regimens. However, this problem is gradually abating due to the more physiologic time-action profiles of the insulin analogs. The new analogs are more predictable than conventional insulins and allow simplified insulin-replacement strategies.[4-8] The pharmacokinetic profiles of these insulin preparations largely determine their role in clinical practice and are intended to mimic a specific component of normal insulin secretion. Rapid- or short-acting insulins counter the postprandial glycemic excursion, and intermediate- or long-acting insulins

Box 29-1. Necessary Features for Basal Insulin

- Twenty-four-hour insulin coverage; flat, peakless profile
- Limited lipolysis and excessive hepatic glucose output (HGO)
- Ability to make simple insulin adjustments to achieve fasting plasma glucose (FPG) < 100 mg/dL
- Reproducibility

replace basal secretion to control mainly nocturnal and fasting hyperglycemia.

The pharmacokinetic characteristics of human insulin and insulin analogs are shown in Table 29–1.[3-10]

Options for Basal Insulin Replacement

The most desirable features of a basal insulin for subcutaneous replacement are listed in Box 29-1. The pharmacokinetics of the ideal basal insulin should provide a peakless profile that allows for the necessary insulin titrations to be made in order to control the postabsorptive nocturnal and fasting period to achieve normal fasting glucose levels of less than 100 mg/dL (5.5 mmol/L) with less risk of nocturnal hypoglycemia. Furthermore, a reproducible protracted 24-hour action also permits a simple once-daily injection regimen for basal insulin coverage given separately from the rapid-acting insulin used for prandial glucose control.

Human NPH, Lente, and Ultralente

Since the 1950s, the intermediate-acting human insulin neutral protamine Hagedorn (NPH) has represented the traditional attempt at basal insulin

replacement therapy. NPH is regular insulin combined with stoichiometric amounts of protein (protamine), producing a poorly soluble insulin–protamine complex. NPH has a peak effect 4 to 6 hours after subcutaneous injection, with a highly variable duration of action of 12 to 16 hours, according to dose, subcutaneous injection site, and—most important—the adequacy of the resuspension prior to administration.

NPH has been used to approximate basal insulin secretion in regimens of 1 or 2 daily doses, but the pronounced peak effect between 4 and 6 hours after each injection requires a rigid mealtime schedule in order for food intake to match the effect of the insulin dose administered several hours earlier. Furthermore, the action of the evening NPH insulin wanes as the physiologic demand for insulin increases in the morning hours before breakfast (dawn phenomenon), thereby increasing the potential for prebreakfast hyperglycemia.

Attempts to correct this limitation by giving NPH at bedtime, thereby delaying the peak action of NPH, increases the risk of nocturnal hypoglycemia, especially if NPH is aggressively titrated against fasting hyperglycemia. Indeed, when administered at bedtime, NPH insulin peaks during early morning hours when the least amount of insulin is needed.[10,11] This nonphysiologic undesirable peak effect is compounded when regular insulin is injected before the evening meal because the action of the prandial insulin extends well into the night, overlapping with the separate basal insulin replacement. The overall result is more risk of episodes of nocturnal hypoglycemia, which accounts for up to 50% of all hypoglycemic events in T1DM patients.[11,12] Similarly, the peak action of the breakfast NPH dose and the short-acting regular insulin overlap, resulting in excessive insulin during the daytime, especially around noon, necessitating between-meal snacks.

The additional insulin suspensions Lente and Ultralente were developed after NPH by combining regular insulin with zinc in an acetate buffer to form a crystalline compound that dissolves poorly in the subcutaneous body fluid.[13] Although intermediate-acting Lente insulin has a slightly longer duration of action than NPH, its effects are also highly variable due to the need for resuspension prior to injection. The long-acting preparation Ultralente has a somewhat longer action than either NPH or Lente. It also has a variable duration of action according to species and dose and substantial day-to-day variability, with erratic peaks 8 to 10 hours after subcutaneous injection, that causes unpredictable hypoglycemia. Indeed, absorption is potentially erratic for NPH, Lente, and Ultralente, largely due to the need for resuspension, resulting in substantial interpatient and intrapatient variability. This lack of reproducibility in lowering blood glucose levels has been and remains a major limitation for most regimens using these old human insulin preparations.

Long-Acting Insulin Analogs: Glargine and Detemir

Recent advances in recombinant DNA technology have resulted in the biosynthetic manufacture of insulin analogs with improved pharmacokinetic properties.

Insulin glargine is a long-acting, once-a-day, human insulin analog distinguished from native human insulin by small alterations to the α- and β-chains. The α-chain has an asparagine-to-glycine substitution at position A21, and two positively charged arginine molecules are added at the C terminus of the β-chain.[14] The resulting molecule has its isoelectric point shifted from a pH of 5.4 to 6.7, making it less soluble at the physiologic pH of subcutaneous tissue. Additionally, the replacement of A21 asparagine by glycine stabilizes the molecule against deamidation in the acidic environment of its pharmaceutical formulation (vial or cartridge).

When injected subcutaneously, glargine forms a suspension or gel-like precipitate at the physiologic pH of the subcutaneous tissue. Slow dissolution of the glargine gel suspension at the injection site results in a relatively constant release with no pronounced peak over a period of up to 24 hours, thereby providing a basal insulin supply comparable to that of nondiabetic persons.[15] The clear solution does not require resuspension before injection, thereby reducing the variability so characteristic of insulin suspensions such as NPH, Lente, and Ultralente.[5,16,17] Short-term studies confirm that glargine is well tolerated in patients with T1DM, with the incidence of adverse events and injection site reactions similar to that of NPH.[18,19] Occasional mild local discomfort was reported in some studies but did not result in discontinuation and it is rarely an issue in clinical practice.

The action profile of insulin glargine in patients with T1DM closely mimics continuous subcutaneous insulin infusion (CSII; insulin pump),[20] the gold standard against which any basal insulin must be compared. In a euglycemic clamp (glucose clamp) study in healthy volunteers to determine the pharmacodynamic properties of insulin glargine, the blood glucose–lowering activity of insulin glargine was found to remain relatively constant throughout the 30-hour study period.[21,22] By comparison, the NPH insulin had its peak action at 4 to 6 hours, then slowly declined over the course of 15 hours.

In another glucose clamp study in persons with T1DM, the mean duration of action of insulin glargine was longer (22 ± 4 h) than that of NPH insulin (14 ± 3 h), but it was similar to that of Ultralente (20 ± 6 h).[16] The peak action of NPH and Ultralente was 4.5 ± 0.5 and 10.1 ± 1.0 hours, respectively, followed by a gradual decline (Fig. 29–2).

Notably, a study comparing the pharmacodynamics of insulin glargine administered via subcutaneous injection in patients with T1DM on the first day and the seventh day showed a slight extension

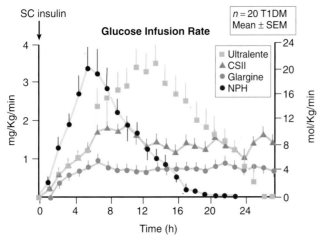

Glargine vs NPH/Ultralente/CSII in Type 1 DM Action Profiles by Glucose Clamp

Figure 29–2. Pharmacodynamic profiles of insulin Ultralente, NPH, and glargine compared to insulin lispro given via continuous subcutaneous insulin infusion (CSII). All four insulins were given at a dose of 0.3 IU/kg. The study was conducted in 20 type 1 diabetic patients, and the profiles were determined using the isoglycemic clamp technique (where data are expressed as the rate of glucose infusion needed to keep the plasma glucose constant at 130 mg/dL). Each subject was studied on four separate occasions, once with each type of insulin. SC, subcutaneous; SEM, standard error of the mean. (From Lepore M, Pampanelli S, Fanelli C, et al: Pharmacokinetics and pharmacodynamics of subcutaneous injection of long-acting human insulin analog glargine, NPH insulin, and Ultralente human insulin and continuous subcutaneous infusion of insulin lispro. Diabetes 49:2142-2148, 2000.)

of its duration of action on day seven compared to day one.[23] After 7 days of glargine administration, the onset of action was earlier, the duration of action was closer to 24 hours (23.2 ± 1.3 h), and the interpatient variability was lower compared with the first subcutaneous injection.

One possible explanation for these findings is the time required for insulin glargine to reach steady state. As is discussed later, these pharmacodynamic properties provide the basis for understanding the clinical trials that have consistently demonstrated lower fasting glucose levels and less hypoglycemia, especially nocturnal hypoglycemia, with insulin glargine when compared with NPH insulin.[15]

Another long-acting insulin analog, detemir, has been approved in Europe and was approved in the US in 2005 by the FDA. Detemir is an acylated derivative of human insulin: LysB29 (Nε-tetradecanoyl)des(B30) human insulin. This preparation is a soluble insulin analog with a neutral pH and a smooth, protracted time-action profile resulting from increased self-association at the injection site and a high degree of albumin binding via the fatty acid chain.[24,25] This high affinity for serum albumin, and its binding in the subcutaneous tissue, circulation, and interstitial

fluid, contributes to its extended duration of action.[25,26] This modification produces a duration of action approximately 14 to 16 hours after subcutaneous injection and therefore makes it more suitable for twice-daily injection as part of a basal–bolus regimen in subjects with T1DM and once or twice daily in subjects with T2DM (as monotherapy or basal–bolus regimen respectively) (see Table 29–1).[26]

Clinical studies have consistently demonstrated that insulin detemir and NPH were equally effective in maintaining control of blood glucose levels, although detemir had to be administered at a higher molar dose.[25] It appears that due to this lower biological potency, a threefold to fourfold higher molar dose is required compared to NPH. Several reports indicate less intrasubject variation as measured by a smaller standard deviation of fasting glucose levels with detemir,[9,27,28] but the clinical implications and the relevance of such a small effect on diabetes management remains to be elucidated. Most clinical studies have demonstrated that there was a reduced risk of hypoglycemia, particularly nocturnal hypoglycemia, with detemir compared with NPH insulin and, interestingly, with little to no weight gain.[9,28,29] It appears from the clinical studies that at therapeutically relevant doses, the duration of action of the analog might not be sufficient to cover 24-hour basal insulin needs, and therefore most patients require a twice-daily administration.[30]

Options for Prandial Insulin Replacement

Short-Acting Human Regular Insulin

Regular insulin has been the standard meal-related insulin since the introduction of insulin therapy, although the purity and species have evolved over the years. The designation of regular insulin as a "short-acting" insulin is only a relative one, because in fact it is relatively slowly absorbed from the subcutaneous tissue into the systemic circulation with a consequent slow onset of action, although the action is more rapid than that of the intermediate-acting insulins like NPH, Lente, and Ultralente.

Subcutaneous regular human insulin has an onset of action within 30 to 60 minutes, a peak effect within 2 to 4 hours, and a duration of action of 6 to 10 hours.[31,32] Because of the relatively slow onset of action of this insulin, subcutaneous injection 30 to 60 minutes before meals is required,[33] but this schedule is rarely achieved in practice. The conventional recommendation for regular insulin administration is inconvenient and unrealistic, and it poses a risk of premeal hypoglycemia if the meal is delayed or early postprandial hyperglycemia if the injection is at mealtime. Consequently, compliance with the required 30-minute lag time following administration of human regular insulin is

Box 29-3. Practical Guidelines for Insulin Therapy in Type 2 Diabetes

Initiation of Basal Insulin

- Continue oral agent (if tolerated and no specific contraindications)
  - Keep metformin dose up to 2000 mg/day *and/or*
  - Reduce pioglitazone to 15 to 30 mg/day or rosiglitazone to 2 to 4 mg/day *and/or*
  - Reduce sulfonylurea to 50% of dose (if using glyburide, consider substituting a different sulfonylurea or meglitinide)
- Start insulin (dose 10 units)
  - Glargine (bedtime or any time, but consistently at the same time of the day)
  - Detemir (bedtime or twice daily)
  - NPH (bedtime or twice daily)
- Adjust insulin dose weekly according to the average of 2 or 3 days of FPG monitoring
  - Increase 2 units if FPG is 100-120 mg/dL (5.5-6.7 mmol/L)
  - Increase 3 units if FPG is 121-140 mg/dL (6.7-7.8 mmol/L)
  - Increase 4 units if FPG is higher than 140 mg/dL (7.8 mmol/L)
- Treat to target FPG lower than 100 mg/dL (5.5 mmol/L)
- Eventually empower patient to continue with ongoing weekly self-insulin adjustments
- Titrate by only 2 units if average FPG is higher than 100 mg/dL

FPG, fasting plasma glucose; MDI, multiple daily insulin injections.

- Reduce insulin if FPG is lower than 72 mg/dL (4.0 mmol/L) or for hypoglycemic symptoms

Advance Basal Insulin plus Prandial Insulin at Main Meal

- Continue basal insulin weekly self-titration
- Consider adding prandial insulin at main meal if:
  - FPG is consistently lower than 100 mg/dL and HbA1c remains higher than 7%
  - Cannot increase further basal insulin without increasing hypoglycemia
  - Basal insulin dose is more than 100 units
- Identify main meal with greatest postprandial excursion
  - Start with 4 to 10 units according to estimated degree of insulin resistance
  - Adjust weekly according to prandial monitoring and carbohydrate intake
  - Twice-daily regimen can consist of insulin glargine moved to a morning dose and lispro, aspart, or glulisine given with the main evening meal

Advance Basal Insulin plus Prandial Insulin at Each Meal

- Advance to full MDI (basal–bolus) regimen, adding the fast-acting analog progressively at each meal according to glucose monitoring and HbA1c targets
- Insulin pens facilitate insulin therapy at any phase of intervention

References

1. Cryer PE: Hypoglycaemia: The limiting factor in the glycaemic management of type I and type II diabetes. Diabetologia 45:937-948, 2002.
2. Cryer PE: Diverse causes of hypoglycemia-associated autonomic failure in diabetes. N Engl J Med 350:2272-2279, 2004.
3. Burge MR, Schade DS: Insulins. Endocrinol Metab Clin North Am 26:575-598, 1997.
4. Barnett AH, Owens DR: Insulin analogues. Lancet 349:47-51, 1997.
5. Bolli GB, Di Marchi RD, Park GD, et al: Insulin analogues and their potential in the management of diabetes mellitus. Diabetologia 42:1151-1167, 1999.
6. Brange J, Volund A: Insulin analogs with improved pharmacokinetic profiles. Adv Drug Deliv Rev 35:307-335, 1999.
7. DeWitt DE, Hirsch IB: Outpatient insulin therapy in type 1 and type 2 diabetes mellitus: Scientific review. JAMA 289:2254-2264, 2003.
8. Becker R, Frick A, Wessels D, et al: Evaluation of the pharmacodynamic and pharmacokinetic profiles of insulin glulisine—a novel, rapid-acting, human insulin analogue. 18th International Diabetes Federation Congress, Paris, France, Auust 24-29, 2003. PS 58:775.
9. Vague P, Selam J-L, Skeie S, et al: Insulin detemir is associated with more predictable glycemic control and reduced risk of hypoglycemia than NPH insulin in patients with type 1 diabetes on a basal-bolus regimen with premeal insulin aspart. Diabetes Care 26:590-596, 2003.
10. Faglia E, Favales F, Brivio M, et al: Comparison of two intensified conventional insulin regimens with three and four daily injections. Diabetes Metab 19:575-581, 1993.
11. Bolli GB, Perriello G, Fanelli CG, De Feo P: Nocturnal blood glucose control in type I diabetes mellitus. Diabetes Care 16:71-89, 1993.
12. Bendtson I: Nocturnal hypoglycaemia in patients with insulin-dependent diabetes mellitus. Dan Med Bull 42:269-284, 1995.
13. Owens DR, Zinman B, Bolli GB: Insulins today and beyond. Lancet 358:739-746, 2001.
14. Levien TL, Baker DE, White JR Jr, Campbell RK: Insulin glargine: A new basal insulin. Ann Pharmacother 36:1019-1027, 2002.
15. Bolli GB, Owens DR: Insulin glargine. Lancet 356:443-445, 2000.
16. Lepore M, Pampanelli S, Fanelli C, et al: Pharmacokinetics and pharmacodynamics of subcutaneous injection of long-acting human insulin analog glargine, NPH insulin, and Ultralente human insulin and continuous subcutaneous infusion of insulin lispro. Diabetes 49:2142-2148, 2000.
17. Rosskamp RH, Park G: Long-acting insulin analogs. Diabetes Care 22(Suppl 2):B109-B113, 1999.
18. Pieber T, Eugene-Jolchine I, Derobert E: Efficacy and safety of HOE 901 versus NPH insulin in patients with type 1 diabetes. The European Study Group of HOE 901 in type 1 diabetes. Diabetes Care 23:157-162, 2000.
19. Rosenstock J, Park G, Zimmerman J, and the US Insulin Glargine Type 1 Diabetes Investigator Group: Basal insulin glargine (HOE 901) versus NPH insulin in patients with

type 1 diabetes on multiple daily insulin regimens. Diabetes Care. 23:1137-1142, 2000.

20. Pickup JC, Keen H, Parsons JA, Alberti KG. Continuous subcutaneous insulin infusion: An approach to achieving normoglycaemia. BMJ 1:204-207, 1978.

21. Rave K, Nosek L, Heinemann L, Frick A, Becker R: Time-action profile of the long-acting insulin analogue insulin glargine in comparison to NPH insulin in Japanese volunteers. Diabetes Metab 29:430-431, 2003.

22. Heinemann L, Linkeschova R, Rave K, et al: Time-action profile of the long-acting insulin analog insulin glargine (HOE901) in comparison with those of NPH insulin and placebo. Diabetes Care 23:644-649, 2000.

23. Fanelli C, Pampanelli S, Procellati F, et al: Pharmacodynamics of subcutaneous injection of insulin glargine after the first as compared to seventh day of its once-daily administration in patients with type 1 diabetes. Diabetologia 4S:A259-802, 2002.

24. Havelund S, Plum A, Ribel U, et al: The mechanism of protraction of insulin detemir, a long-acting, acylated analog of human insulin. Pharm Res 21:1498-1504, 2004.

25. Heinemann L, Sinha K, Weyer C, et al: Time-action profile of the soluble, fatty acid acylated, long-acting insulin analogue NN304. Diabet Med 16:332-338, 1999.

26. Jacobsen L, Popescu G, Plum A: Pharmacokinetics of insulin detemir in patients with renal or hepatic impairment. Diabetes 51:A102, 2002.

27. Heise T, Nosek L, Ronn BB, et al: Lower within-subject variability of insulin detemir in comparison to nph insulin and insulin glargine in people with type 1 diabetes. Diabetes 53:1614-1620, 2004.

28. Home P, Bartley P, Russell-Jones D, et al: Insulin detemir offers improved glycemic control compared with nph insulin in people with type 1 diabetes: A randomized clinical trial. Diabetes Care 27:1081-1087, 2004.

29. Hermansen K, Madsbad S, Perrild H, et al: Comparison of the soluble basal insulin analog insulin detemir with NPH insulin: A randomized open crossover trial in type 1 diabetic subjects on basal-bolus therapy. Diabetes Care 24:296-301, 2001.

30. Pieber T, Plank J, Goerzer E, et al: Duration of action, pharmacodynamic profile and between-subject variability of insulin detemir in subjects with type 1 diabetes. Diabetes 51:A214, 2000.

31. Heinemann L, Chantelau EA, Starke AA: Pharmacokinetics and pharmacodynamics of subcutaneously administered U40 and U100 formulations of regular human insulin. Diabete Metab 18:21-24, 1992.

32. Heinemann L, Richter B: Clinical pharmacology of human insulin. Diabetes Care 3:90-100, 1993.

33. Dimitriadis GD, Gerich JE: Importance of timing of preprandial subcutaneous insulin administration in the management of diabetes mellitus. Diabetes Care 6:374-377, 1983.

34. Sackey AH, Jefferson IG: Interval between insulin injection and breakfast in diabetes. Arch Dis Child 71:248-250, 1994.

35. Lean ME, Ng LL, Tennison BR: Interval between insulin injection and eating in relation to blood glucose control in adult diabetics. BMJ Clin Research Ed 290:105-108, 1985.

36. Kang S, Creagh FM, Peters JR, et al: Comparison of subcutaneous soluble human insulin and insulin analogues (AspB9, GluB27; AspB10; AspB28) on meal-related plasma glucose excursions in type I diabetic subjects. Diabetes Care 14:571-577, 1991.

37. Kang S, Brange J, Burch A, et al: Subcutaneous insulin absorption explained by insulin's physicochemical properties. Evidence from absorption studies of soluble human insulin and insulin analogues in humans. Diabetes Care 14:942-948, 1991.

38. Wilde MI, McTavish D: Insulin lispro: A review of its pharmacological properties and therapeutic use in the management of diabetes mellitus. Drugs 54:597-614, 1997.

39. Whittingham J, Edwards D, Antson A, et al: Interactions of phenol and m-cresol in the insulin hexamer, and their effect on the association properties of B28 Pro Asp insulin analogues. Biochemistry 37:11516-11523, 1998.

40. Kurtzhals P, Schaffer L, Sorensen A, et al: Correlations of receptor binding and metabolic and mitogenic potencies of insulin analogs designed for clinical use. Diabetes 49:999-1005, 2000.

41. Homko C, Deluzio A, Jimenez C, et al: Comparison of insulin aspart and lispro: Pharmacokinetic and metabolic effects. Diabetes Care 26:2027-2031, 2003.

42. Raskin P, Guthrie R, Leiter L, et al: Use of insulin aspart, a fast-acting insulin analog, as the mealtime insulin in the management of patients with type 1 diabetes. Diabetes Care 23:583-588, 2000.

43. Anderson JH Jr, Brunelle RL, Koivisto VA, et al: Reduction of postprandial hyperglycemia and frequency of hypoglycemia in IDDM patients on insulin-analog treatment. Multicenter Insulin Lispro Study Group. Diabetes 46:265-270, 1997.

44. Danne T, Aman J, Schober E, et al: A comparison of postprandial and preprandial administration of insulin aspart in children and adolescents with type 1 diabetes. Diabetes Care 26:2359-2364, 2003.

45. Garg S, Rosenstock J, Ways K: Efficacy and safety of postmeal insulin glulisine (glu) compared with pre-meal regular human insulin (RHI) in a basal-bolus regimen with insulin glargine. Diabetes 53:A125, 2004.

46. Nosek L, Heinemann L, Kaiser M, et al: No increase in the duration of action with rising doses of insulin aspart. Diabetes 52:A128, 2003.

47. Jovanovic L, Acquistapace M, Pettitt D. Postprandial glycemic control is provided by either preprandial or postprandial administration of insulin aspart in type 1 diabetes. Diabetes 51:A102, 2002.

48. Heller SR, Amiel SA, Mansell P. Effect of the fast-acting insulin analog lispro on the risk of nocturnal hypoglycemia during intensified insulin therapy. UK Lispro Study Group. Diabetes Care 22:1607-1611, 1999.

49. Garg SK, Carmain JA, Braddy KC, et al: Pre-meal insulin analogue insulin lispro vs Humulin R insulin treatment in young subjects with type 1 diabetes. Diab Med 13:47-52, 1996.

50. Jacobs M, Keulen E, Kanc K, et al: Metabolic efficacy of preprandial administration of Lys(B28),Pro(B29) human insulin analog in IDDM patients. A comparison with human regular insulin during a three-meal test period. Diabetes Care 20:1279-1286, 1997.

51. Pfutzner A, Kustner E, Forst T, et al: Intensive insulin therapy with insulin lispro in patients with type 1 diabetes reduces the frequency of hypoglycemic episodes. Exp Clin Endocrinol Diabetes 104:25-30, 1996.

52. Holleman F, Schmitt H, Rottiers R, et al: Reduced frequency of severe hypoglycemia and coma in well-controlled IDDM patients treated with insulin lispro. The Benelux-UK Insulin Lispro Study Group. Diabetes Care 20:1827-1832, 1997.

53. Home P, Lindholm A, Hylleberg B, Round P: Improved glycemic control with insulin aspart: A multicenter randomized double-blind crossover trial in type 1 diabetic patients. UK Insulin Aspart Study Group. Diabetes Care 21:1904-1909, 1998.

54. Home PD, Lindholm A, Riis A, and the European Insulin Aspart Study Group: Insulin aspart vs. human insulin in the management of long-term blood glucose control in type 1 diabetes mellitus: A randomized controlled trial. Diabet Med 17:762-770, 2000.

55. Ratner RE, Hirsch IB, Neifing JL, et al: Less hypoglycemia with insulin glargine in intensive insulin therapy for type 1 diabetes. US Study Group of Insulin Glargine in Type 1 Diabetes. Diabetes Care 23:639-643, 2000.

56. Raskin P, Klaff L, Bergenstal R, et al: A 16-week comparison of the novel insulin analog insulin glargine (HOE 901) and NPH human insulin used with insulin lispro in patients with type 1 diabetes. Diabetes Care 23:1666-1671, 2000.

57. Hershon K, Blevins T, Donley D, et al: Beneficial effects of insulin glargine compared to NPH in subjects with type 1 diabetes. Diabetologia 44:A15, 2001.

58. Lalli C, Ciofetta M, Del Sindaco P, et al: Long-term intensive treatment of type 1 diabetes with the short-acting

insulin analog lispro in variable combination with NPH insulin at mealtime. Diabetes Care 22:468-477, 1999.

59. Torlone E, Pampanelli S, Lalli C, et al: Effects of the short-acting insulin analog [Lys(B28),Pro(B29)] on postprandial blood glucose control in IDDM. Diabetes Care 19:945-952, 1996.

60. Rossetti P, Pampanelli S, Fanelli C, et al: Intensive replacement of basal insulin in patients with type 1 diabetes given rapid-acting insulin analog at mealtime: A 3-month comparison between administration of NPH insulin four times daily and glargine insulin at dinner or bedtime. Diabetes Care 26:1490-1496, 2003.

61. Hamann A, Matthaei S, Rosak C, et al: A randomized clinical trial comparing breakfast, dinner, or bedtime administration of insulin glargine in patients with type 1 diabetes. Diabetes Care 26:1738-1744, 2003.

62. Porcellati F, Rossetti P, Pampanelli S, et al: Better long-term glycaemic control with the basal insulin glargine as compared with NPH in patients with type 1 diabetes mellitus given meal-time lispro insulin. Diabet Med 21:1213-1220, 2004.

63. Witthaus E, Stewart J, Bradley C: Treatment satisfaction and psychological well-being with insulin glargine compared with NPH in patients with type 1 diabetes. Diabet Med 18:619-625, 2001.

64. Kolendorf K, Pavlic-Renar I, San-Teusanio F, etal: Insulin detemir is associated with lower risk of hypoglycemia compared to NPH insulin in people with type 1 diabetes. Diabetes 53:A130, 2004.

65. Robertson KJ, Schonle E, Gucev Z, et al: Benefits of insulin detemir vs NPH in children and adolescents with type 1 diabetes: Lower and more predictable fasting plasma glucose and lower risk of nocturnal hypoglycemia. Diabetes 53:A144, 2004.

66. American Diabetes Association: Insulin administration. Diabetes Care 27:106S-107S, 2004.

67. Bode B, Weinstein R, Bell D, et al: Comparison of insulin aspart with buffered regular insulin and insulin lispro in continuous subcutaneous insulin infusion: A randomized study in type 1 diabetes. Diabetes Care 25:439-444, 2002.

68. Weissberg-Benchell J, Antisdel-Lomaglio J, Seshadri R: Insulin pump therapy: A meta-analysis. Diabetes Care 26:1079-1087, 2003.

69. Pickup J, Mattock M, Kerry S: Glycaemic control with continuous subcutaneous insulin infusion compared with intensive insulin injections in patients with type 1 diabetes: Meta-analysis of randomised controlled trials. BMJ 324:705, 2002.

70. Tsui E, Barnie A, Ross S, et al: Intensive insulin therapy with insulin lispro: A randomized trial of continuous subcutaneous insulin infusion versus multiple daily insulin injection. Diabetes Care 24:1722-1727, 2001.

71. Retnakaran R, Hochman J, DeVries JH, et al: Continuous subcutaneous insulin infusion versus multiple daily injections: The impact of baseline HbA1c. Diabetes Care 27:2590-2596, 2004.

72. Bolli G, Capani F, Home PD, et al: Comparison of a multiple daily injection regimen with once-daily insulin glargine basal insulin and mealtime lispro, to subcutaneous insulin infusion: A randomized, open, parallel study. Diabetes 53:A107, 2004.

73. American Diabetes Association: Continuous subcutaneous insulin infusion. Diabetes Care 27:S110, 2004.

74. Rosenstock J, Wyne K: Insulin treatment in type 2 diabetes. In Goldstein B, Müller-Wieland D (eds): Textbook of Type 2 Diabetes. London, Martin Dunitz, 2003, pp 131-154.

75. Ryan EA, Imes S, Wallace C: Short-term intensive insulin therapy in newly diagnosed type 2 diabetes. Diabetes Care 27:1028-1032, 2004.

76. Park S, Choi SB: Induction of long-term normoglycemia without medication in Korean type 2 diabetes patients after continuous subcutaneous insulin infusion therapy. Diabetes Metab Res Rev 19:124-130, 2003.

77. Ilkova H, Glaser B, Tunckale A, et al: Induction of long-term glycemic control in newly diagnosed type 2 diabetic patients by transient intensive insulin treatment. Diabetes Care 20:1353-1356, 1997.

78. Maldonado M, Hampe CS, Gaur LK, et al: Ketosis-prone diabetes: Dissection of a heterogeneous syndrome using an immunogenetic and beta-cell functional classification, prospective analysis, and clinical outcomes. J Clin Endocrinol Metab 88:5090-5098, 2003.

79. Balasubramanyam A, Zern JW, Hyman DJ, Pavlik V: New profiles of diabetic ketoacidosis: Type 1 vs type 2 diabetes and the effect of ethnicity. Arch Intern Med 159:2317-2322, 1999.

80. Banerji MA, Chaiken RL, Huey H, et al: GAD antibody negative NIDDM in adult black subjects with diabetic ketoacidosis and increased frequency of human leukocyte antigen DR3 and DR4. Flatbush diabetes. Diabetes. 43:741-745, 1994.

81. Umpierrez G, Woo W, Hagopian W, et al: Immunogenetic analysis suggests different pathogenesis for obese and lean African-Americans with diabetic ketoacidosis. Diabetes Care 22:1517-1523, 1999.

82. Boden G, Ruiz J, Kim CJ, Chen X: Effects of prolonged glucose infusion on insulin secretion, clearance, and action in normal subjects. Am J Physiol 270:E251-E258, 1996.

83. Brown JB, Nichols GA, Perry A: The burden of treatment failure in type 2 diabetes. Diabetes Care 27:1535-1540, 2004.

84. Wright A, Burden ACF, Paisey RB, et al: Sulfonylurea inadequacy: Efficacy of addition of insulin over 6 years in patients with type 2 diabetes in the U.K. Prospective Diabetes Study (UKPDS 57). Diabetes Care 25:330-336, 2002.

85. Inzucchi SE: Oral antihyperglycemic therapy for type 2 diabetes: Scientific review [see comment]. JAMA 287:360-372, 2002.

86. Dailey GE, Noor MA, Park J-S, et al: Glycemic control with glyburide/metformin tablets in combination with rosiglitazone in patients with type 2 diabetes: A randomized, double-blind trial. Am J Med 116:223-229, 2004.

87. Yale JF, Valiquett TR, Ghazzi MN, et al: The effect of a thiazolidinedione drug, troglitazone, on glycemia in patients with type 2 diabetes mellitus poorly controlled with sulfonylurea and metformin. A multicenter, randomized, double-blind, placebo-controlled trial. Ann Intern Med 134:737-745, 2001.

88. American Diabetes Association: Standards of medical care in diabetes. Diabetes Care 27:S15-S35, 2004.

89. Rosenstock J, Riddle M: Insulin therapy in type 2 diabetes. In Cefalu WT, Gerich JE, LeRoith D (eds): The CADRE Handbook of Diabetes Management. New York, Medical Information Press, 2004, pp 145-168.

90. Schwartz S, Sievers R, Strange P, et al: Insulin 70/30 mix plus metformin versus triple oral therapy in the treatment of type 2 diabetes after failure of two oral drugs: Efficacy, safety, and cost analysis. Diabetes Care 26:2238-2243, 2003.

91. Kilo C, Mezitis N, Jain R, et al: Starting patients with type 2 diabetes on insulin therapy using once-daily injections of biphasic insulin aspart 70/30, biphasic human insulin 70/30, or NPH insulin in combination with metformin. J Diabetes Complications 17:307-313, 2003.

92. Bastyr E, Stuart C, Brodows R, et al: Therapy focused on lowering postprandial glucose, not fasting glucose, may be superior for lowering HbA1c. IOEZ Study Group. Diabetes Care 23:1236-1241, 2000.

93. Rosenstock J, Exubera Phase III Study Group: Mealtime rapid-acting inhaled insulin (Exubera) improves glycemic control in patients with type 2 diabetes failing oral agents: A 3-month, randomized, comparative trial. Diabetes 51:535P, 2002.

94. Shank ML, Del Prato S, DeFronzo RA: Bedtime insulin/daytime glipizide. Effective therapy for sulfonylurea failures in NIDDM. Diabetes 44:165-172, 1995.

95. Holman RR, Steemson J, Turner RC: Sulphonylurea failure in type 2 diabetes: Treatment with a basal insulin supplement. Diabet Med 4:457-462, 1987.

96. Yki-Jarvinen H, Ryysy L, Nikkila K, et al: Comparison of bedtime insulin regimens in patients with type 2 diabetes

mellitus. A randomized, controlled trial. Ann Intern Med 130:389-396, 1999.

97. Riddle MC: Timely addition of insulin to oral therapy for type 2 diabetes. Diabetes Care 25:395-396, 2002.

98. Fonseca V, Bell D, Mecca T: Less symptomatic hypoglycaemia with insulin glargine compared to NPH insulin in patients with type 2 diabetes. Diabetologia 44:A207, 2001.

99. Rosenstock J, Riddle M, HOE901/4002 Study Group: Treatment To Target study: Timing and frequency of nocturnal hypoglycemia. The value of adding bedtime basal insulin glargine over NPH on insulin naive patients with type 2 diabetes on oral agents. Diabetes 51:A482, 2002.

100. Rosenstock J, Schwartz SL, Clark CM, Jr, et al: Basal insulin therapy in type 2 diabetes: 28-week comparison of insulin glargine (HOE 901) and NPH insulin. Diabetes Care 24:631-636, 2001.

101. Yki-Jarvinen H, Dressler A, Ziemen M, HOE Study Group: Less nocturnal hypoglycemia and better post-dinner glucose control with bedtime insulin glargine compared with bedtime NPH insulin during insulin combination therapy in type 2 diabetes. HOE 901/3002 Study Group. Diabetes Care 23:1130-1136, 2000.

102. Riddle MC, Rosenstock J, Gerich J, Insulin Glargine 4002 Study Investigators: The Treat-To-Target Trial: Randomized addition of glargine or human NPH insulin to oral therapy of type 2 diabetic patients. Diabetes Care. 26:3080-3086, 2003.

103. Riddle MC, Rosenstock J: Treatment to Target Study: Insulin glargine vs NPH insulin added to oral therapy of type 2 diabetes. Successful control with less nocturnal hypoglycemia. Diabetes 51:A113, 2002.

104. Rosenstock J, Riddle M, Dailey G, et al: Treatment To Target Study: Feasibility of achieving control with the addition of basal bedtime insulin glargine (Lantus) or NPH insulin in insulin-naive patients with type 2 diabetes on oral agents. Diabetes 50:A520, 2001.

105. Rosenstock J, Sugimoto D, Strange P, et al: Triple therapy in type 2 diabetes (T2DM): Benefits of insulin glargine (GLAR) over rosiglitazone (RSG) added to combination therapy of sulfonylurea plus metformin (SU+MET) in insulin-naive patients. Diabetes 53:A145, 2004.

106. Janka H, Plewe G, Riddle MC, et al: Comparison of basal insulin added to oral agents versus twice daily premixed insulin as initial insulin therapy for type 2 diabetes. Diabetes Care 28:254-259, 2005.

107. Malone J, Bai S, Campaigne B, et al:. Targeting postprandial rather than fasting blood glucose results in better overall glycemic control in patients with type 2 diabetes. Diabetes 53:A137, 2004.

108. Malone J, Holocombe J, Campaigne B, Kerr L: Insulin lispro mix 75/25 compared to insulin glargine in patients with type 2 diabetes new to insulin therapy. Diabetes 53:A137, 2004.

109. Raskin P, Allen E, Hollander P, et al: Initiating insulin therapy in type 2 diabetes. Diabetes Care 28:260-265, 2005.

110. Rosenstock J, Larsen J, Draeger E, et al: Feasibility of improved glycemic control with insulin detemir and insulin glargine in combination with oral agents in insulin naive patients with type 2 diabetes. Diabetes 53:A145, 2004.

111. Monnier L, Lapinski H, Colette C: Contributions of fasting and postprandial plasma glucose increments to the overall diurnal hyperglycemia of type 2 diabetic patients: Variations with increasing levels of HbA1c. Diabetes Care 26:881-885, 2003.

112. Rosenstock J: Insulin therapy: Optimizing control in type 1 and type 2 diabetes. Clinical Cornerstone 4:50-64, 2001.

113. Pratipanawatr T, Cusi K, Ngo P, et al: Normalization of plasma glucose concentration by insulin therapy improves insulin-stimulated glycogen synthesis in type 2 diabetes. Diabetes 51:462-468, 2002.

114. Scarlett J, Gray R, Griffin J, et al: Insulin treatment reverses the insulin resistance of type II diabetes mellitus. Diabetes Care 5:353-363, 1982.

115. Andrews WJ, Vasquez B, Nagulesparan M, et al: Insulin therapy in obese, non-insulin-dependent diabetics induces improvements in insulin action and secretion that are maintained for two weeks after insulin withdrawal. Diabetes 33:634-642, 1984.

116. Garvey WT, Olefsky JM, Griffin J, et al: The effect of insulin treatment on insulin secretion and insulin action in type II diabetes mellitus. Diabetes 34:222-234, 1985.

117. Henry R, Gumbiner B, Ditzler T, et al: Intensive conventional insulin therapy for type II diabetes. Metabolic effects during a 6-month outpatient trial. Diabetes Care 16:21-31, 1993.

118. UK Prospective Diabetes Study (UKPDS) Group: Intensive blood-glucose control with sulphonylureas or insulin compared with conventional treatment and risk of complications in patients with type 2 diabetes (UKPDS 33). Lancet 352:837-853, 1998.

119. Stratton IM, Adler AI, Neil HA, et al: Association of glycaemia with macrovascular and microvascular complications of type 2 diabetes (UKPDS 35): Prospective observational study. BMJ 321:405-412, 2000.

120. Malmberg K, Ryden L, Hamsten A, et al: Effects of insulin treatment on cause-specific one-year mortality and morbidity in diabetic patients with acute myocardial infarction. DIGAMI Study Group. Diabetes Insulin-Glucose in Acute Myocardial Infarction. Eur Heart J 17:1337-1344, 1996.

121. Malmberg K: Prospective randomised study of intensive insulin treatment on long term survival after acute myocardial infarction in patients with diabetes mellitus. DIGAMI (Diabetes Mellitus, Insulin Glucose Infusion in Acute Myocardial Infarction) Study Group. BMJ 314:1512-1515, 1997.

122. Malmberg K, Norhammar A, Wedel H, Ryden L: Glycometabolic state at admission: Important risk marker of mortality in conventionally treated patients with diabetes mellitus and acute myocardial infarction: Long-term results from the Diabetes and Insulin-Glucose Infusion in Acute Myocardial Infarction (DIGAMI) study. Circulation. 99:2626-2632, 1999.

123. Malmberg K, Ryden L, Wedel H, et al: Intense metabolic control by means of insulin in patients with diabetes mellitus and acute myocardial infarction (DIGAMI2): Effects on mortality and morbidity. Eur Heart J 26:650-661, 2005.

124. Steffes MW, Sibley S, Jackson M, Thomas W: β-Cell function and the development of diabetes-related complications in the Diabetes Control and Complications Trial. Diabetes Care 26:832-836, 2003.

125. Hepburn DA, MacLeod KM, Pell AC, et al: Frequency and symptoms of hypoglycaemia experienced by patients with type 2 diabetes treated with insulin. Diabet Med 10:231-237, 1993.

126. The DCCT Research Group: Epidemiology of severe hypoglycemia in the diabetes control and complications trial. Am J Med 90:450-459, 1991.

127. Rosenstock J, Dailey G, Massi-Benedetti M, et al: Reduced hypoglycemia risk with insulin glargine. A meta-analysis comparing insulin glargine with human NPH insulin in type 2 diabetes. Diabetes Care 28:950-955, 2005.

128. Davies M, Storms F, Shutler S, et al, and the AT.LANTUS Study Group: AT.LANTUS trial investigating treatment algorithms for insulin glargine (LANTUS). Results of the type 2 study. Diabetes 53:A473, 2004.

129. Yki-Järvinen H, Hänninen J, Hulme S, et al: Treat To Target simply — the LANMET study. Diabetes 53:2181-2189, 2004.

130. Rosenstock J: Basal insulin supplementation in type 2 diabetes: Refining the tactics. Am J Med 116:10S-16S, 2004.

Chapter 30

Beyond Insulin Therapy

John Crean, David G. Maggs

KEY POINTS

- *Pharmacologic treatments for type 1 and 2 diabetes historically have been based on a monohormonal conceptualization of diabetes: improving glycemic control through restoring or enhancing insulin physiology.*
- *Barriers associated with diabetes medications, including weight gain, edema, and unpredictable day-to-day blood glucose swings, may stem from their singular focus on insulin hormonal mechanisms of action.*
- *Research discoveries since the 1970s have demonstrated the importance of multiple hormones in the regulation of glucose and metabolic homeostasis*
- *Evidence that multiple pancreatic hormones and peptides of the gastrointestinal tract and adipose tissue potently influence glucoregulatory and metabolic processes has led to promising peptide-based therapeutic targets, which are being investigated as treatments for metabolic disorders including diabetes and obesity.*

BACKGROUND

Benefits and Limitations of Intensified Diabetes Treatment Regimens

The Diabetes Control and Complications Trial (DCCT) and the United Kingdom Prospective Diabetes Study (UKPDS) unequivocally showed the importance of establishing glycemic control in patients with type 1 diabetes (T1DM) and type 2 diabetes (T2DM). These landmark clinical trials demonstrated a direct relationship between lowering hemoglobin HbA1c (HbA1c) and reducing the risk of long-term microvascular complications, with no evidence of a glycemic threshold below which the risk of complications was not further reduced.[1-3] The DCCT and UKPDS also revealed that although aggressive intensification of therapy provided initial benefits in improving glycemic control, only a small percentage of patients were able to sustain satisfactory control for an extended period.

In the DCCT, fewer than 5% of the intensively treated patients achieved an average HbA1c at or below the target value by the end of the study.[4] This occurred despite insulin's unlimited potential as a glucose-lowering hormone and the considerable support provided to patients by diabetologists, diabetes educators, and dieticians. Similar outcomes were reported in the UKPDS, where intensive pharmacotherapy, including sulfonylureas or insulin, resulted in an initial improvement in HbA1c. Subsequently, glycemia deteriorated to baseline levels before the study midpoint, and this trend continued such that HbA1c values on study completion were much greater than they were at baseline.[5] The UKPDS results reflect, in part, the progressive nature of T2DM, which is typically characterized by progressive beta cell deterioration, failure of oral medications to produce glycemic control, and eventual need for exogenous insulin.[5]

Despite refinements in insulin and oral agents and heightened awareness of the benefits of optimal glycemic control, the majority of patients with diabetes still fail to meet recommended glycemic targets. Recent epidemiologic data collected from the US health care system reveals that the mean HbA1c among insulin-treated patients with T1DM or T2DM is approximately 9%,[6] which is far in excess of the American Diabetes Association (ADA) recommended target of less than 7%.[7] These outcomes likely reflect barriers and shortcomings associated with intensified diabetes therapies, including weight gain and edema,[8,9] increased risk of severe hypoglycemia,[2,3,10] and the inability to suppress marked day-to-day glucose fluctuations[11,12] and sustain satisfactory glycemic control.[4,5] In the DCCT, for example, patients with T1DM receiving intensive insulin treatment gained an average of 13 pounds more than conventionally treated control subjects.

In the UKPDS, patients with T2DM using insulin also showed greater weight gain compared to conventionally treated patients.[8,9] Intensively treated patients in the UKPDS, regardless of pharmacologic

395

intervention, exhibited signs of beta cell deterioration over the course of the study.[5]

Finally, the advent of continuous glucose monitoring systems (CGMS) has afforded examination of real-world diurnal glucose fluctuations. Studies employing CGMS in patients with T1DM under intensive insulin pump therapy with HbA1c values at or near 7% revealed that many of these patients struggle with extreme diurnal glucose fluctuations, with very little time spent in the euglycemic range.[11,12] A recent investigation has in fact shown that the speed and magnitude of glucose fluctuations are highly predictive of disruptions in mood and cognition.[13]

Beyond Insulin: Glucoregulatory Hormone Systems

Considerable progress has been made in characterizing the challenges and disincentives that patients with diabetes face when adopting intensified treatment regimens, but insights into the physiologic bases of these limitations have been relatively few. Discoveries of endogenous peptides with glucoregulatory roles have highlighted the limitations of the long-held insulinocentric view of diabetes pathophysiology.

An emerging body of evidence has indicated that at least several hormone systems, including peptides of the pancreas, gastrointestinal (GI) tract, peripheral tissues, and the hypothalamic–pituitary axis, contribute to the maintenance of fuel homeostasis and body weight control and are often dysregulated in patients with diabetes. Failure to account for the role of these hormone systems in glucose regulation may explain the shortcomings of current intensive treatment of diabetes. The objective of this chapter is to review these hormone systems and highlight peptides with potential for novel pharmacologic value in the treatment of diabetes.

HORMONE SYSTEMS AND TARGET THERAPEUTIC CANDIDATES

Pancreatic Peptides: Glucagon and Amylin

Discoveries in the 1970s revealed that in addition to insulin, the pancreas synthesizes and secretes metabolically active peptides including the alpha cell hormone glucagon and the beta cell hormone amylin. In healthy persons, these hormones play key roles in maintaining glucose homeostasis. Not surprisingly, their respective secretion is dysregulated in patients with T1DM and T2DM. This section reviews the functional roles of glucagon and amylin in glucose regulation, evidence of their dysregulation in diabetes.

Glucagon
Physiology
Glucagon is a key catabolic hormone, with many actions that oppose those of insulin. This pancreatic hormone primarily stimulates hepatic glucose production during periods of fasting to sustain plasma glucose concentrations. It prevents hypoglycemia, thus preserving normal homeostasis when exogenous sources of energy are unavailable. Glucagon is a 29-amino acid peptide processed from preproglucagon and proglucagon within the pancreatic alpha cells.[14]

The factors mediating glucagon secretion are complex and not fully understood. Autonomic inputs to the alpha cell are activated during hypoglycemia and appear to stimulate glucagon release.[15] In addition, alpha cells possess glucose-sensing properties, secreting glucagon directly in response to low blood glucose independent of autonomic input.[14,16] Elevated glucose concentrations also directly inhibit glucagon secretion, providing further evidence of a cell-based glucose-sensing mechanism.[14] An intraislet feedback loop between alpha cells and beta cells involving insulin, γ-aminobutyric acid (GABA), and glutaminergic signaling may also play a role in stimulating or inhibiting glucagon release.[14,16-18]

Upon binding to its receptor on hepatocytes, glucagon stimulates hepatic glucose production by initiating a series of cellular events. The series begins with activation of G-coupled proteins followed by a subsequent increase in intracellular concentrations of cyclic adenosine monophosphate (cAMP) and activation of protein kinase A (PKA).[16] PKA signaling increases hepatic glucose output through multiple processes, including stimulation of glycogenolysis and inhibition of hepatic glycogen synthesis.[16] Stimulation of PKA pathways also leads to inhibition of pyruvate kinase, resulting in decreased glycolysis and increased gluconeogenesis.[16] Release of glucagon from alpha cells in response to low glucose concentrations represents a key homeostatic mechanism for preserving normoglycemia through glucagon's ability to activate the hepatic signaling pathways necessary for endogenous glucose production and output.[16]

Glucagon Dysregulation and Impaired Glucose Homeostasis
Roger Unger's work in the early 1970s was the first to clearly identify the dysregulation of glucagon secretion as an important manifestation of the pathophysiology of diabetes. This hypothesis was based on studies in which fasting plasma glucagon concentrations were found to be the same in hyperglycemic patients with diabetes and euglycemic healthy subjects, with glucagon concentrations in patients with diabetes nearly double that of control subjects after experimental equilibration of fasting glucose concentrations.[19,20]

The discrepancy between diabetic patients and control subjects was particularly striking immedi-

ately following meal intake: In healthy control subjects, postprandial glucagon concentrations rapidly decreased 25% to 35%, with a correspondingly rapid increase in insulin concentration (Fig. 30–1A). In a patient with diabetes, postprandial glucagon concentrations remained steady or even increased with or without infusion of supraphysiologic doses of insulin. Unger proposed that diabetes was in fact a bihormonal disorder, with the combination of insulin deficiency and glucagon excess.

Subsequent studies have verified that hepatic postprandial glucose production is inappropriately elevated in both T1DM and T2DM, with hyperglucagonemia contributing significantly to the excessive endogenous glucose output, primarily through acceleration of glycogenolysis (see Fig. 30–1B).[21-25] Work by Cherrington and others has revealed that the hepatic sinusoidal insulin-to-glucagon ratio is critical in determining the rate of hepatic glucose production.[26,27] This ratio changes rapidly in response to subtle alterations in prevailing glucose concentrations: When plasma glucose concentrations fall, alpha cells and beta cells respond accordingly (i.e., low insulin-to-glucagon ratio), thus stimulating hepatic glucose output; when concentrations rise, hormone secretion responds in the opposite direction (high insulin-to-glucagon ratio).

In treating diabetes, the inability to administer insulin directly into the portal vein may preclude restoration of the appropriate ratio of these hormones.[28] This may explain the failure of exogenous insulin administration to fully correct postprandial hyperglycemia in patients with diabetes. Consistent with this hypothesis, intensive insulin therapy has been found inadequate to suppress postprandial glycemic excursions.[12,29] For example, in a recent study, adolescents with T1DM receiving intensive insulin treatment, with mean baseline HbA1c of about 7.5%, exhibited extreme diurnal glucose fluctuations, and up to 90% of patients exhibited moderate to severe hyperglycemia following meals.[12]

Although the specific mechanisms underlying glucagon excess during hyperglycemia are not fully understood, chronic exposure to elevated glucose concentrations hypothetically impairs the alpha cell glucose sensing "machinery." There is also evidence that an intraislet feedback loop involving insulin, GABAminergic, and glutaminergic signaling, which is disrupted following beta cell loss, contributes to impaired alpha cell inhibitory control.[17,18,30] Paradoxically, the glucagon counterregulatory response to hypoglycemia is blunted and eventually lost in T1DM and late-stage T2DM, which might also reflect impairment of the alpha cell glucose-sensing capacity.[15]

Taken together, defective glucagon secretion responsiveness can contribute to excessive hyperglycemia and risk of hypoglycemia in diabetes. This issue remains apparent even in patients receiving intensive insulin therapy, in whom, despite supraphysiologic doses of insulin, postprandial glucose excursions remain uncontrolled and the risk for hypoglycemia remains high.[10,29] For example, in the study of intensively treated adolescent patients, although 90% of the subjects experienced postprandial hyperglycemia, up to 70% experienced glucose concentrations in the hypoglycemic range in the overnight period. Thus, as articulated by Unger in the early 1970s, development of a therapeutic approach that corrects the glucagon abnormality can lead to improved metabolic control.

Target Therapeutic Compounds

Antagonizing the action of glucagon has been a heavily researched therapeutic target. Several peptide analogs antagonistic to glucagon have been shown to reduce hepatic glucose output and hyperglycemia in animal models by blocking glucagon-stimulated cAMP production. For example, [1-natrinitrophenylhistidine,12-homoarginine]-glucagon, which disrupts glucagon stimulation of cAMP, significantly decreased endogenous glucose production and hyperglycemia in streptozotocin-induced diabetic rats.[31] Although similar results have been reported with other peptide analogs antagonistic to glucagon, these analogs have yet to undergo testing in humans. Thus, while these peptides are promising candidates for pharmacologic development, the safety and efficacy of these compounds as a potential treatment for diabetes is unknown.

Another strategy for antagonizing glucagon has been the development of nonpeptide receptor antagonists. Bay 27-9955 (Bayer Corporation, Germany) is a nonpeptide, orally administered compound that competitively blocks the interaction of glucagon with its receptor.[32] In healthy subjects, Bay 27-9955 blunted hepatic glucose production and attenuated hyperglycemia during an experimentally induced diabetic state (hyperglucagonemia and hypoinsulinemia).[32]

Skyrin is another nonpeptide compound that has been examined for its glucagon-antagonizing properties. Unlike Bay 27-9955, skyrin does not inhibit the binding of glucagon to its receptor, but it appears to uncouple the receptor from adenylate cyclase activation, thus blocking cAMP production. In primary cultures of human hepatocytes, skyrin reduced cAMP production (55%) and glycogenolysis (27%).[33] These data suggest that compounds that uncouple the glucagon receptor from cAMP production could represent therapeutic targets for treating hyperglucagonemia.

Amylin
Physiology

Amylin is a 37–amino acid peptide hormone that is colocalized and cosecreted with insulin from pancreatic beta cells in response to nutrient stimuli.[34] This polypeptide is structurally similar to calcitonin gene-related peptide (50% identity) and is the product of a discrete gene on chromosome 12.[35,36]

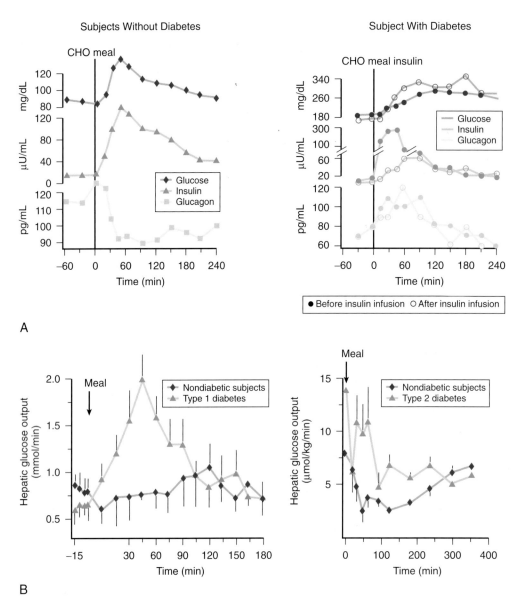

Figure 30–1. A, Failure of glucagon suppression in diabetes. Glucose, insulin, and glucagon concentrations after a carbohydrate (CHO) meal in subjects without diabetes *(left panel)* and a subject with diabetes *(right panel)*. In subjects without diabetes *(left panel)*, a CHO meal results in insulin release and suppression of postprandial glucagon. Concentrations in a subject with diabetes after exogenous insulin administration are also shown *(right panel)*. In patients with type 1 diabetes, there is inappropriate postprandial hyperglucagonemia that is not corrected by administration of insulin. **B,** Hepatic glucose output is abnormally increased after meals in diabetes. Hepatic glucose concentrations after protein ingestion in nondiabetic subjects and patients with type 1 diabetes *(left panel)* as well as after ingestion of a test meal (16% protein, 48% carbohydrate, 36% fat) in nondiabetic subjects and patients with type 2 diabetes *(right panel)*. In patients with type 1 or type 2 diabetes, postprandial hepatic glucose output is abnormally increased. (*A* from Unger RH: Glucagon physiology and patho-physiology. N Engl J Med 285:443-449, 1971. Copyright ©1971 Massachusetts Medical Society. All rights reserved. Reprinted with permission from the Massachusetts Medical Society. *B, left panel,* reprinted from Wahren J, Felig P, Hagenfeldt L: Effect of protein ingestion on splanchnic and leg metabolism in normal man and in patients with diabetes mellitus. J Clin Invest 57:987-999, 1976. Copyright ©1976 by the American Society for Clinical Investigation. Reproduced with permission of the American Society for Clinical Investigation, conveyed through the Copyright Clearance Center. *Right panel* reprinted from Frank JW, Saslow SB, Camilleri M, et al: Mechanism of accelerated gastric emptying of liquids and hyperglycemia in patients with type II diabetes mellitus. Gastroenterology 109:755-765, 1995. Copyright ©1995 with permission from the American Gastroenterological Association.)

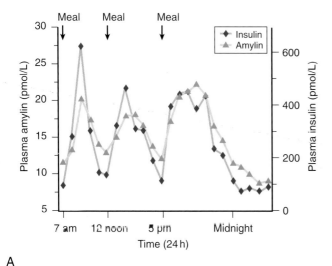

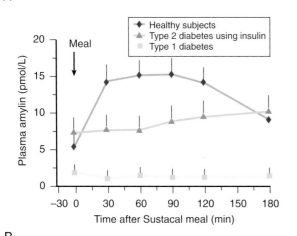

Figure 30–2. **A,** Plasma amylin and insulin concentrations. Amylin and insulin showed similar concentration profiles throughout a 24-hour period in healthy subjects. **B,** Postprandial plasma amylin concentrations. Postprandial amylin concentrations were decreased in both patients with type 1 diabetes and patients with type 2 diabetes who are using insulin, relative to healthy subjects. (From Kruger DF, Gatcomb PM, Owen SK: Clinical implications of amylin and amylin deficiency. Diabetes Educ 25:389-397, 1999. Copyright ©1999 American Association of Diabetes Educators. Reprinted with permission from The American Association of Diabetes Educators.)

Amylin is structurally unrelated to insulin, although it appears to share the same processing enzyme, prohormone convertase, and is copackaged with insulin in secretory granules.[36] The absolute concentrations of circulating plasma amylin (basal state, 4 to 8 pmol/L; postprandial state, 15 to 20 pmol/L) are much like circulating concentrations of other gut peptides, but they are considerably lower than insulin concentrations (molar ratio of 1:30 to 1:50).[34,37] Both hormones increase rapidly following nutrient stimulation and decline to basal concentrations during the postabsorptive period (Fig. 30–2A).[34,37]

Amylin appears to mediate its glucoregulatory properties (discussed later) by binding to its receptor in distinct regions of the brain, particularly the area postrema located in the hindbrain in association with the dorsal vagal complex.[38] The area postrema lies outside the blood–brain barrier and therefore is exposed to changes in plasma peptides, including insulin, amylin, and nutrients such as glucose. The amylin receptor has not been found outside of the central nervous system (CNS).[39]

Amylin Dysregulation and Impaired Glucose Homeostasis

Given the cosecretion of amylin and insulin from the same granules, it is not surprising that amylin is deficient in diabetes when insulin is deficient. Patients with T1DM have an absolute deficiency of both insulin and amylin, whereas insulin-treated patients with T2DM have a relative deficiency with markedly impaired insulin and amylin responses to meals (see Fig. 30–2B).[40]

Numerous preclinical studies have demonstrated that amylin regulates the postprandial rate of glucose entry into the circulation and complements the action of insulin by providing a more precise match between the rate of glucose appearance and insulin-mediated glucose disappearance. This effect appears to be mediated through several mechanisms, including regulation of the rate of gastric emptying,[41] suppression of postprandial glucagon,[42] and regulation of food intake and body weight (Fig. 30–3).[43,44]

In rodents, the specific amylin receptor antagonist AC187 has been shown to increase postprandial glucagon secretion,[45] accelerate the rate of gastric emptying,[46] and disrupt postprandial glucose control.[39] In addition, in rodents administered intracerebroventricular (ICV) infusion of AC187 for 14 days, there was a 14% increase in cumulative food intake and 30% increase in fat mass.[47] In contrast, amylin infusion suppresses postprandial glucagon,[42] slows the rate of gastric emptying,[41] and dose-dependently decreases food intake and reduces body weight.[44]

Preclinical data therefore suggest that amylin is a glucoregulatory hormone with actions that influence the rate of glucose appearance at the time of feeding. Given its absence or deficiency in diabetes, one could speculate that administration of the peptide might offer therapeutic benefit. The administration of naturally occurring amylin is not possible because the peptide is insoluble and self-aggregates. A soluble, nonaggregating analog of human amylin, pramlintide, has been developed by substituting three amino acid residues ([25]Ala, [28]Ser, and [29]Ser) within the human amylin molecule with prolines.[48] In all biochemical and in vivo systems studied to date, pramlintide has elicited a spectrum of actions consistent with those of amylin with at least equal or greater potency.[49] More recently, it was approved for clinical use as an adjunct to insulin in T1DM and T2DM.

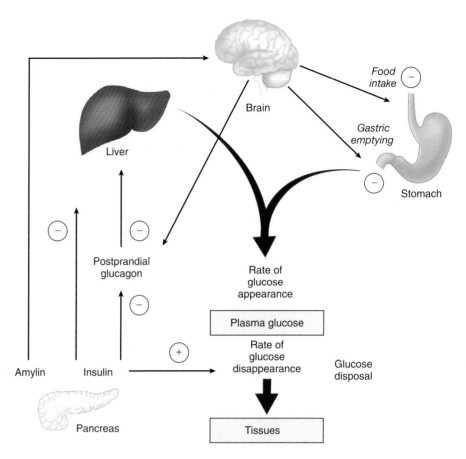

Figure 30–3. Roles of amylin and insulin in glucose homeostasis in a model derived from animal studies. Depicted are multiple mechanisms involving several organs, including regulation of gastric emptying, postprandial glucagon, food intake, and body weight, through which amylin and insulin may maintain glucose balance.

Target Therapeutic Compounds

Studies in patients with T1DM and T2DM have shown that mealtime administration of pramlintide exerts physiologic effects similar to those observed in preclinical studies. The addition of pramlintide to mealtime insulin markedly suppressed excessive postprandial glucagon secretion in patients with T1DM and T2DM without impeding the glucagon response to hypoglycemia.[50,51] Pramlintide, as adjunctive treatment with insulin, has also been shown to slow the rate of gastric emptying of both solid and liquid meals in patients with T1DM, with the half–gastric emptying time prolonged by approximately 60 minutes without carryover effects to the subsequent meal.[52] This indicates that gastric emptying is slowed to the extent that it helps limit postprandial glucose excursions while still allowing a complete emptying of the stomach between meals.

These actions reduce the inflow of exogenous (meal-derived) glucose and the inflow of endogenous (liver-derived) glucose after meals (see Fig. 30–3). The results of several short-term crossover studies examining pramlintide's effect on glucose control following a mixed-meal challenge support this hypothesis: The addition of pramlintide injections to mealtime insulin injections resulted in a significant reduction in the postprandial glucose excursions following standardized mixed meals in patients with T1DM and insulin-using patients with T2DM.[53,54] This effect is apparent with both short-

acting (regular) and rapid-acting (lispro) insulin (Fig. 30–4).[51,55,56] More recently, a study of patients with T1DM treated intensively with insulin pumps revealed that pramlintide also reduced diurnal glucose fluctuations (as assessed by a continuous glucose monitoring system) and postprandial triglycerides.[12]

Long-term (6- to 12-month), randomized, placebo-controlled trials demonstrated overall glycemic improvement following pramlintide treatment relative to placebo (insulin alone). In two 1-year clinical trials, in each of the patients with T1DM and insulin-requiring patients with T2DM, pramlintide treatment resulted in a significant reduction in HbA1c. HbA1c reduction was also accompanied by a decrease in daily insulin requirement and a reduction in body weight in many patients.[57,58]

The most common adverse events reported with pramlintide have been gastrointestinal. Specifically, incidence of mild to moderate nausea was highest upon initiation with pramlintide, especially in patients with T1DM. These side effects were dose dependent and transient, with the incidence between the pramlintide and placebo groups indistinguishable after 4 weeks of therapy.

Overall incidence of severe hypoglycemia was not increased with pramlintide treatment. However, in patients with T1DM, the risk of severe hypoglycemia was increased upon initiation of treatment, but it dissipated after the first 4 weeks. The

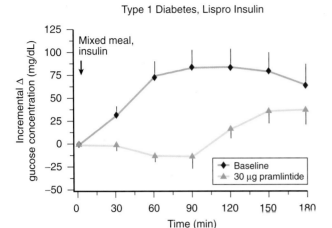

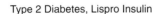

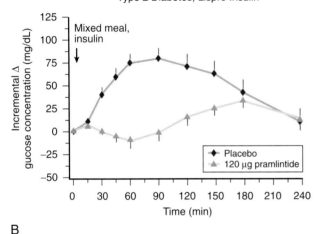

Figure 30–4. Pramlintide used with regular and insulin lispro improved postprandial glucose control. Shown are glucose concentrations in patients with type 1 **(A)** or type 2 **(B)** diabetes (*n* = 16 and 20, respectively) receiving pramlintide or insulin, or both. Glucose concentrations for patients taking pramlintide are decreased relative to glucose concentrations from patients at baseline (for type 1) or receiving placebo (for type 2). (**A** from Levetan C, Want LL, Weyer C, et al: Impact of pramlintide on glucose fluctuations and postprandial glucose, glucagon, and triglyceride excursions among patients with type 1 diabetes intensively treated with insulin pumps. Diabetes Care 26:1-8, 2003. Copyright ©2003 American Diabetes Association. Reprinted with permission from The American Diabetes Asssociation. **B** from Maggs DG, Fineman M, Kornstein J, et al: Pramlintide reduces postprandial glucose excursions when added to insulin lispro in subjects with type 2 diabetes: A dose-timing study. Diabetes Metab Res Rev 20:55-60, 2004.)

increased risk of severe hypoglycemia in T1DM upon initiation of pramlintide treatment may be related to the corresponding increase in mild to moderate nausea. A recent study of patients with T1DM who were intensively treated demonstrated that progressive pramlintide dose titration in combination with an initial 30% to 50% reduction of mealtime insulin reduced the incidence of nausea and mitigated the risk of hypoglycemia upon initiation.[59]

INCRETIN HORMONES: THE ENTERO-INSULAR AXIS

A potential role for intestinal peptides in the regulation of postprandial insulin secretion and glucose regulation was first proposed following the observation that insulin responses to an oral glucose load exceeded those measured after intravenous administration of an equivalent amount of glucose.[60] This phenomenon led to the description of the incretin effect, postulating that gut-derived signals stimulated by oral nutrients promote insulin release (Fig. 30–5).[61]

The incretin concept was further developed by the discovery of two peptides: glucose-dependent insulinotropic polypeptide, also known as gastric inhibitory polypeptide (GIP) and glucagon-like peptide-1 (GLP-1). These peptides are both synthesized and secreted by cells lining the intestinal tract following nutrient intake, and each has insulinotropic properties.[62,63]

The following sections review the insulinotropic, glucoregulatory, and metabolic effects of GIP and GLP-1. Compounds with incretin-mimetic properties (i.e., agents that mimic the enhancement of glucose-dependent insulin secretion and several of the other antihyperglycemic actions of incretins) currently under investigation for use in patients with diabetes are also described.

Gastric Inhibitory Polypeptide and Glucagon-Like Peptide-1
Physiology
GIP is a 42–amino acid peptide hormone synthesized in and secreted from K cells in the intestinal epithelium, the majority of which are located in the proximal duodenum.[64,65] GLP-1 is a 30–amino acid peptide hormone synthesized in intestinal L cells, located predominantly in the ileum and colon.[66] GIP secretion appears to be mediated by direct contact of nutrients, especially fats, with intestinal K cells,[67] whereas the distally located L cells appear to release GLP-1 both by direct nutrient contact and neuronal or neuroendocrine signals that stimulate release in advance of direct contact.[68]

GIP and GLP-1 concentrations rise rapidly following nutrient intake and stimulate insulin secretion in a glucose-dependent fashion. These hormones are insulinotropic only in the presence of glucose concentrations greater than 5 to 6 mmol/L (90 to 108 mg/dL).[69] Specific receptors have been identified for both GIP and GLP-1, and substantial homology exists between the two. Not surprisingly, these peptides enhance insulin secretion by a similar signaling mechanism at their respective receptors. Ligand binding activates

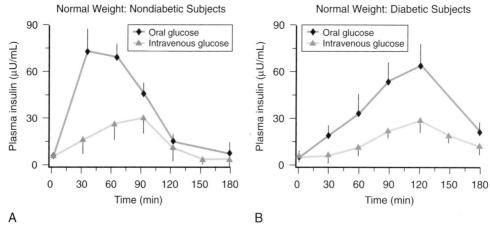

Figure 30–5. The incretin effect: plasma insulin responses to oral and intravenous glucose. Plasma insulin was measured in 18 normal-weight nondiabetic subjects **(A)** and 12 normal-weight diabetic subjects **(B)** after administration of 100 g of either oral or intravenous glucose. The glucose range for nondiabetic subjects was approximately 70 to 120 mg/dL (3.9 to 6.7 mmol/L), and that for diabetic subjects was approximately 85 to 220 mg/dL (4.7 to 12.2 mmol/L). Values are mean (standard error). (Modified from Perley M, Kipnis DM: Plasma insulin responses to oral and intravenous glucose: Studies in normal and diabetic subjects. J Clin Invest 46:1954-1962, 1967. Copyright ©1967 by the American Society for Clinical Investigation. Reproduced with permission of the American Society for Clinical Investigation, conveyed through the Copyright Clearance Center.)

adenylate cyclase and increases intracellular cAMP, with the potentiation of glucose-stimulated and depolarization-stimulated exocytosis from the beta cell mediated by the PKA signaling pathway. GIP and GLP-1 are rapidly inactivated within minutes by dipeptidyl peptidase IV (DPP-IV) after their release into portal circulation.[69]

GLP-1 has also been shown to exert additional pancreatic and extrapancreatic effects: In in vitro and in vivo experiments, GLP-1 has been demonstrated to increase the mRNA concentrations of various beta cell–specific genes including insulin, GLUT-1, and hexokinase-1.[70] GLP-1 also appears to promote glucose competence or responsiveness in beta cells that have lost their sensitivity to glucose.[71] Moreover, several studies in partially pancreatectomized (90% to 95%) rats, intrauterine growth-retarded rats, and aging rats have indicated that GLP-1 might promote expansion of beta cell mass by stimulation of beta cell proliferation and from the differentiation of the ductal epithelium into insulin-secreting cells.[72-75]

With regard to extrapancreatic effects, human and animal investigations have shown that GLP-1 inhibits the postprandial secretion of glucagon, although it is unclear whether this effect stems from direct interaction with pancreatic alpha cells or from an alternate indirect mechanism.[76] GLP-1 also slows the rate of gastric emptying, possibly by a vagally stimulated effect upon binding to GLP-1 receptors located in the hindbrain.[77] Lastly, animal and human studies have indicated that GLP-1 might elicit a postprandial satiety signal, possibly mediated through GLP-1 receptors in the hypothalamus paraventricular nucleus and the amygdala central nucleus.[78-81]

GIP and GLP-1 Dysregulation and Impaired Glucose Homeostasis

The importance of GIP in maintaining normal glucose homeostasis, particularly during the postprandial period, has been demonstrated by several experimental rodent models: blockade of GIP action with a specific antiserum abolished the insulinotropic effect of exogenous GIP and resulted in glucose intolerance.[82] Similarly, in the GIP receptor knockout mouse, the insulin secretory response to an oral glucose load was impaired and associated with glucose intolerance.[83]

In human studies, circulating GIP concentrations were similar in patients with T1DM and in healthy control subjects.[84] However, in patients with T2DM, an exaggerated GIP response to glucose ingestion has been observed.[85] Moreover, infusion of synthetic human GIP in patients with T2DM elicited glucose-stimulated insulin secretion, but at a lesser magnitude than observed in healthy control subjects.[85] Thus, patients with T2DM have features of GIP resistance, and this renders GIP an unattractive therapeutic candidate. In contrast to GIP, studies have demonstrated impaired GLP-1 secretion following meal ingestion in patients with T2DM (Fig. 30–6A).[86] Importantly, the insulinotropic response to GLP-1 is not diminished in patients with diabetes.[87]

Numerous studies have indicated that blocking GLP-1 action by a variety of experimental methodologies disrupts both fasting and postprandial glycemic control. For example, rodents given exendin [9-39], a specific GLP-1 receptor antagonist, exhibit postprandial hyperglycemia and diminished postprandial insulin secretion.[88,89] Similarly, GLP-1 receptor knockout mice have abnormal

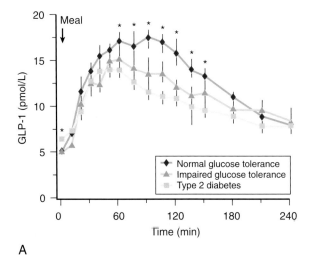

A

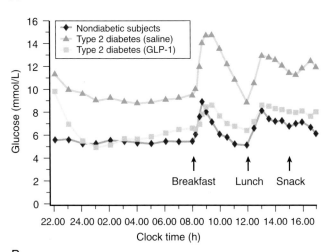

B

Figure 30–6. A, Postprandial glucagon-like peptide-1 (GLP-1) levels are decreased in subjects with impaired glucose tolerance (IGT) and type 2 diabetes. Plasma GLP-1 concentrations in patients with type 2 diabetes (*n* = 54), subjects with normal glucose tolerance (*n* = 33), and subjects with impaired glucose tolerance (*n* = 15) after a mixed breakfast meal (42% fat, 41% carbohydrate, 18% protein) demonstrate the altered levels in impaired glucose tolerance subjects and patients with type 2 diabetes. *Asterisks* indicate *P* < 0.05, normal glucose tolerance versus type 2 diabetes. Values are mean (standard error). **B,** Effect of GLP-1 infusion on glucose concentration in patients with type 2 diabetes (previously taking oral agents). Mean diurnal plasma glucose concentrations in diabetic subjects (*n* = 8) in response to infusion of saline or continuous infusion of GLP-1 compared with nondiabetic control subjects (*n* = 6). GLP-1 infusion restored normal diurnal glucose concentration patterns. (**A** from Toft-Nielsen MB, Damholt MB, Madsbad S, et al: Determinants of the impaired secretion of glucagon-like peptide-1 in type 2 diabetic patients. J Clin Endocrinol Metab 86:3717-3723, 2001. **B** from Rachman J, Barrow BA, Levy JC, et al: Near-normalisation of diurnal glucose concentrations by continuous administration of glucagon-like peptide-1 (GLP-1) in subjects with NIDDM. Diabetologia 40:205-211, 1997. Reprinted with kind permission of Springer Science and Business Media.)

glucose tolerance and attenuated insulin release after glucose ingestion.[90] GLP-1 antagonism has also been found to increase postprandial glucagon concentrations and accelerate gastric emptying.[91] Finally, infusion of exendin [9-39] in healthy subjects resulted in significant increases in fasting glucose concentrations and postprandial glucose and glucagon concentrations.[91]

GLP-1 administration has been shown to substantially improve glycemic control in models of diabetes, further supporting the involvement of this peptide in glucose regulation. Treatment with GLP-1, for example, significantly improved glycemic control in various animal models of diabetes, including db/db and ob/ob mice, ZDF rats, and diabetic rhesus monkeys and pigs.[92-95] As expected, GLP-1 administration enhanced glucose-dependent insulin secretion and corresponding improvements in postprandial and fasting glycemia. Several investigators have also demonstrated that GLP-1 infusion in rodents and other species elicits a glucose-dependent attenuation of glucagon secretion, slowing of gastric emptying, and reductions in food intake and body weight.[96]

GLP-1 and the Treatment of Diabetes

In a study investigating a 4-hour GLP-1 infusion in patients with T2DM, GLP-1 lowered fasting glucose from hyperglycemic to euglycemic concentrations (less than 110 mg/dL).[87] The decline in glucose following GLP-1 infusion corresponded directly with enhancement of insulin secretion. Fasting plasma glucagon concentrations were also reduced.

In a separate 24-hour study, continuous GLP-1 infusion in a group of patients with T2DM resulted in virtually normalized fasting and postprandial glucose concentrations (see Fig. 30–6B).[97] The insulinotropic and glucagonostatic actions of GLP-1 reported in human studies were found to be glucose dependent; thus, when administered alone, GLP-1 should not induce hypoglycemia.

Finally, consistent with actions described in animals, GLP-1 has been reported to slow the rate of gastric emptying[98] and reduce appetite and food intake in both healthy subjects and patients with T2DM.[99] For example, a single subcutaneous (SC) dose of GLP-1 before a liquid meal slowed gastric emptying by up to 45 minutes in patients with T2DM and chronic 6-week SC infusion of GLP-1 reduced body weight by approximately 1.9 kg in obese patients with T2DM.[100]

The collective glucoregulatory actions of GLP-1 make this peptide a potential agent for the treatment of diabetes, but its therapeutic potential is limited by its rapid and extensive degradation by DPP-IV. Thus, sustaining plasma concentrations of GLP-1 long enough to produce a therapeutic effect requires continuous infusion. The next section will review advancements in the development of incretin mimetics, a new class of agents with multiple antihyperglycemic effects that mimic the

effects of incretin hormones and the development of DPP-IV inhibitors.

Target Therapeutic Compounds
GLP-1 Analogs: Rendering the GLP-1 Molecule More Resistant to DPP-IV Breakdown

One approach to mimicking the incretin effect is the development of DPP-IV–resistant GLP-1 analogs. Liraglutide (NN2211) is an acylated DPP-IV–resistant GLP-1 derivative designed for injection.[101] In humans, liraglutide has been reported to exhibit a half-life of approximately 12 hours and is therefore potentially compatible with once-daily injection.[101] The prolonged action of liraglutide is attributed to its binding to serum albumin and its slow release from the injection site. In clinical studies, liraglutide reduced fasting and postprandial glycemia in patients with T2DM after a single 10 μg/kg SC injection.[102] These effects were associated with slowing of gastric emptying, reduced plasma glucagon concentrations, and increased plasma insulin concentrations.

In a study that examined the effect of liraglutide on markers of beta cell function in patients with T2DM, liraglutide treatment reportedly improved first- and second-phase insulin response and increased maximal insulin secretory capacity.[103] In addition, the proinsulin-to-insulin ratio improved following liraglutide administration. These results are consistent with findings in experimental animal models of diabetes, where GLP-1 has been shown to improve beta cell functioning.[71-74]

Finally, data were recently reported from a study that examined the effect of various doses of SC liraglutide administered once daily for 3 months in patients with T2DM (mean baseline HbA1c, 7.6%). Patients receiving the highest dose (0.75 mg) had a 0.75% HbA1c reduction ($P < 0.0001$), a 1.8 mmol/L (32.4 mg/dL) decrease in fasting glucose ($P = 0.0003$), and a significant reduction in the proinsulin-to-insulin ratio (–0.18, $P = 0.0244$) relative to a placebo control group after 3 months of treatment.[104] These glycemic benefits were observed without an increase in body weight, but a higher incidence of dizziness, nausea, vomiting, and diarrhea was observed in liraglutide-treated patients compared to placebo-treated patients.[104]

Another GLP-1 analog, CJC-1131, was engineered with a reactive linker that allows covalent binding to serum albumin.[105] The resultant CJC-1131–albumin drug affinity complex (DAC) appears to retain the actions of GLP-1 along with increased resistance to DPP-IV degradation and prolonged duration of action in vivo.[105,106] In recent phase I and phase II multi-dose clinical trials, SC treatment with CJC-1131 in patients with T2DM resulted in statistically significant reductions in mean daily glucose concentrations.[107,108] In these short-term clinical trials, mild nausea and vomiting occurred in some patients; cases of hypoglycemia and local injection site irritation were not observed.[107] Larger

phase II trials are under way to further evaluate the clinical potential of this GLP-1 analog in patients with T2DM.

Exenatide: Exendin-4

Exendin-4 was originally isolated from the salivary secretions of the lizard *Heloderma suspectum* (Gila monster).[109] Exendin-4 has a 53% amino acid sequence identity with mammalian GLP-1. In the Gila monster, exendin-4 and GLP-1 are not transcribed from the same gene, and therefore, the gene encoding exendin-4 is not the Gila monster homolog of the mammalian proglucagon gene from which GLP-1 is expressed.[110] In mammals, exogenous exendin-4 (exenatide) exhibits antidiabetic activities similar to those of native GLP-1, but it is resistant to degradation by DPP-IV, which contributes to its longer half-life compared with GLP-1.[111,112] In humans, the half-life of exenatide administered SC has been demonstrated to be approximately 2.35 hours.[113]

Exenatide has recently been approved for clinical use as an adjunct to oral agents in the treatment of T2DM. Several short-term phase 2 clinical trials in patients with T2DM have reported that SC exenatide acutely lowered both fasting and postprandial plasma glucose concentrations. In one study, patients receiving SC injections of exenatide for 5 days displayed significant reductions in mean postprandial concentrations of glucose and glucagon compared to placebo-treated control subjects (Fig. 30–7A).[114]

In a separate investigation, patients receiving varying doses of exenatide following an overnight fast showed dose-dependent reductions in plasma glucose concentrations during a subsequent 8-hour period (see Fig. 30–7B, *left panel*).[114] The latter effect occurred with a concurrent dose-dependent and glucose-dependent rise in serum insulin concentrations within the first 3 hours after exenatide administration (see Fig. 30–7B, *right panel*). The rate of gastric emptying, as assessed by acetaminophen appearance rates in plasma, was also slowed in patients treated with exenatide.

With regard to longer-term exposure to exenatide, a 28-day study examined twice-daily exenatide dosing in patients who were unable to attain satisfactory HbA1c goals with oral sulfonylureas or metformin, or both. Mean HbA1c was reduced by approximately 0.9 percentage point from baseline in exenatide-treated patients.[113] This HbA1c reduction occurred without a concomitant increase in body weight.[113] Results from homeostasis modeling of beta cell functioning (HOMA-B) assessed at baseline, day 14, and day 28 suggested improved beta cell secretory function with exenatide therapy.

Additional evidence for the latter effect was reported in a study examining the effect of exenatide on first- and second-phase insulin secretion in patients with T2DM. In this investigation, patients who evidenced severely attenuated first- and second-phase insulin secretion following

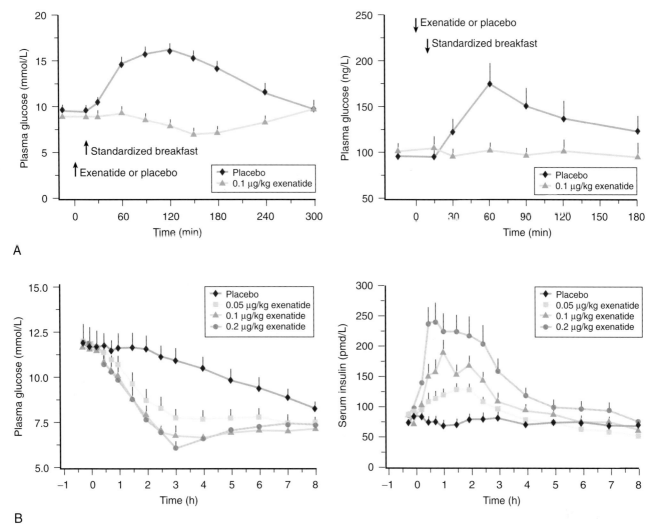

A

B

Figure 30–7. A, Effect of exenatide on postprandial glucose and glucagon in type 2 diabetes. Postprandial plasma glucose *(left panel)* and glucagon *(right panel)* concentration profiles of 20 patients with type 2 diabetes following a single dose of placebo or 0.1 μg/kg exenatide, demonstrating decreased postprandial glucose and glucagon concentrations with exenatide treatment. This followed 4 days of twice-daily treatment with the study medication (placebo or exenatide). Values are mean (standard error). **B,** Effect of exenatide on fasting plasma glucose and insulin in type 2 diabetes. Fasting plasma glucose *(left panel)* and insulin *(right panel)* concentration profiles of 12 patients with type 2 diabetes during the 8 hours following a single dose of placebo or 0.05 μg/kg, 0.1 μg/kg, or 0.2 μg/kg exenatide, demonstrating decreased fasting plasma glucose and increased insulin concentrations with exenatide treatment. Values are mean (standard error). (**A** and **B** from Kolterman OG, Buse JB, Fineman MS, et al: Synthetic exendin-4 (exenatide) significantly reduces postprandial and fasting plasma glucose in subjects with type 2 diabetes. J Clin Endocrinol Metab 88:3082-3089, 2003.)

intravenous glucose infusion (IVGTT) had these responses fully restored upon infusion of exenatide.[115] This result provides further support that incretin mimetic therapy could represent an effective approach for improving beta cell functioning.

Three multi-center, placebo-controlled, phase III clinical trials assessed the safety and efficacy of exenatide (5 μg or 10 μg twice daily) over a 6-month period in patients with T2DM who were unable to achieve glycemic control with oral sulfonylureas or metformin. The first to be published reports that exenatide, when used as an adjunct to oral sulfonylureas, lowered HbA1c. Changes from baseline to week 30 were 0.86 ± 0.11 percentage points in

the 10-μg group, 0.46 ± 0.12 points in the 5-μg group, and +0.12 ± 0.09 points in the placebo group.[116] Subjects in the 10-μg exenatide group also had progressive reduction in weight over the 30 weeks.[116] These findings are consistent with those seen in the earlier phase 2 trials.[116-118]

Exenatide was generally well tolerated in both short- and long-term trials. The most common adverse event was nausea, which occurred with greatest frequency upon initiation of exenatide treatment, was mostly mild to moderate in intensity, and generally subsided with continued exposure to exenatide. A higher incidence of hypoglycemia was also reported in patients treated

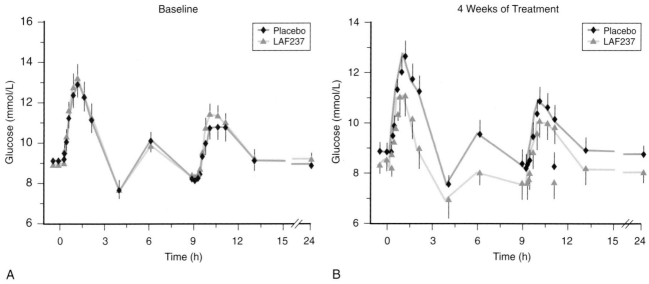

Figure 30–8. Effect of LAF237 on glucose concentrations. Twenty-four-hour glucose concentration profiles at baseline **(A)** and after 4 weeks of daily treatment **(B)** with placebo (*n* = 19) or 100 mg LAF237 (*n* = 19) in patients with type 2 diabetes, showing decreased glucose concentrations after 4 weeks of treatment. Meals were ingested at 0 h, 4 h 15 min, and 9 h. Values are mean (standard error). (From Ahren B, Landin-Olsson M, Jansson, PA, et al: Inhibition of dipeptidyl peptidase-4 reduces glycemia, sustains insulin levels, and reduces glucagon levels in type 2 diabetes. J Clin Endocrinol Metab 89:2078-2084, 2004.)

with exenatide and a sulfonylurea. These episodes were almost exclusively mild to moderate in intensity and occurred less frequently with lower doses of sulfonylurea. However, there was no increase in hypoglycemia when exenatide was used with metformin.

DPP-IV Inhibition

The use of DPP-IV inhibitors to increase endogenous GLP-1 concentrations represents another approach currently being investigated as a treatment for patients with T2DM. LAF237, a DPP-IV inhibitor that rapidly inactivates more than 80% of the pool of circulating DPP-IV, is a compound that has recently entered phase III clinical testing.[119] It is a nonpeptide small molecule and can be administered orally.

In one study, both 4-hour prandial (breakfast) glucose excursions and 24-hour mean glucose concentrations were significantly reduced following 4 weeks of once-daily (100 mg) LAF237 treatment in patients with diet-controlled T2DM (Fig. 30–8).[120] The authors also reported that baseline and postprandial active GLP-1 increased, and postprandial glucagon decreased, following LAF237 treatment.

In a 12-week double-blind, placebo-controlled study examining four separate LAF237 doses in patients with diabetes (baseline HbA1c, 7.7%), there were dose-dependent decreases in HbA1c ranging from 0.3 percentage point (low dose 25 mg once daily) to 0.7 percentage point (high dose 100 mg once daily).[121] In a second double-blind, placebo-controlled 12-week study that assessed LAF237 adjunctive treatment in patients receiving maximally tolerated doses of metformin (baseline

HbA1c, 7.8%), there were dose-dependent decreases in HbA1c of 0.56 percentage point and 0.82 point in the 50-mg and 100-mg once-daily groups, respectively.[122]

To date, adverse events in patients treated with LAF237 have all been mild, with hypoglycemia (10% of patients) and nasopharyngitis (22% of patients) being the most commonly reported events; neither of the latter conditions led to discontinuation of treatment.[122,123] DPP-IV has a broad spectrum of activity and interacts with numerous peptides throughout the body, and therefore attention will be directed to other effects elicited through inhibition of this enzyme's activity.

Gut-Brain Axis: Regulation of Energy Intake

At least several additional peptides produced in the gut have been shown to influence energy homeostasis. Evidence points to peptide neuroendocrine signaling generated by anticipation of meal intake or meal ingestion itself. The peptides represent an enteric signal that communicates short-term energy requirements to the appetite and satiety centers of the brain (Fig. 30–9). Food intake is subsequently activated or inhibited depending on the signal provided by the GI peptide.[123]

Ghrelin

Ghrelin is a gut peptide that has been shown to be a primary signal of acute energy insufficiency. This hormone is a 28-amino acid peptide, which is

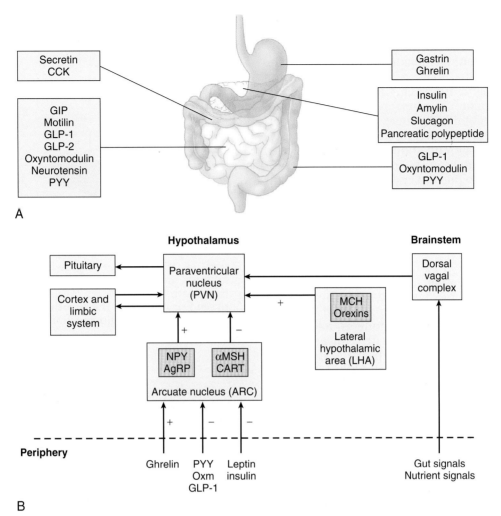

Figure 30–9. Regulation of appetite and weight. **A,** Of the gut hormones shown, cholecystokinin (CCK), glucagon-like peptide-1 (GLP-1), oxyntomodulin, peptide YY (PYY), ghrelin, and pancreatic polypeptide are known to alter food intake and weight. **B,** Appetite regulation occurs via a number of central pathways. AgRP, agouti-related gene product; CART, cocaine- and amphetamine-regulated transcript; GIP, gastric inhibitory polypeptide; MCH, melanin-concentrating hormone; αMSH, α-melanocyte-stimulating hormone; NPY, neuropeptide Y. (From Druce MR, Small CJ, Bloom SR: Minireview: Gut peptides regulating satiety. Endocrinology 145:2660-2665, 2004.)

secreted by endocrine cells in the oxyntic mucosa of the stomach and is a ligand for the growth hormone secreting receptor (GHS-R).[124]

Rodents administered exogenous ghrelin almost triple their food intake.[125] Moreover, with chronic ghrelin treatment, these animals experience weight gain, whereas administration of antighrelin IgG suppresses feeding and reduces weight. In human investigations, concentrations of ghrelin are highest immediately before meals or when meal intake is expected, and they decrease upon nutrient ingestion.[126]

Cross-sectional studies have demonstrated negative correlations between ghrelin concentrations and body weight.[127] In addition, ghrelin increases significantly following diet-induced weight loss.[128] The latter observation may explain rebound weight gain that often occurs following a period of dieting. Ghrelin concentrations are also markedly elevated in patients with Prader-Willi syndrome, a condition associated with voracious appetite and obesity.[127] Finally, exogenous ghrelin infusion in a group of healthy subjects was found to increase food intake by 28% and significantly increase subjective ratings of hunger.[129] Importantly, results from this study support a cause-and-effect relationship between ghrelin and appetite in humans.

The appetite-stimulating effect of this peptide appears to be mediated through activation of neurons that contain neuropeptide Y (NPY) and agouti-related gene product (AgRP) and that exist within the hypothalamic arcuate nucleus (ARC) and colocalize with growth hormone (GH) receptors.[130] Interventions that directly stimulate neuronal release of NPY and AgRP within the ARC result in profound increases in energy intake. Consistent with this hypothesis, intracerebroventricular (ICV) infusion of ghrelin increases the expression of NPY

mRNA and subsequent food intake, whereas ICV administration of an NPY Y1 antagonist suppresses ghrelin-stimulated food intake.[131-133]

The development of therapies antagonistic to the effects of ghrelin may represent a promising approach to regulating energy intake. This may be especially germane in obese patients undergoing diet-induced weight loss, where there is a direct correspondence between weight reduction and resultant increases in ghrelin concentration. In rodents, pharmacologic antagonism of the ghrelin receptor has been found to prevent energy intake and weight gain in lean and obese mice. Thus, ghrelin antagonism may enable patients to avoid rebound weight gain following a successful period of dieting.

PYY (3-36)

Another GI peptide, PYY (3-36), which is expressed by the L cells of the small and large intestines,[134] has also been shown to mediate food intake by an interaction with ARC neurons, with an effect opposite to that of ghrelin. This hormone is released in response to food ingestion, with concentrations rising within 15 minutes and peaking around 60 minutes following meal intake.[135] PYY (3-36) selectively binds to a presynaptic NPY inhibitory autoreceptor (Y2 receptor) and inhibits electrical activity of NPY nerve terminals.[136]

Consistent with this neurochemical action, intraperitoneal injection of PYY (3-36) in freely feeding rats was shown to acutely inhibit food intake, with intraperitoneal administration twice daily for 7 days reducing cumulative food intake by 9% and body weight gain by 18% compared to saline.[135]

In humans, a single infusion of exogenous PYY (3-36) in lean and obese subjects reduced caloric intake by approximately 30% at a buffet lunch administered 2 hours later.[137] Moreover, reduction of cumulative caloric intake was observed for up to 12 hours after PYY infusion. Interestingly, PYY concentrations were reported to be lower in obese subjects relative to lean subjects in both the fasting period and following meal intake, which suggests that PYY deficiency contributes to obesity.

Summary

The release of GI peptides such as ghrelin and PYY (3-36) may represent a gut-derived neurochemical signal that integrates peripheral energy needs with the regions of the brain mediating feelings of satiety and hunger. This hormone system therefore represents a physiologic mechanism through which energy intake and food-seeking behavior are calibrated to accommodate acute changes in energy requirements. Other gut hormones, including cholecystokinin (CCK) and oxyntomodulin (OXM), also have been shown to exert satiety-like effects in a variety of species, including humans. Thus, GI peptides might represent promising therapeutic candidates for the treatment of obesity and other metabolic disorders. PYY (3-36) and CCK agonists

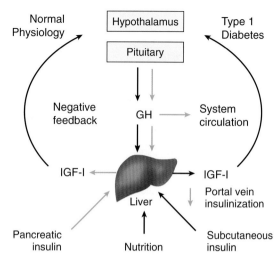

Figure 30–10. Interplay of growth hormone (GH) and insulin-like growth factor-1 IGF-I) for normal persons and patients with type 1 diabetes. (From Holt RI, Simpson HL, Sonksen PH: The role of the growth hormone–insulin-like growth factor axis in glucose homeostasis. Diabet Med 20:3-15, 2003.)

are currently in early-phase clinical development for obesity-related disorders.

The IGF-I and Growth Hormone Axis

Peptides involved in the regulation of the hypothalamic–pituitary axis (HPA) have also been shown to contribute significantly to glucose homeostasis. Numerous studies have demonstrated that the interaction between insulin-like growth factor I (IGF-I) and growth hormone (GH) is particularly important in this regard.[138] These hormones form a delicate feedback loop, which, when disrupted, adversely affects glucose control (Fig. 30–10).[139]

In diabetes, loss of beta cell function and subsequent loss of sufficient portal insulin decreases hepatic IGF-I output. IGF-I appears to function as a negative feedback signal for pituitary GH secretion.[138] Consequently, in patients with diabetes, IGF-I concentrations are often depressed, whereas GH concentrations are abnormally elevated. The latter hormone has potent diabetogenic effects by stimulating the hepatic glucose output, and excessive concentrations have been shown to exacerbate hyperglycemia in diabetes. This section reviews the evidence supporting the involvement of IGF-I–GH dysregulation in the pathophysiology of diabetes and the rationale for IGF-I replacement therapy.

Physiology

IGF-I is a 70–amino acid polypeptide hormone that has approximately 50% amino acid sequence homology with insulin.[138] The majority of IGF-I is derived from the liver, and its synthesis is regulated by GH, portal insulin concentration, and nutri-

tional intake.[140] The interaction of GH with the hepatic GH receptor stimulates expression of the IGF-I gene and the release of IGF-I. In the circulation, IGF-I is bound to one of six IGF binding proteins, with 95% bound to IGF-binding protein 3 (IGF-BP3).[140] The IGF-I receptor is ubiquitously expressed; ligand binding stimulates cellular growth and differentiation.[140]

GH is a single strand of 191 amino acids synthesized in the anterior pituitary cells of the hypothalamus, and it exerts a counterregulatory or diabetogenic effect during periods of fasting, starvation, or stress.[141,142] Infusion of GH in humans increases fasting hepatic glucose output by increasing hepatic gluconeogenesis and glycogenolysis and decreasing peripheral glucose uptake through inhibition of glycogen synthesis and glucose oxidation.[141] In addition, GH stimulates lipolysis and subsequent release of glycerol and nonesterified fatty acids (NEFAs).[143] The latter process contributes to the diabetogenic effect by increasing hepatic glucose output and decreasing peripheral glucose oxidation by the glucose–fatty acid cycle.

IGF-I and Growth Hormone Dysregulation and Impaired Glucose Homeostasis

Animal models and clinical studies have provided evidence for IGF-I–GH dysregulation as a factor contributing to metabolic derangement in diabetes. Transgenic GH mice develop insulin resistance, hyperinsulinemia, hyperglycemia, and hypertriglyceridemia.[144] Glycogen synthase and glycogen phosphorylase activity in muscle and liver tissue is also reduced in these animals and remains unchanged after feeding.

In IGF-I transgenic mice, which have been further manipulated so that hepatic IGF-I gene expression is ablated, serum IGF-I concentrations fall to 15% to 25% relative to controls, while GH increases sixfold.[145] These animals are also hyperinsulinemic and insulin resistant. Persons with acromegaly, which is a disorder caused by hypersecretion of GH, develop peripheral and hepatic insulin resistance, and 40% develop diabetes.[138]

GH concentrations are up to two to three times higher in persons with diabetes compared to healthy subjects. The degree of elevation corresponds to the magnitude of beta cell deterioration.[138] Correspondingly, IGF-I concentrations are typically depressed in patients with diabetes. The derangement in the IGF-I–GH axis has led to the exploration of recombinant IGF-I as a possible treatment for patients with T1DM or T2DM.

Target Therapeutic Compounds
Recombinant IGF-I

Several studies have reported the metabolic changes that occur following acute infusion of IGF-I. In healthy subjects undergoing a euglycemic, hyperinsulinemic clamp, IGF-I improved glucose tolerance, enhanced resting energy expenditure and lipid oxidation, and improved insulin-stimulated oxidative and nonoxidative glucose disposal.[146] Similar outcomes have been reported in patients with T1DM and insulin-using patients with T2DM, in whom acute infusion of IGF-I significantly decreased rates of endogenous glucose appearance while increasing the rate of peripheral glucose disappearance.[147,148]

In short-term clinical trials, SC IGF-I twice-daily adjunctive therapy in patients with T1DM has been reported to significantly decrease overnight GH concentrations, total cholesterol, and triglycerides, resulting in an approximately 45% decrease in daily insulin requirement.[147] Similarly, short-term twice-daily SC IGF-I therapy has been shown to improve fasting and day-long glucose concentrations, decrease endogenous glucose production, and increase whole body insulin-stimulated glucose disposal in patients with poorly controlled T2DM.[149]

Longer-term clinical trials have demonstrated IGF-I's ability to significantly reduce overall glycemia as measured by HbA1c in patients with T1DM or T2DM. For example, in a 3-month trial evaluating the addition of twice-daily SC IGF-I to intensified insulin treatment of patients with T1DM, HbA1c was reduced by an average of 1.2 percentage points, which was statistically superior to the 0.7-point decrease in patients who received intensified insulin therapy alone.[150] In addition, patients receiving IGF-I and insulin reduced their mean total daily insulin dose by more than 12%, whereas patients treated with optimized insulin therapy alone increased their mean total daily insulin dose by 7% during the 3-month trial. There was no increased risk of hypoglycemia or increased weight gain associated with IGF-I treatment in this study.

Similar results were also reported from a study of patients with T2DM who received twice-daily SC IGF-I monotherapy over a 3-month period. In this trial, patients treated with IGF-I had decreases in fasting blood glucose and fasting triglycerides.[151]

However, both of these 3-month studies reported a number of side effects associated with IGF-I therapy, including jaw ache, optic disc swelling, arthralgia, myalgia, headaches, and temporary Bell's palsy. Although these side effects have been shown to be dose-dependent and manageable at lower doses of IGF-I, IGF-I was subsequently withdrawn from development as an adjunctive treatment in diabetes.

IGF-I/IGFBP-3 (SomatoKine)

Although the mechanisms for the side effects associated with IGF-I therapy are not entirely understood, it is possible that the rapid increase in free IGF-I that occurs after SC administration may alter normal dynamics of IGF-I plasma protein binding. This in turn may result in a supraphysiologic rate of IGF-I entry into the extravascular compartment, which might lead to the observed side effects.[152]

Coadministration of IGF-I with IGF binding protein III (IGF-BP-III) is an alternative method to increase IGF-I action while preventing a rapid increase in free IGF-I. Several short-term clinical trials of patients with T1DM and insulin-using patients with T2DM have shown that the combination of IGF-I and IGF-BP-III (SomatoKine, Insmed Inc, Glen Allen, Va) has nearly identical effects in improving glycemia, decreasing nocturnal GH, and lowering insulin requirements as IGF-I but without any of the reported side effects associated with IGF-I monotherapy.[152] Ongoing clinical trials are evaluating SomatoKine as a potential treatment for diabetes.

ENERGY AND METABOLIC HOMEOSTASIS: ADIPOCYTOKINES

In recent years a host of interesting peptides, proteins, and cytokines derived from peripheral tissues, most notably adipose tissue, have been discovered to have potential physiologic and pathophysiologic roles in energy homeostasis. These include leptin, tumor necrosis factor α, interleukin-6, plasminogen activator inhibitor 1, angiotensin II, acylation stimulating protein, resistin, and adiponectin.

Collectively, the adipocytokines have been reported to influence a variety of physiologic functions including energy homeostasis, inflammation, and atherosclerosis, although much of this work has been limited to animal models. Of these factors, leptin and adiponectin have received the most attention as potential therapeutic targets for the treatment of energy and metabolic dysregulation associated with obesity and diabetes.

Leptin

Leptin is primarily an adipocyte-derived hormone that plays an important role in regulating food intake and energy expenditure. This peptide was first described following identification of its mutation as the factor responsible for the obese (ob/ob) mouse.[153] Administration of leptin in ob/ob mice markedly decreased food intake and increased thermogenesis, which led to significant weight reduction. Humans with mutations causing leptin deficiency exhibit marked hyperphagia and severe obesity, conditions that are reversed with small doses of recombinant leptin.[154]

The effects of leptin appear to be mediated centrally in the hypothalamus, at least in part through decreasing NPY mRNA expression and increasing proopiomelanocortin (POMC) mRNA expression.[155] Enhancement of POMC concentrations in the ARC nucleus has been demonstrated to potently suppress food intake.

Several investigators have reported that leptin-induced weight loss in animal models cannot be attributed solely to reduced food intake. Central administration of leptin into the third ventricle of rhesus monkey brains increased circulating concentrations of the sympathetic neurotransmitter norepinephrine.[156] Leptin may therefore also modulate weight loss by increased energy expenditure following activation of the sympathetic nervous system.

Cases of obesity attributable to leptin mutations are rare, however, and the percentage of body fat is actually highly correlated with leptin concentrations. Higher concentrations are associated with more pronounced obesity.[154] In clinical trials, raising circulating leptin to supraphysiologic concentrations only marginally reduces food intake and induces weight loss in obese subjects.[157] In other words, the dose response to increasing leptin concentrations appears to be near maximal at physiologic concentrations.

Increased sensations of hunger during dieting in humans with congenital leptin deficiency, however, have been shown to correspond to the magnitude of decreases of circulating leptin.[158] Moreover, preventing the decline in leptin concentrations during an energy-restricted diet in rats was shown to significantly attenuate food-seeking behavior.[159] Therefore, leptin's primary role appears to lie in its decreased secretion during negative energy balance rather than the peptide itself serving as a signal of positive energy balance. Future studies are needed to determine if prevention of the fall in leptin during dieting and weight loss might prevent rebound weight gain that dieters often experience following successful weight reduction.

Adiponectin

Adiponectin is the most abundant adipose protein, accounting for 0.01% of total human plasma protein.[160] Plasma adiponectin concentrations are decreased in patients with T2DM and obesity, although in a study of Pima Indians and whites, the degree of hypoadiponectinemia was more closely related to the degree of hyperinsulinemia and insulin resistance than adiposity.[161]

Reduced adiponectin concentrations have been reported in rodent models of diabetes, and in rhesus monkeys, weight gain and insulin resistance corresponds to decreased adiponectin concentrations.[162] Similarly, heterozygous and homozygous adiponectin knockout mice become insulin resistant at 6 weeks of age.[163,164] Treatment with recombinant adiponectin in normal and diabetic rodents improves glucose tolerance and insulin sensitivity without stimulating insulin secretion.[165] This effect appears to result from marked enhancement of insulin's ability to suppress hepatic glucose production.[166] Other research has shown that adiponectin may stimulate 5′-AMP-activated protein kinase in skeletal muscle, which may enhance glucose metabolism by increasing fatty acid oxidation and glucose uptake (Fig. 30–11).[167-169]

90. Scrocchi LA, Marshall BA, Cook SM, et al: Glucose home-ostasis in mice with disruption of GLP-1 receptor signaling. Diabetes 47:632-639, 1998.

91. Edwards CM, Todd JF, Mahmoudi M, et al: Glucagon-like peptide 1 has a physiological role in the control of post-prandial glucose in humans: Studies with the antagonist exendin 9-39. Diabetes 48:86-93, 1999.

92. Shen HQ, Roth MD, Peterson RG: The effect of glucose and glucagon-like peptide-1 stimulation on insulin release in the perfused pancreas in a non-insulin dependent diabetes mellitus animal model. Metabolism 47:1042-1047, 1998.

93. Jia X, Elliott R, Kwok YN, et al: Altered glucose dependence of glucagon-like peptide 1(7-36)-induced insulin secretion from the Zucker (fa/fa) rat pancreas. Diabetes 44:495-500, 1995.

94. Young AA, Gedulin BR, Bhavsar S, et al: Glucose-lowering and insulin-sensitizing actions of exendin-4: Studies in obese diabetic (ob/ob, db/db) mice, diabetic fatty Zucker rats, and diabetic rhesus monkeys (Macaca mulatta). Diabetes 48:1026-1034, 1999.

95. Ribel U, Larsen M, Rolin B, et al: NN2211: A long-acting glucagon-like peptide-1 derivative with anti-diabetic effects in glucose-intolerant pigs. Eur J Pharmacol 451:217-225, 2002.

96. Szayna M, Doyle ME, Betkey JA, et al: Exendin-4 decelerates food intake, weight gain and fat deposition in Zucker rats. Endocrinology 141:1936-1941, 2000.

97. Rachman J, Barrow BA, Levy JC, et al: Near-normalisation of diurnal glucose concentrations by continuous adminis-tration of glucagon-like peptide-1 (GLP-1) in subjects with NIDDM. Diabetologia 40:205-211, 1997.

98. Nauck MA, Wollschlager D, Werner J, et al: Effects of sub-cutaneous glucagon-like peptide 1 (GLP-1 [7-36 amide]) in patients with NIDDM. Diabetologia 39:1546-1553, 1996.

99. Drucker DJ: Enhancing incretin action for the treatment of type 2 diabetes. Diabetes Care 26:2929-2940, 2003.

100. Zander M, Madsbad S, Madsen JL, et al: Effect of 6-week course of glucagon-like peptide 1 on glycaemic control, insulin sensitivity, and alpha cell function in type 2 dia-betes: A parallel-group study. Lancet 359:824-830, 2002.

101. Agerso H, Jensen LB, Elbrond B, et al: The pharmacokinet-ics, pharmacodynamics, safety and tolerability of NN2211, a new long-acting GLP-1 derivative, in healthy men. Dia-betologia 45:195-202, 2002.

102. Juhl CB, Hollingdal M, Sturis J, et al: Bedtime administra-tion of NN2211, a long-acting GLP-1 derivative, substan-tially reduces fasting and postprandial glycemia in type 2 diabetes. Diabetes 51:424-429, 2002.

103. Degn KB, Juhl CB, Sturis J, et al: One week's treatment with the long-acting glucagon-like peptide 1 derivative liraglu-tide (NN2211) markedly improves 24-h glycemia and alpha- and alpha cell function and reduces endogenous glucose release in patients with type 2 diabetes. Diabetes 53:1187-1194, 2004.

104. Madsbad S, Schmitz O, Ranstam J, et al: Improved glycemic control with no weight increase in patients with type 2 dia-betes after once-daily treatment with the long-acting glucagon-like peptide 1 analog liraglutide (NN2211): A 12-week, double-blind, randomized, controlled trial. Diabetes Care 27:1335-1342, 2004.

105. Giannoukakis N: CJC-1131. ConjuChem. Curr Opin Investig Drugs 4:1245-1249, 2003.

106. Benquet C, Leger R, Huang X, et al: (DAC:GLP-1) binds covalently in vivo to endogenous albumin: Update on the DAC technology. Diabetes 53:A116, 2004.

107. Guivarc'H P-H, Castaigne J-P, Gagnon C, et al: CJC-1131, a long acting GLP-1 analog safely normalizes postprandial glucose excursion and fasting glycemia in type 2 diabetes mellitus. Diabetes 53:A127, 2004.

108. Wen S, Chatenoid L, Lawrence B, et al: Lack of immuno-genicity of CJC-1311, a long-acting GLP-1 analog for the treatment of type 2 diabetes. Diabetes 53:A151, 2004.

109. Eng J, Kleinman WA, Singh L, et al: Isolation and charac-terization of exendin-4, an exendin-3 analogue from Heloderma suspectum venom. J Biol Chem 267:7402-7405, 1992.

110. Chen YE, Drucker D: Tissue-specific expression of unique mRNAs that encode pro-glucagon-derived peptides or exendin-4 in the lizard. J Biol Chem 272:4108-4115, 1997.

111. Kieffer TJ, McIntosh CH, Pederson RA: Degradation of glucose-dependent insulinotropic polypeptide and trun-cated glucagon-like peptide 1 in vitro and in vivo by dipeptidyl peptidase IV. Endocrinology 136:3585-3596, 1995.

112. Deacon CF, Nauck MA, Toft-Nielsen M, et al: Both subcu-taneously and intravenously administered glucagon like peptide I are rapidly degraded from the NH2-terminus in type II diabetic patients and in healthy subjects. Diabetes 44:1126-1231, 1995.

113. Fineman MS, Bicsak TA, Shen, LZ, et al: Effect on glycemic control of exenatide (synthetic exendin-4) additive to exist-ing metformin and/or sulfonylurea treatment in patients with type 2 diabetes. Diabetes Care 26:2370-2377, 2003.

114. Kolterman OG, Buse JB, Fineman MS, et al: Synthetic exendin-4 (exenatide) significantly reduces postprandial and fasting plasma glucose in subjects with type 2 diabetes. J Clin Endocrinol Metab 88:3082-3089, 2003.

115. Fehse FC, Trautmann ME, Holst JJ, et al: Effects of exenatide on first and second phase insulin secretion in response to intravenous glucose in subjects with type 2 diabetes. Dia-betes 53:A82, 2004.

116. Buse JB, Henry RR, Han J, et al: Effects of exenatide (exendin-4) on glycemic control over 30 weeks in sulfonyl-urea-treated patients with type 2 diabetes mellitus. Diabetes Care 27:2628-2635, 2004.

117. DeFronzo R, Ratner R, Han J, et al: Effects of exenatide (syn-thetic exendin-4) on glycemic control and weight over 30 weeks in metformin-treated patients with type 2 diabetes. American Diabetes Association 64th Annual Scientific Sessions. Orlando, Fla, June 4-8, 2004. Abstract 6-LB.

118. Kendall DM, Riddle MC, Zhuang D, et al: Effects of exe-natide (exendin-4) on glycemic control and weight in patients with type 2 diabetes treated with metformin and a sulfonylurea. American Diabetes Association 64th Annual Scientific Sessions. Orlando, Fla, June 4-8, 2004. Abstract 10-LB.

119. Villhauer EB, Brinkman JA, Naderi GB, et al: 1-[[(3-hydroxy-1-adamantyl)amino]acetyl]-2-cyano-(S)-pyrrolidine: A potent, selective, and orally bioavailable dipeptidyl peptidase IV inhibitor with antihyperglycemic properties. J Med Chem 46:2774-2789, 2003.

120. Ahren B, Landin-Olsson M, Jansson, PA, et al: Inhibition of dipeptidyl peptidase-4 reduces glycemia, sustains insulin levels, and reduces glucagon levels in type 2 diabetes. J Clin Endocrinol Metab 89:2078-2084, 2004.

121. Pratley R, Galbreath E: Twelve-week monotherapy with the DPP-4 inhibitor, LAF237 improves glycemic control in patients with type 2 diabetes (T2DM). Diabetes 53:A83, 2004.

122. Ahren B, Gomis R, Mills D, et al: The DPP-4 inhibitor, LAF237, improves glycemic control in patients with type 2 diabetes (T2DM) inadequately treated with metformin. Diabetes 53:A83, 2004.

123. Druce MR, Small CJ, Bloom SR: Minireview: Gut peptides regulating satiety. Endocrinology 145:2660-2665, 2004.

124. Date Y, Kojima M, Hosoda H, et al: Ghrelin, a novel growth hormone-releasing acylated peptide, is synthesized in a dis-tinct endocrine cell type in the gastrointestinal tracts of rats and humans. Endocrinology 141:4255-4261, 2000.

125. Tschop M, Smiley DL, Heiman ML: Ghrelin induces adi-posity in rodents. Nature 407:908-913, 2000.

126. Cummings DE, Purnell JQ, Frayo RS, et al: A preprandial rise in plasma ghrelin levels suggests a role in meal initia-tion in humans. Diabetes 50:1714-1719, 2001.

127. Haqq AM, Farooqi IS, O'Rahilly S, et al: Serum ghrelin levels are inversely correlated with body mass index, age, and insulin concentrations in normal children and are markedly increased in Prader-Willi syndrome. J Clin Endocrinol Metab 88:174-178, 2003.

128. Cummings DE, Weigle DS, Frayo RS, et al: Plasma ghrelin levels after diet-induced weight loss or gastric bypass surgery. N Engl J Med 346:1623-1630, 2002.

129. Wren AM, Seal LJ, Cohen MA, et al: Ghrelin enhances appetite and increases food intake in humans. J Clin Endocrinol Metab 86:5992, 2001.

130. Willesen MG, Kristensen P, Romer J: Co-localization of growth hormone secretagogue receptor and NPYmRNAin the arcuate nucleus of the rat. Neuroendocrinology 70:306-316, 1999.

131. Luckman SM, Rosenzweig I, Dickson SL: Activation of arcuate nucleus neurons by systemic administration of leptin and growth hormone-releasing peptide-6 in normal and fasted rats. Neuroendocrinology 70:93-100, 1999.

132. Dickson SL, Leng G, Robinson IC: Systemic administration of growth hormone-releasing peptide activates hypothalamic arcuate neurons. Neuroscience 52:303-306, 1993.

133. Hewson AK, Dickson SL: Systemic administration of ghrelin induces Fos and Egr-1 proteins in the hypothalamic arcuate nucleus of fasted and fed rats. J Neuroendocrinol 12:1047-1049, 2000.

134. Adrian TE, Ferri GL, Bacarese-Hamilton AJ, et al: Human distribution and release of a putative new gut hormone, peptide YY. Gastroenterology 89:1070-1077, 1985.

135. Batterham RL, Cowley MA, Small CJ, et al: Gut hormone PYY(3-36) physiologically inhibits food intake. Nature 418:650-654, 2002.

136. Druce M, Bloom SR: Central regulators of food intake. Curr Opin Clin Nutr Metab Care 6:361-367, 2003.

137. Batterham RL, Cohen MA, Ellis SM, et al: Inhibition of food intake in obese subjects by peptide YY3-36. N Engl J Med 349:941-948, 2003.

138. Le Roith D: Seminars in medicine of the Beth Israel Deaconess Medical Center. Insulin-like growth factors. N Engl J Med 336:633-640, 1997.

139. Holt RI, Simpson HL, Sonksen PH: The role of the growth hormone-insulin-like growth factor axis in glucose homeostasis. Diabet Med 20:3-15, 2003.

140. Jones JI, Clemmons DR: Insulin-like growth factors and their binding proteins: Biological actions. Endocr Rev 16:3-34, 1995.

141. Press M: Growth hormone and metabolism. Diabetes Metab Rev 4:391-414, 1988.

142. Wurzburger MI, Sonksen PH: Natural course of growth hormone hypersecretion in insulin-dependent diabetes mellitus. Med Hypotheses 46:145-149, 1996.

143. Bak JF, Moller N, Schmitz O: Effects of growth hormone on fuel utilization and muscle glycogen synthase activity in normal humans. Am J Physiol 260:E736-E742, 1991.

144. Smith LEH, Kopchick JJ, Chen W, et al: Essential role of growth hormone in ischemia induced retinal neovascularization. Science 276:1706-1708, 1997.

145. Yakar S, Liu JL, Fernandez AM, et al: Liver-specific IGF-I gene deletion leads to muscle insulin insensitivity. Diabetes 50:1110-1118, 2001.

146. Boulware SD, Tamborlane WV, Rennert NJ, et al: Comparison of the metabolic effects of recombinant human insulin-like growth factor-I and insulin. Dose-response relationships in healthy young and middle-aged adults. J Clin Invest 93:1131-1139, 1994.

147. Carroll PV, Umpleby M, Ward GS, et al: rhIGF-I administration reduces insulin requirements, decreases growth hormone secretion, and improves the lipid profile in adults with IDDM. Diabetes 46:1453-1458, 1997.

148. Schoenle EJ, Zenobi PD, Torresani T, et al: Recombinant human insulin-like growth factor I (rhIGF I) reduces hyperglycaemia in patients with extreme insulin resistance. Diabetologia 34:675-679, 1991.

149. Moses AC, Young SC, Morrow LA, et al: Recombinant human insulin-like growth factor I increases insulin sensitivity and improves glycemic control in type II diabetes. Diabetes 45:91-100, 1996.

150. Thrailkill KM, Quattrin T, Baker L, et al: Cotherapy with recombinant human insulin-like growth factor I and insulin improves glycemic control in type 1 diabetes. RhIGF-I in IDDM Study Group. Diabetes Care 22:585-592, 1999.

151. RhIGF-I Co-Therapy with Insulin Study Subgroup: RhIGF-I improves glucose control in insulin requiring type 2 diabetes. Proceedings of the 5th Annual Meeting of the American Diabetes Association. San Antonio, Tex, 1997. Abstract 582.

152. Clemmons DR, Moses AC, McKay MJ, et al: The combination of insulin-like growth factor I and insulin-like growth factor-binding protein-3 reduces insulin requirements in insulin-dependent type 1 diabetes: Evidence for in vivo biological activity. J Clin Endocrinol Metab 85:1518-1524, 2000.

153. Chen H, Charlat O, Tartaglia LA, et al: Evidence that the diabetes gene encodes the leptin receptor: Identification of a mutation in the leptin receptor gene in db/db mice. Cell 84:491-495, 1996.

154. Clement K, Vaisse C, Lahlou N, et al: A mutation in the human leptin receptor gene causes obesity and pituitary dysfunction. Nature 392:398-401, 1998.

155. Bjorbaek C, Kahn BB: Leptin signaling in the central nervous system and the periphery. Recent Prog Horm Res 59:305-331, 2004.

156. Satoh N, Ogawa Y, Katsuura G, et al: Satiety effect and sympathetic activation of leptin are mediated by hypothalamic melanocortin system. Neurosci Lett 249:107-110, 1998.

157. Havel PJ: Update on adipocyte hormones: Regulation of energy balance and carbohydrate/lipid metabolism. Diabetes 53:S143-S151, 2004.

158. Keim NL, Stern JS, Havel PJ: Relation between circulating leptin concentrations and appetite during a prolonged, moderate energy deficit in women. Am J Clin Nutr 68:794-801, 1998.

159. Figlewicz DP, Higgins MS, Ng-Evans SB, et al: Leptin reverses sucrose-conditioned place preference in food-restricted rats. Physiol Behav 73:229-234, 2001.

160. Maeda K, Okubo K, Shimomura I, et al: CDNA cloning and expression of a novel adipose specific collagen-like factor, ApM1 (AdiPose most abundant gene transcript 1). Biochem Biophys Res Commun 221:286-289, 1996.

161. Weyer C, Funahashi T, Tanaka S, et al: Hypoadiponectinemia in obesity and type 2 diabetes: Close association with insulin resistance and hyperinsulinemia. J Clin Endocrinol Metab 86:1930-1935, 2001.

162. Stefan N, Stumvoll M: Adiponectin: Its role in metabolism and beyond. Horm Metab Res 34:469-474, 2002.

163. Kubota N, Terauchi Y, Yamauchi T, et al: Disruption of adiponectin causes insulin resistance and neointimal formation. J Biol Chem 277:25863-25866, 2002.

164. Maeda N, Shimomura I, Kishida K, et al: Diet-induced insulin resistance in mice lacking adiponectin/ACRP30. Nat Med 8:731-737, 2002.

165. Berg AH, Combs TP, Du X, et al: The adipocyte secreted protein Acrp30 enhances hepatic insulin action. Nat Med 7:947-953, 2001.

166. Combs TP, Berg AH, Obici S, et al: Endogenous glucose production is inhibited by the adipose-derived protein Acrp30. J Clin Invest 108:1875-1881, 2001.

167. El-Haschimi K, Lehnert H: Leptin resistance—or why leptin fails to work in obesity. Exp Clin Endocrinol Diabetes 111:2-7, 2003.

168. Chandran M, Phillips SA, Ciaraldi T, et al: Adiponectin: More than just another fat cell hormone? Diabetes Care 26:2442-2450, 2003.

169. Yamauchi T, Kamon J, Waki H, et al: The fat derived hormone adiponectin reverses insulin resistance associated with both lipoatrophy and obesity. Nat Med 7:941-946, 2001.

Chapter 31

Pharmacologic Agents and Nutritional Supplements in the Treatment of Obesity

William T. Cefalu and Frank Greenway

KEY POINTS

- *Success with maintaining lifestyle changes to lose weight over the long term is poor.*
- *There are only a limited number of pharmaceutical agents currently approved for use in obesity, and long-term safety clearly is a concern.*
- *Nutritional supplementation with over-the-counter agents to address energy balance represent an attractive and novel approach for obesity.*
- *Very few of the over-the-counter agents promoted for this purpose have delivered on their promise.*

To develop a comprehensive and effective approach to the treatment of obesity, there must be sound scientific evidence in support of and agreement on the pathogenic mechanisms. Fortunately, there has been a rapid and substantive increase in our understanding of underlying physiologic systems and molecular pathways that contribute to the development of obesity because key regulators of energy balance and insulin signaling have been elucidated.

The concept of obesity is simple to grasp: It develops over time when a person takes in more calories than he or she burns. However, insight into the mechanisms behind this observation have revealed systems that are complex and highly integrated. Specifically, the *energy balance equation* implies that food consumption (energy intake) needs to match energy output (energy expenditure) to maintain a stable body weight. Major determinants of energy expenditure are the thermogenic effect of food (TEF), which represents the amount of energy used by ingestion and digestion of food we consume; physical activity; and resting metabolic rate (RMR), which is determined in large measure by the amount of lean body mass.

As outlined in Figure 31–1, ideal body weight for any person is maintained with a balance of energy intake and expenditure. Given the many obesity-promoting changes that have occurred in our environment, including excess energy consumption and reduced physical activity, this balance is shifting in many persons toward being overweight and obese at an alarming rate. It is also clear that many persons manage to resist obesity. The variable susceptibility to obesity in response to environmental factors is undoubtedly modulated by specific genes.[1,2] Further, it is understood that there is a dynamic interplay between the adipose tissue and other key tissues in the body, such as liver, muscle, and regulatory centers of the brain.

Altered regulation of this integrated and coordinated system inevitably leads to accumulation of body fat, insulin resistance, and development of the metabolic syndrome (see Fig. 31–1). Regardless of the underlying etiology, effective treatment of obesity, whether it is from a nonpharmacologic or pharmacologic approach, aims to alter the energy balance equation to one in which expenditure is increased and intake is reduced.

PUBLIC HEALTH SIGNIFICANCE

The public health significance of not treating obesity cannot be understated. Inevitably, obesity leads to the development of traditional and non-traditional risk factors and to the development of the metabolic syndrome. The metabolic syndrome is characterized by coexisting traditional risk factors for cardiovascular disease (CVD) such as hypertension, dyslipidemia, glucose intolerance, obesity, and insulin resistance, in addition to nontraditional CVD risk factors such as inflammatory processes and abnormalities of the blood coagulation system.[2-8] Although the etiology of the metabolic syndrome is not specifically known, it is well established that obesity and insulin resistance are generally present.

The metabolic syndrome contributes greatly to increased morbidity and mortality on several levels. First, the metabolic syndrome can be considered a prediabetic state as demonstrated in Figure 31–2. It is now well accepted that insulin resistance needs to be compensated by hyperinsulinemia in order to maintain normal glucose tolerance.[9,10] In persons who develop diabetes, a progressive loss of the insulin secretory capacity of beta cells appears to

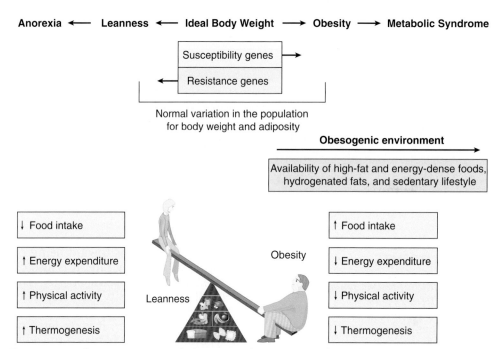

Figure 31–1. Factors contributing to energy balance. In the presence of an obesogenic environment, this balance is shifted to promote obesity.

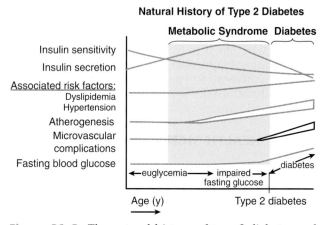

Figure 31–2. The natural history of type 2 diabetes and the importance of the metabolic syndrome in its genesis. The *shaded area* signifies the presence of the metabolic syndrome. (From Cefalu WT. Insulin resistance. In Leahy J, Clark N, Cefalu WT [eds]: The Medical Management of Diabetes Mellitus. New York: Marcel Dekker, 2000, pp 57-75.)

begin years before the clinical diagnosis of diabetes.[10-13] With worsening pancreatic dysfunction and the inability to fully compensate for the degree of insulin resistance, clinically overt type 2 diabetes manifests.[10-13] Thus, obesity and development of the metabolic syndrome figure prominently in the natural history of type 2 diabetes.

A second major reason obesity and the metabolic syndrome contribute to increased morbidity and mortality is the association with cardiovascular disease. Coexisting CVD risk factors such as dyslipidemia, hypertension, inflammatory markers, and coagulopathy are highly associated with the prediabetic state as defined by obesity and insulin resistance.[6,14-16] Each risk factor, considered alone, increases CVD risk, but in combination they provide an additive or synergistic effect.[16] The metabolic syndrome can increase the relative risk of CVD threefold to fourfold.[17] Furthermore, the increase in relative risk for CVD is elevated as much as 15 years before the diagnosis of diabetes is even made.[18]

Because of the CVD significance of the metabolic syndrome, the fact that the metabolic syndrome may be three to four times as common as diabetes, and the observation that obesity and other components of the metabolic syndrome, especially dyslipidemia and diabetes, have become global health epidemics, obesity and its related complications represent a serious public health concern. Approximately 7% to 8% of the population in the United States suffers from the complications of type 2 diabetes, and approximately 40% are obese and might have the metabolic syndrome.[19-21] Minority ethnic groups are at even greater risk.

It is not surprising that the World Health Organization has listed these conditions among the top 10 global health problems in western cultures, and some have considered obesity the most dangerous disease in the world today.[22,23] Strategies for successfully intervening in the development of obesity are urgently needed. Although lifestyle interventions consisting of weight loss and exercise greatly improve insulin sensitivity and can delay the progression to type 2 diabetes,[24] maintenance of lifestyle changes over the long term is poor. This

chapter focuses on the available pharmacologic approaches for treating obesity.

PHARMACOLOGIC AGENTS

Background

Obesity has been recognized as a chronic disease since the NIH Consensus Conference of 1985, but this concept started gaining greater acceptance after the discovery of leptin, when it became clear that the lack of a hormone could be responsible for obesity and replacing that hormone could reverse the obesity.[25,26] As with hypertension and other chronic diseases, medications are used to control the disease and must be given chronically. Medications approved before 1985 were studied and approved for up to 12 weeks as an aid to help reverse bad eating habits. This time limit arose from the belief that obesity was due to bad habits and habits could be retrained over a short period.

The acceptance of chronic medication treatment of obesity has been slow, probably due to two factors. First, obesity is stigmatized in our society, especially in women.[27] The obese are blamed for creating their own problem, and there is a general perception that they could solve the problem by simply pushing away from the table and walking around the block. This attitude ignores evidence that body weight is a controlled variable like blood pressure and is not totally under volitional control. Nevertheless, blaming the victim is common in stigmatized conditions, as is evident with alcoholics and people afflicted with some mental disorders. The second factor is the poor safety record of many obesity medications (Table 31–1).

Thyroid hormone, one of the first treatments for obesity, causes hyperthyroidism.[28] In the 1930s, dinitrophenol as an obesity treatment was associated with cataract formation and neuropathy, prompting its withdrawal from the market.[29] Amphetamine use began in the late 1930s, and the concern regarding addiction still casts a long shadow over all obesity drugs with a similar structure regardless of their addictive potential.[30] In the 1970s aminorex, an obesity drug sold in Europe, was withdrawn due to its association with primary pulmonary hypertension.[31] Fenfluramine, part of the popular phen-fen combination, was withdrawn because of associated cardiac valvular abnormalities.[32] Phenylpropanolamine and ephedra have been withdrawn from the over-the-counter markets due to concerns about hemorrhagic stroke and other cardiovascular events.[33,34]

One can make several generalizations about obesity medications and the studies done to approve them. First, with the exception of topiramate, which gives weight loss for 18 months, all obesity drugs give weight loss for only the first 6 months of use.[35] After the weight-loss period, these

Table 31–1 *Medications No Longer Used to Treat Obesity Due to Safety Considerations*

Drug	Safety Concern	Year
Thyroid hormone	Hyperthyroidism	1890s
Dinitrophenol	Cataracts and neuropathy	1930s
Amphetamine	Drug abuse	1930s
Aminorex	Primary pulmonary hypertension	1970s
Fenfluramine	Heart valve pathology	1990s
Phenylpropanolamine	Hemorrhagic stroke	2000
Ephedra	Cardiovascular events	2004

Table 31–2 *Weight Loss Exceeding Placebo at Time Points in the First Year of Weight Loss Trials Testing Obesity Drugs*

Drug	3 mo	6 mo	12 mo
Phentermine	—	—	7.0 kg
Sibutramine	2.8 kg	—	4.5 kg
Orlistat	—	3.2 kg	3.2 kg
Bupropion	—	2.0 kg	4.9 kg
Topiramate	—	6.5 kg	9.1 kg
Zonisamide	—	5 kg	—
Axokine	—	—	3.3 kg
Rimonabant	—	5 kg	6.5 kg

drugs serve to maintain the lost weight. Being aware of this pattern is important to the treating physician, because patients assume that the drug is no longer working when the weight stops decreasing. One needs to think of these drugs in a manner similar to antihypertensive medications. One does not expect that the blood pressure will keep decreasing indefinitely, and one is not surprised when blood pressure rebounds after antihypertensive medications are stopped. Although obesity medications should be viewed in the same manner, achieving that goal can require an education process.

Obesity drug trials are unique in that they combine more than one obesity treatment. Ethics boards require that the placebo group receive treatment in obesity drug trials. Therefore, the drug and placebo treatments are combined with diet and exercise. The strength of the ancillary weight-loss programs is variable. A more vigorous ancillary weight loss program gives greater weight loss, but the difference between drug and placebo becomes less. European obesity drug trials tend to have greater weight losses, because the criterion for approval is 10% weight loss that is statistically greater than placebo.[36] Obesity drug trials in the United States tend to have a weaker ancillary weight loss program associated with them, give less weight loss, but have greater separation between drug and placebo. This is probably due to the FDA approval criterion that stipulates a 5% greater weight loss than placebo[37] (Table 31–2).

The drugs approved for the treatment of obesity can be divided into two categories, those approved before 1985 and those approved since. The drugs approved before 1985 are chemically related to amphetamine and all are associated with some degree of CNS stimulation. Phentermine and diethylpropion are DEA class IV and are thought to have a lower abuse potential than phendimetrazine and benzphetamine, which also are in DEA class IV, or phenmetrazine, which is in DEA class II.

One might logically ask if these drugs can be useful in a chronic disease when they are all approved for up to 12 weeks of use. There is a study comparing phentermine given continuously to phentermine given every other month and to a placebo in a 36-week trial.[38] The intermittent use of phentermine gave weight loss equivalent to continuous use of phentermine. The intermittent regimen gave lower drug exposure, was less expensive, and allowed phentermine to be used in a way that is consistent with its package insert. Although the long-term studies of these drugs are limited, phentermine gave a 7.9 kg greater weight loss than placebo at 1 year.[39]

Drugs Approved for Long-Term Use

There are only two medications approved for long-term use to treat obesity: orlistat and sibutramine. Orlistat is an inhibitor of pancreatic lipase and causes one third of dietary fat to be lost in the stool.[40] Orlistat is designed for use with a 30% fat diet. It gives approximately 3.2 kg more weight loss than placebo at 6 months and 3.2 kg more weight loss than placebo at 1 year.[41]

The adverse events associated with the use of orlistat can be predicted from its mechanism of action. There is an increased incidence of diarrhea, flatulence, and dyspepsia. Orlistat gives the expected decrease in blood glucose and blood pressure with weight loss, but it gives a reduction in lipids in excess of that expected for the degree of weight loss, probably because it enforces a low-fat diet.

Sibutramine is a reuptake inhibitor of norepinephrine and serotonin. It gives 2.8 kg more weight loss than placebo at 3 months and 4.5 kg more weight loss than placebo at 1 year.[42] The adverse events associated with the use of sibutramine are associated with its adrenergic mechanism of action and include dry mouth, insomnia, and nausea. Sibutramine gives the expected improvement in glucose and lipids with weight loss. Sibutramine is associated with an average increase in pulse rate of 4 beats per minute. The expected improvement in blood pressure is not seen, probably due to noradrenergic stimulation.

Other Drugs

Although only two drugs are approved for the long-term treatment of obesity, some drugs approved for the treatment of epilepsy or depression have been associated with weight loss. Fluoxetine 60 mg daily was evaluated as a potential obesity medication. It gave weight loss for the first 6 months, but while patients were still taking the drug, their weight returned almost to baseline by 1 year.[43] This was presumably the reason that it was not approved for the treatment of a chronic disease.

Bupropion 400 mg has been studied for weight loss in a 6-month trial of depressed patients and in a 1-year trial of obese subjects without depression.[44,45] Weight loss was 2 kg greater in the bupropion group than in the placebo group at 6 months and 4.9 kg greater than placebo at 1 year, suggesting that depressed subjects respond with less weight loss than those without depression. Bupropion is associated with dry mouth and insomnia, but despite its noradrenergic mechanism it does not seem to cause a rise in pulse or blood pressure.

Topiramate and zonisamide are approved for the treatment of epilepsy and have caused weight loss in clinical trials. Topiramate is unique in that it seems to give weight loss for at least 1year rather than only 6 months, as seems to be the case with other drugs that cause weight loss.[46] Topiramate at 192 mg/day gave 6.5 kg greater weight loss than placebo at 6 months, and zonisamide at 400 mg/day gave 5 kg greater weight loss than placebo at 4 months.[47,48] Both of these medications are associated with CNS adverse events such as slowed thinking.

There are two medications in phase III of drug development for long-term treatment of obesity. Axokine, a large protein that works in the leptin pathway distal to leptin, gave 3.3 kg greater weight loss than placebo at 1 year. One third of the subjects developed antibodies to this injectable peptide, and those subjects lost less than 1% of their body weight during the 1-year trial. Adverse events included injection site reactions, nausea, and dry cough. Although this medication was well tolerated, the antibody formation, poor efficacy, and delivery by injections dampen enthusiasm for this medication.

Rimonabant is a cannabanoid-1 receptor antagonist that decreases the intake of highly palatable food. Although a phase II trial in uncomplicated obesity gave marginal weight loss, studies in dyslipidemic subjects gave 5 kg better weight loss than placebo at 6 months and 6.5 kg better weight loss than placebo at 1 year. Adverse events included nausea and diarrhea, but the drug was well tolerated and more dropouts occurred in the placebo group. There was a greater than expected improvement in lipids, and the expected improvement in glucose with weight loss occurred.

Combination drug treatment is standard in the treatment of other chronic diseases. Attempts to

combine sibutramine and orlistat have not resulted in additional weight loss, and other combination treatments for obesity with approved medications other than caffeine and ephedrine have not been reported.[49] Caffeine with ephedrine was an approved obesity drug in Denmark, and it has been used in the United States for the treatment of asthma for decades. Although these drugs are inexpensive, give weight loss similar to the approved obesity drugs', and are available by prescription, they are not approved for treating obesity.[50]

NONPRESCRIPTION OBESITY DRUGS

Nonprescriptions drugs for the treatment of obesity fall into two general categories: drugs with a monograph by the FDA for sale over the counter without a prescription, and dietary herbal supplements. Until recently there were two approved drugs sold under an FDA monograph for obesity, phenylpropanolamine and benzocaine.

Phenylpropanolamine

Phenylpropanolamine is a nonmethylated form of ephedrine that was synthesized in the early 1900s. It was originally used intravenously to raise blood pressure during general anesthesia, but in 1939 Hirsch made uncontrolled observations that it was an effective appetite suppressant. Phenylpropanolamine was marketed as an appetite suppressant beginning in the 1960s, and in 1979 the FDA determined it was safe and effective for this purpose.[51]

Phenylpropanolamine gives weight loss similar to prescription anorectic medications' during the first 4 weeks of treatment.[52] The longest trial with phenylpropanolamine lasted 20 weeks, and at that point the phenylpropanolamine group lost 6.5% of initial body weight compared to 0.5% for the placebo group. This meets the FDA criteria for obesity drug approval, being greater than 5% more weight loss than the placebo.[53] Attempts to add benzocaine to phenylpropanolamine did not result in enhanced weight loss.[54]

In 2000 Kernan and coworkers reported that phenylpropanolamine was associated with an increased incidence of hemorrhagic stroke.[55] Phenylpropanolamine was subsequently removed from the market both as an appetite suppressant and as a component of cough and cold preparations.

Benzocaine

Benzocaine is a topical anesthetic that acts upon nerve endings, affects taste, and decreases the ability to discriminate different degrees of sweetness.[56-59] Plotz treated 50 subjects, 45 of whom had heart disease, in an open-label study with chewing gum containing methylcellulose and benzocaine. This group lost 2.3 pounds per week in the first 3 weeks and 1.8 pounds per week during the remainder of this 10-week trial.[56] Gould performed an open-label study with 100 subjects using diet and benzocaine candy. This group lost 2 pounds per week with a drop in blood pressure during this 11-week trial.[57] Piscano and Lichter reported a 3.8 pound weight loss in 26 children treated with benzocaine candy for 8 weeks with continued normal growth.[59]

McClure and Brusch divided 310 obese subjects into 5 groups of 62 each. The first group was treated with amphetamine, the second was treated with appetite suppressant, the third was treated with diet, the fourth was treated with sucrose hard candy, and the fifth was treated with sucrose hard candy with benzocaine, caffeine, and vitamins. By the end of 4 weeks, the group on benzocaine candy lost 12 pounds, which was twice as much as the group taking amphetamine and 5 times as much as those in the hard candy group. At 21 weeks the benzocaine group was still losing 2 pounds per week, which was greater than any other group.[58]

Collip reported a double-blind placebo-controlled trial in 52 subjects with benzocaine candy. Subjects took 9 to 15 candies a day, each containing 5 mg of benzocaine. The benzocaine group lost 6.7 ± 4.35 pounds compared with 2.54 ± 3.8 pounds in the placebo group over the course of the 6-week trial ($P < 0.001$).[60]

HERBAL SUPPLEMENTS

The use of dietary herbal supplements has increased in the last decade as a result of the Dietary Supplements Health Education Act of 1994, which allows manufacturers to market these products without showing safety or efficacy. Because there is no need to show safety or efficacy, there has been little impetus to do clinical trials with dietary herbal supplements. Many of the dietary herbal supplements are a combination of ingredients to give them brand identity. This makes determining the active ingredient difficult even if clinical trials are done. We will review the herbal supplements that have been used to treat obesity that have some data to support their use.

Metabolic Stimulants

Caffeine and Ephedra
Caffeine and ephedra (also known as ma huang) until recently was the major dietary herbal supplement used for weight loss. In fact, an estimated three billion doses of ephedra-containing supplements were sold in 1999.[61] There are three trials showing that ephedra combined with herbal forms

Table 31–3 *Trials Showing that Ephedra Combined with Herbal Forms of Caffeine Are Effective in Causing Weight Loss*

Author	Start D/P	End D/P	Dose (E/C)	Length	Lost D/P (kg)	Lost D/P (%)
Boozer et al[62]	35/32	24/24	72/240 mg/d	8 wk	4/0.8	4.4/0.9
Boozer et al[63]	83/84	46/41	90/192 mg/d	6 mo	7/3.1	7.9/3.5
Greenway et al[64]	20/20	12/19	72/210 mg/d	12 wk	3/0.8	3.6/1

D/P, drug/placebo; E/C, ephedra plus caffeine.

of caffeine are effective in causing weight loss that is in the range of 8% of initial body weight at 6 months[62-64] (Table 31–3).

There was concern about the quality of these herbal caffeine and ephedra supplements, and some were found to have different amounts of ephedra than were claimed on the label.[65] There were also 31 adverse events reported that were deemed to be definitely or probably related to the use of ephedra-containing products, including hypertension, arrhythmias, stroke, and seizures. Twenty-six percent of these events resulted in death or disability.[66]

Shekelle and colleagues reviewed obesity and athletic performance trials using ephedra or ephedrine, with and without caffeine. Although there were no serious adverse events in the clinical trials, the prevalence of psychiatric, autonomic, or gastrointestinal symptoms and heart palpitations was increased 2.2 to 3.6 times in the ephedra groups.[67] In February 2004 the FDA declared ephedra an adulterant, and this herb was removed from the market.

There is little evidence of efficacy for other dietary herbal supplements sold for weight loss and the treatment of obesity.[68] Nevertheless, we will try to review some of the dietary herbal supplements that have been marketed for this purpose that have supporting evidence.

Green Tea Catechins
Green tea extract is a common ingredient in herbal supplements for weight loss. Catechins in green tea, such as epigallocatechin gallate, inhibit catechol-*O*-methyl transferase, the enzyme that degrades norepinephrine.[69] In vitro brown fat cell experiments have demonstrated that green tea extract containing both catechins and caffeine was more potent in stimulating thermogenesis than equimolar concentrations of caffeine alone.[70]

Because caffeine is contained in green tea extract naturally, it has been difficult to separate the effects of green tea extract from that of caffeine. Dulloo and colleagues gave subjects green tea capsules three times a day, providing a total of 150 mg of caffeine and 375 mg of catechins of which 270 mg was epigallocatechin gallate. The subjects spent three 24-hour periods in a metabolic chamber, during which they received the green tea extract, 150 mg of caffeine, or a placebo. Energy expenditure was higher by 4.5% in the green tea group compared to

the placebo group and 3.2% higher than when the same dose of caffeine was given alone. In addition, fat oxidation was increased. The net effect attributable to green tea was estimated to be 328 kJ/d or about 80 kcal/d.[71]

Although the in vitro studies and metabolic chamber experiments show promise for green tea extract in the treatment of obesity, there is sparse evidence of weight loss from clinical trials. Chantre and Lairon reported a 4.6% weight loss in 12 weeks, but this was an open-label study without a control group, which makes drawing firm conclusions difficult.[72] Kovacs and coworkers evaluated the ability of green tea extract to help maintain a 7.5% weight loss compared to placebo over 13 weeks. Weight regain was similar in both groups.[73] Thus, there is no controlled clinical trial data showing the efficacy of green tea in the treatment of obesity.

Citrus Aurantium
Since ephedra was removed from the market, the use of bitter orange (citrus aurantium) has increased. This herb contains synephrine, phenylephrine, and octopamine, which are α-adrenergic agonists and indirect sympathetic agonists. A study by Colker and colleagues compared an herbal mixture consisting of citrus aurantium extract 975 mg/day, caffeine 528 mg/day, and St. John's wort 900 mg/day with placebo in 23 overweight subjects. Although the herb group lost 1.4 kg more weight than the placebo group, the difference between the groups was not statistically significant.[74]

Case reports have associated supplements containing bitter orange with cardiovascular events.[75] Thus, despite widespread use, this supplement does not have good studies to support its efficacy, and other reports raise questions about its safety.

Red Chili Pepper (Capsaicin)
Three grams of red pepper combined with 200 mg of caffeine decreased food intake and increased energy expenditure compared to the placebo condition, giving a difference in energy balance between the two conditions of 4000 kJ/day.[76] Five grams of fresh chili pepper increased metabolic rate in Thai women.[77] Three milligrams of capsaicin, the active ingredient in red peppers, increased energy expenditure and sympathetic activity in lean, but not obese, young women.[78] Strong soup containing chili peppers decreased subsequent fat intake, but capsules containing the same amount of chili

pepper did not.[79] Red pepper not only increased energy expenditure in women but also increased lipid oxidation.[80]

Another study demonstrated a decrease in energy intake in addition to a decrease in fat and protein intake after ingestion of red pepper.[81] A study in men demonstrated that the increase in energy expenditure after a meal containing red pepper is due to an increase in sympathetic activity that can be blocked by propanolol.[82]

Two clinical trials have evaluated the effect of capsaicin on body weight. The first was a 4-week trial in which the capsaicin was combined with chromium, inulin, phenylalanine, and other ingredients, but there was no difference in weight loss compared to the placebo group.[83] The second trial induced an 8% weight loss with diet and randomized participants to 135 mg of capsaicin per day or to placebo. Weight regain was not different between the groups, but the capsaicin group had a lower respiratory quotient.[84] Thus, although there are encouraging results from acute dosing of red chili peppers and capsaicin, there is no support for capsaicin giving greater weight loss in the trials in which it was compared to placebo.

Fat Metabolism and Nutrient Partitioning

Guggul
Guggul is a resin produced by the mukul mirth tree. Guggulipid is extracted from guggul and contains plant sterols (guggulsterones) that are believed to be its bioactive compounds. There have been four trials comparing guggul or guggal derivatives to placebo for obesity. None gave a statistically superior weight loss compared to placebo.

Bhatt and coworkers in a trial of 58 subjects given guggulipid 1.5 grams three times a day for a month showed only a trend toward weight loss in subjects who weighed more than 90 kg.[85] Shidu and coworkers gave 4 grams per day of guggul gum to 60 subjects for 4 weeks and saw a trend toward weight loss in the guggul group.[86] Koyiyal and coworkers and Antonio and coworkers conducted trials of 85 and 20 subjects, respectively, and neither demonstrated more weight loss in the guggul groups.[87,88] Thus, there is no evidence to support the use of guggul for weight loss.

Evening Primrose Oil
Evening primrose oil contains gamma linolenic acid and has been proposed as a treatment for obesity. Haslett and coworkers compared evening primrose oil and placebo in 100 obese women by giving 2 capsules 4 times a day plus a weight-reduction diet. There was no difference in weight loss over the 12 weeks of the study between the groups.[89] Thus, there is no reason to believe that evening primrose oil is effective in the treatment of obesity.

Congugated Linoleic Acid
Conjugated linoleic acid with the double bonds in the cis-9,trans-11 configuration is formed naturally in the rumen of cattle.[90] Synthetic conjugated linoleic acid is a mixture of cis-9,trans-11 and trans-10,cis-12 isomers.[91]

Clinical trials with synthetic conjugated linoleic acid have shown a reduction in body fat mass at 12 weeks and a reduction in sagittal diameter at 4 weeks.[92,93] Another trial demonstrated a greater regain of lean body mass and a higher metabolic rate with treatment with conjugated linoleic acid after weight loss of 7% of body weight compared to placebo.[94] There was also a decrease in appetite in the conjugated linoleic acid group but no effect on limiting weight regain.[95] In one year-long trial, the conjugated linoleic acid group lost more body fat mass and retained greater lean body mass than the placebo group,[96] but another year-long trial showed no advantage with conjugated linoleic acid for maintaining a 10% to 20% weight loss.[97]

In addition to clinical trials showing marginal advantages for conjugated linoleic acid on body composition, there are trials that raise questions about the long-term safety of conjugated linoleic acid. One trial with cis-9,trans-11 gave increased insulin resistance and increased lipid peroxidation in the conjugated linoleic acid group.[98] Trials with the trans-10,cis-12 isomer also increased insulin resistance and glycemia, reduced high-density lipoprotein (HDL) cholesterol,[99] and increased both oxidative stress and inflammatory markers.[100] Therefore, despite some evidence of beneficial changes in body composition, conjugated linoleic acid seems to worsen insulin resistance. Insulin resistance is associated with the major diseases associated with obesity. Therefore, the use of conjugated linoleic acid for obesity cannot be recommended.

Garcinia cambogia (Hydroxycitrate)
Garcinia cambogia contains hydroxycitric acid, the one isomer out of 16 that inhibits citrate lyase, the first step in fatty acid synthesis outside the mitochondrion. Although hydroxycitrate gave weight loss in rodents,[101] clinical trials have been disappointing. Hydroxycitrate does not seem to increase fat oxidation,[102] decrease food intake, or increase satiety.[103]

One 12-week trial showed a weight loss of 3.7 kg for the hydroxycitrate group, which was significantly greater than the 2.4-kg loss in the placebo group,[104] but two other trials, one with more subjects[105] and the other over 8 weeks,[106] showed no weight loss greater than placebo. Therefore, despite encouraging animal data, there is no evidence that hydroxycitrate is effective for the treatment of obesity in humans.

Dehydroepiandrosterone
Dehydroepiandrosterone is the most abundant steroid in humans. It is a weak androgen but can be converted to estrogens in tissues. Although this

steroid causes weight loss in animals, evidence for weight loss in humans is minimal.

An early study using 200 mg of dehydroepiandrosterone per day showed weight loss in half the women in the trial; the responders were older.[107] Studies in both men and women at 1600 mg/day, however, showed no change in body weight.[108-111] Elderly women treated with 50 mg of dehydroepiandrosterone per day to restore their levels to more youthful values did have a significant decrease in visceral fat and improvement in insulin sensitivity.[112] Thus, dehydroepiandrosterone may be helpful in decreasing the insulin resistance of aging, but there is little evidence for efficacy in the treatment of obesity.

AMINO ACIDS AND AMINO ACID DERIVATIVES

Beta-Hydroxy-Beta-Methylbutyrate

Beta-hydroxy-beta-methylbutyrate is a metabolite of leucine sold to burn fat and build muscle. Although it has been shown at 1.5 to 3 g per day to reduce muscle catabolism and increase fat-free mass in a 2 to 6 week weightlifting program,[113] it has not been evaluated for the treatment of obesity.

5-Hydroxytryptophan and Tyrosine

Supplementation by amino acids or their derivatives has been suggested as a treatment for obesity. 5-Hydroxytryptophan is a precursor of serotonin, and the synthesis of serotonin appears to be substrate limited.

Two small trials have evaluated 5-hydroxytryptophan supplementation. The first trial in 19 subjects showed small but significantly greater weight loss compared to placebo.[114] The second trial was 12 weeks long and studied 28 subjects. The 5-hydroxytryptophan group lost about 5% of body weight and significantly more than placebo.[115]

Tyrosine is the precursor to norepinephrine, but this neurotransmitter is thought to be enzyme limited. In the face of an indirect release of catecholamines, there is evidence in rodents that the reaction may become substrate limited,[116] but trials have not been conducted.

DIETARY FIBER AND ALGAE

Spirulina

Spirulina is a cyanobacterium (also called *blue-green algae*) that grows in warm waters and is usually grown in controlled conditions, which reduces the chances of contamination. A single trial by Becker and colleagues evaluated 200 mg spirulina tablets compared to 200 mg spinach tablets. Fifteen subjects took 14 tablets three times a day for four weeks. There was no difference between the two groups, but there was a statistically significant decrease in body weight from baseline in the spirulina group that did not occur in the placebo group.[117] Thus, although there is no evidence for efficacy with spirulina, it appears that the only study may have been underpowered to detect a difference if it exists.

Dietary Fiber

Epidemiologically, dietary fiber has been inversely related to BMI.[118] The bulk of evidence suggests that dietary fiber decreases food intake and decreases hunger. Water-soluble fiber may be more efficient than water-insoluble fiber in this regard. Dietary fiber supplements of 5 to 40 g/day lead to weight losses 1 to 3 kg more than placebo. Although this amount of weight loss is less than the 5% considered medically significant, the safety of dietary fiber and its other potential benefits for cardiovascular risk factors lead one to recommend its inclusion in weight-loss diets.[119]

Chitosan

Chitosan is deacetylated chitin from the exoskeletons of crustaceans like shrimp and can be considered an animal-derived dietary fiber. Chitosan has been claimed to be a fat blocker and has been advertised in demonstrations in which it precipitates corn oil mixed with water. It is claimed to cause fat malabsorption and weight loss.

Two studies have evaluated the ability of chitosan to cause fat malabsorption. One demonstrated that a combination of chitosan, 2.1 g, and psyllium husk, 300 mg, increased fecal fat excretion by 3 to 4 grams per day, the equivalent of 27 to 36 kcal.[120] A second study compared 2.5 grams of chitosan per day with 360 mg of orlistat per day. There was no increase in fecal fat with chitosan, but there was a 16-gram increase in the orlistat group.[121]

Studies to determine whether chitosan causes weight loss are more numerous. One 6-month trial in 50 obese women with 4.5 grams of chitosan per day saw a 15.9 kg loss in the chitosan group and a 10.9 kg loss in the placebo group, a difference that was significant.[122] Another trial in 68 subjects compared 750 mg of chitosan per day with placebo over 12 weeks and found no difference from placebo.[123] An 8-week trial with 2.4 g chitosan per day in 51 obese women also gave no more weight loss than placebo.[124] A 4-week trial in 30 overweight volunteers gave no difference from placebo as well.[125]

The most convincing study was done by Mhurchu and colleagues.[126] Two hundred fifty over-

weight and obese subjects were randomized to 3g of chitosan per day or placebo for 6 months. The chitosan group lost 0.4kg and the placebo group gained 0.2kg. Due to the large number of subjects, this difference was statistically significant, but is not a clinically significant difference. One would be hard pressed to recommend an obesity treatment that causes less than a 1% difference in weight compared to placebo at 6 months.

CHROMIUM

Several studies have evaluated the effects of chromium supplementation on body weight and composition in persons with and without diabetes. Chromium supplementation has variable effects on body weight and composition in patients with diabetes.[127-136] One study of patients with diabetes indicated no significant effects on either body weight or BMI,[132] but another in elderly subjects with impaired glucose tolerance demonstrated significant reductions in BMI.[131] Of the eight double blind, placebo-controlled trials in subjects without diabetes, chromium supplementation showed decrease in weight and fat in three larger studies.[127-136] Other effects that have been reported include an increase in lean body mass, a decrease in percentage of body fat, and an increase in basal metabolic rate (BMR).[137-138] A meta-analysis of 10 studies in humans showed a small differential effect in favor of chromium.[139]

These results generally support the view that chromium supplementation has at best modest effects on body weight or composition in patients with diabetes and perhaps more consistent positive effects in healthy volunteers. However, most of the studies addressing this question included only small numbers of subjects and were of relatively short duration. In addition, few if any of the studies evaluated redistribution of fat with computed tomography (CT) or magnetic resonance imaging (MRI) or measured parameters assessing alterations in adipocyte function or differentiation. Therefore, there appears to be considerably more work to be done in this area.

CONCLUSIONS

Obesity is, and based on current projections will continue to be, a major public health problem. Although it is well established that lifestyle modification can be successful to decrease weight and effectively improve many of the risk factors associated with obesity and development of the metabolic syndrome, the success of maintaining lifestyle changes over a chronic period is poor. Therefore, strategies to reduce weight by pharmacologic means have represented the traditional approach for clinical medicine.

Unfortunately, there are only a limited number of pharmaceutical agents currently approved for use in obesity, and long-term safety clearly is a concern. Thus, different strategies are urgently needed.

Because of the widespread use of dietary supplements by the general public, nutritional supplementation with over-the-counter agents that effectively address components of the energy balance equation represents a very attractive and novel approach for obesity intervention. However, very few of the over-the-counter agents promoted for this purpose have delivered on their promise.

References

1. Bouchard C: Genetics and the metabolic syndrome. Int J Obes Relat Metab Disord 19 (suppl 1):S52-S59, 1995.
2. Liese AD, Mayer-Davis EJ, Haffner SM: Development of the multiple metabolic syndrome: An epidemiologic perspective. Epidemiol Rev 20:157-172, 1998.
3. DeFronzo RA: Insulin resistance, hyperinsulinemia, and coronary artery disease: A complex metabolic web. J Cardiovasc Pharmacol 20 (Suppl 11):S1-S16, 1992.
4. Reaven GM: Banting lecture 1988. Role of insulin resistance in human disease. Diabetes 37:1595-1607, 1988.
5. Haffner SM: The insulin resistance syndrome revisited. Diabetes Care 19:275-277, 1996.
6. Isomaa B. Almgren P, Tuomi T, et al: Cardiovascular morbidity and mortality associated with the metabolic syndrome. Diabetes Care 24:683-689, 2001.
7. Devaraj S, Rosenson RS, Jialal I: Metabolic syndrome: An appraisal of the pro-inflammatory and procoagulant status. Endocrinol Metab Clin North Am 33:431-453, 2004.
8. Caballero AE: Endothelial dysfunction, inflammation, and insulin resistance: A focus on subjects at risk for type 2 diabetes. Curr Diab Rep 4:237-246, 2004.
9. Kahn SE: The importance of the beta-cell in the pathogenesis of type 2 diabetes. Am J Med 108(Suppl 6a):2S-8S, 2000.
10. Buchanan TA: Pancreatic beta-cell loss and preservation in type 2 diabetes. Clin Ther 25(Suppl B):B32-B46, 2003.
11. Weyer C, Bogardus C, Mott DM, Pratley RE: The natural history of insulin secretory dysfunction and insulin resistance in the pathogenesis of type 2 diabetes mellitus. J Clin Invest 104:787-794, 1999.
12. Weyer C, Tataranni PA, Bogardus C, Pratley RE: Insulin resistance and insulin secretory dysfunction are independent predictors of worsening of glucose tolerance during each stage of type 2 diabetes development. Diabetes Care 24:89-94, 2001.
13. Cefalu WT: Insulin resistance. In Leahy J, Clark N, Cefalu WT (eds): The Medical Management of Diabetes Mellitus. New York, Marcel Dekker, 2000, pp 57-75.
14. McLaughlin T, Allison G, Abbasi F, et al: Prevalence of insulin resistance and associated cardiovascular disease risk factors among normal weight, overweight, and obese individuals. Metabolism 53:495-499, 2004.
15. Shirai K: Obesity as the core of the metabolic syndrome and the management of coronary heart disease. Curr Med Res Opin 20:295-304, 2004.
16. Expert Panel on Detection, Evaluation, and Treatment of High Blood Cholesterol in Adults: Executive Summary of the Third Report of The National Cholesterol Education Program (NCEP) Expert Panel on Detection, Evaluation, and Treatment of High Blood Cholesterol in Adults (Adult Treatment Panel III). JAMA 285:2486-2497, 2001.
17. Lakka HM, Laaksonen DE, Lakka TA, et al: The metabolic syndrome and total and cardiovascular disease mortality in middle-aged men. JAMA 288:2709-2716, 2002.

18. Hu FB, Stampfer MJ, Haffner SM, et al: Elevated risk of cardiovascular disease prior to clinical diagnosis of type 2 diabetes. Diabetes Care 25:1129-1134, 2002.

19. Centers for Disease Control and Prevention: Diabetes prevalence among American Indians and Alaska Natives and the overall population—United States, 1994-2002. MMWR Morb Mortal Wkly Rep 52:702-704, 2003.

20. Mokdad AH, Ford ES, Bowman BA, et al: Prevalence of obesity, diabetes, and obesity-related health risk factors, 2001. JAMA 289:76-79, 2003.

21. Ford ES, Giles WH, Dietz WH: Prevalence of the metabolic syndrome among US adults: Findings from the third National Health and Nutrition Examination Survey. JAMA 287:356-359, 2002.

22. Obesity: Preventing and Managing the Global Epidemic: Report of a WHO Consultation. WHO Technical Report Series, 894. Geneva, World Health Organization, 2000.

23. Evans RM, Barish GD, Wang YU: PPARs and the complex journey to obesity. Nat Med 10:355-361, 2004.

24. Knowler WC, Barrett-Connor E, Fowler SE, and the Diabetes Prevention Program Research Group: Reduction in the incidence of type 2 diabetes with lifestyle intervention or metformin. N Engl J Med 346:393-403, 2002.

25. NIH Consensus Development Conference Statement. Health implications of obesity. Ann Intern Med 103:1973-1977, 1985.

26. Maffei M, Fei H, Lee GH, et al: Increased expression in adipocytes of ob RNA in mice with lesions of the hypothalamus and with mutations at the db locus. Proc Natl Acad Sci U S A 92:6957-6960, 1995.

27. Puhl RM, Brownell KD: Psychosocial origins of obesity stigma: Toward changing a powerful and pervasive bias. Obes Rev 4:213-227, 2003.

28. Putnam JJ: Cases of myxedema and acromegalia treated with benefit by sheep's thyroids: Recent observations respecting the pathology of the cachexias following disease of the thyroid. Clinical relationships of Grave's disease and acromegalia. Am J Med Sci 106:125-148, 1893.

29. Masserman JH, Goldsmith H: Dinitrophenol: Its therapeutic and toxic actions in certain types of psychobiologic underactivity. JAMA 102:523-525, 1934.

30. Lesses MF, Myerson A: Human autonomic pharmacology. XVI. Benzedrine sulfate as an aid in the treatment of obesity. N Engl J Med 218:119-124, 1938.

31. Kramer MS, Lane DA: Aminorex, dexfenfluramine, and primary pulmonary hypertension. J Clin Epidemiol 51:361-364, 1998.

32. Connolly HM, Crary JL, McGoon MD, et al: Valvular heart disease associated with fenfluramine-phentermine. N Engl J Med 337:581-588, 1997.

33. Kernan WN, Viscoli CM, Brass LM, et al: Phenylpropanolamine and the risk of hemorrhagic stroke. N Engl J Med 343:1826-1832, 2000.

34. Shekelle PG, Hardy ML, Morton SC, et al: Efficacy and safety of ephedra and ephedrine for weight loss and athletic performance: A meta-analysis. JAMA 289:1537-1545, 2003.

35. Reiter E, Feucht M, Hauser E, et al: Changes in body mass index during long-term topiramate therapy in paediatric epilepsy patients—a retrospective analysis. Seizure 13:491-493, 2004.

36. European Agency for the Evaluation of Medicinal Products, Committee for Proprietary Medicinal Products: Clinical Investigation of Drugs Used in Weight Control. London, European Agency for the Evaluation of Medicinal Products, 1997.

37. Food and Drug Administration: Guidance for the Clinical Evaluation of Weight Control Drugs. Rockville, Md, Food and Drug Administration, 1996.

38. Munro JF, MacCuish AC, Wilson EM, Duncan LJP: Comparison of continuous and intermittent anorectic therapy in obesity. Br Med J 1:352-356, 1968.

39. Glazer G: Long-term pharmacotherapy of obesity 2000: A review of efficacy and safety. Arch Intern Med 161:1814-1824, 2001.

40. Zhi J, Melia AT, Guerciolini R, et al: Retrospective population-based analysis of the dose-response (fecal fat excretion) relationship of orlistat in normal and obese volunteers. Clin Pharmacol Ther 56:82-85, 1994.

41. O'Meara S, Riemsma R, Shirran L, et al: A systematic review of the clinical effectiveness of orlistat used for the management of obesity. Obes Rev 5:51-68, 2004.

42. Arterburn DE, Crane PK, Veenstra DL: The efficacy and safety of sibutramine for weight loss: A systematic review. Arch Intern Med 164:994-1003, 2004.

43. Darga LL, Carroll-Michals L, Botsford SJ, Lucas CP: Fluoxetine's effect on weight loss in obese subjects. Am J Clin Nutr 54:321-325, 1991.

44. Jain AK, Kaplan RA, Gadde KM, et al: Bupropion SR vs. placebo for weight loss in obese patients with depressive symptoms. Obes Res 10:1049-1056, 2002.

45. Anderson JW, Greenway FL, Fujioka K, et al: Bupropion SR enhances weight loss: A 48-week double-blind, placebo-controlled trial. Obes Res 10:633-641, 2002.

46. Wilding J, Gaal LV, Rissanen A, et al: A randomized double-blind placebo-controlled study of the long-term efficacy and safety of topiramate in the treatment of obese subjects. Int J Obes Relat Metab Disord 28:1399-1410, 2004.

47. Bray GA, Hollander P, Klein S, et al: A 6-month randomized, placebo-controlled, dose-ranging trial of topiramate for weight loss in obesity. Obes Res 11:722-733, 2003.

48. Gadde KM, Franciscy DM, Wagner HR 2nd, Krishnan KR: Zonisamide for weight loss in obese adults: A randomized controlled trial. JAMA 289:1820-1805, 2003.

49. Wadden TA, Berkowitz RI, Womble LG, et al: Effects of sibutramine plus orlistat in obese women following 1 year of treatment by sibutramine alone: A placebo-controlled trial. Obes Res 8:431-437, 2000.

50. Greenway FL: The safety and efficacy of pharmaceutical and herbal caffeine and ephedrine use as a weight loss agent. Obes Rev 2:199-211, 2001.

51. Morgan JP: Phenylpropanolamine: A Critical Analysis of Reported Adverse Reactions and Overdosage. Fort Lee, NJ, Jack K. Burgess, 1986, pp 3-10.

52. Greenway FL: Clinical studies with phenylpropanolamine: A metaanalysis. Am J Clin Nutr 55(1 Suppl):203S-205S, 1992.

53. Schteingart DE: Effectiveness of phenylpropanolamine in the management of moderate obesity. Int J Obes Relat Metab Disord 16:487-493, 1992.

54. Greenway F, Herber D, Raum W, et al: Double-blind, randomized, placebo-controlled clinical trials with non-prescription medications for the treatment of obesity. Obes Res 7:370-378, 1999.

55. Kernan WN, Viscoli CM, Brass LM, et al: Phenylpropanolamine and the risk of hemorrhagic stroke. N Engl J Med 343:1826-1832, 2000.

56. Plotz M: Obesity. Med Times 86:860-863, 1958.

57. Gould WL: Obesity and hypertension: the importance of a safe compound to control appetite. North Carolina Med J 11:327-334, 1950.

58. McClure CW, Brusch CA: Treatment of oral syndrome obesity with non-traditional appetite control plan. J Am Med Womens Assoc 28:239-248, 1973.

59. Piscano J, Lichter H: A matter of taste. NewYork, Frederick Fell Publishers, 1979, pp 42-64.

60. Collipp PJ: The treatment of exogenous obesity by medicated benzocaine candy: A double-blind placebo study. Obes Bariatr Med 10:123-125, 1981.

61. Dietary supplement market view. Chevy Chase, Md, FDC Reports, August 2000.

62. Boozer CN, Nasser JA, Heymsfield SB, et al: An herbal supplement containing ma huang-guarana for weight loss: A randomized, double-blind trial. Int J Obes Relat Metab Disord 25:316-324, 2001.

63. Boozer CN, Daly PA, Homel P, et al: Herbal ephedra/caffeine for weight loss: A 6-month randomized safety and efficacy trial. Int J Obes Relat Metab Disord 26:593-604, 2002.

64. Greenway FL, De Jonge L, Blanchard D, et al: Effect of a dietary herbal supplement containing caffeine and ephedra on weight, metabolic rate, and body composition. Obes Res 12:1152-1157, 2004.

65. Gurley BJ, Gardner SF, Hubbard MA: Content versus label claims in ephedra-containing dietary supplements. Am J Health Syst Pharm 57:963-969, 2000.

66. Haller CA, Benowitz NL: Adverse cardiovascular and central nervous system events associated with dietary supplements containing ephedra alkaloids. N Engl J Med 343:1833-1838, 2000.

67. Shekelle PG, Hardy ML, Morton SC, et al: Efficacy and safety of ephedra and ephedrine for weight loss and athletic performance: A meta-analysis. JAMA 289:1537-1545, 2003.

68. Pittler MH, Ernst E: Dietary supplements for body-weight reduction: A systematic review. Am J Clin Nutr 79:529-536, 2004.

69. Borchardt RT, Huber JA: Catechol O-methyltransferase. 5. Structure-activity relationships for inhibition by flavonoids. J Med Chem 18:120-122, 1975.

70. Dulloo AG, Seydoux J, Girardier L, et al: Green tea and thermogenesis: Interactions between catechin-polyphenols, caffeine and sympathetic activity. Int J Obes Relat Metab Disord 24:252-258, 2000.

71. Dulloo AG, Duret C, Rohrer D, et al: Efficacy of a green tea extract rich in catechin polyphenols and caffeine in increasing 24-h energy expenditure and fat oxidation in humans. Am J Clin Nutr 70:1040-1045, 1999.

72. Chantre P, Lairon D: Recent findings of green tea extract AR25 (Exolise) and its activity for the treatment of obesity. Phytomedicine 9:3-8, 2002.

73. Kovacs EM, Lejeune MP, Nijs I, Westerterp-Plantenga MS: Effects of green tea on weight maintenance after body-weight loss. Br J Nutr 91:431-437, 2004.

74. Colker C, Lalman D, Torina G, et al: Effects of citrus aurantium extract, caffeine and St. John's wort on body fat loss, lipid levels and mood state in overweight healthy adults. Curr Ther Res 60:145-153, 1999.

75. Nykamp DL, Fackih MN, Compton AL: Possible association of acute lateral-wall myocardial infarction and bitter orange supplement. Ann Pharmacother 38:812-816, 2004.

76. Yoshioka M, Doucet E, Drapeau V, et al: Combined effects of red pepper and caffeine consumption on 24 hour energy balance in subjects given free access to foods. Br J Nutr 85:203-211, 2001.

77. Chaiyata P, Puttadechakum S, Komindr S: Effect of chili pepper (Capsicum frutescens) ingestion on plasma glucose response and metabolic rate in Thai women. J Med Assoc Thai 86:854-860, 2003.

78. Matsumoto T, Miyawaki C, Ue H, et al: Effects of capsaicin-containing yellow curry sauce on sympathetic nervous system activity and diet-induced thermogenesis in lean and obese young women. J Nutr Sci Vitaminol (Tokyo) 46:309-315, 2000.

79. Yoshioka M, Imanaga M, Ueyama H, et al: Maximum tolerable dose of red pepper decreases fat intake independently of spicy sensation in the mouth. Br J Nutr 91:991-995, 2004.

80. Yoshioka M, St-Pierre S, Suzuki M, Tremblay A: Effects of red pepper added to high-fat and high-carbohydrate meals on energy metabolism and substrate utilization in Japanese women. Br J Nutr 80:503-510, 1998.

81. Yoshioka M, St-Pierre S, Drapeau V, et al: Effects of red pepper on appetite and energy intake. Br J Nutr 82:115-123, 1999.

82. Yoshioka M, Lim K, Kikuzato S, et al: Effects of red-pepper diet on the energy metabolism in men. J Nutr Sci Vitaminol (Tokyo) 41:647-656, 1995.

83. Hoeger WW, Harris C, Long EM, Hopkins DR: Four-week supplementation with a natural dietary compound produces favorable changes in body composition. Adv Ther 15:305-314, 1998.

84. Lejeune MP, Kovacs EM, Westerterp-Plantenga MS: Effect of capsaicin on substrate oxidation and weight maintenance after modest body-weight loss in human subjects. Br J Nutr 90:651-659, 2003.

85. Bhatt AD, Dalal DG, Shah SJ, et al: Conceptual and methodologic challenges of assessing the short-term efficacy of guggulu in obesity: Data emergent from a naturalistic clinical trial. J Postgrad Med 41:5-7, 1995.

86. Sidhu LS, Sharma K, Puri AS et al: Effect of gum guggul on body weight and subcutaneous tissue folds. J Res Indian Med Yoga Hom 11:16-22, 1976.

87. Kotiyal PJ, Singh DS, Bisht DB: Gum guggulu (Commiphora mukul) fraction "A" in obesity—a double-blind clinical trial. J Res Ayur Siddha 6:20-35, 1985.

88. Antonio J, Colker CM, Torina GC et al: Effects of a standardized guggulsterone phosphate supplement on body composisiton in overweight adults: A pilot study. Curr Ther Res 60:220-227, 1999.

89. Haslett C, Douglas JG, Chalmers SR, et al: A double-blind evaluation of evening primrose oil as an antiobesity agent. Int J Obes 7:549-553, 1983.

90. Griinari JM, Corl BA, Lacy SH, et al: Conjugated linoleic acid is synthesized endogenously in lactating dairy cows by delta(9)-desaturase. J Nutr 130:2285-2291, 2000.

91. Kritchevsky D: Antimutagenic and some other effects of conjugated linoleic acid. Br J Nutr 83:459-465, 2000.

92. Blankson H, Stakkestad JA, Fagertun H, et al: Conjugated linoleic acid reduces body fat mass in overweight and obese humans. J Nutr 130:2943-2948, 2000.

93. Riserus U, Berglund L, Vessby B: Conjugated linoleic acid (CLA) reduced abdominal adipose tissue in obese middle-aged men with signs of the metabolic syndrome: A randomised controlled trial. Int J Obes Relat Metab Disord 25:1129-1135, 2001.

94. Kamphuis MM, Lejeune MP, Saris WH, Westerterp-Plantenga MS: The effect of conjugated linoleic acid supplementation after weight loss on body weight regain, body composition, and restin metabolic rate in overweight subjects. Int J Obes Relat Metab Disord 27:840-847, 2003.

95. Kamphuis MM, Lejeune MP, Saris WH, Westerterp-Plantenga MS: Effect of conjugated linoleic acid supplementation after weight loss on appetite and food intake in overweight subjects. Eur J Clin Nutr 57:1268-1274, 2003.

96. Gaullier JM, Halse J, Hoye K, et al: Conjugated linoleic acid supplementation for 1 y reduces body fat mass in healthy overweight humans. Am J Clin Nutr 79:1118-1125, 2004.

97. Whigham LD, O'Shea M, Mohede IC, et al: Safety profile of conjugated linoleic acid in a 12-month trial in obese humans. Food Chem Toxicol 42:1701-1709, 2004.

98. Riserus U, Vessby B, Arnlov J, Basu S: Effects of cis-9,trans-11 conjugated linoleic acid supplementation on insulin sensitivity, lipid peroxidation, and proinflammatory markers in obese men. Am J Clin Nutr 80:279-283, 2004.

99. Riserus U, Arner P, Brismar K, Vessby B: Treatment with dietary trans10,cis12 conjugated linoleic acid causes isomer-specific insulin resistance in obese men with the metabolic syndrome. Diabetes Care 25:1516-1521, 2002.

100. Riserus U, Basu S, Jovinge S, et al: Supplementation with conjugated linoleic acid causes isomer-dependent oxidative stress and elevated C-reactive protein: A potential link to fatty acid-induced insulin resistance. Circulation 106:1925-1929, 2002.

101. Sullivan C, Triscari J: Metabolic regulation as a control for lipid disorders. I. Influence of (-)-hydroxycitrate on experimentally induced obesity in the rodent. Am J Clin Nutr 30:767-776, 1977.

102. Kriketos AD, Thompson HR, Greene H, Hill JO: (-)-Hydroxycitric acid does not affect energy expenditure and substrate oxidation in adult males in a post-absorptive state. Int J Obes Relat Metab Disord 23:867-873, 1999.

103. Kovacs EM, Westerterp-Plantenga MS, de Vries M, et al: Effects of 2-week ingestion of (-)-hydroxycitrate and (-)-hydroxycitrate combined with medium-chain triglycerides on satiety and food intake. Physiol Behav 74:543-549, 2001.

104. Mattes RD, Bormann L: Effects of (-)-hydroxycitric acid on appetitive variables. Physiol Behav 71:87-94, 2000.

105. Heymsfield SB, Allison DB, Vasselli JR, et al: Garcinia cambogia (hydroxycitric acid) as a potential antiobesity agent: A randomized controlled trial. JAMA 280:1596-1600, 1998.

106. Preuss HG, Bagchi D, Bagchi M, et al: Effects of a natural extract of (-)-hydroxycitric acid (HCA-SX) and a combination of HCA-SX plus niacin-bound chromium and

Gymnema sylvestre extract on weight loss. Diabetes Obes Metab 6:171-180, 2004.

107. Abrahamsson L, Hackl H: Catabolic effects and the influence on hormonal variables under treatment with Gynodian-Depot or dehydroepiandrosterone (DHEA) oenanthate. Maturitas 3:225-234, 1981.

108. Nestler JE, Barlascini CO, Clore JN, Blackard WG: Dehydroepiandrosterone reduces serum low density lipoprotein levels and body fat but does not alter insulin sensitivity in normal men. J Clin Endocrinol Metab 66:57-61, 1988.

109. Mortola JF, Yen SS: The effects of oral dehydroepiandrosterone on endocrine-metabolic parameters in post-menopausal women. J Clin Endocrinol Metab 71:696-704, 1990.

110. Usiskin KS, Butterworth S, Clore JN, et al: Lack of effect of dehydroepiandrosterone in obese men. Int J Obes 14:457-463, 1990.

111. Welle S, Jozefowicz R, Statt M: Failure of dehydroepiandrosterone to influence energy and protein metabolism in humans. J Clin Endocrinol Metab 71:1259-1264, 1990.

112. Villareal DT, Holloszy JO: Effect of DHEA on abdominal fat and insulin action in elderly women and men: A randomized controlled trial. JAMA 292:2243-2248, 2004.

113. Nissen S, Sharp R, Ray M, et al: Effect of leucine metabolite beta-hydroxy-betamethylbutyrate on muscle metabolism during resistance-exercise training. J Appl Physiol 81:2095-2104, 1996.

114. Ceci F, Cangiano C, Cairella M, et al: The effects of oral 5-hydroxytryptophan administration on feeding behavior in obese adult female subjects. J Neural Transm 76:109-117, 1989.

115. Cangiano C, Ceci F, Cascino A, et al: Eating behavior and adherence to dietary prescriptions in obese adult subjects treated with 5-hydroxytryptophan. Am J Clin Nutr 56:863-867, 1992.

116. Hull KM, Maher TJ: L-Tyrosine potentiates the anorexia induced by mixed-acting sympathomimetic drugs in hyperphagic rats. J Pharmacol Exp Ther 255:403-409, 1990.

117. Becker EW, Jakober B, Luft D et al: Clinical and biochemical evaluations of the alga spirulina with regard to its application in the treatment of obesity. A double-blind cross-over study. Nutr Report Internat 33:565-574, 1986.

118. Alfieri MA, Pomerleau J, Grace DM, Anderson L: Fiber intake of normal weight, moderately obese and severely obese subjects. Obes Res 3:541-547, 1995.

119. Greenway FL, Heber D: Herbal and alternative approaches to obesity. In Bray GA, Bouchard C (eds): Handbook of Obesity—Clinical Applications, 2nd ed. New York, Marcel Dekker, 2004, pp 343-345.

120. Barroso Aranda J, Contreras F, et al: Efficacy of a novel chitosan formulation on fecal fat excretion: A double-blind, crossover, placebo-controlled study. J Med 33:209-225, 2002.

121. Guerciolini R, Radu-Radulescu L, Boldrin M, et al: Comparative evaluation of fecal fat excretion induced by orlistat and chitosan. Obes Res 9:364-367, 2001.

122. Zahorska-Markiewicz B, Krotkiewski M, Olszanecka-Glinianowicz M, Zurakowski A: [Effect of chitosan in complex management of obesity.] Pol Merkuriusz Lek 13:129-132, 2002.

123. Ho SC, Tai ES, Eng PH, et al: In the absence of dietary surveillance, chitosan does not reduce plasma lipids or obesity in hypercholesterolaemic obese Asian subjects. Singapore Med J 42:6-10, 2001.

124. Wuolijoki E, Hirvela T, Ylitalo P: Decrease in serum LDL cholesterol with microcrystalline chitosan. Methods Find Exp Clin Pharmacol 21:357-361, 1999.

125. Pittler MH, Abbot NC, Harkness EF, Ernst E: Randomized, double-blind trial of chitosan for body weight reduction. Eur J Clin Nutr 53:379-381, 1999.

126. Mhurchu CN, Poppitt SD, McGill AT, et al: The effect of the dietary supplement, chitosan, on body weight: Randomized controlled trial in 250 overweight and obese adults. Int J Obes Relat Metab Disord 28:1149-1156, 2004.

127. Crawford V, Scheckenbach R, Preuss HG: Effects of niacin-bound chromium supplementation on body composition in overweight African-American women. Diabetes Obes Metab 1:331-337, 1999.

128. Campbell WW, Joseph LJ, Anderson RA, et al: Effects of resistive training and chromium picolinate on body composition and skeletal muscle size in older women. Int J Sport Nutr Exerc Metab 12:125-135, 2002.

129. Lukaski HC, Bolonchuk WW, Siders WA, Milne DB: Chromium supplementation and resistance training: Effects on body composition, strength, and trace element status of men. Am J Clin Nutr 63:954-965, 1996.

130. Hallmark MA, Reynolds TH, DeSouza CA, et al: Effects of chromium and resistive training on muscle strength and body composition. Med Sci Sports Exerc 28:139-144, 1996.

131. Uusitupa MI, Mykkanen L, Siitonen O, et al: Chromium supplementation in impaired glucose tolerance of elderly: Effects on blood glucose, plasma insulin, C-peptide and lipid levels. Br J Nutr 68:209-216, 1992.

132. Anderson RA, Cheng N, Bryden NA, et al: Elevated intakes of supplemental chromium improve glucose and insulin variables in individuals with type 2 diabetes. Diabetes 46:1786-1791, 1997.

133. Amato P, Morales AJ, Yen SS: Effects of chromium picolinate supplementation on insulin sensitivity, serum lipids, and body composition in healthy, nonobese, older men and women. J Gerontol A Biol Sci Med Sci 55:M260-M263, 2000.

134. Volpe SL, Huang HW, Larpadisorn K, Lesser II: Effect of chromium supplementation and exercise on body composition, resting metabolic rate and selected biochemical parameters in moderately obese women following an exercise program. J Am Coll Nutr 20:293-306, 2001.

135. Kaats GR, Blum K, Fisher JA, Adelman JA: Effects of chromium picolinate supplementation on body composition: A randomized, double-masked placebo-controlled study. Cur Ther Res 57:747-756, 1996.

136. Kaats GR, Blum K, Pullin D, et al: A randomized, double-masked, placebo-controlled study of the effects of chromium picolinate supplementation on body composition: A replication and extension of a previous study. Curr Ther Res 59:379-388, 1998.

137. Evans GW: The effect of chromium picolinate on insulin controlled parameters in humans. Int J Biosoc Med Res 11:163-180, 1989.

138. Anderson RA: Essentiality of chromium in humans. Sci Total Env 86:75-81, 1989.

139. Anderson RA: Effect of chromium on body composition and weight loss. Nutr Rev 56:266-270, 1998.

Chapter 32

Physiologic Insulin Replacement with Continuous Subcutaneous Insulin Infusion: Insulin Pump Therapy

Raymond A. Plodkowski and Steven V. Edelman

KEY POINTS

- *An insulin pump involves a minimally invasive catheter that continuously administers insulin to the same subcutaneous site for 3 days.*
- *Insulin pump users can program different basal rates at different times during the day.*
- *The insulin pump can modify the shape of the insulin bolus. Boluses can be immediate, sustained, or a combination depending on the meal composition and timing.*
- *Insulin pump therapy allows for increased flexibility in meal timing and amounts and increased flexibility in the timing and intensity of exercise.*
- *Insulin pump users can enjoy a better quality of life in terms of self-reliance and control.*
- *In the future a continuous glucose sensor will provide real-time data and an algorithm will be used to determine the doses administered by the insulin pump to form a closed-loop system.*

Insulin therapy has rapidly evolved since its discovery in the early 1920s. Bulky needles and syringes have been replaced by narrow-gauge needles and such improved administration devices as insulin pens. These improved methods of delivery have been limited by the kinetics of the available insulins. At first the only short-acting insulin was regular insulin, which did not provide an adequate rapid peak action profile to address prandial glucose surges. Today insulin aspart, insulin lispro, and insulin glulisine are available for better prandial blood glucose control.

There have also been improvements in long-acting basal insulins. In the past, intermediate- and long-acting insulins such as Lente, NPH, and Ultralente had variable kinetics and delayed peaking of action, which could put patients with diabetes at risk for extreme hyper- or hypoglycemia as doses were titrated to achieve an appropriate hemoglobin A1c (HbA1c) goal. Now better long-acting insulins such as insulin glargine are in common use, and soon insulin detemir will also be available. These basal insulins are relatively peakless and can produce a more physiologic basal insulin profile.

In addition to these marked improvements in injectable insulins, continuous subcutaneous insulin infusion (CSII) via an insulin pump offers one of the most physiologic ways to replace insulin. Insulin pumps are an excellent way for many patients to reduce the excursions of daily glucose values, take control of their diabetes, and improve their overall glucose control. Insulin pumps are used primarily with the short-acting insulin analogs aspart and lispro, yielding blood levels of insulin that can be rapidly adjusted by the user.

The insulin pump can administer exact doses of bolus insulin for mealtimes and correction boluses between meals. It can also administer exact basal insulin rates that can be adjusted throughout the day to address the patient's individual needs and lifestyle. Insulin pumps might soon be mated with continuous glucose sensors to create a closed-loop system. Furthermore, intraperitoneal insulin administration via implanted pumps or percutaneous ports are in clinical trials. Thus, the insulin pump has immediate applications and will continue to evolve to help people with diabetes.

In this chapter we discuss the benefits, indications, and practical guidelines for use of insulin pumps in patients with type 1 diabetes mellitus (T1DM) and insulin-requiring type 2 diabetes (T2DM).

PHYSIOLOGIC INSULIN REPLACEMENT VIA INSULIN PUMPS

Bolus Replacement

The goal of insulin pump therapy is to mimic as closely as possible the normal insulin secretion of beta cells. There are two main components to insulin secretion: basal (continuous) secretion and bolus secretion. Persons who do not have diabetes have an insulin surge or bolus after meals that attenuates the postprandial glucose excursion. Patients with diabetes have an inadequate beta cell

response and require short-acting insulin before meals to mimic this physiologic secretion.

The older regular insulin is very nonphysiologic, because it peaks in 2 to 3 hours, leading to uncontrolled postprandial glucose peaks and delayed hypoglycemia. Regular insulin is a "dinosaur" with no advantages over the newer fast-acting insulin analogs. Only in cases of severe gastroparesis is it superior to the analogs.

Insulin lispro and insulin aspart are insulin analogs that have an action onset between 10 and 20 minutes and a peak between 1 and 3 hours, with rapid diminution of activity. Another fast-acting insulin analog, insulin glulisine, has recently become available.[1]

Unfortunately, there is still some amount of variability depending on injection technique and location. In addition, there is no mechanism for adjusting the profile of the insulin bolus once it is administered. An insulin pump involves a minimally invasive catheter that continuously administers insulin to the same subcutaneous site for three days, which limits much of the variability associated with multiple injections. The pump user also can adjust the time action profile of the insulin boluses depending on the type, size, and length of the expected meal.

Basal Replacement

The second component to insulin replacement is the patient's basal insulin requirement. In addition to the prandial surges of insulin, a constant basal insulin level is necessary over the entire 24-hour period to maintain normal metabolic function and prevent diabetic ketoacidosis (DKA) in the fasting state. A common approach to providing a basal insulin level involves the use of an intermediate- or long-acting insulin. The most popular intermediate-acting insulin is neutral protamine Hagedorn (NPH). The insulin is composed of regular insulin mixed with a fish protein (protamine) and zinc. The protamine and zinc slow the absorption of the insulin. NPH has an onset of action of 2 to 4 hours, peak action of 6 to 8 hours, and duration of 10 to 15 hours.[2] For it to serve as a true basal insulin, NPH must be given every 6 hours. However, this is rarely recommended to patients because it is not very convenient.

The newer long-acting insulin analog, insulin glargine, is a 24-hour peakless basal insulin that is less unpredictable, leading to less symptomatic hypoglycemia.[3] There is still some variability depending on injection technique, and its dose cannot be adjusted once it is injected, which is true with any injected insulin. Insulin detemir is in clinical trials and will be another basal insulin analog injected once or twice daily. As seen with insulin glargine, in clinical trials insulin detemir combined with insulin aspart offered greater HbA1c lowering while causing less hypoglycemia compared with traditional multiple daily injection therapy with NPH and regular insulin.[4]

Now that better basal and bolus insulins are available, many patients who would have required insulin pumps in the past can be successfully treated with multiple daily injections (MDI). Thus, patient selection for insulin pumps has become more important. An intermediate step before considering an insulin pump is to initiate intensive physiologic insulin administration with multiple daily injections. Currently we prescribe insulin glargine with insulin lispro or insulin aspart at mealtimes, with an extra injection of insulin lispro or insulin aspart at other times for incidental hyperglycemia. This regimen requires at least four-times-a-day home glucose monitoring, preparing the patient for an easy conversion to an insulin pump if desired and so indicated. A patient who can reliably perform this dosage regimen and frequent home glucose monitoring will do well with insulin pump therapy. If the patient is able to obtain the goal HbA1c level with no significant hypoglycemia on the intensive MDI regimen, insulin pump therapy can be deferred.

POTENTIAL ADVANTAGES OF INSULIN PUMP THERAPY

One of the most important advantages insulin pump therapy offers over multiple daily injections is the elimination of unwanted peaks and valleys that are commonly seen with basal insulin regimens. Insulin administered via a pump often results in lower basal insulin requirements and can be titrated to gain better overall glycemic control while reducing the rate of mild and severe hypoglycemia.[5,6]

Insulin pumps also offer the opportunity to accurately dose preprandial insulin. A study examined the total insulin dose when type 1 diabetic patients use CSII versus MDI therapy and showed that the daily total dose of insulin fell 18% in patients using CSII compared to MDI, while reducing HbA1c from 8.4% to 7.7%.[7] Because it is well established that insulin promotes weight gain, it benefits the patient to use the smallest amount of insulin possible to achieve the desired clinical effect. This study suggests that insulin dosing by pump may be more physiologic and therefore allow for lower insulin doses while maintaining blood glucose control.

Quality of life is also an issue with insulin pump therapy. Insulin pumps may at first appear to be complicated and awkward. However, it has been shown that quality of life scales improve when patients move from traditional insulin injection therapy to insulin pens, and further improvement is seen when patients use insulin pumps.[8]

Several factors contribute to patient satisfaction with insulin pump therapy. From a patient's point

of view, insulin pump therapy has benefits that include a more flexible lifestyle while simultaneously enjoying improved glucose control. Insulin pump therapy allows for increased flexibility in meal timing and amounts, increased flexibility in the timing and intensity of exercise, improved glucose control when traveling across time zones or with variable working schedules, and a better quality of life in terms of self-reliance and control.[9]

There are some distinct practical advantages that the insulin pump maintains over multiple daily injections. Insulin pump users can program different basal rates at different times during the day. For example, some patients experience a significant dawn phenomenon in which the counterregulatory hormone, growth hormone, causes a rise in blood glucose in the early morning prior to waking. The insulin pump user has the option of programming a slightly higher rate of insulin infusion for the early morning hours to address this rise in blood glucose, and patients with overnight hypoglycemia can program the pump to reduce the amount of basal insulin during the night. Patients also have the option to use temporary basal rates during strenuous exercise, illness, or a fast for religious purposes. In addition to the benefits gained by precision control of the basal rates, the pump user has greater flexibility with regard to insulin boluses.

Boluses are easily programmed by the user. Because users have an indwelling subcutaneous catheter, they do not have to inject themselves every time a bolus is needed. Thus, mealtime, snack, and correction boluses are easily facilitated in a timely manner, which has positive results on subsequent glucose values. The insulin pumps can also modify the shape of the insulin bolus. Thus, boluses can be immediate, sustained, or a combination of immediate and sustained administration depending on the meal composition and timing.

POTENTIAL DISADVANTAGES OF INSULIN PUMP THERAPY

Older textbooks list hypoglycemic unawareness as a contraindication to insulin pump therapy because any therapeutic regimen that improves glycemic control typically increases the chances of hypoglycemia as well. Insulin pump therapy is proven to reduce wide fluctuations in blood glucose values, including severe hypoglycemia. If a patient has hypoglycemic unawareness, it is important to set the patient's goals at a higher range to prevent severe hypoglycemia. For example, the goals of glycemic control for a patient with hypoglycemic unawareness should be between 120 and 180 mg/dL instead of the usual 70 to 120 mg/dL range in patients without hypoglycemic unawareness.

Although it is generally accepted that better glucose control is achieved with continuous subcutaneous insulin infusion via insulin pumps, a recent study challenged this assumption. This study compared insulin pump therapy using insulin aspart or insulin lispro with MDI therapy consisting of insulin glargine and insulin aspart or lispro.[10] The study concluded that patients with T1DM could obtain similar glycemic control measured via HbA1c with MDI or CSII. Furthermore, the CSII group had more incidences of DKA (due to pump failure, catheter occlusion, or no insulin remaining in the insulin pump syringe), and cost of therapy was higher than in the MDI group. The study concluded that MDI therapy should be considered before insulin pump therapy. This is a reasonable course of action.

Patients with poor glycemic control may be at risk for frequent skin infections. The presence of a catheter in the subcutaneous tissue for a long period of time increases the chances of infection. Therefore, in patients who have frequent *Staphylococcus* skin infections, insulin pump therapy may be problematic. However, with the improved glycemic control that pump therapy can offer, many patients with a history of frequent skin infections no longer have this problem.

Another potential disadvantage of pump therapy is the risk of sudden extreme hyperglycemia or DKA, especially in type 1 diabetic patients. This is especially true if the patient is using lispro or aspart in the pump. Because only regular or fast-acting insulin is used, a patient can quickly develop extreme hyperglycemia or ketoacidosis if there is a prolonged interruption of insulin delivery. This could occur due to a problem with the infusion line, depletion of a battery pack, an empty insulin reservoir, or pump failure.

The incidence of DKA seems to be decreasing as pump technology improves. A meta-analysis indicated that insulin pump studies prior to 1993 showed a higher incidence of DKA, and studies after 1993 lacked this strong association.[11] Today's pumps are very reliable and failure is unusual. For emergencies, however, pump patients should always carry an extra bottle or insulin pen containing regular, lispro, or aspart insulin.

Financial concerns are always an issue, and the cost of insulin pump therapy together with the accompanying supplies may simply be out of reach if the patient does not have adequate insurance coverage. The pump itself costs $3500 to $5000 and the supplies (which include insulin infusion lines, syringes, tape, and batteries) can total an additional $40 to $50 a month. With appropriately applied pressure by physician and patient, most insurance companies reimburse at least 80%. Representatives from the insulin pump companies also have special staff to help deal with bureaucratic processes.

Finally, to some patients it is wearisome to have something constantly connected to their body. In such cases, a pump vacation is recommended, in which the patient goes back to multiple daily injections for a few days or weeks.

MISCONCEPTIONS REGARDING INSULIN PUMP THERAPY

There are many misconceptions about insulin pump therapy, and physicians and patients should be aware of them. Home glucose monitoring is still important with insulin pump therapy. Patients should understand that frequent blood glucose measurements will be necessary, especially at the time of pump initiation. Later, when the patient is well adjusted to insulin pump therapy, the frequency of home glucose monitoring will depend on the variability of the patient's day-to-day activities, including diet and exercise.

Many patients believe that insulin pump therapy will allow them to eat anything they like at any time. Although insulin pump therapy does allow more flexible meal times and amounts, to maintain or improve glycemic control the patient must maintain some degree of diet discretion. In addition, unwanted weight gain occurs in some patients who start to overliberalize their diets despite good glycemic control.

Insulin pump therapy is not contraindicated for people with hypoglycemic unawareness, and insulin pumps are not only for patients with T1DM.

INSULIN PUMP THERAPY IN TYPE 2 DIABETES

The majority of patients using insulin pump therapy are those with T1DM, who usually do not have insulin resistance and so require low basal rates and smaller insulin boluses. However, insulin pump therapy can also be extremely valuable in patients with insulin-requiring T2DM who have not achieved glycemic control with subcutaneous injections or who are seeking a more flexible lifestyle.

Patients with T2DM who were treated with CSII preferred the pump to their previous injectable insulin regimen for reasons of convenience, flexibility, and ease of use.[12] In addition, many older patients with the diagnosis of insulin-requiring T2DM actually have latent autoimmune diabetes in adults (LADA). When large groups of patients with the diagnosis of insulin-requiring T2DM were tested for anti-GAD antibodies (glutamic acid decarboxylase), 3.7% to 6.3% were positive.[13]

For patients with true T2DM, the underlying metabolic defects are insulin resistance and relative insulin deficiency, which increases insulin requirements. A patient with T2DM should be treated with the minimum amount of insulin necessary to improve glucose control, because excess insulin administration could cause further weight gain. When pump therapy is used, weight gain is less of an issue because patients can generally use less insulin than they were using before the insulin pump. In addition, when the number of hypoglycemic events decreases, there is less overeating to compensate for excessive insulin, which also helps to reduce weight gain. Finally, and theoretically, there may be less strain placed on the pancreatic beta cells of these patients with T2DM. This may help with overall glycemic control, because a functioning beta cell can also autoregulate against hyper- and hypoglycemia, as seen in persons without diabetes.

PATIENT SELECTION

In general, any patient taking insulin who has poor glycemic control or is requesting a more flexible lifestyle could be considered for insulin pump therapy. Obviously, the patient has to be reliable, be able to perform frequent home glucose monitoring, and have a fundamental understanding of diabetes and the importance of good control. However, the patient need not be a rocket scientist or even have a technical background to manage the pump's functions. Menu-driven pump functions have replaced older pumps that used symbols and complex programming algorithms. Today, the patient only has to understand some basic principles of operating and maintaining the insulin pump and related catheter care. The newest pumps interface with glucose meters to make the administration of insulin simpler and more convenient for the user.

Potential pump candidates might benefit from talking to current insulin pump users. The American Diabetes Association (www.diabetes.org) and Juvenile Diabetes Foundation (www.jdf.org) can help patients find local insulin pump support groups. Many of these support groups can be found online by searching for "pumpers." Patients in these groups can inform interested patients about the positive and negative aspects of pump therapy and can give practical tips that are not found in traditional textbooks.

The insulin pump companies have information, including videotapes and manuals, that they can send to patients. Several insulin pump companies have excellent training products (Medtronic MiniMed Inc., 1-800-646-4633, www.minimed.com; Smiths Medical, 1-800-826-9703, www.cozmore.com; Animas Corporation, 1-877-767-7373, www.animascorp.com).

INITIATING INSULIN PUMP THERAPY

Insulin pumps are about the size of a pager or small bar of soap (Fig. 32–1). They weigh approximately four ounces and can be put in a pocket, on a belt, in a specially designed bra, or inside a sock. An insulin pump is an automatic, computerized, mechanical insulin syringe that delivers insulin in a more physiologic fashion. Insulin pumps have a lever that mechanically pushes down a plunger of a large insulin syringe (typically up to 3.0 mL or 300

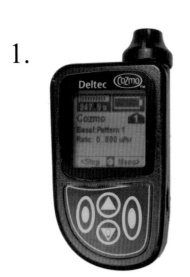

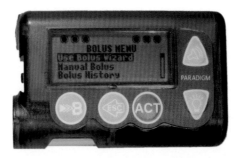

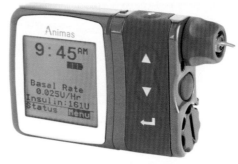

Figure 32–1. Insulin pumps: **1,** Deltec Cosmo insulin pump; **2,** Medtronic Minimed Paradigm insulin pump; **3,** Animas 1200 insulin pump.

units of insulin) automatically 24 hours a day (basal rate), and on demand before meals, (bolus rate). The insulin then travels through a long infusion tube from the insulin syringe that is housed in the insulin pump to the subcutaneous tissue via a flexible catheter (Fig. 32–2). Most pump wearers insert the catheter in the abdominal area, although the upper outer quadrant of the buttocks, upper thighs, or triceps fat pad of the arms can also be used (Fig. 32–3).

The infusion lines have a quick-release mechanism that can be temporarily disconnected from the insertion site (Fig. 32–4). These quick-release catheters make showering, swimming, dressing, and other interfering activities much more convenient. It is recommended that the syringe and the infusion set be filled and changed every 3 days. Many patients, however, use their infusion sets much longer before changing (up to 6 days) without problems.

Prolonged use of the infusion set at a single site longer than 3 days increases the likelihood of irritation or superficial abscess formation that can require antibiotic therapy or incision and drainage. This scenario is infrequent, and most irritated sites improve on their own without the need for antibiotics or other interventions once the infusion set is removed.

Insulin pumps have disposable batteries that last approximately 5 to 8 weeks. All three insulin pump brands have built-in alarms to prevent inadvertent insulin delivery or to warn the patient if the insulin supply is low or the infusion set becomes occluded.

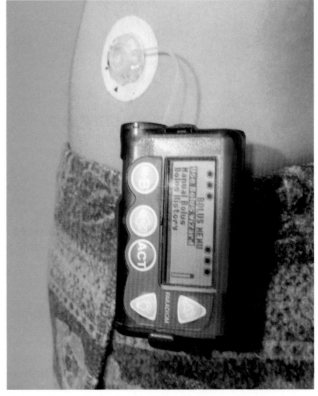

Figure 32–2. Person wearing an insulin pump.

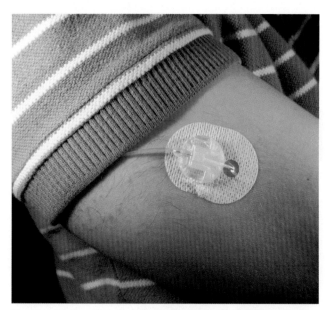

Figure 32–3. Alternate infusion site: upper arm.

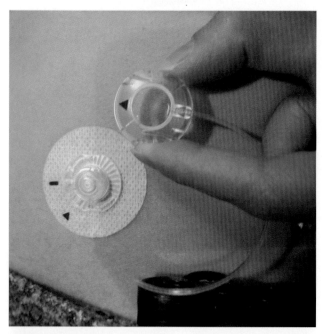

Figure 32–4. Pump infusion catheter with quick-release feature.

There is a choice of insulins for use in pumps. Initially, pumps used regular insulin exclusively. The short-acting insulin analogs lispro, aspart, and glulisine have largely replaced regular insulin because of their rapid onset and short duration of action, allowing them to quickly influence and normalize blood glucose levels. Insulin lispro has been shown to significantly lower HbA1c more than regular insulin with similar basal and bolus doses.[14,15] Additional studies have also shown insulin aspart used in continuous subcutaneous insulin infusion to be efficacious.[16]

In the ideal setting, successful initiation of insulin pump therapy should be orchestrated by an educated and motivated health care team composed of a physician, a diabetes educator, a registered dietician, and a pump counselor. Before beginning insulin pump therapy, it is important to review several topics with the patient. The insulin pump companies have knowledgeable professionals, usually certified diabetes educators, available to help educate patients on these important topics before, during, and after initiation of insulin pump therapy.

Outpatient initiation of insulin pump therapy is feasible, with frequent patient contact required only for the first few days. After the patient has been taught to program and maintain the insulin pump and infusion lines, bolus and basal rates are determined and set. It is sometimes helpful to have patients use saline (instead of insulin) in the pump for a day or two to become accustomed to the controls while they continue to use MDI for their actual insulin administration. Patients are encouraged to follow their usual daily schedule with frequent home glucose monitoring. Blood glucose values should be obtained before each meal, one to two hours after each meal, at bedtime, and at 3 AM. These values help the caregiver adjust the premeal bolus rates as well as the continuous basal rates during a 24-hour period and to assess whether the patient needs any secondary basal rates—for example, to counteract the dawn phenomenon.

The initial bolus and basal rates can be based on the patient's prior insulin regimen or can be determined by the 24-hour insulin requirements. We put most of our patients on an intensive insulin regimen using insulin glargine once daily plus lispro, aspart, or glulisine insulin before each meal. In general, the total 24-hour basal insulin requirements should be in the range of 40% to 60% of the total daily insulin amount used (see later).

INSULIN PUMP BOLUS DOSE MANAGEMENT

When they begin pump therapy, most patients can use the same insulin boluses they were using during MDI therapy. One of the distinct advantages of the insulin pump is the ability to modify the pattern of bolus administration. When patients use multiple daily injections, they are limited by the time-action profile of regular insulin or the fast-acting lispro, aspart, or glulisine once it is injected.

Most pumps can administer different types of boluses (Fig. 32–5).[17] The standard bolus has a quick rise and then fall of insulin administration. The square-wave bolus is characterized by a rapid rise in insulin followed by sustained insulin administration and rapid fall back to baseline. It provides insulin coverage in the event the patient has an extended multicourse meal, buffet, or high-fat or

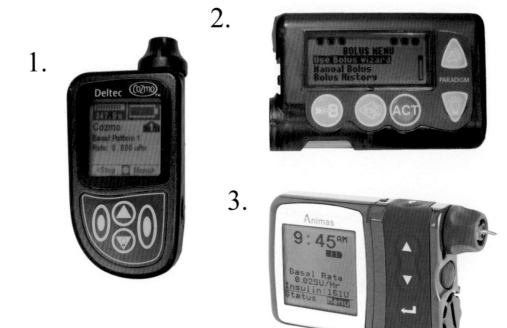

Figure 32–1. Insulin pumps: **1,** Deltec Cosmo insulin pump; **2,** Medtronic Minimed Paradigm insulin pump; **3,** Animas 1200 insulin pump.

units of insulin) automatically 24 hours a day (basal rate), and on demand before meals, (bolus rate). The insulin then travels through a long infusion tube from the insulin syringe that is housed in the insulin pump to the subcutaneous tissue via a flexible catheter (Fig. 32–2). Most pump wearers insert the catheter in the abdominal area, although the upper outer quadrant of the buttocks, upper thighs, or triceps fat pad of the arms can also be used (Fig. 32–3).

The infusion lines have a quick-release mechanism that can be temporarily disconnected from the insertion site (Fig. 32–4). These quick-release catheters make showering, swimming, dressing, and other interfering activities much more convenient. It is recommended that the syringe and the infusion set be filled and changed every 3 days. Many patients, however, use their infusion sets much longer before changing (up to 6 days) without problems.

Prolonged use of the infusion set at a single site longer than 3 days increases the likelihood of irritation or superficial abscess formation that can require antibiotic therapy or incision and drainage. This scenario is infrequent, and most irritated sites improve on their own without the need for antibiotics or other interventions once the infusion set is removed.

Insulin pumps have disposable batteries that last approximately 5 to 8 weeks. All three insulin pump brands have built-in alarms to prevent inadvertent insulin delivery or to warn the patient if the insulin supply is low or the infusion set becomes occluded.

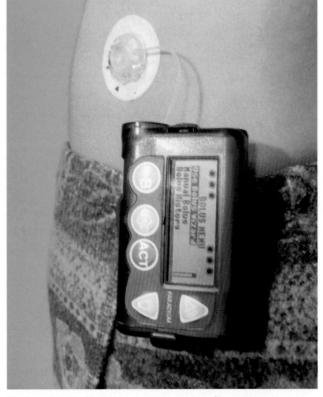

Figure 32–2. Person wearing an insulin pump.

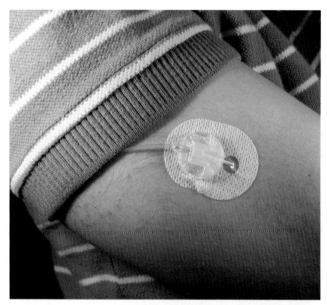

Figure 32–3. Alternate infusion site: upper arm.

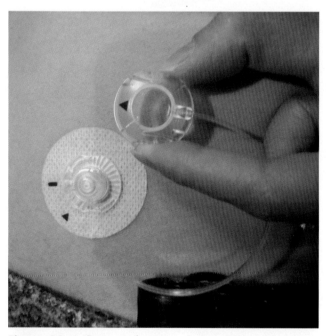

Figure 32–4. Pump infusion catheter with quick-release feature.

There is a choice of insulins for use in pumps. Initially, pumps used regular insulin exclusively. The short-acting insulin analogs lispro, aspart, and glulisine have largely replaced regular insulin because of their rapid onset and short duration of action, allowing them to quickly influence and normalize blood glucose levels. Insulin lispro has been shown to significantly lower HbA1c more than regular insulin with similar basal and bolus doses.[14,15] Additional studies have also shown insulin aspart used in continuous subcutaneous insulin infusion to be efficacious.[16]

In the ideal setting, successful initiation of insulin pump therapy should be orchestrated by an educated and motivated health care team composed of a physician, a diabetes educator, a registered dietician, and a pump counselor. Before beginning insulin pump therapy, it is important to review several topics with the patient. The insulin pump companies have knowledgeable professionals, usually certified diabetes educators, available to help educate patients on these important topics before, during, and after initiation of insulin pump therapy.

Outpatient initiation of insulin pump therapy is feasible, with frequent patient contact required only for the first few days. After the patient has been taught to program and maintain the insulin pump and infusion lines, bolus and basal rates are determined and set. It is sometimes helpful to have patients use saline (instead of insulin) in the pump for a day or two to become accustomed to the controls while they continue to use MDI for their actual insulin administration. Patients are encouraged to follow their usual daily schedule with frequent home glucose monitoring. Blood glucose values should be obtained before each meal, one to two hours after each meal, at bedtime, and at 3 AM. These values help the caregiver adjust the premeal bolus rates as well as the continuous basal rates during a 24-hour period and to assess whether the patient needs any secondary basal rates—for example, to counteract the dawn phenomenon.

The initial bolus and basal rates can be based on the patient's prior insulin regimen or can be determined by the 24-hour insulin requirements. We put most of our patients on an intensive insulin regimen using insulin glargine once daily plus lispro, aspart, or glulisine insulin before each meal. In general, the total 24-hour basal insulin requirements should be in the range of 40% to 60% of the total daily insulin amount used (see later).

INSULIN PUMP BOLUS DOSE MANAGEMENT

When they begin pump therapy, most patients can use the same insulin boluses they were using during MDI therapy. One of the distinct advantages of the insulin pump is the ability to modify the pattern of bolus administration. When patients use multiple daily injections, they are limited by the time-action profile of regular insulin or the fast-acting lispro, aspart, or glulisine once it is injected.

Most pumps can administer different types of boluses (Fig. 32–5).[17] The standard bolus has a quick rise and then fall of insulin administration. The square-wave bolus is characterized by a rapid rise in insulin followed by sustained insulin administration and rapid fall back to baseline. It provides insulin coverage in the event the patient has an extended multicourse meal, buffet, or high-fat or

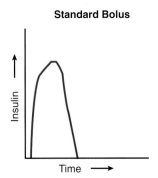
Standard Bolus

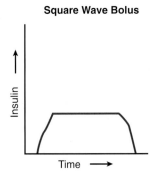
Square Wave Bolus

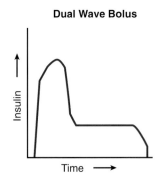
Dual Wave Bolus

Figure 32–5. Insulin bolus waves.

high-protein meal or in patients who have slow gastric emptying due to gastroparesis.

Some pumps also have an option for a dual-wave bolus. This is a rapid peak bolus of insulin followed by lower sustained insulin release over a user-determined period of time. This is helpful in meals that contain both rapidly absorbed nutrients, such as fruit cocktail, followed by a multi-course meal. Patients can experiment and check their postprandial glucose measurements to see which type of bolus matches their eating styles.

Carbohydrate Counting

Another tool that can be used to tailor the bolus dose to a particular meal is carbohydrate counting. Because carbohydrates have a large effect on blood glucose excursions, estimating the amount of carbohydrates allows patients to more accurately approximate the size of the bolus with respect to the expected meal. There are different methods of carbohydrate counting including gram counting and the older exchange system. We prefer the gram-counting method because it yields more-accurate results.[18]

Patients should examine the Nutrition Facts label that is on all food packages as mandated by the Food and Drug Administration. The technique for carbohydrate counting can be easily mastered if it is done with a simple algorithm.[19] First, the patient determines the serving size and decides how many servings he or she is eating. Then the patient looks at the "Total Carbohydrate" section of the label. The number of servings the patient is eating multiplied by the grams of carbohydrate per serving equals the total grams of carbohydrate eaten. When patients are dining at restaurants or eating fast food, they can use lists that give the nutritional content of foods. Several of the pump companies give away these guides, and they can also be purchased at bookstores. They are often extensive and include food items at many common chain restaurants as well as popular meals from various types of cuisines.

The next step is to determine the patient's insulin-to-carbohydrate ratio. Divide the grams of carbohydrate in a meal by the number of insulin units that the patient requires to lower the postprandial blood glucose to less than 180 mg/dL. For example, if a patient eats an 80-gram carbohydrate meal and typically requires 4 units of insulin to lower the blood sugar to the target range, then the insulin-to-carbohydrate ratio is 1 unit of insulin for every 20 grams of carbohydrate. Therefore, if this patient has a 100-gram carbohydrate meal, he or she divides 100 by 20 to find the requirement is 5 units of insulin (Fig. 32–6).

Multiple premeal and postmeal blood glucose measurements are important for determining the most accurate insulin-to-carbohydrate ratio. With practice, patients can become very skilled in estimating the carbohydrate content of foods, and this will be a valuable tool in further refining their insulin bolus regimen.

CALCULATING INSULIN PUMP BASAL RATES

There are three methods for determining the basal rate when initially starting a patient on insulin pump therapy.

The first method uses as a guide the total basal insulin component of the patient's MDI regimen. Approximately 10% to 20% is subtracted from the total dose of insulin glargine, NPH, or Ultralente; this safety factor can be used in all three basal calculation methods. The remainder is divided by 24 to calculate the initial basal rate. For example, if the patient is taking 20 units of insulin glargine at night, then the initial basal rate is:

$$\frac{20\,IU - (0.2 \times 20) = 0.66\,IU \text{ per hour}}{24\,h}$$

or about 0.7 units per hour. If the HbA1c and glucose values are high, then the patient should not subtract the 10% to 20% safety factor, because the patient is probably underinsulinized.

The second method for calculating the basal rate uses the patient's total daily insulin dose as a guide. The basal rate is calculated by taking 50% of the patient's total combined insulin requirements

Nutrition Facts

Serving Size 5 crackers (29g)
Servings per container 9

Amount Per Serving

Calories 130 Calories from Fat 40	
	% Daily Value*
Total Fat 4g	6%
Saturated Fat 1g	5%
Polyunsaturated Fat 0g	
Monounsaturated Fat 1g	
Cholesterol 0mg	0%
Sodium 280mg	12%
Total Carbohydrate 20g	7%
Dietary Fiber 1g	4%
Sugars 3g	
Protein 2g	

*Percent Daily Values are based on a 2,000 calorie diet. Your daily values may be higher or lower depending on your calorie needs.

Insulin-to-Carbohydrate Ratio Calculation

For example: A patient eats 20 small crackers and wants to calculate his or her carbohydrate ratio.

1. First determine the carbohydrate ratio per "Nutrition Facts" to the left:

1. 20 crackers = 4 servings
2. Amount of carbohydrate per serving = 20g
3. 4 servings × 20g carbohydrate per serving = 80 grams of carbohydrate

Divide the carbohydrates consumed at a meal by the insulin bolus taken by the patient at that meal to lower postprandial blood glucose to less than 180 mg/dL.

$$\frac{\text{80g carbohydrate at the meal}}{\text{4 units of premeal bolus insulin}} = \mathbf{20} \text{ grams per unit}$$

(as determined by this patient)

This example's insulin-to-carbohydrate ratio is equal to:

1 unit of insulin for every
20 grams of carbohydrate

2. If the patient intends to eat 5 (instead of 4) servings of the sample food at the left, then:

1 serving = 20g of carbohydrate (from chart to left)

5 servings = 20g × 5 = 100 grams of carbohydrate

$$\frac{\text{100 grams of carbohydrate}}{\text{20 (insulin to carbohydrate ratio)}} = \mathbf{5} \text{ units bolus insulin}$$

Figure 32–6. Insulin-to-carbohydrate ratio calculation.

(including long-acting and short-acting insulins) and dividing it by 24 hours. For example, if a patient uses 19 units of glargine a day and averages 4 units of aspart at breakfast, 5 units of aspart at lunch, and 8 units of aspart at dinner, the total combined daily insulin dose is 36 units. The basal rate would then be 50% of 36 units divided by 24 hours:

$$\frac{36\,\text{IU} \times 0.5 = 0.75\,\text{IU per hour}}{24\,\text{h}}$$

The third basal rate estimation method is based on the patient's body weight. A conservative starting dose for the basal rate can be calculated by using 0.22 units of insulin per kilogram of body weight per day, divided by 24 hours. For example, if a patient weighs 80 kilograms, the basal rate would be calculated by the equation:

$$\frac{80\,\text{kg} \times 0.22 = 0.73\,\text{IU per hour}}{24\,\text{h}}$$

or an approximate basal rate of 0.7 IU per hour.

If there is discrepancy in the estimated basal rate using the three different techniques, the lowest rate should be used for initiating insulin pump therapy to prevent hypoglycemia; the dose can be titrated slowly if needed. It is also important to discontinue the patient's intermediate-acting or long-acting insulin at least 12 to 24 hours before initiating pump therapy.

Verifying the Basal Rate

To verify the overnight basal rate, the patient should avoid eating food after an early dinner and should test the glucose value 2 hours after dinner, at bedtime, at 3 AM, and first thing in the morning. An appropriate basal rate will not lead to hypo- or hyperglycemia in the fasting state.

Some patients need an increased basal rate in the early morning hours to counteract the dawn phenomenon (the early morning resistance to insulin due to circulating growth hormone). In our experience, between 3 AM and 7 AM many patients experience a rise in blood glucose values that requires a 0.1 to 0.4 unit per hour increase during that time period. Occasionally a patient experiences a decrease in basal insulin requirements between the hours of midnight and 3 AM. In patients who are prone to nocturnal hypoglycemia, the basal rate can be decreased during this time period.

The question is often asked by pump patients, "What do you need if you have more than three basal rates?" The answer is, "A new endocrinolo-

gist!" Most pump users achieve excellent glycemic control with three or fewer basal rates per day.

To evaluate the daytime basal rate(s), the patient is instructed to fast from morning until dinnertime. If this is inconvenient, then it is suggested that the patient eat a very early breakfast, skip lunch, and monitor the blood sugars every 2 to 3 hours until dinner. An adequate basal rate will allow for ideal glucose control (between 70 and 110 mg/dL) while in the fasting state during normal daily activities.

Verifying the Bolus Doses

Prior to insulin pump therapy, premeal insulin bolus rates have usually been predetermined based on the patient's prior MDI insulin regimen. The total daily dose of lispro, aspart, or glulisine insulin should be approximately 40% to 60% of the total daily insulin requirements. Carbohydrate counting will help to fine-tune the bolus doses before meals. Many long-term diabetics have a very good sense of how much insulin they need for any particular meal based on years of experience. In general, the premeal insulin dose should be based on experience, carbohydrate counting, the premeal glucose value, and any anticipated exercise after ingestion of the meal.

Correction Factor Bolusing

All insulin users encounter situations where the blood sugar is elevated before and between meals. A correction bolus dose of a fast-acting analog is indicated to help normalize metabolic control back to an adequate baseline glucose value. When suggesting supplemental insulin lispro, aspart, or glulisine to counteract an elevated blood sugar, the *1500 rule* can be used to determine a patient's correction dose. The 1500 rule, or sensitivity factor, gives an estimation of how much the patient's blood sugar will drop when given 1 unit of fast-acting insulin. Add up the patient's total daily insulin requirements and divide that number into 1500.

For example, if a patient uses 30 units of insulin per day, one unit of lispro, aspart, or glulisine insulin will lower the blood sugar by approximately 50 mg/dL (1500 divided by 30). This particular patient would take an additional unit of fast-acting insulin for every 50 mg/dL above the goal glucose value (i.e., 120 mg/dL). For example, if this patient's blood glucose is 220 mg/dL, then the patient needs to take 2 units of insulin to return to the goal 120 mg/dL.

This sensitivity factor can change depending on individual factors such as weight changes and activity levels; therefore, it is meant only as a guide. Some patients have different correction factors for different times of the day and when the blood glucose level is extremely high (glucose toxicity leads to insulin resistance).

Once the patient initiates pump therapy, he or she should make contact with the caregiver at least once every 24-hour period to go over the glucose values and to have any questions answered or concerns addressed. The glucose values could be easily forwarded to the caregiver electronically or by facsimile prior to the phone conversation. In most cases, after 2 or 3 days the bolus and basal rates are fairly close to the ultimate values, and the patient can be seen approximately 2 to 4 weeks after initiating therapy. The support staff from the pump companies are very educated and always willing to help and support patients.

TROUBLESHOOTING EVERYDAY PUMP ISSUES

Unexplained severe hyperglycemia is an indication for immediate evaluation of the insulin pump and infusion line setup. If the delivery of insulin is interrupted during pump therapy, blood sugars will rapidly rise because there is no intermediate- or long-acting insulin in the patient's circulation. This will put the patient at risk for subsequent development of DKA.

The patient should be well trained in troubleshooting. The battery power should be evaluated, the infusion line should be checked for occlusions, air spaces, or leaks, and the insulin reservoir should checked for fullness. Patients using pumps should also always carry a bottle of regular, lispro, aspart, or glulisine insulin with a syringe or insulin pen as a backup should insulin pump abnormalities not be detected or corrected. If there is any question at all, the patient should give the correction bolus via the vial and syringe or pen to ensure insulin delivery.

Temporary pump discontinuation can also lead to loss of glycemic control. The quick release catheters are excellent for showering, bathing, and dressing; however, it should be noted that if a fast-acting analog is used in the pump, temporary pump discontinuation should not be longer than 45 minutes. This is the only disadvantage of switching from the older, regular insulin to the fast-acting analogs. The rapid decline in insulin activity seen with the analogs lessens the practical disconnection time. Many patients disconnect for prolonged periods of time and, although the blood glucose value on reconnection might not be elevated, the patient is relatively insulinopenic, which leads to delayed hyperglycemia for up to several hours.

Placement of the insulin pump during sleeping and sexual intimacy is usually not a problem, with the exception of occasional entanglement in body parts. Many patients use the quick release catheters to free themselves from the insulin pump during any short period of intensive exercise.

Traveling with an insulin pump is very convenient, especially when crossing many time zones and having erratic meal amounts, types, and times. However, with increased airport security there is the potential for delay because airport security personnel might not be familiar with insulin pumps. A doctor's note can facilitate this process. Another alternative is to disconnect the insulin pump temporarily with the quick-release catheter so the pump can be hand inspected by security personnel. Many pumps do not set off the airport security detectors; however, the pump cases may have metal clips and other parts that trip the alarms. In this situation taking the pump out of the case may help.

Some patients benefit from a pump vacation while they are enjoying a water sports weekend or just want to be totally free for a few days or weeks of the mechanical device connected to their body. In this case, we recommend that patients go back to their previous intensive insulin regimen consisting of a long-acting insulin with lispro, aspart, or glulisine insulin before each meal. This is another reason to put the patient on a basal bolus regimen prior to beginning with the pump.

THE UNTETHERED REGIMEN

The *untethered regimen* refers to the therapeutic combination of simultaneously using an insulin pump and insulin glargine to help improve glycemic excursions and overall control in a flexible and user-friendly manner. Why would a patient be on an insulin pump and long-acting insulin at the same time? Although the untethered regimen is not for everyone, using insulin glargine for part of the daily basal insulin dose can offer advantages to many people with diabetes.

It is crucial for long-term success that an insulin regimen be tailored to the patient's needs and lifestyle and not be rigid and inflexible. Insulin glargine used with a multiple daily injection regimen does have some benefits over pump therapy, especially when a patient is physically active in water sports and other activities that are not pump-friendly, such as going to the beach, scuba diving, soaking in a Jacuzzi, or playing basketball. Disconnecting the pump for more than 45 minutes could cause havoc with glucose control, especially if the patient is using fast-acting analogs in the pump. However, a multiple daily injection regimen cannot provide the ease of bolusing throughout the day, before meals, and for between-meal corrections that pump therapy can offer, as well as the square and dual wave bolus features. Thus, the untethered regimen combines the flexibility of basal glargine insulin with the ease of bolus administration via a pump.

To reap the benefits of the best features of both the insulin pump and MDI therapy, a patient should split the basal requirements between the two

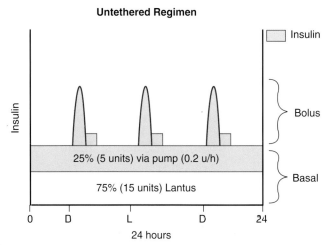

Untethered Regimen

Figure 32–7. The untethered regimen. (Copyright Steve Edelman, MD.)

techniques. For example, 75% of the patient's basal requirements can be given as insulin glargine at bedtime, and the remaining 25% of daily basal insulin can be administered by the pump. A patient whose 24-hour basal requirement is 20 units would take 15 units of Lantus at bedtime and set his or her pump at 0.2 units/hour, which makes up the remaining 25% or approximately 5 units (Fig. 32–7). The pump can be used for standard as well as square-wave and dual-wave bolusing.

In addition, temporary and alternate basal rates can be tailored according to the home glucose monitoring results. Thus, when the patient takes the pump off for extended periods of exercise, the glargine injected the night before will provide a built-in reduced basal rate. The patient does not have to worry about hooking up the pump within 45 minutes or taking frequent injections of insulin to prevent hyperglycemia, because glargine will be present. Nor is there concern about hyperglycemia in case of any sudden, unexpected disruption of insulin delivery from pump therapy.

Weekend warriors who are inactive during the week and on the untethered regimen can build in further flexibility on the weekend. On Friday night the patient can take 100% of the basal requirement as glargine and remove the pump for the weekend, using an insulin pen for meal boluses. On Sunday night the patient would then take 75% of the usual basal requirement and reconnect the pump before going to bed.

This regimen has worked well for many of our young adult and teenage patients who are on sports teams and must disconnect for hours as well as for a handful of elderly patients who are not computer-savvy or mechanically savvy with their pumps. The untethered regimen offers a real buffer safety zone to prevent ketoacidosis for new pumpers or anyone who disconnects frequently.

CLOSING THE LOOP

Insulin pump therapy is an efficacious tool for many people with diabetes. The current technology will continue to evolve, and the ultimate goal will be a closed-loop system where a continuous glucose sensor will provide real-time data to the insulin pump. After verification by the patient, an algorithm would then calculate the proper insulin dosages to be delivered by the pump.

The first continuous glucose sensor, the Continuous Glucose Monitoring System (CGMS, Medtronic MiniMed Inc, Northridge, Calif), uses a minimally invasive glucose oxidase sensor that resides in the subcutaneous fat layer similar to an insulin pump set and measures the glucose level in interstitial fluid.[20] The CGMS system functions continuously for 3 days. Then the patient returns to the doctor's office, and the information is downloaded to the computer for subsequent analysis. Glucose excursions and trends are analyzed and recommendations given to the patient.

The CGMS device had obvious limitations because it was not a real-time device. The FreeStyle Navigator Continuous Glucose Monitor (TheraSense/Abbott Inc, Alameda, Calif), a newer real-time meter that uses a similar electrochemical sensor, is currently in development.[21] In addition to static glucose concentration measurements, the system provides 1-minute updated values, glucose trend information, and glucose alarms with user-chosen values.[22] These features could provide the potential to anticipate, minimize, and even avoid undesirable glycemic excursions.

The Guardian Continuous Glucose Monitoring System (Medtronic MiniMed Inc, Northridge, Calif) is another investigational device that improves on the older CGMS. This system measures real-time glucose levels and has alarms to indicate when blood glucose levels are outside the target range. The glucose oxidase sensor assembly transmits data to a wireless monitor via radio frequency. The transmitter can be placed on a belt, carried in a pocket or purse, or worn discreetly under clothing, as long as it is within six feet of the monitor. The device is calibrated using a home glucose meter at least every 12 hours, and it measures blood glucoses in the range of 40 to 400 mg/dL for up to 72 hours.[23]

Many trials of real-time systems that are implanted within the body are ongoing. One of the limitations of subcutaneous glucose oxidase sensors is that their lifespan is limited to about 3 days because of local inflammation and encapsulation caused by the immune system. This reaction causes the glucose readings to drift, and frequent recalibration is required.

A more durable second-generation implantable glucose oxidase sensor (DexCom, San Diego, Calif) is in clinical trials. In a pilot study, the sensor was implanted subcutaneously in 15 patients and provided accurate continuous blood glucose readings to the user every 5 minutes for several months.[24] When the subjects were able to see the glucose results in real time with a pager-like device receiving the data via telemetry, they experienced fewer glucose values in the high range while enjoying a reduced incidence of hypoglycemia.

Other approaches include near infrared spectroscopy[25] and an intravascular glucose sensor that resides in the superior vena cava or right atrium (Medtronic MiniMed, Inc, Northridge, Calif).[26] Another glucose sensor under development is a viscometric affinity sensor (VAS, Disetronic, Burgdorf, Switzerland), which measures glucose based on its strong effect on the viscosity of a liquid containing Concanavalin A (ConA) and dextran.[27] The dextran molecules are cross-linked by ConA. A probe is placed in the subcutaneous fat layer, which contains a semipermeable membrane. As glucose crosses the membrane it displaces the dextran for the ConA, and the viscosity of the solution decreases. This change in viscosity can be measured by a pressure sensor, and it has a negative linear relationship with the ambient glucose concentration (as glucose level rises, the viscosity decreases).[28] Unlike glucose oxidase sensors, this method does not require recalibrations with finger sticks for up to 2 days.

As sensor technology matures, sensors will be mated with insulin pumps. The current pumps that administer insulin through continuous subcutaneous insulin infusion are limited by the slow absorption of insulin from the subcutaneous tissue. Intraperitoneal infusion promises to overcome the absorption delay. Intraperitoneal infusion can be accomplished by a peritoneal port or an implantable pump.

The Diaport percutaneous intraperitoneal port (Disetronic, Burgdorf, Switzerland) is in clinical trials.[29] It is a titanium port that is inserted through the abdominal wall in a same-day surgical setting. Once it is implanted, one of the currently available external pumps is attached to the percutaneous port. The device is expected to have a lifespan of 5 years after implantation.

The implantable insulin pumps of the mid-1990s showed that intraperitoneal insulin infusion resulted in higher and earlier peak systemic insulin concentrations.[30] These early implantable pumps had reliability issues that have been addressed in reengineered devices and improved, specifically designed insulins.

Forty Medtronic MiniMed model 2001 implantable pumps were consecutively implanted over a 2-month period in volunteers with T1DM. Cumulative experience was 106 patient-years. The systems were equipped with a side port catheter and were refilled at 45-day intervals with an experimental insulin (HOE 21 PH, Aventis Pharmaceuticals Inc, Bridgewater, NJ) that has enhanced physical stability in vitro. This study showed that patients could maintain HbA1c at goal with minimal hypoglycemia.[31] Another small study of 14

patients compared HOE 21PH versus CSII with lispro and suggested that there may be improved HbA1c levels with implantable insulin pumps.[32] As larger populations are studied, the risk–benefit relationship of this new technology will be further defined.

CONCLUSION

Continuous subcutaneous insulin infusion via external insulin pump offers patients with diabetes another option for treatment. Patients who do not have appropriate HbA1c levels or who continue to experience problems with hypoglycemia on MDI therapy may find that CSII offers a solution. The other group of patients with diabetes who benefit from insulin pumps are people who seek a more flexible lifestyle with regard to meal types, timing, and physical activity. The current external pumps will eventually transition to intraperitoneal insulin delivery via percutaneous ports or implanted pumps.

The end of this technological evolution will occur when glucose sensors continuously provide information to insulin pumps, freeing patients from continually making fingersticks and needing to manually enter pump basal rates and bolus doses. For now, the current insulin pump technology is very reliable and offers an excellent option to help improve the lives of many people with T1DM and insulin-requiring T2DM.

References

1. Dreyer M, Prager R, Robinson A, et al: Efficacy and safety of insulin glulisine (GLU) and insulin lispro (IL), combined with insulin glargine (GLAR) in patients with type 1 diabetes. Diabetes 53(Suppl 2):A709, 2004.
2. Skyler JS: Insulin treatment. In Harold Lebovitz (ed): Therapy for Diabetes Mellitus and Related Disorders. 3rd ed. Alexandria, Va, American Diabetes Association, 1998, pp 186-203.
3. Yki-Jarvinen H, Dressler A, Ziemen M et al: Less nocturnal hypoglycemia and better post-dinner glucose control with bedtime insulin glargine compared with bedtime NPH insulin during insulin combination therapy in type 2 diabetes. HOE 901/3002 Study Group. Diabetes Care 23:1130-1136, 2000.
4. Hermansen K, Fontaine P, Kukolja KK et al: Insulin analogues (insulin detemir and insulin aspart) versus traditional human insulins (NPH insulin and regular human insulin) in basal–bolus therapy for patients with type 1 diabetes. Diabetologia 47:622-629, 2004.
5. Zinman B, Tildesley H, Chiasson JL et al: Insulin lispro in CSII: Results of a double-blind crossover study. Diabetes 46:440-443, 1997.
6. Bode BW, Steed RD, Davidson PC: Reduction in severe hypoglycemia with long-term continuous subcutaneous insulin infusion in type 1 diabetes. Diabetes Care 19:324-327, 1996.
7. Crawford LM, Sinha RN, Odell RM, Comi RJ: Efficacy of insulin pump therapy: Mealtime delivery is the key factor. Endocr Pract 6:277-278, 2000.
8. Chantelau E, Schiffers T, Schutze J, et al: Effect of patient-selected intensive insulin therapy on quality of life. Patient Educ Couns 30:167-173, 1997.
9. Norby, D: Intensive Insulin Therapy Using an Insulin Pump: A Guide to Develop a Protocol to Implement Insulin Pump Therapy. Minneapolis, Disetronic Medical Systems, 1995, pp 33-52.
10. Garg SK, Walker AJ, Hoff HK, et al: Glycemic parameters with multiple daily injections using insulin glargine versus insulin pump. Diabetes Technol Ther 6:9-15, 2004.
11. Weissberg-Benchell J, Antisdel-Lomaglio J, Seshadri R: Insulin pump therapy: A meta-analysis. Diabetes Care 26:1079-1087, 2003.
12. Raskin P, Bode BW, Marks JB, et al: Continuous subcutaneous insulin infusion and multiple daily injection therapy are equally effective in type 2 diabetes: A randomized, parallel-group, 24-week study. Diabetes Care 26:2598-2603, 2003.
13. Barinas-Mitchell E, Pietropaolo S, Zhang YJ et al: Islet cell autoimmunity in a triethnic adult population of the Third National Health and Nutrition Examination Survey. Diabetes 53:1293-1302, 2004.
14. Raskin P, Holcombe JH, Tamborlane WV, et al: A comparison of insulin lispro and buffered regular human insulin administered via continuous subcutaneous insulin infusion pump. J Diabetes Complications 15:295-300, 2001.
15. Garg SK, Anderson JH, Gerard LA, et al: Impact of insulin lispro on HbA1c values in insulin pump users. Diabetes Obes Metab 2:307-311, 2000.
16. Bode B, Weinstein R, Bell D, et al: Comparison of insulin aspart with buffered regular insulin and insulin lispro in continuous insulin infusion. Diabetes Care 25:439-444, 2002.
17. Plodkowski RA, Edelman SV: The state of insulin pump therapy: 2002. Curr Opin Endocrinol Diabetes 9:329-337, 2002.
18. Kulkarni K, Fredrickson L, Graff MR: Carbohydrate Counting: A Primer for Insulin Pump Users to Zero in on Good Control. Northridge, Calif, MiniMed, 1999, pp 6-19.
19. Plodkowski RA, Edelman SV: Insulin pump therapy in the management of diabetes. In Meikle AW (ed): Endocrine Replacement Therapy in Clinical Practice, 2nd ed. Totowa, NJ, Humana Press, 2003, pp 235-250.
20. Gross TM, Bode BW, Einhorn D, et al: Performance evaluation of the MiniMed continuous glucose monitoring system during patient home use. Diabetes Technol Ther 2:49-56, 2000.
21. Weinstein R, McGarraugh GV: Accuracy evaluation of the FreeStyle Navigator continuous glucose monitor—detection of hypoglycemia. Diabetes 53:A107, 2004.
22. Bode BW, Feldman B: Clinical utility of the FreeStyle Navigator continuous glucose monitor. Diabetes 53:A709, 2004.
23. Hoss U, Holtzclaw, Kolopp M, et al: Accuracy of the Guardian Continuous Monitoring System under conditions of normal use. Diabetes 53:A462, 2004.
24. Garg SK, Schwartz S, Edelman SV: Improved glucose excursions using an implantable real-time continuous glucose sensor in adults with type 1 diabetes. Diabetes Care 27:734-738, 2004.
25. Cote GL: Noninvasive and minimally-invasive optical monitoring technologies. J Nutr 131:1596S-1604S, 2001.
26. Renard E, Jovanovic G, Costalat G et al: First implications of a long-term glucose sensor connected to insulin pumps in diabetic patients. Diabetologia 44:(Suppl 1):169, 2001.
27. Beyer U, Fleischer A, Kage A, et al: Calibration of the viscometric glucose sensor before its use in physiological liquids—compensation for the colloid-osmotic effect. Biosens Bioelectron 18:1391-1397, 2003.
28. Beyer U, Schafer D, Thomas A, et al: Recording of subcutaneous glucose dynamics by a viscometric affinity sensor. Diabetologia 44:416-423, 2001.
29. Frei T, Liebl A, Renner R, et al: Continuous intraperitoneal insulin infusion (CIPII) via the umbilical vein in type 1 diabetic patients: First results. Diabetologia 43: (Suppl 2):A3, 2000.

30. Kelley DE, Henry RR, Edelman SV: Acute effects of intraperitoneal versus subcutaneous insulin delivery on glucose homeostasis in patients with NIDDM. Diabetes Care 19:1237-1242, 1997.

31. Gin H, Renard E, Melki V et al: Combined improvements in implantable pump technology and insulin stability allow safe and effective long term intraperitoneal insulin delivery in type 1 diabetic patients: The EVADIAC experience. Diabetes Metab 29:602-607, 2003.

32. Catargi B, Meyer L, Melki V et al: Comparison of blood glucose stability and HbA1C between implantable insulin pumps using U400 HOE 21PH insulin and external pumps using lispro in type 1 diabetic patients: A pilot study. Diabetes Metab 28:133-137, 2002.

Chapter 33

Glucose Monitoring of the Present and Future

Satish K. Garg, Leita C. Sharp, and Mary E. Stults

KEY POINTS

- *Home blood glucose monitoring has a huge impact on glycemic control.*
- *Self-monitoring of blood glucose at home must be used to adjust the dose of hypoglycemic agents.*
- *New advances in glucose sensors and continuous glucose monitoring, especially those with hypo- and hyperglycemia alarms, should improve glycemic control and thus promote a better quality of life.*

The goals of appropriate therapy for those with diabetes should include serious effort to achieve levels [of] blood glucose as close to those in the nondiabetic as feasible.

Elliot P. Joslin, 1935

Diabetes mellitus is a group of metabolic diseases characterized by elevated blood glucose resulting from defects in insulin production or insulin action, or both. Diabetes is usually associated with serious acute and long-term complications and premature death, but people with diabetes can take steps to control the disease and lower the risk of complications.[1]

PREVALENCE

Diabetes mellitus, the most common metabolic disease, is increasing in incidence globally. It will affect 216 million persons worldwide by 2010.[2-3] Most of this increase in diabetes prevalence is an increase in type 2 diabetes (T2DM), formerly known as adult-onset diabetes. Type 1 diabetes (T1DM) constitutes about 5% to 10% of all diabetes diagnosed. In 2002, the total prevalence of diabetes in the United States for all ages was estimated to be 18.2 million people, which accounted for 6.3% of the population. Approximately 13 million persons have a formal diagnosis by a health care professional and an estimated 5.2 million persons have undiagnosed diabetes.[4] Another 47 million persons have impaired glucose tolerance (IGT) and are therefore at a very high risk for developing diabetes and cardiovascular disease.

The prevalence of diagnosed diabetes among US adults increased by 40% in 10 years from 4.9% in 1990 to 6.9% in 1999. It is estimated that the number of persons in the United States with diagnosed diabetes will increase by 165% between 2000 and 2050, with the fastest increases occurring in older and minority subpopulations.[5] For children born in the United States in 2000, an estimated lifetime risk of diagnosed diabetes mellitus was roughly 1 in 3 for boys and 2 in 5 for girls.

The risk of diabetes is higher than many people realize. The lifetime risk of diabetes is comparable to or higher than that for many diseases and conditions that are perceived as common, such as breast cancer and coronary heart disease. The prevalence of diabetes is also higher for certain racial and ethnic minority populations. Latin Americans have roughly a 1 in 2 risk at birth and 1 in 3 residual risk at age 60 years of developing diabetes.

COST

Diabetes is a serious and costly disease. Per capita, people with diabetes spend approximately 2.4 times more (more than $13,000 a year) on medical costs compared to people without diabetes.[6] The annual cost of diabetes in the United States in 2002 was estimated to be $132 billion, which is a dramatic increase from $98 billion in 1997. The direct medical costs of diabetes more than doubled in that time, from $44 billion in 1997 to $91.8 billion in 2002 (Fig. 33–1A). Of the direct medical expenditures, 51% were incurred by people older than 65 years of age. Indirect medical expenses were estimated to be $40 billion in 2002 (see Fig. 33–1B).[6] The projected increase in the number of people with diabetes suggests that the annual cost could rise to an estimated $156 billion by 2010 and to $192 billion by 2020.[6]

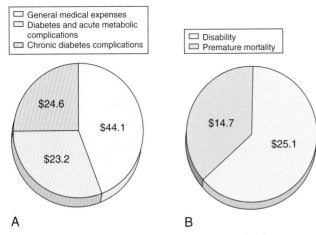

Figure 33–1. A, $91.8 billion in direct medical expenses were attributable to diabetes in 2002. **B,** $39.8 billion in indirect medical expenses were attributable to diabetes in 2002.

PREDIABETES, OBESITY, AND CARDIOVASCULAR DISEASE

> I believe the chief cause of premature atherosclerosis in diabetes is excessive fat, an excess of fat in the body, an excess of fat in the diet, an excess of fat in the blood; with an excess of fat diabetes begins and from an excess of fat diabetics die, formerly of coma, now of atherosclerosis.[7]
>
> *Elliot P. Joslin, 1927*

In response to the Diabetes Prevention Program (DPP), a National Institutes of Health (NIH) sponsored study, the American Diabetes Association (ADA) has recommended that diabetes prevention efforts target people with prediabetes.[8] Prediabetes is a condition in which blood glucose levels are higher than normal but not high enough to be classified as full-blown diabetes. Patients with diagnosed prediabetes have a risk of developing diabetes within 10 years and are at risk for associated heart disease.

Prediabetes is diagnosed by an abnormal fasting plasma glucose (FPG) test or an abnormal oral glucose tolerance test (OGTT). Abnormal results from the FPG test or OGTT indicate impaired fasting glucose if the blood glucose is higher than 100 mg/dL (5.9 mmol/L). The results indicate impaired glucose tolerance if the fasting glucose is higher than 126 mg/dL (7 mmol/L) and the blood glucose level is 140 to 199 mg/dL (7.8 to 11.1 mmol/L) 2 hours after consuming the glucose drink.

Obesity is associated with prediabetes and has a major impact on insulin use in the body. A recent study found that obese children and adolescents with prediabetes had profound peripheral insulin resistance and major defects in the nonoxidative pathway of glucose metabolism. The insulin resis-

tance in these obese young people was found to be associated with increased intramyocellular lipid accumulation along with increased visceral fat mass.[9] The DPP found that overweight persons older than 45 years of age are at increased risk for developing prediabetes and should be screened at their primary health care office. It is also recommended that overweight persons who are younger than 45 years should be screened for prediabetes if they have one or more of the following risk factors:

- Family history of diabetes
- Low HDL cholesterol and high triglycerides
- Hypertension
- History of gestational diabetes or giving birth to a baby weighing more than 9 pounds
- Belonging to certain minority groups, including African American, Asian or Pacific Islander, Native American, or Latin American.

Cardiovascular disease (CVD) is the cause of the majority of diabetic admissions to the hospital as well as 75% to 80% of diabetic death.[8] By the time T2DM is diagnosed in patients, more than half of them will have already experienced a myocardial infarction (MI), suggesting that proatherogenic processes have already been at work for some time.[8] The presence of atherosclerosis and CVD is associated with insulin resistance that is pronounced in the prediabetic state.[10] For this reason, a timely diagnosis of prediabetes is important for controlling CVD. There is also accumulating evidence that inflammation measured by C-reactive protein (CRP) is also associated with increased CVD.

Although prediabetes has a high rate of developing into diabetes, with proper intervention diabetes can be prevented. The DPP study showed that people can reduce their risk for developing diabetes and heart disease by up to 58% through sustained modest weight loss and increased moderate-intensity exercise, such as walking 30 minutes daily.[4] Once a patient develops diabetes, good glycemic control as demonstrated by reaching hemoglobin A1c (HbA1c) goals can drastically decrease micro- and macrovascular complications (Table 33–1).[11-13]

SELF-MONITORING OF BLOOD GLUCOSE

Self-monitoring of blood glucose (SMBG) is essential for guiding the therapeutic plan for diabetes initiated by a health care provider, especially in patients using insulin injections. Self-testing by patients is critical in educating patients about their diabetes status. SMBG is recommended for all patients with diabetes and especially for those who take insulin. The American Diabetes Association (ADA) recommends that intensively managed T1DM patients should perform SMBG at least three times daily. Pregnant women taking insulin for gestational diabetes should test eight to 10 times per day. The ADA does not specify how often

Table 33–1. *Reduction of Diabetic Complications with Increased Glycemic Control*

Improvement in Complication	DCCT	Kumamoto	UKPDS
Decrease in HbA1c	9 ± 7%	9 ± 7%	8 ± 7%
Retinopathy decrease	63%	69%	17-21%
Nephropathy decrease	54%	70%	24-33%
Neuropathy decrease	60%	—	—
Macrovascular disease decrease	41%*	—	16%*

*Not statistically significant.
DCCT, Diabetes Control and Complications Trial; HbA1c, hemoglobin A1c; UKPDS, United Kingdom Prospective Diabetes Study.

people with T2DM should test their blood glucose levels, but testing docs help with their metabolic control.

Individual fluctuations in daily blood glucose levels dictate the frequency of SMBG. SMBG plans direct patients to test their blood glucose levels at different times of the day targeting before meals, 2 hours after meals, bedtime, 3 AM, and any time they experience signs or symptoms of hyper- or hypoglycemia. Patients are advised to test more often when they have a change in their medications, during stress or illness, or in other circumstances such as travel, before and after exercise, and during pregnancy.

Instructions for Performing a Self-Monitored Blood Glucose Test

Blood glucose self-monitoring is an easy test to perform and has come a long way. First the patient must wash the hands with soap and warm water and dry thoroughly. Some health care professionals recommend using alcohol to clean the fingertip that will be used. Next, the patient pricks the finger using a lancet, causing a small drop of blood to appear. It is recommended that this first drop of blood be wiped off and the second drop used for testing. The second drop of blood (1 to 10 μL) is placed on the test strip that is inserted into the SMBG meter. The blood glucose test result can take from 5 to 40 seconds to be displayed on the meter. Patients are often advised to record their SMBG results in a logbook in order to follow their glycemic status closely.

Although SMBG is a good way for patients to have greater control of their own therapy, the time and effort it takes to faithfully perform multiple tests a day at the target times is exhausting for many patients. Also, the multiple invasive fingersticks act as a deterrent to regular testing. For this reason many SMBG tests are missed and blood glucose levels that are out of the euglycemic range are not appropriately treated. This often creates a barrier to therapeutic goals and frustration to both patients and their health care providers. To confront this problem, alternate ways to monitor blood glucose levels, such as continuous glucose monitoring, are under research. Devices that have been approved by the FDA and some currently under development are discussed later.

Eight-Point Profile

Elevated fasting and postprandial glucose levels have been associated with increased risk of microvascular and macrovascular complications. The risk of cardiovascular disease and all-cause mortality has also been found to increase with increasing postprandial blood glucose.[14] Furthermore, the Diabetes Intervention Study demonstrated that postprandial blood glucose was an independent risk factor for mortality in patients with newly diagnosed T2DM.[15] Therefore, 2-hour postprandial blood glucose may be important in reducing diabetic complications and mortality and may be an important focus for therapy.

The best indicator of 2-hour postprandial blood glucose levels is the eight-point profile. The eight-point profile is a series of blood glucose measurements by the patient at the following times: in the morning before breakfast, 2 hours after breakfast, at noon before lunch, 2 hours after lunch, in the evening before dinner, 2 hours after dinner, at bedtime, and at around 3 AM. This profile gives the health care provider a better picture of what the patient's blood sugar levels are throughout the day. This is important for regulating the dose of preprandial insulin that is taken to lower the postprandial blood glucose levels. The frequency with which eight-point monitoring needs to be done can vary from once per week to once per month, depending on the stage of the disease, the medical interventions, and the target HbA1c change undertaken.

Home Blood Glucose Meters

There are many different kinds of SMBG meters available for testing, including fingerstick-only testing meters and dual-site testing meters (fingerstick and alternate site) (Table 33–2). Some meters or personal digital assistants (PDAs) store up to thousands of blood glucose results that can be

Table 33–2. *Examples of Home Blood Glucose Meters*

Manufacturer	Model	Test Site	Testing Time	Results
Abbott	MediSense Precision Xtra	FS	20 seconds	450
Abbott	Freestyle	FS or Alt	15 seconds	250
Bayer	Ascensia Dex 2	FS or Alt	30 seconds	100
BD	BD Logic	FS or Alt	5 seconds	250
Lifescan	One Touch Ultra Smart	FS or Alt	5 seconds	3000
Roche	Accu-Chek Advantage	FS	40 seconds	100

Alt, alternative testing; FS, fingerstick testing.

downloaded at the doctor's office. These meters are helpful for health care providers because they do not depend on the patient's accurate recording of the results to evaluate the recent blood glucose history.

It is the patient's and the health care professional's choice to determine which meter best fits the needs of the patient. However, this selection is often influenced by the brand of meter(s) that the patient's insurance company will cover. Some of the most commonly used meters include Accu-Chek (Roche), One Touch Ultra (Lifescan), Ascencia (Bayer), and Freestyle (Abbott).

Comparing Home Results and Laboratory Results

YSI Glucose Autoanalyzers
YSI glucose autoanalyzers (Yellow Springs Instruments, Yellow Springs, Ohio) are used in the laboratory to measure whole-blood glucose, plasma, serum, and lactate. The analyzers provide fast and accurate results with very high precision. The YSI results are standard measurements for clinical diagnostics against which other blood glucose measurements are judged.

The Clark Error Grid is a graphic way of comparing SMBG results to the YSI standards across the blood-glucose spectrum. Zone A, considered clinically accurate, is ±20% of the standardized value. Values falling into Zone B are clinically inaccurate, but they vary by 20% or more from the standardized values. Zones A and B together are considered the clinically relevant zones. Zone C suggests that an unnecessary overcorrection is possible, and values in Zone D indicate a dangerous failure to detect and treat errors. Zone E signifies erroneous treatment.[16]

HemoCue Glucose 201 Analyzer
The HemoCue blood glucose meter (HemoCue, Inc, Lake Forest, Calif.), which is the size of a paperback book, has been recognized as equivalent in accuracy to the YSI. It has a correlation of $r > 0.98$ when compared to other laboratory methods, with a standard deviation of less than 6 mg/dL. This instrument also has the advantages of displaying results in 40 to 240 seconds and only requiring 5 μL of blood.

To test glucose levels, a blood sample from the fingertip is obtained using a lancet. A microcuvette (stored at 4°C) is then applied to the sample and the necessary amount is drawn into the microcuvette by capillary action. The cuvette is then inserted into the analyzer, and a result is displayed. The time to display depends on the glucose level.[17]

Although not as convenient in size, the HemoCue is a good compromise between the accuracy of the YSI and the ease of use of the other SMBG meters. It is particularly useful for hospital or research use.

Alternative Site Testing

Another choice in SMBG is testing sites other than the fingertip. New meters requiring less blood, combined with the capillary action of some test strips, have allowed alternative sites such as the forearm and thigh to be used. Benefits of alternative site testing include less pain during testing and therefore better compliance for testing multiple times per day. Patients may also prefer alternative site testing when they are using their hands and do not want to worry about continued bleeding.

Unfortunately, the accuracy of alternative sites as compared to fingertip testing is not conclusively proven. During times of rapid change as well as in the hyper- and hypoglycemic ranges, alternative sites tend to react more slowly to fluctuations in blood glucose.[18] A study by Ellison and coworkers suggests that the forearm and thigh may be used for routine fasting (more than 3 hours) measurements, but these locations are not accurate following meals, when glucose levels peak more slowly, so they never reach the same level as fingertip tests do.[19]

GLUCOSE CONTROL PARAMETERS

Glycated Proteins

Virtually all proteins in the body can become glycated. This happens when circulating blood glucose reacts with amino groups on proteins to form covalently bound glycated products. This modification occurs in both circulating and structural proteins.[20]

If hyperglycemia is sustained for long durations, more complicated reactions can occur, yielding advanced glycation end products. These complex compounds include several glucose or glucose-derived products that are covalently bound to proteins.

Advanced glycation end products are nearly irreversibly formed and once created respond very poorly to improvements in metabolic control.[20] An example of an advanced glycated end product is glycated hemoglobin (HbA1c). Hemoglobin (the oxygen-carrying portion of a red blood cell) is a protein that becomes glycated in direct proportion to the ambient concentration of blood glucose.[21-26] Glycated hemoglobin is used as a marker for glucose control in diabetes during the previous 3 months. However, when a patient's HbA1c is extremely elevated (higher than 11%; normal range is 3.5% to 6.2%), it is likely that medical interventions will show a decline sooner (within a month).

Hemolysis

The average life span of an erythrocyte in a person who maintains euglycemia is 120 days. Hyperglycemia decreases the life span of an erythrocyte by damaging the cell membrane, causing cell death.[27] It has been proposed that hyperglycemia causes peroxidation of membrane lipids in red blood cells, causing hemolysis.[28] There is also evidence that the irreversible cross-linking of non-enzymatic glycated proteins contributes to a loss of elasticity that is characteristic of the cells, reducing the deformability and causing a shortened life span.[29]

Hemoglobin A1c Testing

Assay
The HbA1c assay was introduced in 1989 as a replacement for the total glycohemoglobin test. The HbA1c assay is the measurement of glycated hemoglobin and is regarded as the gold standard method for assessing long-term glycemic control. Erythrocytes are freely permeable to glucose, and studies confirm that the rate of formation of glycated hemoglobin is directly proportional to the ambient glucose concentration.[21-26]

When plasma glucose is consistently elevated, there is an increase in the relatively slow, post-translational, largely irreversible, nonenzymatic reaction producing the glycation of hemoglobin. In this reaction, the NH_2-terminal amino acid of the β-chain of hemoglobin forms an unstable Schiff base and then undergoes an Amadori rearrangement to form a stable ketoamine (Fig. 33–2).

Because the average lifespan of an erythrocyte is 120 days, the HbA1c assay reflects the mean blood glucose level over the previous 2 to 3 months.[30] If

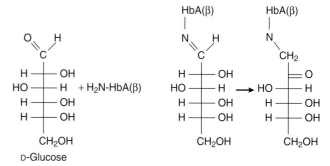

Figure 33–2. Glycation of hemoglobin reaction.

the HbA1c is very high, however, measurements at 1 month can show a significant decline in HbA1c values following medical intervention.

Methodology
The HbA1c assay can be measured by different analytical principles such as immunoassay, ion-exchange chromatography, and affinity chromatography.[31] High-performance liquid chromatography (HPLC) is proven to have a superior specificity and reliability and has therefore become the standard reference method for most HbA1c measurements. When measured by HPLC, a 1% rise in the HbA1c translates into a 1.7-mmol/L (30 mg/dL) increase in the mean glucose.[30] Therefore, an HbA1c of 6% is 6.6 mmol/L (120 mg/dL), 7% is 8.3 mmol/L (150 mg/dL), 8% is 10.0 mmol/L (180 mg/dL), and so on.

Rapid Testing
Other ways to measure HbA1c are by rapid testing methods that can be done in the health care provider's office or at home. Bayer's DCA 2000 instrument and the Aeroset by Abbott are used in the health care provider's office and are NGSP (National Glycohemoglobin Standardization Program) certified. The DCA 2000 is quick and easy, taking only 6 minutes, and is done with a drop of blood from a fingerstick. The Aeroset can run up to 2000 tests per hour.

These clinical tools are valuable to help health care professionals guide their therapeutic decisions. A recent study suggests that clinicians are more likely to advance pharmacologic therapy in patients exhibiting mild hyperglycemia if a rapid HbA1c level is available.[32]

Another way for patients to monitor their HbA1c is by a rapid test made by Metrika. This test uses MODM (micro-optical detection method) technology and is called A1cNow. This test is a portable, single-use device to provide immediate access to quantitative HbA1c status.

Standardization
The Diabetes Control and Complications Trial (DCCT) and the United Kingdom Prospective Diabetes Study (UKPDS) conclusively demonstrated

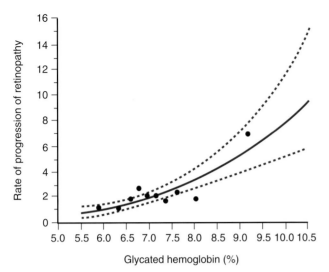

Figure 33–3. Risk of retinopathy progression with increased HbA1c in the Diabetes Control and Complications Trial (DCCT). (From Valle T, Tuomilehto J, Eriksson J: Epidemiology of NIDDM in Europoids. In: Alberti KGMM, Simmet P, DeFronzo RA [eds]: International Textbook of Diabetes Mellitus. Chichester, UK, John Wiley & Sons, 1997, pp 125-142. Copyright © 1997 John Wiley and Sons Ltd. Reproduced with permission.)

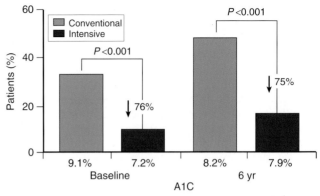

Figure 33–4. The Diabetes Control and Complications Trial (DCCT) substudy Epidemiology of Diabetes Interventions and Complications (EDIC) showed that the benefit in progression of retinopathy lasts beyond the original hemoglobin A1c decrease during EDIC years.

that the risks of complications in diabetic patients were directly related to glycemic control measured by HbA1c.[33] As a result of these findings, the NGSP was implemented. This program certifies laboratories that use approved methods for measuring and reporting DCCT-traceable HbA1c results. The various methods are calibrated with the same set of calibrators and are adjusted to a designated comparison method. There is now widespread acceptance and implementation of the certification process. This standardization allows physicians and patients to relate HbA1c results to DCCT-based treatment goals.[33]

Hemoglobin A1c and Diabetic Complications

The HbA1c test is invaluable in the treatment of patients as a predictor of diabetic complications. Interventions that reduce HbA1c correspondingly reduce the risk of complications.[11-13,34] HbA1c should therefore be measured in all diabetic patients at their initial visit and every 3 months thereafter as part of their routine comprehensive diabetes care. Regular HbA1c measurement allows health care providers to determine whether the patient's metabolic control has been maintained within the target range, and it detects departures from the target range in a timely fashion.[21]

Prolonged elevated HbA1c values are a risk factor for many associated diabetic conditions such as retinopathy (Fig. 33–3), neuropathy, and microvas-

cular complications. The DCCT found that HbA1c was the predominant determinant of risk, but it did not account for the entire risk of retinopathy progression. Other unidentified factors (such as glucose excursions) contributed to a difference between the conventionally treated and the intensively treated groups.[11] Similar results are reported from large studies in subjects with T2DM.[35,13]

Additionally, the benefit of improving HbA1c values may last 6 to 7 years, even when the HbA1c rises, as shown by the Epidemiology of Diabetes Interventions and Complications (EDIC) data (Fig. 33–4). In fact, subjects in the intensively treated group continued to show benefit on progression of diabetic retinopathy and kidney disease at the end of 6 years of follow-up, despite a later elevation in HbA1c.[36]

Fructosamine

The fructosamine test is a rapid, inexpensive assay that provides a measure of nonenzymatic glycated serum proteins.[37-38] This test evaluates glycemic control over the previous 2 to 3 weeks, therefore allowing patients and clinicians to assess more recent changes in glycemic status as compared to HbA1c.[39] Tests for fructosamine can be done in the laboratory, in the office, or by the patient at home with the dual meter. The dual meter can test serum glucose as well as fructosamine using two different strips.

Fructosamine testing may allow for timelier drug titration, making adjustments in medications faster. The acceptance of fructosamine by physicians was evaluated and it was determined that same-day fructosamine concentrations helped with diabetes management due primarily to patients' inadequately monitoring their home blood glucose levels.[40] A recent study published in 2003 by Cohen

and colleagues indicated that there was a correlation between an increased glycosylation gap (the discordance between serum HbA1c and fructosamine levels) and increasing diabetic nephropathy stages.[41]

It has also been suggested that patients presenting with stress hyperglycemia, as identified by raised random serum glucose and a serum fructosamine ≥2.8 mmol/L (60 mg/dL), are associated with having an approximate threefold increased risk of developing diabetes mellitus over 5 years. These patients should therefore be screened for diabetes mellitus on a regular basis.[42] Even though fructosamine testing is a good measure of glucose control over 2 weeks, the long-term glycemic control by measurement of HbA1c values and short-term control with SMBG remains the standard of care.

HYPOGLYCEMIA

Risk of Hypoglycemia

The risk of hypoglycemia is a major issue that is evaluated when treating patients with diabetes. There are different severities of hypoglycemic episodes, including mild, moderate, and severe. With mild hypoglycemia, a patient can recognize accompanying symptoms and treat him- or herself accordingly. With moderate hypoglycemia, a patient might or might not be able to recognize accompanying symptoms and requires the help of another person to treat the symptoms. With severe hypoglycemia, a patient requires the help of another person to treat the symptoms. Symptoms of severe hypoglycemia include seizures and coma and can require administration of glucagon and emergency department visits.

Euglycemia

Maintaining euglycemia is the therapeutic goal for people with T1DM and T2DM. This goal is important because long durations of hyperglycemia can cause microvascular complications such as neuropathy, nephropathy, and retinopathy and macrovascular complications such as cardiovascular disease with associated hyperlipidemia and hypertension.[11]

Hypoglycemia, or glucopenia, acts as a barrier to euglycemia's long-term benefits and is the rate-limiting factor in achieving the glycemic range in patients with diabetes.[43] Hypoglycemia in diabetes is due to endogenous and exogenous hyperinsulinemia caused by insulin, blood glucose–lowering agents such as sulfonylureas, and some other over-the-counter and prescription drugs. When exogenous insulin is given, insulin levels do not decrease as glucose levels fall, therefore causing iatrogenic hypoglycemia. Iatrogenic hypoglycemia is the major form of hypoglycemia in diabetes mellitus, especially T1DM.

Further perpetuating this problem are the altered or absent glucagon, epinephrine, and other counterregulatory responses to low plasma glucose levels. Factors contributing to these altered or absent responses include diabetic autonomic neuropathy, pancreatic alpha cell damage, inflammation of the pancreatic cells due to autoimmune damage, and amyloid deposition in T2DM. These compromised physiologic and behavioral defenses against falling plasma glucose concentrations, compounded by hypoglycemic unawareness, occur in many patients after years with diabetes.[43]

Hypoglycemic Symptoms

Symptoms of hypoglycemia include shakiness, dizziness, sweating, hunger, headache, pale skin, mood swings, and even seizures. The patient who has hypoglycemia awareness can treat the hypoglycemia with glucose tablets or an increase in carbohydrate intake. After a short time the blood glucose levels come back into the euglycemic range and the symptoms subside. On average, subjects with diabetes suffer two episodes of symptomatic hypoglycemia per week and thousands of such episodes in a lifetime.

Asymptomatic Hypoglycemia

Asymptomatic hypoglycemia is experienced in patients as much as 10% of the time and is due to an altered or delayed sympathoadrenal response. When plasma glucose levels are low (usually lower than 50 to 60 mg/dL [2.8 mmol/L]), patients are often unable to treat themselves and help is required from a friend, spouse, or family member. Asymptomatic hypoglycemia can be treated with glucose tablets, an increase in carbohydrate intake, or an external injection or intranasal administration of glucagon. Glucagon counters hypoglycemia by raising the glucose levels through gluconeogenesis in the liver. The glucagon injection is usually given subcutaneously or intramuscularly, and the standard dose is 1 mg (the dose is modified in children). Intranasal administration of glucagon causes a glycemic response similar to that of injected glucagon.

Severe Hypoglycemia

Subjects requiring insulin therapy for the management of diabetes have a higher risk of severe hypoglycemia. Insulin-regulated type 2 diabetics also suffer severe hypoglycemia, but with a lower fre-

quency. Severe hypoglycemic episodes occur when blood glucose levels drop significantly, temporarily disabling the person, which often causes seizure activity or coma. Seizure precipitation is especially common if the patient has an underlying neurologic disease.

Due to the severity of the incident, the patient is often treated in the emergency department or by paramedics at the patient's home. In the hospital, intravenous glucose is the standard treatment followed by oral carbohydrate intake once the patient is able to ingest food safely.[44] Most patients who are treated quickly make a complete recovery, but permanent neurologic deficits can occur, especially in children.[44] An estimated 2% to 4% of deaths of patients with type 1 diabetes have been attributed to hypoglycemia.[43]

Delayed Hypoglycemia

Delayed hypoglycemia usually occurs 6 to12 hours after exercise but has been reported up to 28 hours after exercise.[45] The pathophysiology involves vigorous exercise that severely depletes the body's glycogen stores. If the patient fails to replenish the glycogen stores after exercise by ingesting carbohydrates, then the liver and muscle tissues extract circulating blood glucose to replenish depleted glycogen stores over the next few hours.[46] This causes the blood glucose levels to drop into the hypoglycemic range, and the patient becomes symptomatic.

Nocturnal Hypoglycemia

Nocturnal hypoglycemia is depressed blood glucose levels that occur while the patient is asleep (between the evening injection and getting up in the morning). It is associated with symptoms such as restlessness, nightmares, waking up with bad dreams, and profuse sweating. It has been reported that nocturnal hypoglycemia represents approximately half of all hypoglycemic episodes in insulin-dependent diabetic patients.[11] Asymptomatic nocturnal hypoglycemia is common and can cause morning headache, abnormal or bad dreams, malaise that may result in diminished awareness, reduced responses of adrenaline, and adaptation of cognitive function during the episode.[47-50]

Overtreatment of symptomatic nocturnal hypoglycemia with snacks often results in hyperglycemia the next day. Counterregulatory hormone response with accentuated growth hormone or cortisol release causes a similar rebound in blood sugar levels. Recent nocturnal hypoglycemia can contribute to the vicious cycle of hypoglycemia unawareness and impaired hormonal counterregulation, leading to increased risk for severe hypoglycemia.[51]

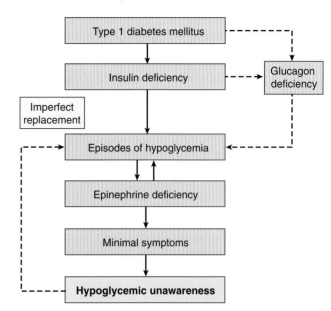

Figure 33–5. Hypoglycemia-associated autonomic failure and hypoglycemia unawareness in type I diabetes. (From Koenig R, Peterson CM, Jones RL, et al: Correlation of glucose regulation and hemoglobin A1c in diabetes mellitus. N Engl J Med 295:417-420, 1976. Copyright © 1976 Massachusetts Medical Society. All rights reserved.)

Hypoglycemia Unawareness

Hypoglycemia unawareness occurs in about 25% of patients with T1DM and is characterized by loss of autonomic warning symptoms before development of neuroglycopenia (Fig. 33–5). Hypoglycemia unawareness is associated with a sevenfold increase in the frequency of severe hypoglycemia, which may be accompanied by seizures and coma. Several risk factors for hypoglycemia unawareness have been identified, including long duration of diabetes, tight glycemic control (low HbA1c values), and repeated episodes of hypoglycemia. It has been thought that altered counterregulatory hormone responses to hypoglycemia are primarily responsible for hypoglycemia unawareness. However, recent studies suggest that impaired β-adrenergic sensitivity might also be involved.[30,44]

NEED FOR CONTINUOUS GLUCOSE MONITORING

Many studies have shown that 24-hour profiles of glucose values can result in better glucose management and a reduction in HbA1c levels.[52,53] Continuous glucose monitoring should provide a convenient and automatic method of monitoring glucose levels with a minimal number of required fingersticks. Improved glycemic control may be achieved by providing additional data to track glucose trends and patterns. Patients can better understand the impact of changes in their diet,

activity, and medications on their glucose levels and evaluate the success of a treatment regimen.

Frequent monitoring, especially during the night when glucose levels are not usually tested, can reveal both hypoglycemic and hyperglycemic excursions in the early morning hours (dawn phenomenon) that could be treated. Decreasing glucose excursions may be beneficial to the quality of life and prevent complications of diabetes as described in the DCCT subanalysis.[11] Even in the intensively treated group in the DCCT, there was a group of patients with higher HbA1c values who had lower risk of diabetic retinopathy onset or progression when compared with the conventionally treated group. Researchers thus concluded that "A1C values may not be the complete picture and glucose excursions may be responsible for diabetes complications."[11]

The availability of continuous glucose monitoring could lead to an improved quality of life due to recognition of hypoglycemic episodes with alarms and reduction of long-term micro- and macrovascular complications of diabetes. It would also make implementation of the DCCT results in clinical practice much easier.

CONTINUOUS GLUCOSE MONITORING SYSTEMS

Invasive Systems

The Medtronic MiniMed Continuous Glucose Monitoring System

The Medtronic MiniMed Continuous Glucose Monitoring System (CGMS) (Medtronic MiniMed, Northridge, Calif) was the first frequent-glucose-monitoring device approved for use in the United States (Fig. 33–6). The system consists of a subcutaneous sensor and an external monitor. The sensor uses interstitial fluid (rather than blood) for evaluating glucose levels.

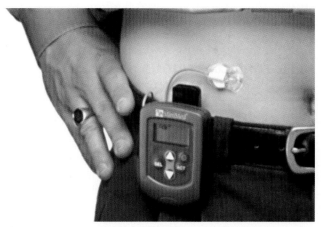

Figure 33–6. Patient wearing the Medtronic MiniMed Continuous Glucose Monitoring System apparatus.

The Medtronic MiniMed sensor continuously monitors interstitial glucose levels by collecting electric signals from the glucose sensor every 10 seconds, converting those signals into glucose values, and storing an average blood glucose value every 5 minutes for up to 72 hours. The sensor is inserted into the skin of the abdomen using an automatic insertion device, similar to an insulin pump catheter insertion, with an introducer needle that is removed immediately after insertion.

The sensor is connected to the monitor by a small wire. The monitor, which is similar in size to a pager, is worn externally. The CGMS system must be initially calibrated by the patient with a fingerstick blood glucose measurement using any home blood glucose monitor. Four fingerstick blood glucose measurements are also required each day for recalibrations. The monitor also allows the patient to enter the time of meals, medication, exercise, and other events the patient might want to recall later.

The glucose values are not displayed on the monitor but rather are sent by the sensor to the monitor and internally stored. The patient takes the sensor back to the health care provider's office to download the data. When the data are downloaded, recorded events appear with their associated glucose levels. Subjects can wear the sensor throughout normal daily activities for up to 72 hours.

In general, the CGMS system may be worn as many times as necessary to evaluate and manage the patient's glucose control. The CGMS system is intended for occasional rather than everyday use, and it is to be used as a supplement to, and not a replacement for, standard blood glucose monitoring.

Rapidly changing glucose levels can create a bigger time lag between blood and interstitial fluid measurements. Studies have shown the time lag between CGMS and blood glucose measured with a fingerstick after a meal to be 4 minutes in the rise and 9 minutes in the fall.[54]

A new Medtronic MiniMed sensor was introduced in November 2002 that is showing improved accuracy in comparison to the previous sensor. The MiniMed Sensor is considered accurate enough to detect trends in glucose values, although the accuracy does not yet approach the level of current home glucose meters, especially in the hypoglycemic regions (lower than 100 mg/dL [5.5 mmol/L]) where it is needed most.[55]

As with any new technology introduced into diabetes management, there are minor obstacles as well as major limitations. Along with the inaccuracies at lower blood glucose levels, patients complain that the CGMS system gives them no real-time data. Patients must wait until they take the sensor back to the health care provider for downloading before they can see the changes and trends in their glucose values. Furthermore, this system is invasive, and the

sensor is inserted using an introducer needle, which can be painful.

Numerous studies on the CGMS have concluded that improved diabetes control and lower HbA1c values can be achieved when patients and their health care providers access the detailed glucose information.[53-57] The effectiveness of the medication in relation to the patient's normal daily activities can be observed and any adjustments made to doses. Other studies have shown there was a significant difference in the number of hypoglycemic episodes detected by the CGMS when compared with SMBG.[53,58-60] Many of the episodes were during the night and were detected only by the CGMS when the patient did not have any symptoms.

The CGMS is currently available for use only by a health care provider for professional use as a Holter monitor. A new MiniMed CGMS system (Guardian) with hypoglycemic and hyperglycemic alarms has been approved by the FDA for professional use. Improvements are being made to the current CGMS system, and new versions may be released that allow patients to see glucose values in real time.

The GlucoWatch Biographer

The GlucoWatch Biographer (Cygnus, San Francisco, Calif) is the first frequent-monitoring device to report real-time glucose values to the patient throughout the day or night (Fig. 33–7A). The device provides a means to obtain painless, automatic, and noninvasive glucose measurements. It consists of two integrated parts, the Biographer and the AutoSensor. The Biographer is a small wristwatch-like device, which is worn on the forearm and contains sampling and detection means, electronic circuitry, and a digital display.[61]

Three separate technologies are incorporated into the GlucoWatch Biographer: glucose sample extraction through reverse iontophoresis, glucose sample measurement by amperometric biosensor, and data verification and conversion using an algorithm leading to the display of the glucose reading.[61]

The AutoSensor is a single-use disposable component that snaps into the Biographer. It is composed of two identical sets of biosensor and iontophoresis electrodes and two hydrogel discs (see Fig. 33–7B). The hydrogel discs serve as the biosensor electrolyte as well as the reservoirs into which the glucose is collected. The glucose oxidase enzyme is dissolved into these hydrogel discs at a concentration sufficient to eliminate enzyme kinetics limitations on the biosensor signal.

The second-generation GlucoWatch Biographer G2 (GWG2) has several improvements over the first-generation Biographer. The most noted improvement is the warm-up time, which was reduced from 3 hours to 2 hours. The GWG2 can display readings as frequently as every 10 minutes rather than every 20 minutes. Other improvements include the ability to store more data values, longer read time, and audible alerts. However, problems

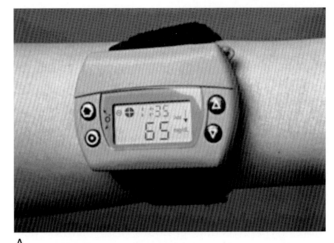

A

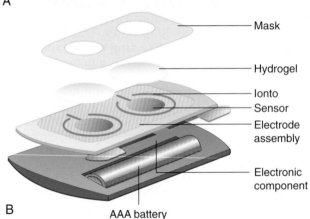

B   AAA battery

Figure 33–7. A, Patient wearing the GlucoWatch biographer. **B,** Diagram of the GlucoWatch biographer electrode assembly. Ionto, ionophoresis.

continue, such as the size of the watch, skin irritation due to reverse iontophoresis, skips during sweating, a warm-up period of 2 hours before calibration, and the need to change the AutoSensor every 14 to 15 hours.

The 2-hour warm-up period is required after the GWG2 is placed on the forearm. During this period a flow of subcutaneous fluid containing solute and glucose is established using reverse iontophoresis.[62] The Biographer must remain securely fastened to the patient's forearm and will not display glucose readings during the 2-hour warm-up period.[63] After the warm-up, the patient must obtain a fingerstick blood glucose reading and enter it into the Biographer to calibrate the system. It is sometimes necessary for the calibration process to be repeated during the wear time. The patient also sets the glucose levels for high and low alarms to sound, such as 300 mg/dL (16.7 mmol/L) for a high alarm and 70 mg/dL (3.9 mmol/L) for a low alarm.

The GWG2 provides up to 12 hours of glucose readings as often as every 10 minutes with up to 6 readings per hour. The readings are the time-averaged measurements of the value 10 minutes

earlier and the current value. Readings may be skipped because of bumping the device, excessive perspiration, and rapid changes in temperature. When a reading is skipped, an alarm sounds. If 6 readings in a row are skipped, the system must be recalibrated with an SMBG or the GWG2 shuts itself off. The glucose readings also lag approximately 17 minutes behind capillary glucose readings.

Clinical studies have shown that accurate and frequent glucose measurements are possible using the GWG2 over a 12-hour period.[64,65] One of the advantages of the GWG2 is its ability to determine glucose patterns and trends.[64,66] The GWG2 can frequently display real-time glucose values and it can detect six times more hypoglycemic episodes and 13 times more hyperglycemic episodes than SMBG performed twice daily.[62] It has an alarm to alert the user if it is predicted that the value will be below the low-alarm level in the next 20 minutes. This alert alarm is particularly helpful in detecting trends, and it can detect up to 90% of rapid falls in glucose levels.

Overall, the GWG2 can provide more real-time data than any other current technology, but it is still not 100% reliable. A glucose reading can be skipped because of excessive perspiration, which is a concern because perspiration can be a symptom of hypoglycemia. Because the GWG2 is worn on the forearm and readings are achieved through iontophoresis, mild to moderate skin irritation occurs.

It is suggested that after removing the AutoSensor the patient apply an over-the-counter hydrocortisone cream to the area to reduce itching or inflammation. Application of hydrocortisone cream might be of concern to the endocrinologist. The wear sites should be rotated. The watch should be removed first and then the sensor. The sensor should be gently removed with Unisolve so as not to tear the skin.

As with the Medtronic MiniMed CGMS, the GlucoWatch is accurate enough to detect trends. A home study showed that HbA1c levels could improve and hypoglycemia could be detected more frequently as a result of wearing the GlucoWatch.[67]

The DexCom Continuous Glucose Monitor

The DexCom Continuous Glucose Monitor (G_1) (DexCom, Inc, San Diego, Calif) consists of a long-term implanted sensor and a pager-size receiver. The sensor is a small cylinder about the size and shape of a AA battery (Fig. 33–8A).[68] The sensor contains a battery, an integrated circuit, a microprocessor, a radio transmitter, and a biosensor covered with a multilayered membrane.[68] An analog-to-digital converter translates the data to digital form, and a radio transmitter sends the data to the receiver. The sensor samples glucose levels every 30 seconds from interstitial fluid in subcutaneous tissue and radio transmits glucose values to the receiver every 5 minutes.

A surgeon implants the sensor in the subcutaneous tissue of the abdomen in an outpatient procedure under local anesthesia. The surgical

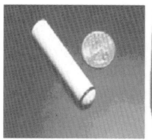 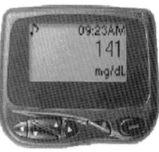

A   B

Figure 33–8. A, DexCom G_1 sensor, which is about the size of a AA battery. **B,** The DexCom receiver, a pager-like device.

technique ensures that the sensor is immobile after implantation. Subjects are instructed to restrict their activities for 72 hours and to avoid vigorous physical activity for 2 weeks following implantation.

The receiver is an externally worn pager-sized device (see Fig. 33–8B). Sensor glucose data are transmitted wirelessly from the sensor to the receiver. After the sensor is implanted, patients are instructed to take a minimum of two SMBG values per day. The blood glucose data are electrically uploaded to the receiver and used to calibrate the transmitted sensor glucose signal. After the sensor start-up period and calibration, the receiver calculates the glucose values using algorithms and displays the glucose values on the receiver every 5 minutes. The data are displayed in real time on the receiver as a number or as 1-hour, 3-hour, or 9-hour glucose trend graphs.

The receiver also provides vibratory and auditory alerts when the glucose levels are high or low. It can store both data from the sensor and data from a blood glucose meter with related time stamps. The sensor-specific receiver is programmed with software that enables the data from the sensor to be stored and uploaded to a personal computer at the clinical site.

In a clinical trial, subjects were allowed to use data from a long-term, implanted, real-time continuous glucose sensor for home use.[68] The study was divided into a blinded control period that lasted 50 ± 16 days and an unblinded period lasting 44 ± 17 days. During the blinded period the calibrated sensor calculated sensor glucose measurements, and the values were stored in the receiver memory. The readings were not made available at any time to the patient or the physician. Patients obtained a minimum of two SMBG values per day and treated their diabetes with insulin as advised by their health care providers. During the unblinded period, patients and their health care providers could see the real-time glucose values and glucose trend graphs. Investigators did not, however, make major therapeutic changes based on the data due to the investigational nature of the device.

There were no serious or unanticipated device-related or procedure-related adverse events during this study. During both the unblinded and blinded study periods, patients visited the clinic with the same frequency, and no additional instruction was provided to the patient on how to use the continuous glucose information during the unblinded period.

Glucose data from the blinded period were compared with data from the unblinded period to see if glucose patterns had changed (Fig. 33–9). During the unblinded period, patients spent 47% less time per day in the hypoglycemic range (lower than 60 mg/dL [3.3 mmol/L] , $P < 0.05$), and 25% less time per day in the hyperglycemic range (higher than 150 mg/dL [8.3 mmol/L], $P < 0.05$) than they did during the blinded period. This result was accompanied by substantially more time per day (88%) spent in the euglycemic zone of 60 to 150 mg/dL (4.4 to 7.8 mmol/L, $P < 0.05$). Results clearly documented improvements in glucose profiles when the patients were able to see the data compared with the blinded period. Therefore, presenting real-time continuous glucose values did help subjects reduce hyperglycemic excursions without increasing the risk of hypoglycemia.[68]

The next generation of DexCom implantable sensor (G_2) is 70% smaller than the original. Early data from this sensor suggests it provides similar decreases in time spent outside of the euglycemic range when compared with the G_1, as well as a decrease in excursion magnitude for blood glucose levels higher than 200 mg/dL (Table 33–3).[69] It is under investigation in a phase II study of 80 patients located at eight sites. Another implantable sensor (G_3) is in development, and it will be at least 50% smaller than the G_2.

The TheraSense Freestyle Navigator Glucose Monitor

The TheraSense Freestyle Navigator (Abbott Laboratories, Abbott Park, Ill.) is another subcutaneous glucose-measuring device that is being developed (Fig. 33–10). The Navigator is intended to be a substitute for current glucose self-monitoring devices, and it continuously monitors glucose levels, provides alarms at predetermined glucose values, and stores the results for analysis by the user or a physician.[70] As with the DexCom monitor, the goal is to provide not only a static glucose reading but also directional data based on analysis taking place at more frequent, fixed time points, therefore allow-

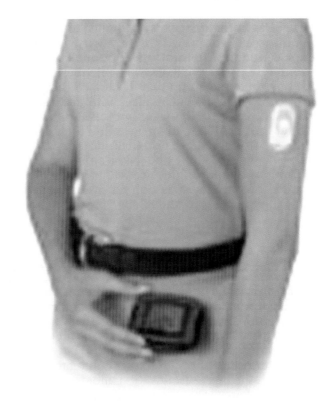

Figure 33–10. Patient wearing the TheraSense Freestyle Navigator.

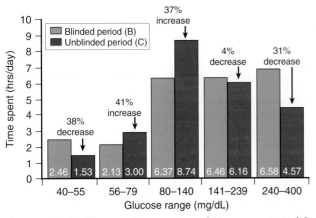

Figure 33–9. Changes in amount of time spent at different blood glucose levels during the DexCom study.

Table 33–3. *DexCom G_2 Results Showing Excursion Duration and Excursion Amplitude*

Blood Sugar Range	Excursion Duration (mean min ± SEM)			Excursion Amplitude (mean mg/dL ± SEM)		
	Blinded	Unblinded	Change	Blinded	Unblinded	Change
Hyperglycemic (≥200 mg/dL)	307 ± 62	215 ± 29	–30%	352 ± 12	332 ± 14	–13%
Hypoglycemic (≤80 mg/dL)	181 ± 15	138 ± 10	–24%	50 ± 3	51 ± 4	+3%

SEM, standard error of the mean.

ing patients to potentially avoid severe hypo- and hyperglycemic events.[70]

The Navigator is a three-part device consisting of a sensor, a transmitter and a monitor. The disposable miniature electrochemical sensor is inserted under the skin with little to no discomfort. This procedure is minimally invasive and can be done by the user with a simple spring-loaded device. The sensor can remain inserted for several days and is comfortable to wear. The sensor does not impair normal physical activities.[70] The sensor takes glucose readings from the interstitial fluid every minute, and the transmitter immediately sends the results to a wireless monitor. The sensor–transmitter unit is worn on the abdomen, upper arm, or an alternative site and can send data to the monitor up to ten feet away by radio frequency. The monitor is approximately the size of a PDA and displays glucose levels and trends and monitors alarm thresholds. The alarms can warn against dangerously high or low glucose levels as well as trends that suggest an impending hyper- or hypoglycemic event.

The Navigator system is calibrated daily on a 1-point scale to provide continuously accurate glucose readings. It uses the Continuous Glucose Error-Grid Analysis (CG-EGA), which was developed by the same group that developed the Clarke Error-Grid Analysis, but it takes into account not only static point accuracy but also directional accuracy, which tells patients whether their glucose levels are rising, falling, or remaining steady.[71] The CG-EGA suggests that the Navigator and other continuous-monitoring devices can provide highly accurate test results. It is not yet available to the public or approved by the FDA.

Noninvasive Methods

Near-Infrared Technology

The Sensys Medical (Sensys Medical, Chandler, Ariz.) device is an investigational device that measures blood glucose noninvasively through the use of near-infrared (NIR) spectroscopy.[63] The methodology measures how NIR light interacts with scattering mediums (solids or colloids) and is a well-studied area. The Sensys Medical device shines low-intensity NIR light onto the forearm. The light is partially absorbed and scattered according to its interaction with body tissue components such as water, fat, protein, and glucose. The portion of light reflected back to the monitor is detected and converted into a blood glucose value through the use of proprietary mathematical algorithms.

The Sensys Medical device is relatively small (slightly larger than a paperback book), weighs less than 1.5 pounds, and is powered by a rechargeable battery (Fig. 33–11). The device includes an LCD display screen as an operator interface using touch-screen data and control inputs. The product

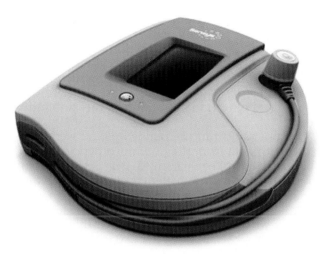

Figure 33–11. The SenSys glucose monitoring device.

contains a tethered fiber-optic sensing head that connects the device to the patient's forearm. The device provides a measurement in 10 seconds using a standardized measurement algorithm.

Before taking measurements, the patient secures a small transparent arm guide, slightly larger than a quarter, onto the forearm using an adhesive patch. The guide remains on the forearm all day. The sensing head assembly attaches to the guide during a measurement. This enables the system to take consistent measurements throughout the day. With the first measurement of the day, the patient also must take a companion glucose reading with a traditional fingerstick and glucose meter. The companion glucose value is used to calibrate the device for that day's use. During each of the day's remaining measurements, the device verifies sensing head and arm placement and the readiness of the internal components, collects a measurement, calculates a glucose value, and presents and stores the value for further analysis.

Depending on the frequency of testing or the limitation of testing on the dorsal aspect of the forearm, it may be necessary for patients to test on the volar aspect of the forearm. A clinical trial testing the physiologic concentration of glucose in the volar and dorsal aspect of the forearm found that the dorsal aspect of the forearm is better perfused than the volar region of the forearm. Capillary glucose determinations of the dorsal aspect of the arm track those of the fingertip better than values from the volar aspect.[72]

Another study, by Monfre and colleagues, found a significant advancement in the state of noninvasive glucose monitoring using NIR through the development and independent testing of standardized calibrations. It was found that standardized calibrations can be used for long-term noninvasive blood-glucose monitoring on patients with diabetes, thus eliminating the need for repeat calibrations.[73]

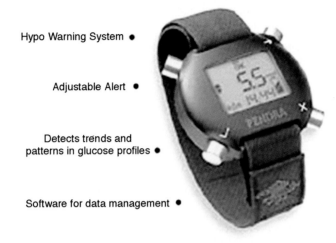

Figure 33–12. The Pendra continuous glucose monitoring device.

Upcoming Monitoring Systems

Many other companies are in the early stages of creating other continuous glucose sensors. A continuous glucose sensor will allow the patient, along with the physician, to micromanage and individualize the care of diabetes. A recent pilot study by Larin and coworkers showed that optical coherence tomography (OCT) is a noninvasive, real-time, and sensitive technique for monitoring blood glucose levels in subjects during an oral glucose tolerance test.[77]

Engineers are studying the possibilities for fluorescent microscale and nanoscale devices for glucose sensing.[78] Other sensors in development include vascular sensors, microdialysis sensors, other optical sensors, and smaller implantable sensors that can be worn for a few days.

Impedance Spectroscopy Technology

The Pendra glucose-monitoring device (Pendragon Medical, Zurich, Switzerland) is a wristwatch-sized monitor worn on the lower forearm. It shows considerable accuracy with optimized fixation.[74] It contains hypoglycemic warning alarms, detects trends and glucose profiles through on-the-minute glucose measurements, and contains software for data management (Fig. 33–12).

Instead of using blood samples or interstitial fluids, the Pendra uses impedance spectroscopy. A change in the electrolyte balance occurs across cell membranes due to specific reactions of blood and tissue cells to different glucose levels. Subtle changes in electrolyte balance because of the sensitive dielectric properties of the tissue relate to variances in glucose level, and they can thus be measured using different frequencies in the radio band. Because frequencies are varied over a specific range, the impedance pattern is measured, and blood glucose concentrations can be monitored.[75]

Unlike the fingerstick method used in home blood glucose monitors, studies have suggested that as the blood glucose values are elevated, no significant differences were found between the different methods or site locations. However, in rapid glucose declines (through IV insulin application), both methods showed slight deterioration in accuracy.[74]

Unlike with the GlucoWatch2 Biographer, there is decreased risk of skin irritation due to using radio waves rather than iontophoresis. Also, readings are taken every minute rather than every 10 to 12 minutes. Neither method is, however, completely accurate.[76] The Pendra is not approved by the FDA and is not currently available for use in the United States.

References

1. Centers for Disease Control and Prevention: National Diabetes Fact Sheet. Available from http://www.cdc.gov/diabetes/pubs/estimates.htm.
2. McCarthy D, Simmet P: Diabetes 1994-2010: Global Estimates and Projections. Melbourne, International Diabetes Institute, 1994.
3. Valle T, Tuomilehto J, Eriksson J: Epidemiology of NIDDM in Europoids. In Alberti KGMM, Zimmet P, DeFronzo RA (eds): International Textbook of Diabetes Mellitus, 2nd ed. Chichester, UK, John Wiley & Sons, 1997, pp 125-142.
4. National Institutes of Health: http://www.niddk.nih.gov.
5. Narayan KM, Boyle JP, Thompson TJ, et al: Lifetime risk for diabetes mellitus in the United States. JAMA 290:1884-1889, 2003.
6. American Diabetes Association: Economic costs of diabetes in the U.S. in 2002. Diabetes Care 26:917, 2003.
7. Plutzky J: Emerging concepts in metabolic abnormalities associated with coronary artery disease. Curr Opin Cardiol 15:416-421, 2000.
8. Zhang P, Engelgau MM, Valdez R, et al: Costs of screening for pre-diabetes among US adults. Diabetes Care 26:2536-2542, 2003.
9. Weiss R, Dufour S, Taksali SE, et al: Prediabetes in obese youth: A syndrome of impaired glucose tolerance, severe insulin resistance, and altered myocellular and abdominal fat partitioning. Lancet 362:951-957, 2003.
10. Haffner S: Pre-diabetes, insulin resistance, inflammation and CVD risk. Diabetes Res Clin Pract 61(suppl 1):S9-S18, 2003.
11. Diabetes Control and Complications Trial Research Group: The effect of intensive treatment of diabetes on the development and progression of long-term complications in insulin-dependent diabetes mellitus. N Engl J Med 329:977, 1993.
12. UK Prospective Diabetes Group: Intensive blood-glucose control with sulphonylureas or insulin compared with conventional treatment and risk of complications in patients with type 2 diabetes (UKPDS 33). Lancet 352:837, 1998.
13. Ohkubo Y, Kishikawa H, Araki E, et al: Intensive insulin therapy prevents the progression of diabetic microvascular complications in Japanese patients with non–insulin dependent diabetes mellitus: A randomized prospective six year study. Diabetes Res Clin Pract 28:103-117, 1995.
14. Liu K, Greenland P, Lowe L, et al: Diabetes, asymptomatic hyperglycemia, and 22-year mortality in black and white men. The Chicago Heart Association Detection Project in Industry Study. Diabetes Care 20:163-169, 1997.

15. Hanefeld M, Fischer S, Julius U, et al: Risk factors for myocardial infarction and death in newly detected NIDDM: The Diabetes Intervention Study, 11-year follow-up. Diabetologia 39:1577-1583, 1996.

16. Garg SK, Potts RO, Ackerman NR, et al: Correlation of fingerstick blood glucose measurements with GlucoWatch Biographer: Glucose results in young subjects with type 1 diabetes. Diabetes Care 22:1708-1714, 1999.

17. Hemocue: Glucose systems. http://www.hemocue.com/hemocueus/sida_20.asp

18. Koschinsky T, Jungheim K, Heinemann L: Glucose sensors and the alternate site testing-like phenomenon: Relationship between rapid blood glucose changes and glucose sensor signals. Diabetes Technol Ther 5:829-842, 2003.

19. Ellison JM, Stegmann JM, Colner SL, et al: Rapid changes in postprandial blood glucose produce concentration differences at fingertip, forearm and thigh sampling sites. Diabetes Care 25:961-964, 2002.

20. Goldman L, Bennet JC (eds): Cecil Textbook of Medicine, 21st ed. Philadelphia, WB Saunders, 2000, pp 611-612.

21. American Diabetes Association: Clinical practice recommendations. Diabetes Care 27(suppl 1):S91-S93, 2004.

22. Bunn H, Haney DN, Kamin S, et al: The biosynthesis of human hemoglobin A1c. J Clin Invest 57:1652-1659, 1976.

23. Fluckiger R, Winterhalter K: In vitro synthesis of hemoglobin A1c. FEBS Lett 71:356-360, 1976.

24. Beach K: A theoretical model to predict the behavior of glycated hemoglobin levels. J Theor Biol 81:547-561, 1979.

25. Higgins P, Bunn F: Kinetic analysis of the nonenzymatic glycation of hemoglobin. J Biol Chem 256:5204-5208, 1981.

26. Derr R, Garrett E, Stacy GA, Saudek CD: Is HbA(1c) affected by glycemic instability? Diabetes Care 26:2728-2733, 2003.

27. Li W, Shen S, Khatami M, Rockey JH: Stimulation of retinal capillary pericyte protein and collagen synthesis in culture by high glucose concentration. Diabetes 33:785-789, 1984.

28. Sushil J: Hyperglycemia can cause membrane lipid peroxidation and osmotic fragility in human red blood cells. The J Biol Chem 264:21340-21345, 1989.

29. Cerami A, Stevens V, Monnier V: Non-enzymatic glycosylation, sulfhydryl oxidation and aggregation of lens proteins in experimental sugar cataracts. Metabolism 28:431-40, 1979.

30. Braunwald E, Fauce AS, Kasper DL, et al (eds): Harrison's Principles of Internal Medicine, 15th edition. New York, McGraw-Hill, 2001.

31. Hoelzel W, Weykamp C, Jeppsson JO, et al, and the IFCC Working Group on HbA₁c Standardization: IFCC reference system for measurement of hemoglobin A₁c in human blood and the national standardization schemes in the United States, Japan, and Sweden: A method-comparison study. Clin Chem 50:166-174, 2004.

32. Miller CD, Barnes CS, Phillips LS, et al: Rapid A1c availability improves clinical decision-making in an urban primary care clinic. Diabetes Care 26:1158-1163, 2003.

33. Little RR, Rohlfing CL, Wiedmeyer HM, et al, and the NGSP Steering Committee: The national glycohemoglobin standardization program: A five-year progress report. Clin Chem 47:1985-1992, 2001.

34. Koenig R, Peterson CM, Jones RL, et al: Correlation of glucose regulation and hemoglobin A1c in diabetes mellitus. N Engl J Med 295:417-420, 1976.

35. Stevens R, Stratton I, Holman R: UKPDS58: Modeling glucose exposure as a risk factor for photocoagulation in type 2 diabetes. J Diabet Complications 16:371-376, 2002.

36. The Diabetes Control and Complications Trial/Epidemiology of Diabetes Interventions and Complications Research Group: Retinopathy and nephropathy in patients with type 1 diabetes four years after a trial of intensive therapy. N Engl J Med 342:381-389, 2000. Erratum in N Engl J Med 342:1376, 2000.

37. Armbruster D: Fructosamine: Structure, analysis and clinical usefulness. Clin Chem 33:2153-2163, 1987.

38. Gebhart SS, Wheaton RN, Mullins RE, Austin GE: A comparison of home glucose monitoring with determination of HbA1c, total glycoHb, fructosamine, and random serum glucose in diabetic patients. Arch Intern Med 151:1133-1137, 1991.

39. Edelman S: Does measuring fructosamine help patients with diabetes: Eff Clin Pract 4:189-190, 2001.

40. Austin GE, Wheaton R, Nanes MS, et al: Usefulness of fructosamine for monitoring outpatients with diabetes. Am J Med Sci 318:316-323, 1999.

41. Cohen RM, Holmes YR, Chenier TC, Joiner CH: Discordance between HbA1c and fructosamine. Diabetes Care 26:163-167, 2003.

42. Wahid ST, Sultan J, Handley G, et al: Serum fructosamine as a marker of 5-year risk of developing diabetes mellitus in patients exhibiting stress hyperglycaemia. Diabet Med 19:543-548, 2002.

43. McCarthy D, Simmet P: Diabetes 1994 to 2010: Global estimates and projections. Melbourne, International Diabetes Institute, 1994.

44. Cryer PE: Glucose homeostasis and hypoglycemia. In Larsen PR, Kronenberg HM, Melmed S, Polonsky KS (eds): Williams Textbook of Endocrinology, 10th ed. Philadelphia, WB Saunders, 2002, pp 1589-1591.

45. MacDonald MJ: Postexercise late-onset hypoglycemia in insulin-dependent diabetic patients. Diabetes Care 10(5):584-588, 1987.

46. Weiland D, White R: Diabetes mellitus: Review article. Clin Fam Pract 4:703-752, 2002.

47. Bendtson I, Gade J, Theilgaard A, Binder C: Cognitive function in type 1 (insulin dependent) diabetic patients after nocturnal hypoglycaemia. Diabetologia 35:898-903, 1992.

48. King P, Kong MF, Parkin H, et al: Well-being, cerebral function, and physical fatigue after nocturnal hypoglycemia in IDDM. Diabetes Care 21:341-345, 1998.

49. Veneman T, Mitrakou A, Mokan M, et al: Induction of hypoglycemia unawareness by asymptomatic nocturnal hypoglycemia. Diabetes 42:1233-1237, 1993.

50. Fanelli CG, Paramore DS, Hershey T, et al: Impact of nocturnal hypoglycemia on hypoglycemic cognitive dysfunction in type 1 diabetes. Diabetes 47:1920-1927, 1998.

51. Cryer P: Iatrogenic hypoglycemia as a cause of hypoglycemia-associated autonomic failure in IDDM. A vicious cycle. Diabetes 41:255-260, 1992.

52. Chase HP, Kim LM, Owen SL, et al: Continuous subcutaneous glucose monitoring in children with type 1 diabetes. Pediatrics 107:222-226, 2001.

53. Kerr D: Continuous blood glucose monitoring: Detection and prevention of hypoglycaemia. Int J Clin Pract 123(suppl):43-46, 2001.

54. Ludvigsson J, Hanas R: Continuous subcutaneous glucose monitoring improved metabolic control in pediatric patients with type 1 diabetes: A controlled crossover study. Pediatrics 111:933-938, 2003.

55. Gross T, Bode B, Einhorn D: Performance evaluation of the MiniMed continuous glucose monitoring system during patient home use. Diabetes Technol Ther 2:49-56, 2000.

56. Salardi S, Zucchini S, Santoni R, et al: The glucose area under the profiles obtained with continuous glucose monitoring system relationships with HbA(1c) in pediatric type 1 diabetic patients. Diabetes Care 25:1840-1844, 2002.

57. Guerci B, Floriot M, Bohme P, et al: Clinical performance of CGMS in type 1 diabetic patients treated by continuous subcutaneous insulin infusion using insulin analogs. Diabetes Care 26:582-589, 2003.

58. Amin R, Ross K, Acerini CL, et al: Hypoglycemia prevalence in prepubertal children with type 1 diabetes on standard insulin regimen: Use of continuous glucose monitoring system. Diabetes Care 26:662-667, 2003.

59. Caplin N, O'Leary P, Bulsara M, et al: Subcutaneous glucose sensor values closely parallel blood glucose during insulin-induced hypoglycaemia. Diabet Med 20:238-241, 2003.

60. Schaffini R, Ciampalini P, Fierabracci A, et al: The Continuous Glucose Monitoring System (CGMS) in type 1 diabetic children is the way to reduce hypoglycemic risk. Diabetes Metab Res Rev 18:324-329, 2002.

61. Tierney MJ, Tamada JA, Potts RO: Clinical evaluation of the GlucoWatch Biographer: a continual, non-invasive glucose

monitor for patients with diabetes. Biosens Bioelectron 16:621-629, 2000.

62. Garg SK, Hoff HK, Chase HP: The role of continuous glucose sensors in diabetes care. Endocrinol Metab Clin North Am 33:163-173, x-xi, 2004.

63. Garg SK, Chase P, Fermi SJ, et al: Evaluation of GlucoWatch Biographer performance during continuous daily wear for six weeks. Diabetes 49(suppl 1):A107, 2000.

64. Garg S, Potts RO, Ackerman NR, et al: Correlation of finger-stick blood glucose measurement with GlucoWatch Biographer glucose results in young subjects with type 1 diabetes. Diabetes Care 22:1708-1714, 1999.

65. Tierney M, Garg S, Ackerman N, et al: Effect of acetaminophen on the accuracy of glucose measurements obtained with the GlucoWatch Biographer. Diabetes Technol Ther 2:199-207, 2000.

66. Tamada J, Garg S, Jovanovic L, et al: Noninvasive glucose monitoring: Comprehensive clinical results. Cygnus Research Team. JAMA 282:1839-1844, 1999.

67. Chase HP, Roberts MD, Wightman C, et al: Use of the GlucoWatch Biographer in children with type 1 diabetes. Pediatrics 111:790-794, 2003.

68. Garg S, Schwartz S, Edelman S: Improved glucose excursions using an implantable real-time continuous implanted glucose sensor in adults with type 1 diabetes. Diabetes Care 27:734-738, 2004.

69. Edelman S, Scott RS, Morrison Z, et al: Early detection of hyper- and hypoglycemic excursions in subjects with Type 1 diabetes using a long-term continuous glucose sensor. Diabetologia 47(suppl 1):A309, 2004.

70. Kovatchev B, Gonder-Frederick LA, Cox DJ, Clarke WL: Evaluating accuracy of continuous glucose-monitoring sensors: Continuous glucose-error grid analysis illustrated by Freestyle Navigator data. Diabetes Care 27:1922-1928, 2004.

71. Clarke W, Cox D, Gonder-Frederick LA, et al: Evaluating clinical accuracy of systems for self-monitoring of blood glucose. Diabetes Care 10:622-628, 1987.

72. Monfre S, Hazen KH, Fischer JS, et al: Physiologic differences between volar and dorsal capillary forearm glucose concentrations and fingerstick glucose concentrations in diabetes. Diabetes 51(suppl 2):A125, 2002.

73. Garg SK, Fischer JS, Ruchti TL, et al: Calibration breakthrough for near-infrared, non-invasive blood glucose monitoring. Diabetes 51(suppl 2):A122, 2002.

74. Forst T, Pfutzner A, Forst S, et al: Accuracy of the non-invasive glucose monitoring device Pendra compared to alternative site testing at the lower forearm during dynamic blood glucose changes in type 1 diabetic patients. Diabetes 53(supplement 2):A102, 2004.

75. Caduff A, Hirt E, Feldman Y, et al: First human experiments with a novel non-invasive, non-optical continuous glucose monitoring system. Biosens Bioelectron 19:209-217, 2003.

76. Caduff A, Dewarrat R, Schrepfer T, et al: Monitoring of Hypoglycemic and Hyperglycemic Excursions in Patients with Diabetes with a Non-invasive, Continuous Glucose Monitoring System. Retrieved October 1, 2004 from http://www.pendramed.ru/downloads/Abstract_DTM_03_San_Francisco_Hypo_Hyper_Study_Profil.pdf

77. Larin KV, Eledrisi MS, Motamedi M, Esenaliev RO: Noninvasive blood glucose monitoring with optical coherence tomography: A pilot study in human subjects. Diabetes Care 25:2263-2267, 2002.

78. McShane ML: Potential for glucose monitoring with nano-engineered fluorescent biosensors. Diabetes Technol Ther 4:533-558, 2002.

Chapter 34

Pancreas, Kidney, and Islet Transplantation: What Every Physician Needs to Know

Jennifer L. Larsen, Gerald C. Groggel, and R. Brian Stevens

KEY POINTS

- *Kidney transplantation should be considered over dialysis for type 1 or type 2 diabetes patients with end-stage renal disease in the absence of contraindications.*
- *A living-donor kidney transplant is preferred over a deceased-donor kidney transplant because of improved patient and graft survival.*
- *Living-donor kidney and simultaneous pancreas–kidney transplantations have the same patient and kidney graft survival in patients with type 1 diabetes, so the risks and benefits of each should be carefully discussed before making a choice.*
- *Diabetic patients who receive either kidney or pancreas transplants require careful long-term follow-up of glucose, blood pressure, and lipids and surveillance for diabetic complications, bone health, and cancer.*
- *Fertility is improved after kidney transplantation. Premenopausal women should be counseled about the potential risks of pregnancy, and any desired pregnancy should be discussed in advance with the transplant team.*
- *Best outcomes after organ transplantation occur when there is regular communication between the transplant team and the practitioner managing diabetic complications and vascular risk factors of the transplant recipient, including changes in medication types and doses, changes in glucose, lipids, or blood pressure, and other new events.*

This chapter describes the indications for kidney transplantation, pancreas transplantation (either in combination with or separate from a kidney transplant), and islet transplantation in the treatment of patients with diabetes. Separately, the consequences of these procedures on patient mortality and diabetic complications as well as expected complications related to the surgery, immune suppression medications, or both, are reviewed. New-onset diabetes after kidney transplantation in nondiabetic recipients, also referred to as posttransplant diabetes, is discussed because its outcomes and management are so similar to those of patients with type 2 diabetes mellitus (T2DM) who undergo kidney transplantation.

KIDNEY TRANSPLANTATION

Indications and Contraindications

Diabetic patients with end-stage renal disease (ESRD) have a higher mortality compared to patients without ESRD, which may depend, in part, on the duration of dialysis itself. Patients with diabetes, who often have greater cardiovascular disease at the time they develop ESRD, also have greater cardiovascular disease mortality while they are on dialysis than do nondiabetic ESRD patients. Other types of morbidity are increased in dialysis patients with diabetes, including peripheral neuropathy and risk of amputation.

It was not until the 1970s that diabetic patients were considered for kidney transplantation.[1] Since that time, the total number of kidney transplants performed continues to increase (Fig. 34–1), and both the number and percentage of kidney transplant patients with diabetes have also increased. Diabetes is now the number one indication for kidney transplantation,[2] and kidney transplantation is the most common transplant procedure performed in diabetic patients.

Kidney transplantation is indicated for the treatment of ESRD of any type, including that of type 1 diabetes (T1DM) and T2DM. Successful kidney transplantation improves patient mortality in both diabetic and nondiabetic ESRD patients. However, diabetic recipients have lower patient and graft survival after a kidney transplant than nondiabetic recipients (Fig. 34–2).[3]

Contraindications to kidney transplantation include active infection, severe cardiovascular disease, other types of end organ failure (e.g., liver or severe pulmonary disease), malignancy (as discussed later in the chapter), current drug or alcohol

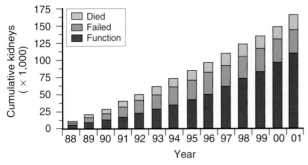

Figure 34–1. Cumulative kidney transplants performed from 1988 to 2001, excluding multiorgan transplants, reported to the UNOS Renal Transplant Registry. Those receiving kidney transplants who have died (Died), who have lost graft function (Failed), and who have presumed intact function (Function) are shown. Those in the Function group include those lost to follow-up and therefore represent an overestimation of those with functioning grafts. (From Cecka JM: The UNOS Renal Transplant Registry. In Cecka JM, Terasaki PI [eds]: Clinical Transplants 2002. Los Angeles, UCLA Immunogenetics Center, 2002, pp 1-20.)

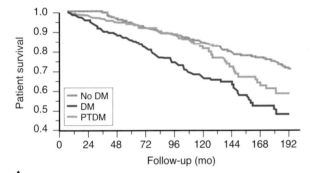

A

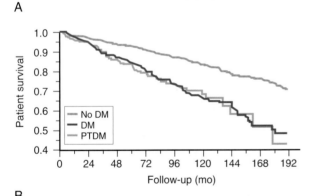

B

Figure 34–2. Kaplan-Meier plot of patient survival after kidney transplant. Three groups are compared: those without diabetes (NoDM, *green line*), those who had diabetes prior to kidney transplant (DM, *red line*), and those who developed diabetes after kidney transplant (PTDM, *blue line*). **A,** Survival was calculated from the day of transplant in all three groups. **B,** Survival was plotted from time of development of diabetes in the PTDM group and compared to survival curves of the NoDM and DM groups shown from time of transplant. Patient survival is similar in both diabetes groups, once diabetes develops. (From Cosio FG, Pesavento TE, Kim S, et al: Patient survival after renal transplantation: IV. Impact of post-transplant diabetes. Kidney Int 62:1440, 2002.)

abuse, and emotional or psychological instability. Morbid obesity and advanced age are relative contraindications.

What constitutes morbid obesity is defined differently from center to center. Because obesity is increasing in the population as a whole, and because it contributes to the risk of T2DM, more and more kidney transplant candidates are also obese, defined as a body mass index (BMI) higher than $30\,kg/m^2$. Obesity makes the kidney transplant procedure more technically difficult, and obese transplant patients have more wound infections and delay in graft function but not greater wound dehiscence.[4] In fact, cadaveric kidney transplantation in those with severe obesity (BMI higher than $41\,kg/m^2$) did not improve patient survival compared to those remaining on the waiting list.[5] Thus, the greater the BMI, the greater the risks, and there might be no benefit.

What constitutes advanced age also varies from center to center. Age 70 was the upper limit of age for kidney transplantation in the past, yet many centers now consider patients older than that age who are in otherwise outstanding health.

Living versus Deceased Donor Kidney Transplant

A kidney graft can be obtained from either a living or a deceased donor. A living donor, related or unrelated, is preferred, whenever possible, because the kidney graft and patient survival are better. The waiting time is shorter for a living than for a deceased donor transplant: The wait can be 2 to 5 years for a deceased-donor kidney, depending on blood type. Grafts from related and unrelated living donors result in the same outcomes, because absence of injury to the kidney might be more important to the outcome than improved matching. Donor nephrectomy can now be performed by laparoscopic surgery, which results in shorter hospitalization time and has contributed to greater numbers of living donor kidney transplants (Fig. 34–3).

However, even a deceased-donor kidney transplant significantly improves patient survival compared to dialysis, particularly in diabetic patients. For this reason, expanded criteria for kidney donors were established to increase the number of kidney grafts available for transplant. Expanded-criteria donor (ECD) grafts include those from older donors (older than 60 years of age) or from younger donors with additional risk factors (hypertension, elevated serum creatinine, or stroke as cause of death). Patients receiving ECD grafts are more likely to have delay in function and may have shorter long-term graft survival, but using these donors has doubled the donor pool in some centers and might prevent death while waiting for a living kidney transplant.[6,7] Commonly, ECD kidney grafts are offered to dia-

betic patients first because diabetic patients appear to have the highest mortality when they remain on the waiting list.

Kidney transplantation is not as arduous a procedure as pancreas–kidney transplantation, so it can be offered to patients with less cardiovascular reserve. Rejection rates are generally low and renal graft survival is excellent overall, more than 90% at 1 year (Table 34–1). As a result, many more patients with T1DM have kidney transplants than simultaneous pancreas–kidney transplants for treatment of ESRD.

PANCREAS TRANSPLANTATION

A total of 18,843 pancreas transplant procedures have been reported to the United Network for Organ Sharing (UNOS) and the International Pancreas Transplant Registry (IPTR) since pancreas transplantation was first performed. Most pancreas transplants have been performed in the United States (Fig. 34–4; December 1966 through October 2002).[8] Three types of pancreas transplant are performed: simultaneous pancreas–kidney (SPK), pancreas after kidney (PAK), and pancreas transplant alone (PTA). Each type has different indications and potentially different complications and outcomes (Fig. 34–5 and see Table 34–1).

Simultaneous Pancreas–Kidney Transplantation

SPK involves the transplant of a pancreas and kidney from the same deceased donor into a matched recipient in one operation. SPK transplant is the most common pancreas transplant procedure; 78% of the pancreas transplants performed in the United States between 1987 and 2002 were transplanted in SPK procedures (see Fig. 34–4).[8]

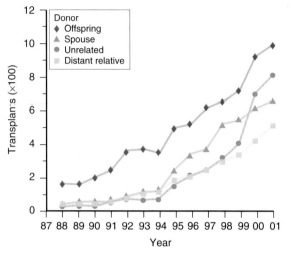

Figure 34–3. Numbers of living donor kidney transplants performed 1987 to 2001, as reported to the UNOS Renal Transplant Registry, including those of offspring, spouses and other unrelated living donors. The number of nonoffspring transplants of all kinds has risen rapidly since 1994. Although parents and HLA-identical siblings are also used as living donors, the rates of these groups have been very consistent: 700 and 500 kidneys, respectively, each year. These data are not shown. (From Cecka JM: The UNOS Renal Transplant Registry. In Cecka JM, Terasaki PI [eds]: Clinical Transplants 2002. Los Angeles, UCLA Immunogenetics Center, 2002, pp 1-20.)

Table 34–1 *Types of Kidney, Pancreas, and Islet Transplantation*

Procedure	Patient Group	1-Year Survival		
		Patient	Pancreas or Islet Graft	Kidney Graft
Kidney transplant, living donor	ESRD with or without diabetes	92% (97% in nondiabetic)	Not applicable	94% to 96% for diabetes patients
Kidney transplant, deceased donor	ESRD with or without diabetes	96% (94% in nondiabetic)	Not applicable	88% to 89% for diabetes patients
Simultaneous pancreas-kidney transplant	Type 1 diabetes with ESRD	95%	84%	92%
Pancreas transplant after kidney transplant	Type 1 diabetes after kidney transplant	94%	76%	78%
Pancreas transplant alone	Type 1 diabetes	98%	77%	Not applicable
Islet transplant	Type 1 diabetes	100%	80% in the best series only reporting those that achieved insulin independence and including those taking oral agents	Not applicable

ESRD, end-stage renal disease.
Kidney patient and graft survival rates are taken from the United Network for Organ Sharing (UNOS) database, 1996-2001,[2] and kidney transplant patient survival data for diabetic patients, 1996-2001, which was obtained per specific UNOS database request and based on Organ Procurement and Transplantation Network (OPTN) data as of May 14, 2004. Pancreas graft survival rates are taken from 1996-2002 data,[22] except for 1-year kidney graft survival following pancreas after kidney transplant, which was obtained through specific UNOS database request (1996-2001) based on OPTN data as of May 14, 2004. Islet data taken from reported University of Alberta data.[45]

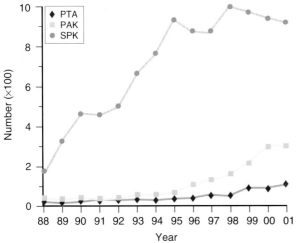

Figure 34-4. Number of pancreas transplants performed by type from 1988-2001, as reported to UNOS. Simultaneous pancreas–kidney (SPK), pancreas after kidney (PAK), and pancreas transplant alone (PTA). (From Gruessner AC, Sutherland DE: Pancreas transplant outcomes for United States [US] and non-US cases as reported to the United Network for Organ Sharing [UNOS] and the International Pancreas Transplant Registry [IPTR] as of October 2002.) (In Cecka JM, Terasaki PI [eds]: Clinical Transplants 2002. Los Angeles, UCLA Immunogenetics Center, 2002, pp 41-77.)

The indication for this procedure at most centers is ESRD secondary to T1DM with no option for a living kidney donor. SPK is also performed in a patient who prefers to receive both organs simultaneously because of the potential benefits of improved glucose control on existing diabetic complications and greater long-term pancreatic graft function compared to a later transplant (see Fig. 34–5B).

Uncommonly, a cadaveric pancreas graft is transplanted at the same time as a living donor kidney to avoid two hospitalizations, improve glucose control, and provide the benefit of improved long-term kidney graft function from a living donor.[9] Even less commonly, a partial or segmental pancreas graft and a kidney from the same living donor are transplanted simultaneously.[10,11] Survival of this pancreas graft is likely to be shorter for this recipient compared to a whole pancreas graft because of the smaller initial islet cell mass. There is also an immediate risk of glucose intolerance for the living donor, which is 33% at 1 year after transplant.[12,13]

One-year patient survival after SPK is comparable to kidney transplant alone (see Table 34–1), and pancreas graft survival after SPK is the best of any pancreas transplant procedure (Figure 34–5B). One-year kidney graft survival rates are equal to or better than those reported for kidney transplant alone,[14] so the success of the kidney graft is not harmed by this procedure (see Table 34–1). Kidney graft and

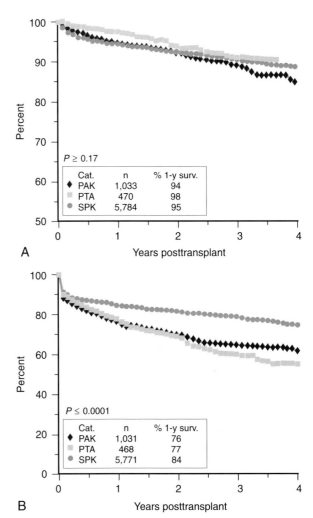

Figure 34–5. Patient and graft survival for all pancreas transplants performed and reported to UNOS from 1996-2002. **A,** Patient survival for simultaneous pancreas–kidney (SPK), pancreas after kidney (PAK), and pancreas transplant alone (PTA). There was no significant difference between the groups ($P \geq 0.17$). **B,** Pancreas graft survival rate for the same three groups. Pancreas graft survival was significantly greater in SPK compared to the other groups, overall ($P \leq 0.0001$). (From Gruessner AC, Sutherland DE: Pancreas transplant outcomes for United States [US] and non-US cases as reported to the United Network for Organ Sharing [UNOS] and the International Pancreas Transplant Registry [IPTR] as of October 2002.) (In Cecka JM, Terasaki PI [eds]: Clinical Transplants 2002. Los Angeles, UCLA Immunogenetics Center, 2002, pp 41-77.)

patient survival are better in patients receiving SPK than a deceased-donor kidney transplant alone or in patients with T1DM who remain on the waiting list.[15-18] Patient and kidney graft survival in SPK recipients is equal to those receiving a living donor kidney transplant alone after 8 to 10 years.[17,18]

African American patients have higher rates of acute and chronic rejection than white patients after a kidney transplant alone,[19] but this pattern has not been observed after SPK for either graft.[20] A

small percentage of SPK procedures are performed in patients with T2DM (6%),[8] and one-year patient and pancreas graft survival are reported to be similar to those for recipients with T1DM. The number of recipients with T2DM who require oral hypoglycemic agents to maintain normal glucose control has not been reported.[8,21,22] Thus, SPK should not be recommended to patients with T2DM outside of a research setting until long-term outcomes of glucose control, weight gain, and cardiovascular disease and mortality are more fully reported.

Pancreas after Kidney Transplantation

PAK transplantation, in which a patient receives a deceased-donor pancreas graft in a different procedure after a kidney transplant, is the second most common pancreas-transplant procedure (17%; see Fig. 34–2 and Table 34–1). The two indications for PAK are a patient with T1DM and ESRD who has either a living donor for a kidney transplant and a desire for a later pancreas transplant or who has had a kidney transplant, has stable renal function, has the cardiac reserve to undergo a pancreas transplant, and is likely to benefit from improved glucose control. The patient survival rate one year after PAK is equal to one-year survival after SPK (see Table 34–1). One-year pancreas graft survival following PAK has greatly improved over time because of improved immunosuppression and less concern about detecting rejection. Pancreas graft survival remains lower after PAK than after SPK (see Table 34–1 and Fig. 34–5).[8,22,23]

Pancreas Transplant Alone

PTA is the least-common pancreas transplant procedure (5% of all pancreas transplants; see Table 34–1). A history of frequent, severe hypoglycemic events is the most common indication, although the American Diabetes Association position statement also includes "frequent, acute and severe metabolic complications (hypoglycemia, hyperglycemia, and ketoacidosis) requiring medical attention" and "clinical and emotional problems with exogenous insulin therapy that are so severe as to be incapacitating; and consistent failure of insulin-based management to prevent acute complications."[24]

Candidates should be evaluated on a case-by-case basis. An endocrinologist should be one of the evaluators, because some patients have improved glycemic control by altering their insulin treatment regimen, increasing glucose testing frequency, and receiving diabetes education. Creatinine clearance must be adequate (preferably greater than 70 mL/min), or renal function could decrease after

transplant, especially with calcineurin inhibitor treatment.[25,26]

One-year pancreas graft survival after PTA is now similar to that for PAK, but it is still less than for SPK (see Fig. 34–5B and Table 34–1).[8] Even with careful patient selection, kidney function can decline and require a kidney transplant within the first year after transplantation (2% to 8%).[22] After 10 years, PTA can improve the pathologic changes of diabetic nephropathy.[27]

Variations in the Pancreas Transplant Procedure

There are variations in how the pancreas transplant procedures are performed, and these variations can affect the types of complications that occur after pancreas transplantation. The two main types of variation involve the location of the exocrine duct (bladder versus enteric placement) and vascular supply of the pancreas graft (systemic versus portal).

Bladder versus Enteric Drainage

Early pancreas transplants were performed by sewing the exocrine duct with a "button" of duodenum to the urinary bladder; this procedure is called *bladder drainage* (BD). With BD, urine amylase can be used to evaluate pancreatic function, and pancreas graft biopsies can be performed through a cystoscope, a distinct advantage when rejection episodes were common and difficult to diagnose without biopsy. Disadvantages of BD include loss of the salt- and bicarbonate-rich exocrine fluid into the urine (normally reabsorbed in the intestine), resulting in volume depletion and metabolic acidosis.

Most patients who receive a BD procedure need sodium bicarbonate replacement therapy, but this does not prevent all episodes of dehydration. BD also results in a variety of urologic complications, including bladder irritation from the exocrine secretions and bleeding from the anastomosis. Both urologic complications result in hematuria, increased episodes of bladder infection, and reflux of urine into the pancreas graft, causing allograft pancreatitis.[28,29]

The alternative to BD is enteric drainage (ED) of the exocrine duct. With ED, the exocrine duct is sewn back into the small intestine directly or with a Roux-en-Y limb, usually the jejunum (see Fig. 34–5).[30,31] ED prevents most volume depletion, metabolic acidosis, and urologic complications described with BD. Even though pancreas biopsies are more difficult to obtain with ED, the need for biopsies has decreased as rates of rejection have also declined. Thus, more transplants use ED at the outset, particularly with SPK (77%) but also with PAK (54%), and PTA (54%).[8] BD can also be converted to ED with ongoing complications.

SPK performed with BD or ED have similar pancreas graft and patient survival. However, with PAK or PTA, pancreas graft survival is better with BD than ED, where more pancreas graft monitoring may be needed.[22] Intra-abdominal sepsis is a serious complication that is more common with ED and can be life-threatening.

Systemic versus Portal Venous Drainage

When BD is used, the graft is too far away to be placed into the portal circulation, so it is placed into the systemic circulation instead, usually using the internal iliac artery and vein. Systemic venous drainage (SVD) results in high circulating systemic concentrations of insulin. Systemic hyperinsulinemia is associated with insulin resistance and increased vascular disease in the general population, but it is less clear whether systemic hyperinsulinemia in this setting has the same consequences, especially because lipids and other markers of vascular disease, including carotid intima media thickness, improve after pancreas transplant performed with SVD.[32,33]

The alternative is portal venous drainage (PVD). When enteric exocrine drainage is used, the surgeon can choose either SVD or PVD. PVD is more physiologic and does not result in systemic hyperinsulinemia. Yet graft survival after PVD transplants is at best similar to SVD, and in some series it is worse. Thus, without a clear-cut imperative to change the technique, most pancreas transplants performed to date continue to use SVD.

THE PRETRANSPLANT EVALUATION

The pretransplant evaluation includes an assessment of specific indications for the procedure; a discussion of the procedure being considered, including possible benefits and risks; a thorough systemic examination for diseases that might affect the success of the transplant, such as unrecognized malignancy or infection; and a psychiatric evaluation. Because vascular disease is common in diabetic patients, and vascular events are the most common cause of morbidity and mortality after transplant, all diabetic candidates require a thorough vascular evaluation, assessing cardiac, carotid, and peripheral vascular disease, as indicated, before transplant. Hypertension can worsen after kidney transplant, so all diabetic recipients should have a retinal exam by an ophthalmologist, if one has not recently been performed, with a plan to perform laser surgery, if indicated, before transplant is considered. Patients waiting for a deceased donor kidney or SPK can remain on the list for 2 to 4 years in some cases. Thus, the transplant team needs to repeat evaluations periodically to exclude intercurrent disease that would preclude transplantation.

INITIAL HOSPITALIZATION AND IMMEDIATE COMPLICATIONS

The patient is generally scheduled to have a transplant with a living donor, or is called to the transplant center when a deceased donor organ becomes available that is a potential match, based on the patient's blood type and HLA status. In both cases, the patient is asked to come to the hospital fasting. After standard laboratory testing and finalizing the match (and establishing the viability of the organ in the case of a deceased donor), the patient is taken to the operating room. The surgery lasts approximately 2 to 4 hours for kidney or pancreas transplant alone and 4 to 6 hours for SPK. Anti-lymphocyte antibody therapy is often used first, either polyclonal antithymocyte globulin (ATG or ATGAM), or monoclonal antibody (e.g., anti-CD 25 antibody). Polyclonal therapy usually depletes T cell number, whereas monoclonal antibody therapy does not. In the past, some centers used both therapies in combination, but combination therapy is uncommon now.

Once stable renal function has been achieved, two or three long-term immune suppression medications are introduced. Higher doses and target concentrations of these agents are used initially, and then they are tapered over time until a maintenance dose and concentration are achieved as guided by blood concentrations checked at specific intervals. The combinations of agents used in each center continue to change based on what agents are available, are proven effective, and have the fewest side effects, as well as, to a certain extent, the center's preference due to past experience. These agents may also be tailored to the individual transplant recipient because of known sensitivities or comorbidities of the patient, which might be affected more by some agents than others (Table 34–2).

The most common immune suppression regimen in most patients for either kidney or pancreas transplant is a combination of tacrolimus and mycophenolate mofetil (MMF), often with low-dose corticosteroids initially. Cyclosporine-based immune suppression regimens are second most common, and although use of rapamycin has been increasing, it remains common overall.

The initial hospitalization is generally 4 to 5 days after kidney transplant and 7 to 12 days after pancreas transplant with or without a simultaneous kidney. The native kidneys may be removed before or after the transplant in cases of polycystic kidney disease, evidence of tumors, bleeding from the native kidney(s), or recurrent infection or kidney stones. The native pancreas is important for its ongoing role in providing digestive enzymes, and only rarely are there indications to remove the native pancreas before or after transplant.

Most complications occur within the first 3 months and can require rehospitalization. After

Table 34–2 *Common Side Effects of Maintenance Immune Suppression Medications*

Side Effect	Relative Severity
Corticosteroids	
Weight gain	+++
Bone loss and osteoporosis	++
Glucose intolerance and insulin resistance	+++
Dyslipidemia	++
Impaired wound healing	+
Cataracts	++
Cyclosporine (Neoral, Sandimmune)	
Renal insufficiency	+++
Hypertension	+++
Dyslipidemia	++
Glucose intolerance	++
Post-transplant lymphoproliferative disease	++
Hypertrichosis	++
Hyperkalemia, especially in combination with ACE inhibitors	++
Hyperuricemia	++
Neurotoxicity	+
Tacrolimus (FK-506, Prograf)	
Renal insufficiency	+++
Dyslipidemia	+
Thrombocytopenia, leukopenia	+
Glucose intolerance	+++
Hypertension	++
Post-transplant lymphoproliferative disease	++
Neurotoxicity	+
Mycophenylate mofetil (MMF; Cellcept)	
Gastrointestinal symptoms, including diarrhea and bleeding	+++
Neutropenia	+++
Post-transplant lymphoproliferative disease	++
Sirolimus (rapamycin, Rapamune)	
Dyslipidemia	+++
Reduced wound healing	+++
Mouth ulcers	++

kidney transplantation, complications include acute allograft dysfunction most often due to acute rejection, delayed graft function often due to injury at time of death (e.g., motor vehicle accident) or preservation injury, acute tubular necrosis due to volume depletion, drug nephrotoxicity including toxicity from the immune-suppression drugs, recurrent disease, and ureteric obstruction. Infections continue to be a cause of morbidity and graft loss during the first year, but after the first year, graft loss is increasingly due to vascular events including cardiovascular death with an intact graft. Drug nephrotoxicity due to tacrolimus and cyclosporine can contribute to both kidney and pancreas graft loss as well.

Acute rejection is also one of the immediate possible complications after pancreas transplantation. If the pancreas and kidney grafts come from the same donor, rejection episodes are usually identified by evaluating kidney function. However, discordant rejection can occur in 5% to 25% of patients, where one organ is rejected independently of the other.[34] If the pancreas and kidney graft donors are different, rejection of the pancreas graft is likely to be independent of kidney rejection.

Other immediate complications after pancreas transplant include thrombosis, pancreatitis, and infection. Although thrombosis is often attributed to technical failure, it can also represent unrecognized acute rejection in many.[35] Exocrine pancreatic duct leaks and allograft pancreatitis are usually due to technical failures, preservation injury, or infection. These leaks can result in fluid collections, pseudocysts, or abscesses around the pancreatic graft that can require multiple operations to resolve or can cause sepsis and death.

With adequate preoperative screening, few acute cardiac events occur as an immediate complication of a transplant procedure. Perioperative infections occur more often with pancreas transplant than with kidney transplant alone. In some cases infections are due to greater immune suppression, additional risk of exocrine duct leaks or pancreatitis, and a greater risk of infection complicating a leak around the exocrine duct. There are more bladder infections in patients who receive pancreas transplant with bladder drainage than with enteric drainage.[29,36]

Overall, early complications, including rejection and infection episodes after pancreas transplant, have decreased since the 1990s. Reoperations, rejection episodes, infections, and total hospitalization time remain greater after SPK than after kidney transplant alone.

ISLET TRANSPLANTATION

Background

Much of the success of the modern era of islet transplantation can be traced back to the work of Paul Lacy.[37] Islet transplant has been a goal for insulin replacement therapy because islets respond to glucose immediately and frequently, which eliminates the need for insulin injections and glucose monitoring and avoids the difficulties of pancreatic exocrine duct management and exocrine drainage of the whole pancreas graft.

However, success in islet transplantation has been elusive. In the 1999 International Islet Transplant Registry report, fewer than 10% of islet transplant recipients were insulin independent for more than a year, and measurable C peptide was considered a

success separate from any documented impact on glucose. In 2000, the University of Alberta group from Edmonton, Canada, first reported insulin independence in 7 of 7 islet transplant recipients,[38] which reinvigorated interest in the field of islet transplantation.

Multiple events have contributed to improved islet transplant success. The Edmonton group used a new steroid-free immune-suppression protocol consisting of the monoclonal antibody daclizumab, tacrolimus, and sirolimus, and they used twice the islet equivalents than previous groups, administered sequentially, from multiple donors.[38] However, other improvements that have affected both the Edmonton group's original report and subsequent advances include a more consistent collagenase preparation for islet separation, greater attention at the time of pancreas graft procurement to prevent injury, and initiation of the two-layer method of pancreas transport with an oxygenated perfluorochemical in addition to University of Wisconsin solution, which decreased preservation injury and improved subsequent islet yields.[39-41]

As a result, the number of islets and pancreas grafts needed to achieve insulin independence after islet transplantation is decreasing, and centers now report insulin independence after islets are transplanted from a single donor.[42,43] The number of islets required varies with recipient weight, BMI, and preexisting insulin resistance as suggested by a daily requirement for insulin (U/kg). As a result, many centers restrict islet transplantation to those with the least resistance based on body size, BMI, or daily units of insulin per kilogram of body weight.

Procedure

Islet transplantation is generally performed by harvesting the islets, suppressing the recipient's immune system, and infusing the islets. First, a pancreas graft is procured, and the pancreas is gently digested into individual islets using a cocktail of enzymes including collagenase. The islets are purified with density centrifugation using a specialized cell processor (Fig. 34–6). The islets are concentrated into a buffer, which can be infused directly, or into culture for 1 to 3 days in some centers. The recipient's immune system is suppressed; depending on the protocol, suppression can occur before, but usually occurs immediately after, the transplant. The islets are infused into the portal vein by gravity, with angiographic visualization. Following the transplant, the recipient receives ongoing immune suppression, with dose adjustment based on concentrations achieved, and is followed up as an outpatient.

Usually islet transplant is performed as an outpatient procedure. In some cases, however, it is performed with direct visualization using minilap-

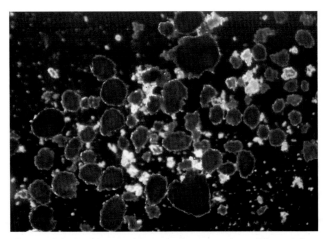

Figure 34–6. Islet preparation for transplant. These islets have been isolated and purified from a whole organ pancreas graft and are now ready for transplantation. (Dithizone stain, islets ranging from approximately 50 to 500 μm in diameter).

arotomy, which then requires a short hospital stay. Insulin treatment is withdrawn as indicated by blood glucose concentrations, but usually not immediately after transplant, to allow time for islet engraftment.

Hypoglycemia episodes and glycemic lability can improve within one month of successful islet transplantation.[44] Because most recipients do not require hospitalization, one of the attractions of islet transplantation is a considerable cost savings as well as less immediate postoperative pain, less need for reoperation, and fewer infections than are often observed with whole-organ pancreas transplantation.

Risks

Islet transplantation is also associated with risks. Transhepatic cannulation of the portal vein, with heparin to prevent thrombosis, can result in bleeding. Bleeding occurred in 10% of the subjects in the first published series. Bleeding may be serious enough to require immediate transfusion or surgery.[45]

Long-term effects of islets engrafted in the liver are unknown. Liver function tests temporarily increase in 46% but return to normal. Observations of fatty change or steatosis around the islets have also been observed, with unknown implications for long-term liver function.[46,47] Despite heparinization, two of 54 subjects experienced a thrombosis event in the liver in one series.[45]

Other potential side effects include increased blood pressure (53%), increased lipids (65%), decreased renal function, and increased proteinuria, possibly all due to the effects of immune-suppression medications. The need for new laser surgery for

diabetic retinopathy also increased (three of 17 in this report).[45] As with kidney and pancreas transplant patients, retinal lesions should be evaluated and treated before islet transplant.

One disadvantage of using a liver infusion site is that no improvement in glucagon response to hypoglycemia has been observed, with either allo- or autotransplant, as compared to whole-organ pancreas transplant.[48,49] Although steroid-free regimens may be an advantage, use of tacrolimus, and possibly sirolimus, can still inhibit insulin secretion or cause islet cell apoptosis, or both, that is likely dose-dependent.[50,51] Finally, recurrent immune-mediated destruction has still been suggested, because titers of anti-islet antibodies can increase.

Outcomes

The best islet graft survival has been published from the Edmonton group. In this center, 80% of recipients were still insulin-independent one year after islet transplant, with a mean hemoglobin A1c (HbA1c) of 6.05%, which includes two patients requiring oral hypoglycemic agent therapy.[45] Because this series only evaluated those who were initially able to achieve insulin independence, this graft survival should not be compared directly to the 1-year graft survival reported after solid-organ pancreas transplant, which includes all transplants, not just those that were successful. However, this series does suggest improvement in islet transplant outcomes compared to previous eras (see Table 34–1).

NEW-ONSET DIABETES AFTER KIDNEY TRANSPLANTATION

The focus of this chapter is on the diabetic patient who is considering transplant, but new-onset diabetes can occur after kidney and other organ transplants. New-onset diabetes after transplant (posttransplant diabetes [PTDM]) is increasing. Prevalence of PTDM after kidney transplant is reported as 5% to 54%, depending on the definition used.[52] Consensus guidelines for diagnosing PTDM were recently established and were based on the American Diabetes Association criteria for diagnosing diabetes outside of the transplant setting.[52]

In some cases, PTDM after kidney or other types of organ transplant represents diabetes that was already present, but unrecognized, prior to transplant. Particularly with ESRD, random or fasting glucose testing might not be sensitive enough to identify diabetes when serum half-life of insulin is markedly prolonged. An oral glucose tolerance test is preferred for evaluating any kidney transplant candidate who has risk factors for developing diabetes including obesity, family history, ethnic background (including and particularly African

Americans), older age, or other features of the metabolic syndrome.[2,3,52,53] Hepatitis C is also a risk factor for PTDM.[54-57]

Risk also depends on the immune-suppression medications chosen. Tacrolimus is associated with greater PTDM than cyclosporine, and both cyclosporine and tacrolimus have greater effects on glucose regulation than mycophenolate mofetil (MMF).

Patients with PTDM have decreased survival and decreased kidney graft survival (see Fig. 34–2).[2,3,58] How, or if, patient or kidney graft survival can be improved in patients who develop PTDM needs to be established, but it could include earlier recognition and treatment of hyperglycemia or more intensive treatment of comorbidities such as hypertension and dyslipidemia.

EVALUATION AND TREATMENT OF HYPERGLYCEMIA AFTER TRANSPLANT

Glucose concentration and insulin requirements often rise immediately after kidney transplantation in diabetic patients because of the stress and pain of surgery, use of immune-suppression medications, and improved renal clearance of administered or endogenous insulin. Although much of this hyperglycemia has been blamed on the use of glucocorticoids, other immune-suppression medications, particularly the calcineurin inhibitors cyclosporine and tacrolimus, also inhibit insulin secretion and can cause structural islet cell changes, including apoptosis.[50,51,59-69]

In contrast, glucose concentration normalizes immediately after successful pancreas transplant of any kind, and HbA1c is often normal by 1 month after transplant.[70] Intermittent or temporary elevations in glucose can accompany high doses of immune-suppression agents, particularly with acute rejection.

Once euglycemia has been achieved after pancreas or islet transplant, the recurrence of blunting of first-phase insulin secretion or impaired glucose tolerance suggests damage to the pancreas graft or increased secretory demand.[71,72] Causes of graft damage include acute or chronic rejection, pancreatitis, thrombosis, islet cell toxicity induced by immune-suppression medication (discussed earlier), or possible immune-mediated islet cell–specific destruction separate from rejection, which is suggested by increased titers of anti-islet antibodies. Causes of increased secretory demand include obesity alone, genetic insulin resistance exacerbated by elevated BMI, and, possibly, immunosuppressant therapy. Although most late hyperglycemia is attributable to chronic rejection, immune-suppression drugs can contribute more than previously appreciated, and islets transplanted into the liver, in particular, can be exposed to higher doses of

immune-suppression medications absorbed from the gastrointestinal tract through the first-past effect.

After pancreas transplant, fasting insulin concentrations are usually 2 to 3 times greater than normal when SVD is used, and they are similar to concentrations in other corticosteroid-treated recipients after PVD.[73-75] Chance of developing or resolving most diabetic complications is tied to normoglycemia. Thus, a fasting glucose and HbA1c is a minimum screen for glucose intolerance at all routine scheduled pancreas or kidney transplant clinic visits. In pancreas or nondiabetic kidney transplant recipients, elevation of HbA1c or fasting glucose higher than 100 mg/dL (based on the most recent guidelines for impaired fasting glucose)[76] should initiate consideration of an oral glucose tolerance test with insulin concentrations to evaluate for graft failure versus new-onset T2DM.

Treatment may be needed if hyperglycemia occurs, but the treatment will vary with the cause. Pancreas graft failure or rejection in patients with T1DM requires insulin. If kidney function is impaired, short-acting insulins are less likely to cause hypoglycemia than are long-acting insulins. There is no established role for oral hypoglycemic agents to forestall reinitiation of insulin with the exception of the diagnosis of new-onset T2DM. Treatment algorithms have been proposed for new-onset T2DM after kidney or pancreas transplant, but what constitutes the best treatment is not known.

Insulin might protect pancreas function until a more specific treatment strategy becomes effective (e.g., antirejection therapy, weight loss, oral hypoglycemic agents, changing doses or type of immune-suppression medication). Unfortunately, there is a disincentive to begin insulin therapy after pancreas transplant, because insulin treatment is the definition of graft failure. Initiation of insulin is also the definition some kidney transplant centers have used to define posttransplant diabetes before the new criteria were developed, so insulin treatment might have been delayed in these patients, as well.

Too often, oral agents are used without adequate follow-up to establish whether or not they control glucose, which can be difficult in the transplant patient. Thiazolidinediones (TZDs) can be effective and safe in transplant patients who are treated with calcineurin inhibitors, but TZDs might only reduce and not replace insulin therapy.[77] There is no contraindication to using sulfonylureas, although risk of hypoglycemia can be increased if there is coexisting renal insufficiency. Metformin should generally be avoided in most transplant recipients because of the contraindications to its use, including high risk of infection, renal insufficiency, and hospitalization, particularly in these patients during the first year. Whether oral hypoglycemic agents are as effective as insulin therapy in the transplant patient has not been well studied.

Regardless of the therapy, glucose should be evaluated frequently by someone comfortable with diabetes management, and insulin should always be used in the hospitalized patient or in any outpatient not achieving rapid glucose control with oral agents and in patients with documented glucose near or higher than 400 mg/dL, unpredictable food intake, ongoing unresponsive infection, or suspected pancreas graft rejection or failure. Well-controlled glucose can decrease time in the intensive care unit (ICU) as well as mortality and the rate of infection in critically ill patients, so there should be no hesitation to use insulin to achieve good glucose control (lower than 150 mg/dL) in any hospitalized transplant patient

MANAGING RISK FACTORS IN VASCULAR DISEASE

Vascular disease is the number one cause of death in the stable pancreas or kidney transplant patient.[78] Evaluation and treatment of vascular disease risk factors are an important part of the long-term management of the kidney and pancreas transplant recipient. These patients should be considered at high risk for vascular disease whether or not any previous vascular disease has been identified.

Screening for risk factors includes assessing smoking status, periodic weight and blood pressure assessments, screening for and treating albuminuria, and measuring lipids with any change in dose or type of immune suppression medication or weight. These assessments should be made at least annually. All diabetic transplant recipients (pancreas, kidney, or islet) and kidney transplant recipients with PTDM should be evaluated with a fasting glucose and HbA1c test at every transplant visit and with onset of any symptoms of hyperglycemia. The patient with diabetes should also perform frequent self-monitoring of blood glucose. The transplant team should reinforce the need for patients to report to the provider who is following their diabetes with any change in their usual values, such as can occur with a change in immune-suppression drug or dose, change in weight, change in eating patterns, new or suspected infection, change in renal function, recent hospitalization, or without a specific known cause.

The optimal frequency of vascular disease testing, noninvasive or invasive, in the transplant patient has not been established, but it should be considered with any change in functional status or suspicious symptoms. Daily low-dose aspirin (88 to 325 mg per day) should be reinitiated beyond the immediate postoperative period, unless there is a specific contraindication.

Lipid treatment goals are the same as for anyone with known vascular disease or diabetes, based on National Cholesterol Education Program Adult Treatment Panel III guidelines and the most recent

ADA guidelines for treatment of lipids in patients with diabetes.[53,79] Dyslipidemia can worsen after kidney or islet transplantation, but it often improves after pancreas transplantation. HMG CoA reductase inhibitors are the first-line agents for treatment of hypercholesterolemia, and they may have other benefits for transplant patients such as decreased graft loss.[80,81] Risk of myositis is greater when HMG CoA reductase inhibitors are used in combination with calcineurin inhibitors. However, starting with a low dose, increasing the dose slowly, and carefully monitoring the calcineurin inhibitor concentrations minimizes risk in most patients. A recent comparison of multiple statins in small, non-randomized groups of renal transplant patients did not demonstrate a particular difference in toxicity between agents.[82]

Dyslipidemia results, in part, from the effects of the immune-suppressant medications themselves, which differ in their impact on lipids, although the mechanism is not well studied in most (see Table 34–2). Thus, changing medications alone can ameliorate dyslipidemia in some, such as switching from cyclosporine to tacrolimus,[83] withdrawing steroids,[84] or removing sirolimus.[85-87] Diet changes, improved insulin delivery or insulin resistance in patients with diabetes, weight control, exercise, and controlling severe proteinuria can also improve lipids in some.

Hypertension management is also important to graft and patient survival. Hypertension is common in kidney and pancreas transplant recipients for many reasons: the direct effects of immune-suppression medications, particularly cyclosporine (see Table 34–2), transplant renal artery stenosis, rejection (acute or chronic), high renin release from the diseased native kidneys when left in place, weight gain, and recurrence of intrinsic renal disease. The presumed blood pressure goal in diabetic patients even after transplant is lower than 130/80 mm Hg, although it can be difficult to achieve and no one has established what the ideal goal should be.

Measures that reduce blood pressure include weight control, salt restriction, exercise, and smoking cessation, because smoking contributes to hypertension and vascular disease progression in transplant patients.[88-91] Patients treated with cyclosporine might benefit by changing to another agent.

Angiotensin converting enzyme (ACE) inhibitors or angiotensin receptor blockers (ARBs) decrease vascular events in nontransplant patients and have few side effects. The ACE inhibitors, in particular, are cost-effective.[92-94] However, ACE inhibitors are more likely to cause hyperkalemia when used with calcineurin inhibitors, and both ACE inhibitors and ARBs are avoided during the first months after kidney transplant because of their effects on renal blood flow. Calcium channel blockers are effective for treating hypertension and specifically protect against the hypertensive effects of the calcineurin inhibitors. However, some, but not all, calcium channel blockers can increase cyclosporine blood levels, which should be monitored.[95]

SURVEILLANCE FOR OTHER DIABETIC COMPLICATIONS

Ongoing surveillance for diabetic complications is necessary in all diabetic patients, even after pancreas transplant. Lifelong annual surveillance eye exams are needed, even after pancreas or islet transplant, because diabetic retinopathy does not always stabilize immediately, corticosteroids can cause or worsen cataracts, opportunistic infections of the eyes are not rare, and if hyperglycemia occurs, eye changes can worsen rapidly.[96]

Often neglected, the feet should still be examined at each visit by the health care team just as before transplant. Neuropathy does not resolve quickly, and peripheral vascular disease may or may not improve, so risk of injury is still increased. Immune suppression medications delay healing and decrease the response to infection. Good foot practices with daily self exam, moisturization as indicated, and protective footwear in those with established neuropathy or peripheral vascular disease should be reinforced at follow-up visits.

INFECTIONS AFTER PANCREAS OR KIDNEY TRANSPLANT

Immune suppression increases the risk for infections of many kinds, and it can increase the speed with which they develop, as well. Infection is one of the most common causes of death after transplant, and it is a common cause of readmission.[97,98] Infections, both minor and major, are still greater in SPK than kidney transplant alone recipients.[99]

Early infections generally result from subclinical infections that were present before surgery and that progress, such as bladder infections or tuberculosis, or they may be related to the surgery itself or placement of intravenous catheters. Bladder infections are greater with BD than ED pancreas transplant procedures.[36] Viral infections, and CMV in particular, are a definite concern in the first 2 to 6 months after transplant. Chemoprophylaxis decreases risk of CMV, which can be a cause of unexplained fever, other opportunistic infections, and possibly vascular disease. CMV infection may also increase risk of acute and chronic rejection.[100-104] Other opportunistic infections and chronic viral infections often occur later, and consequences from some infections, such as West Nile virus or even community-acquired infections, can be worse with immune suppression.[105]

All transplant recipients should receive pneumococcal vaccine, annual influenza vaccinations, and possibly hepatitis B vaccination. Infections of the

feet are particularly common in the diabetic patient after transplant, even with normal blood sugar, because of ongoing neuropathy and peripheral vascular disease. Because progression to osteomyelitis can occur even more quickly, all foot infections should be treated early and watched closely until they resolve.

CANCER SURVEILLANCE

Risk of cancer and cancer progression are also increased in patients receiving chronic immune suppression. More than half of all malignancies reported are due to either cancer of the lip and skin (37%), or lymphoproliferative disease, also called posttransplant lymphoproliferative disease (PTLD; 16%), although overall incidence of cancers, with the exception of skin cancer, is low and is 1% to 2% for PTLD.[106-108]

PTLD is more common in recipients younger than 18 years of age who are male or Caucasian and who have Epstein–Barr virus (EBV) infection.[108] PLTD can occur in a single site or in multiple sites including bone marrow, brain, GI tract, allograft, or liver. Antiviral prophylaxis can prevent EBV infection and associated PTLD, but treatment usually requires decreasing or stopping immune suppression therapy. If graft function is lost, recurrence does not necessarily follow retransplantation.[109]

Hepatitis B and C–associated hepatocellular carcinoma and papillomavirus-associated carcinoma of the cervix, vulva, and perineum are also more common in transplant patients. Although overall risk of death from malignancy, including PTLD, is low in either pancreas or kidney transplant recipients (less than 1%), the relative risk of developing cancer increases with time, from 8% after 5 years to 30% after 15 years.[8,110,111] Thus, death from malignancy can also increase with increased survival of transplant recipients.

All candidates should be screened before transplant for preexisting malignancies using established recommendations, because immunosuppressant medications enhance the growth of any cancers already present. Anyone found to have any kind of cancer prior to transplant, except skin cancer, could require 2 to 5 years of observation before being listed for transplant. A high index of suspicion should be maintained in evaluating any new lesion or suspected new or recurrent malignancy with early biopsy because too often cancer diagnosis is delayed in the transplant patient. Withdrawal of immune suppression may be needed until the cancer is successfully treated.

Other preventive measures that should be discussed with transplant patients and continued indefinitely include consistent use of sunscreens, regular pelvic examinations in women, rectal and prostate examinations in men, and use of barrier contraception in sexually active women to prevent acquisition of papillomavirus. Prophylactic vaccination for hepatitis B might also prevent the development of hepatitis B and its associated hepatocellular carcinoma.

BONE LOSS AFTER ORGAN TRANSPLANTATION

Bone loss and fractures are a common consequence of solid organ transplantation. Whereas the effects of corticosteroids are well known, many are not aware that calcineurin inhibitors also have direct effects on bone.[112-115] Many other factors, including hypogonadism, vitamin D deficiency, adynamic bone disease, previous or ongoing parathyroid disease, previous uncontrolled diabetes, and thyroid function abnormalities, can also contribute to pretransplant bone loss.

Fractures after SPK are common, and 45% to 49% occur within the first two years.[116-118] Factors that predicted the greatest risk of fracture in retrospective, cross-sectional studies of all kidney transplant recipients were increased age, diabetes, long duration of pretransplant kidney failure, history of pretransplant fracture, and female sex.[119-121] Hypogonadism is also associated with greater bone loss in the transplant setting.[115,122-124] Fractures continue to accumulate in some long-term organ transplant studies[121,125]—60% by 15 years for all kidney transplant recipients[120]—but in one study they did not significantly increase after the first year.[126]

Thus, bone density should be assessed before or immediately after transplant and then annually with dual energy x-ray absorptiometry (DEXA). In the absence of hypercalcemia, vitamin D (at least 800 IU/day) and calcium (1200 to 1500 mg/day) should be prescribed daily, and 25-hydroxyvitamin D concentration should be measured periodically to confirm adequate vitamin D replacement because DEXA cannot distinguish osteoporosis from osteomalacia. Parathyroid disease might not resolve for 1 to 2 years after transplant, but if it does not resolve, surgical therapy should be considered for evidence of osteoporosis as well as for hypercalcemia.

Resistance training can be effective in some patients to prevent vertebral osteoporosis,[127] but pharmacologic intervention is required in most patients. There is no agreement about timing of treatment (before, at time of transplant, or upon evidence of bone loss after transplant). The preferred or most effective agent has also not been established. Calcium plus vitamin D, vitamin D alone, oral bisphosphonates (alendronate or etidronate), or intravenous bisphosphonates (pamidronate or zoledronic acid) all reduce bone loss or fractures after kidney transplant. However, most studies are small retrospective trials or nonrandomized, prospective trials, and there are no

published studies of bone loss prevention after pancreas transplant. How long therapy should be given is also not established, but it should not be considered a short-term treatment based on studies to date.

The first prospective, randomized trial of calcitriol versus daily alendronate after cardiac transplant showed both treatments had benefit and there was no significant difference in fracture rates between them.[128] However, bone density was slightly higher with daily alendronate, and hypercalciuria was greater with calcitriol. Calcitonin should not be considered for preventive therapy because it has not been shown to change bone histomorphometry, bone mass, or fracture rate after any kind of transplant.[129,130]

To determine adequacy of vitamin D therapy and evaluate parathyroid disease, all transplant recipients should be screened with DEXA, their calcium, albumin, phosphate, and PTH concentrations should be checked, and their 25-hydroxyvitamin D concentrations should be measured. Most transplant recipients should receive additional therapy, either bisphosphonates or calcium and vitamin D, for prevention. Treatment of established low bone mass or fractures should begin with oral alendronate with adequate calcium and vitamin D replacement therapy until intravenous bisphosphonate therapies are approved for this indication.

HYPOGONADISM, FERTILITY, AND PREGNANCY

Hypogonadism can occur in men and women with ESRD, and it often improves after kidney transplantation. The immune-suppression drugs are not generally associated with oligospermia, with the exception of one case report with rapamycin. In women, the results are not as straightforward.

Menstrual function generally improves after kidney transplantation, although menstrual irregularity is still common after transplant.[131-133] Patients who receive corticosteroids as part of their immune suppression are more likely to experience weight gain (see Table 34–2). Both weight gain and corticosteroids can cause polycystic ovarian syndrome, which can also cause menstrual irregularity and decreased fertility. Cyclosporine, more than tacrolimus, can also contribute to hypogonadism in some women.[113] Other factors that can contribute to menstrual irregularity include pelvic surgery itself, which can compromise ovarian blood supply, and stress, whether from surgeries or infections, which can temporarily disrupt the reproductive system in women.

There are fewer studies evaluating gonad function after pancreas transplant. Few men had hypogonadism before or after pancreas transplant, but 70% of women had abnormal reproductive hormones one year after transplant, including one new case of primary hypogonadism and one case of ovarian hyperstimulation that improved with decreasing the cyclosporine dose. Although changes in reproductive function were unrelated to prolactin concentration, prolactin was still elevated in many patients at 1 year after transplant.[134] Unfortunately, hypogonadism, when it does occur, is often unrecognized and untreated.[122,134]

Fertility also improves in men and women after transplant, but two thirds of transplant recipients receive no instruction about sexuality or fertility after transplant according to a survey.[135] The National Transplant Pregnancy Registry tracks the outcomes of all reported pregnancies of transplant patients and, more recently, paternity after transplant.

Risk to babies fathered by men who are transplant recipients is being monitored, but no adverse effects have yet been reported. Pregnancy in a transplant patient, on the other hand, can have many consequences. Infections in the mother, pre-eclampsia, and graft loss are reported more frequently in SPK recipients than in those with kidney transplant alone, but they are more common with either type of transplant than in the general population.[136] Prematurity is also more common in infants born to SPK recipients than recipients of kidney transplant alone, but low birth weight, spontaneous abortion, and newborn complications are more common for both.[136-138]

Based on these data, pregnancy in a female pancreas or kidney transplant recipient should be treated as a high-risk pregnancy. Women desiring pregnancy after transplant are generally encouraged to wait until immune suppression medication doses are stable, renal function is stable, blood pressure is controlled, and any rejection episode has resolved, preferably after the first year, when lower medication doses are also used. The transplant team should be involved in planning for and managing the pregnancy. Medications should be changed prior to pregnancy in some cases, and doses need to be monitored because sex steroids can change their metabolism.

There is no difference in rates of gestational diabetes or other outcomes between cyclosporine and tacrolimus treatment in pregnancy.[136] There are few reports of patients or babies exposed to newer agents, but of 10 pregnancies exposed to MMF, two babies had congenital malformations.[139] Sirolimus can inhibit cardiac and nerve cell growth in vitro,[140,141] but only one woman has been reported to conceive an infant while taking sirolimus, with a total exposure of 4 weeks in combination with Neoral and prednisone; the baby was born without congenital anomalies.[136]

The impact of immune suppressants on the breastfeeding infant is unknown. The drugs are variably excreted into breast milk, not necessarily at the same concentration as maternal serum levels.[142] Thus, if breastfeeding is practiced or planned, concentrations of the medications should be monitored in the infant.

Long-term risk to the infant of prenatal immune suppression medication exposure is still a concern. White blood cell count in the baby can be low immediately after birth, but it then returns to normal. There is no known long-term risk of prenatal exposure to these medications on the immune system, but a delayed risk, including to the child's offspring, cannot be excluded. Thus, if pregnancy is not desired, a discussion of birth control options should be offered early. Surgical methods of birth control are generally preferred (for the woman or her male partner) because barrier methods might not be effective enough, and the risks of birth control pills (e.g., thromboembolic disease) and intrauterine devices (e.g., infection) may be greater in a transplant than a nontransplant patient.

CONTROVERSIES

- Should the type 1 diabetic patient who has end-stage renal disease and access to a living donor proceed with living donor kidney transplantation or wait for simultaneous pancreas and kidney transplantation?
- Who should be considered for bladder drainage and who should be considered for enteric exocrine drainage with pancreas transplantation?
- Who should be considered for systemic venous drainage and who should be considered for portal venous drainage for pancreas transplantation?
- What is the best immune suppression regimen for long-term graft and patient survival that minimizes long-term complications (e.g., dyslipidemia, hypertension, glucose intolerance, osteoporosis)?
- Who should be considered for pancreas transplant alone or islet transplantation?
- Can post-transplant diabetes be prevented?
- What is the best way to treat hyperglycemia, dyslipidemia, hypertension, and osteoporosis in the transplant patient?

References

1. Kjellstrand CM, Simmons RL, Goetz FC, et al: Mortality and morbidity in diabetic patients accepted for renal transplantation. Proc Eur Dial Transplant Assoc 9:345-358, 1972.
2. Cecka JM: The UNOS Renal Transplant Registry. In Cecka JM, Terasaki PI (eds): Clinical Transplants 2002. Los Angeles, UCLA Immunogenetics Center, 2002, pp 1-20.
3. Cosio FG, Pesavento TE, Kim S, et al: Patient survival after renal transplantation: IV. Impact of post-transplant diabetes. Kidney Int 62:1440-1446, 2002.
4. Espejo B, Torres A, Valentin M, et al: Obesity favors surgical and infectious complications after renal transplantation. Transplant Proc 35:1762-1763, 2003.
5. Glanton CW, Kao TC, Cruess D, et al: Impact of renal transplantation on survival in end-stage renal disease patients with elevated body mass index. Kidney Int 63:647-653, 2003.
6. Stratta RJ, Rohr MS, Sundberg AK, et al: Increased kidney transplantation utilizing expanded criteria deceased organ donors with results comparable to standard criteria donor transplant. Ann Surg 239:688-695, 2004.
7. Gill J, Pereira B: Death in the first year after kidney transplantation: Implications for patients on the transplant waiting list. Transplantation 75:113-117, 2003.
8. Gruessner AC, Sutherland DE: Pancreas transplant outcomes for United States (US) and non-US cases as reported to the United Network for Organ Sharing (UNOS) and the International Pancreas Transplant Registry (IPTR) as of October 2002. In Cecka JM, Terasaki PI (eds): Clinical Transplants 2002. Los Angeles, UCLA Immunogenetics Center, 2002, pp 41-77.
9. Farney A, Cho E, Schweitzer E, et al: Simultaneous cadaver pancreas living-donor kidney transplantation: A new approach for the type 1 diabetic uremic patient. Ann Surg 232:696-703, 2000.
10. Gruessner R, Sutherland D: Simultaneous kidney and segmental pancreas transplants from living related donors—the first two successful cases. Transplantation 61:1265-1268, 1996.
11. Zielinski A, Nazarewski S, Bogetti D, et al: Simultaneous pancreas–kidney transplant from living related donor: A single-center experience. Transplantation 76:547-552, 2003.
12. Kendall DM, Sutherland DE, Najarian JS, et al: Effects of hemipancreatectomy on insulin secretion and glucose tolerance in healthy humans. N Engl J Med 322:898-903, 1990.
13. Robertson RP, Lanz K, Sutherland D, Seaquist E: Relationship between diabetes and obesity 9 to 18 years after hemipancreatectomy and transplantation in donors and recipients. Transplantation 73:736-741, 2002.
14. Cecka JM: The UNOS Scientific Renal Transplant Registry—2000. In Cecka JM, Terasaki PI (eds): Clinical Transplants 2002. Los Angeles, UCLA Immunogenetics Center, 2002, pp 1-18.
15. La Rocca E, Fiorina P, di Carlo V, et al: Cardiovascular outcomes after kidney–pancreas and kidney-alone transplantation. Kidney Int 60:1964-1971, 2001.
16. Venstrom JM, McBride MA, Rother KI, et al: Survival after pancreas transplantation in patients with diabetes and preserved kidney function. JAMA 290:2817-2823, 2003. Erratum in JAMA 291:1566, 2004.
17. Rayhill SC, D'Alessandro AM, Odorico JS, et al: Simultaneous pancreas–kidney transplantation and living related donor renal transplantation in patients with diabetes: Is there a difference in survival? Ann Surg 231:417-423, 2000.
18. Reddy KS, Stablein D, Taranto S, et al: Long-term survival following simultaneous kidney–pancreas transplantation versus kidney transplantation alone in patients with type 1 diabetes mellitus and renal failure. Am J Kidney Dis 41:464-470, 2003.
19. Gjertson D: Multifactorial analysis of renal transplants reported to the United Network for Organ Sharing Registry: A 1994 update. In Terasaki PI, Cecka JM (eds): Clinical Transplants 1994. Los Angeles, UCLA Immunogenetics Center, 1994, pp 519-539.
20. Douzdjian V, Bhaskar S, Baliga P, et al: Effect of race on outcome after kidney and kidney–pancreas transplantation in type 1 diabetic patients. Diabetes Care 20:1310-1314, 1997.
21. Light J, Sasaki T, Currier C, Barhyte D: Successful long-term kidney–pancreas transplants regardless of C-peptide status or race. Transplantation 71:152-154, 2001.
22. Gruessner A, Sutherland D: Analysis of United States (US) and Non-US Pancreas Transplants Reported to the United Network for Organ Sharing (UNOS) and the International Pancreas Transplant Registry (IPTR) as of October 2001. In Cecka and Terasaki E, ed. Clinical Transplants 2001. Los Angeles, UCLA Immunogenetics Center, 2001, pp 41-77.
23. Humar A, Ramcharan T, Kandaswamy R, et al: Pancreas after kidney transplants. Am J Surg 182:155-161, 2001.

24. American Diabetes Association: Pancreas transplantation for patients with type 1 diabetes. Diabetes Care 23:117, 2000.

25. Brennan DC, Stratta RJ, Lowell JA, et al: Cyclosporine challenge in the decision of combined kidney–pancreas versus solitary pancreas transplantation. Transplantation 57:1606-1611, 1994.

26. Lane JT, Ratanasuwan T, Mack-Shipman R, et al: Cyclosporine challenge test revisited: Does it predict outcome after solitary pancreas transplantation? Clin Transplant 15:28-31, 2001.

27. Fioretto P, Steffes MW, Sutherland DE, et al: Reversal of lesions of diabetic nephropathy after pancreas transplantation. N Engl J Med 339:69-75, 1998.

28. Del Pizzo JJ, Jacobs SC, Bartlett ST, Sklar GN: Urological complications of bladder-drained pancreatic allografts. Br J Urol 81:543-547, 1998.

29. Sollinger HW, Messing EM, Eckhoff DE, et al: Urological complications in 210 consecutive simultaneous pancreas–kidney transplants with bladder drainage. Ann Surg 218:561-568, 1993; discussion 568-570.

30. Stephanian E, Gruessner RW, Brayman KL, et al: Conversion of exocrine secretions from bladder to enteric drainage in recipients of whole pancreaticoduodenal transplants. Ann Surg 216:663-672, 1992.

31. Sindhi R, Stratta R, Taylor R: Experience with enteric conversion after pancreas transplantation with bladder drainage. Transplant Proc 27:3014-3015, 1995.

32. Larsen JL, Stratta RJ, Ozaki C, et al: Lipid status after pancreas–kidney transplantation. Diabetes Care 15:35-42, 1992.

33. Larsen J, Ratanasuwan T, Burkman T, et al: Carotid intima media thickness decreases after pancreas transplantation. Transplantation 73:936-940, 2002.

34. Sutherland DE, Gruessner R, Moudry-Munns K, Gruessner A: Discordant graft loss from rejection of organs from the same donor in simultaneous pancreas–kidney recipients. Transplant Proc 27:907-908, 1995.

35. Drachenberg CB, Papadimitriou JC, Farney A, et al: Pancreas transplantation: The histologic morphology of graft loss and clinical correlations. Transplantation 71:1784-1791, 2001.

36. Pirsch JD, Odorico JS, D'Alessandro AM, et al: Posttransplant infection in enteric versus bladder-drained simultaneous pancreas–kidney transplant recipients. Transplantation 66 (12): 1746-1750, 1998.

37. Lacy PE, Kostianovsky M: Method for the isolation of intact islets of Langerhans from the rat pancreas. Diabetes 16:35-39, 1967.

38. Shapiro AM, Lakey JR, Ryan EA, et al: Islet transplantation in seven patients with type 1 diabetes mellitus using a glucocorticoid-free immunosuppressive regimen. N Engl J Med 343:230-238, 2000.

39. Matsumoto S, Rigley TH, Qualley SA, et al: Efficacy of the oxygen-charged static two-layer method for short-term pancreas preservation and islet isolation from nonhuman primate and human pancreata. Cell Transplant 11:769-777, 2002.

40. Matsumoto S, Qualley SA, Goel S, et al: Effect of the two-layer (University of Wisconsin solution–perfluorochemical plus O_2) method of pancreas preservation on human islet isolation, as assessed by the Edmonton Isolation Protocol. Transplantation 74:1414-1419, 2002.

41. Matsumoto S, Rigley TH, Reems JA, Kuroda Y, Stevens RB: Improved islet yields from *Macaca nemestrina* and marginal human pancreata after two-layer method preservation and endogenous trypsin inhibition. Am J Transplant 3:53-63, 2003.

42. Shapiro AM, Ryan EA, Lakey JR: Pancreatic islet transplantation in the treatment of diabetes mellitus. Best Pract Res Clin Endocrinol Metab 15:241-264, 2001.

43. Hering BJ, Kandaswamy R, Harmon JV, et al: Transplantation of cultured islets from two-layer preserved pancreases in type 1 diabetes with anti-CD3 antibody. Am J Transplant 4:390-401, 2004.

44. Ryan EA, Shandro T, Green K, et al: Assessment of the severity of hypoglycemia and glycemic lability in type 1 diabetic subjects undergoing islet transplantation. Diabetes 53:955-962, 2004.

45. Ryan EA, Lakey JR, Paty BW, et al: Successful islet transplantation: Continued insulin reserve provides long-term glycemic control. Diabetes 51:2148-2157, 2002.

46. Markmann JF, Rosen M, Siegelman ES, et al: Magnetic resonance–defined periportal steatosis following intraportal islet transplantation: A functional footprint of islet graft survival? Diabetes 52:1591-1594, 2003.

47. Bhargava R, Senior PA, Ackerman TE, et al: Prevalence of hepatic steatosis after islet transplantation and its relation to graft function. Diabetes 53:1311-1317, 2004.

48. Kendall DM, Teuscher AU, Robertson RP: Defective glucagon secretion during sustained hypoglycemia following successful islet allo- and autotransplantation in humans. Diabetes 46:23-27, 1997.

49. Paty BW, Ryan EA, Shapiro AM, et al: Intrahepatic islet transplantation in type 1 diabetic patients does not restore hypoglycemic hormonal counterregulation or symptom recognition after insulin independence. Diabetes 51:3428-3434, 2002.

50. Paty BW, Harmon JS, Marsh CL, Robertson RP: Inhibitory effects of immunosuppressive drugs on insulin secretion from HIT-T15 cells and Wistar rat islets. Transplantation 73:353-357, 2002.

51. Bell E, Cao X, Moibi JA, et al: Rapamycin has a deleterious effect on MIN-6 cells and rat and human islets. Diabetes 52:2731-2739, 2003.

52. Davidson J, Wilkinson A, Dantal J, et al: New-onset diabetes after transplantation: 2003 international consensus guidelines. Proceedings of an international expert panel meeting. Barcelona, Spain, 19 February 2003. Transplantation 75(10 Suppl):SS3-SS24, 2003.

53. National Cholesterol Education Program (NCEP) Expert Panel on Detection, Evaluation, and Treatment of High Blood Cholesterol in Adults (Adult Treatment Panel III): Third Report of the National Cholesterol Education Program (NCEP) Expert Panel on Detection, Evaluation, and Treatment of High Blood Cholesterol in Adults (Adult Treatment Panel III) final report. Circulation 106:3143-3421, 2002.

54. Yildiz A, Tutuncu Y, Yazici H, et al: Association between hepatitis C virus infection and development of posttransplantation diabetes mellitus in renal transplant recipients. Transplantation 74:1109-1113, 2002.

55. Dosary AA, Ramji AS, Elliott TG, et al: Post-liver transplantation diabetes mellitus: An association with hepatitis C. Liver Transpl 8:356-361, 2002.

56. Bloom R, Rao V, Weng F, et al: Association of hepatitis C with posttransplant diabetes in renal transplant patients on tacrolimus. J Am Soc Nephrol 13:1374-1380, 2002.

57. Kasiske BL, Snyder JJ, Gilbertson D, Matas AJ: Diabetes mellitus after kidney transplantation in the United States. Am J Transplant 3:178-185, 2003.

58. Jindal R, Hjelmesaeth J: Impact and management of posttransplant diabetes mellitus. Transplantation 70(11 Suppl):SS58-SS63, 2000.

59. Nielsen JH, Mandrup-Poulsen T, Nerup J: Direct effects of cyclosporin A on human pancreatic beta-cells. Diabetes 35:1049-1052, 1986.

60. Draznin B, Metz S, Sussman K, Leitner J. Cyclosporin-induced inhibition of insulin release. Biochem Pharm 37:3941-3945, 1988.

61. Gillison SL, Bartlett ST, Curry DL. Synthesis-secretion coupling of insulin: Effect of cyclosporin. Diabetes 38:465-470, 1989.

62. Basadonna G, Montorsi F, Kakizaki K, Merrell R: Cyclosporin and islet function. Am J Surg 156:191-193, 1988.

63. Tamura K, Fujimura T, Tsutsumi T, et al: Transcriptional inhibition of insulin by FK506 and possible involvement of FK506 binding protein-12 in pancreatic beta-cell. Transplantation 59:1606-1613, 1995.

64. Gillison SL, Bartlett ST, Curry DL. Inhibition by cyclosporine of insulin secretion—a beta cell–specific alteration of islet tissue function. Transplantation 52:890-895, 1991.

65. Hirano Y, Mitamura T, Tamura T, et al: Mechanism of FK506-induced glucose intolerance in rats. J Toxicol Sci 19:61-65, 1994.

66. Kneteman NM, Lakey JR, Wagner T, Finegood D: The metabolic impact of rapamycin (sirolimus) in chronic canine islet graft recipients. Transplantation 61:1206-1210, 1996.

67. Fuhrer DK, Kobayashi M, Jiang H: Insulin release and suppression by tacrolimus, rapamycin and cyclosporin A are through regulation of the ATP-sensitive potassium channel. Diabetes Obes Metab 3:393-402, 2001.

68. Drachenberg C, Klassen D, Weir M, et al: Islet cell damage associated with tacrolimus and cyclosporine: Morphological features in pancreas allograft biopsies and clinical correlation. Transplantation 1999; 68:396-402.

69. Neto A, Haapalainen E, Ferreira R, et al: Metabolic and ultrastructural effects of cyclosporin A on pancreatic islets. Transpl Int 1999; 12:208-212.

70. Stratta RJ, Taylor RJ, Zorn BH, et al: Combined pancreas–kidney transplantation: Preliminary results and metabolic effects. Am J Gastroenterol 86:697-703, 1991.

71. Cottrell D, Henry M, O'Dorisio T, Tesi R, Ferguson R, Osei K: Sequential metabolic studies of pancreas allograft function in type 1 diabetic recipients. Diabet Med 9:438-443, 1992.

72. Elmer DS, Hathaway DK, Bashar Abdulkarim A, et al: Use of glucose disappearance rates (kG) to monitor endocrine function of pancreas allografts. Clin Transplant 12:56-64, 1998.

73. Robertson RP, Abid M, Sutherland DE, Diem P. Glucose homeostasis and insulin secretion in human recipients of pancreas transplantation. Diabetes 38(Suppl 1):97-98, 1989.

74. Diem P, Abid M, Redmon JB, Sutherland DE, Robertson RP: Systemic venous drainage of pancreas allografts as independent cause of hyperinsulinemia in type I diabetic recipients. Diabetes 39:534-540, 1990.

75. Osei K, Henry ML, O'Dorisio TM, et al: Physiological and pharmacological stimulation of pancreatic islet hormone secretion in type I diabetic pancreas allograft recipients. Diabetes 39:1235-1242, 1990.

76. Genuth S, Alberti KG, Bennett P, et al: Follow-up report on the diagnosis of diabetes mellitus. Diabetes Care 26:3160-3167, 2003.

77. Baldwin D Jr, Duffin KE: Rosiglitazone treatment of diabetes mellitus after solid organ transplantation. Transplantation 77:1009-1014, 2004.

78. Gaston R, Basadonna G, Cosio F, et al: Transplantation in the diabetic patient with advanced chronic kidney disease: A task force report. Am J Kidney Dis 44:529-542, 2004.

79. Haffner SM, American Diabetes Association: Dyslipidemia management in adults with diabetes. Diabetes Care 27(Suppl 1):S68-S71, 2004.

80. Kobashigawa JA, Katznelson S, Laks H, et al: Effect of pravastatin on outcomes after cardiac transplantation. N Engl J Med 333:621-627, 1995.

81. Katznelson S, Wilkinson AH, Kobashigawa JA, et al: The effect of pravastatin on acute rejection after kidney transplantation—a pilot study. Transplantation 61:1469-1474, 1996.

82. Martinez-Castelao A, Grinyo J, Gil-Vernet S, et al: Lipid-lowering long-term effects of six different statins in hypercholesterolemic renal transplant patients under cyclosporine immunosuppression. Transplant Proc 34:398-400, 2002.

83. McCune TR, Thacker LR II, Peters TG, et al: Effects of tacrolimus on hyperlipidemia after successful renal transplantation: A Southeastern Organ Procurement Foundation multicenter clinical study. Transplantation 65:87-92, 1998.

84. Gruessner RW, Sutherland DE, Parr E, et al: A prospective, randomized, open-label study of steroid withdrawal in pancreas transplantation—A preliminary report with 6-month follow-up. Transplant Proc 33:1663-1664, 2001.

85. Gonwa T, Mendez R, Yang HC, et al: Randomized trial of tacrolimus in combination with sirolimus or mycophenolate mofetil in kidney transplantation: Results at 6 months. Transplantation 75:1213-1220, 2003.

86. Brattstrom C, Wilczek H, Tyden G, et al: Hyperlipidemia in renal transplant recipients treated with sirolimus (rapamycin). Transplantation 65:1272-1274, 1998.

87. Chueh SC, Kahan BD: Dyslipidemia in renal transplant recipients treated with a sirolimus and cyclosporine-based immunosuppressive regimen: Incidence, risk factors, progression, and prognosis. Transplantation 76:375-382, 2003.

88. Aker S, Ivens K, Grabensee B, Heering P: Cardiovascular risk factors and diseases after renal transplantation. Int Urol Nephrol 30:777-788, 1998.

89. Nankivell B, Lau S-G, Chapman J, et al: Progression of macrovascular disease after transplantation. Transplantation 69:574-581, 2000.

90. Naf S, Jose Ricart M, Recasens M, et al: Macrovascular events after kidney–pancreas transplantation in type 1 diabetic patients. Transplant Proc 35:2019-2020, 2003.

91. Sung RS, Althoen M, Howell TA, Merion RM: Peripheral vascular occlusive disease in renal transplant recipients: Risk factors and impact on kidney allograft survival. Transplantation 70:1049-1054, 2000.

92. Yusuf S, Sleight P, Pogue J, et al: Effects of an angiotensin-converting-enzyme inhibitor, ramipril, on cardiovascular events in high-risk patients. The Heart Outcomes Prevention Evaluation Study Investigators. N Engl J Med 342:145-153, 2000. Erratum in N Engl J Med 342:748, 2000.

93. Heart Outcomes Prevention Evaluation Study Investigators: Effects of ramipril on cardiovascular and microvascular outcomes in people with diabetes mellitus: Results of the HOPE study and MICRO-HOPE substudy. Lancet 355:253-259, 2000. Erratum in Lancet 356:860.

94. Ball SG, White WB: Debate: Angiotensin-converting enzyme inhibitors versus angiotensin II receptor blockers—a gap in evidence-based medicine. Am J Cardiol 91(10A):15G-21G, 2003.

95. Tortorice KL, Heim-Duthoy KL, Awni WM, et al: The effects of calcium channel blockers on cyclosporine and its metabolites in renal transplant recipients. Ther Drug Monit 12:321-328, 1990.

96. Scheider A, Meyer-Schwickerath E, Nusser J, et al: Diabetic retinopathy and pancreas transplantation: A 3-year follow-up. Diabetologia 34(Suppl 1):S95-S99, 1991.

97. Stratta RJ, Taylor RJ, Sindhi R, et al: Analysis of early readmissions after combined pancreas–kidney transplantation. Am J Kidney Dis 28:867-877, 1996.

98. Lo A, Stratta RJ, Hathaway DK, et al: Long-term outcomes in simultaneous kidney–pancreas transplant recipients with portal-enteric versus systemic-bladder drainage. Am J Kidney Dis 38:132-143, 2001.

99. Manske CL, Wang Y, Thomas W: Mortality of cadaveric kidney transplantation versus combined kidney–pancreas transplantation in diabetic patients. Lancet 346:1658-1662, 1995.

100. Dittmer R, Harfmann P, Busch R, et al: CMV infection and vascular rejection in renal transplant patients. Transplant Proc 21:3600-3601, 1989.

101. Helantera I, Koskinen P, Tornroth T, et al: The impact of cytomegalovirus infections and acute rejection episodes on the development of vascular changes in 6-month protocol biopsy specimens of cadaveric kidney allograft recipients. Transplantation 75:1858-1864, 2003.

102. Kalil RS, Hudson SL, Gaston RS: Determinants of cardiovascular mortality after renal transplantation: A role for cytomegalovirus? Am J Transplant 3:79-81, 2003.

103. Sageda S, Nordal KP, Hartmann A, et al: The impact of cytomegalovirus infection and disease on rejection episodes in renal allograft recipients. Am J Transplant 2:850-856, 2002.

104. Tenschert W, Dittmer R, Harfmann P, et al: Vascular rejection of renal allografts is linked to CMV IgG–positive organ donor. Transplant Proc 23:2641-2642, 1991.

105. Ravindra KV, Freifeld AG, Kalil AC, et al: West Nile virus–associated encephalitis in recipients of renal and pancreas transplants: Case series and literature review. Clin Infect Dis 38:1257-1260, 2004.

106. Gruessner RW: Tacrolimus in pancreas transplantation: A multicenter analysis. Tacrolimus Pancreas Transplant Study Group. Clin Transplant 11:299-312, 1997.

107. Egidi MF, Trofe J, Stratta RJ, et al: Posttransplant lymphoproliferative disorders: Single center experience. Transplant Proc 33:1838-1839, 2001.

108. Dharnidharka VR, Tejani AH, Ho PL, Harmon WE: Post-transplant lymphoproliferative disorder in the United States: Young Caucasian males are at highest risk. Am J Transplant 2:993-998, 2002.

109. Birkeland SA, Hamilton-Dutoit S, Bendtzen K: Long-term follow-up of kidney transplant patients with posttransplant lymphoproliferative disorder: Duration of posttransplant lymphoproliferative disorder–induced operational graft tolerance, interleukin-18 course, and results of retransplantation. Transplantation 76:153-158, 2003.

110. Pedotti P, Cardillo M, Rossini G, et al: Incidence of cancer after kidney transplant: Results from the North Italy transplant program. Transplantation 76:1448-1451, 2003.

111. Marcen R, Pascual J, Tato AM, et al: Influence of immunosuppression on the prevalence of cancer after kidney transplantation. Transplant Proc 35:1714-1716, 2003.

112. Epstein S, Dissanayake I, Goodman G, et al: Effect of the interaction of parathyroid hormone and cyclosporine A on bone mineral metabolism in the rat. Calcif Tissue Int 68:240-247, 2001.

113. Bowman A, Sass D, Dissanayake I, et al: The role of testosterone in cyclosporine-induced osteopenia. J Bone Miner Res 12:607-615, 1997.

114. Fornoni A, Cornacchia F, Howard G, et al: Cyclosporin A affects extracellular matrix synthesis and degradation by mouse MC3T3-E1 osteoblasts in vitro. Nephrol Dial Transplant 16:500-505, 2001.

115. Stempfle HU, Werner C, Siebert U, et al: The role of tacrolimus (FK506)-based immunosuppression on bone mineral density and bone turnover after cardiac transplantation: A prospective, longitudinal, randomized, double-blind trial with calcitriol. Transplantation 73:547-552, 2002.

116. Weber T, Quarles L: Preventing bone loss after renal transplantation with bisphosphonates: we can . . . but should we? Kidney Int 57:735-737, 2000.

117. Chiu M, Sprague S, Bruce D, et al: Analysis of fracture prevalanece in kidney-pancreas allograft recipients. J Am Soc Nephrol 9:677-683, 1998.

118. Smets YF, van der Pijl JW, de Fijter JW, et al: Low bone mass and high incidence of fractures after successful simultaneous pancreas–kidney transplantation. Nephrol Dial Transplant 13:1250-1255, 1998.

119. Nisbeth U, Lindh E, Ljunghall S, et al: Increased fracture rate in diabetes mellitus and females after renal transplantation. Transplantation 67:1218-1222, 1999.

120. Vautour LM, Melton LJ 3rd, Clarke BL, et al: Long-term fracture risk following renal transplantation: A population-based study. Osteoporos Int 15:160-167, 2003.

121. O'Shaughnessy E, Dahl D, Smith C, Kasiske B: Risk factors for fractures in kidney transplantation. Transplantation 74:362-366, 2002.

122. Stempfle H-U, Werner C, Echtler S, et al: Prevention of osteoporosis after cardiac transplantation: A prospective, longitudinal, randomized, double-blind trial with calcitriol. Transplantation 68:523-530, 1999.

123. Castaneda S, Carmona L, Carvajal I, et al: Reduction of bone mass in women after bone marrow transplantation. Calcif Tissue Int 60:343-347, 1997.

124. Cahill BC, O'Rourke MK, Parker S, et al: Prevention of bone loss and fracture after lung transplantation: A pilot study. Transplantation 72:1251-1255, 2001.

125. Durieux S, Mercadal L, Orcel P, et al: Bone mineral density and fracture prevalence in long-term kidney graft recipients. Transplantation 74:496-500, 2002.

126. Jeffery JR, Leslie WD, Karpinski ME, et al: Prevalence and treatment of decreased bone density in renal transplant recipients: A randomized prospective trial of calcitriol versus alendronate. Transplantation 76:1498-1502, 2003.

127. Mitchell MJ, Baz MA, Fulton MN, et al: Resistance training prevents vertebral osteoporosis in lung transplant recipients. Transplantation 76:557-562, 2003.

128. Shane E, Addesso V, Namerow PB, et al: Alendronate versus calcitriol for the prevention of bone loss after cardiac transplantation. N Engl J Med 350:767-776, 2004.

129. Guichelaar MM, Malinchoc M, Sibonga JD, et al: Bone histomorphometric changes after liver transplantation for chronic cholestatic liver disease. J Bone Miner Res 18:2190-2199, 2003.

130. Hay JE, Malinchoc M, Dickson ER: A controlled trial of calcitonin therapy for the prevention of post–liver transplantation atraumatic fractures in patients with primary biliary cirrhosis and primary sclerosing cholangitis. J Hepatol 34:292-298, 2001.

131. Kim JH, Chun CJ, Kang CM, Kwak JY: Kidney transplantation and menstrual changes. Transplant Proc 30:3057-3059, 1998.

132. Sawamura M, Takao M, Asano T, et al: Female gonadal function after renal transplantation. Transplant Proc 24:1573-1575, 1992.

133. Koutsikos D, Sarandakou A, Agroyannis B, et al: The effect of successful renal transplantation on hormonal status of female recipients. Ren Fail 12:125-132, 1990.

134. Mack-Shipman LR, Ratanasuwan T, Leone JP, et al: Reproductive hormones after pancreas transplantation. Transplantation 70:1180-1183, 2000.

135. Hart LK, Milde FK, Zehr PS, et al: Survey of sexual concerns among organ transplant recipients. J Transpl Coord 7:82-87, 1997.

136. Armenti VT, Radomski JS, Moritz MJ, et al: Report from the National Transplantation Pregnancy Registry (NTPR): Outcomes of pregnancy after transplantation. Clin Transpl 121-130, 2002.

137. Barrou BM, Gruessner AC, Sutherland DE, Gruessner RW: Pregnancy after pancreas transplantation in the cyclosporine era: Report from the International Pancreas Transplant Registry. Transplantation 65:524-527, 1998.

138. Armenti V, Radomski J, Moritz M, et al: Report from the National Transplantation Pregnancy Registry (NTPR): Outcomes of pregnancy after transplantation. In Tersaki CA (ed): Clinical Transplants 2000. Los Angeles, UCLA Immunogenetics Center, 2000, pp 123-134.

139. Armenti VT, Ahlswede KM, Ahlswede BA, et al: National Transplantation Pregnancy Registry—outcomes of 154 pregnancies in cyclosporine-treated female kidney transplant recipients. Transplantation 57:502-506, 1994.

140. Burton PB, Yacoub MH, Barton PJ: Rapamycin (sirolimus) inhibits heart cell growth in vitro. Pediatr Cardiol 1998; 19:468-470.

141. Carreau A, Gueugnon J, Benavides J, Vige X. Comparative effects of FK-506, rapamycin and cyclosporin A, on the in vitro differentiation of dorsal root ganglia explants and septal cholinergic neurons. Neuropharmacology 36:1755-1762, 1997.

142. Moretti ME, Sgro M, Johnson DW, et al: Cyclosporine excretion into breast milk. Transplantation 75:2144-2146, 2003.

Chapter 35

Diabetes and Pregnancy

Emily Lee Albertson, Kristin E. Koenekamp, and Lois Jovanovic

KEY POINTS

- *The prevalence of hyperglycemia during pregnancy may be as high as 13%. Gestational diabetes mellitus affects 14% of pregnant women in the United States each year and appears in weeks 24 to 28 of gestation.*
- *Pregestational diabetic women must achieve normoglycemia before pregnancy in order to minimize the risk of spontaneous abortion or fetal malformation and to prevent progression of diabetic complications during pregnancy.*
- *There is no such thing as a "no-risk" population for gestational diabetes; therefore, universal testing is optimal.*
- *Screening criteria for gestational diabetes is controversial due to lack of consensus in standards. However, the Hyperglycemia and Adverse Pregnancy Outcome study could identify a universal standard.*
- *The Pederson hypothesis predicts the effects of maternal hyperglycemia on the fetus, leading to fetal hyperinsulinemia and fetal hyperglycemia.*
- *Treatment for diabetes in pregnancy includes self-monitoring of blood glucose, frequent hemoglobin A1c testing, carbohydrate restriction, exercise, and insulin therapy if necessary. Pregnant diabetic women should maintain a hemoglobin A1c of less than 5.0% to decrease fetal complications.*
- *Preprandial glucose concentrations during pregnancy should be kept to less than 90 mg/dL and 1-hour postprandial glucose concentrations should be no greater than 120 mg/dL to minimize the risk of macrosomia.*
- *Carbohydrate-restricted diets and exercise can help women with gestational diabetes regulate blood glucose concentrations, especially after meals, and postpone insulin therapy.*
- *Insulin therapy consisting of multiple daily injections can safely help pregnant women with diabetes achieve normoglycemia and reduce the risk of fetal complications. An insulin algorithm takes into account a woman's gestational week and body weight to determine her daily insulin requirements.*

Hyperglycemia is the most common metabolic complication of modern pregnancies.[1] The prevalence of hyperglycemia during pregnancy may be as high as 13%; 0.1% of pregnant women per year have type 1 diabetes mellitus (T1DM), 2% to 3% have type 2 diabetes mellitus (T2DM), and up to 12% have gestational diabetes mellitus (GDM).[2] Although uncontrolled hyperglycemia in all types of diabetes increases potential maternal and fetal risks, it is necessary to distinguish among types, because each type generates different challenges during gestation and distinct developmental outcomes for the fetus.

Pregestational diabetes (T1DM or T2DM) is most threatening because it exists during organogenesis and can have a devastating impact on early fetal development if glucose levels have not been normalized.[3-6] Furthermore, pregestational diabetes places the mother at elevated risk for advancing preexisting diabetic complications.[7] On the other hand, GDM usually appears in the second half of pregnancy and mainly affects fetal growth rate.[8] Infants born to mothers with uncontrolled GDM have greater risks for macrosomia (excessively large neonatal size), subsequent obesity, slower systemic and psychosocial development, and various long-term metabolic consequences.[9,10] There are numerous other serious fetal complications that arise when normoglycemia is not achieved.

In pregnancies complicated by any type of diabetes, near-normal glycemia has been associated with improved outcomes.[11,12] Therefore, clinical treatments should aim to minimize fetal exposure to either sustained or intermittent periods of hyperglycemia.[13] It is especially important to correct 1-hour postprandial glucose elevations.[14] An intensive treatment regimen that encompasses frequent self-monitoring of blood glucose (SMBG), regulated diet and exercise, and insulin therapy, if necessary, is the most effective means to treat diabetes in pregnancy and to optimize fetal outcome.

As new developments within the realm of prenatal diabetes care arise, such as continuous glucose monitoring (CGM)[15] and safe insulin analogs,[16] and as further knowledge is amassed about the deleteri-

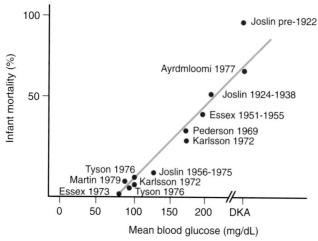

Figure 35–1. Literature review of the relationship between mean maternal blood glucose and infant mortality. Before insulin became commercially available in 1924 and intensive glucose monitoring systems were developed, an infant of a diabetic mother rarely survived. This figure shows studies that found when mean maternal blood glucose concentrations decreased, the percent of infant mortality also decreased. A linear regression line drawn through the points on this figure indicates that at a mean maternal glucose level of 84 mg/dL, there would be no increased risk of infant mortality over the general population (Adapted from Jovanovic-Peterson L, Peterson CM: Turning point in the management of pregnancies complicated by diabetes. Normoglycemia with self blood glucose monitoring of diet and insulin dosing. ASAIO Trans 36:799–804, 1990.)

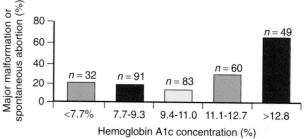

Figure 35–2. Deleterious effect of poor glycemic control on fetal outcome. This figure demonstrates the combined prevalence of major malformation and spontaneous abortion according to hemoglobin HbA1c concentration during the first trimester of pregnancy in 315 women with type 1 diabetes. The risk increases as hemoglobin HbA1c levels rise two to three standard deviations above the mean hemoglobin HbA1c. (Data from Greene MF, Hare JW, Cloherty JP, et al: First trimester hemoglobin HbA1c and risk for major malformation and spontaneous abortion in diabetic pregnancy. Teratology 39:225-231, 1989.)

ous effects of hyperglycemia on the fetus, it will be imperative to implement stricter standards for screening diabetes in pregnancy and to universally apply intensive treatments to achieve normoglycemia and eliminate corresponding fetal complications.

PREGESTATIONAL DIABETES AND PREGNANCY

Pregestational diabetes mellitus is marked by hyperglycemia that exists before pregnancy. Before the introduction of insulin therapy in the 1920s, few women with diabetes even lived to childbearing age. Consequently, fewer than 100 pregnancies were reported in diabetic women before injectable insulin became commercially available in 1924, and these women probably had T2DM, rather than T1DM. Nevertheless, the known cases of diabetes and pregnancy demonstrated an infant mortality rate greater than 90% and a maternal mortality rate of 30% (Fig. 35–1).[17] Even during the 1980s, some physicians still counseled diabetic women to avoid pregnancy altogether.[18]

Since the 1980s, mortality rates of infants born to diabetic mothers have declined as treatment strategies have emphasized better control of maternal plasma glucose levels and SMBG and glycated

hemoglobin (HbA1c) testing have become more widespread among patients with diabetes.[19] Furthermore, new innovations in diabetes technology, such as CGM,[15] are beginning to pave ways for diabetic women to achieve and maintain normoglycemia before and during pregnancy.

Pregestational diabetes complicates roughly 0.2% to 0.5% of pregnancies, or approximately 10,000 to 16,000 pregnancies per year.[20] Epidemiologic studies have revealed that of the pregnant women with pregestational diabetes, 35% had T1DM and 65% had T2DM. This trend is consistent with delayed childbearing age and changes in population demographics.[21] In contrast to GDM, which is discussed in later sections, pregestational diabetes is more serious because it is present before, during, and after pregnancy. Thus, the potential effects of uncontrolled glycemic levels begin at fertilization and implantation, continue throughout pregnancy, and remain as a postpartum threat during critical periods of breastfeeding.[22]

Diabetes and Early Fetal Development

Because fetal organogenesis is nearly complete by 7 weeks postconception, there is an increased risk of spontaneous abortion,[23] congenital abnormalities,[3,4,5] and growth restriction[6] in diabetic women with poor glycemic control during this critical period.[24] Figure 35–2 shows the combined prevalence of spontaneous abortion and major malformations in relation to the HbA1c level during the first trimester of pregnancy. The target range of HbA1c should be less than two standard deviations above the norm range of 5.0% to 6.0%.[25]

Table 35–1. *Testing Protocols Recommended For Women with Pregestational Diabetes*

Test	Frequency
Blood pressure and weight	Before conception and at each visit
Kidney function (creatinine clearance with total microalbumin)	Before conception and then once each trimester
Eye examination (fundus photography and/or dilated examination by ophthalmologist)	Before conception and then once each trimester
Thyroid function (free T$_4$ and TSH)	Before conception and then once each trimester
Hemoglobin A1c	Before conception and then once each month
Self-monitoring of blood glucose (preprandial target, <90 mg/dL; postprandial target, <120 mg/dL)	Before conception and then once each trimester

Note: Ideally, a diabetic woman would plan her pregnancy so that prepregnancy evaluations of diabetic complications can be made and individualized treatment plans can be created. However, if a diabetic woman presents in her first few weeks of pregnancy, rigid protocols must be instituted immediately to begin and maintain optimal control.

Table 35–2. *Risk Classifications Associated with Pregestational Diabetes During Pregnancy*

	Risk Classification	
Complication	With Optimal Glucose Control*	With Suboptimal Glucose Control†
Retinopathy	Minimal	High
Nephropathy	Minimal	High
Neuropathy	Minimal	High
ASCVD	Moderate	High
None	Low	High

ASCVD, atherosclerotic cardiovascular disease.
*Optimal glucose control is defined as follows: fasting blood glucose concentrations, 55 to 65 mg/dL; average blood glucose concentrations, 84 mg/dL; 1-hour postprandial blood glucose concentrations, lower than 120 mg/dL.
†Suboptimal glucose control is defined as failure to meet standards for optimal control.
Adapted from Jovanovic L: Medical Management of Pregnancy Complicated by Diabetes. Alexandria, VA, American Diabetes Association, 1993.

Because many women do not know that they are pregnant during this time of organ formation, prepregnancy counseling and monitoring is vital for diabetic women to achieve normal glycemic levels before conception. In addition, contraception is important for all pregestational diabetic women of childbearing age to prevent unwanted pregnancies that might result in increased risks of early complications.[26,27]

During the second and third trimesters, the most common fetal complications in pregnancies affected by diabetes include stillbirth and fetal macrosomia. Because these complications arise in all types of diabetic pregnancies, they are further discussed in the gestational diabetes section.

Maternal Risks

Prior to insulin therapy, reports showed that maternal survival during pregnancy of women with preexisting diabetes was less than 50%.[28] Today, maternal mortality is rare for both normal and diabetic women.[29] However, pregnant women with uncontrolled pregestational diabetes are at serious risk for progression of diabetic vasculopathy, such as retinopathy and nephropathy.[7] Tables 35–1 and 35–2 show important testing protocols for women with diabetes as they contemplate conception. These protocols are useful for assessing the interplay between current glycemic control and progression of complications.[13]

Diabetic retinopathy progresses for some women during pregnancy, although it is not likely to develop in women who have no evidence of retinal pathology.[30] Among the 140 women in the Diabetes in Early Pregnancy Study (DIEP) who did not have any retinopathy at conception, progression of retinopathy occurred in 10%. In 21% of those with a history of mild retinopathy and in 55% of those exhibiting severe proliferative retinopathy, the retinal status will progress.[31] Five risk factors identify the likelihood that a pregnant diabetic woman will progress to proliferative retinopathy: baseline evidence of retinopathy, elevated HbA1c at conception, elevated HbA1c followed by rapid normalization of blood glucose, a duration of diabetes greater than 6 years, and proteinuria.[22]

Figure 35–3 shows that strict glycemic control has been linked to worsening retinopathy for the mother.[32] Progression may occur because rapidly correcting hyperglycemia lowers the plasma volume and places fragile vessels, such as small retinal blood vessels, at risk for further narrowing.[33-37] Given this occurrence, the best strategy for preserving maternal vision appears to be gradually achieving normoglycemia before pregnancy. For women who have severe preproliferative or proliferative diabetic retinopathy and who are planning pregnancy, laser photocoagulation should be advised.[38]

Pregnancy does not seem to increase the risk of future diabetic nephropathy[39] and will not affect fetal outcome unless preexisting kidney function is greater than 50% impaired.[22] In normal pregnancies, creatinine clearance increases due to increased metabolic rate and increased cardiac output by the 10th and 12th week of gestation. However, this creatinine clearance actually declines in about one third of women with diabetic nephropathy, and another one third does not exhibit the normal pregnancy-induced rise.[40]

Women with proteinuria before pregnancy can witness dramatic rises in urinary protein excretion as pregnancy progresses.[41] Proteinuria greater than

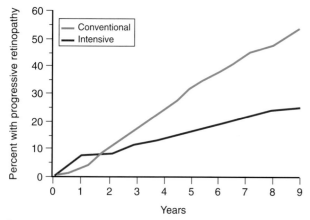

Figure 35–3. Strict glycemic control slows progression of diabetic retinopathy. Incidence of progressive retinopathy in patients with type 1 diabetes and mild to moderate nonproliferative retinopathy who were treated with either conventional *(blue line)* or intensive *(red line)* insulin therapy for 9 years. Although intensive therapy was associated with temporary progression in the first year, there was an overall increasing benefit over time. (Data from The Diabetes Control and Complications Trial Research Group. The effect of intensive treatment of diabetes on the development and progression of long-term complications in insulin-dependent diabetes mellitus. N Engl J Med 329:997-986, 1993.)

250 mg per 24 hours in the first trimester has been linked to nephrotic syndrome during the third trimester. Treatment includes bed rest and, in some cases, replacement of protein losses with albumin supplementation.[42] However, some studies have shown that patients with diabetic nephropathy have a greater than 40% chance of accelerating progression of the complication due to pregnancy.[43] Furthermore, the sample showed a mean serum creatinine increase from 1.8 mg/dL to 2.5 mg/dL, a proteinuria increase in 79% of the 35 patients, and increased hypertension for 73% of the patients. Before becoming pregnant, women with pregestational diabetes should undergo a measurement of urinary protein excretion, serum creatinine levels, and creatinine clearance to prognosticate pregnancy-related risks.[44]

Another risk is maternal hypertension. Fetal complications from maternal hypertension include intrauterine growth restriction and fetal demise. Ideally, all antihypertensive drugs should be stopped before conception if blood pressure remains lower than 130/85 mm Hg (lower than 120/80 if retinopathy exists). This drug elimination is especially important during fetal organogenesis (first 8 weeks of gestation). During the rest of pregnancy, hypertension should be treated by bed rest, followed by medications such as methyldopa and hydralazine, which have been proved safe for the fetus over several generations.[22]

Thyroid autoantibodies occur in about 30% of women with T1DM. Therefore, prepregnancy eval-

uations of diabetic women should include measurements of serum thyrotropin (TSH) and free thyroxine, and treatment should be started immediately if hypothyroidism is detected.[22,44]

GESTATIONAL DIABETES MELLITUS

GDM is defined as glucose intolerance that first manifests during pregnancy. In the United States, 135,000, or 14%, of pregnant women are affected by GDM each year.[45] Although insulin resistance is common to all pregnancies[46] to a certain degree, some women cannot counteract the insulin resistance and consequently develop GDM. The profile of a woman who is at the highest risk for developing GDM is one who is obese, is younger than 25 years of age, has first-degree relatives with diabetes, has a history of abnormal glucose metabolism or poor obstetric outcome, and is a member of an ethnic group with an increased prevalence of diabetes. The ethnic groups with a high prevalence include Hispanic, African American, Native American, South or East Asian, and Pacific Islanders.[47]

The spectrum of risk for GDM varies from 0.1% to 12% (low risk to high risk) based upon the presence or absence of these factors.[48] Women who are in the high-risk category should be tested for GDM as early in pregnancy as possible. Women who are at average risk should be tested at 24 to 28 weeks of gestation. Women at low risk do not have be tested; however, this does not mean that GDM cannot occur in low-risk women.[49] Universal testing is optimal for detecting GDM.

Detection and Diagnosis

In many countries, the World Health Organization (WHO) criteria for GDM is considered the standard. The WHO bases the diagnosis of GDM on a test of impaired glucose tolerance (IGT) with 75 g of oral glucose, which is the same standard for diabetes in nonpregnant adults. This is the lowest glucose load used to identify GDM. Numerous independent studies have shown that the WHO criteria are superior to standards issued by other health organizations when examining undesirable outcomes in pregnancy.[50-52]

In the United States, however, a different two-test method for GDM is used (Fig 35–4). First, a 50-g 1-hour oral glucose challenge test is performed. If the plasma glucose level is less than 140 mg/dL (7.8 mmol/L), GDM is ruled out and no further testing is necessary. However, if the plasma glucose is at least 140 mg/dL (7.8 mmol/L), a 100-g 3-hour oral glucose tolerance test (OGTT) must be administered after the patient has fasted overnight for 8 to 14 hours. From 14% to 18% of all pregnant women require the OGTT.

There is some dispute regarding the cutoff value for the OGTT. The primary criteria that are used clinically come from the National Diabetes Data Group (NDDG) and the American Diabetes Association (ADA).[53] Table 35–3 shows the criteria that these organizations recommend for testing and follow-up and are based on prevalence of diabetes-related complications. For GDM to be diagnosed, the glucose level must be abnormal two or more times in the specified time period. GDM must be diagnosed using the OGTT; fingerstick glucose values are unacceptable.

Currently, the National Institutes of Health (NIH) is conducting the Hyperglycemia and Adverse Pregnancy Outcome (HAPO) study to determine whether the WHO criteria could be instituted as the standard guideline in the United States for diagnosing GDM. Other outcomes that will be examined include the relationship between maternal glycemia and macrosomia and the morbidity associated with fetal hypoglycemia and hyperinsulinemia. Results of the HAPO study are expected in late 2005.[54]

Some controversy has been raised regarding the overall method of testing for GDM. Studies conducted by Buchanan and colleagues in a Hispanic population and further confirmed by Schaefer-Graf and colleagues in the German population confirm that fetal abdominal circumferences could be used to identify women at low risk for fetal macrosomia.[55,56] In these studies, two groups of pregnant women were randomized to one of two protocols. One group underwent monthly ultrasounds and were given insulin therapy only if the fetal circumference reached a certain threshold. The other group monitored their glucose levels and used insulin therapy throughout pregnancy. The results showed there was no difference in the rate of neonatal morbidity between the groups.[55,56] The ultrasound-screening method helps identify and treat the sickest fetuses, which may be cost-effective. However, this method supports secondary and tertiary care instead of prevention.

Fetal Complications

Pregestational and gestational diabetes have many of the same effects on the fetus. However, pregestational diabetes is more commonly associated with congenital anomalies because gestational diabetes does not typically begin until the second trimester, when many structures have already formed. Multiple studies have linked fetal complications to maternal glucose metabolism.[3,12,14,25,27,57-61] These findings have been considered controversial and have been debated because there are cases of neonatal complications even when glucose metabolism was excellent. However, analyses of glucose metabolism in these cases have failed to consider postprandial glucose concentrations.[14,58,59] Elevated postprandial glucose levels have been proposed as the primary etiology for neonatal complications for pregestational T1DM and for GDM.[13,58]

Multiple complications are associated with infants of diabetic mothers. The Pederson hypothesis illustrates the impact of the mother's glucose

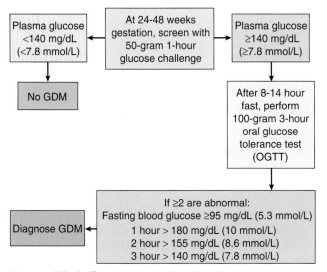

Figure 35–4. Testing procedure for diagnosis of gestational diabetes mellitus (GDM). This figure shows the multistep procedure used to diagnose GDM. After the results of a glucose challenge test are known, subsequent testing is performed on patients who have reached the plasma glucose threshold of 140 mg/dL or more. An oral glucose tolerance test (OGTT) is conducted. When two or more of the results are abnormal, a diagnosis of gestational diabetes mellitus (GDM) is made.

Table 35–3. *Standards for Diagnosing Gestational Diabetes*

Organization	Glucose Load for OGTT	Glucose Fasting Level	1 Hour	2 Hours	3 Hours
National Diabetes Data Group	100 g	105 mg/dL	190 mg/dL	165 mg/dL	145 mg/dL
American Diabetes Association	100 g or 75 g	95 mg/dL	180 mg/dL	155 mg/dL	140 mg/dL*
World Health Organization (IGT)	75 g	n/a	n/a	140 mg/dL	n/a
World Health Organization (Diabetes)	75 g	140 mg/dL	n/a	200 mg/dL	n/a

n/a, not applicable; IGT, impaired glucose tolerance; OGTT, oral glucose tolerance test.
*Not applicable for 75 mg/dL glucose load.
Adapted from Jovanovic L, Pettit DJ: Gestational diabetes mellitus. JAMA 286:2516-2518, 2001.

concentrations on the fetus.[62] Maternal hyperglycemia causes fetal hyperglycemia because glucose easily crosses the placenta. When maternal hyperglycemia occurs earlier than 20 weeks' gestation, congenital anomalies and decreased growth can result.

At 20 weeks the fetus's pancreatic islet beta cells are able to manufacture insulin,[62] and the fetus regulates its own glucose levels. However, as the fetus's pancreas tries to counter the influx of glucose from the mother, fetal hyperinsulinemia can ensue.[62] Hyperglycemia and hyperinsulinemia—individually and in conjunction—have astounding impacts on the development of the fetus in the remaining 20 weeks in utero and subsequently throughout the rest of the child's life.

Periconceptional Period

Infants born to diabetic mothers are four times more likely to have congenital anomalies of the brain, heart, kidney, intestine, and skeleton.[63] Many of these anomalies occur in the periconceptional period (conception to 8 weeks' gestation). HbA1c values at 14 weeks' gestation can be used to determine the risk of congenital defects.

Diabetic pregnant women with an HbA1c greater than two standard deviations from the norm increase their risk for congenital defects. HbA1c values of 7% to 8.5% have been associated with an increased risk of 5% for congenital defects, and when HbA1c values are greater than 10%, the risk jumps to 22%.[64] Central nervous system (CNS) and cardiac anomalies account for more than 50% of the development problems.[63] Some of the most common congenital problems are listed in Box 35-1.

Notably, infants of diabetic mothers are 252 times more likely to exhibit caudal regression, 84 times more likely to have situs inversus, and 4 to 6 times more likely to have renal and cardiac defects.[24] Women with pregestational diabetes must be monitored closely before conception and during gestation to look for congenital abnormalities.

Later Effects on the Fetus

The hyperglycemia associated with pregestational and gestational diabetes exerts similar effects after 20 weeks of gestation. Major risks to the fetus are macrosomia, fetal growth deceleration, small left colon syndrome, erythrocytosis, iron deficiency, hypoglycemia, hypocalcemia, hypomagnesemia, respiratory and cardiac problems, hyperbilirubinemia, and neurologic problems (Fig. 35–5).

Macrosomia

Macrosomia can be defined according to birth weight (4000 g to 4500 g) or based upon a result of 90% or greater growth curve after adjusting for sex, gestational age, and ethnicity. Macrosomia often results from the hyperglycemia the fetus is exposed to from its diabetic mother. The excess glucose and the resulting hyperinsulinemia stimulate fat

---

Box 35-1. Fetal Malformations Associated with Pregestational Diabetes

Neurologic

Failure of neural tube closure

Encephalocele

Anencephaly

Cardiovascular

Atrial septal defects

Left-sided obstructive lesions

Hypoplastic left heart syndrome

Aortic stenosis

Coarctation of the aorta

Transposition of vessels

Ventricular septal defects

Skeletal

Caudal regression syndrome

Spinal abnormalities

Syringomyelia

Renal

Hydronephrosis

Renal agenesis

Cystic kidney

Intestinal

Atresia of the duodenum

Atresia of the rectum

---

storage.[65] Head circumference remains unaffected, but the liver, spleen, and heart can hypertrophy.

The Diabetes in Early Pregnancy (DIEP) investigation studied pregestational pregnant women with T1DM and a control group of nondiabetic pregnant women. One-hour postprandial glucose levels were monitored in each group. Of macrosomic infants born to the diabetic mothers, 28.5% were identified based upon 1-hour postprandial glucose levels.[58]

As Figure 35–6 illustrates, the normal risk of macrosomia is about 10%, but this risk is increased when postprandial glucose levels rise higher than 120 mg/dL. Furthermore, when postprandial glucose concentrations are greater than 120 mg/dL, a linear relationship between macrosomia and postprandial glucose is no longer observed. Therefore, the risk of macrosomia appears to be elevated significantly at blood glucose concentrations higher than 120 mg/dL.[58] Macrosomia is a strong indicator for the cascade of complications that can result from hyperglycemia and hyperinsulinemia.

Birth trauma is associated with macrosomia due to the size differential between the fetus's head and the mother's pelvic region. Erb's palsy (limp or paralyzed arm due to nerve damage), Klumpke's paralysis (paralysis and atrophy of the forearm caused by

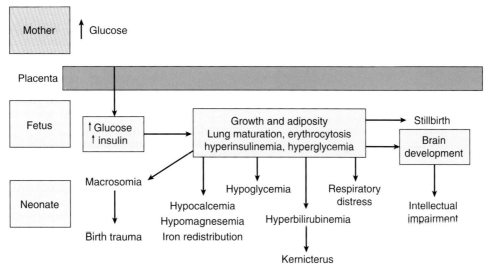

Figure 35–5. Effects of gestational diabetes mellitus on offspring. The basic principle of the Pederson hypothesis is shown. As the maternal glucose levels rise, the fetus also is affected by the glucose that can freely cross the placenta. Fetal hyperglycemia leads to fetal hyperinsulinemia. A cascade of effects occurs as a result of these conditions independently and when combined. ↑, elevated.

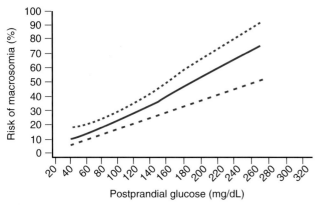

Figure 35–6. The risk of macrosomia versus postprandial glucose levels in the Diabetes in Early Pregnancy Study. In this graph, postprandial glucose levels higher than 120 mg/dL are seen to greatly increase the risk of macrosomia above the normal population risk of 10%. The dotted lines represent 95% confidence intervals. (From Jovanovic-Peterson L, Peterson CM, Reed GF, et al: Maternal postprandial glucose levels and infant birth weight: The Diabetes in Early Pregnancy study. The National Institute of Child Health and Human Development—Diabetes in Early Pregnancy Study. Am J Obstet Gynecol 164:103-111, 1991.)

nerve damage in the neck), diaphragmatic nerve paralysis, and recurrent laryngeal nerve damage can occur when the fetus's neck is stretched as the physician tries to deliver the fetus vaginally.[66]

Cesarean sections are performed in order to avoid birth trauma. However, cesarean section not only subjects the mother to the risks of surgery but can also undermine treatment efforts, and the trend is to do what is necessary to prevent it.[67] Thus the rate of macrosomia, which has been as high as 60%, has decreased to 20% to 35%.[64] This decrease may be due to aggressive treatment of gestational diabetes, which obstetricians have embraced in an attempt to spare the mother and fetus the risks of surgical delivery.

A model for aggressive diabetes diagnosis and treatment to reduce the number of cesarean sections can be seen in Figure 35–7. In Santa Barbara County, the drop in cesarean sections can be correlated with a program that provided universal screening for GDM and treatment of pregnant women to targeted glucose concentrations of 90 mg/dL prandially and 120 mg/dL postprandially or lower. The glucose concentrations were stabilized using diet, exercise, and insulin therapy. As a result of these practices, $2000 was saved per pregnancy for the cost of surgical delivery, and the metabolic problems associated with macrosomia were avoided.[49]

Fetal Growth Deceleration

Diabetic mothers with advanced vascular disease have an increased risk of fetal growth deceleration. This complication occurs in less than 5% of the fetuses and the growth deceleration causes the fetus to be smaller than the fifth percentile for its gestational age.[68,69] Due to placental vascular insufficiency and maternal hypertension, the protein-to-energy ratio does not allow the fetus to maintain adequate oxygen levels. Consequently, fetal growth slows and erythrocytosis occurs to counteract these stresses (see later). Growth deceleration can occur even when the mother's glucose levels are controlled and can lead to complications during birth.[66]

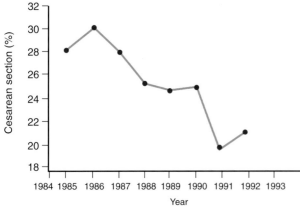

Figure 35–7. Cesarean section percentage versus time in years in Santa Barbara County, Calif. The trend in the graph shows a decrease in the percentage of cesarean sections when universal screening and treatment of postprandial blood glucose levels were normalized. (From Jovanovic, L, Bevier W: The Santa Barbara County Health Care Services Program: birth weight change concomitant with screening for and treatment of glucose-intolerance of pregnancy: A potential cost effective intervention. Am J Perinatol 14:221-228, 1997.)

Organ Development

Glucose levels can affect organ development. The major organ dysgenesis seen in the fetus of a diabetic mother is neonatal small left colon syndrome, in which the diameter of the descending colon, sigmoid flexure, and rectum is small. Intestinal motility is important for the stimulation of growth and differentiation in the fetal gastrointestinal system. Changes in glucose concentrations lead to intestinal hypomotility, which can impair intestinal development.[68]

Erythrocytosis

Erythrocytosis (polycythemia) results from the increased oxygen requirements that stem from hyperglycemia and hyperinsulinemia. Studies have indicated that a fetus in this setting requires 30% more oxygen to account for the increase in metabolic demand caused by excess glucose crossing the placenta.[70,71] Fetal oxygen-carrying capacity is therefore increased by fetal production of additional erythrocytes.[72-74] A study conducted by Green and colleagues has shown that severity of erythrocytosis is clearly correlated with maternal control of glucose levels.[75]

Elevated cord serum erythropoietin is often an indicator of fetal hypoxia.[73] Upon delivery, the hematocrit is not a reliable indicator of hypoxemia because hematocrit is typically elevated in neonates. Therefore, red cell indices are used to measure the risk of hypoxia.

Erythrocytosis can cause stroke, seizures, necrotizing enterocolitis, and renal vein thrombosis. Standard treatment is exchange transfusion.

Iron Deficiency

A corollary complication to erythrocytosis is paradoxical iron deficiency. As the fetus produces more hemoglobin in response to the increased demand for oxygen, iron is redistributed to the new hemoglobin. Although the transferrin receptor expression is increased, the affinity for transferrin decreases because the excess glucose binds to the receptor, blocking the receptor's function.[76,77] The fetus therefore must derive usable iron from stores in the liver, and developing organs such as the heart and brain become iron deficient. These deficiencies can cause myopathies and problems in neurologic development.

Because of iron's role as a growth factor in the body, the overall risk of adverse outcomes in the mother and fetus can be increased. Abnormal cognitive processing may be present at first in the neonate because of the relative iron deficiency during the time it takes for the erythrocytes to release the hemoglobin-bound iron.[78]

Hypoglycemia

When the infant is delivered, the glucose supply from the mother is discontinued. If the fetus was producing extra insulin to counteract the extra glucose from the mother, the infant's insulin levels could be high. The sudden withdrawal of glucose in this setting can result in hypoglycemia. Neonates who are very large or very small for gestational age are more likely to exhibit hypoglycemia than infants whose size is appropriate for gestational age.

Nearly half of infants born to diabetic mothers develop hypoglycemia shortly after birth.[64] The hypoglycemia typically occurs within the first 3 hours of life, and the neonate requires treatment if the blood glucose concentration is 40 mg/dL or less.[79] Hypoglycemia in infants small for gestational age could be due to decreased hepatic storage of glycogen.[66]

Calcium and Magnesium Deficiencies

After birth, the parathyroid glands produce parathyroid hormone (PTH) as necessary to regulate blood levels of calcium and magnesium. The parathyroid glands are inactive in the fetus and do not regulate the fetus's blood calcium and magnesium levels.

The fetus derives its calcium and magnesium supplies from calcium and magnesium that cross the placenta. When the baby is delivered, it must regulate blood levels independently. The parathyroid glands normally are able to regulate blood calcium and magnesium levels within the first 72 hours of life. Hypocalcemia and hypomagnesemia often manifest in infants of diabetic mothers due to a greater delay in the regulation and production of parathyroid hormone.[63,66]

Respiratory and Cardiac Problems

The primary respiratory problem in infants of diabetic mothers is respiratory distress syndrome (RDS). RDS can be caused by surfactant deficiency

or by retained fetal lung fluid. Symptoms include transient tachypnea, intercostal retractions, nasal flaring, apnea, and cyanosis.

RDS occurs more in infants of diabetic mothers due to the lack of maturity in the type II alveolar cells.[66] Hyperinsulinemia in the fetus (in response to excess glucose that crosses the placenta) can suppress the effects of cortisol; cortisol is necessary for production of dipalmitoyl lecithin, and consequently the dipalmitoyl lecithin levels are insufficient for surfactant production.[80] A deficiency in surfactant production, loss of lung volume, and microatelectasis appears to provide the conditions for RDS.[80]

The risk of RDS can be decreased by delivering the fetus after 38 weeks, when the fetus's lungs are mature. In amniotic fluid samples, a 2:1 ratio or greater of lecithin to sphingomyelin (L/S) and a 3% level of phosphatidylglycerol should be observed to minimize the risk of RDS.[81] Because fetal hyperinsulinemia is caused by maternal hyperglycemia, good maternal glucose control can prevent RDS.

Cardiac problems are also common in infants of diabetic mothers. Cardiac function problems occur in about 30% of infants of diabetic mothers. Intraventricular septal hypertrophy and cardiomyopathy can be caused by hyperglycemia and hyperinsulinemia. Heart failure occurs in 10% of infants of diabetic mothers.[64,68]

Hyperbilirubinemia

Hyperbilirubinemia manifests with the symptoms of jaundice.[82] An increase in red cell mass contributes to a 30% increase in the bilirubin that must be metabolized by the liver. Insufficient production of liver enzymes causes increased serum bilirubin levels. Ineffective erythropoiesis provides another source of bilirubin, contributing to the concentration that the liver must regulate. Erythrocytes also add bilirubin to the liver upon degradation.[66]

Hyperbilirubinemia can allow bilirubin to reach the basal ganglia and brainstem nuclei and cause brain damage, a condition known as *bilirubin encephalopathy*. The initial symptoms of bilirubin encephalopathy include lethargy, hypotonia, and poor suck followed by an intermediate phase with symptoms of stupor, irritability, fever, high-pitched cry, and hypertonia.[82,83] Drowsiness and hypotonia may be present intermittently during this period as well. Arching of the neck and trunk may occur. Advanced stages of bilirubin encephalopathy include coma, seizures, and death.[82,83,84,85]

Kernicterus is the chronic form of bilirubin encephalopathy. If bilirubin is sufficiently elevated, the symptoms of bilirubin encephalopathy might not be exhibited before the brain is damaged.[83,84,86] Brain damage associated with kernicterus includes cerebral palsy, auditory dysfunction, dental enamel dysplasia, upward gaze paralysis, intellectual deficits, and other disabilities.[85]

Macrosomic infants are at an increased risk for developing abnormal bilirubin metabolism because poorly controlled maternal glycemia causes the increase in fetal hemoglobin.[75] Bilirubin levels should be monitored for five days after birth. Phototherapy is the standard treatment for elevated bilirubin levels.[85]

Neurologic Problems

Neurologic problems can result from underlying pathology caused by hypocalcemia, hypomagnesemia, hypoglycemia, erythrocytosis, iron deficiency, hypoxia from respiratory complications, and birth trauma. Hypoglycemia tends to affect the infant within 24 hours, and hypocalcemia and hypomagnesemia manifest at 24 to 72 hours.

Symptoms include lethargy, poor feeding, and hypotonicity or jitteriness and hypertonicity. Seizures that result from the underlying pathologies can contribute to long-term cognitive dysfunction and adverse developmental outcomes.[66] Infants with metabolic disturbances (e.g., hypoglycemia, hypocalcemia) that cause seizures have a 10% to 50% risk of neurodevelopmental abnormalities. Hypoxic-ischemic encephalopathy that causes seizures results in developmental delays 80% of the time.[87]

Studies have focused on the long-term effects of infants of diabetic mothers. Although the interpretation of the studies may be difficult due to the time between adverse physiologic events in utero and the manifestation of neonatal (or later) problems, a correlation can be identified between the maternal lipid and glucose concentrations and the intellectual ability of the child up to the age of 11.[88] A trend of poor gestational metabolic management by the mother coincides with the poor level of neurologic functioning of the child.[88]

TREATMENT OF DIABETES IN PREGNANCY

As far back as 1954, Pedersen detected that "the common maternal, fetal, and neonatal complications of a diabetic pregnancy could be diminished by carefully supervised regulation of maternal metabolism."[17] Since 1980, the adoption of *tight*, or normal, glycemic control goals, achieved through careful SMBG and laboratory monitoring of blood glucose, administration of insulin, increased exercise, and regulated diet have been the fundamental treatment components of pregnancies complicated by diabetes.[22]

Blood Glucose Concentrations

Blood glucose is the most important factor to monitor during pregnancies complicated by diabetes because of its significant effect on the health and development of the fetus.[89] The primary benefits of SMBG methods are safety and accuracy in

pregnancy and current use in the majority of diabetic patients. Through SMBG, pregnant diabetic women can allow physicians to personalize treatment plans by maintaining detailed glucose diaries with recorded meals and times, corresponding insulin injections (if on insulin therapy), and both preprandial and postprandial blood glucose measurements.[15] Optimal obstetric outcomes occur when both the preprandial and postprandial blood glucose concentrations stay within the normal range of nondiabetic pregnant women.[89]

Because there is no set standard, controversy exists over the target blood glucose concentrations for diabetic women during pregnancy. In 2001, Parretti and colleagues[90] studied the blood glucose ranges of pregnant women without diabetes, setting a precedent for blood glucose target values during pregnancy. According to Parretti, normoglycemia for nonobese pregnant women without diabetes lies in the range of 54.8 ± 6.2 mg/dL (3.0 ± 0.34 mmol/L) and 105.2 ± 4.9 mg/dL (5.8 ± 0.27 mmol/L) between 28 and 38 weeks' gestation.

Blood glucose goals for pregnant diabetic women should be lowered to reflect the demonstrated norm in nondiabetic pregnant women. However, controversy still remains surrounding optimal blood glucose ranges during pregnancy. The American Diabetes Association identifies targets as a fasting plasma glucose concentration of 105 mg/dL (5.8 mmol/L), a 1-hour postprandial plasma glucose concentration of 155 mg/dL (8.6 mmol/L), and a 2-hour postprandial plasma glucose concentration of 130 mg/dL (7.2 mmol/l).[91] Likewise, Gabbe and Graves recommend target levels of less than 140 mg/dL at 1 hour posprandially and less than 120 mg/dL at 2 hours postprandially.[92] Given evidence on the risk of macrosomia, and its cascading effects, at 1-hour postprandial blood glucose elevations higher than 120 mg/dL,[58] we recommend that pregnant women with diabetes focus on maintaining 1-hour postprandial values at less than 120 mg/dL (6.7 mmol/L) and aim for preprandial blood glucose values less than 90 mg/dL (5.0 mmol/L).[49]

Because SMBG is highly dependent on patient understanding, motivation, and compliance, there are some problems with its usefulness for physicians. Furthermore, new developments with continuous glucose monitoring have revealed postprandial blood glucose elevations that remain undetected with sporadic SMBG values.[93] These results challenge the claim that fetal complications, such as macrosomia, can occur despite excellent metabolic control.[94] New understandings of the relationship between glycemic control and natal outcome are proving that "macrosomia despite normoglycemia" is truly "macrosomia because of undetected hyperglycemia."[95]

HbA1c levels should also be measured frequently in pregnant diabetic women to check the accuracy of self-reported blood glucose values and to track trends that correspond to treatment changes. A constant decrease in blood glucose levels can be statis-

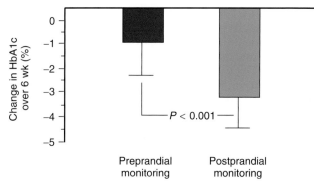

Figure 35–8. Changes in hemoglobin HbA1c (HbHbA1c) over six weeks after monitoring either preprandial or postprandial glucose levels. Over the course of six weeks, HbHbA1c levels were significantly lower in women with gestational diabetes who measured and corrected postprandial glucose levels as compared with women who only monitored preprandial glucose levels. (Adapted from de Veciana M, Major CA, Morgan MA, et al: Postprandial versus preprandial blood glucose monitoring in women with gestational diabetes mellitus requiring insulin therapy. N Engl J Med 333:1237-1241, 1995.)

tically significant in just 3 weeks, instead of 2 to 3 months. Therefore, measuring HbA1c every 2 weeks and comparing it to a patient's previous results can indicate the effectiveness of a treatment.[96] Furthermore, de Veciana and colleagues reported that women who measured both preprandial and postprandial glucose concentrations demonstrated significantly lower HbA1c levels over the course of 6 weeks (Fig. 35–8).[14] The risk of fetal macrosomia decreased from 42% to 12% in women measuring both preprandial and postprandial glucose concentrations.

On average, blood glucose concentrations and HbA1c values fall by 20% in normal pregnant women.[22] One explanation for this phenomenon is that pregnancy is associated with lower blood glucose and higher lactate dehydrogenase concentrations, which cause less glycation.[97] Furthermore, the rate of erythrocyte formation increases during pregnancy. Consequently, the overall volume of erythrocytes is larger, making the fraction of glycated hemoglobin smaller.[96]

There is a consensus that basal glucose concentrations decline during pregnancy because of caloric siphoning from the developing fetus.[98-101] In addition, studies have demonstrated that HbA1c levels are significantly lower in early and late pregnancy in normal women.[102] These findings are of clinical importance when defining a reference range for HbA1c for pregnant diabetic women. Box 35-2 shows the reference intervals that should be used for HbA1c values during pregnancy. Ultimately, diabetic women should aim for HbA1c values less than 5.0% throughout pregnancy to minimize the risk of fetal abnormalities.[103]

Box 35-3. The Jovanovic Diet: An Application for Clinical Use

Ms. R is a 35-year-old Latin American woman in her 14th week of pregnancy. She has a blood glucose level of 250 mg/dL 1 hour after a 50-g glucose challenge test, which indicates gestational diabetes. Ms. R stands 5 ft 4 in tall (1.62 m) and weighed 230 pounds (104.5 kg) before her pregnancy. Her body mass index (BMI) is 39. She was more than 151% heavier than her ideal body weight (120 lbs [54.5 kg]) before pregnancy (Table 35–4).

Ms. R's total daily calorie requirement can be calculated using the first section of Table 35-4. Using her current pregnant weight of 237.5 lbs (108 kg) and the amount of calories needed based on her percentage of ideal body weight (12 to 15 kcal/kg), the number of calories she should consume per day can be determined:

$$12 \text{ kcal} \times 108 \text{ kg} = 1296 \text{ kcal/day}$$

Calories from carbohydrate should be no more than 40% of total calories:

$$1296 \text{ kcal/day} \times 0.4 = 518 \text{ kcal}$$

Therefore, 518 kcal is the maximum amount she should consume from carbohydrate per day.

Now each meal's calorie and carbohydrate amount can be calculated. Ms. R will eat three meals and four snacks throughout the day. The calculation for breakfast is as follows:

$$2/18 \times 1296 \text{ kcal} = 144 \text{ kcal}$$
$$0.10 \times 518 \text{ kcal carbohydrate} = 52 \text{ kcal carbohydrate}$$

We can perform these calculations for other meals and for snacks. Lunch and dinner are each 360 kcal with 155 kcal from carbohydrate; snack after breakfast is 72 kcal with 26 kcal from carbohydrate; snack after lunch is 144 kcal with 52 kcal from carbohydrate; snack after dinner is 144 kcal with 26 kcal from carbohydrate; and bedtime snack is 72 kcal with 52 kcal from carbohydrate.

The snacks all vary in calorie and carbohydrate content to help Ms. R maintain controlled glucose levels. Ms. R knows that if she limits her carbohydrates, particularly potatoes, tortillas, cereal, bread, and pasta, she might be able to avoid insulin injections.

Ms. R calls the dietician, Ms. A, to discuss meal options. She keeps a meal log and monitors her blood glucose levels before meals.

Adapted from Jovanovic L: Controversies in the diagnosis and treatment of gestational diabetes. Cleve Clin J Med 67:481-488, 2000.

Table 35–4. The Jovanovic Diet

Total Daily Calories

Percentage of Ideal Body Weight	Daily Calories per Kilogram Body Weight
80% to 120%	30
121% to 150%	24
>151%	12 to 15

Daily Calorie Distribution

Time	Meal	Fraction of Total Calories	Percentage of Total Daily Carbohydrate
8 AM	Breakfast	2/18	10
10 AM	Snack	1/18	5
12 noon	Lunch	5/18	30
3 PM	Snack	2/18	10
5 PM	Dinner	5/18	30
8 PM	Snack	1/18	5
11 PM	Snack	1/18	10

Adapted from Jovanovic L: Controversies in the diagnosis and treatment of gestational diabetes. Cleve Clin J Med 67:481-488, 2000.

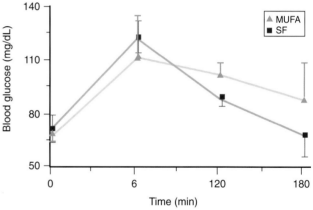

Figure 35–16. Comparison of monounsaturated fat and saturated fat in relation to postprandial blood glucose levels over time. The graph depicts the difference in metabolism of monounsaturated fat (MUFA, *blue line*) and saturated fat *(red line)*. Although the peak values are similar, higher postprandial glucose levels are maintained longer with monounsaturated fats. This may indicate a higher risk of macrosomia associated with higher postprandial values and an increase in insulin dose to decrease postprandial levels when meals with monounsaturated fats are consumed. (Adapted from Ilic S, Jovanovic L, Pettit DJ. Comparison of the effect of saturated and monounsaturated fat on postprandial plasma glucose and insulin concentration in women with gestational diabetes mellitus. Am J Perinatol 16:489-495, 2000.)

would regulate glucose levels and meet the nutrition needs of both mother and fetus.

There has also been a study comparing the effects of saturated fat and monounsaturated fat on postprandial glucose concentrations. Figure 35–16 demonstrates the difference in fats and the duration of glucose concentrations. One-hour postprandial glucose concentrations are about equal in diets containing both types of fat. However, monounsaturated fat intake changes the rate of glucose uptake over longer periods of time: Glucose concentrations remain elevated longer. Given that macrosomia is associated with increased postprandial glucose concentrations, meals containing saturated fat

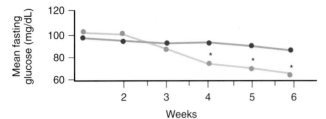

Figure 35–17. Effects of exercise on mean fasting glucose in gestational diabetes patients. This graph depicts a comparison made between gestational diabetes patients treated with medical nutritional therapy *(blue circles)* and those treated with medical nutritional therapy and arm ergometry exercise *(red circles)*. Differences in the glucose levels became noticeable at 4 weeks. (From Jovanovic L, Durak EP, Peterson CM: Randomized trial of diet versus diet plus cardiovascular conditioning on glucose levels in gestational diabetes. Am J Obstet Gynecol 161:415-419, 1989.)

instead of monounsaturated fat could have a superior effect and reduce the dose of insulin required to control postprandial glucose concentrations in GDM.[120]

Exercise

Exercise can also facilitate the treatment of gestational diabetes mellitus. The benefits of exercise in women with pregestational diabetes are not as great. Exercise may be difficult for GDM women due to barriers of obesity and inexperience. These difficulties can be overcome if the motivation to exercise is greater than the desire to take insulin injections. Low-impact exercise is recommended, because it does not provoke contractions or create stress for the fetus.

One study used an arm cycle machine to work the upper body. In this 6-week trial, the group that exercised displayed cardiovascular fitness, normal fasting glucose concentrations, and decreased postprandial glucose levels.[121] A comparison in mean fasting glucose can be seen in Figure 35–17 between the exercise and the control group throughout the duration of the trial.[122] However, once insulin therapy is begun, exercise might not help regulate glucose levels. Similarly, studies have shown that in mothers with T1DM, exercise does not significantly improve glucose levels.[123]

SUMMARY

Diabetes in pregnancy can have adverse effects on both the mother and child. Pregestational diabetic women must control glucose levels prior to and during pregnancy to minimize maternal problems such as nephropathy, retinopathy, and vascular complications.[40] Hyperglycemia in the first 20 weeks of gestation can cause fetal malformations, congenital defects, and spontaneous abortion.[27] However, women who develop GDM are at a lower risk than pregestational diabetic women for fetal structural abnormalities due to its time of onset in the pregnancy.

Medical history, ethnicity, age, and obesity can help identify patients at a high risk for GDM.[47] Universal testing is the ideal form of prevention. GDM is currently diagnosed from two abnormal OGTT results. There is a dispute about which standards to use (NDDG, WHO, or ADA) for the glucose load and what constitutes an abnormal result. The results of the HAPO study could clarify and set specific standards for diagnosing GDM.[54]

Maternal hyperglycemia in either pregestational or gestational diabetic mothers can cause many fetal complications during the growth and maturation of the fetus. Because glucose crosses the placenta, fetal hyperglycemia occurs. According to the Pederson hypothesis, fetal hyperglycemia can lead to fetal hyperinsulinemia.[62] These conditions, independently or combined, can set off a cascade of metabolic, developmental, and growth complications for the fetus. Fetal complications include macrosomia, hypocalcemia, hypomagnesemia, iron redistribution, erythrocytosis, and cardiorespiratory problems. Each of these problems increases the risk for stillbirth, neonatal complications, and birth trauma. There is also increased risk of long-term developmental and neurologic difficulties.[66]

Maternal treatment differs for pregestational and gestational diabetes mellitus, though all efforts are focused on establishing normal preprandial and postprandial glucose levels. Pregestational diabetic mothers must use insulin therapy. GDM mothers may be able to avoid insulin therapy if modifications in diet and exercise are made. Through the use of continuous glucose monitors and frequent HbA1c tests, glucose can be strictly monitored. Studies have suggested that the postprandial glucose concentrations are important indicators for the relative risk of the fetus's developing macrosomia as well as other metabolic complications.[58] Ideally, preprandial glucose should be no more than 90 mg/dL and 1-hour postprandial values should be no greater than 120 mg/dL.[49,58] Because of the increased turnover rate of hemoglobin for women in pregnancy, HbA1c tests can be a valuable tool to recognize trends in glucose control. Ideally, an HbA1c value within two standard deviations of the normal pregnant population can minimize the risk of macrosomia in pregnancies complicated by GDM.[96]

Medical nutrition therapy has been a controversial issue in treating GDM because there is no standard diet recognized or endorsed by the ADA. Carbohydrate-restriction diets have been reported to improve glucose concentration control in GDM.[115] This diet appears to be successful because postprandial glucose levels can be maintained within the recommended levels.[58]

Insulin therapy may be used in the GDM mother to help control glucose levels. Lispro or aspart, rapid-acting insulin analogs, may be used by pregnant women with GDM as a bolus prior to meals in conjunction with a basal insulin (NPH or insulin pump).[108,109]

Exercise also can be used as adjunctive therapy in women with GDM. Precautions must be taken when selecting the appropriate type of exercise to minimize fetal stress and not induce contractions. However, once insulin therapy is started, exercise might not be as beneficial for controlling glucose concentrations.[123]

Pregestational and gestational diabetic mothers have a great responsibility and influence in shaping the futures of their children. Pregestational diabetic mothers must receive proper preparation and management before and during pregnancy to reach optimal glucose levels. The key for success for gestational diabetic mothers is dependent on adequate screening for GDM as well as strict glucose control through diet, exercise, and (if necessary) insulin therapy. If hyperglycemia is prevented in both groups, normal healthy babies will be born.

References

1. American Diabetes Association: Clinical Practice Recommendations 2001: Gestational Diabetes. Diabetes Care 24(Suppl 1):S77-S79, 2001.
2. Hod M, Diamant YZ: Diabetes in pregnancy. Norbert Freinkel Memorial Issue. Isr J Med Sci 27:421-532, 1991.
3. Fuhrmann K, Ruher H, Semmler K, et al: Prevention of congenital malformations in infants of insulin-dependent diabetic mothers. Diabetes Care 6:21-23, 1983.
4. Miller E, Hare JW, Clogerty JP, et al: Elevated maternal hemoglobin HbA1c in early pregnancy and major congenital anomalies in infants of diabetic mothers. N Engl J Med 304:1331-1335,1981.
5. Cousins, L: Etiology and prevention of congenital anomalies among infants of overt diabetic women. Clin Obstet Gynecol 34:484-485, 1991.
6. Petersen M, Pedersen SA, Greisen G, et al: Early growth delay in diabetic pregnancy: Relation to psychomotor development at age 4. BMJ 296:598-601, 1988.
7. van Dijk DJ, Axer-Siegel R, Erman A, Hod M: Diabetic vascular complications and pregnancy. Diabetes Rev 3:632-642, 1995.
8. Catalano PM, Drago NM, Amini S: Maternal carbohydrate metabolism and its relationship to fetal growth and body composition. Am J Obstet Gynecol 172:1464-1470, 1995.
9. Hod M, Diamant YZ: The offspring of a diabetic mother—short- and long-range implications. Isr J Med Sci 28:81-86, 1992.
10. Pettitt DJ, Knowler WC: Long-term effects of the intrauterine environment, birth weight, and breast-feeding in Pima Indians. Diabetes Care 21:B138-B141, 1988.
11. Steel JM, Johnstone FD, Hepburn DA, Smith AF: Can prepregnancy care of diabetic women reduce the risk of abnormal babies? BMJ 301:1070-1073, 1990.
12. Jovanovic L, Druzin M, Peterson CM: The effect of euglycemia on the outcome of pregnancy in insulin-independent diabetics as compared to normal controls. Am J Med 71:921-927, 1981.
13. Jovanovic L: Medical Management of Pregnancy Complicated by Diabetes. Alexandria, VA, American Diabetes Association, 1993; revised 1995 and 2000.
14. de Veciana M, Major CA, Morgan MA, et al: Postprandial versus preprandial blood glucose monitoring in women with gestational diabetes mellitus requiring insulin therapy. N Engl J Med 333:1237-1241, 1995.
15. Thorsell A, Gordon M, Jovanovic L: Continuous glucose monitoring: A stepping stone in the journey towards a cure for diabetes. J Matern Fetal Neonatal Med 15:15-25, 2004.
16. Gamson K, Chia S, Jovanovic L: The safety and efficacy of insulin analogs in pregnancy. J Matern Fetal Neonatal Med 15:26-34, 2004.
17. Pedersen J: Fetal mortality in diabetes in relation to management during the latter part of pregnancy. Acta Endocrinol 15:282-294,1954.
18. Freinkel N: Banting Lecture 1980: Of pregnancy and progeny. Diabetes 29:1023-1035, 1980.
19. Jovanovic L, Peterson CM: Moment in history: Turning point in blood glucose monitoring of diet and insulin dosing. Trans Am Soc Artif Intern Organs 36:799-804, 1990.
20. Connell FA, Vadheim C, Emanuel I: Diabetes in pregnancy: A population-based study of incidence, referral for care and perinatal mortality. Am J Obstet Gynecol 151:598-603, 1985.
21. Engelgau MM, Herman WH, Smith PJ, et al: The epidemiology of diabetes and pregnancy in the US, 1988. Diabetes Care 18:1029-1033, 1995.
22. Jovanovic L: Medical emergencies in the patient with diabetes during pregnancy. Endocrinol Metab Clin North Am 29:771-787, 2000.
23. Mills JL, Simpson JL, Driscoll SG, et al: Incidence of spontaneous abortion among normal women and insulin dependent diabetic women whose pregnancies were identified within 21 days of conception. N Engl J Med 319:1617-1623, 1988.
24. Mills JL, Baker L, Goldman A: Malformations in infants of diabetic mothers occur before the seventh gestational week: Implications for treatment. Diabetes 23:292-295, 1979.
25. Greene MF, Hare JW, Cloherty JP, et al: First trimester hemoglobin HbA1c and risk for major malformation and spontaneous abortion in diabetic pregnancy. Teratology 39:225-231, 1989.
26. Steel JM, Johnstone FD, Hepburn DA, Smith AF: Can prepregnancy care of diabetic women reduce the risk of abnormal babies? BMJ 301:1070-1073, 1990.
27. Kitzmiller JL, Gavin LA, Gin GD, et al: Preconception care of diabetes: Glycemic control prevents congenital anomalies. JAMA 265:726-731, 1991.
28. Hare JW, White P: Pregnancy in diabetes complicated by vascular disease. Diabetes. 26:953-955, 1977.
29. National Center for Health Statistics: Advance report of final mortality statistics, 1991. Mon Vital Stat Rep 42(2 Suppl): 1993.
30. Star J, Carpenter MW: The effect of pregnancy on the natural history of diabetic retinopathy and nephropathy. Clin Perinatol 25:887-916, 1988.
31. Chew EY, Mills JL, Metzger BE, et al: Metabolic control and progression of retinopathy: The Diabetes in Early Pregnancy Study. Diabetes Care 18:631-637, 1995.
32. Early worsening of diabetic retinopathy in the Diabetes Control and Complications Trial. Arch Ophthalmol 116:874-876, 1998.
33. Rand LI, Krolewski AS, Aiello LM, et al: Multiple factors in the prediction of risk of proliferative diabetic retinopathy. N Engl J Med 313:1433, 1985.
34. Jampol LM, Phelps R, Sakol P, et al: Diabetic retinopathy during pregnancy: Role of regulation of hyperglycemia. Ophthalmol Vis Sci 27:4, 1986.
35. Wang PH, Lau J, Chalmers TC: Meta-analysis of effects of intensive blood glucose control on later complications of type 1 diabetes. Lancet 341:1306-1309, 1993.
36. Lauritzen T, Frost-Larsen K, Larsen HW, et al: Effect of 1 year of near normal blood glucose levels on retinopathy in insulin-dependent diabetics. Lancet 1:200-204, 1983.
37. The Kroc Collaborative Study Group: Blood glucose control and the evolution of diabetic retinopathy and albuminuria. A preliminary multicenter trial. N Engl J Med 311:365-372, 1984.

38. Chan WC, Lim LT, Quinn MJ, et al: Management and outcome of sight-threatening diabetic retinopathy in pregnancy. Eye 18:826-832, 2004.

39. Miodovnik M, Rosenn BM, Khoury JC, et al: Does pregnancy increase the risk for development and progression of diabetic nephropathy? Am J Obstet Gynecol 174:1180-1189, 1996.

40. Jovanovic R, Jovanovic L: Obstetric management when normoglycemia is maintained in diabetic pregnant women with vascular compromise. Am J Obstet Gynecol 149:617-623, 1984.

41. Reece EA, Coustan DR, Hayslett JP, et al: Diabetic nephropathy: Pregnancy performance and fetomaternal outcome. Am J Obstet Gynecol 159:56-66, 1988.

42. Kitzmiller JL, Watt N, Driscoll SG: Decidual arteriopathy in hypertension and diabetes in pregnancy: Immunofluorescent studies. Am J Obstet Gynecol 141:773-779, 1981.

43. Irfan S, Arain TM, Shaukat A, Shahid A: Effect of pregnancy in diabetic nephropathy and retinopathy. J Coll Physicians Surg Pak 14:75-78, 2004.

44. Jovanovic L, Hussain Z: Prepregnancy counseling in women with diabetes mellitus. Up to Date, June 30, 2004. Available at http://www.physicians.uptodate.com/topic.asp?file=diabetes/15410.

45. Coustan DR: Gestational diabetes. In Harris MI, Cowie CC, Stern MP, et al (eds): Diabetes in America, 2nd ed. Baltimore: National Institutes of Health, 1995, pp 703-717. [Publication 95-1468.]

46. Xiang AH, Peters RK, Trigo E, et al: Multiple metabolic defects during late pregnancy in women at high risk for type 2 diabetes. Diabetes 48:848-854, 1999.

47. American College of Obstetrics and Gynecology: Gestational diabetes (practice bulletin no. 30). Obstet Gynecol 98:525-538, 2001.

48. Buchanan TA, Unterman T, Metzger BE: The medical management of diabetes in pregnancy. Clin Perinatol 12:625-650, 1985.

49. Jovanovic, L, Bevier W: The Santa Barbara County Health Care Services Program: Birth weight change concomitant with screening for and treatment of glucose-intolerance of pregnancy: A potential cost effective intervention. Am J Perinatol 14:221-228, 1997.

50. Amadin RA, Famuyiwa OO, Adelusi BO: Glycemic RESPONSE to 75gms and 100gms glucose load during pregnancy in Nigerian women. Diabetologia 18:159-161, 1989.

51. Pettit DJ, Bennett PH, Hanson RL, et al: Comparison of World Health Organization and National Diabetes Data Group procedures to detect abnormalities of glucose tolerance during pregnancy. Diabetes Care 17:1264-1268, 1994.

52. Deerochanawong C, Putiyanun C, Wongsuryat M, et al: Comparison of National Diabetes Data Group and World Health Organization criteria for detecting gestational diabetes mellitus. Diabetologia 39:1070-1073, 1996.

53. Metzger BE, Coustan DR: Summary and recommendations of the Fourth International Workshop Conference on Gestational Diabetes Mellitus. Diabetes Care 21(suppl 2):B161-B167, 1988.

54. HAPO Study Cooperative Research Group: The Hyperglycemia and Adverse Pregnancy Outcome (HAPO) Study. Int J Gynaecol Obstet 78:69-77, 2002.

55. Buchanan TA, Kjos SL, Schafer U, et al: Utility of fetal measurements in the management of gestational diabetes mellitus. Diabetes Care 21(Suppl. 2):B99-B106, 1998.

56. Schaefer-Graf UM, Kjos SL, Fauzan OH, et al: A randomized trial evaluating a predominantly fetal growth-based strategy to guide management of gestational diabetes in Caucasian women. Diabetes Care 27:297-302, 2004.

57. Jovanovic L, Saxena BB, Dawood MY, et al: Feasibility of maintaining euglycemia in insulin-dependent diabetic women. Am J Med 68:105-112, 1980.

58. Jovanovic-Peterson L, Peterson CM, Reed GF, et al: Maternal postprandial glucose levels and infant birth weight: The Diabetes in Early Pregnancy study. The National Institute of Child Health and Human Development—Diabetes in Early Pregnancy Study. Am J Obstet Gynecol 164:103-111, 1991.

59. Combs CA, Gunderson E. Kitzmiller JL, et al: Relationship of fetal macrosomia to maternal postprandial glucose control during pregnancy. Diabetes Care 15:1251-1257, 1992.

60. Ylinen K, Aula P, Stenman UH, et al: Risk of minor and major fetal malformations in diabetics with high hemoglobin HbA1c values in early pregnancy. BMJ 289:345-349, 1984.

61. Hanson U, Persson B, Thunell S: Relationship between haemoglobin A1c in early type I (insulin dependent) diabetic pregnancy and the occurrence of spontaneous abortion and fetal malformation in Sweden. Diabetologia 33:100-104, 1990.

62. Pederson J: The pregnant diabetic and her newborn, 2nd edition. Baltimore, Williams and Wilkins, 1977.

63. Kalhan SC, Parimi PS, Lindsay CA: Pregnancy complicated by diabetes mellitus. In Fanaroff AA, Martin RJ (eds): Neonatal-Perinatal Medicine: Diseases of the Fetus and Infant, 7th ed. Philadelphia, Mosby, 2002, p 1357.

64. Kicklighter SD: Infant of diabetic mother. Emedicine October 26, 2001. Available at www.emedicine.com/ped/topic845.htm. Accessed February 25, 2004.

65. Fee B, Weil WM: Body composition of a diabetic offspring by direct analysis. Am J Dis Child 100:718-719, 1960.

66. Nold JL, Georgieff MK: Infants of diabetic mothers. Pediatr Clin North Am 51:619-637, 2004.

67. Naylor, CD, Sermer M, Chen E, Sykora K: Cesarean delivery in relation to birth weight and gestational glucose tolerance. JAMA 275:1165-1170, 1996.

68. Georgieff MK: Therapy of infants of diabetic mothers. In Burg FD, Ingelfinger JR, Wald ER, Polin RA (eds): Current Pediatric Therapy, 15th ed. Philadephia, WB Saunders, 1995, pp 793-803.

69. Creasy RK, Resnik R: Intrauterine growth restriction. In Creasy RK, Resnick R (eds): Maternal–Fetal Medicine, 4th ed. Philadelphia, WB Saunders, 1999, pp 569-589.

70. Milley JR, Papacestas JS, Tabats BD: Effect of insulin on uptake of metabolic substrates by the sheep fetus. Am J Physiol 251:E349-E359, 1986.

71. Phillips AF, Porte PJ, Strabinsky S, et al: Effects of chronic fetal hyperglycemia upon oxygen consumption in the ovine uterus and conceptus. J Clin Invest 74:279-287, 1984.

72. Stonestreet BS, Goldstein M, Oh W, et al: Effect of prolonged hyperinsulinemia on erythropoiesis in fetal sheep. Am J Physiol 257:R1199-R1204, 1989.

73. Widness JA, Susa JB, Garcia JF, et al: Increased erythropoiesis and elevated erthropoietin in infants born to diabetic mothers and in hyperinsulinemic rhesus fetuses. J Clin Invest 67:637-42, 1981.

74. Georgieff MK, Widness JA, Mills MM, Stonestreet BS: The effect of prolonged intrauterine hyperinsulinemia on iron utilization in fetal sheep. Pediatr Res 26:467-469, 1989.

75. Green DW, Khoury J, Mimouni F: Neonatal hemocrit and maternal glycemic control in insulin-dependent mothers. J Pediatr 12:302-305, 1992.

76. Petry, CD Wobken JD, McKay H, et al: Placental transferrin receptor in diabetic pregnancies with increased fetal iron demand. Am J Physiol 267:E507-E514, 1994.

77. Georgieff MK, Petry CD, Mills MM, et al: Increased N-glycosylation and reduced transferrin binding capacity of the transferrin receptor isolated from placentas of diabetic mothers. Placenta 18:563-568, 1997.

78. Bard H, Prosmanne J: Relative rates of fetal hemoglobin and adult hemoglobin synthesis in cord blood of infants of insulin-dependent diabetic mothers. Pediatrics 75:1143-1147, 1987.

79. Schwartz RP: Neonatal hypoglycemia: How low is too low? J Pediatr 131:171-173, 1997.

80. Rooney SA: Regulation of surfactant-associated phospholipids synthesis and secretion. In Polin RA, Fox WW (eds): Fetal and Neonatal Physiology, 2nd ed. Philadelphia, WB Saunders, 1998, pp 1283-1298.

81. Moore, TR: Diabetes in pregnancy. In Creasy RK, Resnik R (eds): Maternal–Fetal Medicine. Philadelphia, WB Saunders,1999, pp 964-995.

82. Ip S, Glicken S, Kulig J, et al: Management of Neonatal Hyperbilirubinemia. Rockville, Md: US Department of Health and Human Services, Agency for Healthcare Research and Quality, 2003. [AHRQ Publication 03-E011]

83. Ip S, Chung M, Kulig J, et al: An evidence-based review of important issues concerning neonatal hyperbilirubinemia. Pediatrics 114:e130-e153, 2004.

84. Johnson LH, Bhutani VK, Brown AK: System-based approach to management of neonatal jaundice and prevention of kernicterus. J Pediatr 140:396-403, 2002.

85. Subcommittee on Hyperbilirubinemia: Management of hyperbilirubinemia in the newborn infant 35 or more weeks of gestation. Pediatrics 114:297-316, 2004.

86. Maisels MJ, Newman TB: Kernicterus in otherwise healthy, breast-fed term newborns. Pediatrics 96:730-733, 1995.

87. Volpe JJ: Neonatal seizures. In Volpe JJ (ed): Neurology of the Newborn, 4th ed. Philadelphia, WB Saunders, 2001, pp 178-216.

88. Rizzo TA, Metzger BE, Dooley SL, et al: Early malnutrition and child neurobehavioral development: Insights from the study of children of diabetic mothers. Child Dev 68:26-38, 1997.

89. Dukes JW, Chen, AC, Jovanovic L: Diabetes in pregnancy. In Gronowski AM (ed): Handbook of Clinical Testing During Pregnancy. Totowa, NJ, Humana Press, 2003, pp 359-390.

90. Parretti E, Mecacci F, Papini M, et al: Third-trimester maternal glucose levels from diurnal profiles in nondiabetic pregnancies. Diabetes Care 24:1319-1327, 2001.

91. American Diabetes Association: Gestational diabetes mellitus. [Practice Guideline] Diabetes Care 27(Suppl 1):S88-S90, 2004.

92. Gabbe SG, Graves CR: Management of diabetes mellitus complicating pregnancy. Obstet Gynecol 102:857-868, 2003.

93. Jovanovic L: The role of continuous glucose monitoring in gestational diabetes. Diabetes Technol Ther 2(Suppl 1):S67-S71, 2000.

94. Viser GHA, van Ballegooie E, Sluiter WJ: Macrosomy despite well-controlled diabetic pregnancy [letter]. Lancet 1:283-285, 1984.

95. Jovanovic L: Gestational diabetes mellitus: The case for euglycemia. Canadian J Diabetes 27:428-432, 2003.

96. Madsen H, Ditzel J, Hansen P: Hemoglobin A1c determinations in diabetic pregnancy. Diabetes Care 4:541-546, 1981.

97. Gunton JE, McElduff A: Hemoglobinopathies and HbA1c measurement. Diabetes Care 23:1197-1198, 2000.

98. Widness JA, Schwartz HC, Kahn CB: Glycohemoglobin in diabetic pregnancy: A sequential study. Am J Obstet Gynecol 136:1024-1029, 1980.

99. Mills JL, Jovanovic L, Knopp R: Physiological reduction in fasting plasma glucose concentration in the first trimester of normal pregnancy: the Diabetes in Early Pregnancy Study. Metabolism 47:1140-1144, 1998.

100. Fadel HE, Hammond SD, Huff TA: Glycosolated hemoglobins in normal pregnancy and gestational diabetes mellitus. Obstet Gynecol 54:322-326, 1979.

101. Jovanovic L: Insulin therapy in pregnancy. In Laehy JL, Cefalu, WT (eds): Insulin Therapy. New York, Marcel Dekker, 2002, pp 139-151.

102. Nielsen LR, Ekbom P, Damm P, et al: HbA1c levels are significantly lower in early and late pregnancy. Diabetes Care 27:1200-1201, 2004.

103. Cefalu WT, Prather KL, Chester DL: Total serum glycosolated proteins in detection and monitoring of gestational diabetes. Diabetes Care 13:872-875, 1990.

104. Piacquadio K, Hollingsworth DR, Murphy H: Effects of in-utero exposure to oral hypoglycemic drugs. Lancet 338:866-869, 1991.

105. Langer O, Conway Dl, Berkus MD, et al: A comparison of glyburide and insulin in women with gestational diabetes mellitus. N Engl J Med 343:1134-1138, 2000.

106. Fineberg SE, Rathbun MJ, Hufferd S, et al: Immunologic aspects of human proinsulin therapy. Diabetes 37:276-280, 1988.

107. Balsells M, Corcoy R, Mauricio D, et al: Insulin antibody response to a short course of human insulin therapy in women with gestational diabetes. Diabetes Care 20:1172-1175, 1997.

108. Fineberg NS, Fineberg SE, Anderson JH, et al: Immunologic effects of insulin lispro [Lys (B28), Pro (B29) human insulin] in IDDM and NIDDM patients previously treated with insulin. Diabetes 45:1750-1754, 1996.

109. Jovanovic L, Ilic S, Pettitt DJ, et al: Metabolic and immunologic effects of insulin lispro in gestational diabetes. Diabetes Care 22:1422-1426, 1992.

110. Bhattacharyya A, Brown S, Hughes S, et al: Insulin lispro and regular insulin in pregnancy. Q J Med 94:m255-m260, 2001.

111. Persson B, Swahn ML, Hjertberg R, et al: Insulin lispro therapy in pregnancies complicated by type 1 diabetes mellitus. Diabetes Res Clin Pract 58:115-121, 2002.

112. Jovanovic L, Knopp RH, Brown Z, et al: Declining insulin requirement in the late first trimester of diabetic pregnancy. Diabetes Care 24:1130-1136, 2001.

113. Jovanovic L, Peterson CM: The art and science of maintenance of normoglycemia in pregnancies complicated by type 1 diabetes mellitus. Endocr Pract 2:130-142, 1996.

114. Peterson CM, Jovanovic L: Percentage of carbohydrate and glycemia response to breakfast, lunch and dinner in women with gestational diabetes. Diabetes 40(Suppl 2):172-174, 1991.

115. Knopp RH, Magee M, Raisys V: Hypocaloric diets and ketogenesis in the management of obese gestational diabetic women. J Am Coll Nutr 10:649-667, 1991.

116. Rizza T, Metzger BE, Urns WJ, et al: Correlations between antepartum maternal metabolism and intelligence of offspring. N Engl J Med 325:911-916, 1991.

117. Jovanovic L, Meztzger B, Knopp RH: Beta hydroxybutyrate levels in type 1 diabetic pregnancy compared with normal pregnancy. Diabetes Care 21:1-5, 1998.

118. King J, Allen L: Nutrition During Pregnancy. Washington, DC, National Academy Press, 1990.

119. Jovanovic L: Nutritional management of the obese gestational diabetic woman [guest editorial]. J Am Coll Nutr 11:246-250, 1992.

120. Ilic S, Jovanovic L, Pettit DJ: Comparison of the effect of saturated and monounsaturated fat on postprandial plasma glucose and insulin concentration in women with gestational diabetes mellitus. Am J Perinatol 16:489-495, 2000.

121. Jovanovic L: Controversies in the diagnosis and treatment of gestational diabetes. Cleve Clin J Med 67:481-488, 2000.

122. Jovanovic L, Durak EP, Peterson CM: Randomized trial of diet versus diet plus cardiovascular conditioning on glucose levels in gestational diabetes. Am J Obstet Gynecol 161:415-419, 1989.

123. Hollingsworth D, Moore T: Postprandial walking exercise in pregnant insulin-dependent (type 1) diabetic women: Reduction of plasma lipid levels but absence of a significant effect on glycemic control. Am J Obstet Gynecol 157:1359-1363, 1987.

124. Jovanovic L, Pettit DJ: Gestational diabetes mellitus. JAMA 286:2516-2518, 2001.

125. Jovanovic L: Time to reassess the optimal dietary prescription for women with gestational diabetes[editorial]. Am J Clin Nutr 70:3-4, 1999.

126. The Diabetes Control and Complications Trial Research Group: The effect of intensive treatment of diabetes on the development and progression of long-term complications in insulin-dependent diabetes mellitus. N Engl J Med 329:997-986, 1993.

KEY POINTS

- *Considerable data link hyperglycemia to poor hospital outcome. Hyperglycemia in hospitalized patients can no longer be ignored or treated retrospectively with regular insulin sliding scales.*
- *All of the oral antidiabetic medications have characteristics that limit their use in hospitalized patients, and thus insulin is the preferred treatment for hyperglycemia in these patients.*
- *The safe and effective use of insulin in hospitalized patients requires that prescribers have a thorough understanding of insulin physiology and the pharmacodynamics of exogenously administered insulin.*
- *A multidisciplinary team approach is needed to establish safe and effective diabetes care pathways for hospitalized patients. The key to success is having a "champion" of each discipline available for questions about all aspects of diabetes care.*

Adults with diabetes are four to six times more likely to be hospitalized than those without diabetes, and nearly two thirds of the $40 billion in direct medical costs related to diabetes is for inpatient care.[1-3] Poor glycemic control is common among hospitalized patients with diabetes for many reasons.[4] The majority of patients are admitted for reasons other than diabetes, and thus diabetes care becomes secondary to care for the primary diagnosis requiring admission. Infection, glucocorticoid therapy, surgical trauma, and general medical stress all contribute to hyperglycemia due to the release of counterregulatory factors that impair insulin action. Additionally, the nutrition intake and activity level of hospitalized patients is often altered or compromised.

Historically, mild to moderate hyperglycemia in the hospitalized patient has been ignored or treated retrospectively with regular insulin sliding scales. The rationale for this practice was based on the assumption that short-term hyperglycemia had minimal impact on the patient's outcome, and the risk of hypoglycemia outweighed the benefit of treating hyperglycemia.[5] In addition, the diabetes regimen used by patients at home was commonly discontinued on admission because of concerns about hypoglycemia in patients who might not be eating their regular diet.

Sliding-scale regular insulin regimens used alone without scheduled insulin have several major limitations that make them unacceptable for routine use. First, they fail to account for the timing of a blood glucose reading, and they give the same predetermined insulin dose regardless of whether the blood glucose reading is preprandial, postprandial, or at bedtime. Second, they fail to consider the insulin sensitivity of the patient. For example, an obese patient with type 2 diabetes (T2DM) admitted for coronary artery bypass grafting (CABG) has a different insulin requirement from a thin patient with type 1 diabetes (T1DM) admitted for a fractured femur. Third, sliding-scale regimens are retrospective, designed to correct inappropriate insulin delivery from the preceding 4 to 6 hours rather than anticipating future requirements. Fourth, sliding-scale regimens typically use regular insulin, which has an onset of 30 to 60 minutes and a duration of 6 to 8 hours in most patients. Thus the cumulative effect of sliding-scale insulin doses sets up the potential to overshoot the desired blood glucose goal and cause a cycle of fluctuating hypo- and hyperglycemia.

Considerable observational data now support a link between hyperglycemia and poor hospital outcome. Capes and colleagues performed a meta-analysis of 15 trials and found that hyperglycemia (blood glucose greater than 110 mg/dL [6.1 mmol/L]), with or without a prior diagnosis of diabetes, increased hospital mortality and congestive heart failure (CHF) in patients admitted for acute myocardial infarction (MI).[6] Bolk and coworkers found similar results in a prospective study of 336 patients admitted for acute MI.[7] Umpierrez and coworkers found that hyperglycemia, fasting blood glucose greater than 126 mg/dL (7.0 mmol/L), or random blood glucose greater than 200 mg/dL (11.1 mmol/L) on general medical and surgical units was associated with increased hospital mortality, a longer length of hospital stay, a greater

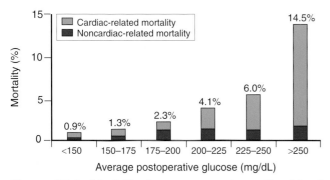

Figure 36–1. Mortality by average postoperative blood glucose for patients after cardiac surgery. The cardiac-related mortality and total mortality increase with increased average blood glucose levels in patients following cardiac surgery. (Reprinted from Furnary AP, Gao G, Grunkemeier GL, et al: Continuous insulin infusion reduces mortality in patients with diabetes undergoing coronary artery bypass grafting. J Thorac Cardiovasc Surg 125:1007-1021, 2003. Reprinted with permission from American Association for Thoracic Surgery.)

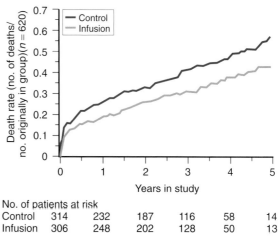

No. of patients at risk

Control	314	232	187	116	58	14
Infusion	306	248	202	128	50	13

Figure 36–2. Actuarial mortality curves for the long-term follow-up DIGAMI (Diabetes Mellitus Insulin-Glucose Infusion in Acute Myocardial Infarction) Trial. Curves are for patients receiving insulin-glucose infusion and for the control group among the total DIGAMI cohort. The absolute reduction in risk was 11%, and reduction in relative risk was 0.72 (confidence interval, 0.55-0.92; P = 0.011). (Reprinted with permission from Malmberg K, for the DIGAMI Study Group: Prospective randomized study of intensive insulin treatment on long term survival after acute myocardial infarction in patients with diabetes mellitus. BMJ 314:1512-1515, 1997.)

risk of infection, and more subsequent nursing home care.[8]

Furnary's group evaluated various insulin regimens and target blood glucose levels in patients with diabetes having cardiac surgery and found that patients with hyperglycemia had greater mortality and increased incidence of deep sternal wound infections (Fig. 36–1).[9,10] Further analysis of this cohort of patients revealed that hyperglycemia on the first and second postoperative days was the single most important predictor of serious infectious complications. A meta-analysis of 26 studies on stroke found increased hospital mortality in patients with admission blood glucose of 110 to 126 mg/dL (6.1 to 7.0 mmol/L). Stroke survivors with admission blood glucoses of 121 to 144 mg/dL (6.7 to 8 mmol/L) had poor functional recovery.[11] Patients with blood glucose greater than 140 mg/dL (7.8 mmol/L) had more severe strokes and greater mortality.

The data support the observation that hyperglycemia is linked to poor patient outcomes, but the bigger question is: Does controlling blood glucose improve outcomes? The Diabetes Insulin Glucose in Acute Myocardial Infarction (DIGAMI) trial was a prospective interventional trial. The investigators found decreased mortality at 1 year for patients with diabetes admitted for acute MI who received intensive therapy with insulin infusion, followed by subcutaneous insulin for 3 or more months compared to patients receiving conventional therapy (18.6% versus 26.1%).[12] Follow-up at 3.4 years revealed continued benefit for intensive therapy compared to conventional therapy (mortality of 33% versus 44%) (Fig. 36–2).[13]

Van den Berge and colleagues found that intensive insulin therapy with a mean blood glucose of

103 ± 19 mg/dL reduced intensive care unit (ICU) mortality as well as overall hospital mortality compared to conventional therapy with mean blood glucose of 153 ± 33 mg/dL in patients receiving mechanical ventilation in a surgical intensive care unit (Fig. 36–3).[14,15] Lazar and colleagues found that tight glycemic control (blood glucose 125 to 200 mg/dL [7.0 to 11.1 mmol/L]), using glucose–insulin–potassium (GIK) infusion in patients with diabetes undergoing coronary artery bypass grafting, reduced the incidence of atrial fibrillation (16.6% versus 42%) and decreased length of hospital stay (6.5 days versus 9.2 days) compared to conventional treatment using intermittent subcutaneous insulin.[16] In addition, patients receiving GIK infusion had a survival advantage during the initial 2 years following surgery (Fig. 36–4), had decreased episodes of recurrent ischemia (5% versus 19%, P = 0.01), and developed fewer recurrent wound infections (1% versus 10%, P = 0.03).

The mechanism by which hyperglycemia worsens clinical outcomes has not been fully elucidated. Studies have shown that hyperglycemia induces phagocyte dysfunction, impairs cardiac ischemic preconditioning with resultant increased infarct size, increases blood pressure, increases natriuretic peptide levels, prolongs the QT interval, increases thromboxane biosynthesis (which causes platelet hyperactivity), increases several markers of inflammation (tumor necrosis factor α [TNF-α], interleukin-6 [IL-6], IL-18), and causes endothelial cell dysfunction.[17-33] Attempts to identify a unifying

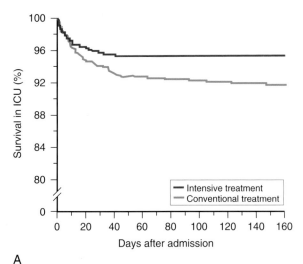

A

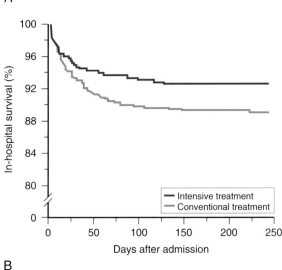

B

Figure 36–3. Kaplan-Meier survival curves for the Van den Berghe trial for patients who received intensive insulin versus conventional treatment in the intensive care unit (ICU). Patients discharged alive from the ICU **(A)** and from the hospital **(B)** were considered to have survived. In both cases, the differences between the treatment groups were significant: ICU survival nominal $P = 0.005$ and adjusted $P < 0.04$; in-hospital survival nominal $P = 0.01$. P values were determined with the use of the Mantel–Cox rank test. (Reprinted with permission from Van den Berghe G, Wouters P, Weelers F, et al: Intensive insulin therapy in critically ill patients. N Engl J Med 345:1359-1367, 2001.)

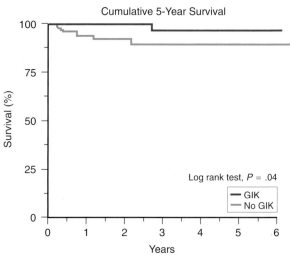

Figure 36–4. Long-term survival for the Lazar trial for patients receiving tight glycemic control with glucose-insulin-potassium (GIK) infusion versus standard therapy with intermittent subcutaneous insulin. Survival was prolonged in patients treated with GIK because of decreased mortality in GIK patients over the initial 2 years after surgery. (Reprinted with permission from Lazar HL, Chipkin SR, Fitzgerald CA, et al: Tight glycemic control in diabetic coronary artery bypass graft patients improves perioperative outcomes and decreases recurrent ischemic events. Circulation 109:1497-1502, 2004.)

basic mechanism for many of the diverse effects of acute hyperglycemia point to the ability of hyperglycemia to produce oxidative stress.[34] Acute experimental hyperglycemia—blood glucose 142 to 300 mg/dL (7.9 to 16.7 mmol/L)—induces generation of reactive oxygen species (ROS).

The data presented support the importance of preventing hyperglycemia; however, the threshold blood glucose, which is associated with increased morbidity and mortality, differs for each of the studies and patient populations, and thus glycemic goals are not well established for hospitalized patients. The focus on in-hospital glycemic control must also be mitigated by attention to the prevention of hypoglycemia. The American College of Endocrinology consensus conference on inpatient diabetes and metabolic control recommend the following glycemic targets: blood glucose no higher than 110 mg/dL (6.1 mmol/L) for critical-care patients, maximum preprandial blood glucose of 110 mg/dL (6.1 mmol/L), and maximum blood glucose levels of 180 mg/dL (10.0 mmol/L) for patients in non–critical-care units.[35] To achieve these glycemia goals without increasing hypoglycemic episodes, all medical professions caring for these patients must collaborate in the form of clinical pathways, treatment algorithms, and appropriate blood glucose monitoring of these patients.

HOW ARE TARGET BLOOD GLUCOSE LEVELS ACIEVED IN THE HOSPITAL?

Oral Agents

None of the oral agents used for diabetes mellitus has been studied for use in hospitalized patients. There are four categories of oral agents: insulin secretagogues (sulfonylureas and meglitinides), α-glucosidase inhibitors, biguanides, and the thiazolidinediones (TZDs). All have characteristics that

limit their use for hospitalized patients. In addition, they do not allow the necessary flexibility to treat hospitalized patients with acutely changing needs.

Secretagogues

The University Group Diabetes Program reported increased cardiovascular mortality among patients treated with the sulfonylurea tolbutamide.[36] A large prospective trial, the United Kingdom Prospective Diabetes Study (UKPDS), found no increase in cardiovascular events, but there was a trend toward fewer cardiovascular events among patients treated with sulfonylureas.[37]

Despite the UKPDS results, questions remain regarding the effect of sulfonylureas on vascular events. Sulfonylureas inhibit adenosine triphosphate–dependent potassium (K_{ATP}) channels in the pancreas, which ultimately leads to insulin release from the beta cells.[38] Similar K_{ATP} channels are found in the heart.[39] During acute myocardial ischemia these K_{ATP} channels open, reducing calcium influx and myocardial contractility, which might protect the heart by reducing oxygen demand.[40] Brief ischemic episodes render the heart more resistant to subsequent ischemia with resultant preservation of myocardial function, called *ischemic preconditioning*.[41] Glyburide blocks the opening of cardiac K_{ATP} in animal models and thus abolishes the protective effect of ischemic preconditioning.[42]

Despite a spectrum of data raising concern about potential adverse effects of sulfonylureas in the inpatient setting, where cardiac or cerebral ischemia is a common problem in an at-risk population, there are insufficient data to specifically recommend against their use in this setting.[34] However, their pharmacokinetic and pharmacodynamic properties limit their use in hospitalized patients. They have a long duration of action, which increases the risk of hypoglycemia in patients who are unable to consume their normal diet. In addition, the long duration of effect makes it difficult to rapidly meet the changing needs of hospitalized patients with sulfonylureas.

The meglitinides are structurally distinct from the sulfonylureas, but they have a similar mechanism of action involving inhibition of K_{ATP} channels on pancreatic beta cells. Both repaglinide and nateglinide have a more rapid onset and shorter duration of action than the sulfonylureas; however, they still do not provide the flexibility necessary for managing acutely ill hospitalized patients. Also, because they inhibit K_{ATP} channels, it is anticipated that they could also abolish the protective effects of ischemic preconditioning.

α-Glucosidase Inhibitors

α-Glucosidase inhibitors block the absorption of dietary carbohydrate and provide a modest decrease in postprandial blood glucose. These agents cause abdominal bloating and gas and thus, given the modest effect on blood glucose, are rarely used.

Biguanides

Metformin, a biguanide, is one of the most commonly used oral agents for T2DM. Metformin is structurally similar to phenformin, which was removed from the market in many countries in the 1970s because of an association with fatal lactic acidosis. Lactic acidosis is a rare complication of metformin use, with fewer than 0.1 cases per 1000 patient-years, despite the relative frequency of risk factors.[43] Predisposing risk factors for lactic acidosis with metformin are hypoperfusion states including congestive heart failure, renal or hepatic insufficiency, chronic pulmonary disease, and advanced age. These risk factors are much more common in hospitalized patients, and coupled with the propensity for acute decompensation in this setting, metformin use should be discouraged for acutely ill hospitalized patients.

Thiazolidinediones

TZDs are another commonly used oral agent for the treatment of T2DM. These agents have a delayed onset of action, on the order of 1 to 3 weeks, which makes them unsuitable for acute management of hyperglycemia in hospitalized patients. In addition, TZDs increase intravascular volume, and preliminary in vitro data suggest that they increase capillary permeability.[44] Both of these effects may have a greater significance in hospitalized patients.

Insulin

Insulin allows for the greatest flexibility and thus is the preferred treatment modality for hospitalized patients with acutely changing clinical situations. In addition, a growing body of literature suggests that it has direct benefits independent of its effect on blood glucose.[45-48] In order to use insulin safely and effectively in hospitalized patients, it is imperative that prescribers have a thorough understanding of its physiology and the pharmacodynamics of exogenously administered insulin.

Insulin Infusion

Continuous intravenous infusion of regular insulin provides the greatest flexibility for titration in hospitalized patients. The onset of action is mere minutes and duration of action is approximately 1 hour, which allows for rapid titration. Continuous insulin infusion is preferred over subcutaneously administered insulin in many clinical situations. These include DKA or a nonketotic hyperosmolar condition; general preoperative, intraoperative, and postoperative care; prolonged (longer than 8 hours) NPO (nothing by mouth) status; acute myocardial infarction; and critical illness in which insulin requirements are rapidly changing and the absorption of subcutaneous insulin may be unpredictable (Fig. 36–5).[34] In addition, intravenous infusions of insulin may be preferred for patients with acute

Blood Glucose (BG) Monitoring: ❏Before meals and at bedtime.   ❏ ____ Hrs after meals.   ❏ 2–3 AM

Goal Premeal BG = _____ (usually 80–150 mg/dL for most patients)

Additional BG Parameters (optional)

Goal Postprandial BG = _____   Goal Bedtime BG = _____

	Breakfast	**Lunch**	**Dinner**	**Bedtime**
Prandial Insulin Orders	Give ____ units of: ❏Lispro (Humalog) ❏Aspart (Novolog) ❏U-100 (Regular)	Give ____ units of: ❏Lispro (Humalog) ❏Aspart (Novolog) ❏U-100 (Regular)	Give ____ units of: ❏Lispro (Humalog) ❏Aspart (Novolog) ❏U-100 (Regular)	
Basal Insulin Orders	Give ____ units of: ❏NPH ❏Lente ❏Ultralente ❏Glargine *		Give ____ units of: ❏NPH ❏Lente ❏Ultralente ❏Glargine *	Give ____ units of: ❏NPH ❏Lente ❏Ultralente ❏Glargine *

* Insulin Glargine cannot be mixed with any other insulin.

Suggested lag times for prandial insulin:

Aspart/Lispro: 0–15 minutes before eating
Regular: 30 minutes before eating

Premeal algorithm for Hyperglycemia: To be administered *in addition* to the scheduled insulin dose to correct premeal hyperglycemia.

❏Lispro (Humalog)
❏Aspart (Novolog)
(Must specify algorithm below)

For blood glucose less than 60 mg/dL, use Hypoglycemia Protocol:

A. If patient can take PO, give 15 g of fast-acting carbohydrate (4 oz fruit juice/nondiet soda, 8 oz nonfat milk, or 3 or 4 glucose tablets)
B. If patient cannot take PO, give 25 ml of D_{50} as IV push
C. Check fingerstick glucose every 15 minutes and repeat A or B if blood glucose is less than 80 mg/dL

❏**LOW-DOSE ALGORITHM**
(For pts requiring less than 40 units of insulin/day)

Premeal BG	Additional Insulin
150–199	1 unit
200–249	2 units
250–299	3 units
300–349	4 units
>349	5 units

❏**MEDIUM-DOSE ALGORITHM**
(For pts requiring 40 to 80 units of insulin/day)

Premeal BG	Additional Insulin
150–199	1 unit
200–249	3 units
250–299	5 units
300–349	7 units
>349	8 units

❏**HIGH-DOSE ALGORITHM**
(For pts requiring more than 80 units of insulin/day)

Premeal BG	Additional Insulin
150–199	2 unit
200–249	4 units
250–299	7 units
300–349	10 units

❏**INDIVIDUALIZED ALGORITHM**

Premeal BG	Additional Insulin
150–199	
200–249	
250–299	
300–349	

General Insulin Dosing Recommendations
Patients with Type 1 Diabetes
These patients must have insulin to prevent ketosis. Even if the patient is not eating, he or she will need at least basal insulin (NPH [neutral protamine Hagedorn], Lente, Ultralente, glargine) to prevent ketosis.
• When admitting a patient with type 1 diabetes, continue the basal insulin that the patient was taking at home at the same dose. If the patient will be taking nothing by mouth, use an insulin drip rather than subcutaneous insulin. The prandial insulin (regular, lispro, aspart) might require adjustment, depending on the patient's situation. *If the patient is eating much less, reduce the prandial insulin.* Many hospitalized patients are under significant metabolic stress (infection, glucocorticoids) and could require larger doses of prandial insulin despite eating less.
• The usual daily insulin requirement for patients with type 1 diabetes is 0.5 to 0.7 U/kg per day. However, patients with newly diagnosed diabetes typically produce some insulin, and thus the daily insulin requirement is 0.3 to 0.5 U/kg per day. Half (50%) should be given as basal insulin and the remainder should be given as prandial insulin.
Patients with Type 2 Diabetes
• If the patient is using insulin at home, continue the outpatient regimen and adjust as needed.
• If the patient was not previously using insulin but will need both prandial and basal insulin, start with a daily insulin requirement of 0.3 U/kg per day. Daily insulin requirements in type 2 diabetes can exceed 1 U/kg per day in some patients

Figure 36–5. Insulin dosing for hospitalized diabetic patients. pts, patients. (Adapted with permission from Trence DL, Kelly JL, Hirsch IB: The rationale and management of hyperglycemia for in-patients with cardiovascular disease: Time for change. J Clin Endocrinol Metab 88:2430-2437, 2003.)

stroke, for patients with hyperglycemia exacerbated by high-dose glucocorticoids, and as a dose-finding strategy for subsequent conversion to subcutaneous insulin.

At our institution, we have developed an insulin-infusion protocol for use throughout the hospital with extensive staff education, which has resulted in significantly better blood glucose control without increasing the incidence or severity of hypoglycemic episodes.[49] Many hospitals restrict use of intravenous insulin infusions to critical care units, because they perceive it as dangerous and requiring close patient monitoring. Although it is true that close monitoring is required for the safe use of insulin infusions, we found that our protocol could be safely initiated in non–critical care units where each nurse typically is in charge of four or five patients. The majority of patients receiving insulin infusions stabilize within the first few hours of therapy, and thus we are able to safely reduce the frequency of blood glucose checks.

Each institution needs to address where and when an intravenous insulin infusion can be administered based on their staffing and experience. Although nursing acuity is high when initiating insulin infusion therapy, it can be viewed as an initial investment in improving blood glucose control and subsequent outcomes.

A variety of insulin-infusion protocols have been published, and there are many more in clinical use that have not been published. Results of studies comparing different intravenous insulin-infusion protocols are not available, and it is likely that different institutions will require different protocols based on their patient populations and staffing. Historically, insulin-infusion protocols have been based solely on the patient's blood glucose, and the infusion was changed by a fixed increment for all patients.[50] An ideal insulin-infusion protocol is based not only on the current blood glucose but also on the rate of change in blood glucose and the patient's insulin sensitivity.

Multiple studies suggest cardiac and neurologic benefits of GIK infusions. The theory promoting this form of therapy is based on the imbalance between low glycolytic substrate in hypoperfused tissue and elevated free fatty acids (FFAs) mobilized through catecholamine-induced lipolysis. The populations included in these studies have often been patients without diabetes or patients with only mild to moderate hyperglycemia. In clinical practice it is difficult to achieve the desired blood glucose control in patients with diabetes using GIK infusions. Adequate nutrition support in the form of glucose is crucial, but it should be administered in a manner that allows for titration of the glucose and insulin separately.

Insulin Requirements

In the ambulatory setting, the daily insulin requirements can be divided into three categories: basal, prandial, and correction. Hospitalized patients

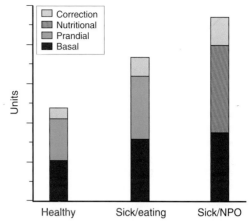

Figure 36–6. Insulin requirements in health and illness. Components of the insulin requirement are divided into basal, prandial or nutritional, and correction insulin. When writing insulin orders, the basal and prandial or nutritional insulin doses are written as programmed (scheduled) insulin, and correction-dose insulin is written as an algorithm to supplement the scheduled insulin. All components of the daily insulin requirement are increased in illness. (Reprinted from Clement S, Braithwaite SS, Magee MF, et al: Management of diabetes and hyperglycemia in hospitals. Diabetes Care 27:553-591, 2004. Copyright © 2004 American Diabetes Association. Reprinted with permission from the American Diabetes Association.)

often do not eat discrete meals, and thus a better categorization is basal, "nutritional insulin," and correction insulin requirements.[34] The *basal insulin requirement* is the amount of exogenous insulin necessary to maintain euglycemia in the absence of nutrition. The *nutritional insulin requirement* is the amount of insulin necessary to cover intravenous dextrose, total parenteral nutrition (TPN), enteral feedings, or discrete meals. The *correction insulin requirement* is the additional insulin required as a result of insulin resistance secondary to counter-regulatory hormone response to stress or the use of corticosteroids, vasopressor agents, or other medications. This classification of the various components of the daily insulin requirement is shown pictorially in Figure 36–6.

Another key component to providing effective insulin therapy is determining whether a patient produces endogenous insulin. Patients with T1DM produce minimal or no endogenous insulin and thus require basal insulin replacement, even if the patient is not eating, in order to prevent iatrogenic DKA. Patients with pancreatic dysfunction, such as pancreatitis, cystic fibrosis, or pancreatic cancer, are also likely to be severely insulin deficient. In contrast, insulin resistance characterizes patients with T2DM and steroid-induced diabetes, with a relative and progressive insulin deficiency. These patients are unlikely to develop ketoacidosis if insulin is withheld.

For most ambulatory patients, the daily insulin requirement is equally divided between basal and prandial insulin. In contrast, for hospitalized patients the nutritional component of the daily insulin requirement may be substantially greater than the basal component. Parenterally administered glucose often requires more insulin than the same amount of glucose given enterally.[51] The mechanisms underlying this observation are not clear, but there are likely gut-related, glucose-lowering peptides as well as gut signaling that are important in pancreatic function for first-phase and total nutrient-related insulin secretion. In addition, glucocorticoids are often administered to hospitalized patients and are well known to affect carbohydrate metabolism. They inhibit glucose uptake into muscle, and to a lesser extent they increase hepatic glucose production[50] and thus have the greatest effect on the nutritional component of the daily insulin requirement.

Determining the daily insulin requirement for hospitalized patients is empirical, because it is difficult to predict the overall effect of several acutely changing factors. The home insulin regimen should be continued for patients who were taking insulin prior to admission and who are able to eat. Only the basal insulin should be continued in patients who will not be eating and in whom enteral or parenteral nutrition has not been started. Supplemental or correction insulin can be given if stress hyperglycemia occurs. Although formal studies have not been done, the rapid-acting insulin analogs—lispro, aspart, and glulisine—are preferred for correction insulin because of their rapid onset and short duration of action.

At our institution we have developed standardized correction algorithms using lispro or aspart and the 1800 rule. The 1800 rule states that 1800 divided by the total daily insulin dose indicates the amount by which a single unit of lispro or aspart will reduce the blood glucose. There are several differences between this approach and the traditional insulin sliding scale. First, basal insulin is given. Second, prandial insulin is given prior to meals even if the premeal blood glucose is within the desired range. Third, the correction insulin dose is based on the patient's insulin sensitivity as determined by the total daily insulin dose and the 1800 rule. Supplemental premeal insulin can also be given to patients treated with oral agents if they experience stress hyperglycemia. However, if diabetes control was poor prior to admission, or if the patient's current condition constitutes a contraindication to continuing oral agents, consideration should be given to changing the diabetes regimen or initiating scheduled insulin therapy.

The daily insulin requirement for patients not previously receiving insulin can be calculated based on body weight and the type of diabetes.[52] Alternatively, if the patient has been receiving an insulin infusion, the total insulin administered over the preceding 24 hours can be used as an estimate. This method must be tempered by the understanding that correction insulin is included in the daily insulin dose in insulin infusion, and parenterally administered glucose requires more insulin than the same amount of glucose given enterally. Thus the daily insulin requirement should be reduced by 20% to 40%. Formal studies addressing this important point would be welcomed. The daily insulin requirement for the majority of patients with T1DM ranges from 0.4 to 0.8 U/kg per day. In contrast, the insulin requirement for patients with T2DM ranges from 0.3 U/kg per day to more than 1 U/kg per day.

Basal Insulin

There are several options for providing basal insulin. The intermediate-acting insulins, NPH and Lente, have traditionally been used. Both NPH and Lente have a pronounced peak. The peak can lead to hypoglycemia if a snack is not consumed or a meal is delayed, and it can lead to insufficient duration of effect, requiring multiple daily injections. Using smaller, more frequent doses of NPH administered every 6 to 8 hours provides more consistent levels, with less of a peak effect.[53]

Ultralente is another option; however, although it has less of a peak effect and a longer duration, it is still not the ideal option due to its marked variability in absorption. Although Ultralente duration of effect is 18 to 24 hours, it is most often used twice daily to provide more consistent insulin levels and to minimize the peak effect.

Insulin glargine, the first long-acting insulin analog, was approved in April 2000. Insulin glargine differs from native insulin in that the 21–amino acid residue on the α-chain has been substituted with a glycine residue, and two arginine residues have been added to the β-chain. When insulin glargine is injected into subcutaneous tissue, these structural alterations shift the isoelectric point, making insulin glargine less soluble at physiologic pH and thus prolonging systemic absorption to approximately 24 hours without a notable peak in most patients.

Prandial Insulin

The options for prandial insulin include regular insulin and the rapid-acting insulin analogs (lispro, aspart, and glulisine). The rapid-acting insulin analogs have a rapid onset of 5 to 20 minutes, attain peak blood levels in about 1 hour, and have a duration of action of 4 to 6 hours. This matches well with the absorption of glucose from low-fat hospital meals. In addition, the rapid onset makes it possible to give the insulin when the food arrives on the hospital unit.

The onset of action for regular insulin is 30 to 60 minutes, it has a peak effect in 2 to 4 hours, and it has a 6 to 8 hour duration of action. The slow onset makes it necessary to inject regular insulin 30 to 60 minutes before the meal is eaten. This is often difficult to do in the hospital setting, when meal delivery times might not be consistent. In practice, most

nurses have learned not to give insulin until the meal arrives on the unit, and thus, if regular insulin is used, there will be a rapid rise in blood glucose because the carbohydrate from the meal is absorbed before regular insulin starts to work. Regular insulin better matches the absorption of carbohydrate from high-fat and high-protein meals, but typically these are not provided in the hospital setting.

Regular insulin may be the preferred prandial insulin in patients with gastroparesis. Patients with gastroparesis have markedly delayed absorption of food, and thus the rapid-acting insulin analogs can cause hypoglycemia before the food is absorbed. We have observed that oncology patients receiving chemotherapy tend to take long periods of time to consume their food, and thus they also tend to do better with regular insulin.

Transition from Infusion to Subcutaneous Insulin

When transitioning a patient from an intravenous infusion of insulin to intermittent subcutaneous insulin administration, subcutaneous insulin should be administered prior to discontinuing the infusion. This allows for the subcutaneous insulin to be absorbed before the intravenous insulin wears off.

If the patient will be eating, the infusion is usually discontinued at the next scheduled meal and after appropriate insulin has been administered subcutaneously. For example, in a patient who uses glargine at bedtime, but in whom the insulin infusion will be stopped at lunch or dinner, an alternative basal insulin will need to be provided until the usual time for glargine administration. If the infusion is to be stopped at lunchtime, a small dose of NPH can be given with the prandial insulin for lunch to provide temporary basal insulin. Alternatively, if the infusion is to be discontinued at dinner, regular insulin has sufficient duration of action to provide basal coverage until the scheduled glargine is given at bedtime.

NUTRITION THERAPY

The caloric needs of most hospitalized patients can be met through provision of 25 to 35 kcal/kg of body weight.[54,55] Protein requirements are increased with physiologic stress. Mildly stressed patients with normal renal and hepatic function require 1.0 g/kg of body weight, and more severely stressed patients can require up to 1.5 g/kg of body weight.

The preferred route for feeding is the oral route. The American Diabetes Association (ADA) does not endorse any single meal plan or percentage of macronutrients and recommends that nutrition therapy should be individualized based on treatment goals, physiologic parameters, and medication use.

The consistent carbohydrate meal planning system provides institutions with a way of provid-ing food service for all patients, not just patients with diabetes. The system is not based on specific calorie levels. The amount of carbohydrate is consistent from meal to meal and day to day. Meals are based on heart-healthy principles, with limited saturated fats and cholesterol and with protein accounting for 15% to 20% of the calories. The majority of the carbohydrate foods should be whole grains, fruits, vegetables, and low-fat milk, but some sucrose-containing foods can be included.

There is no single meal-planning system that meets the needs of all institutions. Budget issues, staff time, local factors, and administrative support affect the choice of meal-planning system. However, given the complexity of nutrition issues, it is recommended that a registered dietitian knowledgeable and skilled in medical nutrition therapy serve as a member of the health care team.

Perhaps more important than the meal plan order is determining what the patient actually consumes. Adjusting insulin or other therapies without confirming what the patient ate is a recipe for disaster. Patients might not eat the food provided by the meal plan and visitors might bring them additional food. It is imperative that these factors be evaluated before making any change in diabetes therapy.

One option we have found useful is withholding the prandial insulin and then having the patient and nursing staff estimate the amount of food eaten and give that fraction of insulin immediately after the food is consumed. If all of the food is eaten, the entire dose is administered; if half is eaten, half the dose is injected, and so forth. With aspart and lispro, this actually works quite well, but it would not be expected to work as smoothly when regular insulin is used as the prandial insulin. Although this system is somewhat cumbersome, we have found it to work best when the correction-dose insulin is provided before the meal, because this prevents the extreme postprandial hyperglycemia that would otherwise occur.

SPECIAL SITUATIONS

Total Parenteral Nutrition

TPN has an extremely high dextrose content and is likely to cause hyperglycemia in patients with diabetes and even in patients without diabetes. In one study of patients with T2DM who were not previously treated with insulin, 77% required insulin while receiving TPN.[56]

There are several strategies for controlling blood glucose in patients receiving TPN. One strategy is to add 10 to 20 units of insulin to the bag of TPN, and increase this amount daily until blood glucose is within the desired range. Another strategy is to use a separate insulin infusion, which allows for more rapid titration and brings most patients within target blood glucose range within 24 hours.[57] Once

the patient's insulin requirement has been established and the patient is stable, the insulin can be added to the TPN and the separate infusion can be discontinued. In one study, this approach resulted in more rapid control of hyperglycemia and fewer wasted bags of TPN.[58]

Glucocorticoid Therapy

Glucocorticoids are well known to alter carbohydrate metabolism. They increase hepatic glucose production, inhibit glucose uptake by muscle, and have a complex effect on beta cell function.[59-61] The inhibition of glucose uptake by muscle appears to be the major defect. This explains the observation that in steroid-induced diabetes, the fasting blood glucose level is often relatively low; however, insulin resistance can lead to marked postprandial hyperglycemia, which worsens over the course of the day. Although glucocorticoid-induced hyperglycemia is common, there are few data to guide the management of this condition.

TZDs may be effective for long-term treatment of mild hyperglycemia resulting from this therapy. They are unlikely to control hyperglycemia if the preprandial blood glucose is greater than 180 mg/dL, and their onset of effect precludes their use for acute management of hospitalized patients.

Insulin is the preferred treatment modality for acute or moderate-to-severe hyperglycemia associated with glucocorticoid use. Given the effect of glucocorticoids on postprandial blood glucose, an emphasis on prandial insulin would be expected to have the best results. There are no trials comparing the use of short-acting analogs to regular insulin for this situation; however, some practitioners prefer regular insulin because of its prolonged action.

When glucocorticoid therapy is initiated in patients with known diabetes, blood glucose should be monitored closely. For patients without a history of diabetes, the fasting blood glucose may give the false impression that there is no hyperglycemia. In this population it is very important to evaluate blood glucose control at various times throughout the day.

Enteral Feeding

Enteral nutrition formulas are generally high in carbohydrate and low in fat and dietary fiber. Carbohydrates contribute 45% to 92% of the calories in enteral feedings.[62] In contrast, the carbohydrate content of typical hospital meals is about 50%,[34] and thus it is not surprising that the insulin requirement is greater when receiving enteral nutrition rather than eating. There are no clinical trials comparing the different strategies of insulin replacement with enteral nutrition, nor is there an optimal enteral nutritional formula for patients with diabetes. For intermittent enteral feedings such as nocturnal tube feeding, NPH insulin with a small dose of regular insulin usually works well. Continuous enteral feedings can be managed several different ways.

One option is to use a small dose of insulin glargine with short-acting correction insulin as needed, while the necessary glargine dose is being determined. The drawback of this strategy is the long duration of insulin glargine. Once the glargine is given it lasts up to 24 hours in most patients, and, if there is any interruption in tube feeding, the patient will be at prolonged risk of hypoglycemia. Alternatively, small doses of NPH and regular insulin can be injected every 6 to 8 hours, to provide consistent insulin levels. The drawback of this strategy is the need for more frequent insulin injections. Another option is to use a continuous insulin infusion to rapidly determine the insulin requirement. Once the insulin requirement has been determined, either glargine or NPH and regular insulin can be used without the need for titration.

FINAL COMMENTS

Insulin misadministration accounts for up to 11% of medication errors in the hospital setting,[63] and thus insulin has been identified as one of several high-alert medications.[64] How can we improve blood glucose control of our hospitalized patients and minimize insulin-related medication errors?

Outcomes using standardized insulin treatment pathways and dose-titration protocols are superior to those achieved with individualization of care.[65,66] A multidisciplinary team approach is needed to establish safe and effective diabetes care pathways for hospitalized patients. The key to success is having a "champion" of each discipline available for questions about all aspects of diabetes care. Furthermore, when system-wide changes are being implemented, it is important to make the changes slowly, perhaps no faster than one unit or floor at a time.

It is also imperative that the patient be part of this team. If a patient has been making sound decisions regarding diabetes self-management prior to admission, he or she should be encouraged to continue these skills in the hospital setting. If the patient's self-management skills are found to be lacking, the hospitalization can be an opportunity to improve them. Clearly, when a patient is acutely ill it is not the ideal time to provide extensive diabetes education; however, at least basic survival skills should be taught, with referral for more extensive education upon discharge.

Implementation of standardized order sets for scheduled and correction-dose insulin can reduce reliance on sliding-scale regimens and improve the transition from insulin infusion therapy to subcu-

taneous insulin administration. Extensive and continual staff education is necessary to ensure the safe and appropriate diabetes management for all hospitalized patients.

CONTROVERSIES

The threshold blood glucose, which is associated with increased morbidity and mortality, differs between studies and patient populations. Glycemic goals are thus not well established for hospitalized patients.

Safety of intravenous insulin infusions might be compromised in patients not receiving one-on-one nursing care in a critical care unit.

PITFALLS/COMPLICATIONS

Hypoglycemia is the primary complication of improved glycemic control. Appropriate patient monitoring, staff education, and standardized treatment pathways are important in order to minimize the incidence and impact of hypoglycemia.

References

1. Roman SH, Harris MI: Management of diabetes mellitus from a public health perspective. Endocrinol Metab Clin North Am 26:443-474, 1997.
2. National Institutes of Health: http://diabetes.niddk.nih.dm/pubs/statistics/index.htm#14
3. American Diabetes Association: Economic costs of diabetes in the U.S. in 2002. Diabetes Care 26:917-932, 2003.
4. Queale WS, Seidler AJ, Brancati FL: Glycemic control and sliding scale use in medical inpatients with diabetes mellitus. Arch Intern Med 57:545-552, 1997.
5. McDonough KA, DeWitt DE: Inpatient management of diabetes. Primary Care 30:557-567, 2003.
6. Capes S, Hunt D, Malmberg K, et al: Stress hyperglycemia and increased risk of death after myocardial infarction in patients with and without diabetes: A systematic overview. Lancet 355:773-778, 2000.
7. Bolk J, van der Ploeg T, Cornel JH, et al: Impaired glucose metabolism predicts mortality after a myocardial infarction. Int J Cardiol 79:201-214, 2001.
8. Umpierrez GE, Isaacs SD, Bazargan N, et al: Hyperglycemia: An independent marker of in hospital mortality in patients with undiagnosed diabetes. J Clin Endocrinol Metab 87:978-982, 2002.
9. Furnary A, Zerr K, Grunkemeier G, et al: Continuous intravenous insulin infusion reduces the incidence of deep sternal wound infection in diabetic patients after cardiac surgical procedures. Ann Thorac Surg 67:352-362, 1999.
10. Furnary AP, Gao G, Grunkemeier GL, et al: Continuous insulin infusion reduces mortality in patients with diabetes undergoing coronary artery bypass grafting. J Thorac Cardiovasc Surg 125:1007-1021, 2003.
11. Capes S, Hunt D, Malmberg K, et al: Stress hyperglycemia and prognosis of stroke in nondiabetic and diabetic patients: A systematic overview. Stroke 32:2426-2432, 2001.
12. Malmberg K, Ryden L, Efendic S, et al: Randomized trial of insulin–glucose infusion followed by subcutaneous insulin treatment in diabetic patients with acute myocardial infarction (DIGAMI study): Effects on mortality at 1 year. J Am Coll Cardiol 26:57-65, 1995.
13. Malmberg K, for the DIGAMI Study Group: Prospective randomized study of intensive insulin treatment on long-term survival after acute myocardial infarction in patients with diabetes mellitus. BMJ 314:1512-1515, 1997.
14. Van den Berghe G, Wouters P, Weekers F, et al: Intensive insulin therapy in critically ill patients. N Engl J Med 345:1359-1367, 2001.
15. Van den Berghe G, Wouters PJ, Bouillon R, et al: Outcome benefit of intensive insulin therapy in the critically ill: Insulin dose versus glycemic control. Crit Care Med 31:359-366, 2003.
16. Lazar HL, Chipkin SR, Fitzgerald CA, et al: Tight glycemic control in diabetic coronary artery bypass graft patients improves perioperative outcomes and decreases recurrent ischemic events. Circulation 109:1497-1502, 2004.
17. Kersten J, Schmeling, T, Orth K, et al: Acute hyperglycemia abolishes ischemic preconditioning in vivo. Am J Physiol 275:H721-H725, 1998.
18. Marfella R, Nappo F, Angelis LD, et al: The effect of acute hyperglycaemia on QTc duration in healthy men. Diabetologia 43:571-575, 2000.
19. Cinar Y, Senyol A, Duman K: Blood viscosity and blood pressure: Role of temperature and hyperglycemia. American J Hypertens 14:433-438, 2001.
20. McKenna K, Smith D, Tormey W, et al: Acute hyperglycaemia causes elevation in plasma atrial natriuretic peptide concentration in type 1 diabetes mellitus. Diabet Med 17:512-517, 2000.
21. Davi G, Catalano I, Averna M, et al: Thromboxane biosynthesis and platelet function in type II diabetes mellitus. N Engl J Med 322:1769-1774, 1990.
22. Knobler H, Savion N, Shenkman B, et al: Shear-induced platelet adhesion and aggregation on subendothelium are increased in diabetic patients. Thromb Res 90:181-190, 1998.
23. Davi G, Ciabattoni G, Consoli A, et al: In vivo formation of 8-iso-prostaglandin f2 alpha and platelet activation in diabetes mellitus: Effects of improved metabolic control and vitamin E supplementation. Circulation 99:224-229, 1999.
24. Sakamoto T, Ogawa H, Kawano H, et al: Rapid change of platelet aggregability in acute hyperglycemia. Detection by a novel laser-light scattering method. Thromb Haemost 83:475-479, 2000.
25. Gresele P, Guglielmini G, DeAngelis M, et al: Acute, short-term hyperglycemia enhances shear stress–induced platelet activation in patients with type II diabetes mellitus. J Am Coll Cardiol 41:1013-1020, 2003.
26. Morohoshi M, Fujisawa K, Uchimura I, et al: Glucose dependent interleukin 6 and tumor necrosis factor production by human peripheral blood monocytes in vitro. Diabetes 45:954-959, 1996.
27. Esposito K, Nappo F, Marfella R, et al: Inflammatory cytokine concentrations are acutely increased by hyperglycemia in humans: Role of oxidative stress. Circulation 106:2067-2072, 2002.
28. Williams S, Goldfine A, Timimi F, et al: Acute hyperglycemia attenuates endothelium dependent vasodilation in humans in vivo. Circulation 97:1695-1701, 1998.
29. Kawano H, Motoyama T, Hirashima O, et al: Hyperglycemia rapidly suppresses flow mediated endothelium-dependent vasodilation of brachial artery. J Am Coll Cardiol 34:146-154, 1999.
30. Shige H, Ishikawa T, Suzukawa M. et al: Endothelium-dependent flow mediated vasodilation in the postprandial state in type 2 diabetes mellitus. Am J Cardiol 84:1272-1274, 1999.
31. Title LM, Cummings PM, Giddens K, et al: Oral glucose loading acutely attenuates endothelium-dependent vasodilation in healthy adults without diabetes: An effect prevented by vitamins C and E. J Am Coll Cardiol 36:2185-2191, 2000.
32. Beckman J, Goldfine A, Gordon M, et al: Ascorbate restores endothelium-dependent vasodilation impaired by acute

hyperglycemia in humans. Circulation 103:1618-1623, 2001.

33. Giugliano D, Marfella R, Coppola L, et al: Vascular effects of acute hyperglycemia in humans are reversed by L-arginine: Evidence for reduced availability of nitric oxide during hyperglycemia. Circulation 95:1783-1790, 1997.

34. Clement S, Braithwaite SS, Magee MF, et al: Management of diabetes and hyperglycemia in hospitals. Diabetes Care 27:553-591, 2004.

35. American Association of Clinical Endocrinologists: Position statement: Inpatient diabetes and metabolic control. www.aace.com/pub/ICC/inpatientStatement.php

36. Meinert C, Knatterud G, Prout T, et al: University Group Diabetes Program: A study of the effects of hypoglycemic agents on vascular complications in patients with adult-onset diabetes II: Mortality results. Diabetes 19:789-830, 1970.

37. UKPDS Study Group: Intensive blood-glucose control with sulphonylureas or insulin compared with conventional treatment and risk of complication in patients with type 2 diabetes (UKPDS 33). Lancet 352:837-853, 1998.

38. Philipson LH, Steiner DR: Pas de deux or more: The sulfonylurea receptor and K^+ channels. Science 268:372-373, 1995.

39. Noma A: ATP-regulated K^+ channels in cardiac muscle. Nature 305:147-148, 1983.

40. Lee C: Gating mechanisms of ATP sensitive potassium channels: Implications in reperfusion injury and pre-conditioning. Cardiovasc Res 28:729-734, 1994.

41. Murray CE, Jennings RB, Reimer KA: Preconditioning with ischemia: A delay of lethal cell injury in ischemic myocardium. Circulation 74:1124-1136, 1986.

42. Toombs CF, Moore TL, Shebuski RJ: Limitation of infarct size in the rabbit by ischemic preconditioning is reversible with glibenclamide. Cardiovasc Res 27:617-622, 1993.

43. Salpeter S, Greyber E, Pasternak G, et al: Metformin does not increase fatal or nonfatal lactic acidosis or blood lactate levels in type 2 diabetes mellitus. Cochrane Database Syst Rev 2:CD002967, 2002.

44. Idris I, Gray S, Donnelly R: Rosiglitazone and pulmonary oedema: An acute dose-dependent effect on human endothelial cell permeability. Diabetologia 46:488-490, 2003.

45. Dandona P, Aljada A, Mohanty P: The anti-inflammatory and potential anti-atherogenic effect of insulin: A new paradigm. Diabetologia 45:924-930, 2002.

46. Dandona P, Aljada A, Bandyopadhyay A: The potential therapeutic role of insulin in acute myocardial infarction in patients admitted to intensive care and those with unspecified hyperglycemia. Diabetes Care 26:516-519, 2003.

47. Das UN: Is insulin an endogenous cardioprotector? Crit Care 6:389-393, 2002.

48. Melidonis A, Stefanidis A, Tournis S, et al: The role of strict metabolic control by insulin infusion on fibrinolytic profile during an acute coronary event in diabetic patients. Clin Cardiol 23:160-164, 2000.

49. Ku S, Sayre CA, Hirsch IB, et al: New insulin infusion protocol improves blood glucose control in hospitalized patients without increasing hypoglycemia. Jt Comm J Qual Saf 31:141-147, 2005.

50. Hirsch IB, Paauw DS, Brunzell J: Inpatient management of adults with diabetes. Diabetes Care 18:870-878, 1995.

51. Hoogwerf BJ: Postoperative management of the diabetic patient. Med Clin North Am 7:339-345, 2001.

52. DeWitt DE, Hirsch IB: Outpatient insulin therapy in type 1 and type 2 diabetes mellitus: Scientific review. JAMA 289:2254-2264, 2003.

53. Lalli C, Ciofetta M, Del Sindaco P, et al: Long-term intensive treatment of type 1 diabetes with the short-acting insulin analogue lispro in variable combination with NPH insulin at mealtime. Diabetes Care 22:468-477, 1999.

54. McMahon MM, Rizza RA: Nutrition support in hospitalized patients with diabetes mellitus. Mayo Clin Proc 71:587-594, 1996.

55. American Diabetes Association: Evidence-based nutritional principles and recommendations for the treatment and prevention of diabetes and related complications (Position Statement). Diabetes Care 26(Suppl 1):S51-S61, 2003.

56. Park RH, Hansell DT, Davidson LE, et al: Management of diabetic patients requiring nutritional support. Nutrition 8:316-320, 1992.

57. Woolfson AM: An improved method for blood glucose control during nutritional support. J Parenter Enteral Nutr 5:436-440, 1981.

58. Sajbel TA, Dutro MP, Radway PR: Use of separate insulin infusions with total parenteral nutrition. J Parenter Enteral Nutr 11:97-99, 1987.

59. Hollingdal M, Juhl CB, Dall R, et al: Glucocorticoid induced insulin resistance impairs basal but not glucose entrained high-frequency insulin pulsatility in humans. Diabetologia 45:49-55, 2002.

60. Boyle PJ: Cushing's disease, glucocorticoid excess, glucocorticoid deficiency, and diabetes. Diabetes Rev 1:301-308, 1993.

61. Lambillotte C, Gilon P, Henquin JC: Direct glucocorticoid inhibition of insulin secretion: An in vitro study of dexamethasone effects in mouse islets. J Clin Invest 99:414-423, 1997.

62. Coulston AM: Enteral nutrition in the patient with diabetes mellitus. Curr Opin Clin Nutr Metab Care 3:11-15, 2000.

63. Cohen MR, Proulx SM, Crawford SY: Survey of hospital systems and common serious medication errors. J Health Risk Manag 18:16-27, 1998.

64. Cohen MR: Medication Errors. Washington, D.C., Institute for Safe Medication Practices, American Pharmaceutical Association, 1999.

65. Rafoth RJ: Standardizing sliding scale insulin orders. Am J Med Qual 17:175-178, 2002.

66. Rozich JD, Howard RJ, Justeson JM, et al: Standardization as a mechanism to improve safety in health care. Jt Comm J Qual Saf 30:5-14, 2004.

Chapter 37

Diabetes Mellitus in Children and Adolescents

Stuart A. Weinzimer and William V. Tamborlane

KEY POINTS

- *Type 1 diabetes is caused by autoimmune-mediated destruction of pancreatic beta cells in genetically susceptible persons after a triggering event, usually a viral infection. The incidence of type 1 diabetes is increasing in the pediatric population, most notably in children younger than 5 years of age.*
- *Pediatric diabetes treatment teams that use a multidisciplinary approach to intensive therapy can be successful in achieving strict treatment goals in children and adolescents.*
- *Type 2 diabetes, which used to account for less than 5% of pediatric diabetes, may now account for up to 45% of new cases of diabetes in children. The differentiation of type 2 diabetes from type 1 diabetes in children at the time of diagnosis may be difficult, and optimal approaches to treatment are currently being investigated.*
- *In both type 1 and type 2 diabetes, hypertension, dyslipidemia, microalbuminuria, and associated comorbidities should be identified and treated effectively.*

Diabetes mellitus is a heterogeneous group of disorders characterized by impaired metabolism of glucose and other energy-yielding fuels, as well as the late development of vascular and neuropathic complications. Diabetes can be divided into at least three subclasses involving distinct pathogenic mechanisms: type 1 diabetes mellitus (T1DM, formerly called insulin-dependent diabetes); type 2 diabetes mellitus (T2DM, formerly called non–insulin-dependent diabetes); and secondary diabetes linked to another identifiable condition or syndrome.

It is important to recognize that not all children with diabetes have T1DM: The prevalence of T2DM is increasing dramatically, especially in obese adolescents of African American, Native American, and Hispanic origin. Regardless of the cause, the disease is associated with insulin deficiency, which in T1DM is usually total and in T2DM partial or

relative when viewed in the context of coexisting insulin resistance. Lack of insulin plays a primary role in the metabolic derangements linked to diabetes, and hyperglycemia, in turn, plays a key role in the complications of the disease.

T1DM in childhood and adolescence presents special challenges to pediatric health care providers. The combination of severe insulin deficiency and the physical and psychosocial changes that accompany normal growth and development make day-to-day management in pediatric patients especially difficult. Moreover, the results of the Diabetes Control and Complications Trial (DCCT) have raised the bar considerably higher with respect to goals of treatment, because intensive treatment has been shown to significantly reduce the risk of progression of retinopathy and the development of microalbuminuria.

Current recommendations mandate that youth with diabetes should aim to achieve glycemic control as close to normal as possible and as early in the course of the disease as possible, while still allowing normal childhood and adolescent psychosocial development. Remarkably, a much greater fraction of young patients are meeting strict standards of care than ever imagined possible only a few years ago, although such intensive care typically requires a specialized pediatric health care team consisting of physicians, nurse practitioners, dietitians, and mental health specialists.

This chapter focuses primarily on T1DM, but it discusses important issues related to pediatric T2DM in the last section.

EPIDEMIOLOGY

Diabetes is the second most common chronic disease in childhood, occurring in about 1 of every 1500 children by the age of 5 and 1 in 350 by age 18 in the United States.[1] There are two peaks in age of presentation, the first at ages 5 to 7 years and second in early puberty. One third of people with diabetes do not present until adulthood. Diabetes affects boys and girls equally.

T1DM is primarily a disease of white persons of Northern European, especially Scandinavian, background. The highest incidence rates of diabetes worldwide are found in Finland, Sweden, and Denmark, where about 30 new cases per 100,000 population are diagnosed annually. For comparison, the annual incidence rate of diabetes in the United States is about 12 to 15 per 100,000 population per year, in Africa is about 5 per 100,000 per year, and in East Asia is less than 2 per 100,000 per year.[2]

CLINICAL PRESENTATION IN CHILDHOOD

Presentation and Symptoms

Classically, children with T1DM present with a triad of polyuria, polydipsia, and polyphagia. However, there is great variation within the spectrum and severity of presentation, and a wide differential diagnosis can exist. Furthermore, the fact that the initial presentation of T1DM is often triggered by an intercurrent illness can also confound the diagnosis.

In children with T1DM, polyuria and compensatory polydipsia result once the renal threshold for glucose has been exceeded (at serum glucose concentrations of about 180 mg/dL), and glucosuria occurs. Hyperglycemia and the resultant hyperosmolar state induce an osmotic diuresis, leading to the polyuria, polydipsia, and enuresis. On presentation, these symptoms have often been present for several weeks.

Progressive insulin deficiency leads to weight loss, fatigue, and general malaise as protein and fat stores are lost. As counterregulatory hormones increase and ketosis worsens, symptoms of acute illness develop, including nausea, anorexia, abdominal pain, and vomiting. At this point the acute worsening of dehydration and acidosis can produce symptoms of lethargy, confusion, stupor, and even coma, and the respiratory compensation for the metabolic acidosis produces hyperpnea, the deep, sighing Kussmaul respirations.

Physical Examination and Laboratory Values

Physical examination findings are typically normal in most children with new-onset T1DM who are not acutely ill upon presentation. Evaluation of the thyroid for goiter and skin for hyperpigmentation allows for the diagnosis of potential comorbidities such as thyroiditis or Addison's disease. Girls should be evaluated for the presence of candidal vulvovaginitis, and both boys and girls should have documentation of height, weight, and sexual maturity rating.

Appropriate laboratory studies begin with the measurement of serum blood glucose. Random casual blood glucose levels are indicated in the setting of a child with symptoms suggestive of diabetes. In the symptomatic child, blood glucose should be checked promptly; children should *not* be instructed to have a fasting blood glucose level measured the next day. In the well-appearing child, minimal laboratory testing is required: electrolytes, blood urea nitrogen (BUN), and creatinine, along with a formal urinalysis for glucose and ketones, may suffice. In children with clinical evidence of more severe dehydration or other organ system signs, the evaluation should be expanded to include blood count with differential, venous or arterial blood gas, and in the setting of fever or shock, blood culture. Other studies depend on the clinical scenario and should be individualized.

Diagnosis and Differential Diagnosis

A careful history, physical examination, and laboratory investigation should allow the diagnosis of diabetes mellitus to be deduced in a rapid, efficient manner. Polyuria, polydipsia, and weight loss in a child should be considered T1DM until proven otherwise. The primary differential diagnosis for T1DM in children is urinary tract infection, due to the symptoms of excessive or frequent urination. Formal urinalysis can easily differentiate diabetes mellitus from diabetes insipidus, because the urine of the former contains glucose, ketones, and osmotically active electrolytes, whereas the urine of the latter is bland and dilute.

Gastroenteritis should be considered in the child with abdominal pain, vomiting, or dehydration, as should streptococcal pharyngitis and pneumonia. Pneumonia or asthmatic exacerbation may also be suggested in the setting of metabolic acidosis and abnormal breathing. In children presenting with fever, vomiting, and abdominal pain, appendicitis or other acute abdominal events may also be possibilities, a situation made more confusing because children in DKA often have leukocytosis.

Other conditions in the differential diagnosis of T1DM include toxic ingestion, pelvic inflammatory disease in a sexually active adolescent, and, in any age, sepsis. Patients with persistent hyperglycemia might also present with various forms of fungal infection. Infants and toddlers can have thrush or diaper candidiasis, and adolescents might present with genital yeast infections. Patients and parents are often unaware that these symptoms are in any way related to diabetes. Thus, a careful genitourinary exam is necessary on admission. In a prepubertal child, the presence of candidiasis should always trigger blood glucose testing by the primary care physician.

It should also be stressed that the diagnosis of diabetes requires measurement of blood glucose; the finding of glucosuria alone is not sufficient. Renal glucosuria, a benign condition in which the threshold for urinary excretion of glucose occurs even at normal blood glucose concentrations, occasionally masquerades as diabetes in the child in whom routine urinalysis is performed in the absence of true symptoms of diabetes.

TREATMENT OF NEW-ONSET TYPE 1 DIABETES IN CHILDHOOD

The goals of management of the child with new-onset T1DM are twofold: metabolic stabilization of the child and education of the family to care for the child after the stabilization has been completed. Treatment of the child with newly diagnosed T1DM depends upon the acuity of the illness at presentation: The ambulatory, well-appearing child without severe dehydration may be handled quite differently from the acutely ill, dehydrated patient who is vomiting.

It is still general practice to admit the child with newly diagnosed T1DM to the hospital, because the frequent monitoring and intense teaching that are required often cannot be accomplished in the ambulatory setting with an untrained family still recovering from the shock of the diagnosis. However, outpatient management of the otherwise well, new diabetic patient may be accomplished by pediatric diabetes treatment teams that have the available resources.[3] The development of diabetes in the sibling of a known patient may be managed in an ambulatory setting, if the child is not acutely ill and the family is well trained in diabetes management. Management of the acutely ill child in diabetic ketoacidosis is discussed separately.

Patients with newly diagnosed diabetes may use a traditional split-mixed regimen, in which combinations of short-acting (regular) and intermediate-acting (NPH or Lente) insulins are given together as two injections daily, with breakfast and dinner. The total dose is divided into two thirds NPH or Lente and one third regular. However, the traditional short-acting regular insulin has now been supplanted by new insulin analogs with a more rapid activity profile.

Lispro and aspart insulins are produced by the substitution of amino acids in the C-terminal region of the β-chain (the reversal of proline at position 28 and lysine at position 29 to Lys28-Pro29 for lispro, and a substitution of aspartic acid for Pro28 for aspart). This bioengineering renders the insulin molecules less likely to aggregate into hexamers in the subcutaneous tissue after injection and thus allows more rapid absorption into the blood stream. The advantages of lispro or aspart over regular insulin include more rapid onset and shorter duration of activity, so that insulin is available immediately to cover meal-related glucose excursions and is not persistent after the complete absorption of the meal.

Clinical trials of lispro and aspart have demonstrated improvements in postprandial hyperglycemia and lower rates of hypoglycemia compared to regular insulin.[4] Because of these improvements, lispro and aspart have essentially replaced regular insulin as the short-acting insulin of choice for most patients with diabetes, and most of our new-onset diabetic children are initiated on a two-shot regimen of lispro or aspart mixed with NPH or Lente, in a one third–to–two thirds ratio.

The NPH and Lente insulins can now also be replaced by another new long-acting insulin analog, insulin glargine. Glargine insulin is an analog of human insulin with C-terminal elongation of the β-chain by two arginine residues and replacement of asparagine in position A21 by glycine. This molecule is soluble in the acidic solution in which it is packaged but relatively insoluble in the physiologic pH of the extracellular fluid. Consequently, microprecipitates of glargine insulin are formed following subcutaneous injection, which markedly delays its absorption into the systemic circulation.

Pharmacokinetic and pharmacodynamic studies have demonstrated that this insulin analog has a very flat and prolonged time-action profile.[5] Results of preliminary studies of the efficacy and safety of glargine in children and adolescents with diabetes showed modestly lower fasting blood glucose levels and reduced risk of nocturnal hypoglycemia with glargine compared to human NPH insulin, although no differences in hemoglobin A1c (HbA1c) were noted.[6,7] Additional studies and more clinical experience need to be accumulated regarding use of this analog in youth with type 1 diabetes. Because glargine cannot be mixed with other insulins, it has to be given by separate injection, which might affect its acceptability by some youngsters. A list of available insulin preparations is shown in Table 37–1.

The rationale for using two rather than three or more injections at onset of diabetes is that with aggressive control of blood glucose levels, most children enter a "honeymoon" or partial remission period after a few weeks of therapy. This remission period is a result of increased insulin secretion by residual beta cells and improved insulin sensitivity with normalization of blood glucose levels.[8] To achieve these effects, most patients are started on a total daily dose of at least one unit per kilogram of body weight per day. Even more important, each component of the insulin regimen is adjusted on the basis of fingerstick blood glucose levels measured at least four times a day. The goal is to obtain premeal blood glucose values within the normal range and is achieved via daily telephone contact with the family for at least the first 3 weeks of treatment. The DCCT data indicate that strict control of diabetes also serves to prolong the period

Table 37–1. *Pharmacodynamic Properties of Common Insulin Formulations*

Category	Onset (h)	Peak (h)	Duration (h)
Rapid Acting			
Insulin Lispro	0.25-0.5	0.5-1	3-4
Insulin Aspart	0.25-0.5	0.5-1	3-5
Short Acting			
Regular	0.5-1	2-4	4-8
Intermediate Acting			
NPH	2-4	4-10	12-18
Lente	3-4	6-12	12-18
Long Acting			
Ultralente	4-6	6-12	18-24
Insulin glargine	2-4	n/a	24+
Premixed			
70/30 (70% NPH / 30% Regular)	0.5-1	2-8	12-18
50/50 (50% NPH / 50% Regular)	0.5-1	2-6	12-18
Mix 25 (75% NPH / 25% Lispro)	0.25-0.5	1-2	12-18
Novolog Mix (70% NPH / 30% Aspart)	0.25-0.5	1-2	12-18

n/a, not applicable.

of residual beta cell function in patients with T1DM.[9]

Infants and young toddlers might require modifications to the standard initial therapy due to greater insulin sensitivity, smaller carbohydrate content of meals, and unpredictability of eating. Total daily insulin doses may be reduced to 0.5 to 0.7 U/kg per day and titrated as necessary. For picky eaters, the rapid-acting insulin may be administered *after* the meal, to minimize hypoglycemia due to missed meals. Infants may require only NPH or Lente and not short-acting meal-related insulin. At present the safety and effectiveness of glargine in infants and toddlers has not been studied.

Prior to discharge, an assessment of the family's overall level of coping and functioning should be made. Special situations, such as blended families or alternate or additional caretakers in the home, should be worked out before hospital discharge. Families typically experience shock and grief at the child's diagnosis, but consideration should be made for referrals for psychosocial counseling if grief, anxiety, or depression appears to be excessive or interferes with diabetes education.

DIABETIC KETOACIDOSIS IN CHILDREN

Definitions

Diabetic ketoacidosis (DKA) is a life-threatening, preventable complication of diabetes mellitus characterized by inadequate insulin action, hyperglycemia, dehydration, electrolyte loss, metabolic acidosis, and ketosis. It is associated with a significant mortality rate and is the most common cause of death in children with T1DM. Children whose diabetes has not yet been diagnosed might present with DKA, so the diagnosis must be considered in any child with confusion or coma of undetermined etiology. Indeed, failure of parents and primary care physicians to recognize the early warning signs of diabetes, leading to more prolonged and severe dehydration and acidosis, often contributes to poor outcomes of treatment of DKA. In children whose diabetes has already been diagnosed, DKA can usually be prevented by patient and family education, frequent monitoring of blood glucose and urinary ketones during intercurrent illness, adequate oral hydration, and supplemental insulin (sick day rules).

Mechanisms

Diabetic ketoacidosis is defined as a blood glucose concentration greater than 200 mg/dL, ketonemia or ketonuria, and a pH less than 7.3. The primary abnormality is insulin deficiency, which leads to hyperglycemia both because of decreased glucose use and increased gluconeogenesis. As glucose levels exceed the renal threshold of 180 mg/dL, an osmotic diuresis occurs, resulting in the loss of extracellular water and electrolytes and worsening of the hyperglycemia. Insulin deficiency also leads to accelerated lipolysis with subsequent conversion of free fatty acids to β-hydroxybutyric and acetoacetic acids. This results in metabolic acidosis. Acetone is also formed and gives a fruity odor to the patient's breath, but it does not contribute to the acidosis.

Potassium, primarily an intracellular ion, is transported out of the cell into the plasma in exchange for hydrogen and is lost in the urine. Thus, virtually all patients with DKA develop a "total body" deficiency of potassium, regardless of their serum potassium level. Phosphate, another predominantly intracellular ion, is handled similarly. Deficiency of 2,3-diphosphoglycerate, a phosphate-containing glycolytic intermediate in red blood cells that facilitates release of oxygen from hemoglobin, may contribute to the development of lactic acidosis, complicating the ketoacidosis. Although insulin deficiency is the principal abnormality, elevations in the counterregulatory hormones (glucagon, cortisol, catecholamines, and growth hormone)

and reduction in circulating free insulinlike growth factor I (IGF-I) contribute to accelerated gluconeogenesis and lipolysis.[10]

Diagnosis

Diabetic ketoacidosis is not difficult to recognize in a child with known diabetes who is dehydrated, hyperventilating, and obtunded. In the child whose diabetes has not yet been diagnosed, however, it may be confused with gastroenteritis, pneumonia, sepsis, toxic ingestion, and central nervous system (CNS) processes. The diagnosis of diabetes (if not already established) is suggested by a history of polyuria, polydipsia, polyphagia, nocturia, or enuresis in a previously toilet-trained child. Weakness and unexplained weight loss may also be presenting features. When the diagnosis of DKA is suspected, an attempt should be made to identify precipitating causes (e.g., infection, stress, or noncompliance). In a child with known diabetes, it is important to briefly review the recent blood glucose history and to ascertain not only the usual insulin dosage but also the quantity and timing of the most recent injection.

Physical Examination
The physical examination should focus initially on the adequacy of the airway, breathing, a thorough assessment of the circulatory status (heart rate, blood pressure, description of mucous membranes, capillary refill, distal pulses, and warmth of extremities), degree of dehydration (including weight if possible), and mental status. A rough estimation of degree of dehydration should be made in order to calculate the fluid deficit and facilitate rehydration therapy, although recent studies have shown that such clinical approximations typically overestimate the actual degree of dehydration.[11] A careful examination and written documentation of the neurologic status is critical, to serve as a baseline in case of deterioration in neurologic status later in therapy.

The general physical examination should include respiratory and abdominal examinations, as well as a search for an intercurrent illness that might have served as the "trigger." Deep, rapid respirations (Kussmaul's breathing) and a fruity odor to the breath are classic signs but are not present in every patient. A careful search should be made for a source of infection that could have precipitated the episode of DKA. Bedside determination of the blood glucose with a glucose monitoring device and evaluation of the urine for glucose and ketones should be performed as quickly as possible, and treatment should be initiated without waiting for the results of the laboratory assessment to become available.

Laboratory Values
The laboratory evaluation of patients suspected to have DKA includes determination of the blood glucose, plasma or urinary ketones, serum electrolyte concentration, BUN, creatinine, osmolarity, and baseline calcium and phosphorus. A baseline blood gas measurement should also be made to determine the pH and partial pressure of carbon dioxide (PCO_2). Although venous blood gas measurements can suffice in milder episodes of DKA, an arterial blood gas measurement should be obtained in patients suspected to have incomplete respiratory compensation or those expected to require bicarbonate therapy (see later). If hypertriglyceridemia is present, the serum sodium concentration may be artifactually lowered. Similarly, the serum sodium will be reduced by approximately 1.6 mEq/L for each 100 mg/dL rise in glucose because of the re-equilibration of the intra- and extracellular compartments at a higher osmolarity.[12] In the presence of ketones (and lactate), a large anion gap acidosis will be present. The degree of elevation of the BUN and creatinine, as well as the hematocrit, could indicate the extent of dehydration and the possibility of renal damage. The initial serum potassium could be low, normal, or high, depending on the degree of acidosis and the quantitative urinary losses.

Management

The acute management of DKA is directed at correction of the dehydration, electrolyte deficits, hyperglycemia, and acidosis (Box 37-1).

Dehydration
Initial fluid therapy is aimed at rapid stabilization of the circulation to correct impending shock, but as in other forms of hypertonic dehydration, too-rapid fluid administration must be avoided. Fluid replacement in excess of 4 L/m² in 24 hours has been associated with the development of potentially fatal cerebral edema in DKA. For this reason, an initial fluid bolus is usually advised to expand the vascular compartment and improve peripheral circulation, but once the patient has been stabilized, subsequent rehydration is accomplished with caution.

Typically, one aims to correct the fluid deficit gradually, over 36 to 48 hours. Gradual correction is particularly important in children at an increased risk for developing cerebral edema. This includes children with altered mental status, history of symptoms longer than 48 hours, pH lower than 7.0, glucose higher than 1000 mg/dL, corrected sodium higher than 155 mEq/L, extreme hyperosmolarity (greater than 375 mOsm/L), or age younger than 3 years. A corrected sodium level that fails to rise with treatment may signify excessive free water accumulation and an increased risk of cerebral edema.

Electrolyte Imbalance
Rehydration fluids should contain at least NaCl 115 to 135 mEq/L to ensure a gradual decline in

Box 37-1. Guidelines for Management of Diabetic Ketoacidosis

Insulin

Continuous intravenous infusion of 0.1 U/kg per hour is typical. For very young or severely acidotic, hyperosmolar patients, 0.05 U/kg hour may be initiated to prevent rapid changes during metabolic stabilization. In hyperglycemic, hyperosmolar, nonketotic coma (which is rarely seen in children except in some adolescents with type 2 diabetes), insulin may be withheld during the first several hours.

Fluids

Infuse 10 to 20 mL/kg 0.9% saline bolus to restore intravascular volume. Repeat as needed to treat shock. Base subsequent fluid administration upon estimated degree of dehydration, and plan to replace deficit evenly over 48 hours.

Sodium

Na^+ deficit at presentation generally resolves with administration of isotonic fluids during resuscitation phase. Measured $[Na^+]$ typically underestimates true Na^+ levels due to effects of hyperglycemia. Calculation and assessment of true $[Na^+]$ over time may decrease risk of cerebral edema.

Potassium

K^+ deficit at presentation requires aggressive therapy. Replacement depends on serum $[K^+]$ at presentation; 20 to 40 mEq (half as KCl and half as KPO_4) added to each liter of rehydration fluid is typical.

Glucose

Glucose is added to rehydration fluids once the blood glucose level falls to less than 300 mg/dL. The goal is generally to reduce blood glucose 50 to 100 mg/dL per hour, although recent evidence suggests that rapid fall in blood glucose might not increase risk of cerebral edema

Bicarbonate

Bicarbonate is considered in extreme acidosis only. Bicarbonate use can increase risk of cerebral edema.

Clinical Monitoring

Assess vital signs, neurologic status, state of hydration, and fluid intake and output at least hourly.

Laboratory Monitoring

Measure blood glucose hourly, electrolytes and pH at least every 2 hours until the patient is stable. Follow blood urea nitrogen (BUN), creatinine, calcium, and phosphate if they are abnormal at presentation.

serum osmolarity and minimize the risk of cerebral edema.[13,14] Early potassium replacement is also important, to correct the potassium depletion that occurs because of the severe initial intracellular losses and the subsequent potassium shift from the extracellular to the intracellular compartment (which occurs when treatment with insulin is initi-

ated and the acidosis is corrected). Potassium is administered only after urine output is ensured to prevent hyperkalemia in the setting of unrecognized renal impairment. Potassium is usually given at a dose of 20 to 40 mEq/L, either as KCl or as combinations of KCl with KPO_4 (which has the additional advantage of replacing the phosphate deficit).

Electrocardiographic monitoring facilitates early recognition of either hyperkalemia (peaked T waves) or hypokalemia (flat or inverted T waves) and the development of potentially dangerous cardiac arrhythmias. Serum calcium should be monitored if phosphate is given, because phosphate administration can precipitate hypocalcemia.

Hyperglycemia

Insulin therapy should be initiated immediately after the patient has been stabilized with an initial fluid bolus, typically at a dose of 0.1 U/kg per hour. As with fluid replacement, the aim of therapy is gradual correction: reduction of the blood glucose by 50 to 100 mg/dL per hour. Usually, the glucose falls significantly with initial rehydration alone.

Dextrose is added to the intravenous solution when the serum glucose level falls below 300 mg/dL, and it is titrated to provide a continued gradual decline in blood glucose to target levels. This is easily accomplished with the simultaneous use of two intravenous solutions, which differ only in the dextrose concentration.

Usually the lowering of the blood glucose concentration precedes the decrease in ketones. Thus, in the situation of continued acidosis with serum glucose concentrations less than 300 mg/dL, it is important not to decrease the rate of insulin infusion, but rather to add dextrose to the rehydration fluids. Determination of urine ketones, though helpful diagnostically, is not an accurate guide to clinical improvement, as only acetoacetate is measured by the usual method and not β-hydroxybutyrate, which predominates early (but not later) in the course of untreated DKA. Newer home glucose meters that also measure serum β-hydroxybutyrate levels by fingerstick samples, however, may be useful in monitoring clinical improvement in DKA.[15]

Acidosis

Bicarbonate therapy for the acidosis of DKA remains controversial. Often, dramatic clinical improvement results simply from initial expansion of extracellular fluid volume, reestablishment of adequate peripheral perfusion, and insulin administration. An elevation in blood pH following bicarbonate administration may be attended by worsening acidosis in the CNS, because carbon dioxide (but not bicarbonate) diffuses across the blood–brain barrier. Furthermore, the organic acids in DKA, in contrast to metabolic acidosis from other causes, are metabolized to bicarbonate. Thus, administra-

promotes weight loss and improves lipid profiles as well, but it is contraindicated in patients with any renal impairment and should be discontinued before radiologic or surgical procedures.

Other oral hypoglycemic agents have had relatively little use in pediatric T2DM. The thiazolidinediones (TZDs) improve insulin resistance through effects on peripheral muscle and adipose tissue, but they have not been adequately studied in children to date. They may be associated with fluid retention and untoward cardiovascular effects. Sulfonylureas and other insulin secretagogues do not target insulin resistance, and they can actually worsen insulin resistance by promoting weight gain. Secretagogues are also associated with higher rates of hypoglycemia. Glucosidase inhibitors such as acarbose are associated with gastrointestinal side-effects that are usually unacceptable to youth. A large-scale, long-term clinical trial sponsored by the National Institutes of Health that will examine different treatment approaches in adolescents with T2DM began recruitment in 2004.

We recommend an intense lifestyle modification program with weight loss and exercise, in conjunction with metformin, as first-line therapy. Metformin may be initiated at 500 mg bid and increased over 1 to 2 weeks to 2000 mg daily as tolerated. TZDs may be added in older adolescents or young adults who have severe insulin resistance. If this regimen is insufficient to reduce the HbA1c to 6.5% or lower, we do not hesitate to add insulin, either as a bedtime injection of Lente or glargine or as a combination rapid–intermediate insulin, such as Humalog Mix 25 (Lilly) or Novolog Mix 70/30 (Novo Nordisk), with breakfast and dinner. An algorithmic approach to medical treatment of pediatric T2DM is illustrated in Figure 37–4.

Although there are no long-term data in children, extrapolation from adult studies such as the United Kingdom Prospective Diabetes Study[58] suggests that aggressive treatment of diabetes comorbidities may be as important as lowering HbA1c levels. Current recommendations from the Task Force on High Blood Pressure in Children and Adolescents[46] mandate that blood pressures above the 90th percentile for age, gender, and height warrant lifestyle interventions (weight loss, exercise, and dietary modification), and above the 95th percentile merit the addition of pharmacotherapy. ACE inhibitors, because of their renoprotective effects on preventing and ameliorating microalbuminuria, should be considered first-line therapy, followed by diuretics and angiotensin II receptor blockers (ARBs).

Complications

Dyslipidemia also commonly accompanies diabetes, and given that cardiovascular disease is the major cause of mortality and morbidity in adults with T2DM, it is advisable to closely monitor and

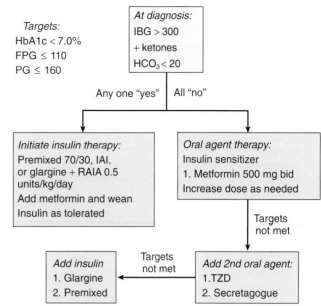

Figure 37–4. Treatment algorithm for children and adolescents with type 2 diabetes. Use of oral agents is as follows: TZDs: pioglitazone, 15-45 mg daily; rosiglitazone, 2-4 mg bid. Secretagogues: glimepiride, 1-4 mg/day; glipizide, 2.5-10 mg bid; nateglinide, 60-120 mg before meals; repaglinide, 0.5-2 mg before meals. *Note:* TZDs and newer secretagogues have not been approved for use in children. FPG, fasting plasma glucose; HbA1c, hemoglobin A1c; IAI, intermediate-acting glucose; IBG, initial blood glucose; PG, preprandial glucose; RAIA, rapid-acting insulin analog; TZD, thiazolinedione.

aggressively treat lipid disorders in pediatric T2DM. As is currently recommended by a consensus panel of the American Diabetes Association, children with T2DM should be screened for dyslipidemia at diagnosis and then every other year thereafter.[47] Optimal lipid levels have been defined as LDL lower than 100 mg/dL, HDL higher than 35 mg/dL, and triglycerides lower than 150 mg/dL. Nonpharmacologic treatments (diet modification and exercise) should be instituted for LDL levels higher than 100 mg/dL, although many children with T2DM require pharmaceutical intervention.

Drug therapy is indicated once LDL levels exceed 130 mg/dL or for triglyceride levels higher than 1000 mg/dL. In the presence of other cardiovascular risk factors (obesity, hypertension, family history of cardiovascular disease), the threshold LDL level for treatment is lowered to 100 mg/dL.[59] As is the case with many of the oral hypoglycemic agents and newer antihypertensive medications, lipid-lowering drugs have not been adequately studied in children. Bile acid binding resins should be considered as first-line therapy, followed by statins as second-line therapy and fibric acid derivatives for hypertriglyceridemia.

Children with T2DM should also meet regularly with dietitians and social workers or psychologists

to reinforce desired behavior and to identify individual or family factors that could complicate adherence.

References

1. Sperling MA: Diabetes mellitus. In Sperling MA (ed): Pediatric Endocrinology. Philadelphia, WB Saunders, 2002, pp 323-366.
2. Karvonen M, Vilik-Kajander M, Moltchanova E, et al: Incidence of childhood type 1 diabetes worldwide. Diabetes Care 23:1516-1526, 2000.
3. Chase HP, Crews KR, Garg S, et al: Outpatient management vs. in-hospital management of children with new-onset diabetes. Clin Pediatr 31:450-456, 1992.
4. Vajo Z, Fawcett J, Duckworth WC: Recombinant DNA technology in the treatment of diabetes: Insulin analogs. Endocr Rev 22:706-717, 2001.
5. Lepore M, Pampanelli S, Fanelli C, et al: Pharmacokinetics and pharmacodynamics of subcutaneous injection of long-acting human insulin analog glargine, NPH insulin, and Ultralente human insulin and continuous subcutaneous infusion of insulin lispro. Diabetes 49:2142-2148, 2000.
6. Schober E, Schoenle E, Van Dyk J, et al: Comparative trial between insulin glargine and NPH insulin in children and adolescents with type 1 diabetes mellitus. J Pediatr Endocrinol Metab 15:369-376, 2002.
7. Murphy NP, Keane SM, Ong KK: Randomized cross-over trial of insulin glargine plus lispro or NPH insulin plus regular human insulin in adolescents with type 1 diabetes on intensive insulin regimens. Diabetes Care 26:799-804, 2003.
8. Yki-Jarvinen H, Koivisto VA: Natural course of insulin resistance in type 1 diabetes. N Engl J Med 315:224-230, 1986.
9. The DCCT Research Group: The effect of intensive diabetes treatment in the DCCT on residual insulin secretion in IDDM. Ann Intern Med 128:517-523, 1998.
10. Attia N, Caprio S, Jones TW, et al: Changes in free insulin-like growth factor-1 and leptin concentrations during acute metabolic decompensation in insulin withdrawn patients with type 1 diabetes. J Clin Endocrinol Metab 84:2324-2328, 1999.
11. Koves IH, Neutze J, Donath S, et al: The accuracy of clinical assessment of dehydration during diabetic ketoacidosis in childhood. Diabetes Care 27:2485-2487, 2004.
12. Katz MA: Hyperglycemia-induced hyponatremia. N Engl J Med 289:843-844, 1973.
13. Harris GD, Fiordalisi I, Harris WL, et al: Minimizing the risk of brain herniation during treatment of diabetic ketoacidemia: A retrospective and prospective study. J Pediatr 117:22-31, 1990.
14. Harris GD, Fiordalisi I: Physiologic management of diabetic ketoacidemia: A 5-year prospective pediatric experience in 231 episodes. Arch Pediatr Adolesc Med 148:1046-1052, 1994.
15. Ham MR, Okada P, White PC: Bedside ketone determination in diabetic children with hyperglycemia and ketosis in the acute care setting. Pediatric Diabetes 5:39-43, 2004.
16. Glaser N, Barnett P, McCaslin I, et al: Risk factors for cerebral edema in children with diabetic ketoacidosis. N Engl J Med 344:264-269, 2001.
17. Duck, SC, Wyatt DT: Factors associated with brain herniation in the treatment of diabetic ketoacidosis. J Pediatr 113:10-14, 1988.
18. Bello FA, Sotos JF: Cerebral edema in diabetic ketoacidosis in children. Lancet 336:64, 1990.
19. Dunger DB, Sperling MA, Acerini CL, et al: ESPE/LWPES consensus statement on diabetic ketoacidosis in children and adolescents. Arch Dis Child 89:188-194, 2004.
20. Diabetes Control and Complications Trial Research Group: The effect of intensive treatment of diabetes on the development and progression of long-term complications in insulin-dependent diabetes mellitus. N Engl J Med 329: 977-986, 1993.
21. Diabetes Control and Complications Trial Research Group: Effect of intensive diabetes treatment on the development and progression of long-term complications in adolescents with insulin-dependent diabetes mellitus: Diabetes Control and Complications Trial. J Pediatr 125:177-188, 1994.
22. Diabetes Control and Complications Trial (DCCT)/ Epidemiology of Diabetes Interventions and Complications (EDIC) Research Group: Beneficial effects of intensive therapy of diabetes during adolescence: Outcomes after the conclusion of the Diabetes Control and Complications Trial (DCCT). J Pediatr 139:804-812, 2001.
23. Grey M, Boland EA, Davidson M, et al: Coping skills training for youth on intensive therapy has long lasting effects on metabolic control and quality of life. J Pediatr 137:107-114, 2000.
24. Ahern JH, Boland EA, Doane R, et al: Insulin pump therapy in pediatrics: A therapeutic alternative to safely lower HbA1c levels across all age groups. Pediatric Diabetes 3:10-15, 2002.
25. Doyle EA, Weinzimer SA, Steffen AT, et al: A randomized, prospective trial comparing the efficacy of continuous subcutaneous insulin infusion with multiple daily injections using insulin glargine. Diabetes Care 27:1554-1558, 2004.
26. Weinzimer SA, Doyle EA, Steffen AT, et al: Rediscovery of insulin pump treatment of childhood type 1 diabetes. Minerva Med 95:85-92, 2004.
27. Zinman B, Tildesley H, Chiasson JL, et al: Insulin lispro in CSII: Results of a double-blind crossover study. Diabetes 46:440-443, 1997.
28. Bode BW, Strange P: Efficacy, safety, and pump compatibility of insulin aspart used in continuous subcutaneous insulin infusion therapy in patients with type 1 diabetes. Diabetes Care 24:69-72, 2001.
29. Boland EA, Grey M, Fredrickson L, et al: CSII: A "new" way to achieve strict metabolic control, decrease severe hypoglycemia and enhance coping in adolescents with type I diabetes. Diabetes Care 22:1779-1784, 1999.
30. Weinzimer SA, Ahern JH, Boland EA, et al: Persistence of benefits of continuous subcutaneous insulin infusion in very young children with type 1 diabetes: A follow-up report. Pediatrics 114:1601-1605, 2004.
31. Attia N, Jones TW, Holcombe J, et al: Comparison of human regular and lispro insulins after interruption of continuous subcutaneous insulin infusion and in the treatment of acutely decompensated IDDM. Diabetes Care 21:817-821, 1998.
32. Celona-Jacobs N, Weinzimer SA, Rearson MA, et al: Insulin pump therapy in children: A cautionary tale. Diabetes 50(Suppl 2):A67, 2001.
33. Bina DM, Anderson RL, Johnson ML, et al: Clinical impact of prandial state, exercise, and site preparation on the equivalence of alternative-site blood glucose testing. Diabetes Care 26:981-985, 2003.
34. Boland EA, DeLucia M, Brandt C, et al: Limitations of conventional methods of self blood glucose monitoring: Lessons learned from three days of continuous glucose monitoring in pediatric patients with type I diabetes. Diabetes Care 24:1858-1862, 2001.
35. Chase HP, Kim LM, Owen SL, et al: Continuous subcutaneous monitoring in children with type 1 diabetes. Pediatrics 107:222-226, 2001.
36. Kaufman FR, Gibson LC, Halvorson M, et al: A pilot study of the continuous glucose monitoring system: Clinical decisions and glycemic control after its use in pediatric type 1 diabetic subjects. Diabetes Care 24:2030-2034, 2001.
37. Chase HP, Roberts MD, Wightman C, et al: Use of the GlucoWatch biographer in children with type 1 diabetes. Pediatrics 111:790-794, 2003.
38. Diabetes Research in Children Network (DirecNet) Study Group: The accuracy of the CGMS in children with type 1 diabetes: Results of the Diabetes Research in Children Network (DirecNet) accuracy study. Diabetes Technol Ther 5:781-789, 2003.
39. Diabetes Research in Children Network (DirecNet) Study Group: The accuracy of the GlucoWatch G2 biographer in children with type 1 diabetes: Results of the Diabetes Research in Children Network (DirecNet) accuracy study. Diabetes Technol Ther 5:791-800, 2003.

40. Diabetes Research in Children Network (DirecNet) Study Group: Accuracy of the GlucoWatch G2 Biographer and the Continuous Glucose Monitoring System during hypoglycemia: Experience of the Diabetes Research in Children Network. Diabetes Care 27:722-726, 2004.

41. American Diabetes Association Task Force for Writing Nutrition Principles and Recommendations for the Management of Diabetes and Related Complications: American Diabetes Association position statement: Evidence-based nutrition principles and recommendations for the treatment and prevention of diabetes and related complications. J Amer Diet Assoc 102:109-118, 2002.

42. Gregory RP, Davis DL: Use of carbohydrate counting for meal planning in type 1 diabetes. Diabetes Educator 20:406-409, 1994.

43. Jones TW, Porter P, Davis EA, et al: Suppressed epinephrine responses during sleep. A contributing factor to the risk of nocturnal hypoglycemia in insulin-dependent diabetes. N Engl J Med 338:1657-1662, 1999.

44. Kordonouri O, Klinghammer A, Lang EB, et al: Thyroid autoimmunity in children and adolescents with type 1 diabetes. Diabetes Care 25:1346-1350, 2002.

45. Freemark M, Levitsky LL: Screening for celiac disease in children with type 1 diabetes: Two views of the controversy. Diabetes Care 26:1932-1939, 2003.

46. National High Blood Pressure Education Program Working Group on High Blood Pressure Control in Children and Adolescents: The fourth report on the diagnosis, evaluation, and treatment of high blood pressure in children and adolescents. Pediatrics 114:555-576, 2004.

47. American Diabetes Association: Management of dyslipidemia in children and adolescents with diabetes. Diabetes Care 26:2194-2197, 2003.

48. Rosenbloom AL, Joe JR, Young RS, et al: The emerging epidemic of type 2 diabetes mellitus in youth. Diabetes Care 22:345-354, 1999.

49. Pinhas-Hamiel O, Dolan LM, Daniels SR, et al: Increased incidence of non–insulin-dependent diabetes mellitus among adolescents. J Pediatr 37:97-102, 1996.

50. Sinha R, Fisch G, Teague B, et al: Prevalence of impaired glucose tolerance among children and adolescents with marked obesity. N Engl J Med 346:802-810, 2002.

51. Travers SH, Jeffers BW, Bloch CA, et al: Gender and Tanner stage differences in body composition and insulin sensitivity in early pubertal children. J Clin Endocrinol Metab 80:172-178, 1995.

52. Guzzaloni G, Grugni G, Mazzilli G, et al: Comparison between beta-cell function and insulin resistance indexes in prepubertal and pubertal obese children. Metabolism 51:1011-1016, 2002.

53. American Diabetes Association: Consensus Statement. Type 2 diabetes in children and adolescents. Diabetes Care 23:381-389, 2000.

54. American Diabetes Association: Type 2 diabetes in children and adolescents. Pediatrics 105:671-680, 2000.

55. Libman I, Pietropaolo M, Arslanian S, et al: Changing phenotype: Are more youngsters with IDDM obese at onset? Diabetologia 44:A257, 2001.

56. Katz LEL, Jawad AF, Ganesh J, et al: Parameters distinguishing childhood type 1 (TIDM) and type 2 diabetes (T2DM) at diagnosis. Diabetes 50(Suppl 2):A55, 2001.

57. Jones KL, Arslanian S, Peterokova VA, et al: Effect of metformin in pediatric patients with type 2 diabetes: A randomized controlled trial. Diabetes Care 25:89-94, 2002.

58. UK Prospective Diabetes Study Group: Tight blood pressure control and risk of macrovascular and microvascular complications in type 2 diabetes: UKPDS 38. BMJ 317:703-713, 1998.

59. Gahagan S, Silverstein J, and the Committee on Native American Child Health and Section on Endocrinology: Prevention and treatment of type 2 diabetes mellitus in children, with special emphasis on American Indian and Alaskan Native children. Pediatrics 112:e328-e347, 2004. Available online at www.pediatrics.org/cgi/content/full/112/4/e328.

KEY POINTS

- *Prevalence of diabetes increases with age.*
- *Nearly 1 in 5 older adults has diabetes mellitus.*
- *Aging is associated with decreased insulin sensitivity, subtle beta cell dysfunction, and altered carbohydrate metabolism.*
- *Older adults with diabetes are at increased risk of physical and cognitive dysfunction.*
- *Age, per se, should not be an excuse for suboptimal glycemic control*
- *Nonpharmacologic management of diabetes in older adults must be individualized.*
- *Physicians must be cognizant of pharmacokinetic and pharmacodynamic changes with age.*
- *Special attention must be paid when using pharmacologic agents in older diabetic adults.*

The incidence and prevalence of diabetes mellitus increase with age, as do the risk of complications from diabetes. Whereas about 6.3% of the total US population has type 2 diabetes (T2DM), this fraction is much higher in those aged 65 to 74.[1,2] According to the Third National Health and Nutrition Examination Survey (NHANES III), more than 18% of people aged 60 years and older have diabetes by the American Diabetes Association fasting plasma glucose criterion,[3] and an equal or slightly higher percentage would have diabetes using criteria based on an oral glucose tolerance test.[3]

With the changing demographics in the United States and worldwide, this incidence has growing implications for older patients and their physicians as well as for the health care economy of the United States and developing countries. Therefore, up-to-date knowledge regarding diabetes mellitus prevention and treatment in the elderly is becoming more important for the practicing physician.

This chapter reviews the pathophysiology of T2DM from an aging perspective, the impact of diabetes on important age-related health outcomes, and updated strategies for managing this complex condition in the context of aging and comorbidity.

SCREENING FOR DIABETES MELLITUS IN OLDER ADULTS

The American Diabetes Association recommends screening every 3 years with a test for fasting plasma glucose level in persons at high risk for developing T2DM. Major risk factors include age 45 years or older, a family history of the disease, obesity, nonwhite race or ethnicity, hypertension, and impaired glucose tolerance. Given the growing number of available therapies, the prevalence of this condition in older people, and the easy access to serum glucose testing and relatively low cost, this recommendation is appropriate for older adults. However, the US Preventive Services Task Force (USPSTF) has also concluded that there was insufficient evidence to recommend for or against screening the general population.

PATHOGENESIS OF TYPE 2 DIABETES IN OLDER ADULTS

Insulin Resistance

Insulin resistance (with reference to glucose homeostasis) is hindrance to the action of insulin on glucose transport from the extracellular space into target tissues. Various methods are used in research (e.g., euglycemic–hyperinsulinemic clamps) and clinical practice (e.g., homeostasis model assessment [HOMA], insulin-to-glucose ratio) to evaluate insulin resistance, and both the research and clinical methods generally correlate well.[4] An enhanced insulin-to-glucose ratio is an indicator of insulin resistance and represents enhanced insulin secretion (due to pancreatic overactivity compensating for the resistance) and with impaired glucose disposal (especially in postabsorptive states).

Several gene mutations have been described to explain insulin resistance; however, they account for barely 5% of all causes of insulin resistance. More is known about the environmental causes of insulin resistance. Examples of environmental causes of insulin resistance include lifestyle-related

522

causes such as obesity and physical inactivity and other physiologic conditions such as pregnancy and aging. Together, these causes account for the vast majority of the cases of insulin resistance and are most commonly associated with development of T2DM. Further, modification of these factors has been shown to improve diabetes and even prevent the onset of T2DM.

Obesity, due to its growing prevalence in the elderly, is notable for its association with insulin resistance. In obese persons, diabetes develops when hyperinsulinemia cannot compensate for obesity-associated insulin resistance. Although the prevalence of obesity progressively decreases after the age of 60 relative to younger ages, the prevalence of obesity within the group of adults older than 65 years has steadily increased (as it has within all age groups since the 1980s). Approximately 42% of both men and women between the ages of 60 and 69, and 37% between the ages of 70 and 79, are overweight (BMI ≥ 25). For persons older than 80 years, 18% of men and 26% of women are overweight. Approximately 15% of older persons entering nursing homes are overweight.

The relation between insulin resistance and aging has also long been recognized. Healthy older adults have higher glucose levels during oral glucose tolerance tests (OGTTs) (Fig. 38–1). The prevalence of diabetes increases with age in ethnically diverse populations. The estimated prevalence of diabetes in adults in the general population in 2002 was 8.7%.[3] However, even by the 1997 American Diabetes Association (ADA) criteria for diabetes, approximately 40% of patients older than 60 years had impaired glucose tolerance, and as many as 50% of these persons met the criteria for diabetes.[2] Furthermore, the incidence of new cases of diabetes diagnosed in elderly persons older than 65 years is almost five times the incidence in their younger counterparts.[5]

Diminished insulin sensitivity has been documented in older hypertensive men.[6] Indeed, epidemiologic studies have revealed an association between hyperinsulinemia and T2DM on the one hand and hypertension on the other.[7] Another hypothesis suggests that insulin resistance is secondary to hypertension and its long-term effects on small blood vessels, causing impaired glucose transport to tissues.[8]

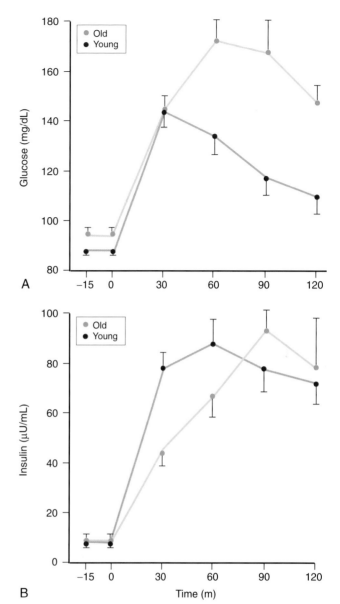

Figure 38–1. Plasma glucose **(A)** and insulin **(B)** levels before and after oral ingestion of 100 g of glucose in 18 healthy old (*blue circles*) and 18 young (*red circles*) subjects matched for relative body weight and socioeconomic group. Subjects were eating an ad libitum diet that, in the older subjects, included approximately 10% fewer total calories and 15% fewer carbohydrate calories than the diet of their younger counterparts. (From Chen M, Halter JB, Porte D Jr: The role of dietary carbohydrate in decreased glucose tolerance of the elderly. J Am Geriatr Soc 35:417-424, 1987.)

Beta Cell Function

Fasting plasma glucose increases approximately 1% per decade after age 20. This is not clinically significant. In contrast, glucose levels following intake of carbohydrates or meals increase 9 to 10 mg/dL per decade at 1 hour and 5 mg/dL per decade at 2 hours. These changes result in a minor increase in glycated hemoglobin (HbA1c) with age. The changes in glucose response to meals are due to a number of alterations but primarily result from a combination of change in body composition and decreased peripheral sensitivity to insulin.

It has been difficult to assess pancreatic beta cell function due to lack of sensitive and specific measures. Also, decrease in insulin clearance with age[9] and coexisting insulin resistance in elderly people further confounds the studies of beta cell function with age. Physiologic feedback in response to

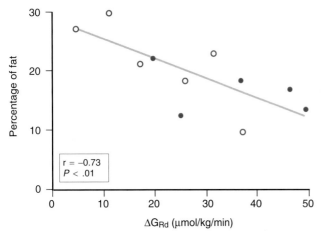

Figure 38–2. Correlation between changes in insulin-stimulated glucose uptake (ΔG_{Rd}) and body fat (% body fat) in elderly (*open circles*) and younger (*solid circles*) men. In elderly and younger men alike, increasing obesity was associated with increasing insulin resistance. (From Boden G, Chen X, De Santis RA, Kendrick Z: Effects of age and body fat on insulin resistance in healthy men. Diabetes Care 16:728-733, 1993; with permission.)

increased insulin resistance should result in hyperinsulinemia. When the degree of insulin resistance has been controlled for, multiple studies report an age-related decline of insulin secretion in humans (see Fig. 38–1).[10-12] Other age-related aberrations in beta cell function include increased levels of proinsulin and proinsulin–insulin,[13] reduced circadian and ultradian oscillations of insulin secretion,[14-16] and diminished enhancement of insulin secretion in response to an eccentric exercise-training program.[17] These data suggest that human aging results in a subtle impairment of beta cell function.

Aging and Carbohydrate Metabolism

Aging is associated with changes in body composition, notably an increase in fat mass and a loss of muscle mass.[18] Indeed, body fat was a determinant of insulin-stimulated glucose uptake independent of age (Fig. 38–2). Increased adiposity is associated with increased free fatty acid (FFA) levels, rate of lipolysis, and rate of lipid oxidation.[19] Overall, most studies suggest an effect of aging on glucose tolerance that is independent of body fat mass.

Calorie restriction and carbohydrate restriction can have different effects on insulin resistance. Calorie restriction can promote weight loss, decrease central adiposity,[20] and ameliorate hyperinsulinemia. However, carbohydrate reduction may in fact promote insulin resistance. Indeed, elderly people had an improved insulin sensitivity and pancreatic beta cell function with an 85% carbohydrate diet, as compared to an ad libitum diet.[21] More research is necessary before dietary carbohydrate

restrictions (especially low-carbohydrate diets) can be recommended to elderly patients with diabetes.

No age-related impairment of insulin-mediated suppression of hepatic glucose production in humans[22] has been reported. However, insulin-mediated total glucose disposal declines with age.[22] In most cells, the Krebs cycle pathway is relatively well preserved; however, the glucose monophosphate pathway and the anaerobic pathways producing lactate are significantly decreased with increasing age. Animal studies have further shown a decrease in glucose transporter expression with aging, suggesting a reduction in glucose transport capacity in fat cells from elderly people.

Physical activity is another confounder in the assessment of effects of aging on carbohydrate metabolism. Physically fit elderly people have less body fat and less central adiposity.[23] These more active people are also more insulin sensitive.[24] Interestingly, when insulin action was assessed using a glycemic clamp, the degrees of physical fitness and of central obesity (body fat distribution) were the most important predictors of the degree of insulin resistance observed, and age was not an important predictor.[24] It should, however, be noted that few data are available on the effects of physical activity on glucose homeostasis in people beyond the seventh decade of life.

Leptin is a peptide hormone that is produced by fat cells. Leptin decreases food intake, alters metabolism, and modulates gonadotrophins.[25] Leptin levels are more strongly correlated with waist (bad) adiposity than hip adiposity. In men, leptin levels show an increase with aging that is strongly related to the fall in testosterone with aging. In women, but not in men, leptin levels are strongly correlated with the development of sarcopenia (loss of muscle mass). Further, increased leptin levels in elderly men are also associated with decline in food intake.[26]

IMPORTANCE OF COMPLICATIONS OF DIABETES IN OLDER ADULTS

The effects of chronic diseases such as diabetes on outcomes such as physical and cognitive function are particularly important when considering prevention and treatment in older persons. Complications of diabetes are numerous and often lead to premature death, but disability and loss of independent function at advanced age is often the more-feared complication for many elderly persons. And because diabetes prevalence rises with age, the impact of diabetes on disability is particularly significant in the aging population, where disability rates are known to be higher than in a younger population.[27,28]

Elderly adults with T2DM are at substantially increased risk of impaired physical and cognitive function.[29,30] Numerous studies have reported

increased associations of diabetes with poor physical performance measured by functional test,[30-36] instrumental activities of daily living limitations,[33-37] and activities of daily living limitations.[31-37] These studies likely underestimate the impact of disease on physical and cognitive function because persons experiencing difficulty in these areas are more likely to be lost to follow-up.[38] And unlike cardiovascular disease events and mortality, data on physical and cognitive function are generally not obtainable from secondary sources such as the Medicare database.

Physical Dysfunction

The primary mechanism for diabetes-associated disability in older adults is thought to be from atherosclerotic and microvascular complications, which alone, apart from diabetes, can result in physical disability.[31,39-41] Additionally, diabetes is a strong predictor of coronary heart disease and cerebrovascular disease, both common precursors to disability in older people.[35] Diabetes is associated with other risks and conditions, including hypertension and dyslipidemia, which increase the risk of vascular diseases. T2DM is also one of the most common causes of blindness, nontrauma amputations, and end-stage renal disease (ESRD) in this and any age group.[29] Therefore, diabetes-related disability is often presumed to be related to the vascular complications of diabetes, such as heart disease, stroke, peripheral vascular disease, and visual disorders. However, recent work has shown that diabetes-related loss of physical function is not dependent on observed vascular diabetic complications alone.[42]

There are several hypotheses regarding why diabetes has such a broad effect on physical functioning. Diabetes has many associated risks, comorbidities, and complications that lead to multiple impairments and a broad impact on functioning. Another hypothesis, a subject of much recent research, is that diabetes and the metabolic syndrome represent a more global underlying disorder, potentially related to inflammatory systemic alterations. Increased inflammatory activity associated with the metabolic syndrome[43] has been associated with T2DM and acute hyperglycemia.[44-47] Similarly, such inflammation is a contributor to loss of muscle mass and physical disability.[48] Thus, diabetes-related inflammation affecting multiple physiologic systems, such as the vascular, nervous, and musculoskeletal systems, could potentially underlie widespread functioning problems.

Cognitive Dysfunction

Cognitive dysfunction represents another serious problem for older people, and a growing body of evidence from several epidemiologic studies suggests that diabetes is a risk factor for cognitive dysfunction.[49-51] Because cognitive dysfunction can impair self-care behavior,[52] and because self-care is crucial for optimal management of diabetes, it is important to clarify the relationship between diabetes and cognitive dysfunction.

People with diabetes have a greater rate of decline in cognitive function and a greater risk of cognitive decline. For reasons stated earlier, the impact of diabetes on cognition longitudinally has very likely been underestimated. Indeed, in one study, which did report diabetes status of patients lost to follow-up, diabetic participants had higher mortality rates or lower follow-up rates, or both, than participants without diabetes.[53]

The Framingham study[54] and the Adult Health study[55] both demonstrated increased cognitive impairment over time in persons with diabetes. In the Framingham study, 2123 subjects aged 55 to 88 completed a neuropsychological test battery during either the 14th or 15th biennial examination. People with diabetes were more likely to achieve scores below the 25th percentile on most tests than were nondiabetic subjects. The Adult Health Study followed a cohort of atomic bomb survivors from Hiroshima and Nagasaki. After 34 to 39 years of follow-up, 1774 participants were screened for dementia. Compared to nondiabetic subjects, diabetes increased the risk for vascular dementia and Alzheimer's dementia 1.3- and 4.4-fold, respectively.

A number of possibilities could explain the association between diabetes and cognitive decline. Again, the relationship between cognitive change and diabetes may be mediated through cerebrovascular disease. Second, and just as with decline in physical function, data show that the inflammation common with diabetes might also be a mediator of cognitive decline.[56] Third, treatment-related hypoglycemia might affect cognitive function. However, there is little evidence to support chronic cognitive impairment secondary to hypoglycemia. Indeed, intensive treatment regimens that were associated with increased hypoglycemic episodes in persons with T1DM did not affect cognition adversely.[57] Fourth, hyperglycemia might also contribute to chronic cognitive impairment. Postmortem studies of senile plaques from the brains of people with Alzheimer's disease demonstrate metabolic oxidation products associated with hyperglycemia.[58,59]

Despite the evidence that diabetes is associated with increased cognitive decline and incident dementia, there is little evidence that diabetes management affects the rate or nature of cognitive dysfunction. Indeed a recent review of the effect of therapy concluded that no studies were appropriate for inclusion in a meta-analysis.[50]

MANAGEMENT OF DIABETES IN OLDER ADULTS

Although epidemiologic and prospective studies have demonstrated the potential benefits of glycemic control,[60-62] clinical trial evidence is lacking regarding the degree to which glycemia should be normalized. Long-term management of glycemia, however, is critical to optimal management of diabetes. Unfortunately, many physicians are reluctant to treat older patients to goal due to the fear of complications arising out of hypoglycemia. Appropriately, the ADA guidelines state that age, per se, should not be the excuse for suboptimal control of blood glucose. The goal of treatment should be to achieve glycemia levels as close to normal as possible so as to prevent or delay the progression of chronic complications while preventing acute symptoms of hyper- and hypoglycemia.

Nonpharmacologic Measures

Diet and Nutrition

The increasing incidence and prevalence of diabetes has substantial economic implications. Cost-effective treatment strategies are needed, and in this context, the role of diet in the treatment of diabetes is increasingly important. Most diet recommendations have focused upon young and middle-aged patients, and few definitive studies have been completed in older populations.[63-65] The ADA's 2004 position statement provides the existing evidence base for recommending diabetes medical nutrition therapy.[3] A clinician trained in diabetes management, such as a nurse or dietitian, is critical to providing high-quality diabetes nutrition therapy. The goals of diet intervention in the elderly are summarized in Box 38-1.

Lack of studies involving large numbers of elderly patients with diabetes has resulted in little to no evidence base for diet recommendations, and the current approach is to extrapolate nutrition recommendations from those for younger patients. However, although calorie restriction is the cornerstone for diabetes management, malnutrition is a common important problem in many elderly persons.[66] In general, calorie intake declines with increasing age, and caution should be exercised when prescribing weight-loss diets in the elderly.

The energy intake of men in the Baltimore Longitudinal Study of Aging and the National Health and Nutrition Examination Study (NHANES) fell from 2700 kcal at ages 23 to 34 to 1800 to 2100 kcal at ages 65 to 80. One third of this decrease was due to a lower metabolic rate. Metabolically active skeletal muscle declined from 45% of body weight in young adults to about 27% by age 70 years; Sixteen percent of persons aged 65 and over eat less than 1000 kcal a day. Two thirds of the reduced energy requirement was due to decreased physical activity, another important variable in diabetes management.

Much controversy has plagued the macronutrient composition of the diet. Historically, a low-fat, high-carbohydrate diet has been recommended. These diets provide up to 60% of total calories from carbohydrates. However, recent diets (e.g., Atkins) have proposed a much lower carbohydrate intake to promote weight loss. The cardiovascular impact of the low-carbohydrate diets remains unclear and, here again, few studies, if any, of the relative benefit of these diets have been done in elderly people. Further, the glycemic index, which has been used to determine the relative glycemic potency of different carbohydrates, may be less important than determining the total quantity of carbohydrates in the meal.

The impact of various levels of protein intake for older diabetics is also unclear. The average protein intake for all ages is 14% to 18% of the daily caloric intake, with approximately 65% from animal sources.[67] High-protein diets may increase glomerular filtration and enhance the progression of diabetic nephropathy.[68] However, a low-protein diet could result in loss of lean body mass, and higher protein requirements are needed in the chronic comorbid and catabolic states typically found in many older adults.

Diet impact on lipid profile is also important. The low-density lipoprotein (LDL) goal in patients with diabetes is now less than 100 mg/dL. Dietary cholesterol should be less than 300 mg/day. Some persons (i.e., persons with LDL cholesterol of 100 mg/dL) may benefit from lowering dietary cholesterol to less than 200 mg/day. To lower LDL cholesterol, energy derived from saturated fat can be

---

Box 38-1. Goals of Medical Nutrition Therapy for Older Adults with Diabetes

- Attain and maintain optimal metabolic outcomes
  - Attain optimal glycemic control.
  - Normalize lipoprotein profile.
  - Normalize blood pressure.
- Prevent and treat chronic complications of diabetes.
  - Minimize risk of long-term microvascular complications.
  - Minimize risk of cardiovascular diseases.
- Prevent and treat obesity.
- Prevent and treat nephropathy.
- Improve health through healthy food choices.
- Encourage physical activity.
- Improve lifestyle and quality of life.
- Address personal and cultural preferences.
  - Improve compliance with nutrition therapy.
  - Provide for nutrition needs to prevent malnutrition.

Box 38-2. American Diabetes Association Recommendations for the Macronutrient Composition of a Diabetic Nutrition Therapy Diet

- Carbohydrates and monounsaturated fats: 60% to 70%
- Proteins: 15% to 20%
- Polyunsaturated fats: approximately 10%
- Saturated fats: 7% to 10%
- Fiber: 20 to 35 grams per day

reduced if weight loss is desirable or replaced with either carbohydrate or monounsaturated fat when weight loss is not a goal. Two or three servings of fish per week provide dietary ω-3 polyunsaturated fat and can be recommended. Advising older patients to replace saturated fats and *trans* fatty acids with mono- and polyunsaturated fats could result in healthier outcomes and better diet adherence than emphasizing a low-fat diet does.

Adequate intake of fiber (20 to 35 g/day) and fruit is also important. Deficiencies of zinc, chromium, magnesium, and potassium can aggravate carbohydrate intolerance, and folate and other vitamins of the B complex might be important in lowering homocysteine levels and preserving beta cell function. A daily multivitamin supplement might be appropriate for older adults, especially those with reduced energy intake. Regardless of diabetes status, older adults should be advised to have a calcium intake of at least 1000 to 1500 mg daily. Box 38-2 shows the ADA recommendations of the macronutrient composition of a diabetic nutrition therapy diet.

Imposing diet restrictions on elderly residents with diabetes in long-term health facilities is not warranted, especially because the primary goal for almost all patients in this setting is comfort. Malnutrition and dehydration can develop because of lack of food choices, poor quality of food, and unnecessary restrictions. Specialized diabetic diets do not appear to be superior to standard (regular) diets in such settings. Therefore, it is recommended that residents be served the regular (unrestricted) menu with consistency in the amount and timing of carbohydrate. There is no evidence to support diets such as "no concentrated sweets" or "no sugar added," which is often served to the elderly in long-term care facilities. Furthermore, it may often be preferable to make medication changes to control blood glucose than to implement food restrictions.

The most reliable indicator of poor nutrition status in the elderly is a change in body weight. In general, involuntary gain or loss of more than 10 pounds or 10% of body weight in less than 6 months indicates a need to evaluate if the reason is nutrition-related. Hypocaloric diets indeed are associated with poorer quality of life, and low body weight has been associated with greater morbidity and mortality in this age group. Hypocaloric diets

should only be recommended to obese elderly insulin-resistant and dyslipidemic patients, and weight gain should be encouraged in underweight malnourished diabetic patients.

Poor dentition (including decayed or missing teeth), periodontal disease, salivary hypofunction, drug-induced dry mouth, and impaired olfaction and taste perception contribute to malnutrition. Hypodipsia and impaired urinary concentrating ability are both part of normal aging and can contribute to dehydration in the absence of adequate fluid intake.

Physical Activity and Exercise

Maximizing mobility and independence is a central mission for geriatric practice and a uniform goal for older people. Physical activity is one of the most effective preventive strategies to increase the percentage of older persons who will be independent in their ninth and tenth decades. Data and outcomes from epidemiologic studies and intervention trials justify the recommendation of physical activity for nearly all older persons.

The Surgeon General and the Centers for Disease Control and Prevention recommend about 150 minutes of physical activity every week, or about 30 minutes of physical activity (not specifically exercise) most or every day of the week. Physical activities need not be sustained: Three walks a day for 10 minutes each is as good as one sustained walk for 30 minutes. This is good news for people who do not enjoy sustained walking or activity.

Beneficial Effects of Exercise

The beneficial effects of regular physical activity have been known since the preinsulin era.[69] Exercise has been demonstrated to improve glucose tolerance in people with diabetes.[69] Aerobic exercise enhances insulin sensitivity acutely[70] and with chronic training.[71-73] Indeed, improvement in long-term glycemic control was seen with regular physical exercise, and this effect is independent of change in body composition.[74,75]

In the young and the elderly, regular physical activity ameliorates insulin resistance, one of the major abnormalities of T2DM.[76] Two large studies found a strong dose-response relationship between exercise and relative risk of developing T2DM in healthy adults. Each incremental increase in volume or intensity of physical activity decreased relative risk of developing T2DM, with the protective effect persisting even after adjustment for BMI.[77,78]

Physical activity unequivocally reduces the risk of developing T2DM in persons with impaired glucose tolerance (IGT).[75,79,80] In the Da Qing IGT and the Finnish Diabetes Prevention Studies, cumulative incidence of diabetes was 20% lower with exercise (equating to 20 to 30 min of daily physical activity) when compared with control subjects.[75,80] The Diabetes Prevention Program found that the cumulative incidence of diabetes was 58% lower in persons

Box 38-3. Beneficial Effects of Exercise in Older Adults with Diabetes

- Improved glycemic control
- Increase in insulin sensitivity
- Improved lipid profile
- Improved blood pressure
- Cardiovascular conditioning
- Increased strength and flexibility
- Maintenance of muscle mass and strength
- Weight loss
- Decreased fat mass
- Improvement in bone density and lower fracture risk
- Improved balance and fewer falls
- Improved sense of well being
- Enhanced quality of life
- Prolonged independence in activities of daily living toward end of life
- Increased longevity

Box 38-4. Risks of Exercise in Older Adults with Diabetes

- Hypoglycemia
- Hyperglycemia after strenuous exercise
- Precipitation of cardiovascular disease
- Vitreous hemorrhage*
- Retinal detachment*
- Increased proteinuria
- Soft tissue and joint injury

*Patients with proliferative retinopathy

Box 38-5. Impediments to Exercise Prescription in Older Adults with Diabetes

- Multiple medical comorbidities (coronary artery disease, chronic obstructive pulmonary disease)
- Osteoarthritis
- Foot abnormalities
- Neurodegenerative diseases
- Sensory deprivation (e.g., visual, auditory)
- Lack of companionship
- Diabetic neuropathy
- Diabetic foot with foot ulcers
- Peripheral vascular disease with claudication

treated with intensive diet and exercise than with placebo. Moreover, overall diabetes incidence was 39% lower with intensive lifestyle intervention than with metformin therapy, and this effect was enhanced with age.[79]

T2DM is associated with coexisting hypertension and dyslipidemia in a majority of older patients, and all these conditions increase the risk of coronary heart disease. Regular physical activity can help improve several of these chronic conditions. Exercise is associated with improvement in hypertension; a decrease in both systolic and diastolic blood pressure of 5 to 10 mm Hg is seen.[81,82] This effect occurs independent of weight loss or changes in body composition, and it may be related to changes in insulin-related renal sodium handling.

Increased lipoprotein lipase activity in the physically trained muscle also results in improvement in lipid profile with exercise.[83] Lowering of serum triglycerides (particularly very-low-density lipoprotein [VLDL]) and an increase in high-density lipoprotein (HDL)[84] contributes to lower atherogenesis in the blood vessels. Exercise is also associated with improvement in endothelial function.[85]

All these effects of regular physical activity cause an improvement in cardiovascular risk factors in the elderly and hence contribute to lower morbidity. Box 38-3 lists the beneficial effects of regular physical activity in elderly patients with diabetes.

Risks of Exercise in Older Adults with Diabetes

Caution is necessary when recommending exercise to older patients, especially patients with T1DM and insulin-receiving T2DM patients (Box 38-4). Hypoglycemia can occur in persons taking insulin or sulfonylureas, and it can occur acutely during exercise or even hours after an exercise session. On the other hand, in patients who do not have enough insulin, unopposed hepatic glucose production during physical activity can lead to hyperglycemia, which can last for hours. Extensive diabetes education is necessary to minimize the risks of these metabolic complications. Complications might be severe and limiting, especially in patients with T1DM and in those with hypoglycemia unawareness.

Exacerbation of previously undiagnosed cardiovascular disease is another potential risk of exercise. A thorough cardiac evaluation should be done in all older patients with diabetes prior to recommending an exercise program. Worsening of degenerative joint diseases may be seen in older patients as well. Box 38-5 lists some of the impediments to prescribing exercise in older adults with diabetes.

Patients with longstanding diabetes should be screened carefully for microvascular complications before they start the exercise program. Patients with proliferative retinopathy can develop vitreous hemorrhage or retinal detachment. Increased proteinuria with physical exercise is seen in patients with nephropathy,[86,87] but no progression of nephropathy has been documented. Peripheral neuropathy increases the risk of injury and can cause trauma to the joints. Autonomic neuropathy may limit cardiac output and aerobic capacity.

Recommendations for Physical Activity in Older Adults with Diabetes

It is recommended that resistance training at least 2 days a week should be included as part of a well-rounded exercise program for older patients with T2DM whenever possible.[88] High-resistance exercises using weights are acceptable for young persons with diabetes but not for older adults and those with long-standing diabetes.[89] Moderate weight-training programs that use light weights and high repetitions can be used for maintenance or enhancement of upper body strength in nearly all patients with diabetes.[89]

Of the endurance activities, walking can be considered the preferred exercise for primary prevention because it provides both endurance and balance stimulus, and it is the primary performance on which many activities of daily living depend. Stair climbing, treadmill walking on an incline, and walking up hills can increase intensity when an exerciser reaches a plateau with brisk walking. Jogging is not recommended for persons who have not run in many years because of the high frequency of musculoskeletal complaints that occur when jogging is initiated.

Endurance walking can increase the risk of falls in patients with impaired gait and balance; injuries are less likely with stationary-bicycle and water-based exercise. Bicycles with reciprocal moving arms are commonly used in cardiac rehabilitation programs. Water-based exercises have been recommended for persons with knee or hip arthritis or foot problems who do not tolerate or enjoy land-based endurance exercise. Water-based exercises include swimming and a wide variety of endurance walking and resistance exercises using paddles attached to arms and legs to increase resistance to movement.

Before starting an exercise program, all patients with T2DM should have a complete history and physical examination (Box 38-6). An exercise stress test is recommended for all persons 35 years of age or older who intend to start a program of moderate or vigorous exercise.[69] Any cardiovascular impairment should be corrected before an exercise program is advised. Patients with microvascular complications should be advised to modify their exercises to minimize risks. Patients with proliferative retinopathy should avoid lifting weights and performing Valsalva's maneuver. Persons with peripheral neuropathy should avoid activities like running and jogging, which can cause trauma to soft tissues and joints.

Pharmacologic Management of Diabetes in Older Adults

With increasing age, diet management of T2DM becomes more challenging, and adequate physical activity is not always possible for the elderly. In this context, addition of medication is necessary.

Box 38-6. Medical Contraindications to Regular Physical Activity

Cardiovascular Contraindications

- Unstable angina
- Angina, hypotension, or arrhythmias provoked by resistance training
- Acute myocardial infarction
- End-stage congestive heart failure (NYHA class IV)
- Severe valvular heart disease
- Malignant or unstable arrhythmias*
- Large or expanding aortic aneurysms
- Known cerebral aneurysm
- Acute deep venous thrombosis
- Acute pulmonary embolism or infarction
- Recent intracerebral or subdural hemorrhage

Musculoskeletal Contraindications

- Significant exacerbation of musculoskeletal pain with resistance training
- Unstable or acutely injured joints, tendons, or ligaments
- Fracture within last 6 months (delayed union)
- Acute inflammatory joint disease

Other Contraindications

- Rapidly progressive or unstable neurologic disease
- Failure to thrive
- Terminal illness
- Uncontrolled systemic disease†
- Symptomatic or large abdominal or inguinal hernias
- Hemorrhoids
- Severe dementia
- Behavioral disturbances
- Acute alcohol or drug intoxication
- Acute retinal bleed or detachment
- Severe proliferative diabetic retinopathy
- Recent ophthalmic surgery
- Severe cognitive impairment
- Uncontrolled COPD
- Prosthesis instability

COPD, chronic obstructive pulmonary disease; NYHA, New York Heart Association.
*Ventricular tachycardia, complete heart block without pacemaker, atrial flutter, junctional rhythms
†For example, uncontrolled diabetes (symptomatic hypo- or hyperglycemia; hemoglobin A1c > 10%), hypertension (untreated systolic blood pressure > 170 mm Hg), thyroid disease, congestive heart failure, sepsis, acute illness, fevers.

As with diet and exercise, pharmacologic management of diabetes in the elderly has to be carefully monitored. When therapy with medications is initiated, self-monitoring of blood glucose is often necessary. Special care should be taken in teaching these techniques. Special attention must also be

Box 38-7. Principles of Appropriate Prescribing for Older Adults

- Maintain an up-to-date list of all of a patient's medications.
- Avoid multiple physicians and pharmacies.
- Inquire about the use of nonprescription medications and supplements.
- Ensure treatment compliance and adherence.
- Discuss care with caregiver.

Box 38-8. Risk Factors for Nonadherence to Treatment

- Poor recall of medication regimen
- Seeing numerous physicians
- Being female
- Having medium income
- Using many medications
- Believing that medications are expensive
- Using numerous pharmacies
- Living alone
- Taking multiple doses daily
- Lack of understanding of the expected regimen
- Lack of instructions on how to use medications
- Cost and financial constraints

paid to the changes in pharmacokinetics and pharmacodynamics with aging. Prescribers need to be especially cognizant of the perils of polypharmacy: drug interactions and adverse drug reactions. Boxes 38-7 and 38-8 list the appropriate prescription principles as well as the risk factors for noncompliance with medications.

Among people aged 65 and older who take prescription drugs, an average of 3.1% of household income is spent on drugs. Among severely disabled elderly persons, outpatient prescription drug costs account for more than half of out-of-pocket expenditures for health care. Hence, cost is a very important factor when choosing medications for management of diabetes in elderly patients, especially those who do not have a prescription benefit program.

Age-Related Pharmacokinetic Changes
Absorption and Bioavailability

Absorption and bioavailability are largely unaltered with aging, although drug absorption might proceed at a slower rate, resulting in lower peak concentrations or an increase in the time to onset of drug effect, or both. Absorption and bioavailability may be an important factor when considering therapy with meglitinides, the short-acting insulin secretagogues. Lifestyle, comorbidity, and the use of other medications affect absorption more than does age alone.

Distribution and Binding

In general, adult weight begins to decline in the seventh or eighth decade. Many frail elderly persons are smaller than average young adults; small size has been suggested as a risk factor for adverse drug events (ADEs). Aging is associated with a decrease in total body water and lean body mass and an increase in body fat, although this is not clinically important with present-day antidiabetic medications. Protein binding is largely unchanged with age.

Hepatic Metabolism and Renal Excretion

Age and gender are among a multitude of factors that affect hepatic metabolism of drugs. Also, glomerular filtration rate (GFR) decreases with aging. Hence, caution should be exercised with respect to drug metabolism and excretion. This is especially true for insulin and insulin secretagogues because the clearance of insulin is reduced in many older people and in many chronic diseases and conditions. A common problem in the older diabetic is failure to match pharmacologic therapy to changes in renal function in frail, poorly nourished patients.

Age-Related Pharmacodynamic Changes

Caution must be exercised in dosing medications because pharmacodynamic differences can result in increased or, rarely, decreased responsiveness to a drug. Pharmacodynamic differences can be due to alterations at the cellular level (e.g., receptors or postreceptor events), at the tissue level (e.g., end-organ sensitivity), or at the level of compensatory or homeostatic mechanisms.

Adverse Drug Events

It is estimated that 5% to 15% of acute geriatric medical admissions are due to ADEs, defined as injury or illness resulting from drug use.[90] Physicians, patients, and family members can misinterpret these adverse events because they appear to be disorders that are prevalent among elderly persons. Further, they differ from ADEs uncovered in younger populations during clinical trials. Few drug safety trials have been done on the older-old, especially among those with multiple medical conditions or with polypharmacy. Pharmacodynamic studies are rare, because they are more difficult to do: they require the intensity of effect to be quantifiable and measurable repeatedly.

Even with the intent to include elderly subjects, the great biological diversity of the elderly age group interferes with recruitment and with the direct clinical applicability of many studies. Of the more than 18,000 patients screened for the Stroke Prevention in Atrial Fibrillation study, only 7% of those enrolled were older than 65. For the Systolic Hypertension in Elderly Persons trial, the corresponding figures are 9% of 52,000. These are among the best trials for answering the clinically relevant questions, yet they represent a minority of patients who have the conditions. Frail elderly persons are

the least likely to be entered in these trials and the most likely to have adverse drug reactions.

New drugs should be prescribed only after older, generally cheaper drugs, whose side-effect profiles are better known, have been tried and have failed. When a new drug is prescribed for an old patient, that patient is entering the postmarketing surveillance phase of the drug's development, and low-frequency side effects should be continually sought and promptly reported to the Food and Drug Administration. A classic example is severe hyperglycemic effects seen to be associated with the use of gatifloxacin in some elderly women.[91]

Medications used in diabetes can cause ADEs by themselves (hypoglycemia, falls, seizures). They can also complicate other illnesses or ADEs, such as hypoglycemia with poor oral intake or anorexia, and overdose with cognitive impairment.

Polypharmacy and changes in pharmacokinetics contribute, along with age, to ADEs. Further, drug interactions can complicate the care of diabetics. Angiotensin-converting enzyme inhibitors increase insulin sensitivity and hence increase the hypoglycemic effect of sulfonylureas. β-Blockers can mask hypoglycemic symptoms, although they rarely cause a major problem. Several drugs increase insulin resistance—for example, niacin, thiazides, and steroids—and hence can increase the requirement of the hypoglycemic agents. Lastly, food can affect drug absorption, and drugs can cause anorexia, altered taste, and other problems that effect food intake.

Special Considerations for Pharmacotherapy in Older Adults

Metformin

Metformin is the most widely used insulin sensitizer. However, few studies of metformin have included elderly patients. Indeed, caution is advised with use in advancing age, and the use is not advised in patients older than 80 years unless measurement of creatinine clearance verifies optimal renal function. In frail elderly people, a normal creatinine can be misleading, and creatinine clearance must be measured prior to using this agent. Use must also be avoided in patients with elevated creatinine or with creatinine clearance less than 60 to 70 mL/min. Use is also avoided in patients with hepatic impairment.

Further, active ischemic heart disease, respiratory failure, septicemia, congestive heart failure, and other uncontrolled medical conditions increase the risk of lactic acidosis. Indeed, some physicians discontinue metformin whenever older-old patients are admitted to the hospital. Metformin must be discontinued 48 hours prior to any contrast study.

Diarrhea and gastrointestinal side effects may be intolerable to some elderly patients. Patients should be monitored for vitamin B_{12} and folic acid deficiency. Ingestion with chromium may induce hypoglycemia.

Sulfonylureas

The insulin secretagogues are the commonest agents used in the management of diabetes. The first-generation sulfonylureas have the potential to cause prolonged hypoglycemia, especially in the elderly, due to their long half-life. Chlorpropamide can also induce hyponatremia and thus is not recommended for use in anyone aged 65 and older. Even with shorter-acting second-generation secretagogues, rapid and prolonged hypoglycemia has been reported. Elderly patients should be started on low doses and the titration must be unhurried. Caution is advised in patients with renal or hepatic impairment

Meglitinides

These newest secretagogues are ultra-short-acting agents and are used most often for postprandial glucose control. No changes in safety and efficacy were seen in patients 65 years old; however, some elderly patients show increased sensitivity to dosing. Due to delayed gastric emptying or slow ingestion of food, or both, hypoglycemia can occur with meglitinides more often in elderly persons than in other populations. No specific dosage adjustment is recommended for patients with renal impairment, although caution is advised in patients with moderate to severe hepatic impairment.

α-Glucosidase Inhibitors

Uncommonly used in the United States, these drugs competitively inhibit pancreatic α-amylase and intestinal brush border α-glucosidases, resulting in delayed hydrolysis of ingested complex carbohydrates and disaccharides and absorption of glucose. No specific problems are reported with use in elderly people besides the usual gastrointestinal side effects.

Thiazolidinediones

These are the newest insulin sensitizers. Anemia and weight gain (with pedal edema) are the commonest side effects. Hypoglycemia is uncommon. However, use is contraindicated in patients with hepatic transaminases more than 2.5 times the upper limit of normal. Further, periodic monitoring of liver function tests is recommended. Use is also contraindicated in patients with advanced congestive heart failure.

Insulin

Insulin is the treatment of choice in T1DM in general and in T2DM when oral hypoglycemic agents and their combinations fail to produce acceptable diabetes control. Many new analogs of insulin with various peaks and durations of action are available.

Diabetes education becomes imperative and much more intense when patients are started on

Box 38-9. Limitations to Use of Insulin in Older Adults with Diabetes

- Inability to draw insulin
- Visual impairment
- Illiteracy
- Sensory impairment
- Hand problems
- Cognitive deficits
- Poor compliance
- Fear of needles

insulin. Often patients can be managed with one shot of insulin daily used at bedtime. With advancing disease, more shots are needed, and eventually an intensive insulin regimen (basal–bolus regimen of 4 shots of insulin per day) is necessary to optimize diabetes management.

Patients need to be informed of the peaks and durations of various insulin analogs to minimize the risk of hypoglycemia. Most hypoglycemic events can be related to a mismatch between the insulin injection and food intake. Optimal control inherently increases the risk of hypoglycemic events, and hence a good regimen maximizes glycemic control while minimizing hypoglycemic events. Box 38-9 lists the limitations to the use of insulin in elderly patients with diabetes.

LIMITATIONS IN DIABETES CARE IN OLDER ADULTS

Care of the older adult with diabetes is a challenge for the clinician, the patient, and the patient's family. Nevertheless, today there are many more satisfactory options for ensuring optimal care. Numerous community organizations are available on the local and national level, and each support should be assessed for possible benefit to a particular patient and the patient's caregivers.

Identifying the best approach to treatment in the context of well-defined goals and including supportive family members and friends is critical to success. The degree of family support to meet the patient's needs, the adequacy of the patient's living situation, and whether the patient's income is sufficient to sustain basic necessities and health care needs are all important factors in diabetic care.

As with many age-related chronic diseases (cognitive impairment, falls, incontinence, coronary heart disease), a team approach is the best model of care. Assistance from mid-level practitioners, referral to a social worker or geriatric case manager, instruction by diabetes educators, and support from other team members is indicated for the most thorough assessment and management. With this structure, treatment can be individualized

and the older diabetic patient can maintain an independent, active life.

References

1. Centers for Disease Control and Prevention: National diabetes fact sheet: General information and national estimates on diabetes in the United States, 2003. http://www.cdc.gov/diabetes/pubs/factsheet.htm.
2. Harris MI, Flegal KM, Cowie CC, et al: Prevalence of diabetes, impaired fasting glucosemia and impaired glucose tolerance in U.S. adults: The Third National Health and Nutrition Examination Survey, 1988-1994. Diabetes Care 21:518-524, 1998.
3. American Diabetes Association: Diabetes mellitus and exercise (position statement). Diabetes Care 27:S58-S62, 2004.
4. Bergman RN, Prager R, Volund A, Olefsky JM: Equivalence of the insulin sensitivity index in man derived by the minimal model method and the euglycemic glucose clamp. J Clin Invest 79:790-800, 1987.
5. Herman WH, Sinnock P, Brenner E, et al: An epidemiologic model for diabetes mellitus: Incidence, prevalence, and mortality. Diabetes Care 7:367-371, 1984.
6. Dengel DR, Pratley RE, Hagberg JM, Goldberg AP: Impaired insulin sensitivity and maximal responsiveness in older hypertensive men. Hypertension 23:320-324, 1994.
7. Reaven PD, Barrett-Connor EL, Browner DK: Abnormal glucose tolerance and hypertension. Diabetes Care 13:119-125, 1990.
8. Julius S, Gudbrandsson T, Jamerson K, et al: The hemodynamic link between insulin resistance and hypertension. J Hypertens 9:983-986, 1991.
9. Halter JB: Aging and carbohydrate metabolism. In Masoro EJ (ed): Handbook of Physiology. Section 11: Aging. New York, Oxford University Press, 1995, p 119.
10. Iozzo P, Beck-Nielsen H, Laakso M, et al: Independent influence of age on basal insulin secretion in nondiabetic humans, European Group for the Study of Insulin Resistance. J Clin Endocrinol Metab 84:863-868, 1999.
11. Dechenes CJ, Verchere CB, Andrikopoulos S, Kahn SE: Human aging is associated with parallel reductions in insulin and amylin release. Am J Physiol 275(5 Pt 1):E785-E791, 1998.
12. Ahren B, Pacini G: Impaired adaptation of first-phase insulin secretion in postmenopausal women with glucose intolerance. Am J Physiol 273(4 Pt 1):E701-E707, 1997.
13. Shimizu M, Kawazu S, Tomono S, et al: Age-related alteration of pancreatic beta-cell function. Increased proinsulin and proinsulin-to-insulin molar ratio in elderly, but not in obese, subjects without glucose intolerance. Diabetes Care 19:8-11, 1996.
14. Frank SA, Roland DC, Sturis J, et al: Effects of aging on glucose regulation during wakefulness and sleep. Am J Physiol 269(6 Pt 1):E1006-E1016, 1995.
15. Scheen AJ, Sturis J, Polonsky KS, Van Cauter E: Alterations in the ultradian oscillations of insulin secretion and plasma glucose in aging. Diabetologia 39:564-572, 1996.
16. Meneilly GS, Ryan AS, Veldhuis JD, Elahi D: Increased disorderliness of basal insulin release, attenuated insulin secretory burst mass, and reduced ultradian rhythmicity of insulin secretion in older individuals. J Clin Endocrinol Metab 82:4088-4093, 1997.
17. Krishnan RK, Hernandez JM, Williamson DL, et al: Age-related differences in the pancreatic beta-cell response to hyperglycemia after eccentric exercise. Am J Physiol 275(3 Pt 1):E463-E470, 1998.
18. Borkan GA, Hults DE, Gerzof SG, et al: Age changes in body composition revealed by computed tomography. J Gerontol 38:673-677, 1983.
19. Bonadonna RC, Groop LC, Simonson DC, DeFronzo RA: Free fatty acid and glucose metabolism in human aging: Evidence for operation of the Randle cycle. Am J Physiol 266(3 Pt 1):E501-E509, 1994.

20. Barzilai N, Banerjee S, Hawkins M, et al: Caloric restriction reverses hepatic insulin resistance in aging rats by decreasing visceral fat. J Clin Invest 101:1353-1361, 1998.

21. Chen M, Halter JB, Porte D Jr: Plasma catecholamines, dietary carbohydrate, and glucose intolerance: A comparison between young and old men. J Clin Endocrinol Metab 62:1193-1198, 1986.

22. Fink RI, Kolterman OG, Griffin J, Olefsky JM: Mechanisms of insulin resistance in aging. J Clin Invest 71:1523-1535, 1983.

23. Ryan AS, Nicklas BJ, Elahi D: A cross-sectional study on body composition and energy expenditure in women athletes during aging. Am J Physiol 271(5 Pt 1):E916-E921, 1996.

24. Coon PJ, Rogus EM, Drinkwater D, et al: Role of body fat distribution in the decline in insulin sensitivity and glucose tolerance with age. J Clin Endocrinol Metab 75.1125-1132, 1992.

25. Morley JE: Anorexia, sarcopenia, and aging. Nutrition 17:660-663, 2001.

26. Morley JE: Decreased food intake with aging. J Gerontol A Biol Sci Med Sci 56(Spec No 2):81-88, 2001.

27. Songer T: Disability in diabetes. In Harris M, Cowie C, Stern MP, et al (eds): Diabetes in America. Bethesda, Md, National Institutes of Health, National Institute of Diabetes and Digestive and Kidney Diseases, 1995, pp 259-283.

28. Resnick HE, Harris MI, Brock DB, Harris TB: American Diabetes Association diabetes diagnostic criteria, advancing age, and cardiovascular disease risk profiles: Results from the Third National Health and Nutrition Examination Survey. Diabetes Care 23:176-180, 2000.

29. Nathan DM: Long-term complications of diabetes mellitus. N Engl J Med 328:1676-1685, 1993.

30. Yaffe K, Blackwell T, Kanaya AM, et al: Diabetes, impaired fasting glucose, and development of cognitive impairment in older women. Neurology 63:658-663, 2004.

31. Gregg EW, Beckles GL, Williamson DF, et al: Diabetes and physical disability among older U.S. adults. Diabetes Care 23:1272-1277, 2000.

32. Guccione AA, Felson DT, Anderson JJ, et al: The effects of specific medical conditions on the functional limitations of elders in the Framingham Study. Am J Public Health 84:351-358, 1994.

33. Miller DK, Lui LY, Perry HM III, et al: Reported and measured physical functioning in older inner-city diabetic African Americans. J Gerontol Med Sci 54:M230-M236, 1999.

34. Moritz DJ, Ostfeld AM, Blazer D II, et al: The health burden of diabetes for the elderly in four communities. Public Health Rep 109:782-790, 1994.

35. Ettinger WH, Fried LP, Harris T, et al: Self-reported causes of physical disability in older people: The Cardiovascular Health Study. CHS Collaborative Research Group. J Am Geriatr Soc 42:1035-1044, 1994.

36. Kishimoto M, Ojima T, Nakamura Y, et al: Relationship between the level of activities of daily living and chronic medical conditions among the elderly. J Epidemiol 8:272-277, 1998.

37. Macheledt JE, Vernon SW: Diabetes and disability among Mexican Americans: The effect of different measures of diabetes on its association with disability. J Clin Epidemiol 45:519-528, 1992.

38. Di Bari M, Williamson J, Pahor M: Missing data in epidemiological studies of age-associated cognitive decline. J Am Geriatr Soc 47:1380-1381, 1999.

39. Klein R, Klein B: Vision disorders in diabetes. In Harris M, Cowie C, Stern MP et al (eds): Diabetes in America. Bethesda, Md, National Institutes of Health, National Institute of Diabetes and Digestive and Kidney Diseases, 1995, pp 293-338.

40. Palumbo P, Melton L III: Peripheral vascular disease and diabetes. In Harris M, Cowie C, Stern MP et al (eds): Diabetes in America. Bethesda, Md, National Institutes of Health, National Institute of Diabetes and Digestive and Kidney Diseases, 1995, pp 401-408.

41. Wingard D, Barrett-Connor E: Heart disease and diabetes. In Harris M, Cowie C, Stern MP et al (eds): Diabetes in America. Bethesda, Md, National Institutes of Health, National Institute of Diabetes and Digestive and Kidney Diseases, 1995, pp 429-448.

42. Maty SC, Fried LP, Volpato S, et al: Patterns of disability related to diabetes mellitus in older women. J Gerontol A Biol Sci Med Sci 59:148-153, 2004.

43. Pickup JC, Mattock MB, Chusney GD, Burt D: NIDDM as a disease of the innate immune system: Association of acute-phase reactants and interleukin-6 with metabolic syndrome X. Diabetologia 40:1286-1292, 1997.

44. Pradhan AD, Manson JE, Rifai N, et al: C-reactive protein, interleukin 6, and risk of developing type 2 diabetes mellitus. JAMA 286:327-334, 2001.

45. Barzilay JI, Abraham L, Heckbert SR, et al: The relation of markers of inflammation to the development of glucose disorders in the elderly: The Cardiovascular Health Study. Diabetes 50:2384 2389, 2001.

46. Ford ES: Body mass index, diabetes, and C-reactive protein among U.S. adults. Diabetes Care 22:1971-1977, 1999.

47. Esposito K, Nappo F, Marfella R, et al: Inflammatory cytokine concentrations are acutely increased by hyperglycemia in humans: Role of oxidative stress. Circulation 106:2067-2072, 2002.

48. Ferrucci L, Harris TB, Guralnik JM, et al: Serum IL-6 level and the development of disability in older persons. J Am Geriatr Soc 47:639-646, 1999.

49. Stewart R, Liolitsa D: Type 2 diabetes mellitus, cognitive impairment and dementia. Diabet Med 16:93-112, 1999.

50. Aerosa S, Evans GJ: Effect of the treatment of type II diabetes mellitus on the development of cognitive impairment and dementia. Cochrane Library, Issue 2, 2005. http://www.cochrane.org/cochrane/revabstr/AB003804.htm.

51. Allen KV, Frier BM, Strachan MWJ: The relationship between type 2 diabetes and cognitive dysfunction: Longitudinal studies and their methodological limitations. Eur J Pharmacol 490:169-175, 2004.

52. Sinclair AJ, Bayer AJ: Cognitive dysfunction in older subjects with diabetes mellitus: Impact on diabetes self management and use of care services. All Wales Research into Elderly (AWARE) study. Diabetes Res Clin Prac 50:203-212, 2000.

53. Tilvis RS, Mervi H, Kahönen-Väre M, et al: Predictors of cognitive decline and mortality of aged people over a 10-year period. J Gerontol 59:M268-M274, 2004.

54. Elias MF, Elias PK, Sullivan LM, et al: NIDDM and blood pressure as risk factors for poor cognitive performance: The Framingham study. Diabetes Care 20:1388-1393, 1997.

55. Yamada M, Kasagi F, Sasaki H, et al: Association between dementia and midlife risk factors: The Radiation Effects Research Foundation Adult Health Study. J Am Geriatr Soc 51:410-414, 2003.

56. Yaffe K, Kanaya A, Lindquist K, et al: The metabolic syndrome, inflammation, and risk of cognitive decline. JAMA 292:2237-2242, 2004.

57. Vlassara H, Bucala R, Striker L: Pathogenic effects of advanced glycosylation: Biochemical, biologic and clinical implications for diabetes and aging. Lab Invest 70:138-151, 1994.

58. Reichard P, Pihl M: Mortality and treatment side effects during long term intensified conventional insulin treatment in the Stockholm diabetes intervention study. Diabetes 43:313-317, 1994.

59. Horie K, Miyata T, Yasuda T, et al: Immunohistochemical localization of advanced glycation end products, pentosidine and carboxymethyllysine in lipofusin pigments of Alzheimer's disease and aged neurons. Biochem Biophys Res Commun 236:327-332, 1997.

60. The Diabetes Control and Complications Trial Research Group: The effects of intensive treatment of diabetes on the development and progression of long-term complications in insulin-dependent diabetes mellitus. N Engl J Med 329:977-986, 1993.

61. Reichard P, Nilsson B-Y, Rosenqvist U: The effects of long-term intensified insulin treatment on the development of microvascular complications of diabetes mellitus. N Engl J Med 329:304-309, 1993.

62. Eschwege F, Richard JL, Thibult N, et al: Coronary heart disease mortality in relation with diabetes, blood glucose

and plasma insulin levels: The Paris Prospective Study, ten years later. Horm Metab Res 15(Supp):41-46, 1985.

63. Fonseca V. Wall J: Diet and diabetes in the elderly. Clin Geriatr Med 11:613-624, 1995.

64. Franz MJ, Horton ES Sr, Bantle JP, et al: Nutrition principles for the management of diabetes and related complications. Diabetes Care 17:490-518, 1994.

65. Reed RL, Mooradian AD: Nutritional status and dietary management of elderly diabetic patients. Clin Geriatr Med 6:883-901, 1990.

66. Porte D Jr, Kahn SE: What geriatricians should know about diabetes mellitus. Diabetes Care 13:Suppl 2, 1990.

67. Henry RR: Protein content of the diabetic diet. Diabetes Care 17:1502-1513, 1994.

68. Brenner BM, Meyer T, Hostetter TH: Dietary protein intake and the progressive nature of kidney disease: The role of hemodynamically mediated glomerular injury in the pathogenesis of progressive glomerular sclerosis in aging, renal ablation, and intrinsic renal disease. N Engl J Med 307:652-659, 1982.

69. Allen FM, Stillman MD, Fitz R: Total Dietary Regulation in the Treatment of Diabetes. New York, The Rockefeller Institute for Medical Research, 1919, Chapter 5.

70. Rogers MA: Acute effects of exercise on glucose tolerance in non–insulin-dependent diabetes. Med Sci Sports Exerc 21:362-368, 1989.

71. Walker K, Piers LS, Putt RS, et al: Effects of regular walking on cardiovascular risk factors and body composition in normoglycaemic women and women with type 2 diabetes. Diabetes Care 22:555-561, 1999.

72. Bogardus C, Ravussin E, Robbins DC, et al: Effects of physical training and diet therapy on carbohydrate metabolism in patients with glucose intolerance and non–insulin-dependent diabetes mellitus. Diabetes 33:311-318, 1984.

73. Trovati M, Carta Q, Cavalot F, et al: Influence of physical training on blood glucose control, glucose tolerance, insulin secretion, and insulin action in non–insulin-dependent diabetic patients. Diabetes Care 7:416-420, 1984.

74. Boule N, Haddad E, Kenny GP, et al: Effects of exercise on glycemic control and body mass in type 2 diabetes mellitus: A meta-analysis of controlled clinical trials. JAMA 286:1218-1227, 2001.

75. Tuomilehto J, Lindstrom J, Eriksson JG, et al: Prevention of type 2 diabetes by changes in lifestyle among subjects with impaired glucose tolerance. N Engl J Med 344:1343-1350, 2001.

76. Defronzo RA, Ferrannini E, Koivisto V: New concepts in the pathogenesis and treatment of non–insulin dependent diabetes mellitus. Am J Med 74:52-81, 1983.

77. Helmrich SP, Ragland DR, Leung RW, Paffenberger RS Jr: Physical activity and reduced occurrence of non–insulin-dependent diabetes mellitus. N Engl J Med 325:147-152, 1991.

78. Hu FB, Sigal RJ, Rich-Edwards JW, et al: Walking compared with vigorous physical activity and risk of type 2 diabetes in women. JAMA 282:1433-1439, 1999.

79. Diabetes Prevention Program Research Group: Reduction in the incidence of type 2 diabetes with lifestyle intervention or metformin. N Engl J Med 346:393-403, 2002.

80. Pan X-R, Li G-W, Hu Y-H, et al: Effects of diet and exercise in preventing NIDDM in people with impaired glucose tolerance: The Da Qing IGT and Diabetes Study. Diabetes Care 20:537-544, 1997.

81. Boyer J, Kasch F: Exercise therapy in hypertensive men. JAMA 211:1668-1671, 1970.

82. Choquette G, Ferguson R: Blood pressure reduction in "borderline" hypertensives following physical training. Can Med Assoc J 108:699-703, 1973.

83. Kiens B, Lithell H: Lipoprotein metabolism influenced by training induced changes in human skeletal muscle. J Clin Invest 83:558-564, 1989.

84. Huttunen JK, Lansimies E, Voutilainen E, et al: Effect of moderate physical exercise on serum lipoproteins. A controlled clinical trial with special reference to serum high-density lipoproteins. Circulation 60:1220-1229, 1979.

85. Roberts CK, Vaziri ND, Barnard RJ: Effect of diet and exercise intervention on blood pressure, insulin, oxidative stress, and nitric oxide availability. Circulation 106:2530-2532, 2002.

86. Mogensen CE, Vittinghus E: Urinary albumin excretion during exercise in juvenile diabetes. A provocation test for early abnormalities. Scand J Clin Lab Invest 35:295-300, 1975.

87. Viberti GC, Jarrett RJ, McCartney M, Keen H: Increased glomerular permeability to albumin induced by exercise in diabetic subjects. Diabetologia 14:293-300, 1978.

88. Albright A, Franz M, Hornsby G, et al: American College of Sports Medicine position stand: Exercise and type 2 diabetes. Med Sci Sports Exerc 32:1345-1360, 2000.

89. American Diabetes Association: Diabetes mellitus and exercise (Position Statement). Diabetes Care 27:S58-S62, 2004.

90. Gurwitz JH, Field TS, Avorn J, et al: Incidence and preventability of adverse drug events in nursing homes. Am J Med 109:87-94, 2000.

91. Arce FCA, Bhasin RS, Pasmantier RM: Severe hyperglycemia during gatifloxacin therapy in patients without diabetes. Endocr Pract 10:40-44, 2004.

Chapter 39

Diabetes in African Americans

Dara P. Schuster and Kwame Osei

KEY POINTS

- *There is greater prevalence of type 2 diabetes mellitus with greater associated morbidity and mortality in African Americans as compared to whites.*
- *African Americans demonstrate greater insulin resistance, decreased hepatic insulin extraction, preserved glucose effectiveness, and rapid decline of beta cell function early in disease evolution when compared to whites.*
- *African Americans demonstrate a greater degree of obesity, and the presence of obesity conveys a greater risk for type 2 diabetes mellitus than in whites.*
- *Cultural, behavioral, and socioeconomic factors and the increased prevalence of hypertension all play a role in worsening health outcomes in type 2 diabetes mellitus in African Americans.*
- *Type 1 diabetes mellitus occurs less frequently in African Americans than in whites, although there is a trend toward increased prevalence in African Americans.*
- *African American women are more likely to have type 1 diabetes mellitus than African American men.*
- *Lifestyle modifications and pharmacologic therapies have been effective in preventing progression of impaired glucose tolerance to type 2 diabetes mellitus in African Americans.*
- *Lifestyle modification and education are priorities for managing type 2 diabetes mellitus.*
- *Early identification and screening of at-risk African Americans is indicated.*
- *Aggressive management of comorbid conditions should help prevent poor health outcomes seen in African Americans.*

African Americans make up the second largest minority population in the United States of America at 38.3 million people or 13.3% of the US population as of March 2002.[1] African Americans are genetically heterogeneous, yet despite the heterogeneity, clear-cut racial and ethnic differences are seen in the presentation and prevalence of certain diseases such as diabetes mellitus. African American adults have a 1.4 times greater prevalence of diagnosed type 2 diabetes mellitus (T2DM) than whites[2] as well as an estimated greater number of undiagnosed cases of T2DM. In contrast, African American children have significantly less incidence of type 1 diabetes mellitus (T1DM) when compared to whites.[2] Regional variations in the prevalence and presentation of T1DM and T2DM are seen across the United States.

Approximately 11.4% of African Americans age 20 years or older have diabetes mellitus, and the percentage increases to 25% by 65 years of age. African American women appear to be adversely affected at an earlier age, with 25% prevalence for women older than 55 years.[3] In addition, African American youth and adolescents are experiencing a disproportionate growth of adolescent T2DM at a rate of 7.2 cases per 1000 population.[4] In fact, according to Pinhas-Hamiel and colleagues,[5] the prevalence of T2DM in the African American youth increased 10-fold in less than a decade.

In addition to greater diabetes prevalence, African Americans also suffer greater morbidity and mortality associated with diabetes. They have 4 to 6 times more end-stage renal disease,[6,7] 2 to 4 times more amputations for nontrauma causes,[8] and 2 to 4 times more retinopathy[9] when compared to whites.

The etiology for these differences in disease prevalence and complication rates is unclear, but it is thought to be related to genetic and environmental differences. Among these are obesity and decreased physical activity. There are clearly unique properties of glucose dysregulation and obesity in African Americans when compared to whites. The purpose of this chapter is to describe the etiopathogenesis, the genetic and environmental factors, and the potential prevention strategies for T2DM in African Americans.

Pathogenesis of Type 2 Diabetes in African Americans

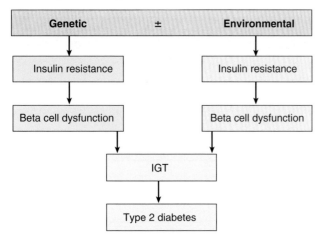

Figure 39–1. Pathogenesis of type 2 diabetes in African Americans. IGT, impaired glucose tolerance.

PATHOGENESIS OF TYPE 2 DIABETES IN AFRICAN AMERICANS

T2DM is characterized by overproduction of glucose by the liver, peripheral insulin resistance, and beta cell dysfunction.[10] Persons with T2DM often manifest any combination of these three abnormalities in varying degrees of severity. It is unknown how the cascade of these abnormalities contributes to the hyperglycemia and diabetes mellitus in African Americans. Pathogenesis of T2DM is shown in Figure 39–1.

Beta Cell Function

All persons with T2DM have some degree of beta cell dysfunction. Beta cell dysfunction has also been demonstrated in the setting of impaired glucose tolerance (IGT). In people of African ancestry, acute first-phase insulin release is diminished, indicating beta cell secretory deficiency in the early, mild T2DM similar to that seen in other populations.[11-15] However, Joffe and coworkers[14] demonstrated prospectively in South African blacks a rapid deterioration of beta cell function when compared to South African whites. Osei and colleagues demonstrated that beta cell function is severely decreased in mild forms of T2DM in Ghanaian immigrants to the United States,[12] native Ghanaians,[16,17] and African Americans.[13] They[17] also showed that normal glucose-tolerant African Americans who are predisposed to T2DM manifest reduced beta cell function 6 to 8 years prior to diagnosis of T2DM.

The presence of significant beta cell dysfunction early in the disease process was also seen in the Insulin Resistance and Atherosclerosis Study.[11,18] Banerji and coworkers[19] reported decreased beta cell

function in African Americans with newly diagnosed T2DM who partially recovered during remission of hyperglycemia. Wing's group[15] studied black patients from South Africa who resided in the United States. They demonstrated that treatment with sulfonylureas resulted in restoration of beta cell function and insulin sensitivity in this African American population.

Similar findings were demonstrated in African American patients who underwent remission and maintained normoglycemia during sulfonylurea therapy.[20] Osei and colleagues[21] demonstrated that beta cell function is modestly improved in African Americans who have IGT and are using a sulfonylurea. The sulfonylurea therapy restored physiologic beta cell secretion following intravenous glucose infusion.

Two other large prospective studies have examined insulin secretion, action, and cardiovascular risk factors. The Bogalusa Heart Study[22] and the CARDIA (Coronary Artery Risk Development in Young Adults) study[23] demonstrated that insulin and cardiovascular risk factors track with aging from puberty to adulthood in nondiabetic African Americans. Because these young adults have not yet developed IGT or diabetes, the magnitude of change in beta cell function is unknown.

Hepatic Insulin Extraction

Insulin action is regulated by the amount of circulating insulin, and circulating insulin, in turn, depends on insulin secretion from the pancreas and insulin clearance from the circulation.

Several studies have documented that nondiabetic and diabetic African Americans have greater insulin resistance or decreased peripheral glucose disposal when compared with whites. The reasons for this are unclear but could be partly ascribed to genetics.

The peripheral hyperinsulinemia found in persons with insulin resistance is due to beta cell hypersecretion and defective insulin clearance. The insulin clearance occurs primarily from the liver, and impaired insulin clearance is closely associated with obesity and altered fat metabolism. In addition to decreased insulin sensitivity, insulin secretion and clearance are also abnormal in the setting of T2DM. Altered hepatic insulin extraction has been noted in several diabetic and nondiabetic ethnic populations when compared to whites.[24]

Osei and colleagues[25] demonstrated decreased hepatic insulin extraction as a very early abnormality in nondiabetic, normal, glucose-tolerant, at-risk African Americans when compared with nondiabetic at-risk whites (Fig. 39–2). In one study, basal and postprandial hepatic insulin extractions were 33% and 45% lower, respectively, in African Americans when compared to whites.[25] Similar findings have been seen in Afro-Caribbeans living

genetic abnormality has been found. In fact, it is unclear whether the concept is universal.

When examining the genetic contribution for increased disease rates, it is important to remember that people of African descent are genetically and phenotypically heterogeneous. In addition, African Americans have at least 25% genetic admixture with Native Americans and whites. These factors might influence metabolic and anthropometric parameters in comparing people of African descent living in a diversity of environments.

Despite the limited metabolic and anthropometric data on recent immigrants from Africa, there are observations that address the thrifty genotype or the thrifty phenotype concept. First, disparity in prevalence rates for T2DM, obesity, and IGT (by 5-fold to10-fold) exist in blacks living in the United States and the United Kingdom when compared to Africans living in their native countries and Afro-Caribbeans living in Jamaica.[78,83]

Second, in the United Kingdom and the United States, black populations demonstrate the prevalence rate for T2DM of 12% versus 0.5% to 2.3% in most African countries, with a total glucose dysregulation burden of 5%.[19,78,83,84] Cameroonians in rural or urban areas have very low rates of diabetes.[85] Cooper and colleagues[83] reported a prevalence rate of diabetes in Nigeria of 2%, which is similar to rates in most parts of Africa. Data on native Ghanaians revealed a prevalence of 5% for T2DM.[86] The rates increase to 5% in Jamaica. These studies found that increasing BMI was closely correlated to increasing rates of T2DM. This association tended to parallel the intensity of westernization and duration of the migration. Similar associations have been seen in Polynesians and Nauruans.

Third, there is no consensus on the metabolic predictors of insulin resistance and hyperinsulinemia, obesity, and T2DM in people of African ancestry. For example, in Pima Indians and whites, insulin resistance and hyperinsulinemia are major risk factors for T2DM; in African Americans the risk is unknown. Banerji and coworkers[19] reported insulin resistance in 40% of African Americans with T2DM, and Haffner's group[18] reported that 14% of their African American population was insulin sensitive in the IRAS study, in agreement with other studies in African Americans. The differences in these studies might reflect the heterogeneity of the study populations, the study design, aerobic capacity, genetic admixture, location, obesity, and definition of insulin resistance.

Presence of obesity tends to correlate with T2DM and hyperinsulinemia, but the relationship between the conventional anthropometric risk factors and insulin sensitivity is very weak in people of African origin, such as African Americans. Finally, in the presence of obesity, there appears to be an attenuated beta cell response to stimulation in people of African ancestry as noted by Osei and colleagues,[12,13,87,88] Joffe and colleagues,[14] and Wing and colleagues[15] when compared to obese white counterparts.

CONTRIBUTORS TO MORBIDITY AND MORTALITY IN AFRICAN AMERICANS WITH TYPE 2 DIABETES MELLITUS

Hypertension

There is greater prevalence of hypertension in African Americans than in whites. Yet the link of hypertension to diabetes and hyperinsulinemia has been variable. In whites, insulin resistance and fasting insulin levels correlate with blood pressure levels with or without hypertension.[89] Although hypertension and hyperinsulinemia and insulin resistance are common in African Americans, the relationship has been weak.

Saad and colleagues[90] and Osei and colleagues[91] found no significant relationship between hypertension and hyperinsulinemia and insulin resistance in African Americans. In the CARDIA study[23] and the Bogalusa Heart study,[22] only a weak relationship was demonstrated between these young adults and adolescent African Americans.

Faulkner and coworkers[92] found a negative relationship between insulin sensitivity and blood pressure in young offspring of African Americans with borderline hypertension. We have found that the rates of hypertension were similar in African Americans and native Ghanaians (30% versus 28%), but the rates of obesity and T2DM were twofold greater in African Americans than in Ghanaians. The reasons for this disparity are unclear.

Heart Disease

Heart disease is seen with increased frequency in the setting of diabetes. The prevalence of heart disease in African Americans has been a topic of debate since the mid-1980s. It was originally thought that the incidence of coronary artery disease was significantly lower in African Americans than in whites. In the NHANES I epidemiologic follow-up, Gillum and coworkers[93] demonstrated a higher incidence of heart disease in African American women aged 25 to 54 than in white women of the same age and a lower incidence in African American men 25 to 74 than in white men of the same age.

The higher rate of coronary heart disease in African American women was explained by a greater number of risk factors. Statistically significant differences in coronary artery disease in ethnic populations have been inconsistently found. Studies have tended to demonstrate lower rates of heart disease in African American men compared to white men,[93] although the rates of coronary heart disease are increasing in both African

American men and women.[94,95] Studies have found that elevated systolic blood pressure, diabetes, cigarette smoking, and, less consistently, cholesterol levels are independent risk factors for coronary heart disease in African American men and women.[11,78,93-95]

In addition to coronary artery disease, Dwyer's group[96] demonstrated that systolic and diastolic dysfunction are common in patients with normal coronary arteries who have hypertension, diabetes, or obesity. Because these risk factors are so common and severe in the African American population, myocardial disease is significantly more common in this segment of the population.

Lipid Abnormalities

Lipid abnormalities and their role in coronary artery disease are well established in several populations.[94,95,97] In general, African Americans manifest higher levels of high-density lipoprotein (HDL) cholesterol with greater apolipoprotein A-II levels and lower triglyceride levels when compared to whites.[97] Fasting serum triglycerides or free fatty acid levels are often found to be low in obese African Americans, especially women, when compared to men.[98] Cook and colleagues[99] found no difference in percentage of low-density lipoprotein (LDL) cholesterol levels in high-, intermediate-, and low-risk categories in African Americans versus whites. However, HDL cholesterol was significantly better in African Americans, with 41%, 33%, and 26% in the high-, borderline-, and low-risk categories, respectively, compared with 73%, 18%, and 9% of whites. Nearly 81% of African Americans had triglycerides that were in the low-risk category compared with 50% of whites.

Despite this favorable lipid profile, the incidence of coronary artery disease and its associated comorbidities in African Americans is increasing. This increase appears to parallel the higher rates of obesity in African Americans, especially in women. Thus, the favorable lipid profile might not confer the same amount of cardioprotection as seen in whites.[93,95]

Hypertension, coronary artery disease, and lipid abnormalities are significant health concerns in African Americans, particularly in the setting of diabetes. Each of these medical issues requires aggressive management, given the deleterious impact of this combination of medical problems. For hypertension, angiotensin converting enzyme (ACE) inhibitors with a thiazide diuretic offer both control of blood pressure and renal protection. But regardless of the medication used, blood pressure management is paramount in the setting of diabetes.

For coronary artery disease, there are no race-specific or ethnicity-specific medications. β-Blockers (even in the setting of diabetes) and aspirin are proven effective. Treatment of hyperlipidemia is evolving. Although there are no race-specific therapies, aggressive lowering of cholesterol, particularly LDL-cholesterol, in the setting of diabetes is recommended. Treatment goals for LDL cholesterol in the setting of diabetes have been lower than 100 mg/dL, but recent data have suggested that lowering LDL cholesterol to less than 80 mg/dL will provide greater cardiovascular protection.

There are limited studies examining the efficacy of HMG-CoA (3-hydroxy-3-methylglutaryl coenzyme A) reductase inhibitors (statins) specifically in African Americans. One such study by Prisant and coworkers[100] demonstrated both efficacy and safety in the use of lovastatin in Africans.

Socioeconomic Factors

In the United States, there is an unequal burden of adverse medical outcomes and inequalities in health care experienced by African Americans,[101-103] and this could play a role in the increased morbidity and mortality seen in diabetes mellitus. In a study by Davis and coworkers,[103] the rate of hospitalization for diabetes among African American men was approximately five times higher than that observed for Asian men and four times higher than that of both white and Hispanic men. African American women exhibited a ninefold higher rate of diabetes hospitalizations than Asian women and an approximately fourfold higher rate than white and Hispanic women, suggesting inequalities in the quality of primary care.

Musey and colleagues[104] reported in an urban African American population that diabetic ketoacidosis (DKA) occurred most often in patients with known diabetes who stopped insulin therapy because of reported lack of money for purchasing insulin or for transportation to the hospital and because of limited self-care skills in diabetes management. In this study population, up to two thirds of the episodes of DKA might have been prevented by better patient education and access to care.

There appears to be a gap in patient education or patient understanding on diagnosis versus ongoing management. In an attempt to understand the barriers in diabetes management in African Americans, Nurss and colleagues[105] formed a discussion group of African Americans with diabetes and their families. The problem areas identified included dietary, habitual, economic, social, and conceptual issues. Diet issues included difficulty following the food-exchange system and analyzing food labels. Recommendations included revising diet strategies to provide appropriate menus, identify low-cost foods, involve patients' families, and teach patients how to make healthy food choices.

These studies emphasize the need to be aware of ethnic diet habits and economic issues in food selection as well as to provide ongoing education about complicated issues such as food exchange.

Finally, it is important for health care providers to identify functional health literacy, which has been found to be deficient in some studies of urban, underserved African Americans, to recognize the barriers to adequate health care, and to provide useful educational materials.

Cultural Factors

Members of various ethnic and racial groups have social norms about desirable body shapes or sizes that are different from norms of middle class Americans or the medical establishment. Studies have demonstrated that Native Americans, African Americans, and Hispanics perceive larger body sizes as healthier, more attractive, and more powerful.[106-108] This cultural attitude may play a role in the acceptance of obesity as a healthy state, yet in African Americans, obesity has been found to have a greater deleterious impact than is seen in whites.

Behavioral Factors

Multiple studies have demonstrated an increased risk of smoking and sedentary lifestyle in the African American population.[109,110] Relative to whites with diabetes mellitus, African Americans with diabetes mellitus were associated respectively with 25% and 58% increased odds of smoking and sedentary lifestyle, adjusting for diagnosed diabetes and other confounding variables. Winckleby and colleagues[109] demonstrated higher rates of smoking, and in this study non-Hispanic black diabetic women had a higher prevalence of smoking and sedentary lifestyle and lower rates of diagnosed diabetes compared with non-Hispanic white women ($P < 0.01$).

Regular physical activity is a protective factor against T2DM and, conversely, lack of physical activity is a risk factor for developing diabetes. Multiple studies have attempted to identify racial differences in lifestyle, exercise, and eating habits in African Americans. Results have been variable. Researchers suspect that a lack of exercise is one factor contributing to the high rates of diabetes in African Americans. In the NHANES III survey, 50% of African American men and 67% of African American women reported that they participated in little or no leisure time physical activity.[74]

Wood and coworkers,[111] studying adults with diabetes, looked at differences in exercise among African Americans, Mexican Americans, and whites. The study demonstrated that the ethnicity of those who did not report exercise in the past month was nearly equally distributed among the three groups, although a higher percentage of African Americans and Mexican Americans did not exercise at all. The ethnic distribution of those participants who did not exercise at all was nearly equal: 34% of whites, 38% of the African Americans, and 39% of the Mexican Americans did not report exercise in the past month.

McNabb, and coworkers[112] demonstrated significant weight loss and improvement in blood glucose control with an 18-week walking program in African Americans with T2DM, although blood glucose control was not maintained at a 1-year follow-up. Lasco's group[113] and Baranowski's group[114] demonstrated variable success in terms of fitness, weight reduction, and blood pressure from exercise programs in nondiabetic African Americans.

Clearly there are modifiable risk factors that could affect the staggering rates of obesity and T2DM in the African American population. Lifestyle modifications such as weight reduction, cessation of smoking, and increasing exercise could play a substantial role in improving outcomes in African Americans with diabetes. Greater education in the community and continued review of these issues with patients in the physician's office on an ongoing basis will be necessary to promote health and overcome some of the lifelong detrimental behavior in African Americans.

OTHER SYNDROMES OF DIABETES IN AFRICAN AMERICANS

Type 1 Diabetes Mellitus

Although the majority of diabetes seen in the African American population is T2DM, there are a significant and increasing number of African Americans with T1DM.[2] However, African American children have lower rates of T1DM than white children, with incidence rates of 3.3 to 11.8 per 100,000 in African Americans versus 13.8 to 16.9 per 100,000 in white children.

The variation in incidence of T1DM in African Americans is thought to be related to environmental as well as white genetic admixture. This has been demonstrated using regional population studies. In a northern area, Allegheny County, Pennsylvania, with a white admixture of 21.2%, the incidence is 11.8 per 100,000 per year. In contrast, in a southern area, Jefferson County, Alabama, the incidence is 4.4 per 100,000 and the white admixture is 17.9%.[2] A racial difference in distribution of cases by gender also exists in the United States, with a female excess in African Americans versus male predominance in white children.[115,116]

Although the prevalence of T1DM is lower in African Americans when compared to whites, the African American group has significantly more problems associated with management of the disease as noted by more hospitalizations,[117,118] worse glucose control in the form of higher hemoglobin A1c,[119,120] and more complications.[121] One report by the DERI Mortality Study Group[121]

reported a twofold excess mortality in African Americans with T1DM when compared to whites with T1DM.

The etiology for the poor outcomes in African Americans appears to be multifactorial and related to lack of education, reduced access to health services, single-parent households, and low economic status. The health care team must be aware of these health care discrepancies and help correct them. Close follow-up and ongoing education are necessary to reverse this trend in diabetes management.

Atypical Diabetes in African Americans

Nonautoimmune ketosis-prone T2DM is a unique form of diabetes seen with increasing frequency in nonwhite populations.[122] This form of atypical T2DM occurs most commonly in young persons of African or Asian descent (male incidence greater than female incidence), with severe ketoacidosis. When compared with T1DM, genetic predisposition is stronger, presentation is older, BMI is greater, ketoacidosis is more severe, and autoimmune markers are absent. Beta cell decline is significantly slower, with 40% of one study cohort remaining insulin independent for 10 years after diagnosis if they had achieved insulin independence after the first relapse.[122] As with T2DM, insulin resistance is present, but unlike with T2DM, insulin resistance is reversible with achievement of euglycemia, beta cells appear to be more sensitive to glucose toxicity, and ketoacidosis is common.

Mauvais-Jarvis and coworkers[122] demonstrated relapse of beta cell failure associated with a 12-month period of increased hyperglycemia. With conventional therapy, the patients typically become insulin independent. In one study cohort, insulin-independent ketosis-prone T2DM was seen in approximately 77%, with 23% of the group demonstrating insulin-dependent, ketosis-prone T2DM. However, the group of insulin-dependent, ketosis-prone T2DM subjects retained 22% of beta cell secretory capacity after 5 years, whereas little to no insulin secretion is seen in T1DM by 1 to 2 years after diagnosis. Although the insulin-independent ketosis-prone T2DM group had long periods of euglycemic remissions, relapse rates of 90% were seen within 10 years.[122]

Obesity is thought to play an important role in the pathophysiology of this form of diabetes. The majority of patients are overweight, and increases in weight precede both initial presentation and subsequent relapses.[123] This is particularly apparent in African American and Hispanic children; 50% of new cases of diabetes are T2DM, yet 25% to 40% of these new patients present in diabetic ketoacidosis.

Another atypical syndrome of diabetes in African Americans is characterized by resistance to ketosis and periods of normal blood glucose followed by subsequent hyperglycemic relapse. This atypical syndrome includes maturity-onset diabetes of youth in African Americans and the syndrome of phasic insulin dependence in Jamaica, which is also reported in the United States.[124,125]

In general, treatment of insulin-deficient diabetes requires the use of insulin regardless of the specific diabetic syndrome. No racial differences have been seen in efficacy of insulin.

PREVENTION OF TYPE 2 DIABETES IN AFRICAN AMERICANS

Investigators[126-128] have previously demonstrated that African Americans with and without IGT and T2DM manifest higher peripheral hyperinsulinemia and greater insulin resistance when compared with their white counterparts. Thus, nondiabetic African Americans with IGT could be targeted for primary diabetes prevention as a means of reducing the burden and complications of diabetes.

The Study to Prevent Non–Insulin-Dependent Diabetes Mellitus (STOP-NIDDM) Trial[129] examined impaired glucose tolerance over the course of 3.3 years. The study demonstrated that acarbose reduced the risk of progression to T2DM by 25% in patients with IGT, although this study did not address particular ethnic groups. STOP-NIDDM participants who received acarbose were later found to have less hypertension and fewer cardiovascular events than those who received placebo, suggesting additional benefit with treatment of IGT.[130]

The Troglitazone in the Prevention of Diabetes (TRIPOD) study[131] demonstrated a 56% risk reduction in development of T2DM over 30 months for Hispanic women with previous gestational diabetes. In this regard, the Diabetes Prevention Program (DPP) demonstrated that lifestyle modification (diet and exercise with 7% weight loss) and metformin reduced the incidence of T2DM in patients with IGT by 58% and 31%, respectively, in all US ethnic populations, including African Americans.[132]

Osei and colleagues[21] studied subjects who were obese, had IGT, and were first-degree relatives of African American patients with T2DM. They demonstrated that chronic low-dose gastrointestinal therapeutic system (GITS) therapy over 24 months in these subjects prevented glycemic deterioration, improved beta cell responses (acute phase and total) to glucose stimulation, and improved disposition index. Chronic GITS therapy was also associated with improved insulin sensitivity. Thus, this preliminary study suggests that chronic GITS could be useful in the primary prevention of T2DM in obese African Americans with IGT (Fig. 39–3).

In a study using troglitazone in normoglycemic African Americans with a first-degree relative with T2DM, Schuster and coworkers[133] found that troglitazone had a modest positive impact on insulin

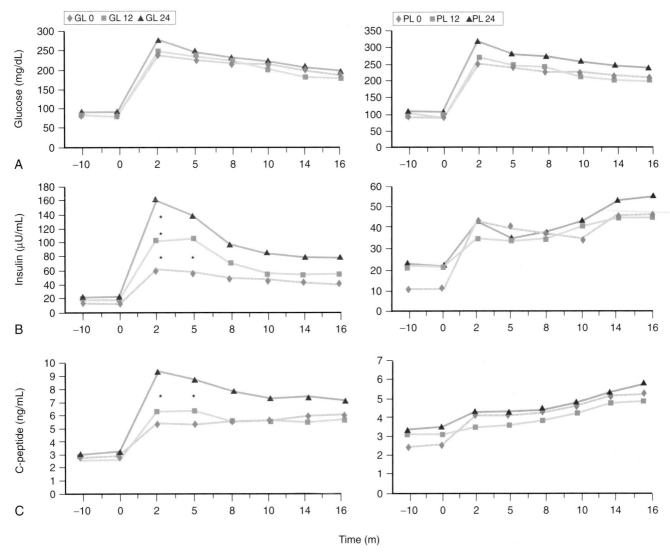

Figure 39–3. Serum glucose **(A)**, insulin **(B)**, and c-peptide **(C)** responses to the intravenous glucose tolerance test in African Americans who have impaired glucose tolerance and were treated with glipizide (GL) or placebo (PL) for 24 months. (Adapted from Osei K, Rinesmith S, Gaillard T, et al: Beneficial metabolic effects of chronic glipizide in obese African Americans with impaired glucose tolerance: Implications for primary prevention of type 2 diabetes. Metabolism 53:414-422, 2004.)

sensitivity and glucose homeostasis, including improvement in overall beta cell response to glucose, pancreatic compensation for insulin resistance, and improved insulin sensitivity. Based on these data, the treatment of normal glucose-tolerant, high-risk African Americans with troglitazone or possibly another thiazolidenedione (TZD) may be beneficial in order to reset and protect glucose metabolism.

These studies demonstrate that pharmacologic therapy using antidiabetic drugs can delay the onset of T2DM in patients with IGT.[129-132] These drugs all lower ambient blood glucose, but each drug class affects the glucose dysregulation of T2DM by a different mechanism.[134-136] It is unclear whether simply lowering mean blood glucose can reduce the risk of developing T2DM or whether it is the drug effect on particular targets of glucose dysregulation or

other unknown drug effects that allow for the decrease in the incidence of T2DM in IGT. Understanding the mechanism of action in nondiabetic patients will be particularly important in the long-term use of these medications.

MANAGEMENT OF DIABETES MELLITUS IN AFRICAN AMERICANS

Given the increased prevalence of T2DM, the significant number of undiagnosed cases, and the propensity for earlier and more-severe complications, early recognition and screening is a necessity in African Americans. Health care professionals should have a low threshold for evaluation of T2DM in African Americans. This need for aggres-

sive screening should also be recognized in obese African American children, given the epidemiologic data indicating epidemic increases in T2DM in young members of some ethnic populations.

Lifestyle modification should be the backbone for the treatment plan of all patients with T2DM. Based on the literature, lifestyle issues are a significant problem in the African American community and others. African Americans have a high propensity for sedentary lifestyle, smoking, and poor diet choices. This issue should be addressed at regular visits to health care professionals, and education should be provided on an ongoing basis. Lifestyle modification, although typically not enough to solely manage T2DM and its associated conditions, should be the cornerstone of therapy. Modest lifestyle modifications have proved to be very effective therapies in African Americans.

Drug therapy for T2DM is now being directed toward the specific defects discussed earlier. Health care professionals are just beginning to tailor drug therapy to the disease process. In particular, we now have drugs that treat peripheral insulin resistance (TZDs, biguanides) and hepatic insulin resistance (biguanides) as well as drugs that stimulate beta cell secretion (sulfonylureas). Early studies using TZDs in rodents demonstrated improvement in beta cell secretion and possibly beta cell regeneration. In the future, drugs that can rejuvenate or regenerate the beta cells themselves could be used to treat the hyperglycemia of T2DM and could also be used in the setting of impaired glucose tolerance or even earlier, when beta cell function is just starting to decline. With the known early decline of beta cell function, drug therapy that treats this defect will be particularly important to the African American population with glucose dysregulation.

Currently there are no race-specific or ethnicity-specific therapies for the management of T2DM, but development of unique treatments based on the defect present in the disease could provide for better blood glucose control and fewer complications. Metformin has been studied in African American adults and children and found to be safe and effective.[137] The TZDs and sulfonylureas have been studied in other ethnic groups and found to be effective in adults. Studies using TZDs are limited in the pediatric population, but as more data emerge on safety, we anticipate increased use of this drug class in children.

As part of the management of T2DM in African Americans, early screening for complications such as microalbuminuria is indicated due to the early presentation and severity of complications in the population. Aggressive management of comorbid conditions such as hypertension, hyperlipidemia, and obesity is encouraged.

Due to the complicated nature of the management of diabetes and associated medical conditions, ongoing education is a priority and needs to be tailored to the cultural and ethnic background of the patients being treated, because many of these disease processes are asymptomatic and treatment can be a financial burden.

CONCLUSION

In a projection of the diabetes burden through 2050, it was noted that African Americans will be the fastest growing ethnic group with diagnosed diabetes.[138] Estimates include a 363% increase in prevalence of diabetes in black men and a 217% increase in black women, as compared with a 148% increase in white men and 107% increase in white women.[138]

Ethnicity and race will continue to play a significant role in predisposition to diabetes. Understanding the impact of race and ethnicity on glucose regulation, insulin sensitivity and insulin metabolism, body composition, and adipose tissue–derived peptides could have profound implications in the prevention and management of diabetes in African Americans.

References

1. McKinnon J: The black population in the United States: March 2002. U.S. Census Bureau, Current Population Reports, Series p20-541. Washington DC, 2003. http://www.census.gov/prod/2003pub5/p20-541.pdf
2. Tull ES, Roseman JM: Diabetes in African Americans. In Harris M (ed): Diabetes in America, 2nd ed. Bethesda: National Institutes of Health, 1995, pp 613-630.
3. Davidson, MB: The disproportionate burden of diabetes in African-American and Hispanic populations. Ethn Dis 11:148-151, 2001.
4. Willi, SM, Egede LE: Type 2 diabetes mellitus in adolescents. Curr Opin Endocr Diabetes 7: 71-76, 2000.
5. Pinhas-Hamiel O, Dolan LM, Daniels SR et al: Increased incidence of non–insulin-dependent diabetes mellitus among adolescents. J Pediatr 128:608-615, 1996.
6. Cowie CC, Port FK, Wolfe RA, et al: Disparities in incidence of diabetic end-stage renal disease according to race and type of diabetes. N Engl J Med 321:1074-1079, 1989.
7. Smith SR, Svetkey LP, Dennis VW: Racial differences in the incidence and progression of renal diseases. Kidney Int 40:815-822, 1991.
8. Reiber GE, Boyko EJ, Smith DG: Lower extremity foot ulcers and amputations in diabetes. In Harris M (ed): Diabetes in America, 2nd edition. Bethesda, Md, National Institutes of Health, 1995, pp 409-428.
9. Harris M, Klein R, Cowie CC, et al: Is the risk of diabetic retinopathy greater in non-Hispanic blacks and Mexican Americans than in non-Hispanic whites with type 2 diabetes? A U.S. population study. Diabetes Care 21:1230-1235, 1998.
10. Harris MI, Flegal KM, Cowie CC, et al: Prevalence of diabetes, impaired fasting glucose, and impaired glucose tolerance in U.S. adults. The Third National Health and Nutrition Examination Survey, 1988-1994. Diabetes Care 21:518-524, 1998.
11. Haffner S, Howard G, Savage P, et al: Insulin sensitivity and acute insulin responses in African Americans, non-Hispanic whites, and Hispanics with NIDDM: The Insulin Resistance and Atherosclerosis Study. Diabetes 46:63-69, 1997.
12. Osei K, Schuster D: Decreased insulin-mediated but not noninsulin-dependent glucose disposal rates in glucose intolerance and type II diabetes in African (Ghanaian) immigrants. Am J Med Sci 311:113-121, 1996.

Chapter 41

Diabetes in Asians

Rajendra Pradeepa and Viswanathan Mohan

KEY POINTS

- *Two thirds of the world's diabetic persons live in the developing world, predominantly in Asia. Type 2 diabetes accounts for more than 90% of all diabetic cases.*
- *By 2030, there are likely to be 366 million diabetic patients globally. Seven of the top 10 countries in the world will be in Asia, with India having the largest number of diabetic patients in the world.*
- *Prevalence of diabetes in China is increasing (greater than threefold increase) with economic development and changes from a traditional to modernized lifestyle. The rise in type 2 diabetes in children has been reported in Japan (seven times more common than type 1 diabetes).*
- *Malaysia and Singapore have shown a striking rise within one to two decades, but studies in Vietnam indicate that the diabetes prevalence rates are still relatively low.*
- *In Asian countries, the prevalence of impaired glucose tolerance is consistently higher than the diabetes prevalence rates, which substantiates the fact that the diabetes pandemic is still rising.*
- *Migrant Asian populations, mostly in people originating from India, have a higher prevalence of diabetes than the native populations of the host countries.*
- *Strong familial aggregation, higher insulin levels, lifestyle changes (especially physical inactivity due to industrialization and urbanization), and adoption of a low-fiber, high-fat diet have been largely responsible for the increasing prevalence rates of obesity leading to type 2 diabetes and associated complications in Asian populations, particularly in Indians.*
- *Future research and prevention strategies for diabetes in Asians should emphasize reducing the impact of this epidemic by focusing on lifestyle changes (increasing physical activity and consumption of traditional high-fiber diets) and prevention of obesity, particularly in highly susceptible populations.*

The epidemiology of diabetes in Asian countries is of prime importance because Asia is comprised of some of the most densely populated countries in the world, including the largest country, China, which contains 20% of the world's population (1.2 billion), India, the second-largest country with a population of 1 billion, Indonesia, the fourth largest country, with a population of about 200 million and Pakistan, the sixth largest with a population of more than 150 million. The people of Asia constitute 60% of the world's population.

Diabetes poses a major health problem globally and is one of the top five leading causes of death in most developed countries. A substantial body of evidence suggests that it could reach epidemic proportions, particularly in developing and newly industrialized countries. Wild and coworkers[1] have projected that the global prevalence of type 2 diabetes (T2DM) will rise from 171 million in 2000 to 366 million by 2030. This figure is 11% higher than the previous estimate of 154 million.[2] The International Diabetes Federation (IDF) independently has made similar estimates.[3]

As shown in Table 41–1, of the predicted top 10 countries in terms of the number of diabetic persons in 2030, seven are in Asia. The figures for India, which currently has the largest numbers of diabetic patients, are predicted to rise from 31.7 million in 2000 to 79.4 million in 2030, and for China the increase is from 20.8 million in 2000 to 42.3 million by 2030.[1]

There are two main forms of diabetes.[4] Type 1 diabetes (T1DM; formerly called *insulin dependent*) is primarily due to autoimmune-mediated destruction of pancreatic beta cells, resulting in absolute insulin deficiency.[5] T2DM (formerly called *non–insulin dependent*) is characterized by insulin resistance or abnormal insulin secretion, or both, either of which may predominate, and accounts for more than 90% of cases globally.[5]

The total number of people with T1DM is on the increase, doubling every decade.[6] T1DM is commonest in Scandinavian populations and is relatively rare in Asians. There is an almost 60-fold difference between the countries with the highest incidence of T1DM and those with the lowest.[7]

Table 41–1. *Top Ten Countries for Estimated Number of Adults with Diabetes, 2000 and 2030*

Rank	Country	2000 (millions)	Country	2030 (millions)
1	India	**31.7**	India	**79.4**
2	China	**20.8**	China	**42.3**
3	United States	17.7	United States	30.3
4	Indonesia	**8.4**	Indonesia	**21.3**
5	Japan	**6.8**	Pakistan	**13.9**
6	Pakistan	**5.2**	Brazil	11.3
7	Russian Federation	4.6	Bangladesh	**11.1**
8	Brazil	4.6	Japan	**8.9**
9	Italy	4.3	Philippines	**7.8**
10	Bangladesh	**3.2**	Egypt	6.7

Note: Numbers in boldface are for countries in Asia.
From Wild S, Roglic G, Green A, et al: Global prevalence of diabetes: Estimates for the year 2000 and projections for 2030. Diabetes Care 27:1047-1053, 2004.

The prevalence of T2DM varies in different geographic regions and in different ethnic groups.[8] According to the World Health Organization (WHO) Ad Hoc Diabetes Report (1993), age-standardized prevalence rates of diabetes were as high as 14% to 20% in migrant Asian Indians, Chinese, and Latin American populations, whereas prevalence is about 3% to 10% in European populations.[9] Also, various epidemiologic studies have shown that the prevalence of diabetes is significantly higher in ethnic minorities (Asians and Hispanics) as compared to those of European descent (whites) even when exposed to similar environmental conditions.[10]

Noteworthy is the finding that between 1990 and 1998, Asian Americans experienced the highest increase in prevalence rates, and immigrants from India, Pakistan, and Bangladesh have the highest predisposition to develop diabetes.[11] Studies since the 1980s have shown that the prevalence of diabetes is rising in astronomical proportions in Asian populations. This chapter discusses the epidemiology and associated risk factors for diabetes in Asians.

EPIDEMIOLOGY OF DIABETES IN ASIANS

The Asian Pacific region is at the forefront of the current epidemic of diabetes,[1,12] and with its large populations it is of major importance in the epidemiology of diabetes. Studies have shown that race, lifestyle changes, level of affluence, industrialization, and urbanization play a major role in the prevalence of T2DM and impaired glucose tolerance (IGT), which varies markedly throughout Asia.[10,13]

Type 2 Diabetes

This section considers the geographic distribution and secular changes in the prevalence of T2DM in the Asian countries. The Asian population is comprised of South Asians who originate from India, Nepal, Pakistan, Bangladesh, and Sri Lanka; Southeast Asians belonging to Myanmar, Thailand, Cambodia, Laos, Vietnam, the Philippines, Indonesia, Malaysia, Singapore, and Brunei; and East Asians from China, Japan, Korea, Hong Kong, and Taiwan.

South Asia

Epidemiologic data for South Asian countries indicate that these countries, particularly India, contain huge populations with a high prevalence of diabetes. With its population of more than 1 billion, India leads the world with the largest number of diabetic persons.[14,15]

India

The first authentic data on prevalence of diabetes in India came from a multicenter study (Ahmedabad, Calcutta, Cuttack, Delhi, Poona, Trivandrum) conducted by the Indian Council of Medical Research (ICMR) in the early 1970s reporting a prevalence of 2.3% in the urban and 1.5% in the rural areas.[16] Another Indian study conducted in Orissa state[17] has also shown that diabetes prevalence was significantly higher in the urban areas compared to the rural areas. A study in the rural Indian population reported a nearly threefold increase in age- and sex-adjusted prevalence of diabetes (from 2.20% to 6.36%) in 2003 when compared with a similar study done 14 years earlier.[18]

A National Urban Diabetes Survey (NUDS) conducted among Indian urban subjects showed that the age-standardized prevalence of diabetes was 12.1% and the prevalence in the southern part of India was found to be higher—13.5% in Chennai, 12.4% in Bangalore, and 16.6% in Hyderabad—than in eastern India (11.7% in Kolkatta, formerly known as Calcutta), northern India (11.6% in New Delhi), and western India (9.3% in Mumbai).[19] The Chennai Urban Population Study (CUPS), involving two residential areas representing the lower-income and middle-income groups in Chennai, found the overall prevalence of diabetes was 12.0%.[20]

Studies in India have also shown that with affluence, the prevalence of diabetes and related disorders tends to increase.[20,21] Thus subjects in the higher socioeconomic group had a higher risk of developing diabetes. This is in marked contrast to the pattern seen in the developed countries, where an inverse relation between socioeconomic status and diabetes is noted and the prevalence of diabetes is higher in the lower socioeconomic groups.[22]

A review that analyzed the trends in diet transition in India revealed a rapid increase in diet-related noncommunicable diseases, including diabetes.[23] In

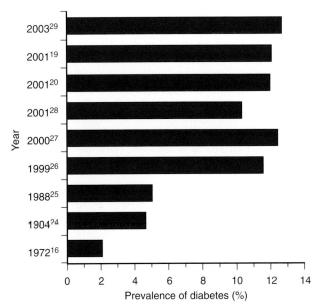

Figure 41–1. Diabetes prevalence in urban India from 1972 to 2003. This graph illustrates the astronomical increase of diabetes from 2.1% to 12.3% during three decades in urban India.

the CUPS study, the age-standardized prevalence of diabetes was significantly higher in the middle-income group than in the low-income group (12.4% versus 6.5%), which clearly demonstrates that with affluence, there is a marked increase in the prevalence rates of diabetes.[20] Figure 41–1 summarizes results of Indian studies that show an escalating prevalence of diabetes even within the Indian subcontinent.[16,19,20,24-29]

Pakistan, Bangladesh, and Sri Lanka
The Pakistan National Diabetes Survey[30] reported that prevalence rates of diabetes in urban and rural men and urban women ranged between 10% and 11%, although a lower prevalence rate was observed in rural women (5%). Although the age-adjusted prevalence of diabetes in 1997[31] in semi-urban Bangladesh was 4.5%, in 2003 in rural areas it was 3.8%.[32] Fernando and coworkers[33,34] reported a diabetes prevalence rate of 5.2% and 6.5% among the suburban Sri Lankan community in 1994 and 2002, respectively.

Southeast Asia
The estimated prevalence of diabetes in Southeast Asians was reported to range between 2% and 5% in 1987.[35]

Malaysia and Indonesia
Studies done in Malaysia and Indonesia also reported similar low estimates for Malays (1% to 2%) in the 1960s and Indonesians (1.5%) in 1976, which could be attributed to the different methodologies and diagnostic criteria used.[36] The national survey conducted in Malaysia in 1997 indicated that the prevalence of diabetes exceeded 8% of the adult population.[37] The prevalence of diabetes in the state of Kelantan in Northeast Peninsular Malaysia (1999) was 10.5%, with no difference in the prevalence between men and women.[38] Studies carried out in different districts of Jakarta, Indonesia, in 1982 and 1992 showed crude prevalence rates of 1.7% and 5.7% respectively, indicating a threefold rise within a decade.[39]

Singapore
Since the 1980s, a rising trend in prevalence of diabetes was observed in the adult population of Singapore, increasing from 1.99% in 1975 to 4.7% in 1984, with a further increase to 9.0% in 1998.[40,41] Both Malaysia and Singapore have shown a striking rise in diabetes prevalence, and studies performed in Singapore also indicate a higher prevalence rate of diabetes among men than women.

Thailand
The first nationwide survey of diabetes conducted in Thailand (1971) by the Diabetic Association of Thailand estimated a prevalence of 2.5% among the 322,953 subjects screened.[42] The International Collaborative Study of Cardiovascular Disease in Asia (2003) estimated the national prevalence of diabetes in Thai adults at 9.6% (2.4 million people), which included 4.8% with previously diagnosed diabetes and 4.8% with newly diagnosed diabetes.[43] However, the prevalence of diabetes in the rural population of Thailand was not low compared to the urban areas. In a study conducted in 13 rural villages of Phon District, Bangkok, the prevalence was 6.7%.[44] The prevalence of diabetes in persons older than 30 years in lower socioeconomic communities of Bangkok in 1990 was 4.5% in slum residents and 5.9% in government apartment residents.[45]

Cambodia, Laos, and Myanmar
No reliable epidemiologic data are available from Cambodia, Laos, or Myanmar, and the magnitude of the problem of diabetes is unknown. Because these countries are in the early stages of epidemiologic transition, it is probable that the diabetes prevalence rates are still relatively low.

Vietnam
Epidemiologic data from Vietnam indicate that the diabetes prevalence rates are quite low. The age-adjusted prevalence rate of diabetes in a survey conducted in Hanoi in 1990 was 1.4%,[46] which was supported by the findings of a survey conducted in Ho Chi Minh City in 1992 reporting a crude prevalence rate of 2.5%.[47] In a cross-sectional study conducted in Ho Chi Minh City in 2001, in 2932 participants aged 15 and older, the crude prevalence of diabetes was 6.6% and prevalence of impaired fasting glucose was 3.2%.[48] This study concluded that aging, a high waist-to-hip ratio, overweight, and a sedentary lifestyle may be important determinants of the increased prevalence of diabetes

during this transition period in Vietnam. Although the prevalence of diabetes in Ho Chi Minh City is lower when compared with some countries in Asia such as Malaysia (10.5%),[38] Indonesia (5.7%),[39] and Thailand (9.6%),[43] the rising trend in prevalence suggests that diabetes will soon be a significant health problem in Vietnam also.

The Philippines
Diabetes was the eighth leading cause of death among Filipinos in 1998.[49] The first national diabetes survey in the Philippines conducted between 1982 and 1983 revealed that the prevalence of diabetes was 4.1%.[50] A survey performed by the Food and Nutrition Research Institute in 1998 reported a 3.9% prevalence of diabetes.[51] In a more recent study of the residents of urban and rural areas in Luzon, the crude diabetes prevalence was 5.1%.[52]

East Asia
Japan
In East Asia, the highest prevalence of T2DM is reported from Japan. Studies on prevalence of diabetes have been conducted in Japan since the early 1960s, and they have reported an adult prevalence rate of 2% to 5%,[53] which increased to 10.2% in 1993.[54] In the rural Funagata area, the prevalence of diabetes (known and newly diagnosed cases combined) in 2000 was 9.1% for men and 10.8% for women.[55] Age-adjusted prevalence of diabetes in men in Hisayama is two times higher than in Funagata (12.8% versus 6.8%).[53,55] It is probable that approximately 7 million people in total have diabetes in Japan,[56] and the incidence rate estimates for T2DM range from 5 to 7 per 1000 person-years.[57]

Recently a rise in T2DM in children has been reported from Japan, and indeed T2DM is reported to be seven times more common than T1DM in children in that country. The incidence of T2DM in children has increased more than 30-fold during the past 20 years.[58]

China
Studies performed in Beijing and Shanghai between 1980 and 1990 reported a consistent prevalence of 1.5% or less.[59,60] However, large-scale epidemiologic studies performed since then indicate a striking increase in prevalence, especially in urban areas. The prevalence of diabetes in China is rapidly increasing with economic development and changes from traditional to modern lifestyle, which is evident from the 10-year prospective study (1986 to 1996) conducted in Da Qing, China. The Da Qing study reported a prevalence of 1% in 1986, but by 1994 the prevalence had risen to 3.5%.[61] In the National Prevalence Survey conducted in 1994, the crude prevalence of diabetes was 2.5%, and the age-standardized prevalence was 2.3%.[62]

Korea
The prevalence of diabetes mellitus in Korea has increased tremendously during the past several

decades. In a recent study conducted in 1108 subjects aged 40 to 99 years living in the Chongup area, adjusted to the Segi world population standard, the prevalence of diabetes was 7.1% by WHO criteria and 7.7% by American Diabetes Association (ADA) criteria.[63] Studies from Hong Kong reported an age-adjusted diabetes prevalence of 7.7%[64] in 1990 and 8.9%[65] in 1995. Although not as high as in Japan, the prevalence of T2DM is also on the increase in adolescents in Hong Kong.[66]

Taiwan
Diabetes is the fifth leading cause of death in Taiwan,[67] and the prevalence was estimated to be between 5.7% and 11.3% in studies conducted in 1980s.[68] A study conducted in Penghu[69] demonstrated an age-adjusted prevalence of T2DM of 16.8%, which is substantially higher than the previously observed prevalence in Chinese populations in mainland China (2%) and Hong Kong (7.7%).[62,64]

Type 1 Diabetes

The incidence of T1DM in Asians seems to be quite low compared to the incidence in other parts of the world. This difference might be attributed to genetic and environmental factors including diet, micronutrient consumption, eating habits, and lifestyle.

India and Pakistan
The incidence of childhood diabetes in Asian populations has been reported to be much lower than that of North American and European populations.[8] Until recently, data on prevalence and incidence of T1DM in Asian countries was sparse. Most of the available data are from the T1DM registries set up in the Asian countries. Based on clinic data, it had been reported that the prevalence of T1DM was low in children in India.[70] In a population-based study conducted in South India in 1991, the prevalence was 0.26 per 1000 (26 per 100,000) children up to 15 years of age.[71] The incidence of T2DM obtained from a registry set up in Chennai for 1991 to 1994 in children in the same age group was 10.5 per 100,000 per year.[72] The incidence of T1DM in Karachi, Pakistan, was estimated to be 0.06 per 100,000 per year.[73]

Thailand
Tuchinda and colleagues[74] reported that 0.08% of children aged birth to 15 years were affected by T1DM in Thailand and that the annual incidence was 0.14 per 100,000 in 1984 and 0.19 per 100,000 in 1985. In northeastern Thailand, the incidence of T1DM in children younger than 15 years was reported as 0.3 per 100,000.[75]

Singapore
In Singapore, the age-standardized incidence rate for the period 1992 to 1994 was 2.46 per 100,000

children birth to 12 years old, which seemed to indicate a rising incidence in that population, the incidence being 1.4 per 100,000 in 1992, 2.4 per 100,000 in 1993, and 3.8 per 100,000 in 1994.[76]

Japan

The prevalence of T1DM in Japanese children is quite low. This was first reported in 1964 by Hososako's group,[77] who found 4 cases among 40,000 children aged birth to 14 years. The prevalence of diabetes from the data of the central registry in Tokyo was 4 or 6 per 100,000 children in 1983.[78] In a population-based epidemiologic study conducted in Hokkaido from 1973 to 1992 (a 20-year study) the mean annual incidence of abrupt-onset T1DM was 1.63 per 100,000 per year.[79]

China

Low prevalence rates of T1DM are also observed in Chinese populations. A nearly 50-fold within-country variation is observed in China, where incidence rates vary from 0.1 per 100,000 per year in Zunyi to 4.6 per 100,000 per year in Wuhan.[80] In a recent survey conducted in the Beijing area, the age-adjusted incidence of T1DM according to the Chinese population census in 2000 was 0.83 per 100,000 in 1988 to 1996 and 0.86 per 100,000 in 1997 to 2000.[81] The age-standardized incidence of T1DM in four districts in Hong Kong during the period 1986 to 1990 was 2.0 per 100,000 per year in children aged younger than 15 years.[82]

Impaired Glucose Tolerance

IGT is defined as plasma glucose values between 141 and 199 mg/dL 2 hours following a 75-g oral glucose load.[5] IGT is considered a stage of prediabetes because persons with IGT are at increased risk for developing diabetes compared with persons who have normal glucose tolerance. Moreover, they are also at greater risk for cardiovascular disease.

In Asian countries, the prevalence of IGT is consistently higher than the diabetes prevalence rates, which suggests that the diabetes pandemic is still rising. A number of epidemiologic studies have been conducted in Asian countries, and these studies have documented high prevalence of IGT among several migrant Asian Indians, lower-income Thais in Bangkok, and Chinese men in Mauritius. Moderate prevalence rates of IGT have been reported in Asian Indians in southern India and in Sri Lankans.[10]

We[20] reported that the age-standardized prevalence rate of IGT was 7.5% in the middle-income group in Chennai in South India, which was significantly higher than the prevalence in the low-income group (2.9%) there. In the National Urban Diabetes Study conducted in India, it was observed that IGT was more prevalent than diabetes

in the younger age group (younger than 40 years).[19] In a study of the Dombivli urban population, the prevalence of IGT was 8.6% in subjects younger than 50 years and 13.4% in subjects older than 50 years. In addition, IGT prevalence increased with age and body mass index (BMI).[83] Patandin and coworkers[84] have reported IGT prevalence (6.6%) to be higher than diabetes prevalence (4.9%) in a rural South Indian population (North Arcot District).

In Bangladesh, Abu Sayeed and colleagues[85] found the age-adjusted prevalence of diabetes to be higher in urban (7.97%) than in rural subjects (3.84%), whereas prevalence of IGT was higher in rural subjects. The higher socioeconomic rural population had a higher prevalence of IGT than their urban counterparts (16.5% versus 4.4%). Higher prevalence of IGT compared to diabetes was also observed in suburban and rural Sri Lanka,[33,86] urban and rural areas of the Philippines,[52] and rural areas of Thailand,[87] Japan,[55] and Korea.[63]

Tan and colleagues[88] have reported the age-standardized prevalence of IGT to be 16.1% in Singapore (Chinese, 16.7%; Malays, 14%; Asian Indians, 13.1%) compared to a diabetes prevalence of 8.4% (Asian Indians, 12.2%; Malays, 10.1%; Chinese, 7.8%). These prevalence rates imply a high risk of IGT in all the three ethnic groups residing in Singapore. In the study conducted in urban and rural areas of Malaysia, the crude prevalence of IGT was higher than the prevalence of diabetes in both of these areas.[89]

However, studies conducted in Japan and China[53,90] have reported a lower prevalence of IGT, implying less risk of IGT in these selected populations. In southern Taiwan, the age-adjusted prevalence of diabetes was 9.2% (men, 10.4%; women, 8.1%) and that of IGT was 15.5% (men, 15.0%; women, 15.9%).[91] The prevalence rate of diabetes and IGT have been compared in selected Asian countries and summarized in Table 41-2.*

EPIDEMIOLOGY OF DIABETES IN MIGRANT ASIANS

Migration (a move from one environment to another, be it external or internal) can lead to an increase in the prevalence of T2DM in a number of ethnic groups in parallel with social and cultural changes.[92] Studies of diabetes in migrant populations thus offer a unique opportunity to observe the effects of genetic and environmental interaction. In addition, the data collected can be useful indicators of potential rates in the country of origin. These studies have provided insights into the importance of environmental factors as determinants of T2DM and could help in planning preventive measures.

*References 19,20,30,33,46,52,54,55,62-64,84-91

Table 41–2. *Prevalence Rate of Diabetes and IGt in Selected Countries in Asia*

Country	Author, Year	Area	Prevalence (%)	
			T2DM	IGT
India	Mohan et al, 2001[20]	Urban*	12.0	5.9
	Ramachandran et al, 2001[19]	Urban‡	12.1	14.0
	Patandin et al, 1994[84]	Rural*	4.9	6.6
Pakistan	Shera et al, 1999[30]	Urban‡	10.8	11.9
		Rural‡	6.5	11.2
Bangladesh	Abu Sayeed et al, 1997[85]	Urban*	8.0	4.8
		Rural*	3.9	11.8
Sri Lanka	Fernando et al, 1994[33]	Suburban‡	5.0	5.3
	Illangasekera et al, 1993[86]	Rural*	2.5	8.0
Vietnam	Quoc et al, 1994[46]	Urban*	1.2	1.6
Thailand	Chaisiri et al, 1997[87]	Rural*	11.9	18.1
Philippines	Baltazar et al, 2004[52]	Urban‡	5.1	8.2
		Rural‡	4.8	7.4
Singapore	Tan et al, 1999[88]	General‡	8.4	16.1
Malaysia	Ali et al, 1993[89]	Urban*	8.2	9.6
		Rural*	6.7	10.5
Japan	Ohmura et al, 1993[54]	General*	10.9	19.8
	Sekikawa et al, 2000[55]	Rural*	10.1	14.5
China	Shi et al, 1998[90]	Urban*	2.3	1.3
	Pan et al, 1997[62]	General*	2.5	3.2
Korea	Park et al, 2000[63]	Rural‡	8.1	12.4
Hong Kong	Cockram et al, 1993[64]	General*	4.5	7.3
Taiwan	Lu et al, 1998[91]	Urban‡	9.2	15.5

*Crude prevalence
‡Age-adjusted prevalence
T2DM, type 2 diabetes mellitus; IGT, impaired glucose tolerance.

Indian Migrants

Many epidemiologic studies of diabetes in migrant Asian populations report a higher prevalence of diabetes than the host populations of those countries.[93-95] Most of these studies are of people originating from India. Asian Indian men had a four times higher prevalence of diabetes than their British counterparts.[94] Similarly, higher prevalence of diabetes in Asian Indians has been reported in Singapore, Malaysia, Mauritius, South Africa, Fiji, Tanzania, and the United States than in the native populations of these countries.[96]

In Singapore, 13.5% of Asian Indians were reported to have diabetes.[34] The age- and sex-adjusted prevalence of diabetes was 13.0% in South African Indians[95] and 9.1% in migrant Hindu Indians in Dar es Salaam, Tanzania.[97] In Fiji, the prevalence for men was 12.1 in urban areas versus 12.9% in rural areas; for women it was 11.3 in urban areas versus 11.0% in rural areas.[93] In Mauritius,[98] the prevalence in Asian Indians was found to be 14%. Figure 41–2 shows the prevalence of diabetes in native and migrant Indian populations.

Bangladeshi Migrants

Bangladeshis residing in east London[99] have a remarkable diabetes prevalence rate of 23.2% compared with 8.3% in non-Asians residing in the same area. In a cross-sectional survey conducted in South Asians (India, Pakistan, and Bangladesh) living in Newcastle, a higher percentage of Pakistani and Bangladeshi men had diabetes (22.4% and 26.6% respectively) than Indians did (15.2%), and South Asians collectively had a five times higher prevalence of diabetes than Europeans (20% versus 4%).[100]

Japanese Migrants

Intergenerational increases in the prevalence of diabetes among Japanese migrants to the West have been reported.[101,102] Hara and colleagues[101] have demonstrated that prevalence of T2DM among persons aged 40 years and older was 2 to 3 times higher in Japanese Americans than in Japanese in Japan: The prevalence of T2DM among Japanese Americans in Hawaii was 18.9%, among Japanese Americans in Los Angeles it was 13.7%, and among Japanese in Hiroshima it was 6.2%. The difference was seen particularly among second- and third-generation Japanese American (Nisei) adults.[103] In Seattle, the prevalence of diabetes was 20% in second-generation Nisei men and 16% in Nisei women 45 to 74 years old, which is an approximately twofold increased risk of developing T2DM for Nisei whose ancestors were from Hiroshima, compared with those who are still residing in Hiroshima.[103] This increase was attributed to the westernization hypothesis, which proposes that a gradual adaptation of a Western lifestyle, including

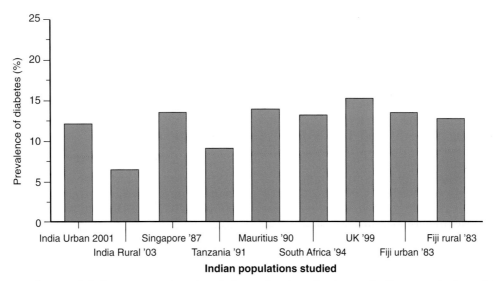

Figure 41–2. Prevalence of diabetes in native *(two leftmost bars)* and migrant Indian populations. Migrant Indian populations have a higher prevalence of diabetes than the native Indians.

a high-fat diet and physical inactivity, contribute to higher rates of diabetes in immigrants.[104.] In 1993, the prevalence of diabetes was 22.6% in first-generation and second-generation Japanese Brazilians, and in 2000, the prevalence was even higher (36.2%).[102,105]

Chinese Migrants

Among the Chinese, the prevalence of diabetes is uniformly higher among Chinese living outside China than in Chinese living in the People's Republic of China. Thai and colleagues[35] reported an age-standardized prevalence of 5.6% in the Chinese population of Singapore. Another study conducted in people of Chinese origin in Mauritius reported a diabetes prevalence of 13% using WHO criteria.[98] In a cross-sectional study conducted by Unwin's group[106] among Chinese and white men and women aged 25 to 64 years residing in the United Kingdom, the prevalence of diabetes in the Chinese population was similar to that of the local population (13%). In Hong Kong Chinese, the age-standardized prevalence of diabetes for the age group 35 to 64 years was 9.5% in men and 10.2% in women, demonstrating a high prevalence of diabetes in this affluent Chinese community.[107]

RISK FACTORS FOR DIABETES IN ASIANS

Environmental and lifestyle changes resulting from industrialization and migration to an urban environment from rural settings may be responsible to a large extent for the epidemic of T2DM in Asians. The various determinants and risk factors for T2DM seem to be common globally. The American Diabetes Association identifies these factors as family history of diabetes, demographic characteristics (age and ethnicity), behavioral and lifestyle factors (obesity and physical inactivity), hypertension, dyslipidemia, IGT or impaired fasting glucose (IFG), and, in women, prior gestational diabetes mellitus (GDM) or polycystic ovary syndrome.[108] The main risk factors for escalation of diabetes in Asian Indians are familial aggregation, high racial susceptibility of T2DM, insulin resistance, and environmental factors that are particularly associated with urbanization. Westernization, coupled with alterations in diet and lifestyle patterns, as well as increased propensity for obesity, also greatly increase the prevalence of T2DM.

Genetic Factors

Genetic susceptibility appears to play an important role in the occurrence of T2DM. However, T2DM is known to be a multifactorial disease caused by a complex interplay of genetic (inheritance) and environmental (diet and lifestyle) factors[109] that influence a number of intermediate traits of relevance to the diabetic phenotype (e.g., beta cell mass, insulin secretion, insulin action, fat distribution, and obesity).[110] The complex interactions between genes and environment complicate the task of identifying any single genetic susceptibility factor for T2DM.

T2DM shows a clear familial aggregation, but it does not segregate in a classic Mendelian fashion. A strong familial aggregation of diabetes is observed among Asian Indians, with high prevalence among the first-degree relatives and vertical transmission through two or more generations. The prevalence

of diabetes increases with increasing family history of diabetes. Comparative studies on migrant Indians and Europeans conducted in the United Kingdom by Mohan and colleagues[111] in the 1980s showed that 10% of Asian Indian diabetic patients had two parents with diabetes, compared to only 1% of European diabetic patients. In CUPS, conducted in South India, the prevalence of diabetes was higher among subjects who had a positive family history of diabetes (18.2%) compared to subjects without a family history of diabetes (10.6%). The overall prevalence of glucose intolerance (diabetes plus IGT) among subjects with two diabetic parents was significantly higher (55%) than among those who had one diabetic parent (22.1%) or those with two nondiabetic parents (15.6%).[112]

In a study conducted by Viswanathan and colleagues[113] to determine the prevalence of T2DM in offspring of two diabetic parents, diabetes was observed in 50% of offspring, and 12% had IGT. Thus 62% of all South Indian offspring of two diabetic parents had abnormal glucose tolerance, which is considerably higher compared to figures of around 25% among Europeans.[113] This might represent an ethnic variation of the genetic factors operating in Indian patients predisposing them to T2DM.

In South African Indians, not only was a prevalence of a positive family history reported in those with T2DM, but also there was a stronger maternal contribution to the putative gene responsible for the disease.[114] Recently, familial aggregation and excess maternal transmission were observed in people with T2DM in Sri Lanka.[115] In the study of 2310 Hong Kong Chinese patients with late-onset T2DM, it was observed that both maternal and paternal factors could be implicated in the development of T2DM in the Chinese population.[116]

Insulin Resistance

Evidence exists that Asian Indians are more insulin resistant than whites and that insulin resistance might play an important role in the pathogenesis of these diseases.[117] Mohan and coworkers[118] first demonstrated that Asian Indians produce higher insulin levels in response to a glucose load than Europeans (hyperinsulinemia). It was later demonstrated by euglycemic clamp studies that insulin resistance is greater among Asian Indians compared to age-, sex-, and BMI-matched Europeans.[119] Retrospective studies have demonstrated that low birth weight is a contributor to insulin resistance among Indians.[120,121] It has been demonstrated that Indian neonates have higher insulin levels and greater adiposity even at birth compared to whites.[121]

The metabolic syndrome, consisting of hyperglycemia, dyslipidemia, insulin resistance, hypertension, and upper body adiposity, is a contributing factor for diabetes in Asian Indians. Studies in India have reported high prevalence of insulin resistance in the general population, and insulin resistance is higher in urban compared to the rural populations.[122,123] The overall prevalence rate of insulin resistance in the CUPS is 11.2%, and the prevalence of insulin resistance in the middle-income group (18.7%) was significantly higher than in the low-income group (6.5%).[122] The prevalence of insulin resistance appears to be higher in Indians (11.2%)[123] than in Japanese (1.6%).[124] Studies have also shown that migrant Asians have a greater propensity for developing insulin resistance compared to host populations.[125,126] Despite similar degrees of hyperglycemia, diabetic Seattle Nisei men had significantly higher insulin levels than diabetic Tokyo men.[126] From these studies it can be hypothesized that increased insulin resistance can at least partly explain the high prevalence of diabetes in both native and migrant Asians.

Environmental Factors

Epidemiologic Transition

Epidemiologic transition is another factor contributing to the current epidemic of T2DM in Asian countries. The epidemiologic transition has occurred in most of the developed countries, but it is at its earliest stages in newly emerging nations and developing countries such as Vietnam. Many industrialized nations in Asia have undergone, or are undergoing, this transition at a very rapid rate and in a diverse and irregular manner.[127] Socioeconomic development since the 1960s has resulted in dramatic changes in lifestyle from traditional to modern, with technologic advancement leading to physical inactivity, affluence leading to consumption of diets rich in fat, sugar, and calories, and the lifestyle changes leading to a high level of mental stress. All of these could adversely influence insulin sensitivity and lead to obesity.

India is undergoing a rapid epidemiologic transition with increased urbanization. The current urbanization rate is 35% compared to 15% in the 1950s, and this could have major implications on the present and future disease patterns in India, with particular reference to diabetes and coronary artery disease.[1] As the epidemiologic transition progresses at different rates in different countries in Asia, we see varying trends in the prevalence rates in different countries within Asia.

Obesity

Obesity is a major risk factor for T2DM. However, when considering obesity as a metabolic risk factor, one needs to take into account the pattern of distribution of body fat. It is believed that central (abdominal) fat distribution, determined by the waist-to-hip ratio, is an important risk factor that acts independently of overall obesity.[128,129] Studies

in native Indians and migrant Indians have demonstrated the association of upper-body adiposity and hyperinsulinemia with T2DM.[117,128] Singh and coworkers[130] reported that the prevalence of central obesity (defined as waist-to-hip ratio greater than 0.85) in the urban North Indian population was 56.2% in men and 51.3% in women, rates higher than the highest rate of overall obesity in Asia. The relationship between central obesity and diabetes is more marked in urban than rural areas and may be of greater importance than overall obesity in Asians with T2DM.[93]

In a study conducted in 2776 randomly selected adults residing in Shanghai, China, the prevalence of diabetes, impaired glucose regulation, and the metabolic syndrome increased progressively in those with a BMI higher than 23 kg/m^2. The authors concluded that although the prevalence of obesity was low in the surveyed Chinese population, higher BMI and waist circumference values are associated with an increasing prevalence of the above-mentioned comorbidities.[131] In Malaysia, obesity is swiftly becoming a major problem and an important contributory factor to diabetes and IGT,[132] which suggests that Malaysia can expect to see a very high rate of diabetes in the near future as a consequence of the high prevalence of overweight and obesity.

The importance of body fat distribution is well illustrated by studies in migrant Asians. Diabetes prevalence has been shown to be much higher in Asians in the United Kingdom than in the European population.[129] It was observed that Asian women had a propensity for increased BMI. Moreover subscapular skin fold was thicker and waist-to-hip ratio was higher in Asian men and women. For any given BMI, it was noted that compared to Europeans, Asians had a higher waist-to-hip ratio.[129] Chandalia and coworkers[117] have shown that for any BMI, migrant Indians had higher body fat, and for any given body fat percentage they also had higher insulin resistance compared to other ethnic groups independent of generalized or truncal adiposity. Studies of migrant Indians in South Africa[133] and Mauritius[98] have shown a positive association of obesity with diabetes, especially among women. The role of obesity might also differ in different ethnic groups as substantiated by reports that migrant Chinese and whites living in the United Kingdom have similar diabetes prevalence rates despite lower BMI values among the Chinese population.[106]

Obesity has been on the increase in children, and this might play a causative role in the escalating prevalence of diabetes in the young.[134] This increased occurrence of overweight in childhood could be the first sign of insulin resistance and future metabolic syndrome. A recent long-term follow-up study carried out in Indians supports this hypothesis and shows that lower birth weight coupled with obesity in childhood and adolescence leads to very high rates of diabetes.[135]

Physical Inactivity

There is sufficient epidemiologic evidence to demonstrate that physical inactivity as an independent risk factor is fuelling the epidemic of T2DM in Asians, predominantly in the urban areas. Migration from rural areas to urban slums in metropolitan cities leads to obesity, glucose intolerance, and dyslipidemia.[28] Adaptation of western lifestyles with decreasing physical activity could be an important contributor.

Several Asian studies have reported that a significant link does exist between the level of physical activity and glucose tolerance.[112,136] The prevalence of diabetes was more than twice as high in those classified as sedentary or undertaking light activity as in those classified as performing moderate or heavy exercise among Melanesian and Indian men in Fiji.[136] In a study conducted in South India, the risk of developing diabetes in the subjects who followed a sedentary lifestyle was three times higher compared to the more physically active subjects.[112] Thus, increased physical activity should form an important management strategy aimed at improvement of insulin sensitivity and prevention of diabetes in high-risk persons.

DIABETIC COMPLICATIONS IN THE ASIAN DIABETIC POPULATION

There are considerable differences in the pattern of diabetes-related complications even within Asia. Indeed, it is difficult to compare the complications between populations due to differences in case mix (T1DM versus T2DM), duration of diabetes, degree of metabolic control, varying criteria used to diagnose complications, and possibly genetic and ethnic differences. In the CUPS study in south India, the prevalence of retinopathy was 19%,[137] neuropathy 17.5%,[138] and microalbuminuria 26.3%.[139] In another study of 500 South Indians with newly diagnosed T2DM, it was observed that 7.3% already had diabetic retinopathy at the time of the diagnosis of diabetes.[140] It has been reported that the prevalence of diabetic nephropathy was 30.3% among 4837 patients with chronic renal failure seen over a period of 10 years.[141] In another large clinic-based study of 1848 T2DM patients, it was observed that 9.4% of subjects had proteinuria.[142]

In the CUPS population, 14.9% of the subjects with IGT and 21.4% of the diabetic subjects had coronary artery disease[143]; the prevalence of peripheral vascular disease was 6.3% among diabetic subjects compared to 2.7% among nondiabetic subjects.[144] In the same population, diabetic subjects had increased carotid intima medial thickness compared to their nondiabetic counterparts.[145] Arterial stiffness was higher among the diabetic subjects compared to their nondiabetic counterparts, and endothelial function was also impaired among diabetic subjects compared to age- and sex-matched nondiabetic subjects.[146]

In a 14-year study conducted in 8793 hospitalized diabetes patients in western India (Mumbai), 81.8% developed complications. Hypertension was observed in 42.2%, ischemic heart disease in 27.2%, cerebrovascular accident in 9.2%, and gangrene and peripheral vascular diseases in 4.2%.[147] In the Diabcare-Singapore project[148] conducted in 22 clinics on 1697 diabetic subjects, retinopathy (12%), cataract (16%), and neuropathy (12%) were commonly reported diabetic complications. Sixteen percent of patients had abnormal levels of protein (higher than 500 mg/24 h) in the urine, 3% had elevated serum creatinine levels, and 36% had microalbuminuria.

In Chinese T2DM patients, peripheral vascular disease was identified in 6.5%, which is lower than the rate in most western countries.[149] In data collected from 10 medical centers in Beijing, Shanghai, Tianjin, and Chongqing,[150] the prevalence rate of diabetic retinopathy was 31.5%, while that of diabetic nephropathy was 39.7% and diabetic neuropathy 51.1%. In the same study, hypertension was observed in 41.8%, coronary heart disease in 25.1%, cerebral vascular disease in 17.3%, and vessel complication of lower limbs was reported in 9.3%.

Studies in the United Kingdom suggest that Asian Indians have higher susceptibility to diabetic nephropathy, the leading cause of end-stage renal disease and morbidity in diabetes. Burden and coworkers[151] reported the incidence rate of end-stage renal failure in diabetic patients of Asian ethnic origin was 486.6 cases per million person-years per year, compared to 35.6 in whites. In another study, which compared the prevalence of complications between Asians and whites, the ischemic heart disease rate was similar in both groups; peripheral vascular disease and retinopathy were lower in Asians, but renal disease was higher in Asians compared to whites (22.3% versus 12.6%).[152] In a cross-sectional study of 583 European and 889 South Asian T2DM clinic patients in the United Kingdom, microalbuminuria, retinopathy, and heart disease were more common in South Asians than in Europeans.[153]

In another study conducted in Asian diabetic patients attending the diabetic clinics in Bradford, adjusting for age and duration of diabetes, the probability of sight-threatening retinopathy was significantly higher in Asians than that in whites. The impact of age and duration was significantly higher in patients of South Asian origin compared to whites.[154] A population-based study carried out in Durban showed that diabetes mellitus was an important risk factor for the high prevalence of ischemic heart disease in Indians.[155]

CONCLUSION

The magnitude of the diabetic epidemic in Asian countries is evident from the available epidemiologic data, with seven Asian countries among the predicted 10 leading countries with diabetic populations. This underscores the need for increased preventive programs and resources. The prevalence of T2DM is increasing rapidly in all ethnic groups in Asia, which could lead to significant morbidity and mortality associated with diabetic complications.

The epidemic of diabetes in Asians may be attributed to strong genetic factors together with urbanization, migration, and lifestyle changes leading to insulin resistance. WHO's predicted estimates for India and China for 2030 shows that diabetes poses a major threat to these countries.

However, the good news is that this is largely preventable. Results from a 6-year randomized, controlled trial, the Da Qing IGT and Diabetes Study[156] conducted among those with IGT in China, demonstrated that diet and exercise interventions led to a significant decrease in the incidence of diabetes. Thus, more preventive programs integrating modified lifestyle with incorporation of physical activity and appropriate nutrition, thereby reducing obesity in adults and children, should be advocated on a wider scale, particularly in populations with a high susceptibility to diabetes.

References

1. Wild S, Roglic G, Green A, et al: Global prevalence of diabetes: Estimates for the year 2000 and projections for 2030. Diabetes Care 27:1047-1053, 2004.
2. King H, Aubert RE, Herman WH: Global burden of diabetes, 1995-2025: Prevalence, numerical estimates, and projections. Diabetes Care 21:1414-1431, 1998.
3. International Diabetes Federation: Diabetes Atlas 2003. Brussels, International Diabetes Federation, 2003.
4. Beverley B, Eveline R: The diagnosis and classification of diabetes and impaired glucose regulation. In Pickup JC, Williams G (eds): Textbook of Diabetes, 3rd ed. Oxford, Blackwell, 2003, p 2.1.
5. American Diabetes Association: Diagnosis and classification of diabetes mellitus. Clinical practice recommendations. Diabetes Care 27:S5-S10, 2004.
6. Zimmet P, Alberti KGMM, Shaw J: Global and societal implications of the diabetes epidemic. Nature 414:782-787, 2001.
7. Scott R, Brown L: Prevalence and incidence of insulin-treated diabetes mellitus in adults in Canterbury, New Zealand. Diabet Med 8:443-447, 1991.
8. Karvonen M, Tuomilehto J, Libman I, et al: A review of the recent epidemiological data on the worldwide incidence of type 1 (insulin-dependent) diabetes mellitus. Diabetologia 36:883-892, 1993.
9. West KM: Diabetes in the tropics: Some lessons for western diabetology. In Podolsky S, Viswanathan M (eds): Secondary Diabetes: The Spectrum of the Diabetic Syndromes. New York, Raven Press, 1980, pp 249-255.
10. King H, Rewers M: WHO Ad Hoc Diabetes Reporting Group: Global estimates for prevalence of diabetes mellitus and impaired glucose tolerance in adults. Diabetes Care 16:157-177, 1993.
11. Simmons D, Williams DAR, Powell MJ: Prevalence of diabetes in different regional and religious South Asian Indian communities in Coventry. Diabet Med 9:428-431, 1992.
12. Mokdad AH, Ford ES, Bowman BA, et al.: Diabetes trends in the U.S.: 1990-1998. Diabetes Care 23:1278-1283, 2000.

Chapter 42

New Drugs and Diabetes Risk: Antipsychotic and Antiretroviral Agents

Samuel Dagogo-Jack

KEY POINTS

- *Antipsychotic-associated diabetes is infrequent and is observed across a wide range of medications.*
- *Retrospective studies suggest that the risk of diabetes is modestly increased with second-generation (atypical) antipsychotic drugs compared with conventional agents.*
- *Weight gain, a common metabolic effect of antipsychotic medications, is a risk factor for type 2 diabetes.*
- *Available data indicate no direct acute effect of atypical antipsychotic drugs on insulin sensitivity or secretion.*
- *Screening includes increased surveillance, documentation of glucose status before drug initiation, periodic measurements of fasting glucose in asymptomatic subjects, and prompt measurement of fasting or random glucose in symptomatic subjects.*
- *Management of patients with hyperglycemia includes diet modification, exercise, and medications (oral antidiabetic agents, insulin).*
- *Human immunodeficiency virus–protease inhibitors are most often implicated in the etiology of antiretroviral-associated diabetes.*
- *The major mechanisms of antiretroviral-associated diabetes involve induction of insulin resistance and concurrent alteration on beta cell function.*
- *Weight gain, body fat redistribution, and lipodystrophy, which are frequent metabolic effects of highly active antiretroviral therapy, are risk factors for type 2 diabetes.*
- *Routine screening for diabetes is recommended in patients with human immunodeficiency virus disease receiving highly active antiretroviral therapy.*
- *Management of patients with hyperglycemia includes diet modification, exercise intervention, and careful selection of antidiabetic agents to minimize toxicities from comorbid conditions and adverse and drug–drug interactions from concurrent medications.*

Millions of people around the world are currently receiving treatment with various antipsychotic medications for major mental disorders. Millions of other patients with the acquired immunodeficiency syndrome (AIDS), which is caused by infection with the human immunodeficiency virus (HIV), are receiving treatment with various antiretroviral agents. Increasingly, reports from the literature in the fields of neuropsychiatry and retrovirology have implicated the use of antipsychotic or antiretroviral agents in the development of unexpected adverse metabolic effects, including diabetes, weight gain, dyslipidemia, and lipodystrophy.

Theoretically, the reports of treatment-emergent diabetes can be explained by increased susceptibility conferred by the underlying disorders, direct toxic effects of the agents used in the treatment of these disorders, or a unique interaction between the pharmacologic agents and the disease states in susceptible persons. Diabetes is reported only in a minority of patients, which suggests that additional host factors must be involved in the expression of antipsychotic-associated diabetes (APAD) or antiretroviral-associated diabetes (ARAD).

This chapter focuses on the issue of diabetes and glucose dysregulation observed during treatment of patients with major psychiatric disorders or HIV–AIDS.

Antipsychotic-Associated Diabetes

The prevalence of type 2 diabetes has been increasing steadily around the world. In the United States, estimates of the prevalence of diagnosed diabetes range from 6% to 10% in the general population and up to 15% or higher in certain demographic groups.[1,2] Similarly, major mental disorders are quite prevalent in society, with estimated lifetime prevalence in the United States of about 10% for major depression, about 1% for schizophrenia, and about 1.2% for bipolar disease.[3,4] Thus, ample

opportunity exists for coincidental concurrence of diabetes and disorders that require antipsychotic therapy.

Nonetheless, the presence of major mental disorders appears to confer increased risk for diabetes: Type 2 diabetes mellitus (T2DM) has been reported to be two to four times more prevalent in patients with schizophrenia, major depression, or bipolar disorder compared with the general population.[5-9] For example, a US national survey in the 1990s showed that the prevalence rate of diabetes in persons aged 45 to 64 years was approximately 6%[1]; a similar survey among patients with schizophrenia aged 45 to 64 years showed a diabetes prevalence rate of approximately 18%.[10] Clearly, several of the conventional risk factors[11] for T2DM identified for the general population (e.g., positive family history, obesity, physical inactivity, ethnicity) must be operating in the psychiatric population also.[12] In addition, the presence of a major mental disorder may be an independent risk factor for the development of T2DM.[13,14]

Although the association between diabetes and mental illness has been recognized for more than a century, case studies published in recent years have led some investigators to focus on the link between exposure to the newer, atypical antipsychotic medications (Table 42–1) and the development of diabetes.[15-18] It must be noted, though, that the increased diabetes risk has been reported even among patients who had not received antipsychotic medication.[5,19] Furthermore, the rate of impaired fasting glucose in first-episode, drug-naive patients with schizophrenia was reported to be 15.4%, compared to 0% in a matched control group of healthy subjects.[19]

Thus, the interpretation of the now numerous reports[5-9,15-18] of APAD is compounded by the increased background risk for diabetes in the psychiatric population, as well as the high prevalence of asymptomatic, undiagnosed diabetes in the general populace.[20,21] These interpretive handicaps make it difficult to prove a cause-and-effect relationship between the antipsychotic agents in question and the occurrence of diabetes. Fortunately, the vast majority of people treated with antipsychotic agents do not develop hyperglycemia.[8] Nonetheless, the etiology and mechanism(s) of APAD need to be elucidated in the few who do develop diabetes.

Table 42–1. *Examples of First- and Second-Generation Antipsychotic Medications*

Drug	Metabolic Side Effects*
First Generation (Typical)	
Chlorpromazine (Thorazine)	Hyperprolactinemia
Perphenazine (Trilafon)	Weight gain
Fluphenazine (Prolixin)	Hyperglycemia
Trifluoperazine (Stelazine)	Insulin resistance
Haloperidol (Haldol)	Poikilothermia
Thiothixene (Navane)	Dyslipidemia
Second Generation (Atypical)†	
Clozapine (Clozaril) (1989)	Weight gain
Risperidone (Risperdal) (1993)	Hyperglycemia
Olanzapine (Zyprexa) (1996)	Insulin resistance
Quetiapine (Seroquel) (1997)	Hyperprolactinemia
Ziprasidone (Geodon) (2001)	Dyslipidemia
Aripiprazole (Abilify) (2002)	ND

*Effects are variable across drug generations. Typical agents tend to induce hyperprolactinemia, whereas atypical agents induce more weight gain and diabetes.
†Years in parentheses indicate FDA approval.
ND, No data.

CLINICAL PRESENTATION

Recent case reports of APAD indicate that the risk is seen across most of the widely used atypical antipsychotic agents.[15-18] Older reports from the last century implicated the first-generation (see Table 42–1) conventional antipsychotic agents.[6,22-26] Thus, both ancient and modern antipsychotic agents have been reported to exacerbate preexisting diabetes or to induce new-onset diabetes. Based on data from postmarketing surveillance reports,[15-17,27-31] the clinical presentation (Table 42–2) of APAD is consistent with T2DM. The mean age at presentation is about 40 years. Two thirds of patients present with new-onset diabetes and 25% present with diabetic ketoacidosis (DKA) or metabolic acidosis, with approximately 7% case fatality. The possibility that some patients with APAD actually have type 1 diabetes (T1DM)

Table 42-2. *Clinical Presentation of Diabetes Associated with the Use of Atypical Antipsychotic Drugs*

Drug	Age (years)	New-Onset Diabetes (%)	Exacerbation (%)	Diabetic Ketoacidosis or Metabolic Acidosis (%)
Clozapine	48.0 ± 14	63.0	14.1	20.8
Olanzapine	40.7 ± 12.9	65.1	15.2	27.7
Risperidone	39.0 ± 17.4	62.9	30.3	27.3
Quetiapine	35.3 ± 16.3	73.9	17.4	45.6*
All	40.8 ± 15.2	64.3	17.2	25.5

Data are based on random 2001-2003 postmarketing FDA MedWatch reports[15-17] of diabetes events on clozapine (n = 384), olanzapine (n = 289), risperidone (n = 132), and quetiapine (n = 46).
*Probably an outlier due to small sample size.

Box 42-1. Putative Mechanisms of Antipsychotic-Associated Diabetes

- Increased penetrance of demographic risk factors for diabetes among patients with serious mental illness
  - Family history of diabetes
  - Obesity or central adiposity
  - Physical inactivity
  - Ethnicity
- Increased background risk for insulin resistance among patients with serious mental illness:
  - Hypothalamic–pituitary–adrenal axis activation[40]
  - Visceral adiposity[39]
  - Mitochondrial dysfunction[117]
- Antipsychotic-induced weight gain
  - Obesity-induced insulin resistance
  - Interaction between obesity and dysglycemia?
  - Host susceptibility or permissive factors?
  - Role of genetic or familial factors?
- Severe acute hyperglycemic crisis following initiation of antipsychotic medication
  - Pharmacogenic or immunologic mechanisms?[119]
  - Antipsychotic induced anti-insulin factor?[26]
  - Role of proinflammatory adipocytokines?[118]
  - Interruption of insulin secretion and insulin action?[118]
  - Interaction with glucose transporter molecules?[70]

has not been excluded, because exhaustive immunologic studies are lacking. It is known that about 15% of adults of European ancestry with apparent T2DM may have circulating pancreatic islet cell autoantibodies. This condition, known as latent autoimmune diabetes of adults (LADA), is associated with severe insulin deficiency and proneness to ketoacidosis.[32]

The frequency of ketoacidosis at presentation with APAD is comparable to the 23% rate reported for the general diabetes population.[33] The mortality rate also is within the 5% to 15% mortality rate for patients with severe hyperglycemic crisis (DKA and nonketotic hyperosmolar syndrome).[34-36] The majority of persons with T2DM show metabolic defects that are characterized by insulin resistance and progressive pancreatic beta cell dysfunction. Thus, studies of insulin sensitivity and beta cell function could help elucidate underlying mechanisms in patients with APAD.

UNDERLYING MECHANISMS

Designing studies to clarify the mechanisms (Box 42-1) that link antipsychotic use to the development or exacerbation of diabetes is problematic. First, of course, is the general barrier related to the informed consent process in mentally compro-

mised research subjects. Second, the ethical dilemma associated with use of placebo in patients with major mental disorders precludes adoption of the gold-standard randomized, placebo-controlled, prospective clinical trial design. Third, in vivo intervention studies are not readily feasible in persons with active mental illness who are clinically unstable. Yet, important mechanistic information may be lost while awaiting clinical stabilization.

Studies performed during acute presentation in incident cases of APAD (ideally, before any therapeutic interventions are instituted) are likely to be most informative. For ethical reasons, however, few such studies exist. One alternative approach has been to study the metabolic effects of selected antipsychotics in healthy subjects. Obviously, such studies are limited by the different *milieu interieur* of the study subjects, as compared with patients with major psychiatric disorders. Differences in neuropsychiatric and neuroendocrine backgrounds certainly limit the extrapolation of studies conducted in healthy subjects to patients with mental disorders. Nonetheless, these studies provide valuable insight into the direct effects of antipsychotic drugs on mechanisms that regulate glucose homeostasis.

Weight Gain, Body Composition, and the Hypothalamic–Pituitary–Adrenal Axis

The link among obesity, insulin resistance, and diabetes[37] is probably mediated by certain secreted products of the adipocytes. Some of these products, collectively known as adipocytokines, adversely affect insulin secretion and insulin action.[38] Many if not most antipsychotics are associated with weight gain, and this side effect has been proposed as a potential link between antipsychotic use and diabetes. It must be noted, however, that psychotic states, such as schizophrenia, may be associated with changes in body composition and fat distribution that predict insulin resistance. For instance, Ryan's group[39] observed greater accumulation of intra-abdominal fat in first-episode, drug-naive patients with schizophrenia.

The centripetal pattern of fat distribution is reminiscent of patients with Cushing's syndrome. Indeed, hypercortisolemia is a hallmark of depression, schizophrenia, and other serious mental illnesses, as a result of activation of the hypothalamic–pituitary–adrenal (HPA) axis.[40] Thus, chronic preconditioning by hypercortisolemia results in abdominal body fat distribution, the pattern usually associated with insulin resistance and the metabolic syndrome, even before antipsychotic medications are employed.[38,40]

Theoretically, induction of remission by antipsychotic therapy should dampen the overactivity of the HPA axis and decrease cortisol output. To the extent that hypercortisolemia is responsible for

redistribution of body fat and insulin resistance, such reduction of cortisol tone ought to reverse the centripetal pattern of adiposity and, perhaps, reduce diabetes risk. Consistent with this notion, studies in diabetic patients with major depression have reported improved glycemic control following treatment with antidepressants.[42,43] Interestingly, treatment with atypical antipsychotic agents (olanzapine and risperidone) for 6 months did not alter visceral adiposity, indicating that longer time frames may be required to demonstrate measurable changes in body composition. Nonetheless, the lack of aggravation of visceral adiposity during 6 months of exposure to these agents is somewhat reassuring.[39]

Obesity alone cannot fully explain APAD because the majority of obese persons in the general population do not develop T2DM.[44] Such persons are able to compensate for obesity-induced insulin resistance by increasing their insulin secretion. Indeed, the decline in insulin sensitivity and insulin secretion during the development of T2DM occurs on a strong background of genetic and environmental determinants.[45,46] Differential expression of, or susceptibility to, genetic and environmental factors might explain why the majority of people do not develop diabetes. If disruption of glucose regulation is an independent (primary or pleitropic) effect of antipsychotic agents, then studies using these agents should demonstrate a propensity to induce insulin resistance with concomitant inhibition of insulin secretion.

Glucose Tolerance, Insulin Sensitivity, and Beta Cell Function

The pathophysiology of T2DM is characterized by concurrent development of progressive insulin resistance and pancreatic beta cell dysfunction.[45,46] Although the frequency of treatment-emergent APAD is low,[8,12] the exact mechanisms remain to be fully elucidated. Theoretically, antipsychotic medications can alter whole-body glucose metabolism through a variety of mechanisms. Ultimately, however, these mechanisms must be funneled through alteration of insulin action and secretion in order for T2DM to result. Therefore, metabolic studies have focused on assessment of glucose tolerance, insulin sensitivity, and beta cell function, as discussed next.

Effects of Atypical Antipsychotics on Glucose Tolerance

A modified oral glucose tolerance test (OGTT) has been used to assess glucose homeostasis in patients with schizophrenia.[47,48] The specific modifications to the standard OGTT protocol that were introduced in this study included use of a 50-gram glucose load (instead of the standard 75 grams), and blood sampling at 0, 15, 45, and 75 minutes (instead of 0, 30, 60, 90, and 120 minutes). The study population comprised patients with schizophrenia ($N = 48$) treated with either typical antipsychotic medications ($n = 17$) or one of the atypical agents, clozapine ($n = 9$), olanzapine ($n = 12$), or risperidone ($n = 10$). None of the subjects showed evidence of diabetes at baseline; the mean fasting plasma glucose levels were less than 100 mg/dL in all groups. Following challenge with 50 grams of oral glucose, plasma glucose values ranged from approximately 130 mg/dL to approximately 180 mg/dL at 45 minutes in patients with schizophrenia as compared to approximately 120 mg/dL in a control group of 31 untreated healthy subjects. After 75 minutes, plasma glucose levels were approximately 110 mg/dL to approximately 160 mg/dL in patients with schizophrenia as compared to approximately 105 mg/dL in healthy subjects.

Notably, the highest postchallenge plasma glucose values observed among the patients with schizophrenia were nondiagnostic for diabetes. A tendency toward higher postload glucose levels was reported for patients treated with atypical antipsychotics compared with those treated with typical agents.[47,48] However, caution is called for in making such inferences, because of the small sample sizes and the cross-sectional, open-label design.

Also, methodologic drawbacks related to the OGTT procedure should further temper conclusions from these studies. Although the sampling intervals adopted during standard OGTT have been at 0, 30, 60, 90, and 120 minutes following glucose ingestion, only the baseline and 120-minute plasma glucose values are interpretable for purposes of assigning glycemic status.[11] There are currently no normative data that would permit valid interpretation of the intervening glucose values obtained between 0 minutes and 120 minutes during the OGTT. Those values tend to be confounded by incomplete and quite variable gastric emptying during the earlier periods of the OGTT.

Insulin Sensitivity

Studies in Healthy Subjects

Some recent studies have used the hyperinsulinemic euglycemic[49] or hyperglycemic[50] clamp techniques to assess the effects of atypical antipsychotic agents on insulin sensitivity. Beasley and colleagues[51] performed a two-step euglycemic clamp at low-dose insulin infusion and high-dose insulin infusion in 55 healthy volunteers with no history of diabetes before and after treatment with antipsychotic agents. Data obtained during low-dose insulin infusion provided measures of insulin sensitivity, and measurements during the high-dose insulin infusion gave estimates of maximum glucose uptake and use. The subjects were random-

ized to three groups: olanzapine treatment ($n = 22$), risperidone treatment ($n = 14$), and placebo ($n = 19$). The euglycemic clamp and the mixed-meal tolerance test were performed at baseline and after 21 to 23 days of drug or placebo treatment. Patients in both antipsychotic groups gained weight compared to the control group (olanzapine, 1.9 kg; risperidone, 1.6 kg; placebo, −0.2 kg).

Glucose disposal rates (mg/kg per minute) at baseline during low-dose insulin infusion were 4.1 ± 1.4 for placebo, 4.8 ± 1.7 for olanzapine, and 4.9 ± 2.1 for risperidone. The corresponding baseline rates of maximum glucose uptake during high-dose insulin infusion were 12.1 ± 2.0, 12.7 ± 2.8, and 13.3 ± 2.9 mg/kg per minute, respectively.[24] There were no significant differences in these baseline parameters. Following drug or placebo treatment, repeat clamp studies showed minimal changes in GDR during low-dose insulin infusion: 0.5 ± 0.8, 0.1 ± 2.0, and -0.6 ± 1.2 mg/kg per minute in subjects treated with placebo, olanzapine, and risperidone, respectively. The changes in maximal glucose uptake were even less impressive: -0.3 ± 1.1, -0.02 ± 2.0, -0.7 ± 1.7 mg/kg per minute in placebo, olanzapine, and risperidone groups, respectively.

These results do not support a major acute or subacute effect of olanzapine or risperidone treatment on insulin sensitivity or maximum insulin-stimulated glucose uptake by tissues. As already noted, there is need for caution in extrapolating studies conducted in healthy subjects to patients with mental disorders. Nonetheless, it is reassuring that two of the most widely prescribed atypical antipsychotics had no significant deleterious effect on glucose homeostasis and insulin sensitivity during approximately 3 weeks of administration in healthy subjects.

Studies in Healthy Subjects and Patients with Schizophrenia

Newcomer and colleagues[52] studied 30 patients with schizophrenia and 28 healthy control subjects. The patients were being treated with antipsychotics and were all overweight or obese, as indicated by their mean body mass index (BMI). The treatment groups were olanzapine ($n = 10$; BMI, 30.8 kg/m^2), risperidone ($n = 10$; BMI, 30.1 kg/m^2), and conventional agents ($n = 10$; BMI, 28.9 kg/m^2). The healthy control subjects were divided into two BMI groups: overweight control (BMI 27.5 kg/m^2) and lean control (BMI 20.5 kg/m^2). All patients and control subjects underwent a single euglycemic clamp procedure to quantitate tissue sensitivity to insulin.

The authors found no cross-sectional differences in insulin sensitivity among patients treated with typical or atypical antipsychotics. Overall, insulin sensitivity among patients receiving drug treatment for schizophrenia was comparable to that of overweight controls and significantly lower than that of lean healthy subjects. A strong effect of BMI rather than drug exposure explained most of the variance

in insulin sensitivity. Increased adiposity indicated by high BMI was strongly associated with decreased insulin sensitivity ($P < 0.0001$).[52]

These interesting data suggest that chronic treatment with antipsychotic agents conferred no independent additional risk for insulin resistance beyond that predicted by BMI. In a sense, these results reinforce the conclusions from the studies by Beasley's group[51] that showed no direct effect of olanzapine or risperidone on tissue sensitivity to insulin.

Effects of Atypical Antipsychotics on Beta Cell Function

The presentation of APAD appears to be consistent with T2DM, although exhaustive immunologic studies have not been undertaken to rule out alternative mechanisms, such as LADA. Indeed, diabetic ketoacidosis and metabolic acidosis may be the initial presentation of APAD in about 25% of patients, which indicates severe insulinopenia in such patients.

Sowell and colleagues[53] used the hyperglycemic clamp method to assess insulin secretory responses before and following treatment with two atypical antipsychotic drugs. In all, 48 healthy volunteers were randomized to treatment with risperidone (4 mg/day, $n = 13$), olanzapine (10 mg/day, $n = 17$), or placebo ($n = 18$) for 15 to 17 days. At the end of the study, body weight increased significantly in the olanzapine (2.8 ± 1.7 kg) and the risperidone (3.1 ± 2.1 kg) treatment groups. The authors also noted an increase (approximately 25%) in insulin secretory response to hyperglycemia and a decrease (approximately 18%) in insulin sensitivity index after treatment with olanzapine and risperidone. The changes in insulin secretion and insulin sensitivity were no longer significant after controlling for changes in weight in a multivariate regression model.[53]

Based on the foregoing data, there is no evidence in support of an acute or subacute inhibitory effect of olanzapine or risperidone on pancreatic beta cell insulin secretory responses. These findings are supported by data from a preliminary study of 25 patients with schizophrenia, using the frequently sampled intravenous glucose tolerance test coupled with Bergman's Minimal Model Analysis.[54] In that study, patients treated with clozapine ($n = 10$; BMI, 27.1 kg/m^2), olanzapine ($n = 9$; BMI, 27.3 kg/m^2), and risperidone ($n = 6$; BMI, 25.7 kg/m^2) had mean fasting insulin levels of 9.97 ± 5.91, 9.19 ± 8.24, and 6.77 ± 5.03 µU/mL, respectively. Following rapid intravenous infusion of glucose (0.3 g/kg body weight), the acute insulin responses to glucose (AIRg) were 639.8 ± 452.8, 704.8 ± 645.4, and 436.9 ± 466.7 µU/mL × min in patients treated with clozapine, olanzapine, and risperidone, respectively. The relatively lower value for AIRg in the

risperidone-treated group is consistent with their lower BMI.

Typical versus Atypical Antipsychotic Agents

As already noted, older-generation antipsychotic agents have long been reported to induce metabolic changes.[6,22-26] The introduction of the atypical antipsychotic medications (see Table 42–1) since the 1990s has been perceived as an advance in the field of psychopharmacology because of their improved efficacy and tolerability over the older typical, or conventional, agents.[3,55-58] Various reports have indicated that use of the atypical antipsychotic agents results in sustained improvements in positive and negative symptoms of schizophrenia, reduced incidence of extrapyramidal syndrome and tardive dyskinesia, improved cognitive function, and decreased relapse rates.[3,55-58] At issue is whether the atypical antipsychotic medications are more liable to induce adverse metabolic effects, particularly diabetes, than the conventional agents.

No direct prospective (head-to-head) comparison studies have been undertaken to address this question. However, a number of cross-sectional studies[59,60] have shown inconsistent results, with a tendency toward a greater propensity for metabolic alterations by atypical antipsychotic agents as compared with older conventional agents. In one study,[59] 157 patients with schizophrenia were randomly assigned to treatment with clozapine, olanzapine, risperidone, or haloperidol and evaluated at baseline and after 8 weeks and 14 weeks of drug treatment. Modest increases (mostly within the normal range) in fasting plasma glucose levels were observed in the groups assigned to either atypical antipsychotics (clozapine, olanzapine, risperidone) or haloperidol, a conventional agent.[59]

In a retrospective cross-sectional study of 1826 patients with schizophrenia treated with the atypical agents (olanzapine, clozapine, risperidone, quetiapine) and 617 patients treated with conventional agents between 1996 and 2001, the crude incidence of diabetes did not differ for atypical antipsychotics and conventional antipsychotics (2.46% versus 2.76%).[17] In Cox proportional hazards models, the atypical agents appeared modestly more likely to be associated with diabetes compared with conventional agents (hazard ratio [HR], 1.17; CI, 1.06-1.30). However, the individual atypical antipsychotics (clozapine, olanzapine, risperidone) did not differ with regard to the risk of diabetes.[17]

In another large cross-sectional study[60] of patients with schizophrenia treated at Veterans Administration (VA) medical centers, the rates of prevalent diabetes were compared between patients receiving atypical agents and those taking conventional agents. The atypical agents evaluated in the study were olanzapine ($n = 10,970$), risperidone ($n = 9903$), and quetiapine ($n = 955$). Clozapine, ziprasidone, and aripiprazole were not included because of small sample size (clozapine) or nonavailability on the formulary. The typical agents included haloperidol, thioridazine, perphenazine, chlorpromazine, fluphenazine, thiothixene, trifluoperazine, loxapine, mesoridazine, and molindone. Patients taking any of these typical agents were classified into one category and compared with patients taking the aforementioned atypical agents.

The authors found that atypical antipsychotic medication was associated with a 9% increased risk for development of diabetes[60] compared with typical antipsychotic agents (HR, 1.09; CI, 1.03-1.15). However, the relative hazard rates were similar for all the individual atypical agents.[60] Despite the limitations inherent in a retrospective nonrandomized study, the findings of the VA study should lead to an increased awareness of possible metabolic risks associated with antipsychotic medications and thus the need for surveillance for treatment-emergent hyperglycemia.

MANAGEMENT

Screening

The increased risks of insulin resistance and T2DM in psychiatric patients[10,61] and the increasing awareness of APAD have led to recommendations[62,63] for diabetes screening. The Food and Drug Administration (FDA) has asked manufacturers of all atypical antipsychotic drugs, including clozapine (Clozaril), risperidone (Risperdal), olanzepine (Zyprexa), quetiapine (Seroquel), ziprasidone (Geodon), and aripiprazole (Abilify), to add a new warning to the drugs' labels about the increased risk of hyperglycemia and diabetes.[62] The FDA warning recommends that patients with diabetes taking atypical antipsychotics be monitored regularly for worsening of glucose control. Patients starting on these drugs who have diabetes risk factors, such as obesity or a family history of diabetes, should have fasting blood glucose testing at the start of treatment and periodically thereafter. Furthermore, all patients treated with atypical antipsychotics should be monitored for symptoms of hyperglycemia, such as excessive thirst, excessive appetite, frequent urination, or weakness.[62]

The American Diabetes Association Consensus panel[63] recommends measuring pretreatment fasting plasma glucose and lipid levels and retesting 12 weeks after introducing an atypical antipsychotic medication. If these screening tests are normal, monitoring of fasting glucose (annually) and fasting lipid profile (quintannually) is recommended.[63] The American Diabetes Association Consensus panel also stresses the need for routine monitoring of weight and blood pressure.[63]

Lifestyle and Pharmacologic Interventions

Patients in whom diabetes is detected should be given standard diabetes management. The therapeutic goals are alleviation of symptoms (if present), achievement of metabolic control, and prevention of acute and long-term complications of diabetes. A regimen that is tailored to individual patients' needs and characteristics and that employs multiple modalities (diabetes education, calorie restriction, physical activity, medications) offers the best chance of accomplishing these goals.[11] Where facilities are available, group counseling and exercise sessions may be an efficient mechanism for delivering lifestyle intervention. The glycemic goal is normalization (or near-normalization) of fasting and postprandial plasma glucose levels, as indicated by a stable hemoglobin A1c (HbA1c) lower than 7%.

The initial choice of medication for control of uncomplicated hyperglycemia is a matter of clinical judgment. Maximal doses of sufonylureas, metformin, and thiazolidinediones (TZDs) give comparable glucose-lowering effects when used as initial monotherapy.[64] Regimens containing metformin are appealing because of the need to minimize weight gain. However, glycemic control must not be compromised on that account. Initial treatment with insulin is indicated for severe hyperglycemia, DKA, and nonketotic hyperosmolar crisis. Insulin also is indicated for persistent hyperglycemia despite maximal doses of oral agents. Large doses (more than 100 units per day) can be required to achieve optimal glycemic control in obese patients presenting with severe APAD.

Switching to Alternative Antipsychotic Drugs

If the hyperglycemia responds readily to these measures, withdrawal or substitution of antipsychotic agents is unwarranted, because of the risk of psychotic relapse. Otherwise, judicious review of antipsychotic medications should be undertaken and alternative agents may be substituted for the agent suspected of triggering the diabetes. Currently, no evidence-based data exist to guide the selection of agents for such substitution, and the metabolic response to switching is unpredictable, so the practice remains empirical. The need for diet modification (and medications for diabetes) often persists, despite change of antipsychotic medication.

Thus, interruption of antipsychotic medication to determine if diabetes will resolve spontaneously is a practice largely driven by curiosity, because prompt resolution of hyperglycemia seldom occurs without specific lifestyle and pharmacologic interventions. Nonetheless, cessation of the incumbent antipsychotic drug may be compelling under certain circumstances (e.g., severe hyperglycemic crisis, DKA, diabetic coma) but must be undertaken in close consultation with a psychiatrist.

CONCLUSIONS

The reports and studies reviewed here indicate that use of atypical antipsychotic drugs is associated with increased risk for diabetes, but there is no evidence that the atypical antipsychotic drugs directly alter insulin secretion or insulin sensitivity. It is plausible that antipsychotic agents (either through weight gain or other unknown effects) uncover latent diabetes tendencies in predisposed subjects.

The effect of weight gain[57] is not to be underestimated, because obesity can significantly increase the risk of development of diabetes in persons with defective beta cell function. Fortunately, weight gain can be managed, as can the hyperglycemia that ensues in some patients.[65] Physicians who treat patients who have major mental disorders should take care to educate their patients regarding the potential for weight gain with antipsychotics. Prophylactic use of behavioral interventions to minimize that risk is strongly advocated.

Several potential targets for future research may be relevant to the elucidation of the key questions. For instance, the role of the central nervous system in regulating circulating glucose and insulin levels needs to be better understood in neuropsychiatric patients.[65,66] Opportunity also exists for an interdisciplinary approach to evaluate the roles of putative metabolic mediators such as leptin,[67,68] the autonomic nervous system,[69] and dopaminergic and histaminergic mechanisms,[70,71] in the regulation of ingestive behavior, body composition, and glucose homeostasis.

Antiretroviral-Associated Diabetes (ARAD)

The introduction of highly active antiretroviral therapy (HAART) has led to dramatic clinical results in people with HIV infection.[72-74] The benefits include suppression of viral load, improvement in CD4 lymphocyte counts, decrease in the number of opportunistic infections and length of hospital stay, and reduction in AIDS-related mortality.[72-74] These advantages of HAART have come at the price of an increased incidence of unanticipated adverse metabolic effects, including insulin resistance, diabetes, dyslipidemia, and lipodystrophy.[75-79] The risk factors, mechanisms, and approach to management of ARAD are discussed in this section.

RISK FACTORS

Inclusion of HIV-1 protease inhibitors (PIs) has been one of the main reasons for the high efficacy of HAART regimens[72-74] and also probably accounts for the adverse metabolic effects. Chronologically, reports of hyperglycemia and other adverse metabolic effects began to appear in the medical literature shortly after clinical deployment of PIs and were nonexistent during the era of nucleoside analog monotherapy. The causal association between PIs and adverse metabolic effects is suggested by the consistency of the pattern of case reports, which, with a rare exception,[79] all cluster within the PI class.[75-78] The association is further strengthened by reports that switching patients to other regimens appears to improve the hyperglycemia and hyperlipidemia observed during use of PI-containing regimens.[80,81]

The exact incidence and prevalence of diabetes in patients treated with PIs are unknown because of lack of population-based studies and possible underreporting bias. In one study of 1230 subjects receiving their first HAART regimen, the adjusted relative hazard rate of hyperglycemia was fivefold higher (95% confidence interval [CI], 1.39-18.16) among patients whose regimens contained PIs compared with patients treated with other regimens.[82] Others have reported that up to 80% of patients treated with PIs develop insulin resistance.[83,84] The risk factors for insulin resistance and diabetes in patients with HIV infection treated with PIs include positive family history of diabetes,[85] weight gain,[85] lipodystrophy,[78] older age,[79] and coinfection with hepatitis C.[82] Clearly, HIV-1 protease inhibitor–associated diabetes or ARAD is a relatively new nosologic entity, the thorough understanding of which could reveal novel insights into metabolic pathophysiology.

UNDERLYING MECHANISMS

Insulin Resistance

The clinical presentation of ARAD is consistent with T2DM, although early use of insulin may be indicated in some patients. Evidence of islet autoimmunity (e.g., glutamic acid decarboxylase antibodies) is distinctly uncommon in patients with ARAD.[85] Yarasheski and colleagues[85] conducted in vivo and in vitro studies in a cross-sectional population of 47 male subjects (39 with HIV infection and 8 healthy, seronegative controls). The HIV-positive patients included those whose diabetes had been diagnosed while they were taking PI-containing regimens (n = 8), patients who did not have diabetes and were not taking PIs (n = 10), and those who did not have diabetes but were taking PI-containing regimens (n = 21). The PI used by subjects in this study was indinavir. Compared with the other groups, the patients with diabetes had higher circulating levels of insulin, C peptide, glucagon, and proinsulin.[85] The proinsulin-to-insulin ratio also was greater in the diabetes group than the others. These and other data[86-91] indicate that insulin resistance rather than primary insulin deficiency is the underlying mechanism for the development of ARAD.

The insulin resistance induced by PIs can be demonstrated acutely following a single dose of indinavir,[86] and it is mediated by inhibition of glucose transport rather than interference with insulin signaling.[87,88] The molecular mechanism of PI-associated insulin resistance could involve alteration in the expression or translocation, or both, of GLUT4 glucose transporters.[89-91] Additional mechanisms for insulin resistance during therapy with PIs include alteration in body composition[92] and development of lipodystrophy.[78,83,84,92,93] Patients with congenital lipodystrophy are severely insulin resistant,[95] as has also been reported for patients with acquired lipodystrophy.[78,83,84,92,93]

As a result of the efficacy of HAART and improved nutrition status, many HIV-infected patients in remission experience significant weight gain, which is a risk factor for insulin resistance and diabetes.[38,44] A tendency to a peculiar pattern of weight gain characterized by a predominantly centripetal or visceral distribution has been reported in HIV-infected patients.[95] This pattern of upper body obesity, even in patients without evidence of lipodystrophy, is a predictor of insulin resistance and the metabolic syndrome.[41,96]

Beta Cell Function

Prospective studies have confirmed that progressive decline in pancreatic beta cell function is necessary for the development of T2DM in persons with insulin resistance.[46,47,65,98] Although circulating insulin levels are higher in patients with ARAD than in controls,[86] the development of hyperglycemia indicates that ambient insulinemia is inadequate for the degree of insulin resistance in these subjects. Moreover, the estimated approximately 80% prevalence of insulin resistance associated with the use of PIs[83,84] does not translate to a similar rate of diabetes, because the majority of patients with HIV infection treated with such regimens do not develop diabetes. Therefore, relative insulin deficiency or beta cell dysfunction must be a permissive factor in persons susceptible to ARAD (Box 42-2). Indeed, minimal modeling predictions of insulin action and insulin secretion during glucose loading in patients with HIV infection treated with indinavir indicate that beta cell dysfunction does contribute to the alteration in glucose disposal.[98]

However, in vitro studies assessing the direct effects of indinavir on cultured pancreatic islets from male Sprague-Dawley rats did not show evi-

Box 42-2. Putative Mechanisms of Antiretroviral-Associated Diabetes

- Induction of insulin resistance
  - Inhibition of glucose transport[87,88]
  - Alteration of GLUT4 expression or translocation[89-91]
  - Increased visceral adiposity[95]
  - Lipodystrophy[92,93]
- Alteration of beta cell function
  - Relative insulin deficiency[98]
  - Decreased glucose uptake and use by beta cells[99]
  - Inhibition of insulin secretion[99]

dence of inhibition of proinsulin conversion to insulin or evidence of glucose-stimulated insulin secretion.[85] In contrast, studies in cultured pancreatic islet cells from mice (C57/Bl×CBA strain) as well as MIN6 insulinoma cell line showed significant and rapid inhibition of glucose-stimulated insulin secretion by indinavir and other protease inhibitors such as amprenavir, nelfinavir, and ritonavir.[99] Indinavir did not affect basal insulin release from the cultured islets, but its inhibitory effect on glucose-stimulated insulin secretion was evident at doses (approximately 2 to 12 μmol/L) within the therapeutic range.[99,100]

Indinavir decreased the rates of glucose uptake and use by cultured MIN6 cells without affecting glucokinase activity. The decreased glucose use provides a mechanism for the inhibition of insulin secretion that is observed following exposure to PIs. Increased intracellular ATP/ADP ratio resulting from glucose use normally serves as a signal for insulin secretion.[101] Thus, interventions that decrease the transport of glucose into the islet cells or its use can be expected to result in decreased insulin output. In vivo, intravenous infusion of indinavir during hyperglycemic clamps in rats decreases first-phase insulin secretion.[99]

MANAGEMENT

Barring evidence to the contrary, standards of care for HIV-infected patients with diabetes should be similar to those applicable to the general diabetes population. The glycemic goals are average preprandial blood glucose values of 80 to 120 mg/dL, bedtime blood glucose of 100 to 140 mg/dL, and HbA1c 7% or lower.[11] A comprehensive approach, tailored to individual needs, using the expertise of diabetes educators, dietitians, and other members of the diabetes care team, is recommended.[63,64]

Nonpharmacologic Interventions

Diet modification through medical nutrition therapy is essential to effective diabetes control.[11]

Broadly, nutrition principles are similar to those advocated for health promotion in the general populace. However, persons with HIV disease and diabetes require individualized diet intervention that is guided by state of glycemic control, body weight, lipid profile, blood pressure, and presence or absence of catabolic drive from opportunistic infections.[46,103,104]

In general, a wholesome, weight-maintaining diet should be offered in the absence of cachexia or overweight. Regular exercise improves cardiovascular fitness, lipid profile, and insulin sensitivity, among other benefits. The safety[105] and beneficial effect of exercise in reducing visceral obesity[106] have been demonstrated in patients with HIV disease.

Medications

The antidiabetic agents used in the general population are effective in controlling hyperglycemia associated with antiretroviral therapy. However, attention must be paid to potential drug interactions and concurrent morbidities when selecting medications for diabetes management in patients with HIV or AIDS. Use of metformin[107,108] or TZDs[109-110] seems a rational approach based on current understanding of the prominent role of insulin resistance in the pathophysiology of ARAD. Patients with HIV nephropathy or abnormal renal function at baseline are not candidates for metformin therapy. Moreover, the gastrointestinal side effects of metformin and the α-glucosidase inhibitors (acarbose, miglitol) may be burdensome in patients with HIV-associated enteropathy.

The potent insulin-sensitizing properties of the TZDs, especially rosiglitazone, which is not significantly metabolized through the CYP 3A4 pathway (used by various antiretrovirals), make them an attractive choice for therapy of ARAD.[109-110] However, potential drug-induced hepatotoxicity, particularly from concurrent antiretroviral medications, can complicate the interpretation of liver function tests. Also, patients with abnormal hepatic function at baseline are not candidates for TZD therapy.

Furthermore, liver enzyme monitoring often is required during therapy with certain PIs and nonnucleoside reverse transcriptase inhibitors.[112] In addition to the above general caveats, it should be noted that nucleoside analogs and other agents used in HAART regimens have specific warnings regarding potential risks of lactic acidosis and severe hepatic dysfunction (Box 42-3).[112] The presence of the latter conditions essentially precludes therapy with biguanide, TZD, or sulfonylurea agents.

As a result of the diverse toxicologic considerations and the need to prevent exacerbation of concurrent risks for lactic acidosis and hepatic dysfunction, exogenous insulin often emerges as

Box 42-3. Antiretroviral Drugs Associated With Lactic Acidosis and Hepatic Dysfunction

Lactic Acidosis or Severe Hepatomegaly

Nucleoside Analogs

Abacavir

Emtricitabine

Lamivudine

Stavudine

Zidovudine

Nucleoside Reverse Transcriptase Inhibitors

Tenofovir

Zalcitabine

Elevated Transaminases

Nonnucleoside Reverse Transcriptase Inhibitors

Delavirdine

Efavirenz

Protease Inhibitors

Fosamprenavir

Lopinavir

Ritonavir

Saquinavir

Table 42–3. *Antiretroviral and Antipsychotic Agents: Parallels and Paradoxes*

HIV-Protease Inhibitors	Atypical Antipsychotics*
Positive Impact on Clinical Measures	
Slow viral replication	Faster onset, higher efficacy
Reduce viral load	Reduce psychiatric symptoms
Increase CD4 counts	Induce clinical remission
Reduce new infections	Prevent relapse
Decrease hospital LOS	Fewer EPS side effects
Decrease AIDS mortality	Improved cognitive function
Unanticipated Adverse Metabolic Effects	
Lipodystrophy, weight gain	Weight gain
Hyperglycemia	Hyperglycemia
Dyslipidemia	Dyslipidemia

*Attributes compared with older conventional antipsychotic agents. AIDS, acquired immunodeficiency syndrome; EPS, extrapyramidal symptoms; LOS, length of stay.

the therapy of necessity. However, sparse subcutaneous tissue in cachetic patients can be a limitation to effective insulin delivery. In addition to glycemic control, care must be taken to optimize the control of comorbid cardiovascular risk factors.[113]

Switching to Alternative Antiretroviral Drugs

It bears stressing that it is not prudent to discontinue otherwise efficacious antiretroviral agents[114] solely because of hyperglycemia. However, if there are other compelling reasons to justify the decision, switching from protease inhibitors to non–PI-containing regimens substituted with nevirapine ameliorates hyperglycemia and dyslipidemia,[80,81] but the effect on lipodystrophy is less certain.[115,116] It is self-evident that any proposed change in antiretroviral medications must be effected by, or undertaken in close consultation with, the appropriate infectious disease or HIV specialist.

CONCLUSIONS

The pathogenesis of ARAD involves complex interactions between components of the HAART regimen (especially HIV-protease inhibitors) and glucoregulatory physiology that result in peripheral

insulin resistance, relative insulin deficiency, and hyperglucagonemia, on a background of improved nutrition and increasing adiposity. Infection with HIV per se does not appear to increase the risk for diabetes. Diabetes in persons with HIV is readily managed by conventional approaches. Routine discontinuation of otherwise efficacious antiretroviral agents is rarely warranted.

There are several conceptual similarities between antipsychotic and antiretroviral agents both in terms of the promise they bring to the target disease states and their unanticipated adverse metabolic effects (Table 42–3). The majority of persons taking these medications do not develop diabetes. The exact mechanisms that trigger diabetes in patients receiving treatment with antipsychotic or antiretroviral agents are incompletely understood. In the case of APAD, the preexisting background of psychotic stress, chronic activation of the HPA axis, and alteration in body composition favors the development of insulin resistance. Additional metabolic stress from drug-induced weight gain and adverse interactions between medications and putative susceptibility factors[117-119] can permit the development of diabetes.

In the case of antiretroviral agents, induction of insulin resistance (and possibly beta cell dysfunction) by HIV protease inhibitors, in susceptible persons, would seem to be the proximate mechanism for the development of diabetes. The approach to management of diabetes associated with antipsychotic and antiretroviral agents is fairly straightforward, although additional vigilance for drug toxicities related to premorbid conditions and concurrent medications is warranted. Increased surveillance for diabetes, including baseline and periodic screening, is recommended in patients receiving therapy with antipsychotic medications or antiretroviral drugs, particularly protease inhibitors.

Clearly, further studies are needed to unravel the exact mechanisms, susceptibility factors, and mediators of the perturbations that trigger diabetes in patients treated with antipsychotic or antiretroviral medications.

Acknowledgment

Dr. Dagogo-Jack is supported in part by NIH Clinical Research Center Grant MO1 RR00211.

References

1. Harris MI, Flegal KM, Cowie CC, et al: Prevalence of diabetes, impaired fasting glucose, and impaired glucose tolerance in US adults. The Third National Health and Nutrition Examination Survey. Diabetes Care 21:518-524, 1998.
2. Mokdad AH, Ford ES, Bowman BA, et al: Diabetes trends in the U.S.: 1990-1998. Diabetes Care 23:1278-1283, 2000.
3. Freedman R: Schizophrenia. N Engl J Med 349:1738-1749, 2003.
4. Rucker L, Dietch JT: Depression in primary care: Evolving concepts and approach to therapy. South Med J 79:215-222, 1986.
5. Mukherjee S, Decina P, Bocola V, et al: Diabetes mellitus in schizophrenic patients. Comp Psych 37:68-73, 1996.
6. Keskiner A, el Toumi A, Bousquet T: Psychotropic drugs, diabetes and chronic mental patients. Psychosomatics 14:176-181, 1973.
7. Mukherjee S, Decina P, Bocola V, et al: Diabetes mellitus in schizophremic patients. Compr Psychiatry 37:68-73, 1996.
8. Buse JB, Cavazzoni P, Hornbuckle K, et al: A retrospective cohort study of diabetes mellitus and antipsychotic treatment in the United States. J Clin Epidemiology 56:164-170, 2003.
9. Cassidy F, Ahearn E, Carroll BJ: Elevated frequency of diabetes mellitus in hospitalized manic-depressive patients. Am J Psychiatry 156:1417-1420, 1999.
10. Dixon L, Weiden PJ, Delahanty J, et al: Prevalence and correlates of diabetes in national schizophrenia samples. Schizophr Bull 26:903-912, 2000.
11. American Diabetes Association: Standards of medical care in diabetes. Diabetes Care 27(suppl 1):S15-S35, 2004.
12. Lamberti JS, Crilly JF, Maharaj K, et al: Prevalence of diabetes mellitus among outpatients with severe mental disorders receiving atypical antipsychotic drugs. J Clin Psychiatry 65:702-706, 2004.
13. Basu R, Brar JS, Chengappa KN, et al: The prevalence of the metabolic syndrome in patients with schizoaffective disorder—bipolar subtype. Bipolar Disord 6:314-318, 2004.
14. Eaton WW, Armenian H, Gallo J, et al: Depression and risk for onset of type II diabetes. A prospective population-based study. Diabetes Care 19:1097-1102, 1996.
15. Koller E, Schneider B, Bennett K, Dubitsky G: Clozapine-associated diabetes. Am J Med 111:716-723, 2001.
16. Koller EA, Doraiswamy PM: Olanzapine-associated diabetes mellitus. Pharmacotherapy 22:841-852, 2002.
17. Ollendorf DA, Joyce AT, Rucker M: Rate of new-onset diabetes among patients treated with atypical or conventional antipsychotic medications for schizophrenia. MedGenMed 6:5, 2004.
18. Haupt DW, Newcomer JW: Risperidone-associated diabetic ketoacidosis. Psychosomatics 42:279-280, 2001.
19. Ryan MC, Collins P, Thakore JH: Impaired fasting glucose tolerance in first-episode, drug-naïve patients with schizophrenia. Am J Psychiatry 160:284-289, 2003.
20. American Diabetes Association: Diabetes Facts and Figures. March 2002. Available at: http://www.diabetes.org/diabetes-statistics/national-diabetes-fact-sheet.jsp.
21. Lowe LP, Liu K, Greenland P, et al: Diabetes, asymptomatic hyperglycemia, and 22-year mortality in black and white men. Diabetes Care 20:163-169, 1997.
22. Hiles BW: Hyperglycemia and glycosuria following chlorpromazine therapy. JAMA 162:1651, 1956.
23. Korenyi C, Lowenstein B: Chlorpromazine induced diabetes. Dis Nerv Syst 29:827-828, 1968.
24. Thonnard-Neumann E: Phenothiazines and diabetes in hospitalized women. Am J Psychiatry 124:138-142, 1968.
25. Heninger GR, Mueller PS: Carbohydrate abnormalities in mania before and after lithium carbonate treatment. Arch Gen Psychiatry 23:310-319, 1970.
26. Meduna LJ, Gerty FJ, Urse VG: Biochemical disturbances in mental disorders. Arch Gen Psychiatry 17:38-52, 1942.
27. Koro CE, Fedder DO, L'Italien GJ, et al: Assessment of independent effect of olanzapine and risperidone on risk of diabetes among patients with schizophrenia: Population based nested case-control study. BMJ 325:243, 2002.
28. Fuller MA, Shermock KM, Secic M, Grogg AL: Fuller comparative study of the development of diabetes mellitus in patients taking risperidone and olanzapine. Pharmacotherapy 23:1037-1043, 2003.
29. Rothbard AB, Kuno E, Foley K: Trends in the rate and type of antipsychotic medications prescribed to persons with schizophrenia. Schizophr Bull 29:531-540, 2003.
30. Sobel M, Jaggers ED, Franz MA: New-onset diabetes mellitus associated with initiation of quetiapine treatment. J Clin Psychiatry 60:556-557, 1999.
31. Wilson DR, D'Souza L, Sarkar N, et al: New-onset diabetes and ketoacidosis with atypical antipsychotics. Schizophr Res 59:1-6, 2003.
32. Groop LC, Bottazzo GF: Genetic susceptibility to non-insulin-dependent diabetes mellitus. Diabetes 35:237-241, 1986.
33. Johnson DD, Palumbo PJ, Chu CP: Diabetic ketoacidosis in a community-based population. Mayo Clin Proc 55:83-88, 1980.
34. Fishbein HA, Palumbo PJ: Acute metabolic complications in diabetes. In National Diabetes Data Group (eds): Diabetes in America, 2nd ed. Washington, DC, National Institute of Diabetes and Digestive and Kidney Diseases, 1995. NIH Publication No. 95-1468, pp. 283-291.
35. Basu A, Close CF, Jenkins D, et al: Persisting mortality in diabetic ketoacidosis. Diabet Med 10:282-289, 1992.
36. Clements RS, Vourganti B: Fatal diabetic ketoacidosis: Major causes and approaches to their prevention. Diabetes Care 1:314-325, 1978.
37. Mokdad AH, Bowman BA, Ford ES, et al: The continuing epidemics of obesity and diabetes in the United States. JAMA 286:1195-1200, 2001.
38. Unger R: Lipotoxicity in the pathogenesis of obesity-dependent NIDDM: Genetic and clinical implications. Diabetes 44:863-870, 1995.
39. Ryan MCM, Flanagan S, Kinsella U, et al: The effects of atypical antipsychotics on visceral fat distribution in first episode, drug-naive patients with schizophrenia. Life Sci 74:1999-2008, 2004.
40. Tsigos C, Chrousos GP: Hypothalamic- pituitary-adrenal axis, neuroendocrine factors and stress. J Psychosomatic Res 53:865-871, 2002.
41. Gold PW, Loriaux DL, Roy A, et al: Responses to corticotropin-releasing hormone in the hypercortisolism of depression and Cushing's disease. Pathophysiologic and diagnostic implications. N Engl J Med 314:1329-1335, 1986.
42. Lustman PJ, Griffith LS, Clouse RE, et al: Effects of nortriptyline on depression and glycemic control in diabetes: results of a double-blind, placebo-controlled trial. Psychosom Med 59:241-250, 1997.
43. Lustman PJ, Freedland KE, Griffith LS, Clouse RE: Fluoxetine for depression in diabetes: A randomized, double-blind, placebo-controlled trial. Diabetes Care 23:618-623, 2000.

44. Lev-Ran A: Thrifty genotype: How applicable is it to obesity and type 2 diabetes? Diabetes Rev 7:1-22, 1999.

45. Weyer C, Tataranni PA, Bogardus C, Pratley RE: Insulin resistance and insulin secretory dysfunction are independent predictors of worsening of glucose tolerance during each stage of type 2 diabetes development. Diabetes Care 24:89-94, 2001.

46. Dagogo-Jack S, Santiago JV: Pathophysiology of type 2 diabetes and modes of action of therapeutic interventions. Arch Intern Med 157:1802-1817, 1997.

47. Haupt DW, Newcomer JW: Hyperglycemia and antipsychotic medications. J Clin Psychiatry 62(Suppl 27):15-26, 2001.

48. Newcomer JW, Haupt DW, Fucetola R, et al: Abnormalities in glucose regulation during antipsychotic treatment of schizophrenia. Arch Gen Psychiatry 59:337-345, 2002.

49. DeFronzo RA, Tobin JD, Andres R: Glucose clamp technique: A method for quantifying insulin secretion and resistance. Am J Physiol 237:E214-E223, 1979.

50. Elahi D: In praise of the hyperglycemic clamp. A method for assessment of beta-cell sensitivity and insulin resistance. Diabetes Care 19:278-286, 1996.

51. Beasley CM, Sowell M, Carlson C, et al: Prospective evaluation of insulin sensitivity by the hyperinsulinemic, euglycemic clamp in healthy volunteers treated with olanzapine, risperidone or placebo. Presented at the 41st American College of Neuropsychopharmacology Annual Meeting, San Juan, Puerto Rico, December 8-12, 2002.

52. Newcomer JW, Haupt DW, Melson AK, Schweiger J: Insulin resistance measured with euglycemic clamps during antipsychotic treatment in schizophrenia. Presented at the Society of Biological Psychiatry 58th Annual Scientific Convention and Program, San Francisco, Calif, May 15-17, 2003.

53. Sowell MO, Mukhopadhyay N, Cavazzoni P, et al: Hyperglycemic clamp assessment of insulin secretory responses in normal subjects treated with olanzapine, risperidone, or placebo. J Clin Endocrinol Metab 87:2918-2923, 2002.

54. Henderson DC, Cagliero E, Borba CP, et al: Atypical antipsychotic agents and glucose metabolism: Bergman's MINMOD analysis. Presented at the 52nd American Psychiatric Association Institute on Psychiatric Services, Philadelphia, October 25-29, 2000.

55. Beasley CM Jr, Tollefson GD, Tran PV: Efficacy of olanzapine: An overview of pivotal clinical trial. J Clin Psychiatry 10:7-12, 1997.

56. Csernansky JG, Mahmoud R, Brenner R: A comparison of risperidone and haloperidol for the prevention of relapse in patients with schizophrenia. N Engl J Med 346:16-22, 2002. [Erratum in N Engl J Med 346:1424, 2002.]

57. Volavka J, Czobor P, Sheitman B, et al: Clozapine, olanzapine, risperidone, and haloperidol in the treatment of patients with chronic schizophrenia and schizoaffective disorder. Am J Psychiatry 159:255-262, 2002.

58. Bilder RM, Goldman RS, Volavka J, et al: Neurocognitive effects of clozapine, olanzapine, risperidone, and haloperidol in patients with chronic schizophrenia or schizoaffective disorder. Am J Psychiatry 159:1018-1028, 2002.

59. Lindenmayer JP, Czobor P, Volavka J, et al: Changes in glucose and cholesterol levels in patients with schizophrenia treated with typical or atypical antipsychotics. Am J Physiol 160:290-296, 2003.

60. Sernyak MJ, Leslie DL, Alarcon RD, et al: Association of diabetes mellitus with use of atypical neuroleptics in the treatment of schizophrenia. Am J Psychiatry 159:561-566, 2002.

61. Dagogo-Jack S: Diabetes and insulin resistance in the neuropsychiatric population. Consultant 43(Suppl):18-23, 2003.

62. Food and Drug Administration: Warning about Hyperglycemia and Atypical Antipsychotic Drugs. FDA Patient Safety News: Show #28, June 2004. Available at http://www.accessdata.fda.gov/scripts/cdrh/cfdocs/psn/printer.cfm?id=229.

63. American Diabetes Association: Consensus development conference on antipsychotic drugs and obesity and diabetes. Diabetes Care 27:596-601, 2004.

64. Moneva M, Dagogo-Jack S: Multiple drug targets in the management of type 2 diabetes mellitus. Curr Drug Targets 3:203-221, 2002.

65. Dagogo-Jack S: Preventing diabetes-related morbidity and mortality in the primary care setting. J Natl Med Assoc 94:549-560, 2002.

66. Craft S, Newcomer J, Kanne S, et al: Memory improvement following induced hyperinsulinemia in Alzheimer's disease. Neurobiol Aging 17:123-130, 1996.

67. Newcomer JW, Selke G, Melson AK, et al: Dose-dependent cortisol-induced increases in plasma leptin concentration in healthy humans. Arch Gen Psychiatry 55:995-1000, 1998.

68. Kraus T, Haack M, Schuld A, et al: Body weight and leptin plasma levels during treatment with antipsychotic drugs. Am J Psychiatry 156:312-314, 1999.

69. Walters JM, Ward GM, Barton J, et al: The effect of norepinephrine on insulin secretion and glucose effectiveness in non–insulin-dependent diabetes. Metabolism 46:1448-1453, 1997.

70. Dwyer DS, Liu Y, Bradley RJ: Dopamine receptor antagonists modulate glucose uptake in rat pheochromoytoma (PC12) cells. Neurosci Lett 274:151-154, 1999.

71. Kroeze WK, Hufeisen SJ, Popadak BA, et al: H-1-histamine receptor affinity predicts short-term weight gain for typical and atypical antipsychotic drugs. Neuropsychopharmacology 28:519-526, 2003.

72. Palella FJ Jr, Delaney KM, Moorman AC, et al: Declining morbidity and mortality among patients with advanced immunodeficiency virus infection. HIV Outpatient Study Investigators. N Engl J Med 338:853-860, 1998.

73. Carpenter CC, Fischl MA, Hammer SM, et al: Antiretroviral therapy for HIV infection in 1997. Updated recommendations of the International AIDS Society–USA panel. JAMA 277:1962-1969, 1997.

74. Hammer SM, Squires KE, Hughes MD, et al: A controlled trial of two nucleoside analogues plus indinavir in persons with human immunodeficiency virus infection and CD4 cell counts of 200 per cubic millimeter or less. N Engl J Med 337:725-733, 1997.

75. Visnegarwala F, Krause KL, Musher DM: Severe diabetes associated with protease inhibitor therapy. Ann Intern Med 127:947, 1997.

76. Flexner C: HIV-protease inhibitors. N Engl J Med 338:1281-1292, 1998.

77. Walli R, Herfort O, Michl GM, et al: Treatment with protease inhibitors associated with peripheral insulin resistance and impaired oral glucose tolerance in HIV-1-infected patients. AIDS 12:F167-F173, 1998.

78. Carr A, Samaras K, Burton S, et al: A syndrome of peripheral lipodystrophy and insulin resistance in patients receiving HIV protease inhibitors. AIDS 12:F51-F58, 1998.

79. Brambilla AM, Novati R, Calori G, et al: Stavudine or indinavir-containing regimens are associated with an increased risk of diabetes mellitus in HIV-infected individuals. AIDS 17:1993-1995, 2003.

80. Martinez E, Conget I, Lazano L, et al: Reversion of metabolic abnormalities after switching from HIV-1 protease inhibitors to nevirapine. AIDS 13:805-810, 1999.

81. Carr A, Thorisdottir A, Samaras K, et al: Reversibility of protease inhibitor (PI) lipodystrophy syndrome on stopping PIs or switching to nelfinavir. Presented at the VI Conference on retroviruses and Opportunistic Infections, Chicago, Ill, January 31–February 4, 1999 (Abstract).

82. Mehta SH, Moore RD, Thomas DL, et al: The effect of HAART and HCV infection on the development of hyperglycemia among HIV-infected persons. J Acquir Immune Defic Syndr 33:577-584, 2003.

83. Hadigan C, Meigs JB, Corcoran C, et al: Metabolic abnormalities and cardiovascular disease risk factors in adults with human immunodeficiency virus infection and lipodystrophy. Clin Infec Dis 32:130-139, 2001.

84. Vigouroux C, Gharakhanian S, Salhi Y, et al: Diabetes, insulin resistance and dyslipidaemia in lipodystrophic HIV-infected patients on highly active antiretroviral therapy (HAART). Diabetes Metab 25:225-232, 1999.

85. Yarasheki KE, Tebas P, Sigmund C, et al: Insulin resistance in HIV protease inhibitor–associated diabetes. J Acquir Immune Defic Syndr 21:209-216, 1999.

86. Noor MA, Seneviratne T, Aweeka FT, et al: Indinavir acutely inhibits insulin-stimulated glucose disposal in humans: A randomized, placebo-controlled study. AIDS 16:F1-F8, 2002.

87. Murata H, Hruz PW, Mueckler M: The mechanism of insulin resistance caused by HIV protease inhibitor therapy. J Biol Chem 275:20251-20254, 2000.

88. Algenstaedt P, Daneshi S, Schwarzloh B, et al: Therapeutic dose of HIV-1 protease inhibitor saquinavir does not permanently influence early insulin signaling. Exp Clin Endocrinol Diabetes 111:491-498, 2003.

89. Murata H, Hruz PW, Mueckler M: Investigating the cellular targets of HIV protease inhibitors: Implications for metabolic disorders and improvements in drug therapy. Curr Drug Targets Infect Disord 2:1-8, 2002.

90. Murata H, Hruz P, Mueckler M: Indinavir inhibits the glucose transporter isoform Glut4 at physiologic concentrations. AIDS 16:859-863, 2002.

91. Nolte LA, Yarasheki KE, Kawanaka K, et al: The HIV protease inhibitor indinavir decreases insulin-and contraction-stimulated glucose transport in skeletal muscle. Diabetes 50:1397-1401, 2001.

92. Lo JC, Mulligan K, Tai VW, et al: "Buffalo hump" in men with HIV-1 infection. Lancet 351:867-870, 1998.

93. Kravcik S: Update on HIV lipodystrophy. HIV Clin Trials 5:152-167, 2004.

94. Garg A, Misra A: Lipodystrophies: Rare disorders causing metabolic syndrome. Endocrinol Metab Clin North Am 33:305-331, 2004.

95. Kosmiski L, Kuritzkes D, Hamilton J, et al: Fat distribution is altered in HIV-infected men without clinical evidence of the HIV lipodystrophy syndrome. HIV Med 4:235-240, 2003.

96. Bjorntorp P: Metabolic abnormalities in visceral obesity (editorial). Ann Intern Med 24:3-5, 1992.

97. Weyer C, Bogardus C, Mott DM, Pratley RE: The natural history of insulin secretory dysfunction and insulin resistance in the pathogenesis of type 2 diabetes. J Clin Invest 104:787-794, 1999.

98. Dube MP, Edmondson-Melancon H, Qian D, Aqeel R, et al: Prospective evaluation of the effect of initiating indinavir-based therapy on insulin sensitivity and B-cell function in HIV-infected patients. J Acquir Immune Defic Syndr 27:130-134, 2001.

99. Koster JC, Remedi MS,Qui H, et al: HIV protease inhibitors acutely impair glucose-stimulated insulin release. Diabetes 52:1695-1700, 2003.

100. Anderson PL, Brundage RC, Bushman L, et al: Indinavir plasma protein binding in HIV-1 infected adults. AIDS 14:2293-2297, 2000.

101. Cook DL, Hales CN: Intracellular ATP directly blocks K channels in pancreatic β-cells. Nature 311:271-273, 1984.

102. Wanke CA, Falutz JM, Shevitz A, et al: Clinical evaluation and management of metabolic and morphologic abnormalities associated with human immunodeficiency virus. Clin Infect Dis 34:248-259, 2002.

103. Grundy SM: Dietary therapy in diabetes mellitus. Is there a single best diet? Diabetes Care 14:796-801, 1991.

104. Bouvier G: Nutrition counseling is important for HIV-infected diabetics. HIV Clin 16:9, 2004.

105. Roubenoff R, Skolnik PR, Shevitz A, et al: Effect of a single bout of acute exercise on plasma human immunodeficiency virus RNA levels. J Appl Physiol 86:1197-201, 1999.

106. Roubenoff R, Weiss L, McDermott A, et al: A pilot study of exercise training to reduce trunk fat in adults with HIV-associated fat redistribution. AIDS 13:1373-1375, 1999.

107. Saint-Marc T, Touraine J: Effects of metformin on insulin resistance and central adiposity in patients receiving effective protease inhibitor therapy. AIDS 13:1000-1002, 1999.

108. Hadigan C, Corcoran C, Basgoz N, et al: Metformin in the treatment of HIV lipodystrophy syndrome: A randomized controlled trial. JAMA 284:472-477, 2000.

109. Walli R, Michl M, Bogner J, Goebel F: Effects of the PPAR-gamma activator troglitazone on protease inhibitor associated peripheral insulin resistance [abstract 673]. In Program and Abstracts of the 6th Conference on Retroviruses and Opportunistic Infections (Chicago). Alexandria, Virginia: Foundation for Retrovirology and Human Health, 1999.

110. Sutinen J, Kannisto K, Korsheninnikova E, et al: Effects of rosiglitazone on gene expression in subcutaneous adipose tissue in highly active antiretroviral therapy–associated lipodystrophy. Am J Physiol Endocrinol Metab 286:E941-E949, 2004.

111. Gelato MC, Mynarcik DC, Quick JL, et al: Improved insulin sensitivity and body fat distribution in HIV-infected patients treated with rosiglitazone: A pilot study. J Acquir Immune Defic Syndr 31:163-70, 2002.

112. PDR Staff: Physicians Desk Reference 2004. Montvale, NJ, Thompson PDR, 2003, pp 481, 496, 1114, 1392, 1467, 1489, 1493, 1608, 2630, 2905, 2913.

113. Penzak SR, Chuck SK: Management of protease inhibitor-associated hyperlipidemia. Am J Cardiovasc Drugs 2:91-106, 2002.

114. Powderly WG: Lessons learned from switching antiretrovirals [abstract]. Antivir Ther 5(Suppl 5):17, 2000.

115. Martinez E, Garcia-Viejo MA, Blanco JL, et al: Impact of switching from human immunodeficiency virus type 1 protease inhibitors to efavirenz in successfully treated adults with lipodystrophy. Clin Infect Dis 31:1266-1273, 2000.

116. Yarasheski KE, Tebas P, Claxton S, et al: HIV-protease inhibitor switch to nevirapine improves insulin tolerance but does not correct adipose maldistribution [abstract P93]. Antivir Ther 5(Suppl 5):78, 2000.

117. Odawara M, Isaka M, Tada K, et al: Diabetes mellitus associated with mitochondrial myopathy and schizophrenia: A possible link between diabetes mellitus and schizophrenia (letter). Diabet Med 14:503, 1997.

118. Tsuchiyama N, Ando H, Sakurai M, Takamura T: Modulating effects of olanzapine on the development of diabetic ketoacidosis [letter]. Diabet Med 21:300-301, 2003.

119. Holden RJ, Pakula IS: The link between diabetes and schizophrenia: An immunological explanation (letter). Aust N Z J Psychiatry 33:286-287, 1999.

Chapter 43

Running a Diabetes Clinic

Anne L. Peters

KEY POINTS

- *Diabetes centers cannot exist without institutional and community support.*
- *Multiple approaches need to be employed to ensure long-term success.*
- *The patient must be an empowered participant in his or her care.*
- *Primary care providers must be a key part of any diabetes approach and must be given the resources to succeed.*
- *A computerized infrastructure for maintaining a database, tracking patients, and following outcomes is invaluable.*
- *Improved outcomes and associated cost savings have been demonstrated in individual programs. The current challenge is to extend high-quality care across populations.*

Most people with diabetes in America are treated by their primary care providers. Diabetologists tend to be located in large cities, so many patients with diabetes do not have the option of being treated by a specialist. Therefore, the concept of the *diabetes clinic* has been changing. The notion of population-based chronic disease management, along with focused centers where diabetes experts are available, has replaced the prior clinic-based model. However, many models of care require the existence of specialty centers for management of the most complex cases.

In order for diabetes centers of any sort to survive, they must exist within an institutional and societal infrastructure that provides financial and programmatic support. This review discusses the composition and effectiveness of individual centers as well as the dissemination of quality diabetes care through chronic-care programs.

HISTORY

In the past, our efforts to treat diabetes patients have not resulted in success. If they had, diabetes would not be the leading cause of adult blindness, kidney failure, and nontrauma-based lower extremity amputation in the United States.[1] Average hemoglobin A1c (HbA1c) levels in patients treated for diabetes in the United States are far higher than the targets required to prevent the complications of diabetes: The mean HbA1c in diabetic patients is 9%, but the target is lower than 7%.[2] Studies looking at the achievement of the three major risk-reduction targets—lowering HbA1c, lowering blood pressure, and lowering low-density lipoprotein (LDL) cholesterol levels—find that results are even worse at achieving all three.[3]

To combat this problem, many organizations have implemented diabetes disease management programs. By 1998 it was reported that 79% of HMOs offered diabetes disease management programs.[4] These programs often vary in definition, scope, and availability to patients, but clearly they are proliferating and offer the opportunity for a coordinated approach to diabetes care.

Diabetes is particularly well suited to using a comprehensive approach for managing multiple risk factors. With a comprehensive approach, outcomes are easily measured and care can be integrated, which is critical for preventing the microvascular and macrovascular complications of the disease.[5] Criteria for assessing how well diabetes care is being provided was developed as part of the Diabetes Quality Improvement Project (DQIP).[6] The DQIP measure set is shown in Table 43-1.

Assessing outcomes is not enough, however. Outcomes must be improved and sustained over time. These changes must occur at the most basic level—interaction between patient and provider—in order to be successful. The chronic care model, discussed next, attempts to assess what is good and what is lacking in the dynamic between patient and health care provider.

Table 43-1. *HEDIS Guidelines for the Diabetes Quality Improvement Project Initial Measure Set**

Accountability Set

1. Percentage of patients taking more than 1 HbA1c test per year
2. Percentage of patients with the highest-risk HbA1c level (HbA1c > 9.5%)
3. Percentage of patients assessed for nephropathy
4. Percentage of patients receiving a lipid profile once in 2 years
5. Percentage of patients with LDL† less than 130 mg/dL
6. Percentage of patients with blood pressure† <140/90 mm Hg
7. Percentage of patients receiving a dilated eye exam

Quality Improvement Set

1. HbA1c levels of all patients reported in six categories: <7.0%, 7.0% to 7.9%, 8.0% to 8.9%, 9.0% to 9.9%, >10.0%, no value documented
2. Distribution of LDL values† (<100 mg/dL, 100 to 129 mg/dL, 130 to 159 mg/dL, >159 mg/dL, no value documented)
3. Distribution of blood pressure values† (systolic: <140 mm Hg, 140 to 159 mm Hg, 160 to 179 mm Hg, 180 to 209 mm Hg, >209 mm Hg; diastolic: <90 mm Hg, 90 to 99 mm Hg, 100 to 109 mm Hg, 110 to 119 mm Hg, >119 mm Hg, no value documented)
4. Fraction of patients receiving a well-documented foot exam to include a risk assessment

*Some of the measures have exclusions based on comorbidity or based on the results from a previous examination. All measures apply to diabetic patients between 18 and 75 years of age, regardless of type of diabetes. Measures 1, 2, and 7 can be applied to children 10 to 17 years old as well. See http://www.ncqa.org/Programs/HEDIS/HEDIS%202005%%20Info.htm for details.
†For all measures requiring a value (e.g., LDL cholesterol, blood pressure), the most recent test result is used.
  HbA1c, hemoglobin A1c; HEDIS, Health Plan Employer Data and Information Set; LDL, low-density lipoprotein.

Box 43-1. Components of the Chronic Care Model

- Self-management support
- Decision support: educational materials and meetings for physicians
- Delivery system design: use of case managers, multidisciplinary teams, and scheduling of planned diabetes follow-up visits
- Clinical information systems: reminder systems and feedback on physician performance

THE CHRONIC CARE MODEL

To understand the treatment of diabetes, it is necessary to understand it in the context of the overall management of chronic disease. The chronic care model was developed by Edward Wagner as a guide for dealing with chronic illness in primary care. The model was derived from efforts to improve chronic illness management at Group Health Cooperative of Puget Sound in Washington, from literature reviews, and from suggestions of an advisory panel to Group Health's MacColl Institute for Healthcare Innovation. In a series of articles published in the *Journal of the American Medical Association*,[7,8] the basic tenets of the chronic care model are discussed, and specific examples are provided of how this type of care can affect the health of specific patients with chronic illness.

The model looks at the entire health care system and how it affects the care of patients with chronic disease. Interventions used in the chronic care model to improve process and outcomes measures,

as well as to lower the costs of care and improve quality of life, include self-management support, decision support, delivery system design, and clinical information systems (Box 43-1).[7] The model predicts that improvement in its four interrelated components can lead to system reform in which knowledgeable and empowered patients interact with prepared, proactive practice teams to provide better care for chronic disease.

One particularly successful example of the chronic care model was the Danish study of primary care disease management for diabetes.[9] This was a randomized trial of 970 patients with diabetes treated by 474 general practitioners. Usual care was compared with a program involving decision support, regular follow-up, reminder systems, and self-management support based on individualized goal setting. After 6 years of follow-up, patients in the intervention group had significantly lower HbA1c, blood pressure, and cholesterol levels than those in the control group. This study shows the benefits of providing the tools and education opportunities for practitioners in primary care to enhance outcomes in their patients with diabetes.

Bodenheimer and colleagues performed a meta-analysis to evaluate the published studies on the use of interventions to improve diabetes care.[8] The chronic care model components that were necessary for inclusion in the meta-analysis were support, delivery system design, and clinical information systems. At least one of these components had to be included in the intervention. Of the 39 studies that fit the criteria for the meta-analysis, 32 of them found at least one process or outcomes measure improved by using one or more chronic care model components. Eighteen of the 27 studies available to evaluate cost showed reduced health care cost or lower use of health care services for the treatment of heart failure, asthma, and diabetes. Therefore, the principles of the chronic care model clearly can be effective in the setting of diabetes care.

In 1999 a conference on chronic care and behavioral science research in diabetes was held,[10] sponsored by the National Institute on Diabetes and Digestive and Kidney Diseases. The participants addressed the status of research on quality of care, patient–provider interactions, and health care

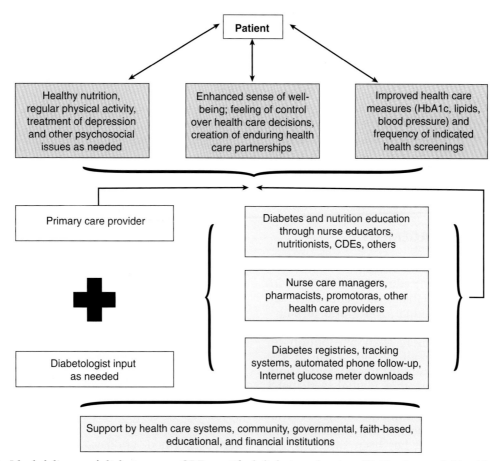

Figure 43–1. Ideal delivery of diabetes care. CDE, certified diabetes educator; HbA1c, hemoglobin A1c.

systems' innovations related to improved diabetes outcomes. It was concluded that although the quality of care provided to the vast majority of diabetic patients is problematic, it was not primarily the fault of either individual patients or health care professionals. Rather, it was a systems issue because our health care system is based on a model of care for acute illness, rather than chronic disease management. As described by Tom Bodenheimer, it is the "tryanny of the urgent" that short-changes chronic disease management. When office visits are limited, most patients want the health care provider to address their acute concerns, rather than spend time on the management of a chronic disease that is largely asymptomatic.

Another area in which diabetes management differs from the treatment of other illnesses is that patients and their families, not health care professionals, are largely responsible for the management of the disease.[11-14] Providers need to work with patients to develop collaborative approaches to care that patients feel are appropriate so they can follow through once they leave the office.[10] This shift in view from the provider to the patient as the active decision maker and problem solver is central to productive patient–provider interactions for management of diabetes and other chronic illnesses. Figure

43–1 illustrates the multifaceted care required by patients with diabetes.

DESIGNING THE DIABETES CARE SYSTEM

In addition to needing time to focus on diabetes management in patient appointments and patients' participation in their care, diabetes clinics must be designed to provide patients with regular care and follow-up over extended periods of time. This can be done in the setting of the primary care office, an endocrinology office, or some hybrid of the two (where patients are seen by a diabetes team for evaluation and then sent back to the primary care provider for ongoing management). In any case, patients need access to diabetes education, both initially and on an ongoing basis, as is discussed later. Similarly, patients need to be given access to a nutritionist, who can help define nutrition targets and design an approach to food that meshes with the patient's metabolic needs and lifestyle.

To provide consistent ongoing care, a diabetes registry or database is an indispensable tool. With it data can be analyzed and evaluated to assess how patients are doing, but it also serves a vital tracking

role. It allows patients to be notified to come in for appointments or laboratory tests and it continues to notify both provider and patient when visits have not occurred. It is virtually impossible for busy clinicians to track patients and make sure they return with appropriate frequency. In a diabetes center for the underserved in East Los Angeles it is the patients with the highest HbA1c levels who are most often lost to follow-up.[15] These are often the patients who need the most help and who will be lost from care if they are not tracked in some way.

DIABETES SELF-MANAGEMENT EDUCATION

Diabetes self-management education (DSME) is an integral component of diabetes care. Education can be provided in an individual or a group format.[16] Either approach can work, and in many cases it is useful to provide more than one option for education, because not all people learn in the same way. It is the accessibility to education, both initially and in follow-up, that is vital to diabetes management.

Although it has been difficult to prove that DSME, in isolation, improves outcomes, as part of a treatment program it has been shown to enhance psychosocial and health outcomes.[17-19] In these studies, education occurred in the setting of a primary care practice and was associated with improved processes of care and better health.

Two very important elements of DSME are medical nutrition therapy (MNT) and exercise. A review of studies on MNT has shown significant improvements in weight and HbA1c levels in patients who participate in the education process provided by a registered dietitian.[20] Another review[21] evaluated the effectiveness of diet interventions in patients with chronic disease as reported in 92 independent studies. Most studies were similarly successful in reducing intake of total and saturated fat (7.3% reduction in the percentage of calories from fat), and increasing fruit and vegetable intake (an average increase of 0.6 servings per day). The two intervention components seemed to be particularly promising in modifying diet behavior—goal setting and small groups. Interventions designed to improve diet behavior are effective, although it is impossible to conclude which interventions are the most effective because the interventions are heterogeneous.

The National Standards for Diabetes Self-Management Education Programs were developed to limit variation in educational interventions[22] and to provide basic standards for care. The key elements of self-management education are presented in Box 43-2. These standards stress the need for patients with diabetes to acquire both knowledge and skills to manage their disease, which should result in

> ### Box 43-2. DSME Written Curriculum Guidelines
>
> A written curriculum, with criteria for successful learning outcomes, shall be available. Assessed needs of the individual will determine which content areas listed below are delivered.
>
> - Describing the *diabetes disease process* and treatment options
> - Incorporating appropriate *nutritional management*
> - Incorporating *physical activity* into lifestyle
> - Using *medications* (if applicable) for therapeutic effectiveness
> - *Monitoring* blood glucose, monitoring urine ketones when appropriate, and using the results to improve glycemic control
> - Preventing, detecting, and treating *acute complications*
> - Preventing (through *risk reduction* behavior), detecting, and treating chronic complications
> - *Goal setting* to promote health, and *problem solving* for daily living
> - Integrating *psychosocial adjustment* to daily life
> - Promoting *preconception care*, management during *pregnancy*, and *gestational diabetes management* (if applicable)

better-informed choices and more-desirable behavior. The focus is shifted from simply providing knowledge to assisting patients in developing strategies for behavior change. Education programs that meet the National Standards for Diabetes Self-Management Education Programs are recognized by the ADA as programs of excellence.[22a]

The National Diabetes Education Program (NDEP) was started in 1997 through a joint effort by the National Institutes of Health (NIH) and the Centers for Disease Control and Prevention (CDC).[23] It is a public–private partnership that now includes more than 200 additional organizations. The goal of the NDEP is to promote early diagnosis and to improve the treatment and outcomes for people with diabetes.

Initially the NDEP focused on therapies that improved glucose control, but it has recently expanded to include an initiative to promote optimal control of lipids and blood pressure in addition to optimal control of blood glucose. The audience for the initiative includes people with diabetes and their families (with special emphasis given to those who are members of high-risk minority groups), the general public, health care providers, and health care payers, purchasers, and policy makers.

The NDEP's messages and approaches are consistent with ADA and other national guidelines, as well as national outcome-focused programs such as the Diabetes Quality Improvement Program (DQIP), and they are designed to improve health care provider practice and patient outcomes. The guide-

Box 43-3. National Diabetes Education Program Guidelines

- Practice goal-oriented management of blood glucose, lipids, and blood pressure to help prevent or delay diabetes complications.
- Ensure that people with diabetes receive diabetes self-management education, including self-monitoring of blood glucose as necessary.
- Ensure proper food intake and physical activity to help achieve target values, including body weight.
- Use the HbA1c test for monitoring blood glucose control and for guiding therapy to achieve blood glucose target levels.
- Use combination drug therapy as necessary to achieve and maintain target values.
- Use a coordinated team approach to patient care.

lines are listed in Box 43-3. Information regarding participating in the NDEP can be found on their Web site.[23]

USING NONTRADITIONAL PROVIDERS

In addition to the traditional diabetes team, consisting of a physician, diabetes nurse educator, and nutritionist, other health care providers can and should be included in patient care. In essence, at every step in the health care system patients should be encouraged to take an active role in their health, and self-management behavior should be reinforced.

Pharmacists

Pharmacists are members of the health care team who can play a vital role in patient care. In several studies[24,25] pharmacists have been shown to enhance the treatment of hyperglycemia and hypertension.

In one study,[25] a comprehensive pharmacist-led, primary care–based diabetes management program for patients with type 2 diabetes and poor glucose control was implemented in an academic general internal medicine practice. Clinic-based pharmacists helped provide support through teaching, telephone follow-up, medication adjustment (following algorithms) and use of a diabetes tracking database. Although the study was not controlled, a significant fall in HbA1c levels (the major outcomes measure) was seen in the pharmacist-treated group. In another study, a team of pharmacists was able to help treat hypertension in a group of patients followed for their diabetes in a nurse-based disease management program.[24]

In a small study of pharmacist-managed diabetes care in a free medical clinic, process and outcomes measures were improved in the population followed under the disease management program.[26] Data from 89 patients treated by pharmacists following algorithms were compared to 92 diabetic patients receiving routine care. The experimental patients had higher baseline HbA1c levels (8.8% versus 7.9%) and had more complications. However, during the study there was an increased frequency of HbA1c and lipid measurements, an increase in compliance with recommended foot and retina exams, and a significant reduction in HbA1c levels (–0.8 percentage points versus –0.05 points).

Promotoras

Promotoras, laypersons with diabetes, have been trained to lead classes and provide diabetes care. They were used quite effectively in Project Dulce,[27] which is a comprehensive diabetes management program for the underserved poor in San Diego. (The outcomes from this study are discussed under "Program Design.") The participants in Project Dulce are primarily Latin American patients with type 1 and 2 diabetes, from six community clinic sites in North San Diego County, California. The patients were covered by state Medicaid (Medi-Cal) or the San Diego County Medically Indigent Adult (MIA) health services program or they were completely uninsured and had incomes below the federal poverty level. In this program, in addition to diabetes nurse case managers, the traditional role of community health workers was expanded by providing them with extensive training to be effective diabetes peer educators. Patients with diabetes who were thought to have leadership traits were chosen from the clinic's patient population and trained using a program developed by the Latino Health Access Program (Orange County, Calif).

After the initial training, the promotoras completed a Project Dulce–specific training program. The comprehensive diabetes curriculum consisted of 12 weekly 2-hour sessions. In addition to traditional diabetes education content, classes included interactive sessions in which the patient-trainees discussed their personal experiences, fears, and beliefs about diabetes. Visual demonstrations were employed to further enhance the training. The use of these peer educators was a vital part of Project Dulce, and it helped in their outreach efforts to involve the local communities. Use of such peer educators, chosen based on leadership skills as well as the structure of the communities (for example, using schools, local government, and religious communities to help in outreach efforts) is a vital part of extending the diabetes clinic into areas where ongoing care can occur.

USING TECHNOLOGY TO PROVIDE DIABETES CARE

Recent advances in technology have made it increasingly possible to electronically monitor patients and provide care when patients are out of the office. This extends the concept of the diabetes clinic to a much broader entity of ongoing support and encouragement that can affect patient behavior on a much more frequent basis than can occur in episodic visits to a clinic.

Balas and colleagues performed a meta-analysis of randomized clinical trials of computer-assisted interventions in diabetes care.[28] Studies were grouped into three categories: computerized prompting of diabetes care, use of home glucose records in computer-assisted insulin dose adjustment, and computer-assisted diabetes patient education. In many of the studies improvement in blood glucose levels was seen when the technology was employed. Such components as prompting follow-up procedures, computerized insulin therapy adjustment using self-monitoring of blood glucose levels, remote feedback, and counseling had documented benefits in improving diabetes-related outcomes.

Electronic modalities have also been employed to enhance behavioral change as part of primary care practices. One review[29] describes examples of a variety of interactive behavior change technologies such as the Internet, clinic-based CD-ROMs, and interactive voice-response telephone calls, which have been shown to be useful adjuncts to clinic-based behavioral counseling. Use of such technology can increase the effectiveness of behavioral counseling provided in a clinic visit and can help to sustain the improvements over time.

One barrier to computerized monitoring and diabetes follow-up is the current visit-based reimbursement structure. Nurses who provide telephone follow-up or responses to e-mail queries or electronically transmitted data do not generate revenue although these activities take provider time. In capitated settings in which improved diabetes outcomes and avoidance of emergency room visits and hospital visits result in lower costs, some of the cost savings can be used to provide care. However, in the traditional fee-for-service model, often little time is available for encounters that do not generate revenue, such as telephone calls and e-mails.

Registries

A diabetes registry is the most basic form of diabetes management, whether it involves management of a small group of patients seen in a diabetes center or patients treated throughout a larger population base. A diabetes registry tracks patient outcomes and provides feedback to primary care providers. The registry can be further enhanced with decision support tools and nurse case managers who can provide intensive care for patients who need it.[7]

In a large community internal medicine practice, a diabetes registry was created and some of the patients in the registry received direct letters regarding their need for care. Patients who received letters had improved HbA1c levels and lower LDL cholesterol levels.[30]

Web-Based Programs

The Internet provides instant access to information about disease treatment strategies and individual patient data. Although concerns about patient confidentiality and computer viruses have slowed some of the growth of the Internet in medicine, it is a tool that is increasingly used.

One study, done at the Massachusetts General Hospital in Boston, assessed the efficacy of a Web-based decision support tool for diabetes management.[31] The system was studied in a hospital-based internal medicine practice and provided interactive patient-specific clinical data, treatment advice, and links to other Web-based care resources. Intervention and control groups were compared. Process measures (such as how often HbA1C and LDL cholesterol levels were measured) increased, and outcomes measures improved slightly. These results suggest that a Web-based tool for information management and decision support could be useful in managing diabetes.

Telemedicine

Different types of telemedicine have been employed in diabetes management. In one study,[32] an indigent population (largely Hispanic) was treated through a telemedicine diabetes disease management program. Using the telemedicine tools, patients monitored their blood sugars daily at home and nurses were alerted if patients reported any abnormalities. After 1 year, reductions in health care system resource use and charges, as well as improvements in quality of life, were demonstrated. Researchers concluded that many of the improvements occurred because of the nurse's ability to intervene quickly if needed.

In a study in Department of Veterans Affairs (VA) clinics, a system using automated telephone disease management (ATDM) with nurse follow-up was effective for improving diabetes outcomes.[33] In this study, patients received biweekly ATDM health assessment and self-care education calls. Nurses followed up depending on the response to the ATDM reports.

DESIGNING SYSTEMS

Given the limited resources available for diabetes care, clinics may need to be structured to treat those

at greatest risk first. Kaiser-Permanente in Northern California implemented a stratification system.[7] Patients with chronic diseases, such as diabetes, are divided into three levels: patients with stable conditions (Level 1), patients with poorly controlled conditions (Level 2), and patients who have complex multiple diagnoses or who are high-use patients (or both) (Level 3). Patients in Level 3 are assigned a nurse case manager or medical social worker. Patients in Level 2 are seen by care managers (nurses, pharmacists, dietitians), who work intensively with patients for 6 to 15 months until the patient's condition stabilizes and the patient returns to Level 1.

Underserved and minority populations can also benefit from a well-designed diabetes management system. Clinica Campesina,[7] in Denver, provides care to a largely uninsured Hispanic population. As part of the diabetes collaborative, the clinic used primary care teams, a diabetes registry, physician reminders, diabetes group visits, and a focus on diabetes self-management education to improve outcomes. From October 1998 the average HbA1c level was 10.5%; it had decreased to 8.6% by March 2000. The percentage of patients with self-management goals increased from 3% to 65%, and the percentage having retina examinations increased from 7% to 51%.

In Atlanta, in a large public hospital treating a primarily low-income African American population, a diabetes treatment program has been implemented.[34,35] The structured care program consists of intensive education in lifestyle modification, self-management training, and diet, coupled with intensification of medical therapy when needed to control hyperglycemia. The overall treatment approach has resulted in significantly lower HbA1c levels with a fall from a baseline of 9.3% to 8.2% at one year ($P < 0.001$).

In Southern California, programs for lower-income underserved minority groups have been quite successful. Project Dulce, in San Diego,[27] used nurse case managers and peer empowerment groups (promotoras) to treat patients and showed a decrease in HbA1c levels from 12% to 8.3%. Decreases in blood pressure and LDL cholesterol and an increase in knowledge and treatment satisfaction were also seen.

A Southern California (Santa Barbara, Los Angeles, San Diego) nurse case-management program for Medi-Cal patients showed an improvement in outcomes, as well.[36] A randomized study compared the diabetes management program to standard care. During 1 year, a progressive reduction in HbA1c was seen in both groups: from 9.54% to 7.66% (a reduction of 1.88 percentage points) in the intervention group and from 9.66% to 8.53% (a reduction of 1.13 points) in the control group. Two programs in Los Angeles in two underserved communities also showed improvements in diabetes outcomes[37,38] through diabetes case management.

Although these programs are effective, none look at long-term (5 to 10 years) sustainability of the improvements. In one study, patients did well when followed intensively, but once they returned to their primary care providers for ongoing care in combination with yearly evaluations in the diabetes clinic, HbA1c levels increased back to preprogram levels.[15] Interestingly, LDL and blood pressure lowering persisted after program discharge, as did use of medication, including aspirin, angiotensin-converting enzyme (ACE) inhibitors, and statins.[15] Another limitation is that these are not population-based programs. Although all of these programs were successful, they included only a few hundred patients with diabetes in health care systems where thousands of persons need access to good preventive health care.

COST ANALYSIS

Diabetes is a costly disease. In the United States the 2002 estimated annual economic cost of diagnosed cases of diabetes was $132 billion.[39] This total includes $91.8 billion in direct medical and treatment costs and $39.8 billion in indirect costs attributed to disability and premature mortality. The per capita health care cost for these patients was about $13,243 compared to a per capita cost of $2,560 for persons without diabetes.

The majority of health care costs ($40.3 billion) are associated with inpatient hospital care; outpatient services account for about 24% of costs. A relatively small amount (9.6%) of expenditures is related to pharmacy costs.[40] Chronic diabetic complications account for nearly 27% of total health care costs, with 64% of these costs being related to cardiovascular disease. About half of total health care expenditures is related to general medical conditions such as liver disease, septicemia, respiratory failure, and affective disorders. Patients with diabetes have a longer length of hospital stay and a higher readmission rate compared to patients without diabetes.[41,42] Therefore, targeting the inpatient period as well as the postdischarge interval can help reduce costs and improve outcomes.

Increasingly, studies of diabetes disease management have included cost data. One study[43] shows improvement in the frequency of HbA1c testing (44.9%) through implementation of a diabetes disease management program. In addition, a drop was seen in every dimension of use of medical services. Inpatient admissions fell by 391 per 1000 and total medical costs were also reduced. Another, much larger study[44] was performed from 1992 to 1997 in a staff model health maintenance organization in Washington state. Data were collected on a total of 4744 patients. Patients were characterized as improved if the HbA1c level fell by at least 1 percentage point and that level was sustained for at least a year. Out of the total, 732 patients were considered improved. Those who did not improve had a much higher baseline HbA1c level (10%) than

those who did (7.7%). Mean total health care costs were $685 to $950 less each year in the improved cohort. Additionally, use of medical services was consistently lower in the improved cohort. These cost savings were seen within 1 to 2 years of improvement of glycemic control.

Sidorov and colleagues performed a retrospective review of health care claims and other measures of health care use over 2 years among 6799 patients continuously enrolled in the Geisinger Health Plan.[45] Data on patients enrolled in an opt-in disease management program (n = 3118) were compared to those who were not enrolled (n = 3681). Per-member per-month paid claims averaged $394.62 for program patients compared with $502.48 for nonprogram patients (P < 0.05). Program patients had lower inpatient health care use (mean of 0.12 admissions per patient per year and 0.56 inpatient days per patient per year) than did nonprogram patients (0.16 admissions and 0.98 inpatient days per year, P < 0.05). Program patients also experienced fewer emergency department visits than nonprogram patients but had a higher number of primary care visits.

Other large studies include a retrospective review of the effect of the Diabetes Treatment Center of America (DTCA) model[46] using data from 7000 members treated in one of seven managed care plans. Compliance with national guidelines for process measures increased: Annual rates increased from 34% to 76% for assessing HbA1c levels, from 23% to 40% for retina exams, and from 2% to 25% for documented foot exams. However, average HbA1c levels decreased only from 8.9% to 8.5%. Overall, these changes resulted in a total cost decrease of $44 per diabetic member per month, largely due to a reduction in inpatient costs. In another study,[47] a computer system was developed to guide and track the care provided to diabetic patients. Of 8200 diabetic patients, the 30% considered to be at highest risk were entered into the system. Measures of compliance with annual diabetes process and outcomes measures were higher in the computer-managed group. Use of inpatient services also decreased.

At Group Health, Inc., a managed care program, patients were encouraged to participate in a diabetes disease management program (Disease Management Solutions [DMS]).[48] More than 8000 patients participated in the program over 2.5 years. Claims data showed that participation in the program increased use of primary care services, but the increase in costs was lower than for those not enrolled. Self-reported compliance with diabetes process measures and tests increased, and patients reported fewer missed days of work when followed in the program.

A program called Diabetes Decisions was implemented in a managed care organization.[49] A major intervention in the program was outbound calls by specialized trained nurses. Outcomes included diabetes process measures, financial parameters, and participant satisfaction. By year three, there were 422 continuously active participants. From baseline to the third year of the program, significant increases in frequency of HbA1c testing (21.3% to 82.2%), dilated retina exams (17.2% to 70.7%), and performance of foot exams (2.0% to 75.6%) were noted. For 166 participants with five HbA1c determinations, HbA1c values dropped from 8.89% to 7.88%. Participants experienced a 36% drop in inpatient costs. Without adjusting for medical inflation, total medical costs decreased by 26.8% from the baseline period, dropping to $268.63 per diabetes participant per month by year three, a gross savings of $98.49 per diabetes patient per month. After subtracting the fees paid to Diabetes Decisions, a total net savings of $986,538 was realized. This yielded a return on investment of 3.37%, thereby creating a positive financial model for diabetes management.

As part of the cost of medical care, it is important to remember that when patients have to pay for certain aspects of their care out of pocket, such as for medication, adherence to prescribed therapies can decrease. This may be particularly true when treating the elderly, who are often taking many expensive medications without pharmacy benefits and who may be struggling to live on a fixed income. In one study of adults treated with oral antidiabetes medication, 19% reported cutting back on medication use in the prior year because of cost.[50]

A cost analysis of the landmark United Kingdom Prospective Diabetes Study (UKPDS) showed that although pharmacy costs increase in intensively treated patients,[51] this cost is more than offset by the lower costs of treating chronic complications (largely due to hospitalizations) found with stricter glycemic control. The UKPDS trial did not include aggressive lipid lowering in its study design, which would likely further reduce the costs of chronic complications. Studies such as Action to Control Cardiovascular Risk in Diabetes (ACCORD),[52] which is combining intensive glycemic and hypertension control and aggressive lipid lowering, should provide us with more data over time for outcomes and cost.

DISABILITY COSTS

Work disability and quality of life are two areas that can be substantially affected by adequate diabetes treatment. Rates of disability in patients with diabetes have been high: Rates are 25.6% in patients with diabetes compared to 7.8% in patients without diabetes.[39] Annually this translates to a loss of nearly 88 million disability days, with 74,927 workers reported to be permanently disabled.[53] On average, diabetic persons aged 18 to 64 years lost 8.3 days from work as compared with 1.7 days for persons without diabetes.

Work disability can be reduced if patients with diabetes are appropriately treated.[54] This is clearly an important issue to employers, who often pay for health insurance. In a randomized, controlled study of 569 patients with type 2 diabetes, glycemic control was improved using long-acting glipizide (glipizide GITS [gastrointestinal therapeutic system]).[54] As expected, after 12 weeks, glycemic parameters were better in the treated patients. In addition, however, quality of life was improved, as were a number of health economic outcomes. The glipizide GITS group had higher retained employment, less absenteeism, fewer bed-days, and less disability.

THE FUTURE OF DIABETES CARE

The increasing number of patients with diabetes will require increased attention to providing appropriate, efficient diabetes care in order to improve outcomes and lower rates of complications. Due to a lack of diabetes specialists, the bulk of the diabetes care provided will be in the primary care setting, where chronic disease management has long been hard to deliver consistently. Electronic registries and patient tracking systems could make it easier to identify patients who need further care, but it remains up to the providers to help patients employ the therapies that can modify the course of their disease.

Nonphysician health care providers, such as diabetes educators, nutritionists, pharmacists, mental health professionals, and promotoras, should play an increasingly large role, because much of the care of the patient with diabetes involves education and a health partnership that inspires the patient to adopt new, healthier behavior. A diabetes clinic might not look much like the typical physician's office of the past, but it can be a hub for patient outreach. A variety of providers can interact with patients by telephone or using Internet-based technology, and patients can send data electronically and can return for classes or individual sessions as needed. A relatively small number of physicians can oversee a much larger staff who are devoted to tracking and treating patients as they are followed in their primary care provider's office.

Some patients, however, need a close and ongoing relationship with a diabetes specialist and ideally a team of diabetes health care providers who offer a full range of services for the patient with diabetes. As technology and treatment become more complex, specialists will need to be available to guide patients in using the new technology.

Regardless of the setting, we currently have treatments for diabetes that can help patients live longer, healthy lives. Programs are effective in patients from all socioeconomic groups, which is particularly important because diabetes occurs more commonly in persons from minority groups. In addition to lowering blood sugar levels, however, all programs for diabetes management must include measures to lower lipid and blood pressure levels, which lower the risks for vascular and neuropathic complications. Designing and implementing programs that include all patients with diabetes is a challenge for all of us who provide preventive health care.

Multiple models for care will be required; which model is most effective depends on the prevailing fiscal, institutional, and political environment. All programs must incorporate the primary care physician as a partner in chronic care delivery. Emerging computerized technologies must be incorporated into systems of care for tracking patients and providing a solid infrastructure for patient care. With appropriate partnerships of patients with their health care team and of health care team members with each other, great benefits can be achieved for all concerned.

References

1. American Diabetes Association: National Diabetes Fact Sheet. http://www.diabetes.org/diabetes-statistics/national-diabetes-fact-sheet.jsp
2. Saaddine JB, Engelgau MM, Beckles GL, et al: A diabetes report card for the US: Quality of care in the 1990s. Ann Int Med 13:565-74, 2002.
3. McFarlane SI et al: Control of cardiovascular risk factors in patients with diabetes and hypertension at urban academic medical centers. Diabetes Care 25:718-723, 2002.
4. Thomas JL: Pharmacy Benefit Report: Trends and Forecasts. East Hanover, NJ, Novartis, 1998.
5. Peters AL: Diabetes disease management: Past, present and future. The Endocrinologist 11:86-93, 2001.
6. National Committee for Quality Assurance: Diabetes Quality Improvement Project Initial Measure Set. Available at: http://www.ncqa.org/dprp/dqip2.htm.
7. Bodenheimer T, Wagner E, Grumbach K: Improving primary care for patients with chronic illness: The chronic care model. JAMA 288:1775-1779, 2002.
8. Bodenheimer T, Wagner EH, Grumbach K: Improving primary care for patients with chronic illness: The chronic care model, part 2. JAMA 288:1909-1914, 2002.
9. Olivarius NF, Beck-Nielsen H, Andreasen AH, et al: Randomised controlled trial of structured personal care of type 2 diabetes mellitus. BMJ 323:970-975, 2001.
10. Glasgow RE, Hiss RG, Anderson RM, et al: Report of the Health Care Delivery Work Group: Behavioral research related to the establishment of a chronic disease model for diabetes care. Diabetes Care 24:124-130, 2001.
11. Greineder DK, Loane KC, Parks P: Randomized controlled trial of a pediatric asthma program. J Allergy Clin Immunol 103:436-440, 1999.
12. Pieber TR, Holler A, Siebenhofer A, et al: Evaluation of a structured teaching and treatment programme for type 2 diabetes in general practice in a rural area of Austria. Diabet Med 12:349-354, 1995.
13. de Weerdt I, Visser AP, Kok GJ, et al: Randomized controlled multicentre evaluation of an education programme for insulin-treated diabetic patients. Diabet Med 8:338-345, 1991.
14. Dougherty G, Schiffrin A, White D, et al: Home-based management can achieve intensification cost-effectively in type I diabetes. Pediatrics 103:122-128, 1999.
15. Mathur R, Roybal GM, Harmel AP: Are the benefits of a diabetes disease management program sustainable over time? Diabetes 53(Suppl 1):A51, 2004.

16. Rickheim PL. Weaver TW, Flader JL, Kendall DM: Assessment of group versus individual diabetes education. Diabetes Care 25:269-274, 2002.

17. Brown SA: Studies of educational interventions and outcomes in diabetic adults: A meta-analysis revisited. Patient Educ Counsel 16:189-215, 1990.

18. Norris SL, Engelgau MM, Narayan KMV: Effectiveness of self-management training in type 2 diabetes: A systematic review of randomized controlled trials. Diabetes Care 24:561-587, 2001.

19. Wagner EH, Grothaus LC, Sandhu N, et al: Chronic care clinics for diabetes in primary care: A system-wide randomized trial. Diabetes Care 24:695-700, 2001.

20. Pastors JG, Warshaw H, Daly A, et al: The evidence for the effectiveness of medical nutrition therapy in diabetes management. Diabetes Care 25:608-613, 2002.

21. Ammerman AS, Lindquist CH, Lohr KN, Hersey J: The efficacy of behavioral interventions to modify dietary fat and fruit and vegetable intake: A review of the evidence. Prev Med 35:25-41, 2002.

22. Mensing C, Boucher J, Cypress M, et al: National standards for diabetes self-management education. Standards and review criteria. Diabetes Care 25:S140-S147, 2002.

22a. American Diabetes Association: Education Recognition Program. Available at: http://www.diabetes.org/for-health-professionals-and-scientists/recognition/edrecognition.jsp.

23. National Institutes of Health: National Diabetes Education Program. Available at: http://ndep.nih.gov.

24. Patel PV, Mathur R, Gong WC, et al: Results of a pharmacist run protocol drive blood pressure clinic in Latino patients with type 2 diabetes mellitus. Diabetes 53(Suppl 1):A50, 2004.

25. Rothman R, Malone R, Bryant B, et al: Pharmacist-led, primary care-based disease management improves hemoglobin A1c in high-risk patients with diabetes. Am J Med Qual 18:51-58, 2003.

26. Davidson MB, Karlan VJ, Hair TL: Effect of a pharmacist-managed diabetes care program in a free medical clinic. Am J Med Qual 15:137-142, 2000.

27. Philis-Tsimikas A, Walker C, Rivard L, et al, for Project Dulce: Improvement in diabetes care of underinsured patients enrolled in Project Dulce: a community-based, culturally appropriate, nurse case management and peer education diabetes care model. Diabetes Care 27:110-115, 2004.

28. Balas EA, Krishna S, Kretschmer RA, et al:. Computerized knowledge management in diabetes care. Med Care 42:610-621, 2004.

29. Glasgow RE, Bull SS, Piette JD, Steiner JF: Interactive behavior change technology: A partial solution to the competing demands of primary care. Am J Prev Med 27(Suppl 2):80-87, 2004.

30. Stroebel RJ, Scheitel SM, Fitz JS, et al: A randomized trial of three diabetes registry implementation strategies in a community internal medicine practice. Jt Comm J Qual Improv 28:441-450, 2002.

31. Meigs JB, Cagliero E, Dubey A, et al: A controlled trial of Web-based diabetes disease management: The MGH Diabetes Primary Care Improvement Project. Diabetes Care 26:750-757, 2003.

32. Cherry JC, Moffatt TP, Rodriguez C, Dryden K: Diabetes disease management program for an indigent population empowered by telemedicine technology. Diabetes Technol Ther 4:783-791, 2002.

33. Piette JD, Weinberger M, Kraemer FB, McPhee SJ: Impact of automated calls with nurse follow-up on diabetes treatment outcomes in a Department of Veterans Affairs Health Care System: A randomized controlled trial. Diabetes Care 24:202-208, 2001.

34. Ziemer DC, Goldschmid M, Musey VC, et al: Diabetes in urban African Americans, III. Management of type II diabetes in a municipal hospital setting. Am J Med 101:25-33, 1996.

35. Cook CB, Ziemer DC, El-Kebbi I, et al: Diabetes in urban African Americans. XVI. Overcoming clinical inertia improves glycemic control in patients with type 2 diabetes. Diabetes Care 22:1494-1500, 1999.

36. The California Medi-Cal Type 2 Diabetes Study Group: Closing the gap: Effect of diabetes case management on glycemic control among low-income ethnic minority populations. The California Medi-Cal Type 2 Diabetes Study. Diabetes Care 27:95-103, 2004.

37. Mathur R, Roybal GM, Harmel ALP: Global risk reduction through diabetes disease management in an underserved Latino population. Diabetes 52(Suppl 1):A266, 2003.

38. Davidson MB: Effect of nurse-directed diabetes care in a minority population. Diabetes Care 26:2281-2287, 2003.

39. American Diabetes Association: Economic costs of diabetes 2002. Diabetes Care 26:917-932, 2003.

40. Selby JV, Ray GT, Zhang D, Colby CJ: Excess costs of medical care for patients with diabetes in a managed care population. Diabetes Care 20:1396-1402, 1997.

41. Ossorio RC, Peters AL, Chen LS, et al: Development of a diabetes registry in an IPA setting—outpatient and inpatient applications. Diabetes 48(Suppl 1):A419, 1999.

42. Aro S, Kangas T, Reunanen A, et al: Hospital use among diabetic patients and the general population. Diabetes Care 17:1320-1329, 1994.

43. Berg GD, Wadhwa S: Diabetes disease management in a community-based setting. Manag Care 11:42, 45-50, 2002.

44. Wagner EH, Sandhu N, Newton KM, et al: Effect of improved glycemic control on health care costs and utilization. JAMA 285:182-189, 2001.

45. Sidorov J, Shull R, Tomcavage J, et al: Does diabetes disease management save money and improve outcomes? A report of simultaneous short-term savings and quality improvement associated with a health maintenance organization–sponsored disease management program among patients fulfilling health employer data and information set criteria. Diabetes Care 25:684-689, 2002.

46. Rubin RJ, Dietrich KA, Hawk AD: Clinical and economic impact of implementing a comprehensive diabetes management program in managed care. J Clin Endo Metab 83:2635-2642,1998.

47. Domurat ES: Diabetes managed care and clinical outcomes: The Harbor City, California, Kaiser Permanente Diabetes Care System. Am J Manag Care 5:1299-1307, 1999.

48. Lynne D: Diabetes disease management in managed care organizations. Dise Manag 7:47-60, 2004.

49. Synder JW, Malaskovitz J, Griego J, et al: Quality improvement and cost reduction realized by a purchaser through diabetes disease management. Dis Manag 6:233-241, 2003.

50. Piette JD, Heisler M, Wagner TH: Problems paying out-of-pocket medication costs among older adults with diabetes. Diabetes Care 27:384-391, 2004.

51. Gray A, Raikou M, McGuire A, et al: Cost effectiveness of an intensive blood glucose control policy in patients with type 2 diabetes: Economic analysis alongside randomized controlled trial (UKPDS 41). BMJ 320:1373-1378, 2000.

52. Action to Control Cardiovascular Risk in Diabetes (ACCORD): http://www.accordtrial.org/public/index.cfm.

53. Mayfield JA, Deb P, Whitecotton L: Work disability and diabetes. Diabetes Care 22:1105-1109, 1999.

54. Testa MA, Simonson DC: Health economic benefits and quality of life during improved glycemic control in patients with type 2 diabetes mellitus. JAMA 280:1490-1496, 1998.

Chapter 44

Using Computers and Information Technology in Diabetes Care

Lawrence Blonde, Jayant Dey, and Kevin Peterson

KEY POINTS

- *Health care professionals must manage large amounts of disease-specific and patient-specific information.*
- *Health care professionals who care for patients with diabetes have particularly large and complex information-management tasks.*
- *Use of information technology to help communicate, manage information, provide decision support, and prevent errors is becoming an essential skill for diabetes practitioners.*
- *Information technology can also help patients to manage their diabetes.*
- *The Internet is a key component of diabetes information technology.*

Health care professionals are information managers. They manage both disease-specific and patient-specific information and must integrate both types of information to provide the best possible care for their patients. Information management needs are especially great for health care professionals who care for people with complex chronic diseases like diabetes mellitus.

Diabetes is a disease of details. Recommended clinical visits, monitoring, multiple performance measures, and a myriad of clinical parameters challenge the health care professional to deliver care that is complete and current. To deliver optimal care, health care professionals need to integrate information storage and retrieval with disease tracking and performance. The Institute of Medicine (IOM) recommendation on physician core competencies urges health care professionals to use "information technology to communicate, manage knowledge, mitigate error and support decision making."[1]

The uses of information technology and computers in diabetes care are listed in Box 44-1. This chapter reviews some of these potential information technology contributions to diabetes care.

USING COMPUTERS TO IMPROVE DIABETES CARE

The Need for Clinical Information Systems

As other chapters in this book have detailed, there is a genuine and growing epidemic of diabetes mellitus in this country and around the world. Today there are an estimated 18.2 million Americans with diabetes,[2] and this country spends $132 billion annually in their care.[3] Much of this cost is related to the chronic microvascular, neuropathic, and macrovascular complications of diabetes.

Landmark randomized, controlled clinical trials have demonstrated that treatment of hyperglycemia, as well as the hypertension and dyslipidemia that often accompany diabetes, can markedly reduce the development and progression of these complications. Moreover, in the last decade many new therapeutic agents have become available with which to better treat diabetes patients. Yet most patients do not achieve treatment targets advocated by the American Diabetes Association (ADA), the American College of Endocrinology, and other guideline-setting organizations. One study[4] has noted that fewer than 40% of the adults with diabetes achieve treatment goals for cardiovascular (CV) risk factors and only 7% achieved recommended targets for hemoglobin A1c, blood pressure, and cholesterol.

These and other findings reflect a need for better education of both health care professionals and patients. However, there is also a growing awareness that education alone will not solve this problem. The lack of optimal diabetes care is also related to flaws in our systems of care for complex, chronic diseases. Indeed, the American health care delivery system too often is fragmented, lacks clinical information capabilities, often duplicates services, and is poorly designed for delivering chronic care. In addition, much information is locked in older "legacy" systems that do not provide information exchange with other systems, which isolates information from both the health care professional and the patient.

Most physicians or systems of care cannot easily look across their patient populations and identify the patients who are not attaining treatment goals. Without this ability to examine a population, health care professionals cannot implement prospective measures to improve quality of care and outcomes. Instead, they have to wait for each patient to visit and then make reactive evaluations and therapy adjustments. Should the patient present with a problem that takes precedence over his or her chronic illness, the opportunity may be missed and necessary evaluations and changes might not be made at all. This lack of an organized system of care contributes to suboptimal diabetes control and outcomes as well as increased costs.

In contrast, a more systems-based approach provides population-based care guided by an understanding of the history of the disease and accompanied by well-timed interventions to prevent exacerbations and complications. Wagner and coworkers have proposed a chronic care model as a guide to higher-quality management of chronic illness.[5] This model highlights clinical information systems, delivery systems redesign, and decision support among the interrelated components of improved care. The ability to deliver information to the members of the care delivery team is fundamental to a successful implementation of the model.

The IOM has called for action to provide care that is evidence based, patient centered, and systems oriented and that takes advantage of information technologies that could contribute to better and continuous quality improvement.[6]

Clinical Information Systems

One of the key components of a systems approach is a clinical information system. This can range from a patient registry containing patient demographic, diagnosis, laboratory, and medication information to a full-featured electronic medical records system (EMR). The system does not have to be electronic, and a simple rotary file (such as Rolodex) or paper-based system can be effective. However, a registry—ideally electronic—organizes patient information so that the health care professional can rapidly see across her or his entire practice population or can look longitudinally into an individual patient's history. It can also serve as the basis for scheduling follow-up appointments, tests, reminders, and interventions and for continuous quality improvements. Also vital are the use of clinical practice guidelines, which ideally are supported through electronically generated reminders.[7]

Registries

Computer-based disease registries are software database applications that contain disease-specific information about a patient population. Information in a registry is structured to allow sorting, analysis, and retrieval of subsets that meet certain criteria. A review of chronic disease registries can be downloaded from the California HealthCare Foundation.[8] The Virginia Health Quality Center has assembled a comparison spreadsheet (http://www .vhqc.org/inc/pdf/regprodgrid.doc) for registry software for preventive health and chronic disease management used in different regions.

Registries can be used to identify patients with diabetes who have not achieved target HbA1c, blood pressure, or lipid levels, or to report population-based information such as the mean HbA1c for all patients, for patients of specific health care professionals, or for patients receiving certain treatments. Registries can also aggregate information about individual patients, which can be used during and between patient visits to optimize care by facilitating targeting of high-risk groups or by initiating reminders. Population-level registry information can demonstrate the quality of care delivered to diabetic patients by an individual physician or other health care professional, by groups of health care professionals, or by an entire system of care. Registries often have a variety of components, including storage, reporting functions, data entry, data access and management, and import and export functions.

Electronic Medical Records

In the early 1990s, the IOM called for a nationwide electronic medical records system by the end of the decade.[9,10] Almost halfway through the succeeding decade this goal is not much closer to being achieved. Nevertheless, the potential of EMRs even within a solo medical practice is enormous, and health care professionals who care for people with diabetes mellitus, as well as their patients, are among those likely to derive the greatest benefit from their use. This is because people with diabetes have many comorbidities and are often treated by

many different health care professionals and prescribed a large number of medications.

EMRs allow the capture, organization, and analysis of health care services including examination and laboratory results. They can facilitate direct patient care services by providing continually up-to-date problem lists, medication lists, and easily retrievable, readable, and problem-specific progress notes. Moreover, EMRs have many advantages over paper medical records, including less expensive, more secure chart storage and retrieval, remote access to patient information, and the ability to rapidly find specific information items.

EMRs can allow multiple authorized health care professionals to access records simultaneously, even from disparate locations, and to share information and incorporate diagnostic and therapeutic decision support tools. Computerized records can automatically calculate a body mass index (BMI) value when a patient's height and weight are entered. One can generate reports of all patients whose HbA1c, blood pressure, or lipid values are not at goal or demonstrate the quality of care that is being delivered for regulatory purposes or contract negotiations. When a medication has a labeling change requiring an alteration in monitoring or when an indication is changed or withdrawn an EMR can allow rapid identification of patients taking that medication. Moreover, using patient demographic information stored in an EMR or registry one can quickly generate personalized mail-merge letters communicating to patients what has occurred and how they need to proceed to address the issue.[11]

Both registries and EMRs can support population management quality improvement initiatives that have been demonstrated to enhance diabetes care. One can use these resources to identify patients within a practice or system who have diabetes, to risk stratify those patients, and to implement risk-specific strategies to improve care and then regularly reassess the effects of the interventions.[12] Ideally such programs include information technology approaches to identify patients who have not achieved recommended therapy targets as well as decision-support tools suggesting appropriate therapeutic perturbations.[13]

Implementing Registries and Electronic Medical Records

Computerized registries and EMRs can improve the organization and efficiency of diabetes health care delivery. Studies have demonstrated that such systems can improve the processes of care. Improvement in outcomes has been inconsistent. However, the marked improvements in care outcomes among people with diabetes treated through the Veterans Health Administration System can be attributed at least in part to their adoption of a system-wide electronic health record.[14] Other large systems are also investing in such technology.[15]

Barriers to implementing EMRs or registries in practice settings include security and confidentiality concerns; the cost of hardware and software; the cost of acquiring, implementing, updating, and maintaining the technology; and perceived cost of data entry. Yet implementation of an EMR system can result in a positive financial return on investment to the health care organization.[16,17] Purchasing a registry application or an EMR is a complex process, and appropriate choices must take into account individual characteristics of the practice or system in which it will be used.

The National Diabetes Education Program has a relatively new Web site (www.betterdiabetescare .nih.gov) that can help health care professionals who want to enhance the organization and systems of diabetes health care delivery in their practices.[18] Included on this Web site is information from the Health Disparities Collaboratives Tools for Diabetes,[19] which addresses such issues as clinical information systems, including constructing a registry; decision support, including diabetes care chart audit, flow sheet, protocol checklist, and patient encounter form; and delivery system design, including group visit starter kit, sample registry report, and standing orders.

Some EMRs have incorporated specific diabetes-related features. For example, CliniPro's Diabetes Management System[20] features direct data transfer from 15 different glucose meters; health analysis charts and graphs to track vital factors, such as blood glucose and medication, and compare results to recommended levels identified in the patient's care plan; and assessment screens to help identify, record, and monitor behavior goals, such as nutrition.

The Diabetes Education Management Module[21] has tools to help manage an organization's diabetes education program and collect data required for submission to the ADA's Education Recognition Program. Features include patient evaluations, class and individual consultation scheduling, customizable course descriptions, and patient attendance and progress reports.

The Delphi Diabetes Manager[22] (www .delphihealth.com/sol_ddm_overview.shtml) software provides the ability to monitor and analyze clinical results on an ongoing basis. Delphi developed the software in collaboration with the American Diabetes Association (ADA). This and other registry software products can assist with tracking, abstraction, and analysis of data needed for application for the National Committee for Quality Assurance (NCQA) and ADA Provider Recognition and ADA Education Recognition programs. A number of other products are also focused on diabetes or have diabetes-specific modules.[23]

DiaTrends (Overlook Software, Greensboro, NC), is another registry program for health care professionals to track and improve diabetes management

outcomes.[24] Practicing clinical endocrinologists were involved in the development of the system.

USES OF CLINICAL INFORMATION SYSTEMS

Electronic Medication Information

Patients with diabetes, especially those with type 2 diabetes (T2DM), often are prescribed many medications so that information about indications, contraindications, dosing, and drug interactions are needed by their health care professionals. A number of electronic sources of information about medications can be viewed on the Internet or installed on a personal computer or personal digital assistant (PDA). Handheld resources were recently reviewed.[25] ePocratesRx[26] and mobile PDR[27] are two good examples that offer very good functionality and have free versions.

ePocratesRx provides medication information by class or by drug, provides drug interaction for 2 to 20 medications, and has an insulin dosing calculator adapted from an algorithm developed at the Diabetes Research Institute at the University of Miami School of Medicine by Dr. Luigi Meneghini. It also has MedMath,[28] developed by Dr. Phillip Cheng, which includes formula calculations including BMI, anion gap, basal energy expenditure, ideal body weight, LDL cholesterol, osmolality, number needed to treat, water deficit, and many others.

Electronic Prescribing

Electronic prescribing offers a number of advantages over conventional prescribing, including generation of active medication lists for all patients. These lists can be made available to all authorized personnel and make it easy to identify potential drug interactions. A number of systems offer wireless access via PDA, tablet, or laptop computer. Electronic prescribing can dramatically reduce the time it takes to authorize refills and can reduce potential medication errors.[29] It can also be cost effective.[30-36]

eHealth Initiative has an extensive discussion of this topic.[37] Its report on electronic prescribing[38] reflects the collective wisdom of a diverse group of experts who began work in early 2003 with the objective of determining what action is needed to accelerate the adoption of electronic prescribing in ambulatory care.

Diabetic Retinopathy Screening

Diabetic retinopathy screening cameras can be installed in clinical settings frequented by diabetes patients, such as primary care offices and endocrinologists' offices. Retinal photographs can be sent via an organizational intranet or the Internet to retina specialists for reading.

A report[39] of one institution's use of this approach demonstrated that in images of 830 eyes of 415 patients, most of whom had T2DM, macular hard exudates were observed in 50 eyes (6.0%), non-proliferative diabetic retinopathy was noted in 14.1%, and proliferative diabetic retinopathy in 1.8%. Overall, 10% of the patients were referred to a retina specialist based on the screening photographs.

The main difficulty encountered with the screening program was image inconsistency. Overall, 35% of the images graded were of poor quality, usually (84.4%) because of poor exposure. The quality of the images improved significantly over the study period. A systematic review[39a] comparing the effectiveness of screening and monitoring tests for diabetic retinopathy concluded the most effective strategy for testing is the use of mydriatic retinal photography with the additional use of ophthalmoscopy for cases where photographs are ungradable.

Computerized Prompts for Diabetes Management

As early as 1976, reports demonstrated that computer-generated suggestions regarding tests and medication changes could have a significant impact on physician behavior.[40] Use of well-designed and implemented technology in diabetes management can potentially improve outcomes, increase efficiency and access to care, and reduce system errors. Empowering increasingly sophisticated patients with technology-based diabetes self-management tools can enhance their involvement in disease management.

As noted earlier, there is discordance between targets recommended by guidelines and those achieved in clinical practice. Using computer-based algorithms and clinician prompting at the point of patient care could help bridge the difference between what is known and what is done.

Prompts can be separated into passive, active, and patient-specific prompts. Reminders can also be active and passive. For example, a passive prompt, such as a wall poster listing clinical targets, can be effective as long as the doctor looks at it periodically. Active reminders mean that the doctor has responded to the prompt; for example, after performing the foot exam, the doctor puts a check by the foot exam. Finally, the patient-specific prompt is a recommendation for a given patient; for example, "Today you need to perform this patient's annual microalbuminuria screen."

The use of diabetes guideline recommendations printed on the patient encounter forms was com-

pared to usual clinical practice in a randomized manner in a family practice setting in the United States over a 6-month period.[41] Although adherence to physical examination guidelines increased significantly, no significant difference was noted in HbA1c assessment, foot examination, or ophthalmologic examination guidelines. In a clinic-based trial of 2 years' duration, patient-specific reminders regarding tests and physical examinations were compared with usual care over 2-year periods in the United Kingdom.[42] Routine diabetic clinic visits and physician reviews increased in both studies along with increased assessments of HbA1c, but there were no significant differences in HbA1c levels in either group during the studies.

Meigs and colleagues[43] assessed the effects of a Web-based decision support tool by conducting a randomized, controlled trial of 12 intervention and 14 control staff providers and 307 intervention and 291 control patients with T2DM in a hospital-based internal medicine clinic. The decision support tool displayed interactive patient-specific clinical data, treatment advice, and links to other Web-based care resources. The number of HbA1c tests obtained per year increased significantly in the intervention group, as did the number of LDL cholesterol tests and the fractions of patients undergoing at least one foot examination per year. Levels of HbA1c decreased by 0.2 percentage points in the intervention group and increased by 0.1 points in the control group ($P = 0.09$). Fractions of patients with LDL cholesterol levels lower than 130 mg/dL increased by 20.3% in the intervention group and 10.5% in the control group ($P = 0.5$). Thus the improvements in glycemic and lipid control seen with this intervention were not statistically significant.

The authors concluded that Web-based patient-specific decision support has the potential to improve evidence-based parameters of diabetes care. However, an accompanying editorial by O'Connor[44] expressed disappointment that key care outcomes such as HbA1c and LDL levels did not improve by a statistically significant amount. Another study also showed increased rates of test ordering but no improvement in metabolic parameters such as HbA1c, lipids, or blood pressure levels.[45] O'Connor suggests that reminders to physicians that tests are due or patients are not yet at their clinical goals are important but not sufficient. Rather, clinicians need information systems that suggest specific clinical interventions for a particular patient at a particular time.

In contrast, Balas and colleagues[46] found evidence that what they termed *computerized knowledge management* could be associated with improvements in follow-up procedures, insulin dose adjustment, and diabetes-related outcomes. They identified reports of randomized clinical trials of computer-assisted interventions in diabetes care and grouped them into three categories: computerized prompting of diabetes care, use of home glucose records in computer-assisted insulin dose adjustment, and computer-assisted diabetes patient education.

Among 40 eligible studies, HbA1c and blood glucose levels were significantly improved in 7 and 6 trials, respectively. In 6 of 8 studies of computer prompting, guideline compliance was improved. Overall compliance with recommended diabetes care procedures was 71% to 227% higher when physicians were prompted compared to usual care. Three of four studies of small insulin-dosage computers were associated with reduced hypoglycemic events and insulin doses. Meta-analysis of studies using home glucose records in insulin dose adjustment demonstrated a significant mean decrease in blood glucose and HbA1c. Several computerized educational programs were associated with improvement in diet and metabolic indicators.

Computer-Assisted Self-Monitored Blood Glucose Management

The advent of blood glucose monitors for patient use has greatly assisted diabetes management. Self-monitoring of blood glucose (SMBG) facilitates medication adjustments, identification and prompt treatment of hyper- and hypoglycemia, and enhanced ability to assess the impact of lifestyle choices and medication.

Computer-based clinical algorithms interfacing with patient-reported blood glucose results have been employed to assist in titration and adjustment of insulin therapy. Patients with type 1 diabetes (T1DM) who used memory glucose meters and had glucose data analyzed with software were compared systematically with those using glucose meters without memory for SMBG. The first group reported significant improvement in their understanding of diabetes and improvement in their interaction with the health care provider.[47] Similarly, use of a computerized recording of 7-day food intake in T1DM patients was found to be easy, reliable, and time saving as opposed to manual entries in a diary.[48]

A number of computer-assisted insulin-dose calculation programs have been studied and tried in clinical settings. Many of these are now available for use in handheld devices and personal computers.[49-53] Using such data as food intake, blood glucose, physical activity, and insulin regimen, these programs have been shown to effectively improve glycemic control and decrease insulin dosage. Most studies evaluating use of home glucose records in computer-assisted insulin dose adjustment have had a positive impact on HbA1c levels.

The second group of studies reviewed by Balas comprised 25 investigations involving 1286 adults and 197 children.[46] Glucose measurements taken at home were subjected to computerized analysis and reporting for insulin dose and therapy adjustment by clinicians. The computerized analysis of home

glucose records was associated with significant improvements in A1C for the intervention group patients in these studies. Some computer-assisted insulin-dose calculation programs may be more time consuming for the clinician to implement and run and may be most efficiently used as a component of team treatment of diabetes patients.

Although most such programs have not been adopted for standard use by most diabetes patients or their health care providers, computer analysis of SMBG readings can nevertheless provide significant benefits. One benefit is increased accuracy of SMBG data compared to log books in which patients enter data manually.[54-56] Of equal importance is the advantage that analysis of downloaded SMBG meter readings confers on the ability to recognize glycemic patterns that can inform therapeutic decisions. Nevertheless, this technology should be viewed as complementary to rather than a substitute for written logs, which might contain information that cannot currently be input into the meter and can help identify occasional faulty time-and-date stamping of meter readings.

Computer software available for modern glucose meters allows blood glucose data to be organized and structured into information that persons with diabetes and their health care providers can analyze and synthesize to facilitate adjustments in therapy and improvements in glycemic control. These programs can average all readings and in some cases do so by time of day, day of the week, or meal period. For example, presenting the means of several days' blood glucose values at specific times of the day with standard deviations shows both glycemic patterns and their variability.[57]

SMBG software can plot graphs and create charts of glucose trends over time. Some newer meters can show blood glucose averages by time of day for the past several days and present the information to users directly on the meter itself without requiring downloading to a computer. Patients who take insulin can have information immediately available to guide insulin adjustments. Some meters allow the entry of additional data, such as insulin doses administered, meals or snacks eaten, grams of carbohydrate consumed, and physical activity.

Glucose meter software can help to visually transform SMBG data into useful information. However, use of this technology remains modest. Because each company has its own proprietary software, one has to learn several different, often fairly complex programs and match each meter with its software. This presents a barrier in a busy practice. Increased use might result if all or most meters could download to a generic common program that allowed data to be presented in the most commonly used reports and graphs. Companies could still compete by developing proprietary software whose special features might provide an incentive for their use. Despite present barriers, greater use of this technology could help improve glycemic control of diabetic patients.

Glucose meter software can present extensive blood glucose data in diverse numerical and graphic displays. In addition to tabular displays, results can be presented in pie charts, histograms, or plots of glucose values over a modal or average day or week. Some applications can relate glycemia to nutrition, physical activity, and insulin therapy. With this information, achievement of glycemic goals can be assessed, and pattern recognition can identify explanations for failure to achieve targets and suggest treatment modifications to address them.

Computer programs vary in their displays and reports. Hirsch recently summarized the technologic features and computer requirements of the most popular commercial diabetes management software.[57] Most data management systems have a logbook screen with a table of glucose readings by date and time. Some have reports with the average blood glucose value and average number of blood glucose tests per day; the distribution of values including the percentage above, below, and within goal; the frequency of SMBG testing at different times; and a modal or average day for a set period of time giving the mean values for different times of the day over the period, often with standard deviations providing a measure of glycemic variability. Hirsch has proposed that twice the standard deviation should be less than the average blood glucose level for a given time period as an initial goal for glycemic variability.

As an example of the utility of glucose meter software, consider the case of a 65-year-old retired engineer with T2DM who is taking a mixture of NPH and regular insulin twice daily (before breakfast and before the evening meal). He performed SMBG only before breakfast and before his evening meal. His SMBG values averaged approximately 130 mg/dL, but his HbA1c was approximately 8%. He was asked to perform SMBG 2 hours after lunch and communicate the results (Fig. 44–1). Graphs of pre- and postmeal average by day demonstrate increased postprandial values each day. Graphs of a modal day show that the daily postlunch glucose readings are responsible for most of the hyperglycemic values. The carbohydrate content of his lunch was not markedly greater than that at other meals. His current insulin regimen fails to provide adequate coverage for his noon meal, which was only revealed by more appropriate SMBG testing.

Some meters allow users to manually insert insulin doses, although automated capture of this information would be even more helpful. Ultimately one would like software presentation of the relationship between insulin dose and glucose response in individual patients and groups of patients. Similarly, one would like to be able to determine the blood glucose excursion after specific foods or meals. Such presentations would really transform data into information and knowledge that could inform therapeutic approaches and increase their likelihood of success.

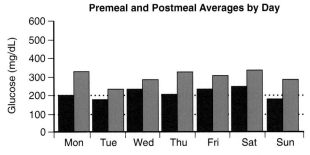

Premeal and Postmeal Averages by Day

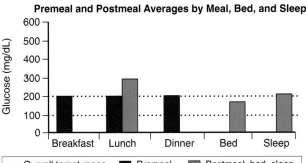

Premeal and Postmeal Averages by Meal, Bed, and Sleep

··· Overall target range ■ Premeal ▨ Postmeal, bed, sleep

Highest value:	390	Premeal target		Postmeal target	
Lowest value:	63	Within target:	8%	Within target:	0%
Average:	207	Above target:	92%	Above target:	100%
Standard dev.:	79	Below target:	0%	Below target:	0%

Overall target range is defined as the low and high end of the premeal and postmeal target ranges. Some blood glucose readings have been edited.

Figure 44–1. Graphs of premeal and postmeal average by day.

The Internet can be used to enhance the value of SMBG by increasing contact between patients and their health care providers. Kwon's group[58] investigated the effectiveness of an Internet-based blood glucose monitoring system on control of HbA1c levels. Physicians could view each of their patients' blood glucose levels, medication, and other data such as BMI, blood pressure, and baseline laboratory data. Physicians sent recommendations back to each patient. Patients were able to see their physicians' recommendations as well as the laboratory data. After 12 weeks, HbA1c levels were significantly decreased from 7.59% to 6.94% within the intervention group ($P < 0.001$) and were significantly lower than in the control group after adjusting for the baseline HbA1c (6.94% versus 7.62%; $P < 0.001$).

Other Diabetes Management Software

In addition to software offered by meter companies, many personal computer, Web-based, and PDA resources allow people with diabetes to track blood glucose data and other parameters including insulin doses, food consumption, and exercise. Some programs allow this information to be shared with the health care professionals. Other applications provide management assistance to patients or health care professionals, or both. An extensive listing of these resources can be found at Jean-François Yale's site (www.mendosa.com), which also has formal reviews of some resources. Some examples are discussed next to provide information about functionality of resources in this category.

Spreadsheets and Databases

Several downloadable spreadsheets are available. Jean-François Yale has a log sheet[59] that accommodates entry of blood glucose readings, insulin dosages, carbohydrate grams, and exercise at any hour of the day. A spreadsheet template to track blood glucose readings, insulin dosages and ratio, carbohydrate grams, and exercise is available for Microsoft Excel[60] as a spreadsheet application. You can also download it as a portable document format (PDF) file[61] for Adobe Acrobat.

Nagykaldi and Mold[62] described how physicians in their practice-based research network implemented a PDA-based diabetes management system. Implementation of the Diabetes Patient Tracker resulted in a significant improvement ($P < 0.05$) in nine of 10 diabetic quality of care measures compared with preintervention levels in 20 primary care practices. The number of foot examinations and retina examinations performed in the last year also increased ($P = 0.03$ and $P = 0.02$, respectively).

With Diabetes Partner PC (www.numedics.com), patients can create and maintain a point-and-click electronic record of blood glucose levels, medications, and food intake. Diabetes Partner PC interfaces with seven different blood glucose meters to download and store an unlimited number of daily readings. Patients can also manually enter test results and identify factors (such as exercise, stress, or illness) that might have influenced particular readings. The program includes an electronic log book for recording doses of insulin or oral agents administered at established time slots each day. The program log can also record and store daily nutritional intake facilitated by a USDA database with the nutritional breakdown of more than 6000 food items and a repository for personal recipes and favorite meals, as well as a corresponding breakdown of carbohydrate, protein, fat, and calorie counts. Diabetes Partner PC can create color-coded charts and graphs to identify blood glucose levels that are above, below, or on target as well as track medication and diet information. Health analysis charts and graphs can be printed for evaluation by patients' health care professionals.

Diabetes Self-Management Reminders

Best 4 Diabetes (www.best4diabetes.com) can automatically (or manually) upload readings from many glucose meters. Users can also enter diet and medication information. The program can incorporate individual care plans and remind patients when values are out of the recommended ranges or when

they fail to record medication, meals, or blood glucose readings.

iMetrikus (www.imetrikus.com) is a health care technology company that provides services for diabetes patients and clinicians. MediCompass, the company's health management system, lets patients and health care professionals jointly monitor the patient's health by recording daily activities, medications, self-testing results, and health care visits. The program supports diabetes as well as asthma, chronic obstructive pulmonary disease, hypertension, heart failure, cardiovascular disease, HIV and AIDS, and weight management. iMetrikus software for clinicians lets them create a population registry, gather patient information between health care encounters, identify and track important patient trends, and access patient records from any browser-enabled desktop computer.

MetrikLink is a service of iMetrikus that allows information sharing within the health care team. MetrikLink connects to 30 personal monitoring tools, such as blood glucose monitors, and transmits data to authorized members of the health care team using standard telephone lines. The iMetrikus Web site provides information about their chronic disease management products.

AIDA Online Web-based Glucose–Insulin Diabetes Simulator (www.2aida.org) contains a model of the glucose–insulin interaction that occurs in the human body. The software allows the user to see how insulin and diet interact to affect blood glucose levels for typical insulin-dependent diabetic patients. AIDA runs on Windows platforms (including Virtual PC or SoftWindows for the Macintosh), and the simulations can also be run over the Web from AIDA Online. More than 400,000 visits have been logged at the AIDA Web pages, and more than 80,000 copies of the program have been downloaded free-of-charge.[63]

AIDA is intended for educational, teaching, and demonstration purposes. Because of the complexity of the human glucoregulatory system, one simple model cannot accurately predict each individual patient's blood glucose profile. Therefore, the software should not be used for creating treatment plans. Forty standard case scenarios are provided, and further case scenarios can be generated by users.

Insulin Dose Calculators

There is evidence that computers can help with insulin dose adjustments for real-life patients.[46,64]

Insulin Dose Calculator, an online service based in Latvia (juri.dia-club.ru/eng), analyzes foods to be eaten and recommends an insulin dose based on the analysis of dietary protein, fat, and carbohydrate values and the glycemic index as well as information that users provide about themselves. The site links to discussion forums about the program and other diabetic issues.

Insulin Helper (www.mistebar.com) is another Web-based resource offering insulin dose assis-

tance. Other resources are reviewed by Balas and colleagues.[46]

Lehmann[65] has pointed out the need for validation studies of information technology resources that have been developed as advisory tools, especially those intended to help patients and their health care professionals to optimally adjust insulin dosing. Patients should certainly engage their health care professionals in a discussion of these resources before starting to use them.

Food and Nutrition Information Technology

A number of information technology resources address food and nutrition. Both nutritionsoftware.org and www.mendosa.com are good resources for finding some of these.

The US Department of Agriculture's National Nutrient Database (www.nutrition.gov) is available online. A user-friendly, searchable version of this authoritative nutrition database can be downloaded onto personal computers.

With nearly 70,000 members, the American Dietetic Association is the nation's largest organization of food and nutrition professionals. Their site, www.eatright.org, serves the public by promoting optimal nutrition, health, and well-being for those with diabetes as well as the general population.

The Diabetes Exercise and Sports Association (DESA) (www.diabetes-exercise.org) provides information to enhance the quality of life for people with diabetes through exercise and physical fitness.

Calorieking.com has an extensive food nutrition database and several commercial applications to track daily calorie consumption and exercise on both Palm and PocketPC devices.

Computer Planned Nutrition from Nutritional Computing Concepts (www.ncconcepts.com) analyzes food intake and recipes and plans menus from an extensive food database. Glucose data can be transferred from Bayer, LifeScan, and TheraSense meters.

CarbCheck (www.carbcheckhome.com) provides a free carbohydrate, fat, and protein database that runs on a Palm PDA.

Computer Applications for Clinical Questions

Although prospective learning will always be important for health care professionals, it is not possible to prospectively obtain all of the knowledge required to appropriately treat all patients. Therefore, clinicians must be able to access knowledge at the point of care that answers clinical questions and provides diagnostic and therapeutic decision support. A number of available computer applications address this need. Three of these are

highlighted here. Many Internet sites can provide valuable information to clinicians, and the applications discussed in this section can be accessed on the Internet. However, Internet information resources are discussed separately in the section that follows this one.

UpToDate
www.UpToDate.com

UpToDate is a subscription-based clinical information resource available to physicians on an individual, group, or institutional basis. UpToDate gets physicians concise, practical answers at the point of care. Content covers internal medicine and its subspecialties, obstetrics and gynecology, family medicine, and pediatrics. Content is comprehensive yet concisely written and is extensively referenced.

UpToDate has extensive information about diagnosis, evaluation, and management of diabetes mellitus and its complications and comorbidities. More than 355 topic documents are devoted specifically to diabetes mellitus, and many more address related issues. Despite the large amount of information, UpToDate uses a sophisticated controlled vocabulary to search for information, which allows users to quickly navigate to information that answers specific, focused questions. Some examples are "the most appropriate treatment of hypertension and/or dyslipidemia in patients with T2DM," "the effects of exercise in people with diabetes," and "ACE inhibition or angiotensin receptor antagonism in patients at high risk for a cardiovascular event."

UpToDate offers personal, workstation, and enterprise subscription options. Content can be accessed on the Web, through a CD-ROM, or on Windows Pocket PC PDAs. A Palm version is in development.

InfoPOEMs and InfoRetriever
www.infopoems.com

This subscription service is not a diabetes-specific application but rather a more general medical application resource. It does include diabetes-specific information, and because people with diabetes are likely to have other medical problems, it can be helpful in their care. The system identifies and summarizes new medical evidence that is deemed valid and clinically significant. (POEMs is an acronym for "Patient-Oriented Evidence that Matters.")

Daily InfoPOEMs point out relevant research to subscribers via daily e-mail synopses every Monday through Friday. Monthly, the complete set is compiled and sent for additional summary review. Each InfoPOEM is also added to the InfoRetriever database for easy future reference. Editors review more than 1200 studies monthly from more than 100 medical journals, although a number of diabetes journals are not included. The POEMs process applies specific criteria for validity and relevance to clinical practice. About 1 in 40 studies qualifies.

InfoRetriever allows simultaneous searching of the complete InfoPOEMs database along with six additional evidence-based databases. Search results come from all InfoPOEMs, all Cochrane Systematic Review abstracts, more than 200 decision rules, 2200 predictive calculators, more than 700 summaries of evidence-based practice guidelines, and the full 5-Minute Clinical Consult.

Other features include an International Classification of Diseases, 9th Revision (ICD-9), look-up, an evaluation and management (E/M) coding assistant for payments, guided searches of Medline and other Internet references, and hundreds of indexed links to patient-education materials on the Web.

American College of Physicians
pier.acponline.org

The PIER (Physicians Information and Education Resource) site is an electronic medical resource for members of the American College of Physicians (ACP). It provides evidence-based clinical guidance presented electronically in a unique layered and telegraphic format designed for rapid access to clinical information at the point of care by physicians and allied health care providers, as well as managers, insurers, policy makers, and others. This continually updated resource encompasses adult medicine, but significant content focuses on diabetes as well as on medical conditions that occur commonly in people with diabetes including hypertension, dyslipidemia, cardiovascular disease, and stroke.

PIER is available as a free-standing resource on the Web and on PDAs. It integrates with EMRs, order-entry systems, hospital information systems, and practice-management systems.

PIER includes recommendations based on all levels of medical evidence including randomized, controlled trials, cohort and observational studies, case reports, and expert opinion. Recommendations in PIER include strength-of-recommendation ratings based on the quality of underlying evidence, and each cited reference is graded according to level of evidence. All PIER content is rigorously peer reviewed and updated continually by editorial consultants with the support of periodic searches of the medical literature performed by experts in evidence-based medicine. After initial release, modules are updated on a quarterly basis by either the author or an editorial consultant.

Contents of PIER include disease modules (evidence-based guidance on diagnosis and management of more than 320 diseases), screening and prevention modules (best evidence to support rational use of screening and prevention measures in healthy people), complementary and alternative medicine (CAM) modules (overview of modalities often used by patients and CAM management of common medical problems), ethical and legal issues modules (background and guidance in approaching common legal and ethical dilemmas that arise in daily practice), procedures modules

(details of commonly ordered diagnostic and therapeutic tests and interventions), and drug resource (a comprehensive third-party database of pharmacologic agents).

The disease-based modules are PIER's core. Each disease module presents a series of succinct practice recommendations that are supported by rational and pertinent evidence. Disease modules also include links to a comprehensive drug resource, which is accessible directly and through drug therapy tables; PubMed abstracts and the full text of selected references; other ACP knowledge resources including guidelines, Medical Knowledge Self-Assessment Program, Annals of Internal Medicine, and ACP Journal Club; other resources such as Clinical Evidence; Cochrane Reviews; and other guidelines and Web resources.

PIER source files are in XML, ensuring their ability to be integrated into virtually any EMR or electronic medical resource. Use of PIER in conjunction with EMRs can be tracked to measure performance and document real-time, clinically relevant continuing medical education. PIER is available at no charge to members of the American College of Physicians. There is an annual charge to members for the PDA version.[66] PIER has recently also become available via the STAT!Ref Electronic Medical Library.[67]

Data Privacy and Confidentiality

In 1996 HIPPA created a health information privacy rule to safeguard privacy and confidentiality.[68] HIPAA regulations must be met and access must always be limited to providers of care who have been trained in the expected standards of confidentiality. For all providers, signed statements protecting the rights of the individual patient regarding data (both in print as well as electronic format) should be on file.

Obviously data privacy becomes an increasingly important problem as more and more patient information is in electronic form, such as with electronic medical records and registries. The liability for loss of data or inadvertent release of data is magnified by how much information is compromised. Every practice must have adequate firewall protections, data security, secure information backup, identified access roles, and other policies related to responsible computer management.

THE INTERNET AND DIABETES CARE

Few innovations in history have had the potential to so profoundly change our lives as the Internet. What began in 1969 as a Department of Defense initiative and then evolved to a communications network for educational institutions and computer junkies has now metamorphosed into a vast network of networks and the subject of endless treatises in the poplar media. In the midst of the Cold War, Defense Department scientists developed a technology known as *packet switching* that could ensure data movement from one point to another even in the face of war-related interruptions to some parts of the network. The technology is called TCP/IP.

Linked information on World Wide Web pages allows users to click on a link and navigate to other information on the same page, on other pages of the same document, on other files on the same computer or on other computers linked to the Internet anywhere in the world. Moreover, the navigation requires no knowledge of arcane, difficult-to-remember commands. Hypertext links have the great utility of allowing users to navigate though information according to their own interests and information needs as opposed to those predetermined by an author. The Web also allows authors to link to other sources of information rather than having to recreate it themselves.

Increasingly prevalent and easy access to the World Wide Web has dramatically reduced the barriers to publication of information, because it is much easier and much less expensive to place information on the Web than it is to publish and distribute it in hard copy form. This ease of publication has led to an incredible proliferation of information on the Web, including extensive diabetes information for the public, people with diabetes, and their health care professionals.

Information on the Web is largely not peer reviewed, and there are no standardized criteria for assessing quality or validity; thus, information seekers need to be cautious. One can use the credibility of the provider as a surrogate for validity. Thus, information from not-for-profit disease-specific organizations, government sources, and specialty-specific organizations can be considered reliable. Examples of such organizations are listed in Box 44-2. One should always check the date of Web-based information.

This section reviews a variety of valuable Internet sites for diabetes health care professionals in their clinical, research, and education roles and provides a number of examples of each. Some Web sites with particular information of value to patients and the public are also noted. Many of these sites have been described in a section of Web Alerts published in the journal, Current Diabetes Reports (http://www.current-reports.com/).[69]

American Diabetes Association

www.diabetes.org
The ADA Web site is an essential resource for anyone with an interest in diabetes. Patient and public information includes clear, easy-to-understand descriptions of prediabetes, the different categories of diabetes, and their treatment approaches.

- American Association of Clinical Endocrinologists, www.aace.com
- American Association of Diabetes Educators, www.aade.net
- American Diabetes Association (ADA), www.diabetes.org
- Centers for Disease Control and Prevention (CDC), www.cdc.gov
- Endocrine Society, www.endocrine-society.org
- National Diabetes Education Program (NDEP), www.ndep.nih.gov
- National Institute of Diabetes, Digestive and Kidney Diseases (NIDDK), www.niddk.nih.gov
- BioCritique, www.biocritique.com/
- Children with Diabetes, www.childrenwithdiabetes.org
- Council for the Advancement of Diabetes Research and Education, www.cadre-diabetes.org/home.asp
- Diabetes Physician Recognition Program, www.ncqa.org/DPRP
- Glucagon.com, www.glucagon.com
- MDLinx, www.mdlinx.com/EndoLinx
- Medscape Diabetes and Endocrinology from WEBMD, www.medscape.com/diabetes-endocrinologyhome
- National Diabetes Information Clearinghouse, www.diabetes.niddk.nih.gov
- The Texas Diabetes Council, www.tdh.state.tx.us/diabetes/healthcare/

There is a diabetes risk test, a tip of the day, and a recipe of the day. People can find ADA-recognized diabetes education programs and NCQA/ADA-recognized physicians through the site.

ClubPed is a new Web initiative of the American Diabetes Association designed to help those with and at risk for diabetes mellitus to get the many health benefits that can be gained from walking. The Web site features My Tracker, which lets people set a goal for the number of steps they plan to walk. They can set a goal for the number of times each week they plan to walk, the number of steps each week, and the total number of steps that they plan to walk by a certain date. After this, every time people sign on to the site they can track the steps walked and what percentage of the goal they have achieved. A full progress report function provides detailed information on progress including graphs of current and historical progress. Virtual rewards are even available for those meeting targets.

People can join or donate to the ADA and order ADA materials or products on the Web site. Sections focused on ADA volunteer activities are included.

There is also extensive diabetes-related news coverage. Health care professionals can freely view ADA practice guidelines or download them to their computer or PDA, They are also available at no charge in full text or PDF. This compilation contains all current ADA position statements related to clinical practice. It is a convenient and important resource for all health care professionals who care for people with diabetes.

Abstracts of all ADA journals can also be viewed or downloaded to computers or PDAs, and subscribers can access the full text of manuscripts from ADA journals. One can view the program and register for association meetings. For the Annual Scientific Sessions, a scheduling application and abstracts can be viewed online. Increasingly, some meeting contents are being posted as Webcasts during or following the meetings. Continuing education for physicians and nurses is available for some of these offerings.

Diabetes PHD (Personal Health Decisions www.diabetes.org/phd/profile/default.jsp) is a new interactive ADA Web-based tool that makes it easier for people with diabetes—and anyone at risk for developing diabetes, heart disease, or stroke—to better manage their health. Diabetes PHD is a unique health-risk profiling program that is available free to the public and can be used to explore the effects of a wide variety of health care interventions, including losing weight, stopping smoking, and taking certain medications. Diabetes PHD enables users to enter personal health parameters such as age, sex, height, weight, health history, and medications; in return, users receive a health-risk profile. The application also demonstrates how the individual can change their risk by changing modifiable health parameters such as weight, blood pressure, or cholesterol. The tool can be used to help both patients and health professionals make informed choices about how best to reduce a patient's risk for diabetes and/or its complications.

The software underpinning for Diabetes PHD is Archimedes, which was developed by Kaiser Permanente's Drs. David Eddy and Leonard Schlessinger with support from a grant to the American Diabetes Association (ADA) from Bristol-Myers Squibb Co. Archimedes is an extremely comprehensive model that simulates the biological processes underlying the development of diabetes.

American Association of Clinical Endocrinologists

www.aace.com

The Web site of the American Society of Clinical Endocrinologists (AACE) provides innumerable resources to health care professionals interested in clinical endocrinology. Although significant components of the content are limited to members, many resources are available for other health care professionals, patients with endocrinology problems, and the general public. AACE Medical Guidelines for Clinical Practice are posted on the Web site and include guidelines for the treatment of diabetes mellitus, dyslipidemia, and atherosclerosis, as well as the use of dietary supplements and neutraceuti-

cals. In addition there are AACE position statements on such topics as obesity, the insulin resistance syndrome, the metabolic and cardiovascular consequences of polycystic ovary syndrome, and inpatient diabetes.

A link to the AACE Power of Prevention site provides resources to patients and others at risk for a number of endocrine disorders including diabetes and the metabolic syndrome. Other resources on the AACE site can help people learn about endocrine problems, alert them when they might be at risk, and help them to find an endocrinologist if they so desire.

The organization has held a number of consensus conferences and published several white papers focusing on comprehensive diabetes care, the insulin resistance syndrome, and management of hyperglycemia in hospitalized patients. AACE guidelines are also available on the Web site.

For example, the AACE/ACE (American College of Endocrinology) conference on the insulin resistance syndrome, an epidemic condition that dramatically increases risk for T2DM, coronary heart disease, and stroke, and is estimated to affect one in three Americans, extended the concept of the metabolic syndrome (NCEP/ATP III). The conference addressed the underlying pathophysiology of insulin resistance, which leads not only to CVD but also to diabetes and other disorders and recognized additional associated disorders, such as polycystic ovary syndrome (which affects one in 10 US women of child-bearing age) and nonalcoholic fatty liver disease.

Another example is the 2004 American College of Endocrinology Consensus Conference on Inpatient Diabetes and Metabolic Control, which reviewed data on the impact of hyperglycemia on hospitalized patients and made specific recommendations about appropriate therapeutic targets and strategies. All final consensus conference statements are posted on the AACE Web site as is the full text (for members and subscribers) of Association publications.

American Association of Diabetes Educators

www.aadenet.org

The American Association of Diabetes Educators (AADE) is a multidisciplinary organization representing more than 10,000 health care professionals who provide diabetes education. The site has news issues of interest to diabetes educators, including reimbursement for educational services, association guidelines, advanced credentials, and new diabetes products and services. The site also includes a career network allowing one to post or search for a job, a document fax service, and articles and abstracts from *The Diabetes Educator*. An extensive section is devoted to legislation and reimbursement, including a Guide to Medicare Coverage of Diabetes Education and Supplies and information about insurance reimbursement by state. The site provides information about the association's annual meeting and other educational programs and courses, including continuing education online. There is also a link to the site of the National Certification Board for Diabetes Educators. AADE membership is required for access to some of the information.

Centers for Disease Control and Prevention

www.cdc.gov

The CDC National Center for Chronic Disease Prevention and Health Promotion Diabetes Public Health Resource provides extensive, regularly updated information about diabetes.

The National Center for Health Statistics (NCHS, www.cdc.gov/nchs) is a rich source of information about America's health.[70] As the nation's principal health statistics agency, it compiles statistical information to guide actions and policies to improve the health of the US population. The NCHS is a unique public resource for health information.

The site has a list of frequently asked questions (FAQ), diabetes statistics, state-based diabetes control programs, and publications and products. The CDC provides information about state laws related to diabetes. Information about a broad spectrum of other health topics is available in a section called Health Topics A to Z. These resources all support one of the CDC's missions to help translate research into improved treatment and health outcomes for patients.

National Institute of Diabetes and Digestive and Kidney Diseases

www.niddk.nih.gov

This major branch of the National Institutes of Health (NIH) provides extensive information about many diabetes topics, research issues, diabetes statistics, and other important diabetes content. There is comprehensive information about National Institute of Diabetes and Digestive and Kidney Diseases (NIDDK) research funding opportunities. The NIDDK laboratories section includes information on senior scientists' projects, research and training opportunities, scientific databases and resources, and the Office of Technology Development. Descriptive information is provided about each of the basic laboratories and clinical research branches of the Institute. The Office of Technology Transfer works to convey inventions made in Public Health Service laboratories to the private sector for development to benefit the public health, and the site lists technologies available for licensing.

A Diabetes Dictionary[71] defines, in alphabetical order, terms used when talking or writing about diabetes. It is designed for people with diabetes, their family members, and the public. It also can assist health care professionals to better communicate

with their patients and the public. The dictionary provides basic information about diabetes, its consequences, and care.

There are links to different, but complementary, assembled views of the human genome, along with useful browsing tools, posted by the National Center for Biotechnology Information, the University of California at Santa Cruz, and the European Bioinformatics Institute. Clinical trials information includes links to ClinicalTrials.gov, NIDDK-funded clinical trials, and the NIDDK data and safety monitoring policies. The site has links to easy-to-read publications for patients, their families, the public, and Spanish-speakers. Health topics include information about the HbA1c test, currently recommended and alternative therapies for diabetes, complications of diabetes, hypoglycemia, Medicare coverage, questions to ask your doctor about diabetes, principles for controlling diabetes for life, and pancreatic islet cell transplantation.

www.diabetes.niddk.nih.gov

The National Diabetes Information Clearinghouse (NDIC) is an information service of the NIDDK. Congress established the NDIC in 1978 to increase knowledge and understanding about diabetes among patients, health care professionals, and the public. The NDIC works closely with professional and patient-advocacy organizations, other government health organizations, NIDDK's Diabetes Research and Training Centers, the National Diabetes Education Program (NDEP), and the scientific staff of the NIDDK to identify and respond to the need for information about diabetes and its management. People can contact NDIC with their questions by phone, fax, e-mail, or postal mail. NDIC provides general information to support and foster the relationship between patients and their health care providers. Spanish-speaking information specialists are also available.

The NDIC publications about diabetes are developed by certified diabetes educators, reviewed by nationally recognized researchers and experts, tested for ease of comprehension, and published free of copyright. Their easy-to-read publications are translated into Spanish. Single copies are free, and low-cost bulk copies are available for clinics, practices, health fairs, and community events. All NDIC publications are posted online in downloadable formats.

Thousands of Web sites link to NDIC materials. NDIC refers people to health advocacy organizations and other sources of diabetes expertise and assistance. They maintain a Web-based directory of government and nonprofit organizations dedicated to diabetes, and they link to myriad services provided by the National Library of Medicine, including Medline and MedlinePlus.

www.chid.nih.gov

The NDIC also maintains a free public database of health education media, the diabetes section of the Combined Health Information Database, which includes thousands of references to materials produced by organizations for patients and health care professionals, including fact sheets, brochures, posters, foreign-language materials, and audiovisual materials. The NDIC also provides warehousing and distribution services for the NDEP.

National Diabetes Education Program

ndep.nih.gov

The NDEP is sponsored by the U.S. Department of Health and Human Services' National Institutes of Health and the Centers for Disease Control and Prevention and includes over 200 public and private partner organizations at the national, state, and local levels, working together to reduce the morbidity and mortality associated with diabetes. NDEP strives to improve outcomes for people with diabetes by promoting early diagnosis, more effective treatment of hyperglycemia and diabetic co-morbidities, and ultimately the prevention of the onset of diabetes. The NDEP's target audiences include people with diabetes and their families, the general public, minority populations (including African Americans, Asian Americans, Hispanic Americans, Native Americans, and Pacific Islanders), health care professionals, and health care payers, purchasers, and policy makers.

The NDEP has created program partnerships with other organizations concerned with diabetes and the health status of their constituents. They have developed and implemented ongoing diabetes awareness and education activities and identified, developed, and disseminated educational tools and resources, including those that address the needs of special populations. They have developed and disseminated guiding principles that promote quality diabetes care and promoted policies and activities to improve the quality of and access to diabetes care.

The NDEP Web site has extensive information about diabetes as well as the awareness campaigns and materials developed by the NDEP. NDEP has materials in English, Spanish, and many Asian languages. Each of the campaigns has abundant online information and other materials for health care professionals, patients, and the public. There are also order forms for printed materials. For example, the Foot Care Kit for Diabetes includes "Feet Can Last a Lifetime: A Health Care Provider's Guide to Preventing Diabetes Foot Problems," flyers for the examination rooms, and a document called "Steps for Preventing Diabetes Foot Problems." NDEP materials are not copyrighted, and individual users and organizations have permission to copy and distribute them. Most of these materials are in PDF, allowing easy downloading and reprinting. Materials for patients in this area include "Take Care

of Your Feet for a Lifetime," foot care tips, and a "To Do List."

Other materials include "Team Care: Comprehensive Lifetime Management of Diabetes"; "Making a Difference: The Business Community Takes on Diabetes"; "Medicare Coverage of Diabetes"; and "Tools for Working with the Media." Public service announcements focus on a variety of target audiences including a general audience, African American audience, American Indian audience, Asian American and Pacific-Islander audience, Hispanic audience, and older American audience.

NDEP has launched the first national multicultural diabetes prevention campaign, "Small Steps. Big Rewards: Prevent Type 2 Diabetes," to take action against the growing diabetes epidemic. This initiative is designed to translate the results of the Diabetes Prevention Program (DPP) Study, which provided scientific evidence that people at high risk could prevent or at least delay the onset of diabetes by losing 5 to 7 percent of body weight and getting 30 minutes of physical activity such as brisk walking on most days.[72] The NDEP campaign is especially focused on high-risk multicultural and older adult audiences. Campaign materials include motivational tip sheets for consumers as well as print and radio public service ads. Each set of materials is specifically tailored for one of the high-risk groups: African Americans, Hispanic Americans, American Indians and Alaska Natives, Asian Americans and Pacific Islanders, and adults aged 60 years and older.

The "Small Steps. Big Rewards. Your Game Plan for Preventing Type 2 Diabetes" resource allows people to learn about their risk for developing type 2 diabetes and how to start a game plan to prevent or delay the onset of the disease. It provides tips on how to set goals, track progress, start a walking program, and where to get more help. The "Game Plan Food and Activity Tracker" can be used to record food and drink intake and the time spent on physical activity. One can print copies of the tracker that people can keep with them at all times. Patients can use the "Game Plan Fat and Calorie Counter" booklet to look up the number of calories and fat grams in the foods and drinks consumed each day. This fat and calorie counter lists hundreds of food items, including restaurant, ethnic, and regional foods.

There are also links to the Diabetes Prevention Program Web sites.[73] The lifestyle manuals of operations are available at this site in PDF. The manuals may be downloaded, duplicated, transmitted, and otherwise distributed for educational or research purposes only, provided proper credits are given to the DPP Research Group.

NDEP has created a truly superb Web site with extremely valuable materials for anyone with an interest in diabetes.

NDEP's Better Diabetes Care: www.betterdiabetescare.nih.gov
The NDEP believes that this new Web site will help users to implement improved systems of care with features that include patient-centered care, self-management support, community partnerships, a focus on evidence-based decision-making, effective information systems, and meeting the needs of diverse populations. Primary health care professionals, specialists, diabetes educators, and virtually all health care professionals who participate in diabetes care should be able to benefit from the information on this site, as would administrators, planners, employers, and other purchasers of health care.

The site is divided into sections that include the needs and priorities for systems change; the basic concepts behind systems change; how to implement systems change; the components of patient-centered care, team care, and community partnerships; and issues to address such as reimbursement, cultural competency, professional training, and resistance to change and how to evaluate the progress of change and its effects. An extensive toolbox of resources includes clinical practice recommendations, risk-assessment tools, algorithms, patient-education and clinical-management support tools, information about computer registries and data abstraction tools, and cost of diabetes assessment tools.

www.diabetesatwork.org
Another NDEP Web resource is Diabetes at Work (www.diabetesatwork.org) a business and managed-care diabetes and health resource kit that is hosted by the National Business Group on Health. Diabetes at Work was developed by a collaboration of NDEP, the National Business Group on Health, America's Health Insurance Plans, and the National Business Coalition on Health.

Diabetesatwork.org lets companies assess their need for diabetes education and benefits and services for employees. It provides employers with more than 30 educational lesson plans and more than 20 fact sheets on diabetes-related health issues. These materials can be used to inform employees about how to best prevent or manage their diabetes while at work and how to reduce their risk for further complications. Materials are available in Spanish to assist employers in reaching the growing Hispanic workforce who are also at increased risk for diabetes. Information is also provided on the close association between diabetes and heart disease and tips on what diabetes services and benefits health plans can offer employees.

Diabetes Physician Recognition Program

www.ncqa.org/DPRP
To support the goal of providing comprehensive, high-quality health care to people with diabetes, the Diabetes Physician Recognition Program (DPRP), cosponsored by the National Committee for Quality Assurance (NCQA) and the ADA, assesses physicians on their performance on 11 key measures of care

for adult patients and eight key measures of care for pediatric patients.

The DPRP is a voluntary program for individual physicians or physician groups that provide care to people with diabetes. Physicians in all settings can achieve recognition by submitting data that demonstrate they are providing high-quality diabetes care. The program assesses key measures that were carefully defined and tested for their relationship to improved care for people with diabetes. Program measures are part of the NCQA's Health Plan Employer Data and Information Set (HEDIS). The ADA and the NCQA believe that care will improve if physicians know what processes and outcomes are essential and if they collect data on what they do and are able to review aggregate data from their patient populations.

Aggregate performance results indicate that DPRP-recognized physicians provide high-quality care. The DPRP Web site provides a listing of recognized physicians, frequently asked questions and answers about the measures, aggregate performance results of recognized physicians (compared to that achieved by average health plans and in the Medicare fee-for-service population) and a downloadable PowerPoint presentation about DPRP. One can also obtain DPRP materials online.[74]

BioCritique

www.biocritique.com

The BioCritique Forums provide free-access educational experience for medical professionals. Expert panelists post, rate, and critique important research papers. Papers are then linked to useful related resources such as educational slides, structured PubMed queries, clinical practice guidelines, teaching assessments, and applicable drug and patient information.

An exclusive sponsorship is offered for each major therapeutic area. The diabetes component of BioCritique is sponsored by AstraZeneca and GlaxoSmithKline. At present, over 400 papers in this section can be sorted chronologically, by key topics, by user ratings, or by a user's customized profile. Each paper has the citation and a concise critique by a content expert. One can link to the full abstract of the paper, to related articles or other papers from the author via PubMed, to clinical guidelines (not yet available for some of the papers), and to other clinical trials via www.clinicaltrials.gov. Users can also e-mail critiques to colleagues.

Continuing medical education (CME) credit is available for clinicians who participate in courses based on some of the papers. Many papers have associated slide presentations that can be viewed or downloaded. Sponsored educational programs based on BioCritique abstracts may appear as BioDiscussions, for which there are e-mail invitations. If a registered user does not see slide icons to the left of some of the papers on the BioCritique list of abstracts, he or she can contact the help desk to request permission to view this useful content.

Council for the Advancement of Diabetes Research and Education

www.cadre-diabetes.org

The Council for the Advancement of Diabetes Research and Education (CADRE) provides educational programs and resources to further expand knowledge about diabetes mellitus and its treatment. The CADRE Web site provides information about CADRE regional and national medical education programs. Health care professionals can register for many of these programs and sign up at no charge to be a member of CADRE on the Web site. CADRE membership benefits include access to extensive educational resources, the vast majority of which can be downloaded from the Web site. These resources include educational reprint slide kits; information about CADRE symposia at national medical association meetings; educational monographs, including the recently published CADRE Handbook; automatic subscription to the CADRE newsletter and other CADRE publications; and access to a downloadable extensive collection of diabetes slides, issues of the CADRE newsletter, and diabetes news.

CADRE reprint lecture kits are available on the site. Each CADRE reprint lecture kit includes reprints of one or more seminal articles on diabetes, slide images, and lecture notes printed on four-color 4×6 cards, and a summary card reviewing key points from each article. The slides can be viewed or downloaded in PowerPoint format. Lecture notes can be downloaded in PDF. The site also contains a section called Diabetes Tactics, which consists of case studies presenting challenging diabetes treatment scenarios that practitioners are likely to encounter. These brief case studies explore controversies or dilemmas in diabetes management and offer practical suggestions for dealing with management challenges. CADRE's Web site provides access to diabetes news and a section devoted to key features of diabetes treatment options. There are also links to various agencies and associations that provide diabetes information and resources.

The CADRE Core Slide Kit presents approximately 310 slides in nine sections: Pathogenesis and Classification of Glycemic Disorders; Insulin Deficiency and Insulin Resistance; Microvascular and Macrovascular Complications: Epidemiologic Studies; Evidence for Benefits of Tight Metabolic Control: Intervention Studies; Therapeutic Options: Secretagogues, Sensitizers, and Prandial Regulators; Therapeutic Options: Insulins; and Therapeutic Tactics; The Management of Diabetes in Pregnancy; Type 1 Diabetes Mellitus. A PowerPoint file for each section

can be downloaded along with a PDF file of notes for the slides. This slide set should be very helpful to diabetes health care professionals, especially those who participate in diabetes-related CME activities.

CADRE programs are supported by unrestricted educational grants from several pharmaceutical companies. Registration (which is free) is required for access to some of the content.

Children with Diabetes

www.childrenwithdiabetes.org

This is an excellent resource for children with diabetes, their parents, and health care professionals, as well as for teachers and others who interact with children. Despite the extensive contents, the Web designers have thoughtfully made navigation through the site extremely easy, including clear directions for first-time users.

Key sections for children include: Kids' Voices, which contains home pages of kids with diabetes including photos and a brief story about each child; the Family Support Network, an interactive database containing the names and e-mail addresses of kids with diabetes and their parents; Parents' Feelings, which tries to explain to kids what their parents are feeling; Camps for Kids with Diabetes, which identifies camps that have an on-line presence; and Message Board, which is for posting messages for kids to read on the Web.

There are also sections for parents. Parents Place is the home for parent-specific information; Parents Voices contains home pages of parents with kids with diabetes, describing their experiences with diabetes. The Adults section contains the wisdom of adults with T1DM explaining how they have come to terms with diabetes and offering words of encouragement to children and parents alike.

Ask the Diabetes Team allows parents to submit questions about diabetes to the site's team of diabetes specialists. Diabetes Basics offers some basic medical information about diabetes, insulin. and research. The Products section contains descriptions and reviews of various diabetes products including blood glucose meters, books, and videos for children with diabetes. On-Line Links is a list of links to other sites on the Web that contain information about or related to diabetes. There are also chat rooms for users to interact with others.

The Search page allows free-form text searches. To find information about carbohydrate counting, for example, one can just type in the term and click on the Find Documents button to retrieve a list of each page in the Web site that contains the words "carbohydrate counting."

The Texas Diabetes Council

http://www.dshs.state.tx.us/diabetes/default.shtm

The Texas Diabetes Council Web site has resources for both health care professionals and patients. Site resources include Minimum Standards for Diabetes Care in Texas, which reflects the consensus that these standards should be met under all types of health care plans and delivery systems. They are used to define minimum benefits for health plans regulated by the Texas Department of Insurance and include two downloadable Microsoft Word files: Minimum Practice Recommendations Flow Sheet (28 kb) and Macrovascular Risk Reduction in Diabetes: Antiplatelet Therapy (14 kb).

There are also diabetes treatment algorithms to assist in the delivery of primary care practice. They have been developed by a panel of experts through an open, peer-reviewed process to ensure that they are complete, accurate, and consistent with the current state of knowledge on diabetes treatment. They include a disclaimer that they should not be interpreted as prescribing an exclusive course of management and that every professional using these guidelines is responsible for evaluating the appropriateness of applying them in any particular clinical situation. Specific algorithms include:

- Glycemic Control Algorithm for Type 2 Diabetes Mellitus in Children and Adults
- Insulin Algorithm for Type 1 Diabetes Mellitus in Children and Adults
- Insulin Algorithm for Type 2 Diabetes Mellitus in Children and Adults
- Initial Insulin Therapy for Type 2 Diabetes Mellitus in Children and Adults: A Simplified Approach
- IV Insulin Infusion Protocol for Critically Ill Adult Patients in the ICU Setting
- Exercise Algorithm IFG/Type 2 Diabetes Prevention & Therapy
- Hypertension Algorithm for Diabetes Mellitus in Adults
- Lipid Treatment Algorithm for Type 1 and Type 2 Diabetes Mellitus in Adults
- Medical Nutrition Algorithm IFG/Type 2 Diabetes Prevention & Therapy
- Weight Loss Algorithm for Overweight and Obese Adults
- Prevention and Delay of Type 2 Diabetes in Children and Adults with Impaired Fasting Glucose (IFG) and/or Impaired Glucose Tolerance (IGT)
- Diabetic Foot Care/Referral Algorithm
- Weight Management Algorithm for Overweight Children and Adolescents

Medscape Diabetes and Endocrinology from WEBMD

www.medscape.com/ diabetes-endocrinologyhome

Medscape offers specialists, primary care physicians, and other health professionals extensive and integrated medical information and education tools. Medscape delivers to users specialty-specific content according to a user-designated profile. Each of the specialty areas, including diabetes-endocrinology, has CME activities, extensive conference coverage that summarizes key data and presentations from major medical meetings; daily professional medical news in each specialty from Reuters, Medscape Medical News, and medical news journal publishers; MedPulse, a weekly email newsletter that highlights what is new in each specialty on Medscape; and content from more than 50 medical journals. Druginfosearch provides comprehensive drug information, searchable by drug or disease.

An Ask the Expert section provides helpful information from expert clinicians. Topics have included New Data on Insulin Glargine and CSII, Diabetes and Stress, and Treating Hypertension and Dyslipidemia in Diabetes Patients. Medscape provides information from major conferences including the American Diabetes Association 63rd Scientific Sessions, the Endocrine Society 85th Annual Meeting, and the 18th International Diabetes Federation Congress. These include daily news from the conference, commentary, and clinically focused overviews. CME credit for physicians, nurses, and pharmacists is often obtainable from reading the conference overviews and completing a posttest.

Resource Centers are collections of Medscape's key clinical content, selected by Medscape editors. Some of those relevant to health care professionals caring for people with diabetes include Insulin Pump Therapy, ALLHAT, Diabetic Microvascular Complications, Erectile Dysfunction, Combination Therapy for Type 2 Diabetes, Nutrition, Chronic Kidney Disease, Heart Failure, and Weight Management. Access requires registration. There is no charge.

MDLinx

www.mdlinx.com/EndoLinx

MDLinx owns and operates a network of 34 Web sites and more than 700 daily e-mail newsletters that provide highly focused content to 255,000 physicians and health care professionals, as well as to a growing number of patients. MDLinx has created a network of comprehensive sites for each medical specialty and therapeutic category that helps provide information health care professionals need to stay current. MDLinx recently launched PatientLinx, a free Web site that provides reliable clinical updates for patients.

The endocrinology section, called EndoLinx, provides access to news and summaries of literature articles in many areas including diabetes, atherosclerosis and lipids, hypertension, and obesity. Many summaries provide links to the abstract of the paper.

Glucagon.com

www.glucagon.com

Glucagon.com is devoted to the study of the glucagon-like peptides and is maintained by Dr. Daniel J. Drucker at the University of Toronto. Sections on the site are devoted to Dr. Drucker's lab, dipeptidyl peptidase IV (DPP-IV), exenatide, gastric inhibitory polypeptide (GIP), glicentin, glucagon, the glucagon gene, glucagon-like peptides 1 and 2 (GLP-1, GLP-2), gut endocrine cells, islet alpha cells, links, liraglutide, meetings, oxyntomodulin, patents, receptors, research reagents, and reviews. Each section has a written overview of the topic with a number of links to other related information as well as links to PubMed references and to full-text PDF files for some of the references. Slides in PDF color format are available for some topics. For example, one can download slides on phase II data obtained with the Novartis DPP-IV inhibitor.

Practitioner Sites

Increasingly, health care professional organizations and practices are using the World Wide Web to market their practices and to communicate with patients. Practice Web sites can provide existing and prospective patients with information about services offered and allow patients to schedule appointments, find educational resources, and get answers to frequently asked questions about the practice and about health problems. Some sites even allow patients to sign in to a secure area and find out some test results.

NuWeb (www.numedics.com/products/nuweb) is a Web hosting service for diabetes practices provided by the developer of CliniPro and Diabetes Partner PC. NuWeb provides access to educational materials and information to patients and the public through posted documents such as press releases.

COMPUTER-AIDED PATIENT EDUCATION

Diabetes education is a multifaceted task involving instruction on various aspects of self care. The availability of computerized diabetes education in such content areas as meal planning, glucose monitoring, exercise, and diabetes complications increases patient access and can improve the effectiveness of the clinical intervention. Significant improvements

in HbA1c, glucose levels, and serum cholesterol have been documented in studies comparing these systems with usual care. Nebel and colleagues[75] showed that adaptive interactive computer-based education programs that can be personalized to patients' needs and skills achieved significantly better results as compared to a conventional one in teaching patients about hypoglycemia.

CONCLUSION

Diabetes mellitus is a common, serious, and costly disorder. What started as an American epidemic is in danger of becoming a worldwide pandemic. Complex treatment is needed for the more than 18 million persons in this country with diabetes, and efforts are required to attempt to prevent the 41 million persons with prediabetes from progressing to diabetes. Treatment requires patient education, lifestyle measures, and pharmacologic agents to treat glycemia as well as the often accompanying comorbidities such as hypertension and dyslipidemia. The complexity of the task is magnified by the wealth of new information generated continually by research efforts.

Computers can help the public, patients with diabetes, their families and their health care professionals to prospectively learn about this condition and to identify information at the point of care that can enhance treatment and outcomes. Moreover, patients and their health care professionals also need to manage information about their individual medical condition and its treatment. Health care professionals and health systems need to access information about the population with diabetes in their care. Such information can identify people needing services and support continuous quality improvement efforts for the entire system. Moreover, information technology could potentially remind both patients and health care professionals of needed assessments and therapy.

Indeed, Bodenheimer and Grumbach[76] have suggested that computer use could be a spark to revitalize primary care by enhancing medical records, communication between physicians and patients, information sharing among health care providers, and rapid access to reliable medical information for both physicians and patients. Their message seems applicable to many areas of medicine that provide evaluation and management services for people with chronic medical problems. The authors note the barriers to broader adoption of information technology in medical practice and note the need for the redesign of some systems of clinical processes to facilitate the implementation and value of technology.

Although it is not possible to even mention much less provide details about all resources, this chapter has attempted to identify the categories of diabetes-related information technology and to reference some sources for further information about them.

References

1. Peterson C. Health professions education: A bridge to quality. Tar Heel Nurse 65:12, 2003.
2. Centers for Disease Control and Prevention: National Diabetes Fact Sheet. http://www.cdc.gov/diabetes/pubs/factsheet.htm.
3. Hogan P, Dall T, Niilov P: Economic costs of diabetes in the US in 2002. American Diabetes Association. Diabetes Care 26:917-932, 2003.
4. Saydah SH, Fradkin J, Cowie CC. Poor control of risk factors for vascular disease among adults with previously diagnosed diabetes. JAMA 291:335-342, 2004.
5. Wagner EH, Glasgow RE, Davis C, et al. Quality improvement in chronic illness care: A collaborative approach. Jt Comm J Qual Improv 27:63-80, 2001.
6. Committee on Quality of Health Care in America: Crossing the Quality Chasm: A New Health System for the 21st Century. Washington, DC, Institute of Medicine, 2001.
7. Blonde L: CADRE. Curr Diabetes Pract 2:1-2, 2002.
8. Simon J, Powers M: Chronic Disease Registries: A Product Review. Oakland, California HealthCare Foundation, 2004. PDF downloadable at: http://www.chcf.org/
9. Institute of Medicine: The Computer-Based Patient Record: An Essential Technology for Health Care, rev ed. Washington, DC, National Academies Press, 1997.
10. Bakke, K: The Clinically Related Information System (CRIS): A CPR Pilot Using Primary Care Advice Rules and Reminders. Second Annual Nicholas E. Davies CPR Recognition Symposium. Bethesda, Md, Computer-based Patient Record Institute, 1996.
11. EMR Update: http://www.emrupdate.com/.
12. Clark CM Jr, Snyder JW, Meek RL, et al: A systematic approach to risk stratification and intervention within a managed care environment improves diabetes outcomes and patient satisfaction. Diabetes Care 24:1079-1086, 2001.
13. Grant RW, Cagliero E, Sullivan CM, et al: A controlled trial of population management: Diabetes mellitus: Putting evidence into practice (DM-PEP). Diabetes Care 27:2299-2305, 2004.
14. Graham G, Nugent L, Strouse K: Information everywhere: How the EHR transformed care at VHA. J AHIMA 74:20-24, 2003.
15. Kaiser Permanente gets ready to roll out automated medical records system nationwide. Qual Lett Healthc Lead 15:12, 2003.
16. Wang SJ, Middleton B, Prosser LA, et al: A cost-benefit analysis of electronic medical records in primary care. Am J Med 114:397-403, 2003.
17. Antoine, W: Electronic miracle. Memorial Hermann put its patient files online and watch its revenue grow. Health Forum J 45:34-35, 2002.
18. National Diabetes Education Program: Better diabetes care. http://www.betterdiabetescare.nih.gov
19. Health Disparities Collaboratives: Tools: Diabetes, all elements. Available at: http://www.healthdisparities.net/.
20. NuMedics: CliniPro Diabetes Management System. http://www.numedics.com/clinipro/.
21. American Diabetes Association: Education Recognition Program. www.diabetes.org/for-health-professionals-and-scientists/recognition/edrecognition.jsp#applying
22. Delphi Health Systems: Delphi Diabetes Manager. http://www.delphihealth.com/sol_ddm_overview.shtml
23. Virginia Health Quality Center: Diabetes: Resources for improving care. http://www.vhqc.org/index/diabetes.
24. Overlook Software: DiaTrends diabetes management software. http://overlooksoftware.com/.
25. Liu D: Drug information on the handheld computer in 2004: An update. Medical Software Reviews March–April:14-16, 2004.
26. ePocrates: http://www2.epocrates.com/index.html
27. PDR.net: http://www.pdr.net/pdrnet/librarian
28. Cheng P: MedMath 2.01: Download and documentation. http://smi-web.stanford.edu/people/pcheng/medmath/.

29. Miller SR: Scrip for success. Kentucky family practice uses electronic prescriptions to improve efficiency, revenue and customer service. Health Manag Technol 24: 20-21, 2003.

30. Corley ST: Electronic prescribing: A review of costs and benefits. Top Health Inf Manage 24:29-38, 2003.

31. eHealth Initiative: Electronic prescribing. http://www .ehealthinitiative.org/initiatives/erx/

32. Allscripts: Clinical information systems: Electronic prescribing. http://www.allscripts.com/slnsClncInfoEPrscrb.aspx

33. Bluefish: BluefishRx prescription writer. http://bluefishwireless.com/eprescribing/eprescribing.htm

34. ePocrates: ePocrates Rx online. http://www2.epocrates.com/products/rxonline/

35. Caremark: iScribe electronic prescribing. http://www.iscribe .com/index.html

36. Zix Corporation: PocketScript. http://www.zixcorp.com/ehealth/eprescribing.php.

37. eHealth Initiative: http://www.ehealthinitiative.org/.

38. eHealth Initiative. Electronic Prescribing: Towards Maximum Value and Rapid Adoption. http://www .ehealthinitiative.org/initiatives/erx/

39. Choremis J, Chow DR: Use of telemedicine in screening for diabetic retinopathy. Can J Ophthalmol 38:575-579, 2003.

40. McDonald CJ: Protocol-based computer reminders, the quality of care and the non-perfectability of man. N Engl J Med 295:1351-1355, 1976.

41. Lobach DF, Hammond WE: Computerized decision support based on a clinical practice guideline improves compliance with care standards. Am J Med 102:89-98, 1997.

42. Hurwitz B, Goodman C, Yudkin J: Prompting the clinical care of non–insulin dependent (type II) diabetic patients in an inner city area: One model of community care. BMJ 306:624-630, 1993.

43. Meigs JB, Cagliero E, Dubey A, et al: A controlled trial of Web-based diabetes disease management: The MGH diabetes primary care improvement project. Diabetes Care 26:750-757, 2003.

44. O'Connor PJ: Electronic medical records and diabetes care improvement: Are we waiting for Godot? Diabetes Care 26:942-943, 2003.

45. Montori VM, Dinneen SF, Gorman CA, et al, and the Translation Project Investigator Group: The impact of planned care and a diabetes electronic management system on community-based diabetes care: The Mayo Health System Diabetes Translation Project. Diabetes Care 25:1952-1957, 2002.

46. Balas EA, Krishna S, Kretschmer RA, et al: Computerized knowledge management in diabetes care. Med Care 42:610-621, 2004.

47. Marrero DG, Kronz KK, Golden MP, et al: Clinical evaluation of computer-assisted self-monitoring of blood glucose system. Diabetes Care 12:345-350, 1989.

48. Rivellese AA, Ventura MM, Vespasiani G, et al: Evaluation of new computerized method for recording 7-day food intake in IDDM patients. Diabetes Care 14:602-604, 1991.

49. Chiarelli F, Tumini S, Morgese G, et al: Controlled study in diabetic children comparing insulin-dosage adjustment by manual and computer algorithms. Diabetes Care 13:1080-1084, 1990.

50. Danne T, Kordonouri O, Casani A, et al: Recent advances on the pathogenesis and management of both diabetic retinopathy and nephropathy with particular reference to children and adolescents with type 1 diabetes. Diabetes Nutr Metab 12:136-144, 1999.

51. Peters A, Rubsamen M, Jacob U, et al: Clinical evaluation of decision support system for insulin-dose adjustment in IDDM. Diabetes Care 14:875-880, 1991.

52. Peterson CM, Jovanovic L, Chanoch LH: Randomized trial of computer-assisted insulin delivery in patients with type I diabetes beginning pump therapy. Am J Med 81:69-72, 1986.

53. Schrezenmeir J, Sturmer W, Gobel D, et al: Brockmann-bodies in hollow fibres may solve availability problems for islet transplantation. Life Support Syst 3(Suppl 1):666-669, 1985.

54. Gonder-Frederick LA, Julian DM, Cox DJ, et al. Self-measurement of blood glucose. Accuracy of self-reported data and adherence to recommended regimen. Diabetes Care 11:579-585, 1988.

55. Ziegler O, Kolopp M, Got I, et al: Reliability of self-monitoring of blood glucose by CSII-treated patients with type I diabetes. Diabetes Care 12:184-188, 1989.

56. Mazze RS, Shamoon H, Pasmantier R, et al: Reliability of blood glucose monitoring by patients with diabetes mellitus. Am J Med 77:211-217, 1984.

57. Hirsch I: Blood glucose monitoring technology: Translating data into practice. Endocr Pract 10:67-76, 2004.

58. Kwon HS, Cho JH, Kim HS, et al: Establishment of blood glucose monitoring system using the Internet. Diabetes Care 27:478-483, 2004.

59. Yale JF: Log sheet in PDF. Automatically download at: http://www.mendosa.com/logsheet.pdf

60. Yale JF: Blood glucose spreadsheet for Microsoft Excel. Automatically download at: http://www.mendosa.com/BGspreadsheet.xls.

61. Yale JF: Blood glucose spreadsheet in PDF. Automatically download at: http://www.mendosa.com/BGspreadsheet.pdf.

62. Nagykaldi Z, Mold JW: Diabetes Patient Tracker, a personal digital assistant–based diabetes management system for primary care practices in Oklahoma. Diabetes Technol Ther 5:997-1001, 2003.

63. Lehmann ED: British Diabetic Association review of the AIDA v4 diabetes software simulator program. Diabetes Technol Ther 6:87-96, 2004.

64. Boukhors Y, Rabasa-Lhoret R, Langelier H, et al: The use of information technology for the management of intensive insulin therapy in type 1 diabetes mellitus. Diabetes Metab 29:619-627, 2003.

65. Lehmann ED: Computerised decision-support tools in diabetes care: Hurdles to implementation. Diabetes Technol Ther 6:422-429, 2004.

66. American College of Physicians: PIER PDA. http://www .acponline.org/catalog/pierpda/pier_pda.htm?php

67. STAT!Ref: ACP PIER Physician's Information and Education Reference. http://www.statref.com/ourproducts/ebm/ebm.htm

68. Department of Health and Human Services: The Health Insurance Portability and Accountability Act (HIPAA). Downloads available at: http://aspe.hhs.gov/admnsimp and http://www.hhs.gov/ocr/hipaa.

69. Current Diabetes Reports (http://www.current-reports.com/home_journal.cfm?JournalID=DR).

70. Centers for Disease Control and Prevention, National Center for Health Statistics: Health and Stats: http://www.cdc.gov/nchs/products/pubs/pubd/hestats/hestats.htm.

71. National Center for Health Statistics: NCHS Health and stats. http://www.cdc.gov/nchs/products/pubs/pubd/hestats/hestats.htm

72. Knowler WC, Barrett-Connor E, Fowler SE, et al, and the Diabetes Prevention Program Research Group. Reduction in the incidence of type 2 diabetes with lifestyle intervention or metformin. N Engl J Med 346:393-403, 2002.

73. http://www.bsc.gwu.edu/dpp/manuals.htmlvdoc/

74. http://www.ncqa.org/communications/Publications/dprppubs.htm.

75. Nebel IT, Klemm T, Fasshauer M, et al: Comparative analysis of conventional and an adaptive computer-based hypoglycaemia education programs. Patient Educ Couns 53:315-318, 2004.

76. Bodenheimer T, Grumbach K: Electronic technology: A spark to revitalize primary care? JAMA 290:259-264, 2003.

Pearls from Major Clinical Trials: Approaches to Improving Outcome of Persons with Diabetes

Zachary Bloomgarden

KEY POINTS

- *Glycemic control is associated with reduction in neuropathy, nephropathy, retinopathy (microvascular disease), and atherosclerotic complications of diabetes, with no evidence of a threshold below which further benefit is not attained.*
- *There is at present no satisfactory evidence that any one form of glucose-lowering therapy is to be preferred, although there is a suggestion of particularly favorable effects of metformin.*
- *Blood pressure treatment is important for persons with diabetes because it leads to reduction in cardiovascular disease and microvascular disease. Some studies suggest particular benefit of therapies directed at angiotensin II.*
- *Lipid treatment is important for persons with diabetes. Therapy directed at triglycerides and high-density lipoprotein cholesterol with fibrates and at low-density lipoprotein cholesterol with statins has benefit.*
- *Combination therapy is of particular benefit in reducing risk of complications in persons with diabetes.*

Cardiovascular disease (CVD) mortality among adults without diabetes in the United States declined by 36% among men and 27% among women in the 10 years leading to the period 1982-1984. During the same period, the decline in age-adjusted CVD mortality for diabetic men was 13%, and CVD mortality of diabetic women increased 23%.[1] Levels of diabetes are predicted to double over the coming decades, from 171 million patients in 2000 to 366 million in 2030 (Fig. 45–1),[2] and the health and economic burden of the disease looms ever larger. It is clear, then, that the development and validation of approaches to improve CVD outcome among persons with diabetes is an urgent clinical goal. Fortunately, there has been an immense growth of clinical information to aid us in determining appropriate therapies for persons with diabetes. This chapter summarizes the findings of major randomized clinical trials of glucose, blood pressure (BP), and lipid treatment, both separately and in combination, for persons with diabetes.

GLYCEMIA TRIALS

The relationship between blood glucose and clinical outcome in retinopathy, nephropathy, neuropathy, and CVD is consistently found in studies of persons with type 1 diabetes (T1DM) and type 2 diabetes (T2DM) across a range of levels of glycemia (Table 45–1).

Diabetes Control and Complications Trial

A number of previous studies had shown benefits of improved glycemic control,[3] but with the Diabetes Control and Complications Trial (DCCT) it became widely appreciated that persons with T1DM receiving intensive therapy guided by frequent blood glucose monitoring have improved outcome. In 1993 the DCCT began studying 1441 patients with T1DM. One group received intensive therapy and the other received conventional therapy. Outcomes for the intensive group were generally superior to those for the conventional group.

The 6.5-year mean hemoglobin A1c (HbA1c) in the intensively treated group was 2 percentage points lower than that with conventional insulin therapy. The primary prevention cohort of 726 participants had no retinopathy at baseline, and the secondary prevention cohort of 715 subjects had mild retinopathy. Intensive therapy reduced the adjusted mean risk for the development of retinopathy in the primary prevention cohort by 76%, slowed the progression of retinopathy in the secondary intervention cohort by 54%, and reduced the development of proliferative or severe nonproliferative retinopathy by 47%. In the two cohorts combined, intensive therapy reduced the occurrence of microalbuminuria by 39% and of macroalbuminuria by 54%.[4]

Intensive therapy reduced the development of clinical neuropathy in both cohorts by 64% after 5 years. Nerve conduction velocities increased significantly in patients receiving conventional therapy but remained generally stable for those following the intensive regimen.[5]

The initial level of HbA1c observed at eligibility screening and the duration of T1DM were the dominant baseline predictors of the risk of progression. In each treatment group, the mean HbA1c during the trial was the dominant predictor of retinopathy progression. Each lowering of HbA1c by one tenth of a percentage point was associated with a 43% to 45% lower risk. Similar results also apply to nephropathy and neuropathy progression.[6] Extrapolated to 1 million persons with T1DM in the United States, achievement of an HbA1c of 7.2% would lead to a gain of close to 8 million person-years of sight, close to 6 million person-years free of end-stage renal disease (ESRD), and more than 5 million person-years of additional survival.[7]

Analysis of the DCCT data showed that in addition to glycemia there were individual differences in clinical characteristics leading to greater or lesser difficulty in a given person's achieving improved glycemic control, with consequent change in outcome. Subjects who maintained C peptide at low but sustained levels, evincing greater level of preservation of endogenous insulin, showed reduced incidence of long-term complications as well as improved ability to avoid hypoglycemia.[8] The level of HbA1c in the DCCT varied as a function of mean glucose concentration, but there were also important differences between study participants in the degree of hemoglobin glycation for a given mean glucose level, based on capillary glucose collected before and 90 minutes after each meal and at bedtime every 3 months during the study. Subjects in the highest tertile of hemoglobin glycation had threefold and sixfold greater development of retinopathy and of nephropathy, respectively, a phenomenon seen particularly in participants with low mean glucose concentrations.[9]

Part of the importance of the DCCT was its demonstration of the need for behavior change and of the value of teamwork in patient care. There are, however, difficulties with intensive treatment. It is expensive (costing approximately $4500 per patient per year for DCCT participants, although there is no evidence that comparable costs are encountered by experienced clinicians offering intensive diabetes treatment). Particularly on initiation, intensive

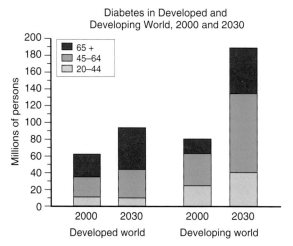

Figure 45–1. Prevalence of diabetes in developed and developing world, 2000 and 2030. (Redrawn from data in Wild S, Roglic G, Green A, et al: Global prevalence of diabetes: Estimates for the year 2000 and projections for 2030. Diabetes Care 27:1047-1053, 2004.)

Table 45-1. *Relationship between Hemoglobin A1c and Risk of Diabetic Complications*

Study and Type	Population	Complications	Decrease per 1% Decrease in HbA1c
DCCT: RCT (see text)	Type 1 diabetes, N = 1440	Retinopathy, nephropathy, neuropathy	30% to 35%
Kumamoto*: RCT	Type 2 diabetes, N = 110	Retinopathy, nephropathy, neuropathy	30% to 38%
UKPDS: RCT and epidemiologic analysis (see text)	Type 2 diabetes, N = 4209	Retinopathy, CVD	28%
Joslin Clinic†: epidemiologic analysis	Type 1 diabetes, N = 1795	Nephropathy	30% to 70%
WESDR‡	Type 2 diabetes	Retinopathy, nephropathy, neuropathy, CVD	20% to 50%
Elderly Japanese Study§: epidemiologic analysis	Type 2 diabetes, N = 123	Nephropathy	20% to 40%

CVD, cardiovascular disease; DCCT, Diabetes Control and Complications Trial; HbA1c, hemoglobin A1c; RCT, randomized, controlled trial; UKPDS, United Kingdom Prospective Diabetes Study; WESDR, Wisconsin Epidemiologic Study of Diabetic Retinopathy.
*Ohkubo Y, Kishikawa H, Araki E, et al: Intensive insulin therapy prevents the progression of diabetic microvascular complications in Japanese patients with non-insulin-dependent diabetes mellitus: A randomized prospective 6-year study. Diabetes Res Clin Pract 28:103-117, 1995.
†Warram JH, Manson JE, Krolewski AS: Glycosylated hemoglobin and the risk of retinopathy in insulin-dependent diabetes mellitus. N Engl J Med 332:1305-1306, 1995.
‡Klein R: Hyperglycemia and microvascular and macrovacular disease in diabetes. Diabetes Care 18:258-268, 1995.
§Tanaka Y, Atsumi Y, Matsuoka K, et al: Role of glycemic control and blood pressure in the development and progression of nephropathy in elderly Japanese NIDDM patients. Diabetes Care 21:116-120, 1998.

treatment is associated with an increase in the frequency of hypoglycemia, both in the DCCT and in community studies.[10]

Similar to findings in studies of persons with type 2 diabetes (discussed later), participants in the intensive treatment group experienced a 73% greater likelihood of becoming overweight, and the frequency of hypoglycemia was threefold greater with intensive than with conventional therapy,[11] both factors that might actually increase risk of adverse cardiovascular outcome. Indeed, analysis of quartiles of weight gain shows that the top quartile of weight gain of the intensively treated group gained 7 BMI units, for a 29% increase in body weight. The weight gain was associated with an increase in LDL cholesterol and triglycerides and a reduction in HDL cholesterol, the triglyceride and HDL changes suggesting development of insulin resistance.[12]

The Epidemiology of Diabetes Intervention and Complications (EDIC) follow-up study of patients who had been enrolled in the DCCT reported that the 7% versus 9% differential in HbA1c levels between the intervention and control groups of the DCCT was not maintained after these patients were returned to community care: Both groups showed HbA1c of approximately 8% during the first 4 years of follow-up. Surprisingly, however, the cumulative incidence of further progression of retinopathy remained different, approximately 2% versus 8% at 2 years and 6% versus 18% at 4 years following the conclusion of the formal study comparing the former intensive treatment with the control group. Similarly, microalbuminuria developed in 5% versus 11%, and progression from micro- to macroalbuminuria was seen in 8% versus 31%, respectively.[13] This memory effect suggests that aggressive management of glycemia early in the course of diabetes is particularly important in preventing later complications.

United Kingdom Prospective Diabetes Study

The findings of the 22-year United Kingdom Prospective Diabetes Study (UKPDS) give insight into to the efficacy and safety of treatment of T2DM in preventing macrovascular and microvascular complications. At the time of diagnosis of diabetes, 5102 patients who did not have T1DM, severe CVD, renal disease, retinopathy, or other severe illness and who could be randomized to insulin treatment were entered in the study. During a 3-month run-in period the patients were treated with diet; mean HbA1c was 6.9%. A group of 4209 patients whose fasting blood glucose (FBG) was 110 to 270 mg/dL and who were not symptomatic, allowing randomization to a control group, also entered the study. Of these, 1138 were entered into a control group with conventional treatment, which initially was only continued attention to diet.

Glycemic Control

By 3 years, 26% of the control patients were found to require pharmacologic intervention based on symptoms or on FBG higher than 270 mg/dL.[14] The intensive treatment group, whose treatment was initiated at the time of diagnosis, included 342 obese patients randomized to metformin and another 2729 patients either given insulin, with multiple doses if required for increasing degrees of hyperglycemia, or one of the sulfonylureas—glyburide or chlorpropamide—with metformin and then insulin added if required. At 3 years, 87% of those in the chlorpropamide group, 93% of the glyburide group, 89% of the metformin group, and 73% of the insulin group were taking the initially prescribed monotherapy. Furthermore, 9% to 13% of those on one of the oral agents required an additional oral agent or insulin, and 14% of insulin-treated patients required multiple doses, showing the complexities of diabetes management.

The glucose level was not stable through the study either in the control or the intensive intervention group. The FBG of participants in the control group fell from 207 mg/dL at the time of randomization to 144 mg/dL at 3 months with the diet intervention, but it increased at 3 years to 162 mg/dL and at 9 years to 180 mg/dL. Of participants in the control group, then, FBG remained below 270 mg/dL in 90% at 1 year, in 40% at 7 years, and in only 20% at 12 years. The mean FBG in the intensively treated group was 122 mg/dL at 1 year, 135 mg/dL at 6 years, and 144 mg/dL at 12 years.

HbA1c was 7.0% at baseline in the intensive group, decreasing to 6.2% at 1 year, and subsequently increasing by 0.2 to 0.3 percentage points per year, so that it returned to the baseline level of 7.0% at 5 years and increased to 8.0% at 11 years. In contrast, the control group patients began with average HbA1c of 6.9%. HbA1c increased to 8.0% at 6 years, with a slower subsequent increase to 8.5% at 11 years (Fig. 45–2). The 10-year average HbA1c was 7.0% for the intensive treatment group and 7.9% for the control group.

The more rapid increase in HbA1c than in FBG in the intensive group has been taken to suggest that there was a relatively greater increase in postprandial glucose levels, so that this less readily determined measure of control might be important in attaining long-term glycemic stability. Body weight in control group participants increased by 2.5 kg over baseline at 6 years and was subsequently stable through 10 years. In the intensive group, body weight increased by 5 kg over baseline at 6 years and reached a level 3.1 kg over the conventionally treated group at 10 years.[15]

Endpoints

There were 3277 nonfatal and 927 fatal endpoints during the study period, occurring in 1401 (36%) of the patients. Diabetes-related endpoints including death, myocardial infarction (MI), congestive heart failure (CHF), angina, stroke, amputation, renal

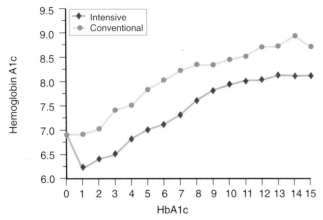

Figure 45–2. Hemoglobin A1c with intensive versus conventional treatment in the United Kingdom Prospective Diabetes Study (UKPDS). (Redrawn from data in UK Prospective Diabetes Study Group: Intensive blood-glucose control with sulphonylureas or insulin compared with conventional treatment and risk of complications in patients with type 2 diabetes [UKPDS 33]. Lancet 352:837-853, 1998.)

failure, cataract, blindness, and retinal photocoagulation occurred 12% less often in the intensively treated group. Total microvascular endpoints were decreased 25%, cataract 24%, retinopathy progression 21%, and microalbuminuria 33% by the intensive intervention. The risks of requiring photocoagulation and of loss of vibratory sensation were also significantly decreased. The relative risk of myocardial infarction (MI) was decreased 16%. Although some have questioned the latter finding because of its borderline statistical significance (P = .052), both an epidemiologic analysis of the study and a post-UKPDS follow-up similar to the EDIC study of the DCCT show robust statistically significant evidence that the decline in this macrovascular endpoint was a real phenomenon.[16] There was no significant difference between the groups in diabetes-related deaths. The investigators concluded that one can "reduce the risk of the diabetic complications that cause both morbidity and premature mortality" with "an intensive glucose-control treatment policy."[15]

Pharmacologic Therapy

An important question addressed by the UKPDS was the assessment of whether there was a difference in outcome between insulin and sulfonylurea treatments. In this study, 896 patients were randomized to the control group, 619 were treated with chlorpropamide, 615 with glyburide, and 911 with insulin. At 10 years, FBG levels were 175 mg/dL in the control group, 160 mg/dL with chlorpropamide, 155 mg/dL with glyburide, and 140 mg/dL with insulin. The HbA1c was 9.0% for control, 7.9% for chlorpropamide, 8.1% for glyburide, and 7.7% for insulin. Weight had increased from baseline by 2.5

kg, 5 kg, 5 kg, and 7.5 kg, respectively. Severe hypoglycemia requiring assistance of another person did not occur with conventional treatment but was seen in approximately 0.5% of the two sulfonylurea groups and in around 2% of the insulin-treated patients annually. With chlorpropamide, 4 mm Hg higher systolic and 2 mm Hg higher diastolic BP were seen during the study period. No significant differences were seen between the sulfonylurea and insulin groups in total diabetes-related endpoints, diabetes-related mortality, MI, microvascular endpoints, retinopathy, or microalbuminuria.[15]

Metformin was used as monotherapy only in obese patients in the UKPDS.[17] Weight gain was greater with insulin and sulfonylureas than with conventional treatment or with metformin. Fasting insulin levels increased with insulin and sulfonylureas, were stable with diet, and fell with metformin, confirming metformin's action as an insulin sensitizer. Hypoglycemia occurred rarely with metformin.

In the metformin substudy of obese patients, BMI was 31.6 kg/m^2, and other baseline characteristics, including FBG and HbA1c, were similar to those of the overall group. Weight gain with metformin was similar to that in the control group and less than that with sulfonylureas or insulin. The incidence of total diabetes-related endpoints with metformin decreased 32% in comparison to that in the conventional-treatment group, which was significantly lower than the 7% reduction in the other intensive treatment groups. There was similarly a 42% lower diabetes-related mortality with metformin compared to 20% reduction in the other intensive-treatment groups, 36% lower total mortality with metformin compared to 8% reduction in the other intensive treatment groups, and 39% lower MI rate with metformin compared to 21% reduction in the other intensive treatment groups.

This gives a strong evidence base favoring use of this agent as initial treatment of overweight persons with diabetes. Indeed, the study authors concluded, "metformin treatment appears to be advantageous as a first-line pharmacological therapy in diet-treated overweight patients with T2DM." The situation is complex, however, because an additional group of 268 UKPDS patients already treated with sulfonylureas for whom metformin was added, compared with 269 treated with sulfonylureas alone, showed an unexpected and significant 60% higher mortality in the combination group. The authors suggested that this represented one of the "extremes of the play of chance" rather than true evidence that the combination is disadvantageous, and preliminary reports of the post-UKPDS analysis suggest that combined metformin–sulfonylurea treatment did not show a significant disadvantage with longer follow-up.[16]

Another substudy in the UKPDS administered acarbose for 3 years. The study randomized 973 patients to this treatment and 973 to placebo, with a protocol increasing the dose to 50 mg three times

daily over 3 weeks, then to 100 mg three times daily over the subsequent 4 months. Subjects were divided into 52% treated with sulfonylureas, insulin, or metformin, 34% treated with a combination of sulfonylureas plus metformin, multiple insulin injections, or sulfonylureas plus insulin, and 14% treated with diet alone. The FBG was 160 mg/dL with placebo throughout the 3-year period, 140 mg/dL in the intention-to-treat acarbose group at 1 year, and 150 mg/dL in the acarbose group at 3 years. HbA1c was 0.2 percentage points lower in the acarbose group. However, compliance was a problem, with 32% of placebo patients and 39% of acarbose patients failing to take the recommended tablets during the 3-year period. Discontinuation was associated with symptoms of flatulence and diarrhea. In patients actually on treatment, HbA1c was 0.5 percentage points lower than in the placebo group at 1, 2, and 3 years, comparable to the benefit seen with metformin. In this shorter substudy, there was no effect of the intervention on outcome.[18]

Glycemic Effect on Vascular Disease

An important question is the extent to which the association between diabetes and vascular disease is mediated by hyperglycemia. Epidemiologic analysis of the UKPDS, adjusted for age, sex, and ethnicity, examined 4585 patients. The analysis showed that an increase in HbA1c from 6% to 11% more than doubled the risk of MI and was associated with a 10-fold increase in risk of microvascular disease. Several important observations can be made from these data. At HbA1c levels less than 6%, the risk of a macrovascular event is more than three times that of a microvascular event; microvascular events exceed macrovascular events only at HbA1c greater than 10%.

This result suggests that the burden of diabetes differs for persons with poor versus good glycemic control. Furthermore, it is apparent that hyperglycemia might not increase macrovascular disease to the same extent as it does microvascular disease (Fig. 45–3).[19] Relative to an HbA1c of 6%, and correcting in multivariate analysis for sex, age, ethnic group, smoking, and baseline HDL and LDL cholesterol, triglyceride, presence of albuminuria, and systolic blood pressure (BP), each 1 percentage point increase in HbA1c was associated with an increase in total diabetes endpoint development by 21%, diabetes-related and total mortality by 25% and 17%, and MI, heart failure, and stroke by 14%, 16%, and 12%, respectively. There are indeed strong associations between glycemia and CVD endpoints, although the magnitude of increase in microvascular events per 1% increase in HbA1c was greater at 37%. All of these outcomes were highly significant, concordant with the results of the intention-to-treat group analysis, and without a specific threshold of benefit. Based on a related economic analysis, the UKPDS showed that persons in the intensive group could expect a mean of 15.08 event-

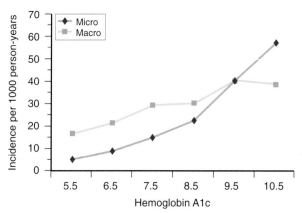

Figure 45–3. Epidemiologic analysis of relationship between hemoglobin A1c and microvascular *(red lozenges)* or macrovascular *(blue squares)* endpoints in the United Kingdom Prospective Diabetes Study (UKPDS). (Redrawn from data in Stratton IM, Adler AI, Neil AW, et al: Association of glycaemia with macrovascular and microvascular complications of type 2 diabetes (UKPDS 35): Prospective observational study. BMJ 321:405-412, 2000.)

free years, and those in the control group would expect 13.94 event-free years, for a net gain of 1.14 such years.[20]

Progression of Diabetes

The UKPDS showed that T2DM is a progressive disease with declining beta cell function, leading over time to a requirement for multiple drugs for optimal control of glycemia.[21] Two additional analyses performed as part of this fascinating and huge trial shed further light on approaches that can be used as glycemia worsens. In a study analyzing combined use of insulin with oral agents, 339 persons whose FBG exceeded 108 mg/dL despite maximal sulfonylurea treatment (53% of sulfonylurea-treated persons by 6 years) were given the long-acting insulin Ultralente administered once daily before the evening meal. Regular insulin was added before meals if preprandial home blood glucose levels remained higher than 126 mg/dL. This approach optimized glycemic control: 47% of those receiving sulfonylurea plus insulin (but 35% of those randomized to insulin alone) attained HbA1c lower than 7% at 6 years, despite somewhat lower total insulin doses (0.24 U/kg body weight versus 0.3 U/kg body weight per day). Major hypoglycemia, however, occurred in 1.6% of patients per year with sulfonylurea plus insulin; hypoglycemia was seen in 3.2% of patients per year with insulin treatment alone.[22]

Another interesting observation in the UKPDS was that of the frequency and associations of islet cell autoimmunity among subjects presenting with clinical evidence of T2DM. Either islet cell antibodies or glutamic acid decarboxylase antibodies were present at baseline in 35% of those age 25 to 34 years, 16% of those age 35 to 44 years, 11% of those

age 45 to 54 years, and 9% of those age 55 to 65 years. Among 1538 patients not assigned insulin, 94% with islet cell antibodies and 84% with positive glutamic acid decarboxylase antibodies required insulin therapy by 6 years, compared with 14% of those without the antibodies. This observation suggests that an appreciable number of persons initially thought to have T2DM actually have features of T1DM, with clinical implication for therapeutic management.[23]

University Group Diabetes Program

The University Group Diabetes Program (UGDP) was initiated in 1959, and patients were recruited from 1961 to 1966. In this study, 1027 patients were treated with placebo, a constant insulin dose, a variable insulin dose, phenformin, or tolbutamide. The 9-year follow-up study showed that despite leading to better glycemic control, insulin failed to improve mortality over that seen with placebo.[24]

Fasting plasma glucose levels were maintained at 121 mg/dL in the variable-dose insulin group; these levels were 30 to 40 mg/dL lower than in the placebo or fixed insulin treatment group. No significant differences were found, however, in the final prevalence or the cumulative incidence of total deaths, CVD deaths, or MI among the three treatment groups, even when outcomes were adjusted for baseline cardiovascular risk factors. There was a suggestion only from post hoc analysis that patients in both insulin treatment groups with good glucose control had fewer cardiovascular events than did those with fair or poor control.

Administration of the sulfonylurea tolbutamide was, however, found to increase CVD mortality with a relative risk more than 2.5 times that seen in the insulin or placebo groups. The tolbutamide arm of the study was discontinued, with the authors stating "the findings suggest that Tolbutamide and diet may be less effective than diet alone or than diet and insulin at least in so far as cardiovascular mortality is concerned."[25] Subsequently the biguanide phenformin was also found to be associated with increased CVD mortality and its use was also discontinued, leading to withdrawal of this agent from use in the United States.[26]

The UGDP has been subject to intense scrutiny and controversy. A lawsuit culminated in a determination by the US Supreme Court that the UGDP raw data should not be released to scientists who believed that its analysis was biased and wanted to study the raw data themselves. A detailed audit conducted by the Biometrics Society concluded that the UGDP results were fairly analyzed and reported, and the court accepted this conclusion.[27] Those who argue against the UGDP conclusions believe that it was flawed by confounding factors that included inadequate power, insufficient separation of glycemic levels, ignorance of smoking history, and

---

Box 45-1. Statement Mandated by the Food and Drug Administration for Sulfonylurea Package Inserts

SPECIAL WARNING ON INCREASED RISK OF CARDIOVASCULAR MORTALITY

The administration of oral hypoglycemic drugs has been reported to be associated with increased cardiovascular mortality as compared to treatment with diet alone or diet plus insulin. This warning is based on the study conducted by the University Group Diabetes Program (UGDP), a long-term prospective clinical trial designed to evaluate the effectiveness of glucose-lowering drugs in preventing or delaying vascular complications in patients with T2DM. The study involved 823 patients who were randomly assigned to one of four treatment groups (Diabetes, 19, SUPP. 2: 747-830, 1970). UGDP reported that patients treated for 5 to 8 years with diet plus a fixed dose of tolbutamide (1.5 grams per day) had a rate of cardiovascular mortality approximately 2½ times that of patients treated with diet alone. A significant increase in total mortality was not observed, but the use of tolbutamide was discontinued based on the increase in cardiovascular mortality, thus limiting the opportunity for the study to show an increase in overall mortality. Despite controversy regarding the interpretation of these results, the findings of the UGDP study provide an adequate basis for this warning. The patient should be informed of the potential risks and advantages of [name of sulfonylurea] and of alternative modes of therapy. Although only one drug in the sulfonylurea class (tolbutamide) was included in this study, it is prudent from a safety standpoint to consider that this warning may also apply to other oral hypoglycemic drugs in this class, in view of their close similarities in mode of action and chemical structure.

---

variation in distribution of complications among study centers.[28] The most recent statistical reanalysis of the study concludes, however, that the intervention groups were adequately balanced for measured risk factors, and that those taking tolbutamide indeed had increased CVD mortality.[29]

The strongest argument against the UGDP is the UKPDS finding that subjects randomized to sulfonylureas did not show an increase in adverse outcome over that seen with insulin treatment, and they showed lower rates of adverse events than seen in the conventionally treated group. Indeed the UGDP controversy was one of the important motivations that led the UKPDS to be organized. The study should not, however, be forgotten. Indeed, based on the UGDP results, the package insert for all sulfonylureas sold in the United States contains a warning mandated by the Food and Drug Administration (Box 45-1).

A biological mechanism for the adverse CVD findings with tolbutamide may be the effect of sulfonylureas on cardiac adenosine triphosphate (ATP)-sensitive potassium channels (K_{ATP}), potentially blocking the endogenous cardioprotective ischemic preconditioning process.[30] This hypothesis has led some to recommend that these agents be

discontinued prior to elective bypass surgery or angioplasty or when patients present with coronary ischemia.[31]

Diabetes Insulin–Glucose in Acute Myocardial Infarction Study

Recognizing that diabetes mellitus is common among patients with acute MI, that the condition is associated with poor short-term and long-term prognosis, and that poor metabolic control is common among diabetic patients with MI, the Diabetes Insulin–Glucose in Acute Myocardial Infarction (DIGAMI) Study[32,33] was conducted. Subjects were 306 patients with MI and blood glucose levels higher than 198 mg/dL (or higher than 234 mg/dL for those not known to have diabetes). The subjects were randomized to intravenously administered insulin and glucose, and 314 comparable patients were randomized to a control group without intensive glycemic treatment.

Patients were stratified based on prior MI and prior insulin treatment (those with both had a 41% 1-year mortality rate versus 13% for those with neither). Age, sex, history of prior MI, congestive heart failure, and cigarette use were similar in both groups. In the study population, 40% had had a prior MI, 50% had prior angina, 20% had heart failure, 50% had hypertension, and 20% had cigarette use. Mean HbA1c at randomization was 8%. The initial blood glucose was 283 mg/dL, decreasing at 24 hours to a greater degree in the insulin group. HbA1c reduction was greater in the infusion group than in the control group: At 3 months HbA1c was reduced in the infusion group by 1.1 percentage points, and in the control group it was reduced 0.4 percentage points. At 12 months the reductions were 0.9 points versus 0.4 points. At discharge, 90% of those randomized to the infusion group received insulin, and at 1 year 72% continued with this. In the control group, 44% were discharged on insulin, with some increase at 1 year, perhaps reducing the effect of the intervention.

Almost half of the patients had thrombolysis, and most were treated with aspirin, β-adrenergic blocking agents, and ACE inhibitors. At 1-year follow-up, mortality was 19% in the intervention group and 26% in the control subjects. Mortality at 3.4 years was 33% for the intervention group versus 44% for control subjects, an absolute decrease in mortality of 11% and a relative decrease of 28%. The most common cause of death was CHF in the control group, with no effect of the intervention on nonfatal reinfarction. Multivariate analysis of 1-year mortality revealed that administration of insulin, treatment with β-adrenergic blocking agents, and thrombolytic therapy all contributed to an improved outcome.[34]

Interestingly, subgroup analysis showed the infusion treatment had particular benefit in patients younger than age 65 years who had no prior insulin treatment and no history of MI. Improvements were seen in 81% of this group versus 15% of controls with similar initial characteristics receiving insulin treatment at discharge; the frequencies of insulin treatment were 66% in the treatment group versus 24% in control subjects at 1 year. Glycemic improvement was greater in this subset than in the overall group, with HbA1c decreasing 1.3 percentage points at 3 months and at 12 months in those assigned insulin treatment versus 0.6 points and 0.5 points, respectively, in the controls. This group's mortality rate was lowered to 5% (versus 12% in the control group) at 1 year, and at 3.4 years absolute mortality was decreased by 15%. There has therefore been speculation that some of the benefit found in the study might, in fact, be due to withdrawal of sulfonylureas in patients at risk of recurrent myocardial ischemia,[35] perhaps supporting the UGDP findings with tolbutamide.

In DIGAMI 1, a glucose–insulin infusion was started at the time of acute myocardial infarction. Glucose control improved and long-term mortality decreased 30% to 50% for persons not previously receiving insulin, with decreased mortality of subsequent myocardial infarction. The control group with T2DM had 35% to 40% overall mortality after several years. HbA1c decreased 0.9 percentage points in the intervention group and 1.5 points among patients not previously receiving insulin.

A follow-up DIGAMI study was presented in September 2004 at the European Association for the Study of Diabetes meeting in Munich. The follow-up study also compared glucose–insulin infusion and insulin treatment with conventional treatment. Although the goal of the glucose–insulin infusion was to decrease the blood glucose to 126 mg/dL from the baseline level of 230 mg/dL, the infusion group only achieved a level of 164 mg/dL, a significant but not clinically great difference from the 24-hour glucose level of 180 mg/dL in the conventional treatment group. Although at least three insulin doses daily were recommended for maintenance treatment, only 45% of intensively treated participants received this, and 15% in the conventional treatment groups received 3 or more insulin doses daily.

Extensive conventional treatment was used, including revascularization for 40%, thrombolytics for 35%, heparin for 75%, β-blockers for more than 80%, aspirin for 90%, ACE inhibitors for 65%, and lipid treatment for 60% of patients in all groups. HbA1c showed a small difference at 3 months but no difference subsequently, and FBG levels during follow-up were similar in all the groups. However, body weight increased 4.7 kg with intensive insulin treatment but 0.4 kg with conventional treatment.

There was no mortality benefit, but it is difficult to argue that a study that failed to show benefit of glycemic control is meaningful if, in fact, the degree of improvement in glycemic control was minimal.

It would be unfortunate—and premature—to conclude from this recent report that efforts to aggressively treat diabetes in persons with acute myocardial infarction are unnecessary. The baseline FBG was an independent predictor of mortality, with the rate increasing 20% per 54 mg/dL glucose increment and 10% per 1 percentage point higher HbA1c. Highly significant effects were seen for β-blockers, which were associated with 35% lower mortality, and for statins, with 44% lower mortality.

HYPERTENSION AND BLOOD PRESSURE–RELATED TRIALS

Hypertension Optimal Treatment Study

The Hypertension Optimal Treatment (HOT) study randomized 18,790 patients with diastolic BP between 100 mm Hg and 115 mm Hg, of whom 1501 had diabetes, to goal diastolic BPs of 90, 85, and 80 mm Hg. Achieved mean diastolic pressures in the three groups were 85.2, 83.2, and 81.1 mm Hg, respectively. The calcium channel blocker (CCB) felodipine was the initial therapeutic choice and was administered at the end of the study in 77%, 78%, and 79% of patients in the three groups. β-Blockers were given to 25%, 28%, and 32%, angiotensin converting enzyme (ACE) inhibitors to 35%, 42%, and 45%, and diuretics to 19%, 22%, and 24%, respectively.

Despite the small degree of BP separation, the risk of a major CVD event was reduced with greater intensiveness of treatment. This risk reduction was particularly seen among the subgroup with diabetes. The diabetic subjects had 24.4, 18.6, and 11.9 major CVD events, respectively, per 1000 patient-years, and CVD mortality was 11.1, 11.1, and 3.7, respectively, per 1000 patient-years.[36]

United Kingdom Prospective Diabetes Study

In the hypertension substudy of the United Kingdom Prospective Diabetes Study, 1148 persons with diabetes and hypertension were randomized to "tight" or "less tight" BP control. The tight-control group had a 9-year mean level of 144/82 mm Hg, and the less-tight group had a mean level of 154/87 mm Hg.

Effects on Endpoints
In subjects randomized to the lower BP level, the heart failure endpoint was decreased 56%, the stroke endpoint was decreased 44%, diabetes-related death was decreased 37%, and overall diabetes-related endpoints were decreased 24%. It is fascinating that microvascular endpoints such as need for laser photocoagulation were reduced 37%, and two-step retinopathy progression decreased from 36.7% to 27.5% at 4.5 years and from 51.3% to 34% at 7.5 years.[37]

Epidemiologic analysis of the relationship between systolic BP and coronary artery disease (CAD) events in the overall UKPDS population of patients with diabetes showed that compared to subjects with systolic BP lower than 125 mm Hg, subjects whose systolic BP was 125 to 142 mm Hg had a 1.52-fold increase in risk of CAD events, and those with systolic BP levels higher than 142 had a 1.82-fold increase. Each 10 mm Hg decrease in BP was associated with a reduction in total diabetes endpoint development by 12%, in diabetes-related mortality by 15%, in total mortality by 11%, in MI by 11%, in stroke by 17%, in microalbuminuria by 13%, and in CHF by 15%. There was no evidence of a J-shaped curve or threshold effect.[38]

Hypertension and Hyperglycemia
The UKPDS showed evidence of interaction between BP and glycemic treatments. In the group with the highest HbA1c, BP had greater deleterious effects, so that subjects who had HbA1c higher than 8% and systolic BP higher than 170 had a ten-fold increase in total endpoints. In contrast, subjects who had systolic BP lower than 140 had little risk of MI regardless of HbA1c, underscoring the need for careful treatment of both factors.

To prevent 1 retinal or renal endpoint in the UKPDS, 14 patients needed to be treated for 10 years with tight control of hypertension, compared with 36 patients treated with tight glycemic control. The number needed to treat (NNT) to prevent any diabetes endpoint was 6 with tight control of hypertension versus 20 with tight control of hyperglycemia. The authors of the UKPDS suggested that target organ damage in diabetes may be more strongly dependent on hypertension than on hyperglycemia.

The glycemia study was not designed to treat to a glycemic goal, but rather to analyze two different treatment strategies, immediate versus delayed. Both sulfonylureas and insulin showed similar decreases in total and microvascular events and in MI.

In the BP substudy, in contrast, a treat-to-target approach was taken, with 5 mm Hg and 10 mm Hg separations in diastolic and systolic BPs. At least three drugs were required in 29% of patients. By trial design, the majority of patients in the glycemic intervention only received one therapeutic agent for diabetes, with consequent gradual loss of glycemic control, suggesting that the intensiveness of care of hypertension was greater than that of diabetes.[39]

Perhaps the correct approach to comparing treatment for hyperglycemia and hypertension in the UKPDS, then, is to realize that as both HbA1c and BP increase, adverse outcomes increase in an addi-

tive fashion. Illustrating this, diabetes mortality in the intensive BP treatment group was 8 per 1000 patient-years in the insulin group and 11 per 1000 patient-years in the glycemic control group. Diabetes mortality in the less-tight BP treatment group was 12 per 1000 patient-years in the insulin group and 19 per 1000 patient-years in the glycemic control group.

In the hypertension substudy, the intensively treated subset received either atenolol or captopril as primary treatment. Cumulative diabetes-related endpoints and specific outcomes including total and fatal MI, heart failure, angina, stroke, and retinopathy were similar in the two intensive treatment groups. However, 35% of subjects treated with atenolol and 22% of subjects treated with captopril discontinued the initial antihypertensive treatment. Claudication, bronchospasm, and erectile dysfunction occurred more commonly with atenolol. There were also metabolic differences: Mean HbA1c was 7.5% in the atenolol group but 7% in the captopril group during the first 4 years of follow-up, although 25% more persons who were treated with atenolol received additional glucose-lowering treatment. Weight gain was significantly greater with atenolol at 3.4 kg versus 1.6 kg with captopril.[40]

An epidemiologic analysis of the relationship between BP and endpoints in the UKPDS showed a linear increase in events with increasing BP. Total diabetes-related event rates increased from 36 to 76 per 1000 patient-years comparing systolic BP lower than 120 versus higher than 160. Diabetes-related mortalities were 10 and 30 per 1000 patient-years for the respective groups.[41]

Heart Outcomes Prevention Evaluation

The Heart Outcomes Prevention Evaluation (HOPE) study randomized 9297 patients from 267 sites in 19 countries to ramipril 10 mg daily or to placebo.[41] All subjects had increased risk of CVD, and 3658 of them had diabetes. The study was not actually designed to lower BP; rather, it addressed the question of whether ACE inhibitors have direct protective effects in reducing the development of atherosclerosis.

Among those without diabetes at baseline, diabetes developed in 3.6% of those randomized to ramipril versus 5.4% of those in the placebo group, and there was a 44% decrease in the likelihood of requiring glucose-lowering therapy.[42] In those with diabetes at the outset, administration of ramipril was associated with a 20% decrease in CVD events, 24% decrease in all-cause mortality, 37% decrease in CVD mortality, and 33% decrease in stroke. Development of macroalbuminuria decreased 22%.[42]

Five-year event rates in subjects with diabetes ranged from 11% in those without CVD at baseline to 26.5% in those with CVD, so that the number of diabetic patients who must be treated for 5 years to prevent one adverse event is approximately 15 with CVD and 40 without, making this a highly effective form of treatment. Furthermore, outcome appeared to progressively improve with longer duration of treatment.

There was a fall in BP of 1 to 2 mm Hg in the ramipril group. Although the decrease in BP potentially contributed to the benefit seen, it did not in itself appear sufficient to explain the reported effect, suggesting that there was indeed specific benefit of angiotensin-directed treatment.

Losartan Intervention for Endpoint Reduction in Hypertension

Losartan was shown to decrease CVD mortality by 13% when compared to atenolol in the Losartan Intervention For Endpoint Reduction in Hypertension (LIFE) study. Subjects were 9193 patients with 44,119 patient-years of follow-up; all had essential hypertension (baseline BP 174/98 mm Hg) and signs of left ventricular hypertrophy (LVH) on electrocardiogram.[43] Patients were assigned to treatment with losartan or atenolol 50 mg daily. Hydrochlorothiazide 12.5 mg daily was added, then the losartan or atenolol was increased to 100 mg, and finally the dose of hydrochlorothiazide was increased to 25 mg daily to reach a target BP of less than 140/90 mm Hg.

BP decreased to 144/81 mm Hg in the losartan group and 145/81 mm Hg in the atenolol group. Heart rate decreased by 2 beats per minute (BPM) in the losartan group and 8 BPM in the atenolol groups. In the losartan group, 4019 subjects did not have diabetes at baseline, and new-onset diabetes developed in 241 (6%). In the atenolol group, 3979 persons did not have diabetes at the outset, and new-onset diabetes was seen in 319 (8%). Other findings reported significantly less frequently with losartan were bradycardia, cold extremities, sexual dysfunction, albuminuria, fatigue, dyspnea, peripheral edema, and pneumonia, although higher rates of development of hypotension and back pain were reported.

The 1195-patient subgroup with diabetes displayed greater benefit than those without diabetes, including 40% lower CVD mortality for the losartan group versus 10% for the atenolol group and 11% total mortality with losartan versus 17% with atenolol. In the losartan group, 5% were hospitalized for CHF versus 9% in the atenolol group. The losartan group had a greater reduction in LVH, although both groups had similar levels of angina and requirements for revascularization. A difference particularly marked among study participants with diabetes was the rate of developing higher than 300 mg albuminuria per 1 g urinary creatinine: In the losartan group the rate was 7% versus 13% in the atenolol group.[44]

The two agents differed in effect on sudden death among persons with diabetes: Death occurred in 14 of 586 persons (2.4%) treated with losartan but in 30 of 609 (4.9%) treated with atenolol. Sudden death rates were not different with losartan versus atenolol among persons without diabetes. Among persons with diabetes and atrial fibrillation, despite the lesser decrease in heart rate, 5 of 86 receiving losartan but 14 of 105 treated with atenolol had sudden death,[45] suggesting a particularly high risk group for which the usual approach with β-blockers might not offer optimal protection.

Benefit of losartan in reducing sudden death was seen following a 12-month lag, suggesting that the antiarrhythmic effect might be due to structural change. Such structural change is perhaps caused by regression of left ventricular hypertrophy and atrial fibrosis, which could lessen the abnormalities in QT dispersion and heart rate variability that contribute to development of repolarization abnormalities. Angiotensin II facilitates sympathetic tone, suggesting another potential beneficial effect of ACE inhibitors and ARBs.

Reduction of Endpoints in NIDDM with the Angiotensin II Antagonist Losartan

The Reduction of Endpoints in NIDDM with the Angiotensin II Antagonist Losartan (RENAAL) trial showed significant renal benefits with administration of losartan 50 to 100 mg daily versus placebo to 1513 patients with T2DM and nephropathy. Nephropathy was defined as more than 300 mg albuminuria per 1 g creatinine or more than 500 mg/day proteinuria, or both, plus serum creatinine 1.3 to 3.0 mg/dL. Blood pressure decreased from 153/82 mm Hg at baseline to 146/78 mm Hg with losartan versus 150/80 mm Hg with placebo at 1 year. At later points, the levels were similar: 144/77 mm Hg at 2 years and 141/74 mm Hg at study end.

Over a mean period of 3.4 years, the composite endpoint of doubling of serum creatinine, development of end stage renal disease (ESDR), or death, occurred 16% less often with losartan; the decrease was 15% after adjusting for the lower BP with this agent. Proteinuria decreased approximately 40% with losartan but showed little change in the placebo group. Eight percent of patients in the losartan group had doubling of serum creatinine versus 10% who took placebo, and ESRD developed in 7% of treated patients versus 9% of placebo patients. Heart failure occurred 32% less often with losartan; the trend began immediately following institution of treatment, with an initial hospitalization for heart failure reported in 11.9% of losartan-treated subjects versus 16.7% of placebo-treated subjects.

One case of ESRD was prevented for every 16 patients treated, and losartan decreased the number of days with ESRD by 32%, at a savings of $5300 per patient. Additional antihypertensive treatment—CCB, 75 to 300 mg daily— was given to 87% to 90% of patients, suggesting that these agents apparently did not interfere with the benefits of losartan.[46]

Irbesartan Diabetic Nephropathy Trial

The related Irbesartan Diabetic Nephropathy Trial (IDNT) randomized 1715 patients to irbesartan, amlodipine, or placebo. Subjects had T2DM, proteinuria (greater than 900 mg/day), and creatinine between 1.0 and 3.0 (women) or between 1.2 and 3.0 (men). The target BP was 135/85 mm Hg, and BP decrease was from 159/87 mm Hg at baseline to 140-144/77-80 mm Hg in the three treatment groups. Time to doubling of serum creatinine was 33% longer with irbesartan. Patients assigned to receive amlodipine had a higher rate of CHF than either the placebo or irbesartan group, although those receiving this agent had a 41% lower nonfatal MI rate than that among the patients assigned to receive placebo, suggesting some benefit with this agent as well.

Adjustment for BP did not change the significant benefits of irbesartan on renal end points. However, each 1 mm Hg lowering of BP was associated with a 3% decrease in the rate of progression to renal end points.[47] There is a particular association between diabetic nephropathy and heart failure: 20% of the 1715 diabetic persons with moderate renal insufficiency developed heart failure over a $2\frac{1}{2}$ year period,[48] and the CHF hospitalization rate was 23% lower with irbesartan.

Antihypertensive and Lipid-Lowering Treatment to Prevent Heart Attack Trial

The largest investigation to date of treatment of hypertension is the Antihypertensive and Lipid-Lowering Treatment to Prevent Heart Attack Trial (ALLHAT). The study enrolled 42,418 hypertensive persons, 36% with diabetes. Subjects were randomized to regimens based on chlorthalidone, amlodipine, or lisinopril.[49] BP decreased from 146/84 mm Hg to 137/79 mm Hg with chlorthalidone, 138/79 mm Hg with amlodipine, and 140/80 mm Hg with lisinopril at 1 year and to 134/75 mm Hg with chlorthalidone, 135/75 mm Hg with amlodipine, and 136/75 mm Hg with lisinopril at 5 years; the chlorthalidone group had significantly lower systolic levels.

Cumulative event rates for the primary outcome (fatal CHD or nonfatal MI) were similar in all groups, both in the overall study and among the

diabetic subset. Among the subset of patients with diabetes, those treated with chlorthalidone versus amlodipine showed no difference in total mortality, total CHD, total CVD, or stroke, although the development of heart failure was 42% lower with chlorthalidone. Comparing chlorthalidone versus lisinopril in the diabetic subset, there was no difference in total mortality, total CHD, or stroke, but there was an 8% greater total CVD and 22% greater heart failure rate with lisinopril.

Analysis correcting for the greater degree of BP lowering with chlorthalidone has not been reported. A further difficulty in the interpretation of the study is the frequent need for multiple BP-lowering treatment among persons with hypertension. Diuretics were excluded from their typical position as second agents after lisinopril and after amlodipine. Patients in the lisinopril group were not allowed to have CCBs, and those randomized to amlodipine were not allowed to have ACE inhibitors. These restrictions could have compromised the antihypertensive benefit of the nondiuretic-based treatment regimens. The particular increase in heart failure is thus not surprising in view of the well-known role of diuretics in prevention of heart failure symptoms. A further caveat in the interpretation of the study is that at 5 years 20% of patients randomized to chlorthalidone were not taking a diuretic, 20% of those randomized to amlodipine were not taking a CCB, and 27% of those randomized to lisinopril were not taking an ACE inhibitor.

Chlorthalidone was associated with higher cholesterol and glucose and lower potassium levels than the other two agents. Analysis of FBG showed that 11.6% of initially nondiabetic patients receiving chlorthalidone, but 8.1% of those receiving lisinopril, developed diabetes at 4 years. Preliminary reports suggest that this adverse consequence was particularly prominent among persons without diabetes but with impaired fasting glucose, who made up 9% of the nondiabetic study population[50] and showed particularly high risk of development of diabetes in the diuretic group.

Diabetes-Preventive Effects of Angiotensin Antagonist Therapy

In view of the evidence of protection against diabetes development in the HOPE, LIFE, and ALLHAT studies, it has been of interest to determine whether the phenomenon has been generally observed in studies of ACE-inhibitor and ARB treatment in persons with hypertension or CVD, or both, who are at relatively high risk of developing diabetes. This question can be addressed using the statistical method of meta-analysis.[51] Across nine studies comparing angiotensin-directed treatment with a variety of other treatments of persons without diabetes at baseline, the likelihood of development

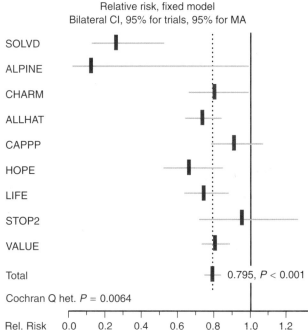

Figure 45–4. Relative risk of development of diabetes reduction among persons receiving ARB or ACEI therapy in comparison to control. ALLHAT, Antihypertensive and Lipid-Lowering Treatment to Prevent Heart Attack Trial; ALPINE, Antihypertensive Treatment and Lipid Profile in a North of Sweden Efficacy Evaluation; CAPPP, Captopril Prevention Project; CHARM, Candesartan in Heart failure: Assessment of Reduction in Mortality and morbidity; CI, confidence interval; Cochran Q het., Cochran's Q test for heterogeneity between trials; HOPE, Heart Outcomes Prevention Evaluation; LIFE, Losartan Intervention For Endpoint reduction in hypertension; MA, meta-analysis; SOLVD, Studies Of Left Ventricular Dysfunction; STOP2, Swedish Trial in Old Patients with Hypertension 2; VALUE, Valsartan Antihypertensive Longterm Use Evaluation. (Data from references 43, 45, 51, 62-67.)

of diabetes is reduced by 20% (Fig. 45–4). This figure is remarkably consistent in most studies, suggesting this to be an important effect. Two randomized, controlled studies in progress, the Diabetes Reduction Approaches with Ramipril and Rosiglitazone Medications (DREAM) and Nateglinide and Valsartan in Impaired Glucose Tolerance Outcomes Research (NAVIGATOR) trials, will further assess the degree of protection conferred by an ACE inhibitor or ARB on persons at risk for developing diabetes.

LIPID TRIALS

A number of studies have addressed the effects of dyslipidemia in persons with diabetes. It is intriguing to note that although there is currently a therapeutic emphasis on the administration of HMG-CoA reductase inhibitors (statins) for CVD

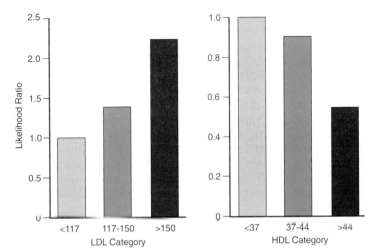

Figure 45–5. Lipid levels for persons with diabetes in the United Kingdom Prospective Diabetes Study (UKPDS). (Redrawn from data in Turner RC, Millns H, Neil HA, et al: Risk factors for coronary artery disease in non–insulin dependent diabetes mellitus: United Kingdom Prospective Diabetes Study (UKPDS: 23). BMJ 316:823-828, 1998.)

endpoint reduction, virtually across the board there is a substantial literature suggesting similar benefit among persons with diabetes treated with peroxisome proliferator-activated receptor α (PPARα) agonists (fibrates).

Epidemiology of Dyslipidemia among Persons with Diabetes

In the UKPDS, LDL cholesterol levels in persons with diabetes were similar to those seen in a non-diabetic population among men, whereas levels were slightly elevated among women.[52] Although no lipid-related intervention was performed, analysis of the effects of various risk factors showed that for diabetic subjects, LDL cholesterol, HDL cholesterol, HbA1c, systolic BP, cigarette use, age, and gender were significant risk factors for CVD. LDL and HDL cholesterol levels contributed more to CVD risk than high HbA1c and high BP did (Fig. 45–5).[53]

In the Multiple Risk Factor Intervention Trial (MRFIT), the adverse effect of hypercholesterolemia among 5163 subjects with diabetes versus 342,815 subjects without diabetes was analyzed over 12 years of follow-up. The analysis suggests that although risk increases with increasing cholesterol in both groups, at any cholesterol level the likelihood of developing CVD is approximately threefold greater for persons with diabetes. The absolute risk of CVD increases more steeply, with worsening risk factor levels among diabetic persons than persons without diabetes, supporting the importance of lipid treatment in this population (Fig. 45–6).[54]

Veterans Affairs HDL Cholesterol Intervention Trial

The Veterans' Affairs HDL Intervention Trial (HIT)[55] studied a group of 2531 men, 25% of whom had

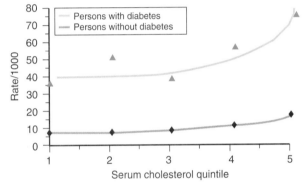

Figure 45–6. Relationship between rate of development of diabetes and quintile of total cholesterol level among persons with and without diabetes in the Multiple Risk Factor Intervention Trial. (Redrawn from data in Stamler J, Vaccaro O, Neaton JD, Wentworth D: Diabetes, other risk factors, and 12-yr cardiovascular mortality for men screened in the Multiple Risk Factor Intervention Trial. Diabetes Care 16:434-444, 1993.)

diabetes. The study addressed the treatment of lipids. Subjects had low HDL cholesterol averaging 32 mg/dL, elevated triglyceride levels averaging 161 mg/dL, and LDL cholesterol levels averaging 111 mg/dL. Gemfibrozil was compared with placebo, and there was a 5-year follow-up.

There was a 22% decrease in cardiac mortality and nonfatal MI with the intervention. Patients with and without diabetes had identical relative CVD rate reduction, but the 5-year absolute event rate was twice as great among persons with diabetes, and they had a correspondingly doubled absolute reduction in CVD events. The degree of benefit was greatest for those who achieved HDL cholesterol higher than 35 mg/dL and triglycerides lower than 160 mg/dL. The triglyceride level was an independent risk factor for the subgroup with the lowest HDL levels. Decreased stroke, transient ischemic attack, and carotid endarterectomy, as well as

surgery for peripheral arterial insufficiency and hospitalization for CHF, were also seen, although there was no change in the frequency of development of angina.

Multivariate analysis adjusted for age, hypertension, diabetes, and BMI showed that for each 5 mg/dL increase in HDL there was an 11% decrease in risk.[55a] Separately analyzing the CHD event rate by HDL quintile achieved on therapy showed that at a given level of HDL, patients who were receiving gemfibrozil had fewer events than those who were receiving placebo, suggesting that the agent might have direct benefits (i.e., not mediated by HDL cholesterol).

When the study participants were reanalyzed for evidence of insulin resistance, 53% had waist measurement larger than 100 cm, 57% had hypertension, and mean fasting plasma glucose was 115 mg/dL. Average fasting insulin was 42 μU/mL, and 32% of participants had insulin levels above the 90th percentile of the Framingham study; this group had the highest CVD event rate. In addition to the 25% of participants with a history of diabetes, another 6% of participants had fasting glucose higher than 126 mg/dL, and 16% had average glucose 103 mg/dL but insulin levels in a range comparable to that of the diabetic group, so that in total approximately 50% had diabetes or hyperinsulinemia.

When the expanded diabetes group was analyzed, risk reduction was 28%, and the reduction of relative risk was similar in diabetic subjects with and without hyperinsulinemia and in the nondiabetic group with hyperinsulinemia. For a given level of hyperglycemia, those with hyperinsulinemia had a higher 5-year event rate. Although there was no significant decrease in mortality in the overall study population, the subgroup with either diabetes (based on history or on fasting glucose) or hyperinsulinemia did show a significant reduction in all-cause mortality.

Diabetes Atherosclerosis Intervention Study

The Diabetes Atherosclerosis Intervention Study (DAIS) involved 418 patients with diabetes treated with fenofibrate or placebo. Triglyceride levels fell 40% and 25% in the highest and middle tertiles, respectively (27% overall, versus 2% increase with placebo). HDL increased 8% and 10% in the lowest and middle tertiles (7% overall, compared with a 1% increase with placebo). LDL cholesterol fell 6% in the treated group and increased 2% with placebo, and apolipoprotein B fell 11% in the treated group and increased 1% with placebo, suggesting a decrease in the LDL particle number and implying a change from the atherogenic small, dense LDL phenotype to larger, more buoyant, and less atherogenic particles. The study showed a 40%

reduction in angiographic progression of coronary disease.[56]

Scandinavian Simvastatin Survival Study

A dramatic decrease in major CVD events was reported in the subgroup of 202 patients with diabetes who had a prior history of MI or other CVD treated in the statin versus placebo Scandinavian Simvastatin Survival Study (4S).[57] CVD events were decreased by 55% in diabetic subjects who were treated with simvastatin; CVD events decreased by 32% in nondiabetic subjects who were treated with simvastatin. CHD events decreased by 43% versus 29%, respectively, in these groups. These results were achieved even though patients with triglycerides higher than 350 mg/dL or with poor diabetic control were excluded from the study.

Similar benefit was found for 281 patients with diabetes diagnosed on the basis of FBG higher than 126 mg/dL and for 678 subjects who had impaired FBG levels from 110 to 125 mg/dL.[58] This was a population with baseline LDL cholesterol averaging 180 mg/dL, and so these subjects should not be considered representative of the typical diabetic patient group with considerably lower LDL cholesterol levels.

Heart Protection Study

The Heart Protection Study (HPS) showed benefit of simvastatin 40 mg daily in persons with diabetes, both at LDL cholesterol levels currently considered to require treatment and at levels less than 100 mg/dL.[59] This was a large trial of 20,536 persons who had evidence of CVD or hypertension, or both. The simvastatin-treated group included 2978 subjects and the control group 2985 subjects who also had diabetes. Of these, 601 treatment-group subjects and 748 control-group subjects had a CVD event. The reduction in relative risk was 20% and the reduction in absolute risk was 5% for diabetic subjects with a CVD event who were in the treatment group.

COMBINATION TREATMENT

One trial to date was specifically designed to address the combination of a number of therapeutic modalities in persons with T2DM.

Steno Diabetes Center Study

Given the benefits of glucose-lowering treatment, BP-lowering treatment, and lipid treatment, it

appears that persons with diabetes should have aggressive multifactorial intervention to address all of these abnormalities. In the small but important Steno Diabetes Center study, 160 patients aged 40 to 65 years who had T2DM and microalbuminuria (urinary albumin between 30 and 300 mg in at least four of six 24-hour urine collections) were randomized to intensive treatment by a physician–nurse–dietician team or to standard treatment by general practitioners.[60,61] Treatment goals were HbA1c 6.5% for the intensive group versus 7.5% for the standard group, total cholesterol 193 mg/dL versus 250 mg/dL, HDL higher than 42 mg/dL versus 35 mg/dL, triglyceride 151 mg/dL versus 195 mg/dL, and BP 140/85 versus 160/95.

Treatment

The intensive group was instructed in a diet with 30% fat and high vegetable intake and encouraged to exercise at least 30 minutes three times weekly. They were given smoking-cessation counseling, and nicotine replacement was provided for patients and spouses. Only modest lifestyle improvement was obtained despite the more aggressive team approach.

The diabetes treatment regimen started with sulfonylureas for nonobese patients and metformin for obese patients. Both treatments were subsequently combined, and NPH insulin was added once daily to one oral agent. Regimens were changed to a multiple-dose insulin treatment without oral agents when patients required more than 80 units of insulin daily. This approach might not be currently considered optimal for glycemic control in T2DM, and indeed only modest glycemic control was obtained.

Statins or fibrates were given for dyslipidemia. ACE inhibitors were given to all patients, and subsequent BP treatment was with thiazides, then CCBs, and then β-blockers. Aspirin was given to all patients who had evidence of CVD, and all intensive-treatment patients were given vitamin E 100 units and vitamin C 250 mg daily.

Endpoints

Development of macroalbuminuria (urinary albumin excretion greater than 300 mg/day) was the primary endpoint of the first 4-year component of the study. Retinopathy and neuropathy were secondary endpoints.[62]

Results

At 4 years, diabetes treatment in the intensive versus standard groups used diet or oral agents alone in 33 versus 43 patients. ACE inhibitors were given to 69 versus 36 patients and statins were given to 33 versus 2 patients. The fasting glucose was 135 mg/dL in the intensive group versus 180 mg/dL in the standard group, HbA1c was 7.6% versus 9.0%, BP was 136/76 mm Hg versus 144/81 mm Hg, LDL-cholesterol was 112 mg/dL versus 124 mg/dL, triglyceride was 159 mg/dL versus 239 mg/dL, and

urine albumin excretion was 51 mg/day versus 104 mg/day. The intensive treatment group's risk for developing nephropathy, retinopathy, and autonomic neuropathy was reduced by 27%, 45%, and 32%, respectively, and overall they had a 50% reduction in development of complications. Although there was no reduction in the overall CVD event rate at this point, evidence of peripheral arterial insufficiency (based on arm to toe BP gradient) developed in 10 intensively treated versus 26 conventionally treated patients.

After 7.8 years of follow-up, HbA1c was 7.9% in the intensively treated group versus 9% in the conventionally treated group, BP was 131/73 mm Hg versus 146/78 mm Hg, LDL cholesterol was 81 mg/dL versus 128 mg/dL, and mean urine albumin was 26 mg per 24 hours versus 126 mg per 24 hours. The cholesterol goal had been attained by 70% of intensively treated patients versus 20% of conventionally treated patients, and 50% versus 20% attained the systolic BP goal. Adverse effects of the more intensive treatment were not seen. There was no significant increase in hypoglycemia in the intensively treated group and similar weight gain in the two groups.

The intensively treated group had a 53% lower likelihood of developing CVD, with 85 events occurring among 35 patients (44%) of the conventional group but 33 events among 19 patients (24%) of the intensively treated group. There were 17 nonfatal MIs in the conventional group versus 5 in the intensive group, 10 versus 5 coronary artery bypass grafts, 5 versus no coronary angioplasties, 12 versus 6 peripheral vascular surgeries, and 20 versus 3 nonfatal strokes. Microvascular endpoints remained significantly lower: The likelihood of nephropathy was 39%, retinopathy 42%, and autonomic neuropathy 37%. A multivariate analysis suggested that cholesterol treatment was of greatest importance, BP treatment (including use of ACE inhibitors and ARBs) of next importance, and aspirin of third importance in efficacy of preventing endpoints. All three of these treatments appeared to be of greater benefit than the glycemic intervention.

SUMMARY

There is now substantial evidence from randomized, controlled trials that treatment of hyperglycemia, hypertension, and dyslipidemia are crucial elements of care of persons with diabetes. This is, of course, a field with constant ongoing investigation, with studies of thousands of persons expected to give a great deal more information on a multiplicity of approaches to diabetes management over the coming years. The DREAM, NAVIGATOR, Fenofibrate Intervention and Event Lowering in Diabetes (FIELD), Carotid Intima-Media Thickness in Atherosclerosis Using Pioglitazone (CHICAGO), Pioglitazone Effect on Regression

of Intravascular Sonographic Coronary Obstruction Prospective Evaluation (PERISCOPE), Bypass Angioplasty Revascularization Investigation in Type 2 Diabetes (BARI-2D), and Action to Control Cardiovascular Risk in Diabetes (ACCORD) trial results are eagerly awaited.

References

1. Gu K, Cowie CC, Harris MI: Diabetes and decline in heart disease mortality in US adults. JAMA 281:1291-1297, 1999.
2. Wild S, Roglic G, Green A et al: Global prevalence of diabetes: Estimates for the year 2000 and projections for 2030. Diabetes Care 27:1047-1053, 2004.
3. Wang PH, Lau J, Chalmers TC: Meta-analysis of effects of intensive blood-glucose control on late complications of type I diabetes. Lancet 341:1306-1309, 1993.
4. The Diabetes Control and Complications Trial Research Group: The effect of intensive treatment of diabetes on the development and progression of long term complications in insulin-dependent diabetes mellitus. N Engl J Med 329:977-986, 1993.
5. The Diabetes Control and Complications Trial Research Group: The effect of intensive diabetes therapy on the development and progression of neuropathy. Ann Intern Med 122:561-568, 1995.
6. The Diabetes Control and Complications Research Group: The relationship of glycemic exposure (HbA1c) to the risk of development and progression of retinopathy in the Diabetes Control and Complications Trial. Diabetes 44:968-983, 1995.
7. The DCCT Research Group: Lifetime benefits and costs of intensive therapy as practices in the DCCT. JAMA 276:1409-1415, 1996.
8. Steffes MW, Sibley S, Jackson M, Thomas W: β-Cell function and the development of diabetes-related complications in the Diabetes Control and Complications Trial. Diabetes Care 26:832-836, 2003.
9. McCarter RJ, Gomez R, Hempe JM, Chalew SA: Biological variation in HbA1c predicts risk of retinopathy and nephropathy in type 1 diabetes. Diabetes Care 27:1259-1264, 2004.
10. Chase HP, Lockspeiser T, Perry B: The impact of the DCCT and humalog insulin on glycohemoglobin levels and severe hypoglycemia in type 1 diabetes. Diabetes Care 24:430-434, 2001.
11. The Diabetes Control and Complications Trial Research Group: Adverse events and their association with treatment regimens in the Diabetes Control and Complications Trial. Diabetes Care 18:1415-1427, 1995.
12. Purnell JQ, Hokanson JE, Marcovina SM, et al: Effect of excessive weight gain with intensive therapy of type 1 diabetes on lipid levels and blood pressure: Results from the DCCT. Diabetes Control and Complications Trial. JAMA 280:140-146, 1998.
13. The Diabetes Control and Complications Trial/Epidemiology of Diabetes Interventions and Complications Research Group: Retinopathy and nephropathy in patients with type 1 diabetes four years after a trial of intensive therapy. N Engl J Med 342:381-389, 2000.
14. United Kingdom Prospective Diabetes Study (UKPDS) 13: Relative efficacy of randomly allocated diet, sulphonylurea, insulin, or metformin in patients with newly diagnosed non–insulin dependent diabetes followed for three years. BMJ 310:83-88, 1995.
15. UK Prospective Diabetes Study Group: Intensive blood-glucose control with sulphonylureas or insulin compared with conventional treatment and risk of complications in patients with type 2 diabetes (UKPDS 33). Lancet 352:837-853, 1998.
16. Bloomgarden ZT: Glycemic treatment. Control of glycemia. Diabetes Care 27:1227-1234, 2004.
17. UK Prospective Diabetes Study Group: Effect of intensive blood-glucose control with metformin on complications in overweight patients with type 2 diabetes (UKPDS 43). Lancet 352:854-865, 1998.
18. Holman RR, Cull CA, Turner RC: A randomized double-blind trial of acarbose in type 2 diabetes shows improved glycemic control over 3 years. Diabetes Care 22:960-964, 1999.
19. Stratton IM, Adler AI, Neil AW, et al: Association of glycaemia with macrovascular and microvascular complications of type 2 diabetes (UKPDS 35): Prospective observational study. BMJ 321:405-412, 2000.
20. Gray A, Raikou M, McGuire A, et al: Cost effectiveness of an intensive blood glucose control policy in patients with type 2 diabetes: Economic analysis alongside randomised controlled trial (UKPDS 41). BMJ 320:1373-1378, 2000.
21. Turner RC, Cull CA, Frighi V, Holman RR, for the UK Prospective Diabetes Study Group: Glycemic control with diet, sulfonylurea, metformin, or insulin in patients with type 2 diabetes mellitus: Progressive requirement for multiple therapies (UKPDS 49). JAMA 281:2005-2012, 1999.
22. Wright A, Burden ACF, Paisey RB, et al: Sulfonylurea inadequacy: Efficacy of addition of insulin over 6 years in patients with type 2 diabetes in the U.K. Prospective Diabetes Study (UKPDS 57). Diabetes Care 25:330-336, 2002.
23. Turner R, Stratton I, Horton V, et al: UKPDS 25: autoantibodies to islet-cell cytoplasm and glutamic acid decarboxylase for prediction of insulin requirement in type 2 diabetes. Lancet 350:1288-1293, 1997.
24. Knatterud GL, Klimt CR, Levin ME, et al: Effects of hypoglycemic agents on vascular complications in patients with adult-onset diabetes. VII. Mortality and selected nonfatal events with insulin treatment. JAMA 240:37-42, 1978.
25. The University Group Diabetes Program: A study of the effects of hypoglycemic agents on vascular complications in patients with adult-onset diabetes. Diabetes 19(suppl 2):747-839, 1970.
26. The University Group Diabetes Program: A study of the effects of hypoglycemic agents on vascular complications in patients with adult-onset diabetes. V. Evaluation of pheniformin therapy. Diabetes 24 Suppl 1:65-184, 1975.
27. Audit confirms conclusions of UGDP study on oral diabetes drugs. FDA Drug Bull 8:34-36, 1978-1979.
28. Genuth S: Exogenous insulin administration and cardiovascular risk in non–insulin-dependent and insulin-dependent diabetes mellitus. Ann Intern Med 124(1, pt 2):104-109, 1996.
29. Blume JD: Tutorial in biostatistics: Likelihood methods for measuring statistical evidence. Statist. Med 21:2563-2599, 2002.
30. Brady PA, Terzic A: The sulfonylurea controversy: More questions from the heart. J Am Coll Cardiol 31:950-956, 1998.
31. Meier JJ, Gallwitz B, Schmidt WE, et al: Is impairment of ischaemic preconditioning by sulfonylurea drugs clinically important? Heart 90:9-12, 2004.
32. Malmberg K, Ryden L, Efendic S, et al: Randomized trial of insulin-glucose infusion followed by subcutaneous insulin treatment in diabetic patients with acute myocardial infarction (DIGAMI study): Effects on mortality at 1 year. J Am Coll Cardiol 26:57-65, 1995.
33. Malmberg K: Prospective randomised study of intensive insulin treatment on long term survival after acute myocardial infarction in patients with diabetes mellitus. BMJ 314:1512-1515, 1997.
34. Malmberg K, Rydén L, Hamssten A, et al (DIGAMI Study Group): Effects of insulin treatment on cause-specific mortality and morbidity in diabetic patients with acute myocardial infarction. Eur Heart J 17:1337-1344, 1996.
35. Mühlhauser I, Sawicki PT, Berger M: Possible risk of sulfonylureas in the treatment of non–insulin-dependent diabetes mellitus and coronary artery disease. Diabetologia 40:1492-1493, 1997.
36. Hansson L, Zanchetti A, Carruthers SG, et al: Effects of intensive blood-pressure lowering and low-dose aspirin in patients with hypertension: Principal results of the Hypertension Optimal Treatment (HOT) randomised trial. HOT Study Group. Lancet 351:1755-1762, 1998.

37. UKPDS Group: Tight blood pressure control and risk of macrovascular and microvascular complications in type 2 diabetes: UKPDS 38. BMJ 317:703-713, 1998.

38. Turner RC, Millns H, Neil HA, et al: Risk factors for coronary artery disease in non–insulin dependent diabetes mellitus: United Kingdom Prospective Diabetes Study (UKPDS: 23) BMJ 316:823-828, 1998.

39. Adler AI, Stratton IM, Neil HA, et al: Association of systolic blood pressure with macrovascular and microvascular complications of type 2 diabetes (UKPDS 36): Prospective observational study. BMJ 321:412-419, 2000.

40. UK Prospective Diabetes Study Group: Efficacy of atenolol and captopril in reducing risk of macrovascular and microvascular complications in type 2 diabetes: UKPDS 39. BMJ 317:713-720, 1998.

41. The Heart Outcomes Prevention Evaluation Study Investigators: Effects of ramipril on cardiovascular and microvascular outcomes in people with diabetes mellitus: Results of the HOPE study and MICRO-HOPE substudy. Lancet 355:253-259, 2000.

42. Yusuf S, Gerstein H, Hoogwerf B, Pogue J, et al, for the HOPE Study Investigators: Ramipril and the development of diabetes. JAMA 286:1882-1885, 2001.

43. Dahlof B, Devereux RB, Kjeldsen SE, et al: Cardiovascular morbidity and mortality in the Losartan Intervention For Endpoint reduction in hypertension study (LIFE): A randomised trial against atenolol. Lancet 359:995-1003, 2002.

44. Lindholm LH, Ibsen H, Dahlof B, et al: Cardiovascular morbidity and mortality in patients with diabetes in the Losartan Intervention For Endpoint reduction in hypertension study (LIFE): A randomised trial against atenolol. Lancet 359:1004-1010, 2002.

45. Lindholm LH, Dahlöf B, Edelman JM, et al: Effect of losartan on sudden cardiac death in people with diabetes: data from the LIFE study. Lancet 362:619-620, 2003.

46. Brenner BM Cooper ME, de Zeeuw D, et al, for the RENAAL Study Investigators: Effects of losartan on renal and cardiovascular outcomes in patients with type 2 diabetes and nephropathy. N Engl J Med 345:861-869, 2001.

47. Lewis EJ, Hunsicker LG, Clarke WR, et al: Renoprotective effect of the angiotensin-receptor antagonist irbesartan in patients with nephropathy due to type 2 diabetes. N Engl J Med 345:851-860, 2001.

48. Berl T, Hunsicker LG, Lewis JB, et al, for the Irbesartan Diabetic Nephropathy Trial Collaborative Study Group: Cardiovascular outcomes in the Irbesartan Diabetic Nephropathy Trial of patients with type 2 diabetes and overt nephropathy. Ann Intern Med 138:542-549, 2003.

49. The Antihypertensive and Lipid-Lowering Treatment to Prevent Heart Attack Trial (ALLHAT) Officers: Major outcomes in high-risk hypertensive patients randomized to angiotensin-converting enzyme inhibitor or calcium channel blocker vs. diuretic. JAMA 288:2981-2997, 2002.

50. Barzilay JI, Jones CL, Davis BR, et al: Baseline characteristics of the diabetic participants in the Antihypertensive and Lipid-Lowering Treatment to Prevent Heart Attack Trial (ALLHAT). Diabetes Care 24:654-658, 2001.

51. Cucherat M: EasyMA 2001, Software for meta-analysis of clinical trials. Posted 8/05/2002. http://www.spc.univ-lyon1.fr/easyma/dos.

52. UK Prospective Diabetes Study (UKPDS) XI: Biochemical risk factors in type 2 diabetic patients at diagnosis compared with age-matched normal subjects. Diabet Med 11:534-544, 1994.

53. Turner RC, Millns H, Neil HA, et al: Risk factors for coronary artery disease in non–insulin dependent diabetes mellitus: United Kingdom Prospective Diabetes Study (UKPDS 23) BMJ 316:823-828, 1998.

54. Stamler J, Vaccaro O, Neaton JD, Wentworth D: Diabetes, other risk factors, and 12-yr cardiovascular mortality for men screened in the Multiple Risk Factor Intervention Trial. Diabetes Care 16:434-444, 1993.

55. Rubins H, Robins SJ, Collins D, et al: Gemfibrozil for the secondary prevention of coronary heart disease in men with low levels of high-density lipoprotein cholesterol. N Engl J Med 341:410-418, 1999.

55a. Robins SJ, Collins D, Wittes JT, et al: VA-HIT Study Group: Veterans Affairs High-Density Lipoprotein Intervention Trial. Relation of gemfibrozil treatment and lipid levels with major coronary events: VA-HIT: A randomized controlled trial. JAMA 285:1585-1591, 2001.

56. Effect of fenofibrate on progression of coronary-artery disease in type 2 diabetes: The Diabetes Atherosclerosis Intervention Study, a randomised study. Lancet 357:905-910, 2001.

57. Pyorala K, Pedersen TR, Kjekshus J, et al: Cholesterol lowering with simvastatin improves prognosis of diabetic patients with coronary heart disease: A subgroup analysis of the Scandinavian Simvastatin Survival Study (4S). Diabetes Care 20:614-620, 1997; erratum in Diabetes Care 20:1048, 1997.

58. Haffner SM, Alexander CM, Cook TJ, et al: Reduced coronary events in simvastatin-treated patients with coronary heart disease and diabetes or impaired fasting glucose levels: Subgroup analyses in the Scandinavian Simvastatin Survival Study. Arch Intern Med 159:2661-2667, 1999.

59. MRC/BHF Heart Protection Study of cholesterol lowering with simvastatin in 20,536 high-risk individuals: A randomised placebo-controlled trial. Lancet 360:7-22, 2002.

60. Gaede P, Vedel P, Parving HH, Pedersen O: Intensified multifactorial intervention in patients with type 2 diabetes mellitus and microalbuminuria: The Steno type 2 randomised study. Lancet 353:617-622, 1999.

61. Gaede P, Vedel P, Larsen N, et al: Multifactorial intervention and cardiovascular disease in patients with type 2 diabetes. N Engl J Med 348:383-393, 2003.

62. Vermes E, Ducharme A, Bourassa MG, et al: Enalapril reduces the incidence of diabetes in patients with chronic heart failure: Insight from the Studies Of Left Ventricular Dysfunction (SOLVD). Circulation. 107:1291-1296, 2003.

63. Lindholm LH, Persson M, Alaupovic P, et al: Metabolic outcome during 1 year in newly detected hypertensives: Results of the Antihypertensive Treatment and Lipid Profile in a North of Sweden Efficacy Evaluation (ALPINE study). J Hypertens 21:1563-1574, 2003.

64. Pfeffer MA, Swedberg K, Granger CB, et al, and the CHARM Investigators and Committees: Effects of candesartan on mortality and morbidity in patients with chronic heart failure: The CHARM-Overall programme. Lancet 362:759-766, 2003.

65. Hansson L, Lindholm LH, Niskanen L, et al: Effect of angiotensin-converting-enzyme inhibition compared with conventional therapy on cardiovascular morbidity and mortality in hypertension: The Captopril Prevention Project (CAPPP) randomised trial. Lancet 353:611-666, 1999.

66. Hansson L, Lindholm LH, Ekbom T, et al: Randomised trial of old and new antihypertensive drugs in elderly patients: Cardiovascular mortality and morbidity the Swedish Trial in Old Patients with Hypertension–2 study. Lancet 354:1751-1756, 1999.

67. Julius S, Kjeldsen SE, Weber M, et al, and the VALUE Trial Group: Outcomes in hypertensive patients at high cardiovascular risk treated with regimens based on valsartan or amlodipine: The VALUE randomised trial. Lancet 363:2022-2031, 2004.

Index

Note: Page numbers followed by the letter b refer to boxed material; those followed by the letter f refer to figures, and those followed by t refer to tables.

629